ENDOCRINOLOGY
ADULT AND PEDIATRIC

ENDOCRINOLOGY

ADULT AND PEDIATRIC   6TH EDITION

THE PARATHYROID GLAND AND BONE METABOLISM

Volume Editor

John T. Potts, Jr, MD

Jackson Distinguished Professor of Clinical Medicine
Harvard Medical School;
Director of Research and Physician-in-Chief Emeritus
Department of Medicine
Massachusetts General Hospital
Boston, Massachusetts

ELSEVIER
SAUNDERS

SAUNDERS

1600 John F. Kennedy Blvd.
Ste 1800
Philadelphia, PA 19103-2899

Endocrinology, Adult and Pediatric: The Parathyroid Gland
and Bone Metabolism

ISBN: 978-0-323-09098-8
POD ISBN: 978-0-323-24063-5

Notice

Knowledge and best practice in this field are constantly changing. As new research and experience broaden our knowledge, changes in practice, treatment, and drug therapy may become necessary or appropriate. Readers are advised to check the most current information provided (i) on procedures featured or (ii) by the manufacturer of each product to be administered to verify the recommended dose or formula, the method and duration of administration, and contraindications. It is the responsibility of the practitioner, relying on their own experience and knowledge of their patients, to make diagnoses, to determine dosages and the best treatment for each individual patient, and to take all appropriate safety precautions. To the fullest extent of the law, neither the Publisher nor the authors, contributors, or editors assume any liability for any injury and/or damage to persons or property arising out of or related to any use of the material contained in this book.

The Publisher

Content for this eBook is derived from a book that may have contained additional digital media. Media content is not included in this eBook purchase.

Library of Congress Cataloging-in-Publication Data
Endocrinology / senior editors, Leslie J. De Groot, J. Larry Jameson ; section editors Ashley Grossman ... [et al.].—6th ed.
    p. ; cm.
Includes bibliographical references and index.
ISBN-13: 978-1-4160-5593-9 (v.1 & v.2 : hardback : alk. paper)
ISBN-13: 978-9996074479 (v.1 : hardback : alk. paper)
ISBN-10: 9996074471 (v.1 : hardback : alk. paper)
ISBN-13: 978-9996074417 (v.2 : hardback: alk. paper)
[etc.]
1. Endocrine glands–Diseases. 2. Endocrinology. I. De Groot, Leslie J. II. Jameson, J. Larry.
[DNLM: 1. Endocrine System Disease. 2. Endocrine Glands. 3. Hormones. WK 140 E5595 2010]
RC648.E458 2010
616.4—dc22

Acquisitions Editor: Helene Caprari
Developmental Editor: Mary Beth Murphy
Publishing Services Manager: Anne Altepeter
Project Manager: Jennifer Nemec
Design Direction: Ellen Zanolle

Transferred to Digital Printing in 2013

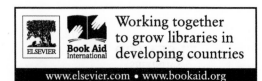

Senior Editors

J. Larry Jameson, MD, PhD

Professor of Medicine, Dean
Northwestern University Feinberg School of Medicine
Northwestern University
Chicago, Illinois

David de Kretser, AO, FAA, FTSE, MD, FRACP

Emeritus Professor
Monash Institute of Medical Research
Monash University
Clayton, Melbourne, Victoria, Australia

Ashley Grossman, BA, BSc, MD, FRCP, FMedSci

Professor of Neuroendocrinology
Endocrinology
St. Bartholomew's Hospital
London, United Kingdom

John C. Marshall, MD, PhD

Andrew D. Hart Professor of Internal Medicine
Director, Center for Research in Reproduction
Department of Medicine
University of Virginia School of Medicine
Charlottesville, Virginia

Shlomo Melmed, MD

Senior Vice President, Academic Affairs and Dean of
   the Faculty
Cedars Sinai Medical Center
Los Angeles, California

Leslie J. De Groot, MD

Research Professor
Cellular and Life Sciences
University of Rhode Island, Providence Campus
Providence, Rhode Island

John T. Potts, Jr, MD

Jackson Distinguished Professor of Clinical Medicine
Harvard Medical School;
Director of Research and Physician-in-Chief Emeritus
Department of Medicine
Massachusetts General Hospital
Boston, Massachusetts

Gordon C. Weir, MD

Head, Section on Islet Transplantation and Cell Biology
Diabetes Research and Wellness Foundation Chair
Joslin Diabetes Center;
Professor of Medicine
Harvard Medical School
Boston, Massachusetts

Harald Jüppner, MD

Professor of Pediatrics
Endocrine Unit and Pediatric Nephrology Unit
   Massachusetts General Hospital and Harvard Medical
   School
Boston, Massachusetts

Contributors

Murat Bastepe, MD, PhD
Assistant Professor of Medicine
Endocrine Unit, Department of Medicine
Massachusetts General Hospital and Harvard
  Medical School
Boston, Massachusetts

John P. Bilezikian, MD
Professor of Medicine
Division of Endocrinology
Columbia University
New York, New York

Roger Bouillon, MD, PhD, FRCP
Professor of Medicine and Chair of Endocrinology
Experimental Medicine and Endocrinology
Katholieke Universiteit Leuven
Leuven, Belgium

F. Richard Bringhurst, MD
Associate Professor of Medicine, Harvard Medical
  School
Physician, Massachusetts General Hospital
Senior Vice President for Medicine and Research
  Management
Massachusetts General Hospital
Boston, Massachusetts

Edward M. Brown, MD
Professor of Medicine Division of Endocrinology,
Diabetes, and Hypertension
Department of Medicine
Brigham & Women's Hospital
Boston, Massachusetts

Roland D. Chapurlat, MD, PhD
Professor of Rheumatology;
Head, Division of Rheumatology;
Director, INSERM Research Unit 831;
Director, National Reference Center for Fibrous
  Dysplasia of Bone
Lyon, France

Leslie J. De Groot, MD
Research Professor
Cellular and Life Sciences
University of Rhode Island, Providence Campus
Providence, Rhode Island

Pierre D. Delmas, MD, PhD†
Professor of Medicine
Claude Bernard University of Lyon;
Chief of Department, Rheumatology
Hôpital E. Herriot;
Director, Research Unit (Pathophysiology of
  Osteoporosis) INSERM
Lyon, France;
President, International Osteoporosis Foundation
Nyon, Switzerland

Marie B. Demay, MD
Professor of Medicine
Massachusetts General Hospital
Harvard Medical School
Boston, Massachusetts

Michael J. Econs, MD
Glenn W. Irwin, Jr. Professor of Endocrinology and
  Metabolism
Director, Division of Endocrinology and
  Metabolism
Professor of Medicine and Medical and Molecular
  Genetics
Indiana University School of Medicine
Indianapolis, Indiana

David M. Findlay, PhD
Professor of Orthopaedic Research
Department of Orthopaedics and Trauma
University of Adelaide
Adelaide, South Australia, Australia

Thomas J. Gardella, PhD
Associate Professor in Medicine
Department of Medicine, Endocrinology Unit
Massachusetts General Hospital and Harvard
  Medical School
Boston, Massachusetts

Harry K. Genant, MD
Professor, Emeritus
Radiology, Medicine and Orthopaedic Surgery;
Executive Director, Osteoporosis and Arthritis
  Research Group
Department of Radiology
University of California, San Francisco;
Chairman, Emeritus and Member, Board of
  Directors
Synarc, Inc.
San Francisco, California

Francis H. Glorieux, MD, PhD
Professor
Departments of Surgery, Pediatrics, and Human
  Genetics
McGill University, and Shriners Hospital for
  Children
Montreal, Québec, Canada

Mara J. Horwitz, MD
Assistant Professor of Medicine
Department of Medicine, Division of
  Endocrinology
University of Pittsburgh
Pittsburgh, Pennsylvania

J. Larry Jameson, MD, PhD
Professor of Medicine, Dean
Northwestern University Feinberg School of
  Medicine
Northwestern University
Chicago, Illinois

Harald Jüppner, MD
Professor of Pediatrics
Endocrine Unit and Pediatric Nephrology Unit
Massachusetts General Hospital and Harvard
  Medical School
Boston, Massachusetts

Stephen M. Krane, MD
Persis, Cyrus and Marlow B. Harrison
  Distinguished Professor of Clinical Medicine
Harvard Medical School;
Center for Immunology and Inflammatory
  Diseases
Massachusetts General Hospital
Boston, Massachusetts

Henry M. Kronenberg, MD
Chief, Endocrine Unit and Professor of Medicine
Department of Medicine
Massachusetts General Hospital and Harvard
  Medical School
Boston, Massachusetts

Christa Maes, PhD
Senior Postdoctoral Fellow
Department of Experimental Medicine
Katholieke Universiteit Leuven
Leuven, Belgium

T. John Martin, MD, DSc
Professor of Medicine
St Vincent's Institute
University of Melbourne
Melbourne, Victoria, Australia

Jeffrey A. Norton, MD
Professor of Surgery
Stanford University
Stanford, California

John T. Potts, Jr, MD
Jackson Distinguished Professor of Clinical
  Medicine
Harvard Medical School;
Director of Research and Physician-in-Chief
  Emeritus
Department of Medicine
Massachusetts General Hospital
Boston, Massachusetts

James H. Rosing, MD
Chief Resident
General Surgery
Stanford University Hospital and Clinics
Stanford, California

Isidoro B. Salusky, MD
Distinguished Professor of Pediatrics
Pediatrics
David Geffen School of Medicine at UCLA
Los Angeles, California

Patrick M. Sexton, BSc(Hons), PhD
NHMRC Principal Research Fellow
Professor of Pharmacology
Monash Institute of Pharmaceutical Sciences
Department of Pharmacology
Monash University
Parkville, Victoria, Australia

†Deceased.

Frederick R. Singer, MD
Director, Endocrine/Bone Disease Program
John Wayne Cancer Institute
Santa Monica, California;
Clinical Professor of Medicine
David Geffen School of Medicine at University of
    California Los Angeles
Los Angeles, California

Shonni J. Silverberg, MD
Professor of Medicine
Division of Endocrinology and Metabolism
Columbia University College of Physicians and
    Surgeons
New York, New York

René St-Arnaud, PhD
Professor and Senior Investigator
Genetics Unit
Shriners Hospital for Children;
Professor of Medicine, Surgery, and Human
    Genetics
Department of Human Genetics
McGill University
Montreal, Québec, Canada

Andrew F. Stewart, MD
Chief, Division of Endocrinology, and Professor of
    Medicine
Division of Endocrinology, Department of
    Medicine
University of Pittsburgh School of Medicine
Pittsburgh, Pennsylvania

**Rajesh V. Thakker, MD, FRCP, FRCPath,
FMedSci**
May Professor of Medicine
Nuffield Department of Medicine
University of Oxford
Oxford, Oxon, United Kingdom

Katherine Wesseling-Perry, MD
Assistant Professor of Pediatrics
Department of Pediatric Nephrology
David Geffen School of Medicine
University of California Los Angeles
Los Angeles, California

Michael P. Whyte, MD
Professor of Medicine, Pediatrics, and Genetics
Division of Bone and Mineral Diseases
Washington University School of Medicine,
Medical-Scientific Director
Center for Metabolic Bone Disease and Molecular
    Research
Shriners Hospital for Children
St. Louis, Missouri

Preface

The sixth edition of *Endocrinology, Adult and Pediatric* has been a standard but comprehensive and authoritative text in the field. In each of the areas a thorough discussion of basic research is coupled with careful attention to the pathophysiology of endocrine disorders, as well as detailed clinical diagnostic and therapeutic approaches.

Recognizing the comprehensive nature of the text, we are now pleased to offer a derivative edition that features for our colleagues separate sections in each of the fields covered in the text. We believe that the ability to access each of the sub-areas as a separate topic will appeal particularly to practicing endocrinologists. Hence this section deals with the field of calciotropic hormones and bone and mineral metabolism. In recent editions we have broadened our coverage of pediatric disorders as well as major diseases common to the aging population such as osteoporosis. The sixteen chapters in this ebook offer the reader an opportunity to understand the advances in genetics that have clarified features of many disorders involving calciotropic hormones, as well as newer diagnostic approaches and effective therapies for bone diseases ranging from osteoporosis to Paget's disease.

John T. Potts, Jr., MD

Contents

Contents

PARATHYROID HORMONE AND PARATHYROID HORMONE–RELATED PEPTIDE IN THE REGULATION OF CALCIUM HOMEOSTASIS AND BONE DEVELOPMENT

THOMAS J. GARDELLA, HARALD JÜPPNER, EDWARD M. BROWN, HENRY M. KRONENBERG, and JOHN T. POTTS, JR.

Parathyroid hormone (PTH) and PTH-related peptide (PTHrP), along with other calciotropic hormones, play critical roles in calcium homeostasis and bone biology. First discovered as a calcium-regulating hormone in the 1920s,[1-3] PTH is secreted by the parathyroid glands and is one of the most important regulators of blood calcium concentration in all terrestrial vertebrate species, from amphibians to mammals. PTHrP, a slightly larger molecule than PTH, was discovered more recently through efforts to identify the factor that causes, when produced in excess by certain tumors, the humoral hypercalcemia of malignancy syndrome. In contrast to PTH, which is produced by discrete endocrine glands, PTHrP is produced as a paracrine/autocrine factor in many different adult and fetal tissues and has, unlike PTH, multiple functions (Fig. 1-1).[4-6]

PTH and PTHrP most likely evolved from a common ancestral precursor. Despite this common evolutionary origin, both peptides share only limited overall amino acid sequence identity, yet at least their N-terminal regions are sufficiently homologous to enable them to bind to and activate a common G protein–coupled receptor, the PTH/PTHrP receptor (also referred to as PTH1R).[7-9] This receptor mediates the most important biological actions of both peptides: PTH-dependent regulation of calcium and phosphorous homeostasis and PTHrP-dependent regulation of endochondral bone formation.[10-14]

This chapter reviews (1) the comparative chemistry of PTH and PTHrP, their genes, and their interactions with the PTH1R; (2) the current molecular models of productive interactions of the two ligands with their common receptor; and (3) the different biological roles of both peptides on target tissues, such as the role of PTH in calcium homeostasis and bone turnover, the role of PTHrP in bone and cartilage development, and the role of PTH in regulating renal phosphate excretion (see Fig. 1-1). However, the chapter does not review the potentially numerous and still incompletely characterized biological roles of PTHrP outside the field of mineral ion homeostasis and bone biology. The evolutionary history of the principal PTH/PTHrP receptor is reviewed,

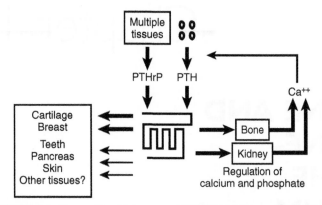

FIGURE I-I. The parathyroid hormone (PTH)/PTH-related peptide (PTHrP) receptor interacts with indistinguishable efficiency and efficacy with PTH and PTHrP, and it activates at least two distinct second messenger systems, cyclic adenosine monophosphate and Ca^{2+}/inositol 1,4,5-triphosphate. The receptor is abundantly expressed in bone and kidney, where it mediates the endocrine actions of PTH, and in the metaphyseal growth plate and numerous other tissues, where it mediates the autocrine/paracrine actions of PTHrP.

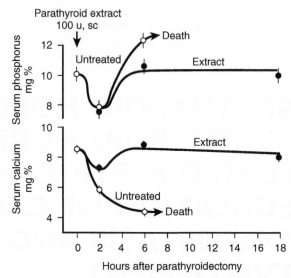

FIGURE I-2. Rate of change in blood phosphorus and calcium levels in rats with stressed calcium homeostasis (low-calcium diet) after parathyroidectomy without treatment or with 100 U of parathyroid hormone extract given in addition at the time of parathyroidectomy. Rapid and usually fatal hypocalcemia and hyperphosphatemia result within hours unless hormone is given. (Data from Munson PL: Studies on the role of the parathyroids in calcium and phosphorus metabolism, Ann N Y Acad Sci 60:776–796, 1955.)

as well as the functional characteristics of two novel, closely related receptors and the pharmacologic and physicochemical evidence for several additional, still incompletely characterized, receptors for PTH and PTHrP.

Regulation of Mineral Ion Homeostasis— General Considerations

To ensure a multitude of essential cellular functions, the extracellular concentration of calcium (Ca^{2+}_o) is maintained within narrow limits.[15,16] In terrestrial vertebrates, calcium is necessary for adequate mineralization of the skeleton, which provides mechanical support and protection for internal organs and acts as levers for the various muscle groups involved in locomotion. Because of its high calcium content, 99% of the body's supply, the skeleton also serves as the most important reservoir from which calcium can be rapidly mobilized. Because food intake and thus the nutritional supply of calcium are usually discontinuous, intestinal calcium absorption occurs only intermittently. Maintenance of a constant blood calcium concentration thus constitutes a major homeostatic challenge, which during evolution led to the development of highly efficient mechanisms to increase intestinal calcium absorption, reduce urinary calcium losses, and facilitate, if necessary, rapid mobilization of calcium from the skeletal reservoir (see Chapter 5).[16]

In contrast to these environmental challenges of most terrestrial vertebrates, marine animals, which are usually exposed to the high environmental calcium concentration of seawater (10 mM) had to adopt mechanisms by which extracellular calcium could be reduced.[17,18] Unlike the diet of terrestrial animals, seawater provides only a very limited supply of phosphate, and this environmental deficiency resulted in the development of mechanisms to conserve phosphate. It thus appears plausible that the efficient intestinal absorption of phosphate and the impressive capacity of the mammalian kidney to retain phosphate[15,19] are remnants of earlier evolutionary adaptations to life in the low-phosphate environment of the oceans. To reduce blood calcium concentrations, fish use stanniocalcin, which is produced by the corpuscles of Stannius, as well as several other hormonal factors.[17,18,20] Some data indicate that the mammalian

homologue of stanniocalcin has similar properties when tested in rodents, but it remains uncertain whether this peptide hormone has a significant physiologic role in mammalian mineral ion homeostasis.[21] A widely expressed mammalian peptide, stanniocalcin 2, that was discovered because of its structural homology with stanniocalcin, appears to inhibit phosphate uptake in renal epithelial cells.[22] However, newer data (see later) indicate that fibroblast growth factor-23 (FGF-23) and perhaps soluble frizzled-related protein 4 (sFRP4), dentin matrix protein 1 (DMP-1), and matrix extracellular phosphoglycoprotein (MEPE)[23] are more likely to be involved physiologically in the regulation of mammalian phosphate homeostasis (see Chapter 6). Calcitonin, made by the ultimobranchial bodies in fish, has a calcium-lowering function in these vertebrate species, but its biological role in mammals remains uncertain (for review, see Chapter 2).[24]

Parathyroid Hormone

PTH and the active form of vitamin D, 1,25-dihydroxyvitamin D_3 [1,25(OH)$_2$D$_3$], are the principal physiologic regulators of calcium homeostasis in humans and all terrestrial vertebrates.[11,25,26] Synthesis and secretion of PTH are stimulated by any decrease in blood calcium, and conversely, secretion of the hormone is inhibited by an increase in blood calcium.[27-29] This rapid negative feedback regulation of PTH production, along with the biological actions of the hormone on different target tissues, represents the most important homeostatic mechanism for minute-to-minute control of calcium concentration in the extracellular fluid (ECF) (Fig. 1-2).[30-32] In contrast to the rapid actions of PTH, 1,25(OH)$_2$D$_3$ is of critical importance for long-term, day-to-day, and week-to-week calcium balance (see Chapter 3). The actions of both hormones are coordinated, and each influences the synthesis and secretion of the other. Calcitonin, the third of the calciotropic hormones known to be important in the regulation of vertebrate mineral ion homeostasis (see

Chapter 2), may be vestigial in humans with respect to calcium homeostasis and will not be discussed in this brief review of physiology.

At least three distinct but coordinated actions of PTH increase the flow of calcium into the ECF and thus increase the concentration of blood calcium (see Fig. 1-2).[27-29] Through its rapid actions on the kidney and bone, which are all mediated through the PTH/PTHrP receptor and subsequent secondary messages in specific and highly specialized cells, PTH increases the release of calcium from bone, reduces the renal clearance of calcium, and stimulates the production of $1,25(OH)_2D_3$ by activating the gene encoding 25-hydroxyvitamin D-1α-hydroxylase (1α-hydroxylase) in the kidney. The relative importance of the first two actions of PTH on the rapid, minute-to-minute regulation of calcium is not definitively resolved, but most physiologists have stressed the importance of the effects of PTH on bone in maintaining hour-to-hour calcium homeostasis in the ECF. Several lines of evidence, such as that provided by calcium kinetic analysis, indicate a transfer between ECF and bone of as much as 500 mg of calcium daily, which is equivalent to one-fourth to one-half the total ECF calcium content.[15] Besides regulating this transfer of calcium from bone through direct breakdown of bone tissue (mineral and matrix), PTH influences the rates of exchange of calcium adsorbed to the surface of bone; this exchangeable calcium pool can be stimulated to provide a rapid and substantial rate of entry of calcium into blood. In addition to these PTH-dependent actions on bone, actions of PTH on the kidney may also be extremely important in the precise hourly regulation of ECF calcium. The third action of PTH on calcium homeostasis—namely, enhancement of intestinal calcium absorption—is indirect and involves the synthesis of $1,25(OH)_2D_3$ from the biologically inactive precursor $25(OH)D_3$. However, it is difficult to quantitatively analyze or to proportionately contrast the relative physiologic importance of the direct and indirect actions of PTH on the three principal target tissues: kidney, bone, and intestine.

The complexity of bone as a tissue and the many detectable rates of exchange of calcium between the skeleton and the ECF have made the action of PTH on the skeleton difficult to analyze. The state of calcium in blood is complex; much of the calcium is present as chelates or is bound to plasma proteins (for detailed review, see Chapter 5). Because actual filtered loads depend on the ratio of free and bound forms of calcium, it is difficult to calculate renal calcium clearance accurately. The different PTH-dependent actions to promote calcium entry into the ECF are most clearly defined in conditions of deficiency or excess of PTH, such as during experiments in animals or during controlled observations in patients with disorders of parathyroid gland function. The experimental data in these extremes abundantly affirm the crucial calcium homeostatic role of PTH. However, because of continuous and rapid adjustments in mineral ion concentration, it can be difficult to observe the consequences of hormone action under normal physiologic conditions. For example, the rate of PTH secretion changes continually and rapidly so that the controlled variable, calcium, remains constant, and it may therefore be difficult to experimentally detect small corrective changes.

Teleologically, the action of PTH on the regulation of blood phosphate concentration in terrestrial species is best understood as a secondary, rather than a homeostatic, action. Phosphate is abundant in the food chain in terrestrial existence. Phosphate deficiency, unlike calcium deficiency, in the absence of specific organ dysfunction is, therefore, an unlikely environmental challenge (see Chapter 6 for detailed review of the regulation of phosphate homeostasis). To correct a deficiency in calcium, mineral stores in bone can be rapidly dissolved; such activity results, however, in the simultaneous liberation of ionic calcium and phosphate. Because a high blood phosphate level tends to lower the calcium concentration through multiple mechanisms, the rise in blood calcium that occurs after bone dissolution (desirable homeostatically) is beneficial only if the concomitant increase in blood phosphate concentration (undesirable) can be rapidly corrected. To maximize the control of calcium homeostasis, PTH thus has divergent actions on renal tubular handling of the two mineral ions: It increases the retention of calcium and at the same time diminishes reabsorption of phosphate. Through these mechanisms—namely, increased renal phosphate clearance to prevent hyperphosphatemia and increased tubular calcium reabsorption—PTH guarantees that an elevation in blood calcium results from the increased release of calcium from bone. The renal action of PTH on phosphate homeostasis is biologically predominant over the increased phosphate flux from bone. Consequently, parathyroidectomy (experimentally, in animals) or renal resistance to PTH, as in patients with pseudohypoparathyroidism or renal failure, leads not only to hypocalcemia but also to an increase in blood phosphate and a marked reduction in urinary phosphate excretion (see Fig. 1-2). This finding demonstrates the importance of the PTH-dependent action on phosphate homeostasis in the kidney, which becomes particularly important in disease states when high bone turnover is the result of dietary calcium deficiency or lack of biologically active vitamin D.

CHEMISTRY

The first extracts from bovine parathyroid glands were described in 1925, and the content of biologically active PTH was assessed by their hypercalcemic and phosphaturic properties.[2,3] However, it was not until 1959, when Aurbach[33] and Rasmussen and Craig[34] developed improved extraction procedures, that it became possible to isolate and purify sufficient quantities to determine the primary structure of bovine, porcine, and human PTH through the protein sequence determination methods.[35-40] Two groups independently determined the sequences of human and bovine hormones.[35-40] Shown in Fig. 1-3A are the sequences of the bovine, porcine, and human hormones determined by one group.[36,37,39,40] Discordant sequences for the human PTH polypeptide, and in one position for the bovine hormone, published by the other group,[35,38] are not shown in Fig. 1-3A, since nucleotide sequence analysis of genomic and complementary DNA confirmed the amino acid sequences of the first group (the only exception was residue 76 in human PTH, which was determined to be glutamine instead of glutamic acid).[36,37,40] Based on these amino acid sequences, the PTH(1–34) fragments of the different species were synthesized, and their biological activities were compared in vitro and in vivo with those of highly purified intact PTH from the same species (Table 1-1). Molecular cloning techniques then led to the deduction of the amino acid sequences of rat, chicken, and dog PTHs,[41-44] followed more recently by the identification of PTH molecules in other mammals and fish, as shown in Fig. 1-3A and discussed later. The synthetic peptides used in parathyroid hormone research today are based largely on the (1–34) regions of the mammalian hormone sequences shown in Fig. 1-3A.[45,46]

Extensive sequence homology is present in the mammalian PTH species (see Fig. 1-3A and D); these molecules consist of a single-chain polypeptide with 84 amino acids and a molecular

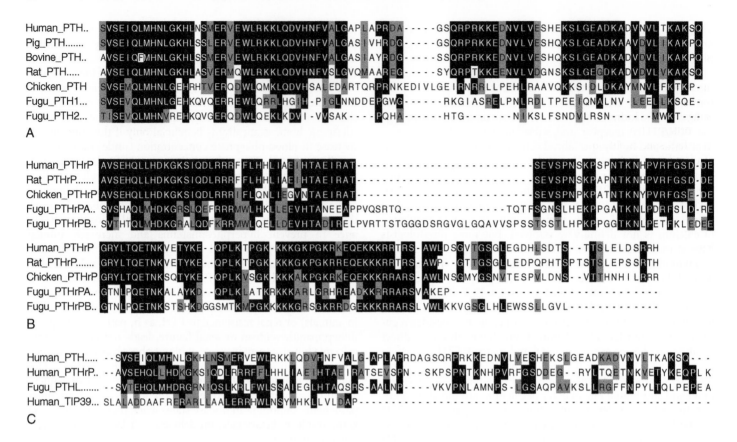

A

B

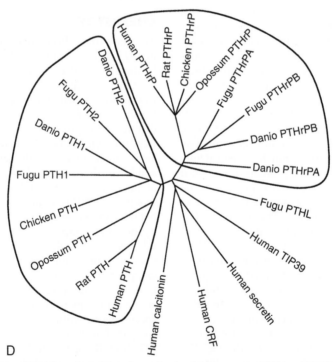

D

FIGURE 1-3. Sequence Relationships in PTH and PTHrP peptides. Comparisons of amino Acid sequences of PTH and PTHrP peptides from different species are shown in **A** and **B,** respectively. Comparison of human TIP39 and a PTH-Like peptide from the puffer fish *(Takifugu rubripes)* to human PTH and PTHrP (the (1–84) region only) is shown in **C.** In **A-C,** amino acid identities are shown on black field and similarities on gray field. A phylogenetic tree of the ligands is shown in **D,** with other family B receptor ligands, secretin, calcitonin, and cotricotropin-releasing factor (CRF) included as marginally homologous ligands. Fugu PTHL is speculated to be a precurssor to PTH and PTHrP.

weight of approximately 9400 daltons (that of human PTH[1–84] is 9425 D). The N-terminal region of PTH, which is necessary and sufficient for the regulation of mineral ion homeostasis, shows high sequence conservation among all the vertebrate species (see Fig. 1-3A). The middle portions of the different molecules exhibit the most structural variation, which could suggest that this region of PTH is only of limited functional importance. The nonmammalian PTH homologues of chicken[42,43] and fish species *Danio rerio* (zebrafish)[47] and *Takifugu ruberipes* (puffer fish)[48,49] diverge considerably from the mammalian hormones C-terminal of amino acid residue His32. Interestingly, both fish species have two distinct genes encoding two separate PTH molecules, called *PTH1* and *PTH2*.[47,48] The zebrafish peptides are considerably shorter than mammalian PTH (67 and 68 residues), while fugu PTH1 is predicted to be 81 residues in length and fugu PTH2 is predicted to be 63 residues.[48]

After the original work establishing that the first 34 amino acids of mammalian PTH were sufficient to produce a fully active synthetic peptide,[45,46] much work has centered on defining the minimum pharmacophore essential for biological activity. In a following section, we describe how sites of ligand interaction with the PTH/PTHrP receptor were defined by performing assays with products of various combinations of shortened and modified PTH ligands and mutagenized receptors. Furthermore, a fusion protein consisting of ligand substituted for most of the receptor amino-terminal extracellular domain was generated, and this helped define a much smaller minimum chain length of PTH peptide needed for biological activity.[50] As also discussed later in the section on hormone/receptor interactions, it has been determined that substitutions of non-naturally occurring amino acids (e.g., α-aminoisobutyric acid at positions 1 and 3 in the

primary ligand structure) favoring formation of an α-helix, even in short peptides, such as PTH(1–14), produce peptides that are highly potent when tested in vitro using cell-based assays and have highly stabilized helical structure in solution[51-55] (Fig. 1-4).

The in vitro activity of the native PTH(1-14), which is quite weak, is improved about 100,000-fold by the modifications indicated in Fig. 1-4. Shorter PTH peptides have also been shown to be active in vivo, since some cause hypercalcemia and are anabolic on bone, although their potency is much less than that of PTH(1-34) due to a more rapid clearance.[56] Replacement of valine-2 in these peptides with bulky amino acids, such as tryptophan or *para*benzoyl-L-phenylalanine (Bpa), results in competitive antagonist peptides defective for AC/cAMP and PLC/IP₃/Ca²⁺ signaling, thus confirming the critical role that this conserved valine plays in receptor activation.[57] Other longer-length PTH or PTHrP analogs having residue-1 (serine or alanine) replaced by glycine,[58] Bpa,[59] or tryptophan[60] exhibit signal-selective properties in that they efficiently stimulate the cAMP cellular pathway but not the inositol tri-phosphate/intracellular Ca²⁺ pathway.

The three-dimensional structures of intact PTH(1-84) and the N-terminal biologically active fragments of both PTH and PTHrP have been analyzed by various solution-based methods, including nuclear magnetic resonance (NMR) spectroscopy. Interpretation of these results in terms of biological mode of action is not straightforward, because the ligand interacts with a membrane-embedded receptor, and the biophysical properties of this environment, as well as the receptor-induced conformational changes that occur, are mostly unknown. However, the bioactive (1-34) portions of the ligands are generally found to contain helical structure within their N-terminal and especially C-terminal portions, with some flexibility in the midregion.[61-64] An x-ray crystallographic study of PTH(1-34) revealed α-helical structure extending nearly the full length of the peptide.[65] A persisting question is thus whether the ligand bound to the receptor adopts a linear and extended[62] or "U-shaped" folded structure, the latter suggested by tertiary interactions seen in some solution-phase biophysical studies.[61,63,64] Of particular interest has been the question of whether common structural features would be discerned for PTH and PTHrP that could explain their use of apparently overlapping binding sites on the common PTH/PTHrP receptor; to some extent, the helical propensities of at least the C-terminal domains of the peptides are consistent with this possibility.[62,66,67]

Therefore, consistent with their rather limited homology in primary structure (see Fig. 1-3), convincing evidence has not yet been provided for the conclusion that the N-terminal fragments of PTH and PTHrP display a similar secondary structure in solution. Because of their generally demonstrated similar potencies at the PTH/PTHrP receptor, it seemed likely that both ligands would adopt very similar conformations when part of the active

Table 1-1. Comparison of the Biological Activity of Parathyroid Peptides from Different Species

Peptide	Potency (MRC mmg)*	
	In Vitro Rat Renal Adenyl Cyclase Assay	**In Vivo Chick Hypercalcemia Assay**
Native hormones		
Bovine 1-84	3000 (2500-4000)	2500 (2100-4000)
Porcine 1-84	1000 (850-1250)	4800 (3300-7000)
Human 1-84	350 (275-425)	10,000 (9060-13,400)
Synthetic fragments		
Bovine 1-34	5400 (3900-8000)	7700 (5200-11,100)
Human 1-34	1700 (1400-2150)	7400 (5200-9700)
[Ala¹]-human 1-34	4300 (3400-5400)	—

From Rosenblatt M, Kronenberg HM, Potts JT Jr: Parathyroid hormone. In DeGroot L (ed): Endocrinology, ed 2, Philadelphia, 1989, WB Saunders, p 853.

*Values are expressed as mean potency with 95% confidence intervals and are based on Medical Research Council research standard A for parathyroid hormone.

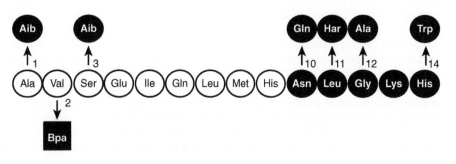

FIGURE 1-4. The native (rat) PTH(1-14) sequence and activity-modifying substitutions. The six substitutions shown *above* the sequence, when combined, enhance activity by as much as 100,000-fold; the Bpa² substitution shown *below* confers antagonist properties to the peptide. The (1-9) region (*nonshaded circles*) is thought to be the minimum-length agonist pharmacophore. Nonencoded amino acids include: α-amino-isobutyric acid (Aib), homoarginine (Har), and *para*-benzoyl-L-phenylalanine (Bpa).

hormone-receptor complex. However, recent data (discussed later) suggest that each ligand selectively binds to or induces a distinct receptor confirmation. Ideally, each hormone should be co-crystallized with the PTH/PTHrP receptor to permit analysis by x-ray diffraction of those intermolecular interactions that are characteristic of the biologically active hormone-receptor complexes. G protein–coupled receptors such as the PTH/PTHrP receptor have multiple membrane-embedded domains and are likely to have complex three-dimensional structures. Interaction with either PTH or PTHrP appears to involve several distinct receptor domains (see later discussion) that may undergo significant conformational changes after ligand binding has occurred, which makes it even more challenging to conduct x-ray or multidimensional NMR analyses. Recent advances, however, have been made it possible to co-crystallize the extracellular portion of the PTH/PTHrP receptor with the carboxyl end of the PTH (1-34) peptide[68] and to crystallize the membrane-spanning portion of a distantly related GPCR, the β2-adrenergic receptor.[69]

EVOLUTION

To maintain extracellular calcium and phosphate concentrations within narrow limits, the intricate regulatory system outlined, in which PTH plays the most important role, developed in the terrestrial animals. In mammals, PTH is produced almost exclusively by the parathyroid glands (only small amounts of its messenger RNA [mRNA] have been detected elsewhere[70,71]). During evolution, these glands first appear as discrete organs in amphibians, that is, with the migration of vertebrates from an aquatic to a terrestrial existence, and their appearance most likely represents an evolutionary adaptation to an environment that is, by comparison to seawater, low in calcium.[17,18,72] Parathyroid glands have not been identified in fish or invertebrate species, but earlier immunologic and RNA hybridization data from fish provided evidence for expression of PTH proteins in several tissues, including pituitary,[17,18,73] plasma, brain, kidney, spinal cord, ultimobranchial gland, as well as in the ventral neural tube and mineralizing jaw during development.[48,74] Now, with the rapid advances in characterization of complete genomes of multiple species, we have definitive proof of the earlier evolutionary origin of both PTH and PTHrP (see Fig. 1-3). Gene analyses of several teleost fish species, including the zebrafish, *Danio rerio*, and the puffer fishes *Takifugu rubripes* and *Tetraodon fluviatilis*, reveal the duplication of the *PTH* gene in each case.[48,75] Both the PTH1 and PTH2 peptides derived from the zebrafish activate the PTH/PTHrP receptors from different species,[49,75] and indeed, a fugu PTH(1-34) peptide has been shown to induce bone anabolic effects in osteopenic ovariectomized rats.[76]

In addition to PTH, the teleost fish also express PTHrP, again encoded by duplicate genes.[75,77-80] Furthermore, PTHrP immunoreactivity has been detected in the cartilaginous sharks and rays[81] and in a more primitive agnathan, the lamprey.[82] The teleost PTHrPs contain some amino acid residues characteristic of mammalian PTH; for example, fish PTHrP contains Met at position 8, Trp at position 23, and Leu at position 28, which are amino acid residues found in mammalian PTH. However, there is only one amino acid residue, Gln(Q)25, in fish PTH that is found in some mammalian PTHrP species but not in mammalian PTH (see Fig. 1-3). This pattern suggests that the fish proteins may be phylogenetically closer to a common PTH/PTHrP precursor than are the mammalian proteins (see later). Indeed, in addition to duplicate copies of PTH and PTHrP genes, the puffer fish genome contains a fifth gene that encodes a protein containing

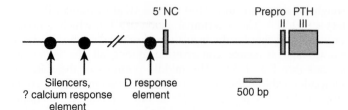

FIGURE 1-5. Schematic of the parathyroid hormone (PTH) gene along several thousand base pairs (approximate length shown by the scale marker for 500 bp). The three exons in the mRNA are represented as numbered rectangles. Control elements are identified in the 5' noncoding region (5' NC). A region responsive to vitamin D is within a few hundred base pairs of exon 1. Far upstream are silencers involved in calcium regulation.

amino acid residues characteristic of both PTH and PTHrP. This gene, called *PTH-L*, is phylogenetically an intermediary to PTH and PTHrP and may thus represent first definitive evidence for an ancestral gene from which the two divergent ligand forms evolved (see Fig. 1-3C and D).[48,75]

THE *PTH* GENE AND ITS mRNA

The human *PTH* gene consists of three exons located on chromosome 11p15.[83-86] The first exon is 85 nucleotides in length and is noncoding (Fig. 1-5). Exon 2 (90 bp) encodes most amino acids of the prepropeptide sequence, whereas the third exon (612 bp) encodes the remainder of the propeptide sequence and all amino acids of the mature peptide, and it constitutes the 3' noncoding region.[87] Several frequent intragenic polymorphisms (TaqI and PstI[88]; BstBI[89]; DraIII[90]; XmnI[91]), and a tetranucleotide repeat ([AAAT]n;[92]) have been identified in the human *PTH* gene, and some were shown to be informative in genetic linkage studies.[93-95] Two mRNAs that are 822 and 793 bp in length are derived in the human gene from the two transcriptional start sites, which follow two different functional TATA boxes that are separated by 29 bp.[87] Two closely spaced TATA boxes and two distinct transcripts are also derived from the bovine PTH gene, while rat and chicken PTH genes give rise to only one transcript; as a consequence of a long 3' noncoding region, the transcript from the chicken PTH gene is unusually long and comprises 2.3 kb.[25,96] The genes encoding zebrafish PTH1 and PTH2 have a similar overall organization as the mammalian PTH genes.[47]

PTH BIOSYNTHESIS AND INTRAGLANDULAR PROCESSING

During the synthesis of the preproPTH molecule, the signal sequence, which comprises the 25-amino-acid-containing "pre" sequence, is cleaved off after entry of the nascent peptide chain into the intracisternal space bounded by the endoplasmic reticulum. A heterozygous mutation in this leader sequence, which changes a cysteine to an arginine at position −8 and thus impairs processing of preproPTH to proPTH, has been identified as the most plausible molecular cause of an autosomal dominant familial form of hypoparathyroidism.[97,98] The mutant hormone was found to be trapped intracellularly, predominantly in the endoplasmic reticulum (ER), leading to a marked up-regulation of ER stress-responsive proteins (BiP and PERK) and the proapoptotic transcription factor, CHOP, indicating that apoptosis-mediated parathyroid cell death is the likely cause of the observed hypoparathyroidism.[99]

Subsequent to the removal of the pre-sequence, the propeptide is transported to the trans-Golgi network, where the pro-sequence (amino acid residues −6 through −1) is removed.[100]

This latter process may involve furin (paired basic amino acid cleaving enzyme) and/or proprotein convertase-7 (PC-7), which are both expressed in parathyroid tissue; their expression levels do not appear to be regulated by either calcium or $1,25(OH)_2D_3$.[101,102] After removal of the basic pro-sequence, the mature polypeptide, PTH(1-84), is packaged into secretory granules. Two proteases, cathepsins B and H, are subsequently involved in the intraglandular generation of carboxyl-terminal PTH fragments from the intact hormone; no amino-terminal PTH fragments appear to be released from the gland.[103-105] Since small or intermediate-size carboxyl-terminal fragments of PTH are unlikely to be involved in the regulation of calcium homeostasis, the intraglandular degradation of intact PTH is thought to represent an inactivating pathway, at least with regard to the regulation of mineral ion homeostasis. Consistent with this conclusion, hypercalcemia results in a substantial decrease in PTH secretion and, furthermore, favors the secretion of carboxyl-terminal PTH fragments, including a previously undetected large molecular species that are truncated at the amino-terminus (see following section).[105-108] However, recent studies have shown that some amino-terminally truncated PTH fragments, such as PTH(7-84), have hypocalcemic properties in vivo and can furthermore reduce the formation of osteoclasts in vitro.[109]

The pool of stored, intracellular PTH is small, and the parathyroid cell must therefore have mechanisms to increase hormone synthesis and release in response to sustained hypocalcemia. One such adaptive mechanism is to reduce the intracellular degradation of the hormone, thereby increasing the net amount of intact, biologically active PTH that is available for secretion. During hypocalcemia, the bulk of the hormone that is released from the parathyroid cell is intact PTH(1-84).[103-105,107,108] As the level of Ca^{2+}_o increases, a greater fraction of intracellular PTH is degraded, and with overt hypercalcemia, most of the secreted immunoreactive PTH consists of biologically inactive C-terminal fragments.[10,25,26]

REGULATION OF *PTH* GENE EXPRESSION

Another adaptive mechanism of the parathyroid cell to sustained reductions in Ca^{2+}_o is to increase cellular levels of PTH mRNA, a response that takes several hours. A reduction in Ca^{2+}_o increases, whereas an elevation in Ca^{2+}_o reduces the cellular levels of PTH mRNA by affecting both its stability and the transcriptional rate of its gene.[11,26,110,111] Available data suggest that phosphate ions also regulate, directly or indirectly, *PTH* gene expression. In the rat, hypophosphatemia and hyperphosphatemia, respectively, lower and raise the levels of mRNA for PTH through a mechanism that is independent of changes in Ca^{2+}_o or $1,25(OH)_2D_3$. An elevated extracellular phosphate concentration could thus contribute importantly to the secondary hyperparathyroidism frequently encountered in patients with end-stage renal failure, who often have chronically elevated serum phosphate concentrations.

Metabolites of vitamin D, principally $1,25(OH)_2D_3$, also play an important role in the long-term regulation of parathyroid function and may act at several levels: by affecting the secretion of PTH and regulation of its gene, by regulating transcriptional activity of the genes encoding the calcium-sensing receptor (CaSR; see later) and the vitamin D receptor (VDR), as well as by regulating parathyroid cellular proliferation.[11,26,110,112] $1,25(OH)_2D_3$ is by far the most important vitamin D metabolite that modulates parathyroid function. It acts through a nuclear receptor, the VDR, often in concert with other such receptors (i.e., those for retinoic acid or glucocorticoids), on DNA sequences upstream from the *PTH* gene (see Chapter 3).[113,114] $1,25(OH)_2D_3$-induced upregulation of VDR and CaSR expression in the parathyroid could potentiate its inhibitory action(s) on PTH synthesis and secretion.[11,26,110] Noncalcemic or less calcemic analogs of $1,25(OH)_2D_3$ inhibit PTH secretion while producing relatively little stimulation of intestinal calcium absorption and bone resorption[115-117] and may thus be attractive candidates for treating the hyperparathyroidism of chronic renal insufficiency.

Adjustment of the rate of parathyroid cellular proliferation is the third adaptive mechanism contributing to changes in the overall secretory activity of the parathyroid gland. Under normal conditions, parathyroid cells have little or no proliferative activity. The parathyroid glands, however, can enlarge greatly during states of chronic hypocalcemia, particularly in the setting of renal failure, probably because of a combination of hypocalcemia, hyperphosphatemia, and low levels of $1,25(OH)_2D_3$ in the latter condition.

REGULATION OF PARATHYROID HORMONE SECRETION

A large number of factors modulate PTH secretion in vitro,[11,26,118] but most of these factors are not thought to control hormonal secretion in vivo in a biologically relevant manner. Therefore, we focus in this section principally on factors that are the most physiologically meaningful regulators of PTH secretion—that is, the extracellular ionized calcium concentration itself (Ca^{2+}_o), $1,25(OH)_2D_3$, and the level of extracellular phosphate ions. Of these three, Ca^{2+}_o is most important in the minute-to-minute control of PTH secretion. Indeed, the actions of $1,25(OH)_2D_3$ and phosphate ions on the secretion of PTH probably result at least in part from their effects on hormonal biosynthesis rather than secretion per se.[11,26,118] Ca^{2+}_o also modulates several other aspects of parathyroid function that indirectly affect PTH secretion, including *PTH* gene expression, the hormone's intracellular degradation, and parathyroid cellular proliferation, as described previously. Recent data have shown that novel factors playing key roles in phosphate homeostasis, especially FGF-23 and α-klotho (a coreceptor for FGF receptors), also modulate parathyroid function, inhibiting[119,120] and enhancing[121] parathyroid function, respectively. Our rapidly improving understanding of how these factors participate in phosphate homeostasis is described in detail in Chapter 6.

Physiologic Control of PTH Secretion by Ca^{2+}_o

As illustrated in Fig. 1-6A, the relationship between PTH and Ca^{2+}_o is represented by a steep inverse sigmoidal curve that can be quantitatively described by four parameters.[122-124] These are the maximal rate of PTH secretion at low Ca^{2+}_o (parameter A); the slope of the curve at its midpoint (parameter B); the value of Ca^{2+}_o at the midpoint (e.g., the "set point" or the level of Ca^{2+}_o half-maximally suppressing PTH release; parameter C); and the minimal secretory rate at high Ca^{2+}_o (parameter D) (see Fig. 1-6B). Parameter A in vivo is the sum of the maximal rates of PTH release from all individual parathyroid chief cells, as reflected by the resultant, maximally stimulated level of circulating PTH. Because of the steepness of the Ca^{2+}_o-PTH relationship, small alterations in Ca^{2+}_o evoke large changes in PTH release, thereby contributing importantly to the near constancy of Ca^{2+}_o in vivo. Indeed, parathyroid cells can readily detect reductions in Ca^{2+}_o of a few percentage points,[123] and the percent coefficient of variation in Ca^{2+}_o in humans is less than 2%.[125] The set point of the parathyroid gland is the key determinant of the level at which Ca^{2+}_o is "set" in vivo, although the parathyroid set point

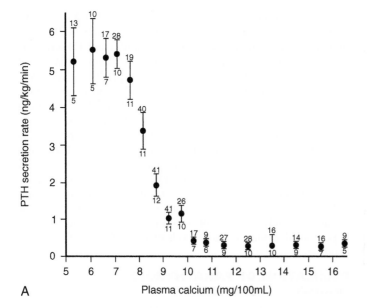

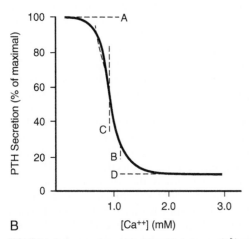

FIGURE I-6. Inverse sigmoidal relationship between Ca^{2+} and parathyroid hormone (PTH) release and the four-parameter model describing these curves. **A,** Secretory response of bovine parathyroid glands to induced alterations in plasma calcium concentration. Calves were infused with calcium or ethylenediaminetetraacetic acid, and PTH secretion was assessed by measuring PTH levels in the parathyroid venous effluent. The *symbols and vertical bars* indicate the secretory rate (mean ± SE) in calcium concentration ranges of 1 or 0.5 mg/100 mL. The number of calves and samples are indicated, respectively, by numbers below and above. **B,** Sigmoidal curve generated by the equation $Y = [(A - D)/(1 + (X/C^B)] + D$; the significance of A, B, C, and D are described in the text. (**A,** Data from Hurst JG: Sigmoidal relationship between parathyroid hormone secretion rate and plasma calcium concentration in calves. Endocrinology 10:10, 1978; **B,** Data from Brown EM: PTH secretion in vivo and in vitro, Miner Electrolyte Metab 8:130–150, 1982.)

is usually slightly lower than the ambient blood Ca^{2+}.[126] Thus, the parathyroid cell is normally more than half-maximally suppressed at normal levels of Ca^{2+}_o and has a large secretory reserve for responding to hypocalcemic stress. Nevertheless, PTH levels in vivo also fall dramatically (e.g., by 80%) when Ca^{2+}_o rises to frankly hypercalcemic levels,[122,123] which is thought to contribute importantly to the mineral ion homeostatic system's defense against hypercalcemia.[126] Furthermore, elevating Ca^{2+}_o also decreases the proportion of secreted intact PTH because of increased intraglandular degradation to inactive fragments (see the earlier section, PTH Biosynthesis and Intraglandular Processing, and the later section, Metabolism of PTH).[106,127] Even with severe hypercalcemia, however, some residual release of intact

PTH(1-84) still occurs in vivo and persists at a level approximately 5% of that observed with a maximal hypocalcemic stimulus[29,108,128] (see Fig. 1-6A). This nonsuppressible basal component of PTH release may contribute to the hypercalcemia caused by hyperparathyroidism when the mass of abnormal parathyroid tissue is very great (e.g., in patients with renal failure).[124,129-131]

The parathyroid cell has a temporal hierarchy of responses to low Ca^{2+}_o that permits it to secrete progressively larger amounts of hormone during prolonged hypocalcemia.[11,26,118] To meet acute hypocalcemic challenges, PTH is released within seconds from preformed secretory vesicles by exocytosis as dictated by the sigmoidal curve (see Fig. 1-6). Sufficient PTH is stored in the parathyroid chief cell to sustain maximal, low Ca^{2+}_o-stimulated PTH release for about 60 to 90 minutes.[126] Another rapid response of the parathyroid cell to hypocalcemia that enhances its net synthetic rate of PTH is reduced intracellular hormonal degradation—the opposite of what occurs at high levels of Ca^{2+}_o—which occurs within minutes to an hour.[106,127] Hypocalcemia persisting for hours to days elicits increased *PTH* gene expression, whereas that lasting for days to weeks or longer stimulates parathyroid cellular proliferation.[11,26,118,132] A greater secretory capacity for PTH on a per-cell basis (e.g., as a result of enhanced *PTH* gene expression) increases maximal hormonal secretion in vivo, as does an increase in cell number as a result of parathyroid cellular proliferation (see Fig. 1-6). In severe secondary hyperparathyroidism, very large increases in parathyroid cellular mass can elevate circulating PTH levels by 100-fold or more.

In addition to responding to changes in Ca^{2+}_o per se, the parathyroid cell also appears to sense the rate of change in Ca^{2+}_o such that rapid decrements in calcium promote more vigorous secretory responses than do changes of a similar magnitude occurring more slowly.[133] Furthermore, during dynamic testing of parathyroid function in vivo by induced increases or decreases in Ca^{2+}_o, PTH in blood is higher at a given serum calcium concentration when Ca^{2+}_o is falling than when it is rising (e.g., hysteresis is occurring in this relationship).[134,135] The latter results in an apparent direction dependence of the secretory response, which when combined with the rate dependence just described, may allow for a physiologically appropriate, more vigorous secretory response to large rapid decrements in Ca^{2+}_o. Also present are circadian[136] (for review, see Diaz et al.[26]) and more rapid (i.e., occurring at rates of one to six pulses per hour) phasic changes in circulating PTH levels,[26,137] but the physiologic significance of these changes is not known.

Mechanism of Ca^{2+}_o Sensing by Parathyroid Cells and Other Cells Involved in Mineral Ion Homeostasis

The molecular mechanism underlying Ca^{2+}_o-regulated PTH secretion involves a G protein–coupled, cell surface Ca^{2+}_o-sensing receptor (CaSR).[138] The CaSR was first isolated from bovine parathyroid glands[139] and subsequently from human parathyroid and several other tissues and species.[140] The receptor exhibits the characteristic "serpentine" motif (seven membrane spanning domains) of the superfamily of G protein–coupled receptors (Fig. 1-7). Its long, N-terminal extracellular domain contains the major, but not all, determinants of Ca^{2+}_o binding.[141-143] Changes in Ca^{2+}_o modulate a number of second messenger systems via coupling of CaSR through its intracellular domains to the relevant G proteins regulating these signaling pathways.[138] These functions include activation of phospholipases C, A_2, and D,[144] stimulation of several mitogen-activated protein kinases,[145] and

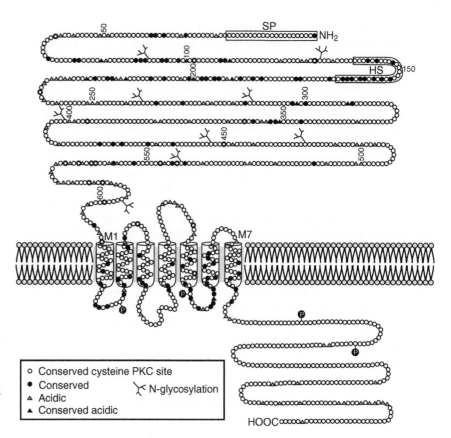

FIGURE 1-7. Schematic representation of the predicted topology of the calcium-sensing receptor cloned from human parathyroid gland. *HS,* Hydrophobic segment; *SP,* signal peptide; △, acidic residues (▲, conserved among species); *branched markers,* sites of glycosylation; *P,* sites of phosphorylation. (From Brown EM, Gamba G, Riccardi D, et al: Cloning and characterization of an extracellular Ca^{2+}-sensing receptor from bovine parathyroid, Nature 366:575–580, 1993.)

○ Conserved cysteine PKC site
● Conserved
△ Acidic
▲ Conserved acidic
⋎ N-glycosylation

inhibition of adenylyl cyclase.[146] Despite numerous studies conducted over the past 25 years, a full understanding of the major second messenger pathways through which changes in Ca^{2+}_o, acting via the CaSR, regulate various aspects of the function of parathyroid and other CaSR-expressing cells remains elusive (discussed later). Recent evidence, however, indicates key roles for the G proteins, G_q and G_{11}, but their downstream transduction pathways participating in the control of parathyroid function are uncertain.[147] In the parathyroid, the CaSR mediates the inhibitory actions of Ca^{2+}_o on PTH secretion and gene expression as well as parathyroid cellular proliferation.[138,148]

The CaSR is also expressed in several additional tissues involved in systemic mineral ion homeostasis, including the calcitonin-secreting C-cells of the thyroid,[149] diverse cells within the kidney,[150] bone cells and/or their precursors,[110] and intestinal epithelial cells. In the C cell, the CaSR mediates the stimulatory action of high Ca^{2+}_o on calcitonin secretion, a Ca^{2+}_o-lowering hormone. In the kidney, the CaSR in the cortical thick ascending limb of the nephron mediates direct high-Ca^{2+}_o-induced inhibition of the tubular reabsorption of Ca^{2+} and Mg^{2+}.[150,151] Therefore, raising Ca^{2+}_o both directly inhibits renal tubular reabsorption of Ca^{2+} via actions on the CaSR expressed in nephron segments involved in hormonal regulation of Ca^{2+} reabsorption (e.g., by PTH) and indirectly inhibits it by reducing PTH secretion (see the later section, Renal Calcium Reabsorption). The CaSR probably also mediates the long-recognized but poorly understood inhibitory effect of hypercalcemia on renal water conservation, probably exerting this action by inhibiting vasopressin-stimulated water flow in the distal collecting duct.[138] A possible physiologic relevance of this action is to prevent the development of excessively high concentrations of calcium in the distal collecting system, thereby perhaps mitigating the risk of renal stone formation.[151] Elevating Ca^{2+}_o stimulates osteoblastic bone forma-

tion and inhibits osteoclastic bone resorption.[110,152] The CaSR is expressed by chondrocytes as well as by osteoblasts and osteoclasts and/or their precursors,[110] and recent data suggest that it plays key roles in skeletal development.[153] It is not currently known whether the CaSR expressed in intestinal epithelial cells plays any role in regulating $1,25(OH)_2D_3$-mediated absorption of calcium.

The identification of hypercalcemic (e.g., familial hypocalciuric hypercalcemia and neonatal severe hyperparathyroidism)[154] and hypocalcemic (i.e., autosomal-dominant hypocalcemia)[155] disorders caused by inactivating and activating mutations of the CaSR, respectively, has provided incontrovertible proof of the receptor's central, nonredundant role in setting the serum calcium concentration.[156,157] Patients with these disorders have characteristic abnormalities in parathyroid and renal Ca^{2+} sensing/handling that have clarified the receptor's normal role in these tissues, outlined previously. Targeted disruption of the *CASR* gene has also enabled the generation of mouse models of familial hypocalciuric hypercalcemia and neonatal severe hyperparathyroidism via inactivation of one or both alleles of the CaSR[158], further supporting its importance in Ca^{2+}_o homeostasis.

$1,25(OH)_2D_3$, Phosphate, and Other Factors Regulating PTH Secretion

In addition to directly inhibiting *PTH* gene expression, $1,25(OH)_2D_3$ also reduces PTH secretion[159,160] (for review, see[11,26,118]). It is not known whether this latter action is solely secondary to the effect of $1,25(OH)_2D_3$ on biosynthesis of the hormone and/or represents a direct action on the secretory process per se. Increasing the ambient level of phosphate in vitro, independent of concomitant changes in Ca^{2+}_o, enhances parathyroid cellular proliferation, PTH gene expression, and hormonal secretion.[161-163] Phosphate-induced changes in PTH secretion, however, take several hours and may result secondarily from changes in hormonal biosynthesis rather than secretion per se.[163] Finally, Mg^{2+}_o clearly functions as a CaSR agonist in vitro when tested in cells containing an endogenous CaSR[164] (e.g., parathyroid cells) or expressing the cloned CaSR,[139] although it is twofold to threefold less potent than Ca^{2+}_o on a molar basis. Because levels of serum ionized Mg^{2+}_o are lower than those of Ca^{2+}_o, it is presently unclear whether Mg^{2+}_o acts as a physiologically relevant CaSR agonist at the parathyroid gland in vivo under normal circumstances. Patients with inactivating or activating CaSR mutations, however, can exhibit mild hypermagnesemia or hypomagnesemia,[156] respectively, thus suggesting that the CaSR does contribute to setting Mg^{2+}_o in vivo, as previously suggested.[165] It may do so, at least in part, in the kidney, where Mg^{2+}_o in the tubular fluid of the thick ascending limb exceeds that in blood and may be sufficient to activate the CaSR that regulates tubular reabsorption of Ca^{2+}_o and Mg^{2+}_o in this nephron segment.[138,151,166,167] In addition to the inhibitory effect of elevated Mg^{2+}_o on PTH secretion, low concentrations of Mg^{2+}_o—as in patients with overt magnesium deficiency—also reduce PTH secretion.[168] The mechanism(s) underlying this effect of hypomagnesemia has recently been suggested to involve increased activity of G proteins to which the CaSR normally couples, probably G_i and $G_{q/11}$, thereby leading to increased intracellular signaling and inhibition of PTH secretion.[169]

METABOLISM OF PARATHYROID HORMONE

Studies performed over more than 3 decades by several laboratories have focused on the heterogeneity of circulating forms of PTH, which was first identified by Berson and Yalow in 1968 (Fig. 1-8).[170] From these investigations, it is now apparent that in addition to the full-length polypeptide PTH(1-84), which is the biologically active hormone, much of the circulating hormone lacks an intact N-terminus, and most of these fragments are

thus devoid of biological activity, at least with regard to the PTH/PTHrP receptor-mediated regulation of mineral ion homeostasis.[25] C-terminal PTH fragments are produced in and released from the parathyroid gland, but they are also derived from circulating intact hormone by efficient, high-capacity degradative systems in the liver and kidney and most likely at other peripheral sites (Fig. 1-9). However, some PTH fragments, such as PTH(7-84), appear to be generated within the gland and to have some biological activity.[171-173]

Direct measurement of arterial and venous differences in parathyroid effluent blood (with vigorous conditions to prevent any ex vivo cleavage of hormone after sample collection) were performed in cattle and confirmed that smaller C-terminal fragments and intact hormone, but not N-terminal fragments, are secreted into the circulation. The relative concentration of these C-terminal fragments released from the gland increases under conditions of systemic hypercalcemia, when overall secretion rates of intact hormone are lower.[105,174] The C-terminal PTH fragments are similar to those generated by peripheral metabolism (see later) but were not chemically characterized.

The peripheral metabolism of PTH has been analyzed by injecting intact hormone into the circulation of test animals. Such experiments have not been performed in human subjects, but it is assumed that the similar metabolism of PTH in rats, dogs, and cows is reflective of its metabolism in humans.[175] Clearance of intact PTH from plasma was found to be very rapid (half-life, 2 to 4 minutes),[176,177] the major sites of clearance being the liver and kidney. Clearance by the liver predominates over clearance by the kidney; the two organs together account for virtually all clearance of intact hormone. Hepatic clearance of intact hormone has been estimated to be 40% to 75% and renal clearance 20% to 30%.[25]

In summary, current evidence indicates that intact PTH and multiple C-terminal fragments (which are derived from glandu-

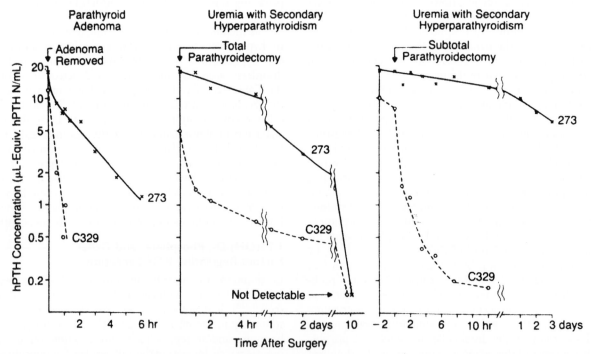

FIGURE 1-8. Disappearance of immunoreactive parathyroid hormone (PTH) from plasma after parathyroidectomy in patients with primary or secondary hyperparathyroidism. Plasma samples were assayed with antiserum C329 and antiserum 273, with an extract of a normal human parathyroid gland used as a standard (hPTH N) and ^{125}I-bPTH used as a tracer. Plasma concentrations of hormone are given as microliter equivalents of the plasma standard of hPTH (see the text). (Data from Berson SA, Yalow RS: Immunochemical heterogenicity of parathyroid hormone in plasma, J Clin Endocrinol Metab 28:1037–1047, 1968.)

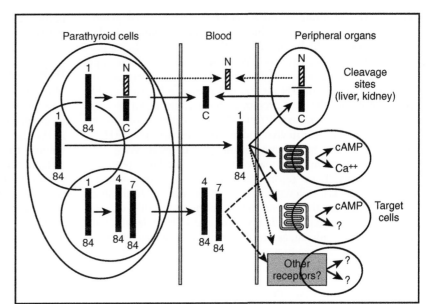

FIGURE I-9. Scheme of parathyroid hormone (PTH) cleavage and the interaction of PTH with the PTH/PTH-related peptide receptor (PTHIR) and with other putative receptors on target cells. Within parathyroid cells, secretory vesicles (circles) and in peripheral organs various patterns of cleavages of PTH (1–84) occur, resulting in multiple circulating fragments including N-terminal (N) (diagonal stripes), suggesting rapid degradation, and C-terminal fragments (C) (solid bars). The carboxyl end of intact PTH and possibly some C fragments interact with a putative C-terminal receptor and, as well, inhibit actions of PTH on the PTHIR. cAMP, Cyclic adenosine monophosphate.

lar and peripheral cleavage and may not be identical) are the principal circulating hormonal forms (however, recent data suggest the presence of a previously unrecognized large N-terminally truncated form of the hormone [discussed later]). Biologically active N-terminal fragments of PTH, if found in the circulation at all, are likely to circulate only at extremely low concentrations (<10-13 to 10-14 mol/L). More recent in vivo evidence regarding the renal clearance and metabolism of intact PTH (as distinct from C-terminal fragments) indicates a peritubular uptake process, rather than glomerular filtration followed by uptake from the tubular lumen and subsequent cleavage.[178] Furthermore, other studies indicate that megalin, a multifunctional endocytic receptor expressed in the proximal renal tubules, can mediate the reuptake and subsequent degradation of the fraction of PTH that is subject to glomerular filtration.[179] Megalin-mediated uptake depends on an intact N-terminus of PTH; C-terminal fragments that are eliminated by glomerular filtration are not recognized by megalin. The potential significance, quantitatively and biologically, of glomerular filtration and megalin-mediated uptake of intact PTH therefore remains uncertain. However, megalin-ablated mice excrete fourfold more N-terminal PTH in the urine than do wild-type animals.[179]

Because of the lack of evidence of circulating forms of biologically active, N-terminal fragments, it was feasible to introduce immunometric assays that use two different antibodies: an immobilized capturing antibody directed against the C-terminal portion of PTH(1-84) and a radiolabeled or enzyme-labeled detection antibody directed against an epitope within the N-terminal portion of the intact molecule[180,181] (see Fig. 1-9).

Although these two site assays have been clinically useful and provided a great improvement over earlier assays,[180] recent studies have demonstrated the presence of circulating PTH fragments that are different in character and composition from any of the hormone fragments discussed previously.[108,128,182] The studies that led to the detection of these PTH species were at least partly stimulated by the clinical observations that two-site immunometric assays to measure intact PTH frequently gave high levels of nonsuppressible PTH in patients with end-stage renal disease, yet the patients had clinical and/or histologic evidence of a dynamic bone disease[108,183-186] (see Chapter 14).

High-performance liquid chromatography analysis of blood samples from such uremic patients and from patients with other forms of hyperparathyroidism revealed two distinct immunoreactive peaks in column effluent that were detectable (although with differing sensitivity) by different commercial assays. One peak corresponded to intact PTH(1-84), whereas the other peak migrated close to the position occupied chromatographically by synthetic PTH(7-84).[108,128] This finding suggested that the epitope of the detection antibody in these assays did not require the presence of the first six or more amino acids of PTH(1-84).[128,129] The results were interpreted as being consistent with the view that the molecular entity or entities detected besides PTH(1-84) are N-terminally truncated forms of the intact molecule that are similar, but not necessarily identical, to synthetic PTH(7-84).[128] In fact, more detailed chromatographic studies performed with one of these "intact" PTH assays showed significant variation in the ratio of the N-terminally truncated PTH to PTH(1-84). Individuals with normal renal function showed a lower ratio than did patients with uremia; furthermore, the percentage of immunoreactivity representing N-terminally truncated forms of PTH (PTH[7-84]) rose in both groups when hypercalcemia was present.[108]

The newer immunoradiometric assays that have N-terminal epitopes at the extreme amino-terminus of PTH(1-84) show significantly lower PTH concentrations in patients with chronic renal failure during stimulation and suppression of glandular activity with alterations in calcium, a result consistent with the conclusion that only full-length and therefore biologically active PTH(1-84) is detected by these assay systems.[173,182,187]

The findings outlined previously were expected to have considerable significance for the management of patients with parathyroid dysfunction, especially in the presence of renal failure. Treatment of patients with end-stage renal disease with large amounts of vitamin D and/or calcium (or calcimimetics) has been associated with adynamic bone disease, which can be deleterious, particularly in growing children.[188-190] Particularly during hypercalcemia, N-terminally truncated forms of PTH become a significant, if not the dominant, PTH species.[191,192] Measurement of "intact" PTH by earlier assays[180] therefore overestimated the concentrations of biologically active PTH and could result in the overtreatment of uremic patients with vitamin D-analogs and/or calcium. The resulting suppression of the parathyroid gland, even without evoking an inhibitory effect of a fragment similar to PTH(7-84), could be acting together to excessively reduce PTH-dependent bone turnover. When secretion of PTH is suppressed, as in hypercalcemia, and the fractional concentration of the large N-truncated PTH increases, however, inhibition of the actions of native PTH on calcium or bone could occur. Recent experiments with synthetic PTH(7–84) support the conclusion that such actions occur in vivo and in vitro. For example, PTH(7-84) was shown to have hypocalcemic properties in vivo,[171,173] and it reduces, presumably via receptors specific for C-terminal PTH fragments, bone resorption that may be partly due to impaired osteoclast differentiation.[109,171] It is not yet established clinically whether the newer radioimmunoassays that do not detect large but amino-terminally truncated PTH molecules will have a decisive advantage in diagnosis and management of primary and secondary hyperparathyroidism[187] (see Chapters 7 and 14).

By contrast to the extensive metabolism of PTH, recent evidence suggests that intact FGF23, which is most likely the most important phosphate-regulating hormone,[23] does not appear to undergo significant metabolism.[193] In fact, immunoreactive FGF23, which can be extraordinarily elevated in patients with end-stage renal disease, appears to be largely intact and biologically active. This makes it unlikely that FGF23, unlike PTH, is metabolized in peripheral organs.

PTH-Dependent Regulation of Mineral Ion Homeostasis Mediated Through the PTH/PTHrP Receptor (Type I Receptor)

PTH is, as outlined earlier, the most important peptide regulator of mineral ion homeostasis in mammals. Through its actions on the kidney and bone, PTH maintains blood calcium concentration within narrow limits. In bone it stimulates the release of calcium, and in the kidney it enhances renal tubular reabsorption of calcium (and diminishes tubular reabsorption of phosphate). Furthermore, in the kidney it increases the synthesis of renal 1α-hydroxylase, which stimulates $1,25(OH)_2D_3$ production and thus increases, albeit indirectly, intestinal absorption of calcium (and phosphate). These direct and indirect endocrine actions of PTH are mediated through the PTH/PTHrP receptor (PTH1R), a G protein–coupled receptor that is abundantly expressed in both major target tissues of PTH action.

ACTIONS OF PARATHYROID HORMONE ON KIDNEY

In addition to regulating renal calcium and phosphate transport, PTH modifies the tubular handling of magnesium, sodium, potassium, bicarbonate, and water and stimulates renal gluconeogenesis. Specific regions of the nephron that are involved in each of the PTH-dependent actions have been defined through in vivo micropuncture analyses and through in vitro studies with nephron segments that have been dissected from the remainder of the kidney. Furthermore, cell lines from specific regions of the kidney have also been used. However, interpretation of these results has to take into account the complexity of the organization of the kidney as an organ (for example, the complex anatomic relationship involving different renal tubular segments spanning both the cortex and medulla and the effects of countercurrent distribution that modify solute and water transport), particularly since certain in vivo features of renal tubules are not readily imitated in vitro through the use of isolated tubules or cells.

RENAL CALCIUM REABSORPTION

Most of the calcium in the glomerular filtrate is reabsorbed. The bulk of this reabsorption (65%) occurs via passive, paracellular mechanisms, both in the proximal tubules and, to a lesser extent, in the thick ascending limb of Henle's loop and the distal convoluted tubule.[194-198] As noted by Diaz and colleagues,[26] the calcium-sensing receptor plays an important PTH-independent role in the adjustment of renal calcium reabsorption in the cortical thick ascending limb. The physiologically important stimulation of renal calcium reabsorption by PTH occurs almost entirely in the distal nephron. In the cortical thick ascending limb, PTH increases the magnitude of the lumen positive potential that drives the passive paracellular reabsorption of calcium and magnesium. In the distal convoluted tubule, in contrast, PTH promotes increased transcellular Ca^{2+} reabsorption by coordinate up-regulation of molecular components of this transcellular pathway.[199] PTH enhances uptake of Ca^{2+} into the tubular cells via the (luminal) plasma membrane channel, TRPV5,[200,201] as well as its active extrusion against a steep electrochemical gradient at the basolateral membrane. This latter process of extrusion involves two types of transporters. One is the plasma membrane calcium pump (Ca^{2+}, Mg^{2+}-ATPase, PMCA) and the second is a Na^+/Ca^{2+} exchanger (NCX1), which in turn is indirectly regulated by NA^+/K^--ATPase(s), which maintains the transcellular Na^+ gradient. Studies performed with membrane vesicles from the distal region of the kidney show increased activity of the Na^+/Ca^{2+} exchanger in response to PTH.[202] PTH also stimulates the translocation of preformed Ca^{2+} channels sequestered within the interior of certain distal tubular cells, presumably TRPV5, apical surface (Fig. 1-10),[203] which translocate to the apical (i.e., luminal) surface of the renal tubular epithelial cell and mediate increased cellular Ca^{2+} uptake. Because PTH simultaneously enhances the activity of Na^+/Ca^{2+} exchangers in the basolateral (antiluminal) membrane, the overall process promotes an increase in transcellular Ca^{2+} uptake from the lumen to blood, that is, from the apical to the basolateral membrane.

REGULATION OF 1α- AND 24-HYDROXYLASE ACTIVITY

PTH is a major inducer of the activity of proximal tubular 1α-hydroxylase, a microsomal cytochrome P-450 enzyme that synthesizes biologically active $1,25(OH)_2D_3$ from the substrate $25(OH)D_3$.[204-206] This effect of PTH on synthesis of the renal enzyme shows longer lag times than its effect on renal Ca^{2+} transport and is mediated, at least in part, by the protein kinase A (PKA) signaling pathway of the PTH/PTHrP receptor.[207,208] Although 1α-hydroxylase activity has been detected in several nonrenal tissues, its mRNA was found in abundant concentrations only in the kidney, thus confirming that this organ is the most important site for the generation of $1,25(OH)_2D_3$. PTH-dependent synthesis of new 1α-hydroxylase protein requires several hours and is blocked by $1,25(OH)_2D_3$ and actinomycin D, a blocker of protein synthesis.[208-210] PTH administration increases the mRNA encoding the 1α-hydroxylase.[208] Hypophosphatemia is, similar to PTH, a major inducer of 1α-hydroxylase, whereas hypercalcemia, as would be generated by sustained increases in circulating levels of PTH or PTHrP, suppresses synthesis of the enzyme, thus limiting overall $1,25(OH)_2D_3$ synthesis in a homeostatic manner. The molecules $25(OH)D_3$ and

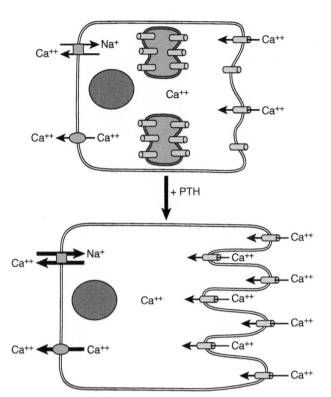

FIGURE 1-10. PTH regulation of calcium transport in renal distal tubule cells. Parathyroid hormone (PTH) triggers the translocation of preformed voltage-dependent calcium channels from sites of intracellular sequestration to the apical membrane, which also undergoes rapid morphologic changes that greatly increase its surface area. Intracellular free calcium levels rise significantly, and increased net transepithelial calcium transport occurs, mainly via enhanced Na^+/Ca^{2+} exchange at the basolateral membrane, supported in turn by Na^+/K^+-ATPase.

$1,25(OH)_2D_3$ can also be hydroxylated by the 24-hydroxylase, but the resulting metabolites, $24,25(OH)_2D_3$ and $1,24,25(OH)_3D_3$, appear to have no major role in the regulation of mineral ion homeostasis (see Chapter 3). However, PTH has an inhibitory effect on the 24-hydroxylase, thus reducing the inactivation of $1,25(OH)_2D_3$; in contrast, $1,25(OH)_2D_3$ stimulates the synthesis of 24-hydroxylase, thereby inducing its own metabolism.[211,212]

RENAL PHOSPHATE TRANSPORT

PTH is of major importance for maintaining normal blood calcium levels, but it is not the principal regulator of the serum phosphate concentration, which appears to depend on specific phosphaturic factors, particularly FGF-23 (see Chapter 6).[19,23,213] However, when PTH causes an increase in bone resorption (as might occur with prolonged dietary calcium deprivation), calcium and phosphate increase simultaneously in the blood. Although calcium is needed, phosphate is best excreted, which is mainly accomplished by a PTH-stimulated increase in renal phosphate clearance.

PTH acts directly on proximal tubular cells, where it regulates expression of NPT2a and NPT2c in the brush border membrane. Whereas NPT2a is expressed in segments S1 through S3 of the proximal tubule, NPT2c is expressed only in the S1 segment. NPT2a protein undergoes internalization in response to PTH,[214] followed by lysosomal degradation[215]; in contrast, recent evidence suggests that NPT2c can be recycled and reinserted into the brush border membrane.[216] In the proximal renal tubules, PTH furthermore enhances the production of biologically active $1,25(OH)_2$ vitamin D.[217-220] All these actions of PTH are mediated

through the PTH/PTHrP receptor (PTH1R), which is expressed at the basolateral membrane (BLM) and at much higher levels at the apical brush border membrane (BBM) of the proximal renal tubules.[217,221-223]

The PTH-dependent renal actions probably involve cAMP/PKA-dependent and $Ca^{2+}/IP_3/PKC$-dependent signaling events at the BLM, and both pathways appear to contribute to the reduction in proximal tubular phosphate reabsorption.[217,218,220] In contrast to these dual signaling properties of the PTH1R at the BLM, there is considerable evidence to suggest that the inhibition of phosphate uptake mediated through the PTH1R at the BBM involves predominantly, if not exclusively, a pertussis-toxin-sensitive, PKC-dependent pathway.[217,224-227] PTH thus activates both major signaling pathways via PTH/PTHrP receptors located at either the BLM or the BBM, and it induces phosphaturia by reducing expression of the type II sodium-phosphate cotransporters, NPT2a and NPT2c.

Activation of the cAMP/PKA pathway down-stream of the PTH1R is undoubtedly involved in the PTH-dependent regulation of NPT2a expression.[226-228] In fact, patients affected by pseudohypoparathyroidism type Ia (PHP-Ia), a disease caused by inactivating mutations in GNAS, the gene encoding the alpha subunit of the stimulatory G protein ($G_{s\alpha}$), develop hyperphosphatemia due to a lack of functional $G_{s\alpha}$ in the proximal tubules and consequently show impaired urinary cAMP and phosphate excretion in response to PTH (see Chapter 6). However, the phosphaturic response stimulated by PTH is not totally absent, since PHP-Ia patients have a small but delayed increase in urinary phosphate excretion after challenge with PTH, which suggests that signaling molecules other than cAMP could also be involved in promoting phosphate excretion.[229-231]

Besides regulating NPT2a expression, PTH also affects expression of the second kidney-specific sodium-dependent phosphate cotransporter, namely NPT2c.[227] The mRNA encoding NTP2c is about 10-fold less abundant than that encoding NPT2a, which initially suggested that NTP2c plays only a minor biological role limited to some period during postnatal development.[232] It was then found, however, that homozygous and compound heterozygous mutations in NPT2c cause hereditary hypophosphatemic rickets with hypercalciuria (HHRH), an autosomal-recessive disorder.[233-236] This disease linkage makes it certain that NPT2c serves important functions in biology and is not redundant with NPT2a.[218-220] Nevertheless, it is so far unknown how the two transporters differ in their functional roles. Both proteins are internalized at the BBM in response to treatment with PTH, but the time courses of these agonist-dependent processes differ, raising the possibility that different scaffolding proteins regulated by PTH underlie the differential regulation of NPT2a and NPT2c. Furthermore, activation of different signaling pathways down-stream of the PTH1R—namely, the cAMP-dependent activation of PKA or the Ca^{2+}/IP_3-dependent or Ca^{2+}/IP_3-independent activation of PKC—may have different roles in the regulation of NPT2a and NPT2c expression (Fig. 1-11).

These differences may involve "signalsomes," that is, specialized intracellular domains in which proteins involved in a specific biochemical process or pathway are brought into close proximity by binding to "scaffold" proteins, thereby limiting their diffusion and altering receptor-mediated downstream signaling pathways.[237] In renal proximal tubules, the sodium/hydrogen exchanger regulatory factors 1 and 2 (NHERF1/2) are prominent scaffold proteins that contain two PDZ (psd-95, discs large, ZO-1)-binding domains and a C-terminal ERM (ezrin, radixin, moesin)-binding motif (see review[238]). The PTH1R inter-

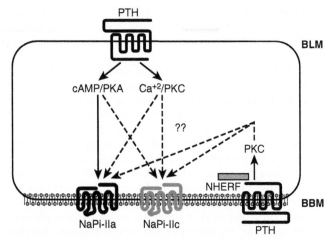

FIGURE 1-11. PTH regulation of renal phosphate transport. A proximal convoluted tubule cell is depicted. The type II sodium-dependent phosphate cotransporters NaPi-IIa and NaPi-IIc (also referred to as NPT2a and NPT2c) reabsorb phosphate from the tubule lumen. NHERF-1 promotes apical localization of NaPi-IIa (but not NaPi-IIc) and establishes a regulatory complex for PTH-mediated inhibition of phosphate reabsorption. PTH inhibits phosphate reabsorption by reducing expression of both transportes. PTH1 receptors (PTH1R) located on both the basolateral and luminal surfaces reduce NaPi-IIa and NaPi-IIc expression via signaling pathways involving protein kinase A (cAMP/PKA) (solid arrow) and other pathways (dotted arrows), still less characterized, including PLC/PKC. (Courtesy Dr. Matthew Mahon.)

acts with NHERF proteins through a C-terminal PDZ-binding motif [239,240] (see Fig. 1-11), which leads in some cell lines to NHERF-dependent suppression of PTH-stimulated cAMP accumulation.[239] In opossum kidney cells (OK), NHERF1 enhances PTH1R signaling through intracellular calcium and PLC.[240] In fact, anchoring the receptor to the BBM of proximal tubules appears to promote signaling through the IP$_3$/PKC pathway, illustrating how domain-specific factors can influence receptor-dependent signaling.

Similar to the PTH1R, NPT2a also contains a C-terminal motif that binds to PDZ domains of NHERF1,[241] and NHERF1-null mice display phosphate wasting due to a reduction in NPT2a expression at the BBM of proximal tubules. Thus, this transporter requires a NHERF1-assembled scaffold for proper membrane expression.[242] Furthermore, NHERF1 has been shown to be an essential factor for PTH-mediated regulation of NPT2a expression in OK cells and in primary proximal tubular cell cultures isolated from NHERF1-null mice. Combined, these findings demonstrate that NHERF1 not only establishes NPT2a surface expression but also aids in the formation of a regulatory complex necessary for PTH-elicited phosphaturia. In vitro, NHERF1-assembled complexes consisting of PTH1R and NPT2a are present in apical domains of OK cells and in genetically modified LLC-PK1 cells developed for studying phosphate transport.[243]

The PTH fragment peptide, PTH(3-34), has been frequently used in efforts to discern the signaling events at the BBM from those at the BLM which regulate NPT2a and NPT2c; some data suggest that this analog may selectively activate the PKC signaling pathway[244-246] and thus should act only at the BBM. There are, however, no data demonstrating that PTH(3-34) can directly activate the PLC-dependent formation of IP$_3$, and in fact substitutions or deletions at positions 1 and 2 of PTH result in markedly and/or selectively impaired activation of the PLC/IP$_3$/Ca^{2+} signaling response.[58-60,247] PTH(3-34) has been shown to activate PKC via a non-PLC/IP$_3$-dependent mechanism, perhaps involving another phospholipase such as PLA$_2$.[246] In any case, several investigators have shown that PTH(3-34), as well as other PTH and PTHrP fragments truncated at the amino-terminus, can

inhibit the uptake of phosphate by opossum kidney cells (which do not express significant amounts of NPT2c) in the apparent absence of significant cAMP accumulation.[248-252] Furthermore, PTH(3-34) was shown to promote, at least partially, urinary phosphate excretion in animals.[253] This raises the possibility that PTH fragments such as PTH(7-84) and PTH(4-84), which are found in the circulation of patients with primary or secondary hyperparathyroidism, could induce phosphaturic effects.[172,191,192,254,255] PTH(7-84), however, does not appear to have phosphaturic activity when tested in vivo, or in some in vitro systems. In addition, PTH(3-34) can activate at least partially the cAMP-dependent PKA in cells.[256,257] This makes it plausible that the capacities of amino-terminally truncated PTH or PTHrP analogs to promote the urinary excretion of phosphate arise at least to some extent from partial activation of the cAMP/PKA pathway at the BLM.

As mentioned, PTH treatment leads to the reduction of NPT2a and NPT2c in the kidney, but effects of the hormone on the two cotransporters appear to differ, as shown in thyro-parathyroidectomized rats.[218-220,227] NPT2a is expressed in the segments S1-S3 of the proximal renal tubules, whereas NPT2c is present only in S1.[218-220,227] NPT2a is the more abundantly expressed cotransporter, and it handles (in the mouse) 70% to 80% of renal phosphate reabsorption, with NPT2c accounting for the remaining 20% to 30%. In response to PTH, NPT2a disappears rapidly from the BBM and translocates to lysosomes where it undergoes degradation, whereas NPT2c disappears from the BBM surface at a much slower rate and does not seem to undergo lysosomal degradation but rather may recycle back to the BBM surface.[216] The mechanisms underlying these diverse response profiles are uncertain at present, but the generation of engineered LLC-PK1 cells that show PTH-dependent inhibition of phosphate transport via reductions in either NPT2a or NPT2c expression[243] will likely lead to important new insights into the molecular and cellular processes involved.

ACTIONS OF PARATHYROID HORMONE ON BONE

PTH affects a wide variety of the highly specialized bone cells, including osteoblasts, osteoclast/stromal cells, and osteocytes, the latter being the most numerous cell type in bone. Some of these effects reflect direct actions of PTH; others are indirect and mediated in an autocrine/paracrine manner through factors released by cells (osteoblasts) expressing PTH/PTHrP receptors that regulate the activity of yet other cells (osteoclasts) that lack these receptors.[258-260]

PTH action on bone cells can be considered from at least five distinct perspectives. First is its major physiologic role—the maintenance of calcium homeostasis. As noted in Fig. 1-2, this action can be analyzed most clearly in experimental animals through parathyroidectomy, with resultant hypocalcemia. Renal losses of calcium are significant contributors to the severe, sometimes fatal hypocalcemia, but the loss of PTH action on bone cells is the predominant cause. The traditional explanation is that the hypocalcemia is due principally to the loss of PTH stimulation of osteoclastic bone resorption, but other mechanisms may be involved (see later). A second perspective is the action of PTH when administered pharmacologically, resulting in elevation of serum calcium, immediately preceded by a short-lived fall in calcium. It is still unclear which specific cellular actions explain the physiologic actions known to follow PTH administration to animals in vivo. Earlier studies had shown that the administration of PTH leads within minutes to a transient lowering of blood calcium caused by uptake of the mineral by bone cells,[261] which is rapidly followed by increased mobilization of calcium from the mineral phase into the bloodstream.[261,262] Although there continues to be uncertainties regarding the cellular/anatomic basis of these rapid responses to PTH, considerable progress has been made in elucidating the mechanisms through which bone cells respond to PTH and to other autocrine/paracrine factors such as cytokines (see Chapters 4 and 12). A major pathway for calcium release from bone involves osteoclasts; these cells undergo multiple cellular changes involving the activation of cellular transporters and pumps, as well as the secretion of enzymes such as cathepsin K and collagenases, but other mechanisms of calcium release are proposed.[261,262]

A third perspective regarding PTH action on bone cells can be appreciated through results seen when PTH is used as a therapy for osteoporosis. Chronic administration of PTH, if given intermittently, stimulates bone formation, an action that involves a complex set of cellular responses in bone, affecting principally stromal cell/osteoblast proliferation, differentiation, and cellular actions.[263-267] It is also clear that actions on osteocytes are involved in PTH actions on bone[267,268]; together, PTH effects on the two cell types, osteoblasts and osteocytes, stimulate bone matrix formation and bone mineral deposition, as well as bone mineral mobilization (see Chapters 4 and 5).

Fourthly, pathophysiologic actions of PTH are seen in hyperparathyroidism with chronic excess levels of PTH. In this situation, both bone formation and bone resorption are stimulated, the latter effect being predominant (see Chapters 4 and 7).

Finally, one must consider parathyroid hormone action on bone (and that of the closely related PTHrP) from the important role played, along with multiple other hormones and cytokines, in the complex system biology of embryonic bone formation and bone formation and remodeling in the adult. Numerous other hormones and autocrine/paracrine-acting cytokines interact with PTH and PTHrP in this still incompletely understood complex cellular biology of bone.

Effects on Osteoblasts

Osteoblasts express the PTH/PTHrP receptor abundantly and show vigorous responses to the hormone. PTH stimulates the generation of cAMP, inositol triphosphate, and diacylglycerol in cells expressing the cloned PTH/PTHrP receptor.[8,9,269] A remarkable number of cellular activities of osteoblasts are influenced by PTH, including cellular metabolic activity, ion transport, cell shape, gene transcriptional activity, and secretion of multiple proteases (see Chapters 4 and 12). Continuous PTH administration in vivo results in decreased bone mass, whereas intermittent administration of PTH leads to an increase.[25,270,271] Osteoblast synthetic activity is strongly stimulated in both situations, but osteoblast/stromal cell increased production of RANK ligand and suppression of osteoprotegerin secretion[272,273] dominate through stimulation of osteoclastic activity in chronic PTH administration.

PTH administration leads to multiple osteoblastic responses, including reduced rates of cell apoptosis,[263] increased expression and activity of Runx 2,[274,275] and increased rates of osteoblastic cell differentiation.[264,276]

The exact cellular mechanisms whereby intermittent PTH administration selectively enhances bone formation remain unclear at present, as are correlations between in vivo and in vitro responses. Further exploration of these mechanisms is clearly of great interest for understanding the hormone's therapeutic potential as a bone anabolic agent.[277]

Effects on Osteoclasts

It is generally agreed that osteoclasts lack PTH receptors, and hence actions of PTH are indirect, largely through stimulation of cytokines elaborated from osteoblasts/stromal cells. These molecules include osteoclast-differentiating factor, now usually called *RANK-L*,[278,279] a membrane-associated protein with homology to the family of tumor necrosis factors (TNFs) that induces—upon cell-to-cell contact and in the presence of macrophage colony-stimulating factor—the differentiation of osteoclast precursors into mature bone-resorbing osteoclasts.[280-282] These effects of RANK-L are likely to be mediated through RANK, a member of the TNF receptor family that is expressed on osteoclast precursors.[279,280] However, RANK-L also interacts with osteoprotegerin, a soluble decoy receptor with homology to the TNF receptor family.[283] Transgenic expression of osteoprotegerin in mice leads to impaired osteoclastogenesis and thus to osteopetrosis,[284,285] whereas ablation of the osteoprotegerin gene through homologous recombination in mice results in osteoporosis associated with arterial calcifications.[286] Ablation of the gene for RANK-L results in severe osteopetrosis due to lack of osteoclasts, a defect in tooth eruption, and a complete lack of lymph nodes, but without obvious abnormalities in mineral ion homeostasis.[274] Similarly, ablation of the RANK-L receptor (RANK), leads to osteopetrotic changes similar to those observed in RANK-L-ablated mice, but also to hypocalcemia and secondary hyperparathyroidism and to renal phosphate wasting.[275] It appears plausible that challenging the homeostatic control mechanisms of either of these knockout mice, in particular, through dietary calcium and vitamin D deficiency will further aggravate the degree of hypocalcemia and urinary phosphate excretion. However, despite the absence of such experimental data, the outlined findings further illustrate the importance of osteoclastic bone resorption for maintaining blood calcium concentrations.

Some of the factors previously noted to have an important role in the paracrine stimulation of osteoclast formation, such as interleukin 6, interleukin 11, prostaglandin E2, $1,25(OH)_2D_3$, and other peptides, including PTH,[287-289] were shown to directly stimulate the production of RANK-L by osteoblasts.[290] Other cellular responses involved in bone resorption include the development of vitronectin-mediated anchorage of osteoclasts to the bone surface, acidification of the circumscribed and sealed-off extracellular environment that is created between the osteoclast and bone, and in addition, the secretion of a variety of proteases and other enzymes (see Chapter 4).

Effects on Osteocytes

Osteocytes, long neglected in bone cell biology, are the most numerous cell type in bone, and there is a growing appreciation that they play a central biological role with a myriad of functions ranging from transducing mechanical signals into bone growth and increased bone mineral density to hitherto completely unappreciated roles in phosphate homeostasis.[272,273,277]

Osteocytes contain abundant parathyroid hormone receptors, and there is now a clearly defined, biologically significant series of responses to parathyroid hormone action that have been described.[266-268,291] Chapters 4, 5, and 6 outline the roles of the osteocyte in bone turnover and the complex, still incompletely defined role of multiple interacting factors within osteocytes or secreted by them, including matrix extracellular phosphoglycoprotein (MEPE), dentin matrix protein 1 (DMP-1), and fibroblast growth factor 23 (FGF-23), in the regulation of renal phosphate clearance.[23,292]

The clearly defined effect of PTH to reduce sclerostin (SOST) production by osteocytes in turn enhances osteoblastic activity by blocking the suppressive effects of SOST on osteoblast activity and the Wnt signaling pathway.[266-268] Chapter 4 provides a more detailed review of the role of osteocytes as mechanosensors and sources of humoral factors in bone biology (see also Chapter 6).

Parathyroid Hormone–Related Peptide

Analysis of the physiologic actions of PTH and the molecular basis of its biological activity requires consideration of the functions of PTHrP. This peptide, discovered and characterized several decades after discovery of PTH, undoubtedly shares an evolutionary origin with PTH. PTHrP has (see Fig. 1-3), at least in mammals, both chemical and functional overlaps with PTH, but many of its biological roles are quite different. When secreted in large concentrations (e.g., by certain tumors), PTHrP has PTH-like properties. Typically, however, it functions as an autocrine/paracrine rather than an endocrine factor. PTHrP is a larger, more complex protein than PTH and is synthesized at multiple sites in different organs and tissues. The still-evolving story of this protein and its proteolytic fragments is beyond the scope of this chapter (for comprehensive review, see[4,6,293]). However, selective functions in the regulation of mineral ion homeostasis and bone development are reviewed here.

A substance with biological properties similar to those of PTH was first proposed in the early 1940s, when Albright discussed a patient with malignancy-associated humoral hypercalcemia.[294] The clinical and biochemical characterization of similarly affected patients subsequently established the syndrome of humoral hypercalcemia of malignancy[295] and eventually led to the amino acid sequence analysis and molecular cloning of PTHrP from several different tumors.[296-298] It is now generally accepted that PTHrP is the most frequent humoral cause of hypercalcemia in malignancies.[4,293,299] PTHrP interacts with the same receptor used by PTH, and when large amounts of the peptide are released from certain tumors, it mimics some or all of the effects of excess PTH. However, PTHrP is also expressed in a remarkable variety of normal fetal and adult tissues,[4,293,298,300-304] which suggested soon after its discovery that it has additional biological role(s)

that are unrelated to calcium and phosphorus homeostasis and that these role(s) are distinct from those mediated by PTH. One of its most prominent functions is the regulation of chondrocyte proliferation and differentiation and consequently bone elongation and growth.[12,13,305,306]

THE *PTHrP* GENE IN COMPARISON TO THE *PTH* GENE

The human PTHrP gene is located on chromosome 12p12.1-11.2,[298] which has a region analogous to that containing the human PTH gene on chromosome 11p15.[83-85] Both the PTH and the PTHrP genes have a similar organization, including equivalent positions of the boundaries between some of the coding exons and the adjacent introns[11,87,298,307] (Fig. 1-12).

Like the PTH gene, the PTHrP gene contains a single exon that encodes most amino acid residues of the prepropeptide sequence, and both genes have an exon that encodes the remainder of the propeptide sequence, that is, two basic residues (Lys and Arg) that are required for endoproteolytic cleavage of the mature peptide, and either all or most of the amino acids of the secreted peptides. The similarities in their protein sequence and in the structure of their genes, as well as the overlap in some of their functional properties, confirmed that both peptides are derived from a common ancestor.[4,6,293] By now, both mammalian genes have diverged considerably; for example, in contrast to the less complex PTH gene, which gives rise to a single gene product, the PTHrP gene uses at least three different promoters and alternative splice patterns that lead to the synthesis of several different mRNA species encoding peptides with different C-terminal ends.[6,293,298,307] A polymorphic dinucleotide repeat sequence that has been used for genetic linkage studies is located downstream of exon 4 (which is exon 6 according to a different nomenclature) of the human PTHrP gene[308] (see Fig. 1-12); thus far, no human disorder has been discovered that is caused by mutations in the PTHrP gene.

When compared with each other, chicken PTHrP and the known mammalian species of PTHrP show strong amino acid sequence homology within the first 111 residues; the degree of amino acid sequence conservation of PTHrP is considerably higher than that of the known PTH species (see Fig. 1-3). The amino acid sequence homology between both peptide families is restricted to the N-terminal portion, where 6 of the first 12

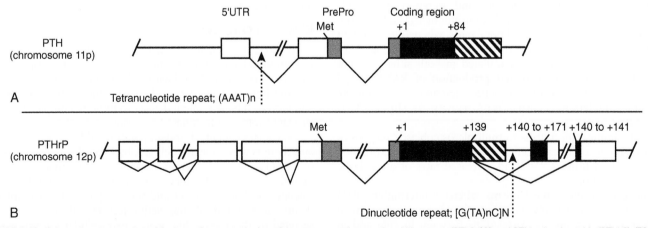

FIGURE 1-12. Schematic representation of the intron/exon organization of the genes encoding parathyroid hormone (PTH) **(A)** and PTH-related peptide (PTHrP) **(B)**. The introns are represented by a *solid line*, and the coding and noncoding exons are shown *(boxes)*; Met indicates the initiator methionine of the prepropeptide sequences *(shaded boxes)*, and numbers indicate the first and the last amino acid residues of the secreted peptides that are encoded by the different exons *(filled boxes)*. The approximate locations of frequent microsatellite polymorphisms in either the PTH[92] or the PTHrP[308] gene are indicated.

Table 1-2. Selective Characteristics of Other Potential Receptors for PTH and/or PTHrP Distinct from the PTH1R and PTH2R

Receptor	Target Tissue	Ligand Specificity	Function	Signaling Properties	References
PTH-specific receptors	Bone, kidney, cartilage, parathyroid gland-derived fibroblasts	Carboxyl-terminal fragments of PTH—i.e., 7-84, 19-84, or 39-84	Hypocalcemic actions, inhibition of osteoclast activity, and unknown functions	Unknown	109,171,173,482,487-489,495
	Bone, cartilage	Mid-regional fragments of PTH	Cell proliferation	PL-C	244,471-473
PTHrP-specific receptors	Placenta	Mid-regional fragments of PTHrP—i.e., (38-94)NH$_2$ or (67-86)NH$_2$	Transplacental calcium transfer	Unknown	309,325
	Keratinocytes, squamous cell carcinoma	Mid-regional fragments of PTHrP—i.e., (38-94)NH$_2$ or (67-86)NH$_2$	Unknown	Ca^{2+}, IP$_3$	324
	Bone cells	PTHrP(107-139)NH$_2$, PTHrP(107-111)NH$_2$, and other peptides	Inhibition of osteoclasts Stimulation of osteoblast	Unknown	317-320,482
	Hippocampus	PTHrP(107-139)NH$_2$	Unknown	Ca^{2+}	491
	Supraoptic nucleus	Amino-terminal fragments of PTHrP; PTH is considerably less active	Vasopressin-release	cAMP	496,497
PTH3R	Unknown (isolated thus far only from zebrafish and chicken)	For zebrafish PTH3R: PTH(1-34) and PTHrP(1-36) For chicken PTH3R: unknown	Unknown	cAMP	398
Other receptors that interact with PTH and PTHrP	Pancreatic cells, keratinocytes, squamous cell carcinoma	Amino-terminal fragments of PTH or PTHrP	Unknown	Ca^{2+}	

amino acid residues are conserved in all PTH and PTHrP species (see Fig. 1-3); the middle and C-terminal regions of both peptides share no recognizable similarity.

PTHrP is likely to undergo extensive posttranslational processing, resulting in peptide fragments, some of which may have biological properties distinct from those of PTHrP(1-34) on calcium and bone metabolism. The N-terminal PTHrP fragment functionally homologous to PTH is derived through cleavage at amino acid residue Arg37.[309,310] PTHrP(1-36) interacts efficiently with the PTH1R,[7-9,311] and it has an in vivo efficacy similar to that of PTH(1-34).[312-314] Longer, glycosylated fragments of N-terminal PTHrP were also described; however, these forms appear to be generated predominantly by skin-derived cells, and their biological role, if different from that of PTHrP(1-34) or PTHrP(1-36), remains to be established.[315]

In addition to the biologically active N-terminal PTHrP fragment, different C-terminal fragments are generated and accumulate in patients with end-stage renal disease.[316] A PTHrP fragment consisting of amino acids 107 to 139 and a shorter peptide, PTHrP(107-111), may be relevant to the control of bone metabolism because both fragments were shown to inhibit osteoclastic bone resorption[317,318] and to stimulate osteoblast activity and proliferation.[319] Although some investigators, using modified experimental conditions, were unable to confirm the in vitro findings with osteoclasts,[320] more recent data indicate that PTHrP(107-139) reduces the number of osteoclasts and inhibits bone resorption in vivo.[321] Taken together, these findings suggest that C-terminal PTHrP fragments may have a role in regulating bone resorption and/or formation (Table 1-2).

Cleavage at amino acid residue Arg37 also generates PTHrP(38-94) amide, a PTHrP fragment that could be of considerable importance in maintaining fetal calcium homeostasis.[309,322] This peptide is found in the circulation[323] and appears to interact with a distinct receptor that signals through changes in intracellular free calcium and is likely to be an important regulator of transplacental calcium transfer.[309,322,324-326] Studies with PTHrP(38-94) amide and PTHrP(67-86) amide have shown that these fragments increase the blood calcium concentrations of parathyroidectomized fetal lambs and PTHrP-ablated murine fetuses, respectively[309,325,326] (see later). These results confirmed earlier data that had provided the first evidence for an important role of PTHrP in the regulation of fetal calcium homeostasis.[327]

FUNCTIONS OF PTHrP

The first actions of PTHrP to be defined were the PTH-like actions associated with the humoral hypercalcemia of malignancy.[4,6,293] In this pathologic circumstance, PTHrP acts like a hormone, that is, it is secreted from the tumor into the bloodstream and then acts on bone and kidney to raise calcium levels (see Chapter 7). Whether PTHrP circulates at high enough levels in normal adults to contribute at all as a hormone to normal calcium homeostasis is an unanswered question; the levels are certainly low, and patients with congenital or acquired hypoparathyroidism are hypocalcemic despite the presence of PTHrP. Although incomplete and somewhat conflicting, growing evidence suggests, however, that PTHrP may act as a hormone in two special circumstances: during fetal life and during lactation as outlined in the next sections.

Role of PTHrP in Placental Calcium Transport

During intrauterine life, fetal blood calcium is higher than maternal blood calcium, at least partly because of active transport of calcium across the placenta. In fetal life, in contrast to adulthood, PTHrP is made in easily detectable amounts in the parathyroid gland. Parathyroidectomy lowers the blood level of calcium in fetal sheep and abolishes active calcium transport across the experimentally perfused placenta. PTHrP from human tumors and synthetic PTHrP(1-84), PTHrP(1-108), PTHrP(1-141), and PTHrP(67-86) amide acutely restored placental transport of calcium in a perfused placenta preparation.[328,329] PTHrP with an intact N-terminus, PTHrP extracts, or synthetic peptides such as PTHrP(1-34) or PTHrP(1-36), as well as intact PTH and PTH(1-34), had no effect on placental calcium transport. These results suggest that PTHrP secreted from the fetal parathyroids acts on the placenta to induce calcium transfer from the mother to the fetus.

The role of PTHrP in placental calcium transport is also supported by studies in mice missing both alleles of the PTHrP gene. The blood calcium of fetal PTHrP-ablated mice is identical to maternal blood calcium, that is, the transport of calcium from the mother into the fetus is diminished.[325] The defect in placental calcium transport can be corrected acutely by injecting PTHrP(1-86) or PTHrP(67-86) into the fetal blood circulation but not by injecting PTHrP(1-34) or PTH(1-84). These studies in mice and sheep suggest that a receptor distinct from the cloned PTH/PTHrP receptor mediates the action of PTHrP on placental calcium transport. Consistent with this hypothesis, placental calcium transport is actually increased in mice missing the PTH/PTHrP receptor.[325] The possible role of the fetal parathyroid gland as the crucial source of the PTHrP is suggested by the mentioned experiments in sheep,[328,329] but no measurements of PTHrP in fetal sheep blood have been made.

Role of PTHrP in Lactation

The second possible setting for humoral actions of PTHrP is during pregnancy and lactation. During lactation, transfer of calcium from bone into milk results in a measurable decline in bone mineral content.[326] In experimental animals, PTH and $1,25(OH)_2D_3$ have been eliminated as possible agents responsible for directing this transfer.[330,331] Furthermore, the lactating breast secretes PTHrP into the circulation,[332] and urinary cAMP rises in response to suckling.[333] Postpartum lactating women have elevated levels of PTHrP in the bloodstream,[334-337] and hypoparathyroid patients who are maintained normocalcemic by treatment with $1,25(OH)_2D_3$ can become hypercalcemic during lactation. Thus, PTHrP in the bloodstream may act on bone to release calcium and on the kidney to increase reabsorption of calcium from the urine, thus retaining the calcium for transport into milk. Consistent with this hypothesis, mice missing PTHrP production specifically in breast tissue have decreased bone turnover and preservation of bone mass.[338] PTH alone cannot effectively serve these roles, because the slight elevation in ionized calcium during lactation suppresses PTH levels.[334-337,339] An exaggeration of this lactational elevation of PTHrP may explain the rare occurrence of hypercalcemia and high PTHrP levels in pregnant and lactating women.[340,341]

However, PTHrP was shown to have additional roles in the breast, and it has a major role in breast development, acting through the PTH1R.[342,343] PTHrP is synthesized by breast tissue and is excreted in enormous amounts into breast milk. Thus, PTHrP in the breast appears to have both paracrine and endocrine roles. These roles may be subverted in breast cancer, a setting in which PTHrP may facilitate the growth of metastases in bone[344] and also cause humoral hypercalcemia. The lactating mammary gland can sense extracellular calcium through the calcium-sensing receptor, thereby adjusting calcium and PTHrP secretion into milk. Further, in fetal life, PTHrP, acting through the PTH/PTHrP receptor, is required for the normal development of breast tissue.[338,343]

PTHrP in Bone and Tooth Development

PTHrP has an essential role in bone development. This role is best illustrated by the phenotype of mice missing both copies of the PTHrP gene.[305,345,346] These mice die at birth and have diffuse abnormalities in all bones that form by the replacement of a cartilage mold with true bone (endochondral bone formation).

The original cartilage molds form normally, but the chondrocytes within the molds stop dividing prematurely and differentiate into hypertrophic chondrocytes at an accelerated pace. Consequently, the growth plates of these bones show dramatically truncated columns of proliferating chondrocytes. The resultant bones are short and mineralize sooner than normal. Growth plates of mice missing the PTH/PTHrP receptor look similar to those of the PTHrP knockout mouse,[12] which suggests that the PTH/PTHrP receptor mediates the actions of PTHrP on chondrocytes. PTHrP is made by perichondrial cells, particularly those at the ends of bones near the joint surfaces and to a lesser extent by chondrocytes, again particularly those at the ends of bones. The PTH/PTHrP receptor is expressed at low levels in adjacent chondrocytes in the proliferating columns and is dramatically expressed in chondrocytes just leaving the proliferative pool and becoming hypertrophic. The PTHrP made by the perichondrial cells and some chondrocytes thus acts on proliferating chondrocytes to keep cells in the proliferative pool to slow differentiation into hypertrophic chondrocytes, and to also slow the subsequent death of hypertrophic chondrocytes by apoptosis. This hypothesis is further supported by the phenotypes of transgenic mice that express the PTHrP gene at high levels in chondrocytes.[306] In these mice, chondrocyte differentiation is dramatically slowed. An analogous phenotype is demonstrated by transgenic mice in which chondrocytes express a constitutively active PTH/PTHrP receptor.[347] Both these transgenes can at least temporarily reverse the growth plate abnormalities in PTHrP knockout mice and allow the mice to live for several months postnatally.[347,348] In the developing tooth bud, PTHrP via the PTH1R appears to mediate transmission of important cell-differentiation signals at the mesenchymal/epithelial interface.[349]

Mice with abnormal PTHrP genes or abnormal PTH/PTHrP receptors have helped clarify the pathogenesis of two human diseases: Blomstrand's lethal chondrodystrophy, in which homozygous or compound heterozygous inactivating PTH/PTHrP receptor mutations are found,[350-353] and Jansen's osteochondrodystrophy, in which heterozygous constitutively active PTH/PTHrP receptors lead to hypercalcemia and short stature.[354-357] Both these diseases are discussed in detail in Chapter 5.

The potent effects of locally produced PTHrP on bone development and the abnormalities associated with too little or too much PTHrP action suggest a need for careful local regulation of PTHrP production (Fig. 1-13). One major determinant of PTHrP production in the growth plate is Indian hedgehog (Ihh) (see Chapter 4 for details). Ihh belongs to the hedgehog family of secreted proteins that are important for embryonic patterning[358] and acts through Patched, a receptor with 12 membrane spanning helixes that associates physically with Smoothened and thereby suppresses its constitutive activity.[359,360] In growth plates, expression of Ihh is restricted to the transition zone within the growth plate, where proliferating chondrocytes differentiate into hypertrophic cells.[13] Ihh, directly or indirectly, stimulates the production of PTHrP by perichondrial cells and chondrocytes near the ends of long bones. This PTHrP then slows the differentiation of chondrocytes and slows the differentiation of cells capable of synthesizing Ihh. Thus, a negative feedback loop controlled by Ihh and PTHrP ensures proper pacing of the proliferation and differentiation of chondrocytes. Ihh also has actions on chondrocytes independent of the effects of PTHrP; Ihh is a powerful stimulator of chondrocyte proliferation. For a more comprehensive review of the control of the growth plate, the role of Ihh, and PTHrP, as well as their interacting cytokines, see Chapter 4.

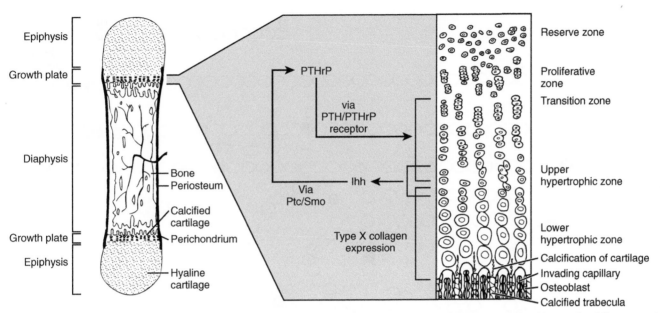

FIGURE 1-13. Schematic regulation of chondrocyte differentiation within the metaphyseal growth plate by a paracrine feedback loop involving parathyroid hormone-related peptide (PTHrP) and Indian Hedgehog (Ihh). *Ptc,* Patched; *Smo,* smoothened.

PTHrP is made by normal cells of the osteoblast lineage[361] and is likely to have a number of functions in normal osteoblast development and function. Mice missing one copy of the PTHrP gene are osteopenic. Thus, PTHrP appears to increase osteoblastic bone formation.[362] One function of PTHrP in the bones adjacent to developing teeth has been clarified. The mice described earlier, in which transgenic production of PTHrP or a constitutively activated PTH/PTHrP receptor by chondrocytes reverses the growth plate abnormalities of PTHrP-ablated mice and allows postnatal survival, have failure of normal tooth eruption.[347,348] Normally, the developing tooth elicits PTHrP production in the bone in which the tooth is embedded. This PTHrP then stimulates cells of the osteoblast lineage, which in turn stimulate the development and activity of osteoclasts, the bone-resorbing cells. This stimulation of bone resorption allows the tooth to erupt normally. PTH, a circulating endocrine factor, is unable to compensate for the lack of high local concentrations of PTHrP and thus cannot adequately stimulate the local bone resorption needed for tooth eruption.

It is likely that the local actions of PTHrP in the growth plate and bone are representative of the local actions of PTHrP to control cellular differentiation and proliferation in a number of organs. Still not fully characterized is the amount of cross-talk between the distinct ligands PTH and PTHrP, which can both activate the PTH/PTHrP receptor. Just as such cross-talk certainly explains PTHrP-mediated hypercalcemia of malignancy, it is likely that normally PTH and PTHrP both activate the PTH/PTHrP receptor in a number of tissues in a way that allows integration of the signals from locally produced PTHrP and systemically provided PTH (see Ligand-Induced Conformational Changes later).

Other Paracrine Actions of PTHrP

Most of the actions of PTHrP are not thought to be hormonal, but rather to be paracrine or autocrine.[363] PTHrP is synthesized at one time or another during fetal life in virtually every tissue. This widespread expression of PTHrP in fetal life probably explains the extensive expression of PTHrP in a great variety of malignancies. Malignant tissues often revert to a fetal pattern of gene expression; synthesis of PTHrP may be part of this pattern. PTHrP is also synthesized by many adult tissues.[4,293,363] In tissues such as skin and hair, it is likely that PTHrP regulates cell proliferation and differentiation.[364] PTHrP is also synthesized widely in the smooth muscle of blood vessels and in the gastrointestinal tract, uterus, and bladder, and transgenic expression of PTHrP in smooth muscle cells leads to severe defects in cardiac development.[365,366] In these tissues, PTHrP is synthesized in response to stretch and acts on smooth muscle in an autocrine fashion to relax the muscle.[367] PTHrP is also widely expressed in neurons of the central nervous system; its function in the brain is unknown. In mice missing the PTHrP gene, widespread degeneration of neurons occurs postnatally; as explained earlier, these mice survive postnatally through expression of PTHrP only in cartilage cells.[348]

Receptors for PTH and PTHrP

Because of the diverse actions of PTH, which were shown to be either direct or indirect and to involve multiple signal transduction mechanisms, it was initially thought that several different receptors would mediate the pleiotropic actions of this peptide hormone. Although some of these actions were subsequently shown to be PTHrP-dependent rather than PTH-dependent, it was somewhat surprising that the initial cloning approaches led to the isolation of complementary DNAs (cDNAs) encoding only a single G protein–coupled receptor, the common PTH/PTHrP receptor, also called the *PTH1R* (Fig. 1-14). The recombinant PTH/PTHrP receptor was shown to interact about equivalently with PTH and PTHrP ligands and to activate at least two distinct second messenger pathways, the adenylyl cyclase/cAMP/PKA and phospholipase C (PLC)/IP$_3$, Ca^{2+}, DAG/PKC pathways, mediated by G$_{\alpha s}$ and G$_{\alpha q/11}$, respectively.[7-9,368,369] It is now clear that depending on cell type, the PTH/PTHrP receptor can activate various other signaling cascades, including the extracellular signal-regulated kinase (ERK) cascade[60,370-372] and the phospho-

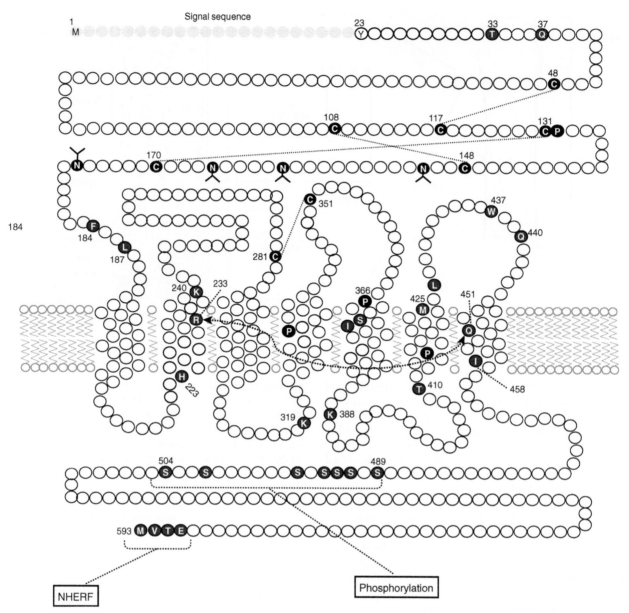

FIGURE 1-14. The PTH/PTHrP receptor: location of some key residues and crosslinking analysis. The schematic of the PTH/PTHrP receptor shows some of the residues believed to play key roles in the structure and/or function of the receptor. These include the conserved extracellular cysteines (C), which form a disulfide linkage network (*dashed lines*)[68]; the asparagines (N), modified with glycosyl groups (forks)[498]; Thr33 and Gln37, which contribute to PTH(15-34) binding affinity; Phe184 and Leu187, which contribute to PTH(1-14) agonist activity[429]; Arg233, Ser370, Ile371, Met425, Leu427, Trp437, and Gln440, which contribute to the agonist/antagonist responses mediated by residues 1 and/or 2 of the ligand[430,450]; a putative interhelical interaction between Arg233 and Gln451 (*dashed connector*)[430]; conserved prolines (P), including Pro132, the site of an inactivating mutation (Leu) in Blomstrand's chondrodysplasia[351]; His223, Thr410, and Ile458, the sites of activating mutations in Jansen's chondrodysplasia[357]; Lys319 and Lys 388, at which mutations impair G_q and G_s/G_q coupling, respectively[499,500]; serine (S) residues in the carboxy-terminal tail that are phosphorylated upon agonist activation[501,502]; and four C-terminal residues (Glu590–Met593) that mediate binding to members of the sodium-hydrogen exchanger regulating factor (NHERF) family of proteins.[239,503] The first 23 residues of the receptor (*shaded*) represent the signal sequence and are not present in the mature membrane-embedded receptor.

lipase D/rho A cascade, [373] the former potentially involving in addition to $G_{\alpha s}$, β-arrestins[60] or transactivation of ERK via extracellularly released epidermal growth factor,[371] the latter through activation of the $G_{\alpha 12/13}$ subtype of heterotrimeric G proteins.[373]

The initial finding that both PTH and PTHrP could activate the recombinant PTH/PTHrP receptor confirmed earlier studies using different clonal cell lines or renal membrane preparations that had shown that PTH and PTHrP bind to and activate a common G protein–coupled receptor with similar efficiencies and efficacies.[311,374-376] Based on these and subsequent findings, such as the similar phenotypes observed in mice that are null for either PTHrP or the PTH/PTHrP receptor,[12,13] it is very likely that

most of the endocrine actions of PTH and most of the paracrine/autocrine actions of PTHrP are mediated through the PTH/PTHrP receptor.

THREE PARATHYROID HORMONE RECEPTOR SUBTYPES

Subsequent to cloning of the PTH/PTHrP receptor, or the *PTH1R*, different efforts led to the identification of two novel receptors closely related to the initially isolated receptor. One of these receptors, called the *PTH2 receptor* (PTH2R), was obtained from a human brain cDNA library[377] and found to have reactivity towards PTH but not towards PTHrP.[377-380] The

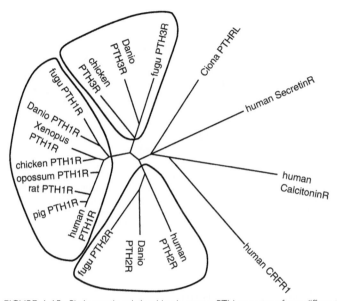

FIGURE 1-15. Phylogenetic relationships between PTH receptors from different species and other secretin receptor family members. Receptor amino acid sequences, with predicted signal peptides and exon E2-encoded segments of mammalian PTH1Rs removed, were aligned using the ClustalW(1.83) program, and an unrooted tree in which branch distances indicate amino acid sequence divergence was generated using the Phylip(3.67) DrawTree program.

PTH2R from rat, however, responded poorly to both PTH and PTHrP.[381,382] A search for the true ligand for this PTH2 receptor led to the isolation of a hypothalamic peptide of 39 amino acids (TIP39) called *tubular infundibular peptide* which efficiently binds to and activates both rat and human PTH2Rs.[383] TIP39 shows weak amino acid sequence homology to the N-terminal 34 amino acids of PTH and PTHrP, as well as some overlap in secondary structure (see Fig. 1-3).[384] Intact TIP39 binds relatively weakly to the PTH1R, but deletion of the first seven residues results in a high-affinity PTH1R antagonist.[385-387] The peptide TIP39 is produced at the hypothalamus and within the testes,[383,388] and together with the PTH2R appears to play an autocrine/paracrine role in germ cell development, inasmuch as mice lacking the gene for TIP39 are sterile due to a failed formation of spermatatids.[389]

The second novel PTH receptor variant isolated, the PTH3 receptor (PTH3R), has so far been found in fish[390] and birds (see NCBI chicken genome website) but not in mammals (Fig. 1-15). Functional and phylogenetic analyses indicate that the PTH3R is more closely related to the PTH1R than to the PTH2R.[390] In addition to the three identified PTH receptor subtypes, there are functional and physicochemical data suggesting that there may be additional receptors that interact with portions of either PTH or PTHrP which are C-terminal of the principal bioactive region defined by the (1–34) segment (see following and Table 1-2). As of yet, however, no gene or cDNA encoding such a novel receptor has been identified.

THE PTH/PTHrP RECEPTOR TYPE-1— EVOLUTION, GENE STRUCTURE, AND PROTEIN TOPOLOGY

The PTH1R belongs to a distinct subgroup of G protein–coupled receptors called the *class B*, or *secretin family* GPCRs. The first cDNAs encoding the PTH/PTHrP receptor were isolated through expression cloning techniques from two different model cell lines: OK cells, an opossum kidney–derived proximal tubule-like cell, and ROS 17/2.8 cells, a rat osteosarcoma-derived osteoblast-like cell.[7,8] Subsequently, cDNAs encoding the human,[9,391,392] mouse,[393] rat,[394] chicken,[13] porcine,[395] dog,[396] frog,[397] and fish PTH/PTHrP receptors[398] were isolated through hybridization techniques from different tissue sources, i.e., kidney, osteoblast-like cells, brain, embryonic stem cells, and/or whole embryos. Northern blot and in situ studies[304,399,400] and data provided through available public EST (expressed sequence tag) databases confirmed that the PTH/PTHrP receptor is expressed in a wide variety of fetal and adult tissues. The tetraploid African clawed frog, *Xenopus laevis*, expresses two nonallelic isoforms of the PTH/PTHrP receptor,[397] whereas all other investigated species have only one copy of the receptor gene per haploid genome.

The possible existence of PTH/PTHrP receptor subtypes with distinct, organ-specific characteristics had been suggested by distinct ligand binding properties[401-403] or by the activation of distinct second messenger pathways in different clonal cell lines.[251,404,405] However, the cloning of identical PTH/PTHrP receptors from human kidney, brain, and bone-derived cells[9,391,392] indicated that the previously observed pharmacologic differences could likely be explained by species-based variations in receptor primary sequence, rather than to tissue-based differences in expression of various receptor subtypes.

The gene encoding the human PTH/PTHrP receptor is located on chromosome 3p (within the region 3p21.1-3p24.2). Its intron/exon structure[406-408] is largely preserved in the genes encoding the rat and mouse receptor homologs.[409,410] The gene spans at least 20 kb of genomic DNA and consists of 14 coding exons and at least three noncoding exons. The size of the coding exons in the human gene ranges from 42 bp (exon M7) to more than 400 bp (exon T), and the introns vary in length from 81 bp (intron between exons M6/7 and M7) to more than 10,000 bp (intron between exons S and E1). Two promoters for the PTH/PTHrP receptor, P1 and P2, have been described in rodents.[409-412] The activity of P1 (also referred to as *U3*) is mainly restricted to the adult kidney, while that of P2 (also referred to as *U1*) is detected in several fetal and adult tissues, including cartilage and bone. In humans, a third promoter (P3, also referred to as *S*) appears to control PTH/PTHrP receptor expression in some tissues, including kidney and bone.[408,413,414]

The expressed human PTH/PTHrP receptor protein is 593 amino acids in length, including the 22-amino-acid N-terminal signal peptide sequence that is removed in the mature receptor. The predicted topology is defined by a relatively large amino-terminal extracellular domain (~160 amino acids in the human PTH1R), a juxtamembrane, or J, region containing seven membrane spanning helices and interconnecting loops, and a carboxy-terminal tail of about 110 amino acids (see Fig. 1-14). In mammals, the PTH1R N-domain is encoded by five exons: S, E1, E2, E3, and G. Exon S and G encode the signal peptide and a glycosylated segment,[415] respectively. Exons E1, E3, and G encode segments that include a number of conserved residues that are likely required for proper folding of the protein, surface expression, and/or ligand binding. These residues include six cysteine residues that form a disulfide bond network that stabilizes the N-domain structure.[68,416,417] Exon E2 encodes a nonconserved 41-amino-acid segment that is not essential for receptor function, since it can be targeted for deletion or large insertions, such as with green fluorescent protein (GFP), without a major loss in ligand binding affinity or surface expression.[416-418] Indeed, an equivalent of exon E2 is absent in the PTH1Rs from all nonmammalian species, as well as in other members of this GPCR subfamily (mammalian and nonmammalian), including the PTH2R.[390,397,419] The E2 segment of the mammalian *PTH1R* gene might thus reflect an evolutionarily recent genetic insertion event[390] or perhaps an atavistic genomic remnant. In any event, the E2 segment appears to form a nonfunctional loop that is conformationally flexible; a recent x-ray crystallographic analysis of the *PTH1R* N-terminal domain structure found this segment to be disordered in the crystal and hence unresolved.[68]

The initial cloning of the PTH1 receptor, cDN,[7,8] along with the cDNAs for the receptors for secretin[420] and calcitonin,[421] led to the realization that these receptors form a distinct GPCR subfamily, now called the *class B* or *secretin family* receptors.[419,422,423] These family B receptors share a similar overall structural topology, which is defined by the large N-terminal extracellular domain containing the conserved disulfide bond network, as well as a number of other conserved amino acids dispersed throughout the receptor protein.[419] Protein alignment analyses reveal virtually no amino acid sequence homology between the family B GPCRs and the receptors comprising the four other major GPCR subgroups, including the well studied β_2-adrenergic receptor and rhodopsin, representing the family A GPCRs.[422] The structural similarity between these groups of receptors is therefore limited to the common use of a heptahelical domain organization for the membrane-spanning J region.[422,424] As an evolutionary protein class, the secretin receptor family appears to have arisen during the divergence of the metazoans. Representatives of the receptor family are found in the genomes of a variety of invertebrate species, including the insect *Drosophila melanogaster,* and the nematode *Caenorhabditis elegans,* but not in yeast or bacteria.[419] A plausible PTH/PTHrP receptor homolog is present in the genome of the tunicate sea squirt *Ciona intestinalis* (see Fig. 1-15) pointing to a much earlier evolutionary origin of the PTH receptor than previously known.[419,425]

The three-dimensional molecular structures of the receptors in the secretin family are still only poorly defined because none has been adequately isolated or crystallized in an intact form. For several members of these receptors, however, including the PTH1R,[68] the CRFR1,[426] the CRFR2,[427] and the PACR1,[428] high-resolution three-dimensional structures of the isolated N-terminal domain in complex with a cognate peptide ligand have recently been obtained, either by solution-phase NMR[427,428] or x-ray crystallography.[68,426] These studies reveal a similar overall fold composed of three layers of secondary structure: an upper layer formed by an N-terminal α-helix, a middle layer of β sheet, and a lower layer formed by a β strand and short C-terminal α-helix (Fig 1-16). The overall fold is stabilized by the three conserved disulfide bonds and an extensive array of hydrophobic and electrostatic packing interactions.[68] The ligand, represented by the PTH(15-34) domain, binds as an amphipathic α-helix within a central groove in the structure, as described further later. The membrane-spanning helical regions of the class B receptors may be predicted to at least generally follow the heptahelical domain topology used by the class A receptors, which is now revealed by three-dimensional crystal structure of the β_2-adrenergic receptor.[69]

MECHANISMS OF LIGAND BINDING AND ACTIVATION AT THE PTH1R

The ligand-binding mechanisms used by the PTH receptor have been extensively analyzed by a combination of approaches, including functional methods that are based on receptor site–directed mutagenesis and ligand analog design strategies[50,51,429-434]

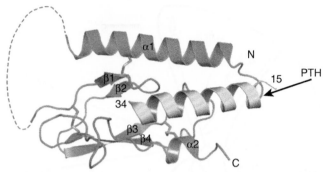

FIGURE 1-16. Crystal structure of the PTH1R amino-terminal domain in complex with PTH(15-34). The tertiary fold of the receptor N domain is defined by an upper layer of N-terminal α-helix (α1), a middle layer of beta sheet (β1, β2), and a lower layer of beta sheet (β3, β4) and short C-terminal α-helix (α2). The ligand lies as an amphipathic α-helix in a groove formed along the center of the structure. The 41-amino-acid exon E2-encoded segment is not resolved in the crystal structure and indicated here as a *dashed line.*[68]

and biophysical methods that are based on the use of photoreactive cross-linking analogs of the ligand that permit direct identification of sites of intermolecular proximity by protein fragmentation and mapping analysis. The cross-linking analogs used in these studies have been labeled at various positions with a photoreactive benzophenone group, incorporated either directly into the peptide chain, as *para*benzoyl-L-phenylalanine (BPA),[434-437] or attached to the epsilon amino function of lysine-13 (BpLys).[438] The combined functional and cross-linking data suggest that the ligand, as represented by the bioactive PTH(1-34) peptide, binds to the receptor via a two-step mechanism that involves two principal and somewhat autonomous components of the overall interaction.[439-442] The C-terminal portion of the ligand representing the principal binding domain[443,444] first contacts the N-terminal domain of the receptor to establish initial docking interactions,[417] and subsequently the N-terminal portion of the ligand interacts with the J domain portion of the receptor to produce the holo-enzyme bimolecular complex that can couple to and activate G proteins (Fig. 1-17). The overall interaction is certain to be more complex than indicated here, but this general scheme of interaction is now believed to extend to most of the class B family of peptide hormone–binding G protein–coupled receptors.[440,441,445,446]

Specific contacts to the receptor's N-domain have now been elucidated by the recent crystal structure of the PTH1R N-domain in complex with PTH(15-34) (see Fig. 1-16).[68] The PTH(15-34) domain binds as an amphiphilic α-helix, with the hydrophobic face of the helix formed by Trp23, Leu24, and Leu28, making extensive contacts with a hydrophobic surface formed on the floor of the central groove that runs through the N-domain structure. The guanidinium side chain of highly conserved Arg20 of the ligand makes additional contacts with at least five receptor residues that form an intricate pocket at the end of the groove. Binding studies performed using both the intact receptor and the isolated N-domain confirm the importance of the identified contacts to the development of ligand-binding affinity.[68]

The ligand interactions that occur with the receptor's J domain are known with far less certainty, but these appear to principally involve ligand residues extending from position 1 to about position 19.[436,441,442] This portion of the ligand contains the activation pharmacophore, which has minimally been defined by peptide functional studies as the PTH(1-9) segment.[50] A contact site for conserved valine-2 in the ligand, which plays a critical role in receptor activation,[57,447] has been mapped by cross-linking

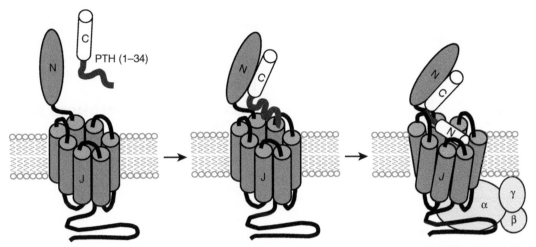

FIGURE 1-17. Two-site ligand-binding mechanisms for the PTH/PTHrP receptor. The ligand, PTH(1-34), first interacts with the PTH1R N-domain via its C-terminal helical portion and then engages the juxtamembrane (J) region via its N-terminal segment to induce the conformation changes involved in receptor activation and G-protein coupling.

methods to Met425 at the extracellular end of the transmembrane domain (TM) 6.[448,449] This interaction site is supported by functional data,[448,449] however, other sites in the receptor (e.g., Ser370 and Ile371) have also been implicated by mutagenesis approaches to be likely contact sites for Val2.[450] Other cross-linking studies identified proximities between residue 19 in the ligand and Lys240 at the extracellular end of TM2,[451] and between residue 13 in the ligand and Arg186 at the boundary of the N-domain and TM1.[438] These and other data combined suggest that the ligand's N-terminal domain binds as an α-helix to lie in a groove formed at the extracellular surface of the receptor's juxtamembrane region and in the same plane as the outer layer of the cell membrane.[441,451] Such a binding mode could allow Val2, as well as other key ligand residues that define the agonist pharmacophore, such as Ile5 and Met8,[50,452] to make intimate contacts with the membrane embedded core region of the receptor and thereby induce the conformational changes involved in receptor activation.[59,453]

The cognate interaction pocket in the receptor's juxtamembrane region that accommodates and responds to the key pharmacophoric elements in the ligand have only been approximately defined. The development of highly potent N-terminal PTH fragment analogs, based on the weakly active native PTH(1-14) peptide scaffold, provides a class of minimized ligand structures that can used to specifically probe this component of the interaction process more effectively than is possible with PTH(1-34) (see Fig. 1-4). These minimized ligands, referred to generally as the *M class* of PTH ligands, maintain affinity and efficacy on the PTHR, as well as on a PTHR construct that lacks the N-terminal domain.[50-53,57,429] Furthermore, the M-PTH analogs have highly stabilized N-terminal helical backbone structures, in part due to the incorporation of conformationally constrained amino acid analogs, such as α-amino-isobutyric (Aib), at positions 1 and 3.[51,54,55,454] A recent use of such modified M-PTH(1-14) analogs for compound screening resulted in the identification of a new class of PTH nonpeptide mimetic ligands that bind specifically to the PTH1R J domain.[455,456] Although these compounds bind with micromolar affinities and function as competitive antagonists, they represent potential leads towards new mimetic compounds that function as PTH1R agonists and are orally active.

LIGAND-INDUCED CONFORMATIONAL CHANGES

Given the absence of a high-resolution, three-dimensional molecular structure for the intact PTH/PTHR bimolecular complex, it is difficult to describe the conformational changes that occur in the complex upon ligand binding, receptor activation, and G-protein coupling. Problems that need to be solved include determining how the N and J domains of the receptor are oriented relative to each other, whether PTH(1-34) adopts a linear or U-shaped structure as it is bound to the receptor,[62-65] and the molecular movements that occur in the complex during the ligand binding, activation, and G-protein coupling cycle. Several new approaches, however, are beginning to help illuminate these aspects of PTH receptor function.

Kinetic binding assays performed in membranes with various PTH and PTHrP radioligand analogs has revealed that the PTH1R can adopt different conformations that display differential affinities for structurally diverse ligands and are differentially coupled to heterotrimeric G proteins.[439,457] In particular, the studies show that PTH(1-34) can form a complex with the receptor that remains stable upon the addition of GTPγS, a reagent that at the high concentrations used is expected to fully activate the G protein and hence dissociate the receptor–G protein heterotrimer complex and thus shift the receptor into a low-affinity state.[457] Moreover, the ligand can bind efficiently to the receptor in membranes prepared from cells lacking G$_{\alpha s}$. In contrast, PTH(1-14) forms a complex that rapidly dissociates upon GTPγS addition and binds only poorly in the absence of G$_{\alpha s}$.[457]

The data thus suggested that certain ligands (e.g., PTH[1-34]) preferentially bind to or induce a novel high-affinity PTH1R conformation, called R^0,[458] that can stably hold the ligand in place even upon G-protein activation/dissociation, whereas other ligands (e.g., M-PTH[1-14]) preferentially bind to or induce a different high-affinity conformation, called *RG*, that is dependent on G-protein coupling and thus reverts to a low-affinity form upon G-protein activation/dissociation. These findings predicted that ligands that bind to the R^0 conformation would produce protracted signaling responses, owing to multiple or prolonged rounds of G-protein coupling. This prediction was indeed supported by data showing that PTH(1-34) produced extended

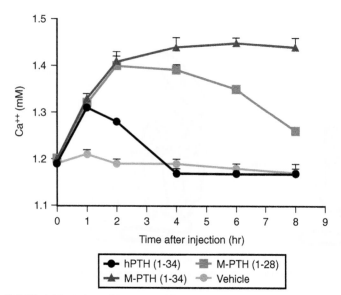

FIGURE 1-18. Actions of long-acting PTH analogs in vivo. PTH analogs were injected into mice to assess acute effects on blood ionized calcium levels. The modified ligand, M-PTH(1-34), which binds to the R^0 PTHR conformation with higher affinity than does unmodified PTH(1-34), induces a markedly prolonged increase in blood ionized Ca^{2+}. These prolonged effects were not explainable by a prolonged half-life of the modified peptide in the circulation, and they were paralleled by prolonged cAMP-stimulating activity in MC3T3 osteoblastic cells in culture. Thus, high-affinity binding to the R^0 PTHR conformation can lead to prolonged PTHR signaling actions in vitro and in vivo. (Data from Okazaki M, Ferrandon S, Vilardaga JP, et al: Prolonged signaling at the parathyroid hormone receptor by peptide ligands targeted to a specific receptor conformation, Proc Natl Acad Sci U S A 105:16525–16530, 2008.)

cAMP responses after ligand washout, as compared to M-PTH(1-14).[457] It was also found that PTHrP(1-36), in contrast to PTH(1-34), binds with relative selectivity to the RG versus R^0 conformation.[459] These observations suggested the hypothesis that altered modes of receptor conformational selectivity at the PTH1R, as exhibited by different ligands, may translate into altered biological actions for those ligands in vivo and may even explain the relatively deficient capacity of PTHrP(1-36), versus PTH(1-34), to induce vitamin D synthesis and increase blood calcium levels when injected into human subjects.[460] This general hypothesis was tested further using a new analog, M-PTH(1-34), that has even stronger selectivity for the R^0 conformation than does PTH(1-34). The analog indeed produced markedly prolonged cAMP responses in cells and markedly prolonged, even as compared to PTH(1-34), hypercalcemic (Fig. 1-18) and hypophosphatemic responses when injected into mice.[461]

That the PTH1R can adopt multiple conformational states and thereby display altered modes of biological action is consistent with the finding of certain PTH ligand analogs that have capacities to selectively activate one signal pathway over another[58-60,247] or, when altered by certain point mutations, to mediate ligand-independent signaling activity.[462] The notion of multiple PTH1R conformations and altered signaling directionality is also in line with the generally accepted views of how most if not all G protein–coupled receptors operate in their respective biological milieus.[463] The recent use of fluorescent (Forster) resonance energy transfer (FRET) methodologies, utilizing PTH receptors tagged with spectral variants of green fluorescent protein together with fluorescently labeled PTH ligands, has opened new routes for defining with high temporal resolution and precision the kinetics of receptor conformational change and ligand-receptor

interaction processes. Such studies show that indeed the structurally different ligands, such as PTH(1-34), PTHrP(1-36), and M-PTH(1-14), form kinetically distinguishable complexes with the PTH1R and confirm the differences in dissociation rates seen in the radioligand-based membrane binding studies (Fig. 1-19A).[418,453,459]

MECHANISMS OF PROLONGED SIGNALING AT THE PTH1R

The subcellular mechanisms and pathways that underlie the differences in the duration of the signaling responses seen for the different analogs remains to be established, but it has been found, again using the FRET approach as well as fluorescence confocal microscopy methods, that these long-acting ligands induce long-lived complexes of ligand, receptor, and G protein (see Fig. 1-19B) that remain intact and associated with adenylyl cyclase, even as the proteins move to the intracellular endosomal domain.[464] This raises the intriguing possibility that in addition to, or as an extension of, the receptor-phosphorylation and arrestin-dependent internalization, desensitization and recycling processes that are known to regulate PTH1R actions,[59,465-468] there may be a component of the mechanism by which the ligand•receptor•G-protein complex formed by PTH but not PTHrP remains assembled within the endosomes and catalytically active for longer time intervals than previously appreciated.[464] Further studies are needed to test this hypothesis. The results could provide additional clues for designing new PTH analogs that have time-limited or prolonged actions on the PTH1R; such ligands could have improved efficacy, compared to PTH(1-34), as therapies for the diseases of osteoporosis[277,469] and hypoparathyroidism,[470] respectively.

OTHER RECEPTORS FOR C-TERMINAL PTH OR PTHrP

There is evidence for the presence of additional receptors and/or binding proteins that interact with portions of PTH or PTHrP C-terminal of the PTH(1-34), but thus far no cDNA encoding such a receptor has been identified. Considerable information has accumulated that indicates that regions of PTH(1-84) other than the N-terminal residues may be responsible for novel biological actions (see Table 1-2), although many of these effects are still largely limited to in vitro studies. A series of synthetic peptides forming the central region of PTH were reported to delineate a core domain, PTH(30–34), that stimulates the proliferation of chondrocytes but does not appear to involve the cAMP/PKA pathway.[244,471-474] Early competition binding assays with renal plasma membranes and rat osteosarcoma cells demonstrated binding sites for C-terminal PTH(53-84) that are discrete from those that bind PTH(1-34).[475-478] The observation that N-terminal and C-terminal fragments of PTH elicited contrasting effects on alkaline phosphatase activity[479-481] supports the existence of a receptor with specificity for the C-terminal portion of PTH. Considerable evidence suggests that the C-terminal portion of PTH(1-84) has biological activity. For example, C-terminal PTH fragments such as PTH(39-84) and PTH(53-84) stimulate the formation of bone-resorbing osteoclasts from precursor cells,[482] and the same PTH fragments were shown to enhance the influx of ^{45}Ca into SaOS-2 cells.[483] Several different clonal cell lines, including bone- and cartilage-derived cells in which the common PTH/PTHrP receptor had been deleted through homologous recombination, showed increased proliferative activity in response to intact PTH and C-terminal fragments.[484,485] Furthermore, PTH(1-84) was more potent than PTH(1-34) in increasing

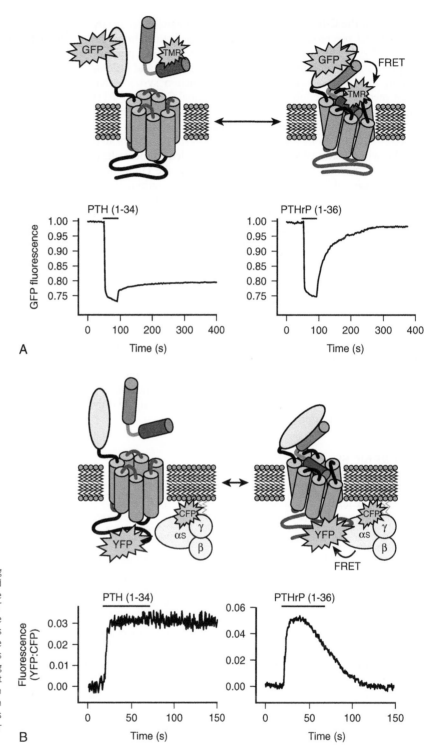

FIGURE 1-19. Differential receptor binding and G protein coupling kinetics induced by PTH and PTHrP. **A,** The binding of PTH and PTHrP analogs labeled on lysine13 with tetramethylrhodamine (TMR) to GFP-PTH1R was monitored using single-cell FRET recording. Upon binding, GFP fluorescence emission is reduced due to FRET-based quenching by the TMR group. The ligand was applied for 20 seconds (black bar), and then washed out. Over the time course studied, PTH remains bound to the receptor whereas PTHrP dissociates. **B,** Coupling to G proteins was monitored using a PTHR tagged in the cytoplasmic tail with yellow-fluorescent protein (YFP) and a Gγ subunit tagged with cyan fluorescent protein (CFP). The ratiometric FRET response (YFP emission:CFP emission upon CFP excitation) increases upon R-G coupling. The recordings show that R-G coupling following ligand wash-out is prolonged for PTH but not for PTHrP.[459,464]

the concentration of fibronectin in vivo,[486] and C-terminal PTH fragments increased type I procollagen expression.[487]

In direct support of a biological role for C-terminal PTH fragments, ROS 17/2.8 cells, rat PT-r3 cells, osteolytic cell lines lacking the PTH1R were shown to specifically interact with the C-terminal portion of PTH.[488,489] With the use of radiolabeled [Tyr34]hPTH(19-84), which does not bind to cells that express high concentrations of the PTH/PTHrP receptor, these cells were shown to bind PTH(1-84) and PTH(19-84) with equivalent high affinity, whereas fragments of PTH(19-84) that were truncated at the N-terminal end showed a progressive loss of binding affin-

ity.[488] However, even PTH(53-84) showed some displacement of the radiolabeled [Tyr34]hPTH(19-84), whereas the midregional fragment PTH(44-68) failed to do so. Other studies using ROS 17/2.8 cells, but with [35S-Met]hPTH(1-84) instead of 125I-labeled [Tyr34]hPTH(19-84), showed similar binding characteristics of C-terminal PTH fragments, and these studies indicated that residue 84 contributes to the overall ligand-binding affinity.[489] Photoaffinity cross-linking experiments led to the identification of approximately 80-kD and 30-kD proteins that show high-affinity interaction with the C-terminal portion of PTH but not with the N-terminal PTH(1-34).[488] These findings suggest that the C-terminal portion of PTH interacts specifically with a novel receptor/binding protein that is distinct from the PTH1R. Complementary DNA clones encoding this putative receptor/binding protein have not yet been isolated, and little or nothing is known about the signal transduction systems that might mediate the actions of these midregional/C-terminal PTH fragments.

The development of antibodies that can distinguish truly intact PTH(1-84) from variants that are N-terminally truncated or otherwise posttranslationally modified has led to the realization that such PTH variants can be present in the circulation, and, in cases of primary or secondary hyperparathyroidism, potentially at levels exceeding those of PTH(1-84).[172,191,192,255] How such PTH variants might affect calcium homeostasis and other physiologic processes remains to be determined, but in a rat model study, N-terminally truncated PTH was shown to effectively inhibit the capacity of PTH(1-34) to stimulate synthesis of $1,25(OH)_2$-vitamin-D_3.[173,490]

There is also evidence to suggest that non-PTH1R receptors can mediate actions induced by the midregion of PTHrP and may thus play an important role in placental calcium transport[309,325] (see earlier discussion), as well as modulate biological functions in skin.[324] Likewise, actions of the C-terminal PTHrP portion on osteoclasts and osteoblasts[317-319,321] and on the central nervous system[491] appear to be mediated through a specific receptor, and other receptors have been characterized that interact equivalently with the N-terminal portions of PTH and PTHrP but signal only through changes in intracellular free calcium.[492-494]

Summary

The actions of the amino-terminal portion of PTH and PTHrP (or fragments of this region) are mediated through a single receptor, the PTH/PTHrP receptor, or PTH1R, which belongs to a distinct family of G protein–coupled receptors. The PTH1R mediates the actions of at least the amino-terminal regions of PTH and PTHrP and signals through multiple second messenger pathways, including the cAMP/PKA and inositol triphosphate/Ca^{2+}/diacylglycerol/PKC pathways. The *PTH1R* gene is expressed in a large variety of fetal and adult tissues, but the receptor is most abundant in kidney and bone, where it mediates the endocrine actions of PTH in mineral ion homeostasis, and in the metaphyseal growth plate, where it mediates the autocrine/paracrine actions of locally synthesized PTHrP. Gene deletion studies demonstrate a critical role for the PTH1R and PTHrP in embryonic and postnatal development of cartilage and bone, but the biological role of this PTHrP-PTH1R paracrine interaction system in the adult remains incompletely understood. The PTH1R is thus used by two ligands for distinct biological functions, endocrine-homeostatic versus paracrine/autocrine-developmental, and it adopts multiple conformational states to support these disparate modes of action. The biological roles of other receptors, such as the PTH-2 receptor, which binds TIP39, or the still hypothetical receptors that specifically interact with more C-terminal regions of PTH or PTHrP, also remain undefined.

REFERENCES

1. Hansen AM: The hydrochloric x sicca: a parathyroid preparation for intramuscular injection, Mil Surg 54:218–219, 1924.
2. Collip JB: Extraction of a parathyroid hormone which will prevent or control parathyroid tetany and which regulates the level of blood calcium, J Biol Chem 63:395–438, 1925.
3. Albright F, Bauer W, Ropes M, et al: Studies of calcium and phosphorus metabolism. Iv. The effect of the parathyroid hormone, J Clin Invest 7:139–181, 1929.
4. Broadus AE, Stewart AF: Parathyroid hormone-related protein: structure, processing, and physiological actions. In Bilezikian JP, Levine, MA, Marcus R, editors: The parathyroids. Basic and clinical concepts, New York, 1994, Raven Press.
5. Moseley JM, Martin TJ: Parathyroid hormone-related protein: physiological actions. In Bilezikian JP, Raisz LG, Rodan RA, editors: Principles of bone biology, New York, 1996, Academic Press.
6. Yang KH, Stewart AF: Parathyroid hormone-related protein: the gene, its mRNA species, and protein products. In Bilezikian, JP, Raisz LG, Rodan RA, editors: Principles of bone biology, New York, 1996, Academic Press.
7. Jüppner H, Abou-Samra AB, Freeman MW, et al: A G protein-linked receptor for parathyroid hormone and parathyroid hormone-related peptide, Science 254:1024–1026, 1991.
8. Abou-Samra AB, Jüppner H, Force T, et al: Expression cloning of a common receptor for parathyroid hormone and parathyroid hormone-related peptide from rat osteoblast-like cells: a single receptor stimulates intracellular accumulation of both camp and inositol triphosphates and increases intracellular free calcium, Proc Natl Acad Sci U S A 89:2732–2736, 1992.
9. Schipani E, Karga H, Karaplis AC, et al: Identical complementary deoxyribonucleic acids encode a human renal and bone parathyroid hormone (PTH)/PTH-related peptide receptor, Endocrinology 132:2157–2165, 1993.
10. Potts JT Jr, Jüppner H: Parathyroid hormone and parathyroid hormone-related peptide in calcium homeostasis, bone metabolism, and bone development: the

proteins, their genes, and receptors. In Avioli L, Krane S, editors: Metabolic bone disease, New York, 1997, Academic Press.
11. Silver J, Kronenberg HM: Parathyroid hormone—molecular biology and regulation. In Bilezikian JP, Raisz LG, Rodan RA, editors: Principles of bone biology, New York, 1996, Academic Press.
12. Lanske B, Karaplis AC, Luz A, et al: PTH/PTHRP receptor in early development and Indian hedgehog-regulated bone growth, Science 273:663–666, 1996.
13. Vortkamp A, Lee K, Lanske B, et al: Regulation of rate of cartilage differentiation by Indian hedgehog and PTH-related protein, Science 273:613–622, 1996.
14. Kronenberg HM, Lanske B, Kovacs CS, et al: Functional analysis of the PTH/PTHRP network of ligands and receptors, Recent Prog Horm Res 53:283–301, 1998.
15. Bringhurst FR: Calcium and phosphate distribution, turnover, and metabolic actions. In DeGroot LJ, editor: Endocrinology, ed 2, Philadelphia, 1989, Saunders.
16. Neer RM: Calcium and inorganic phosphate homeostasis. In DeGroot LJ, editor: Endocrinology, ed 2, Philadelphia, 1989, Saunders.
17. Wendelaar-Bonga SE, Pang PK: Control of calcium regulating hormones in the vertebrates: parathyroid hormone, calcitonin, prolactin, and stanniocalcin, Int Rev Cytol 128:139–213, 1991.
18. Pang PTK, Pang RK: Hormones and calcium regulation in vertebrates: an evolutionary and overall consideration. In Pang PKT, Schreibman MP, editors: Regulation of calcium and phosphate, San Diego, 1989, Academic Press.
19. Drezner MK: Phosphorus homeostasis and related disorders. In Bilezikian JP, Raisz LG, Rodan RA, editors: Principles in bone biology, New York, 1996, Academic Press.
20. Wagner G, Dimattia G, Davie J, et al: Molecular cloning and cDNA sequence analysis of Coho salmon stanniocalcin, Mol Cell Endocrinol 90:7–15, 1992.
21. Olsen H, Cepeda M, Zhang Q, et al: Human stanniocalcin: a possible hormonal regulator of mineral metabolism, Proc Natl Acad Sci U S A 93:1792–1796, 1996.

22. Ishibashi K, Miyamoto K, Taketani Y, et al: Molecular cloning of a second human stanniocalcin homologue (stc2), Biochem Biophys Res Commun 250:252–258, 1998.
23. White KE, Larsson TE, Econs MJ: The roles of specific genes implicated as circulating factors involved in normal and disordered phosphate homeostasis: frizzled related protein-4, matrix extracellular phosphoglycoprotein, and fibroblast growth factor 23, Endocr Rev 27:221–241, 2006.
24. Martin JT, Findley DM, Moseley JM, et al: Calcitonin. In Avioli LV, Krane SM, editors: Metabolic bone disease, ed 3, New York, 1998, Academic Press.
25. Potts JT Jr, Bringhurst FR, Gardella TJ, et al: Parathyroid hormone: physiology, chemistry, biosynthesis, secretion, metabolism, and mode of action. In DeGroot LJ, editor: Endocrinology, ed 3, Philadelphia, 1995, Saunders.
26. Diaz R, El-Hajj GF, Brown E: Regulation of parathyroid function, New York, 1998, Oxford University Press.
27. Nordin BEC, Peacock M: Role of kidney in regulation of plasma calcium Lancet 2:1280–1283, 1969.
28. Peacock M, Robertson WG, Nordin BEC: Relation between serum and urinary calcium with particular reference to parathyroid activity, Lancet 1:384–386, 1969.
29. Mayer G, Habener J, Potts JT Jr: Parathyroid hormone secretion in vivo. Demonstration of a calcium-independent nonsuppressible component of secretion, J Clin Invest 57:678–683, 1976.
30. Parsons JA, Potts JT Jr, editors: Physiology and chemistry of parathyroid hormone, Philadelphia, 1972, Saunders.
31. Potts JT Jr, Deftos LJ: Parathyroid hormone, calcitonin, vitamin D, bone and bone mineral metabolism. In Bondy PK, Rosenberg LE, editors: Duncan's disease of metabolism, ed 3, Philadelphia, 1974, W. B. Saunders.
32. Rasmussen H, Bordier P: The physiological and cellular basis of metabolic bone disease, Williams & Wilkins, 1974, Baltimore.
33. Aurbach GD: Isolation of parathyroid hormone after extraction with phenol, J Biol Chem 234:3179, 1959.

34. Rasmussen H, Craig LC: Purification of parathyroid hormone by use of counter-current distribution, J Am Chem Soc 81:5003, 1959.
35. Brewer HB Jr, Ronan R: Bovine parathyroid hormone: amino acid sequence, Proc Natl Acad Sci U S A 67:1862, 1970.
36. Niall HD, Keutmann HT, Sauer RT, et al: The amino-acid sequence of bovine parathyroid hormone, Hoppe Seylers Z Physiol Chem 351:1586–1588, 1970.
37. Sauer RT, Niall HD, Hogan ML, et al: The amino acid sequence of porcine parathyroid hormone, Biochemistry 13:1994, 1974.
38. Brewer HB Jr, Fairwell T, Ronan R, et al: Human parathyroid hormone: amino acid sequence of the amino-terminal residues 1–34, Proc Natl Acad Sci U S A 69:3585, 1972.
39. Niall HD, Sauer RT, Jacobs JW, et al: The amino acid sequence of the amino-terminal 37 residues of human parathyroid hormone, Proc Natl Acad Sci U S A 71:384, 1974.
40. Keutmann HT, Sauer MM, Hendy GN, et al: The complete amino acid sequence of human parathyroid hormone, Biochemistry 17:552, 1978.
41. Heinrich G, Kronenberg HM, Potts JT Jr, et al: Gene encoding parathyroid hormone: nucleotide sequence of the rat gene and deduced amino acid sequence of rat preproparathyroid hormone, J Biol Chem 259:3320–3329, 1984.
42. Khosla S, Demay M, Pines M, et al: Nucleotide sequence of cloned cDNAs encoding chicken preproparathyroid hormone, J Bone Miner Res 3:689–698, 1988.
43. Russell J, Sherwood LM: Nucleotide sequence of the DNA complementary to avian (chicken) preproparathyroid hormone mRNA and the deduced sequence of the hormone precursor, Mol Endocrinol 3:325–331, 1989.
44. Rosol TJ, Steinmeyer CL, McCauley LK, et al: Sequences of the cDNAs encoding canine parathyroid hormone-related protein and parathyroid hormone, Gene 160:241–243, 1995.
45. Potts JT Jr, Tregear GW, Keutmann HT, et al: Synthesis of a biologically active N-terminal tetratriacontrapeptide of parathyroid hormone, Proc Natl Acad Sci U S A 68:63–67, 1971.
46. Tregear GW, Van Rietschoten J, Greene E, et al: Bovine parathyroid hormone: minimum chain length of synthetic peptide required for biological activity, Endocrinology 93:1349–1353, 1973.
47. Gensure R, Ponugoti B, Gunes Y, et al: Isolation and characterization of two PTH-like molecules in zebrafish, Endocrinology 145:1634–1639, 2004.
48. Guerreiro PM, Renfro JL, Power DM, et al: The parathyroid hormone family of peptides: structure, tissue distribution, regulation, and potential functional roles in calcium and phosphate balance in fish, Am J Physiol Regul Integr Comp Physiol 292:R679–696, 2007.
49. Danks J, Ho P, Notini A, et al: Identification of a parathyroid hormone in the fish *Fugu rubripes*, J Bone Miner Res 18:1326–1331, 2003.
50. Shimizu M, Carter P, Gardella T: Autoactivation of type 1 parathyroid hormone receptors containing a tethered ligand, J Biol Chem 275:19456–19460, 2000.
51. Shimizu N, Guo J, Gardella T: Parathyroid hormone (1–14) and (1–11) analogs conformationally constrained by α aminoisobutyric acid mediate full agonist responses via the juxtamembrane region of the PTH-1 receptor, J Biol Chem 276:49003–49012, 2001.
52. Shimizu M, Carter P, Khatri A, et al: Enhanced activity in parathyroid hormone (1–14) and (1–11): novel peptides for probing the ligand-receptor interaction, Endocrinology 142:3068–3074, 2001.
53. Shimizu M, Potts JJ, Gardella T: Minimization of parathyroid hormone: novel amino-terminal parathyroid hormone fragments with enhanced potency in activating the type-1 parathyroid hormone receptor, J Biol Chem 275:21836–21843, 2000.
54. Shimizu N, Dean T, Khatri A, et al: Amino-terminal parathyroid hormone fragment analogs containing α,-α-dialkyl amino acids at positions 1 and 3, J Bone Miner Res 19:2078–2086, 2004.
55. Tsomaia N, Pellegrini M, Hyde K, et al: Toward parathyroid hormone minimization: conformational studies of cyclic PTH(1–14) analogues, Biochemistry 43:690–699, 2004.
56. Shimizu M, Shimizu N, Okazaki M, et al: Parathyroid hormone(1–14) fragments increase bone mass in ovx rats. Advances in skeletal anabolic agents for the treatment of osteoporosis meeting abstracts, M15, 2004.
57. Shimizu N, Dean T, Tsang JC, et al: Novel parathyroid hormone (PTH) antagonists that bind to the juxtamembrane portion of the PTH/PTH-related protein receptor, J Biol Chem 280:1797–1807, 2005.
58. Takasu H, Gardella T, Luck M, et al: Amino-terminal modifications of human parathyroid hormone (PTH) selectively alter phospholipase C signaling via the type 1 PTH receptor: implications for design of signal-specific PTH ligands, Biochemistry 38:13453–13460, 1999.
59. Bisello A, Chorev M, Rosenblatt M, et al: Selective ligand-induced stabilization of active and desensitized parathyroid hormone type 1 receptor conformations, J Biol Chem 277:38524–38530, 2002.
60. Gesty-Palmer D, Chen M, Reiter E, et al: Distinct beta-arrestin- and G protein-dependent pathways for parathyroid hormone receptor-stimulated erk1/2 activation, J Biol Chem 281:10856–10864, 2006.
61. Barden JA, Kemp BE: NMR solution structure of human parathyroid hormone(1–34), Biochemistry 32:7126–7132, 1993.
62. Pellegrini M, Royo M, Rosenblatt M, et al: Addressing the tertiary structure of human parathyroid hormone-(1–34), J Biol Chem 273:10420–10427, 1998.
63. Marx U, Adermann K, Bayer P, et al: Solution structures of human parathyroid hormone fragments HPTH(1–34) and HPTH(1–39) and bovine parathyroid hormone fragment BPTH(1–37), Biochem Biophys Res Commun 267:213–220, 2000.
64. Chen Z, Xu P, Barbier J-R, et al: Solution structure of the osteogenic 1–31 fragment of the human parathyroid hormone, Biochemistry 39:12766–12777, 2000.
65. Jin L, Briggs S, Chandrasekhar S, et al: Crystal structure of human parathyroid hormone 1–34 at 0.9 Å resolution, J Biol Chem 275:27238–27244, 2000.
66. Barden JA, Kemp BE: NMR study of a 34-residue N-terminal fragment of the parathyroid-hormone-related protein secreted during humoral hypercalcemia of malignancy, Eur J Biochem 184:379–394, 1989.
67. Klaus W, Dieckmann T, Wray V, et al: Investigation of the solution structure of the human parathyroid hormone fragment (1–34) by ^{1}h NMR spectroscopy, distance geometry, and molecular dynamics calculations, Biochemistry 30:6936–6942, 1991.
68. Pioszak AA, Xu HE: Molecular recognition of parathyroid hormone by its G protein-coupled receptor, Proc Natl Acad Sci U S A 105:5034–5039, 2008.
69. Kobilka B, Schertler GF: New g-protein-coupled receptor crystal structures: insights and limitations, Trends Pharmacol Sci 29:79–83, 2008.
70. Fraser RA, Kronenberg HM, Pang PK, et al: Parathyroid hormone messenger ribonucleic acid in the rat hypothalamus, Endocrinology 127:2517–2522, 1990.
71. Nutley MT, Parimi SA, Harvey S: Sequence analysis of hypothalamic parathyroid hormone messenger ribonucleic acid, Endocrinology 136:5600–5607, 1995.
72. Roth SI, Schiller AL, editors: Comparative anatomy of the parathyroid glands, vol. VII, Washington, DC, 1981, American Physiological Society.
73. Fraser RA, Kaneko T, Pang PKT, et al: Hypo- and hypercalcemic peptides in fish pituitary glands, Am J Physiol 260:R622-R626, 1991.
74. Hogan BM, Danks JA, Layton JE, et al: Duplicate zebrafish PTH genes are expressed along the lateral line and in the central nervous system during embryogenesis, Endocrinology 146:547–551, 2005.
75. Canario AV, Rotllant J, Fuentes J, et al: Novel bioactive parathyroid hormone and related peptides in teleost fish, FEBS Lett 580:291–299, 2006.
76. McManus JF, Davey RA, Maclean HE, et al: Intermittent fugu parathyroid hormone 1 (1–34) is an anabolic bone agent in young male rats and osteopenic ovariectomized rats, Bone 42:1164–1174, 2008.
77. Danks JA, Devlin AJ, Ho PMW, et al: Parathyroid hormone-related protein is a factor in normal fish pituitary, Gen Comp Endocrinol 92:201–212, 1993.
78. Devlin AJ, Danks JA, Faulkner MK, et al: Immunochemical detection of parathyroid hormone-related protein in the saccus vasculosus of a teleost fish, Gen Comp Endocrinol 101:83–90, 1996.
79. Danks JA, McHale JC, Martin JT, et al: Parathyroid hormone-related protein in tissues of the emerging frog *(Rana temporaria)*: immunohistochemistry and in situ hybridization, J Anat 190:229–238, 1997.
80. Trivett M, Officer R, Clement J, et al: Parathyroid hormone-related protein (PTHrP) in cartilaginous and bony fish tissues, J Exp Zool 284:541–548, 1999.
81. Trivett MK, Walker TI, Macmillan DL, et al: Parathyroid hormone-related protein (PTHrP) production sites in elasmobranchs, J Anat 201:41–52, 2002.
82. Trivett MK, Potter IC, Power G, et al: Parathyroid hormone-related protein production in the lamprey *Geotria australis*: developmental and evolutionary perspectives, Dev Genes Evol 215:553–563, 2005.
83. Antonorakis SE, Phillips JA, Mallonee RL, et al: S-globin locus is linked to the parathyroid hormone (PTH) locus and lies between insulin and PTH loci in man, Proc Natl Acad Sci U S A 80:6615–6619, 1983.
84. Naylor SL, Sakaguchi AU, Szoka P, et al: Human parathyroid hormone gene (pth) is on short arm of chromosome 11, Somat Cell Gene 9:609–616, 1983.
85. Mayer H, Breyel E, Bostock C, et al: Assignment of the human parathyroid hormone gene to chromosome 11, Hum Genet 64:283–285, 1983.
86. Zabel BU, Kronenberg HM, Bell GI, et al: Chromosome mapping of genes on the short arm of human chromosome 11: parathyroid hormone gene is at 11p15 together with the genes for insulin, c-Harvey-ras 1, and β-hemoglobin, Cytogenet Cell Genet 39:200–205, 1985.
87. Kronenberg HK, Igarashi T, Freeman MW, et al: Structure and expression of the human parathyroid hormone gene, Recent Prog Horm Res 42:641–663, 1986.
88. Schmidtke J, Pape B, Krengel U, et al: Restriction fragment length polymorphism at the human parathyroid hormone gene locus, Hum Genet 67:428–431, 1984.
89. Gong G, Johnson M, Barger-Lux M, et al: Association of bone dimensions with a parathyroid hormone gene polymorphism in women, Osteoporos Int 9:307–311, 1999.
90. Kanzawa M, Sugimoto T, Kobayashi T, et al: Parathyroid hormone gene polymorphisms in primary hyperparathyroidism, Clin Endocrinol (Oxf) 50:583–588, 1999.
91. Mullersman J, Shields J, Saha B: Characterization of two novel polymorphisms at the human parathyroid hormone gene locus, Hum Genet 88:589–592, 1992.
92. Parkinson D, Shaw N, Himsworth R, et al: Parathyroid hormone gene analysis in autosomal hypoparathyroidism using an intragenic tetranucleotide (aaat)n polymorphism, Hum Genet 91:281–284, 1993.
93. Ahn TG, Antonarakis SE, Kronenberg HM, et al: Familial isolated hypoparathyroidism: a molecular genetic analysis of 8 families with 23 affected persons, Medicine (Baltimore) 65:73–81, 1986.
94. Miric A, Levine MA: Analysis of the preproPTH gene by denaturing gradient gel electrophoresis in familial isolated hypoparathyroidism, J Clin Endocrinol Metab 74:509–516, 1992.
95. Bilous R, Murty G, Parkinson D, et al: Brief report: autosomal dominant familial hypoparathyroidism, sensorineural deafness, and renal dysplasia, N Engl J Med 327:1069–1074, 1992.
96. Kronenberg HM, Bringhurst FR, Nussbaum S, et al: Parathyroid hormone: biosynthesis, secretion, chemistry, and action. In Mundy GR, Martin TJ, editors: Handbook of experimental pharmacology: physiology and pharmacology of bone, Heidelberg, Germany, 1993, Springer-Verlag.
97. Arnold A, Horst SA, Gardella TJ, et al: Mutation of the signal peptide-encoding region of the preproparathyroid hormone gene in familial isolated hypoparathyroidism, J Clin Invest 86:1084–1087, 1990.
98. Karaplis AC, Lim SK, Baba H, et al: Inefficient membrane targeting, translocation, and proteolytic processing by signal peptidase of a mutant preproparathyroid hormone protein, J Biol Chem 270:1629–1635, 1995.
99. Datta R, Waheed A, Shah GN, et al: Signal sequence mutation in autosomal dominant form of hypoparathyroidism induces apoptosis that is corrected by a chemical chaperone, Proc Natl Acad Sci U S A 104:19989–19994, 2007.
100. Habener JF, Rosenblatt M, Potts JT Jr: Parathyroid hormone: biochemical aspects of biosynthesis, secretion, and metabolism, Physiol Rev 64:985–1053, 1984.

101. Hendy GN, Bennett HP, Gibbs BF, et al: Proparathyroid hormone is preferentially cleaved to parathyroid hormone by the prohormone convertase furin. A mass spectrometric study, J Biol Chem 270:9517–9525, 1995.
102. Canaff L, Bennett HP, Hou Y, et al: Proparathyroid hormone processing by the proprotein convertase-7: comparison with furin and assessment of modulation of parathyroid convertase messenger ribonucleic acid levels by calcium and 1,25-dihydroxyvitamin D_3, Endocrinology 140:3633–3642, 1999.
103. MacGregor RR, Hamilton JW, Kent GN: The degradation of proparathormone and parathormone by parathyroid and liver cathepsin b, J Biol Chem 254:4428–4433, 1979.
104. MacGregor RR, Hamilton JW, Shofstall RE, et al: Isolation and characterization of porcine parathyroid cathespin b, J Biol Chem 254:4423–4427, 1979.
105. Mayer GP, Keaton JA, Hurst JG, et al: Effects of plasma calcium concentration on the relative proportion of hormone and carboxyl fragments in parathyroid venous blood, Endocrinology 104:1778–1784, 1979.
106. Habener JF, Kemper B, Potts JT Jr: Calcium-dependent intracellular degradation of parathyroid hormone: a possible mechanism for the regulation of hormone stores, Endocrinology 97:431–441, 1975.
107. D'Amour P, Palardy J, Bahsali G, et al: The modulation of circulating parathyroid hormone immunoheterogeneity in man by ionized calcium concentration, J Clin Endocrinol Metab 74:525–532, 1992.
108. Brossard JH, Clouthier M, Roy L, et al: Accumulation of a non-(1–84) molecular form of parathyroid hormone (PTH) detected by intact PTH assay in renal failure: importance in the interpretation of PTH values, J Clin Endocrinol Metab 81:3923–3929, 1996.
109. Divieti P, John MR, Juppner H, et al: Human pth-(7–84) inhibits bone resorption in vitro via actions independent of the type 1 PTH/PTHrP receptor, Endocrinology 143:171–176, 2002.
110. Yamaguchi T, Chattopadhyay N, Brown EM: G protein-coupled extracellular Ca^{2+} ($Ca^{2+}{}_o$)-sensing receptor (CAR): roles in cell signaling and control of diverse cellular functions. In O'Malley B, editor: Hormones and signaling, San Diego, 1998, Academic Press.
111. Moallem E, Kilav R, Silver J, et al: RNA-protein binding and post-transcriptional regulation of parathyroid hormone gene expression by calcium and phosphate, J Biol Chem 273:5253–5259, 1998.
112. Brown A, Zhong M, Finch J, et al: Rat calcium-sensing receptor is regulated by vitamin D but not by calcium, Am J Physiol 270:F454-F460, 1996.
113. Russell J, Sherwood L: The effects of 1,25-dihydroxyvitamin d_3 and high calcium on transcription of the pre-proparathyroid hormone gene are direct, Trans Assoc Am Physicians 100:256–262, 1987.
114. Okazaki T, Igarashi T, Kronenberg HM: 5′-flanking region of the parathyroid hormone gene mediates negative regulation by $1,25(oh)_2$ vitamin D_3, J Biol Chem 263:2203–2208, 1989.
115. Slatopolsky E, Finch J, Ritter C, et al: A new analog of calcitrol, 19-nor-1,25-$(OH)_2D_2$, suppress parathyroid hormone secretion in uremic rats in the absence of hypercalcemia, Am J Kidney Dis 26:852–860, 1995.
116. Slatopolsky E: The role of calcium, phosphorus and vitamin d metabolism in the development of secondary hyperparathyroidism, Nephrol Dial Transplant 13(Suppl 3):3–8, 1998.
117. Llach F, Keshav G, Goldblat M, et al: Suppression of parathyroid hormone secretion in hemodialysis patients by a novel vitamin d analogue: 19-nor-1,25-dihydroxyvitamin D_2, Am J Kidney Dis 32(Suppl 2):S48–S54, 1998.
118. Silver J, Moallem E, Epstein E, et al: New aspects in the control of parathyroid hormone secretion, Curr Opin Nephrol Hypertens 3:379–385, 1994.
119. Ben-Dov IZ, Galitzer H, Lavi-Moshayoff V, et al: The parathyroid is a target organ for FGF23 in rats, J Clin Invest 117:4003–4008, 2007.
120. Krajisnik T, Bjorklund P, Marsell R, et al: Fibroblast growth factor-23 regulates parathyroid hormone and 1-alpha-hydroxylase expression in cultured bovine parathyroid cells, J Endocrinol 195:125–131, 2007.
121. Imura A, Tsuji Y, Murata M, et al: Alpha-klotho as a regulator of calcium homeostasis, Science 316:1615–1618, 2007.
122. Mayer GP, Hurst JG: Sigmoidal relationship between parathyroid hormone secretion rate and plasma calcium concentration in calves, Endocrinology 102:1036–1042, 1978.
123. Brent GA, LeBoff MS, Seely EW, et al: Relationship between the concentration and rate of change of calcium and serum intact parathyroid hormone levels in normal humans, J Clin Endocrinol Metab 67:944–950, 1988.
124. Brown EM: Four-parameter model of the sigmoidal relationship between the parathyroid hormone release and extracellular calcium concentration in normal and abnormal parathyroid tissue, J Clin Endcrinol Metab 56:572–581, 1983.
125. Parfitt AM: Bone and plasma calcium homeostasis, Bone 8(Suppl. 1):1–8, 1987.
126. Brown EM: Extracellular Ca^{2+} sensing, regulation of parathyroid cell function, and role of Ca^{2+} and other ions as extracellular (first) messengers, Physiol Rev 71:371–411, 1991.
127. Hanley D, Takatsuki K, Sultan J, et al: Direct release of parathyroid hormone fragments from functioning bovine parathyroid glands in vitro, J Clin Invest 62:1247–1254, 1978.
128. Lepage R, Roy L, Brossard JH, et al: A non-(1–84) circulating parathyroid hormone (PTH) fragment interferes significantly with intact PTH commercial assay measurements in uremic samples, Clin Chem 44:805–809, 1998.
129. Parfitt AM: Hypercalcemic hyperparathyroidism following renal transplantation: differential diagnosis, management, and implications for cell population control in the parathyroid gland, Min Electrol Metab 8:92–112, 1982.
130. Gittes RF, Radde IC: Experimental model for hyperparathyroidism: effect of excessive numbers of transplanted isologous parathyroid glands, J Urol 95: 595–603, 1966.
131. Lewin E, Olgaard K: Influence of parathyroid mass on the regulation of PTH secretion, Kidney Int Suppl, S16–21, 2006.
132. Levi R, Silver J: Pathogenesis of parathyroid dysfunction in end-stage kidney disease, Pediatr Nephrol 20:342–345, 2005.
133. Grant FD, Conlin PR, Brown EM: Rate and concentration dependence of parathyroid hormone dynamics during stepwise changes in serum ionized calcium in normal humans, J Clin Endocrinol Metab 71:370–378, 1990.
134. Conlin PR, Fajtova VT, Mortensen RM, et al: Hysteresis in the relationship between serum ionized calcium and intact parathyroid hormone during recovery from induced hyper- and hypocalcemia in normal humans, J Clin Endocrinol Metab 69:593–599, 1989.
135. Cunningham J, Altmann P, Gleed J, et al: Effect of direction and rate of change of calcium on parathyroid hormone secretion in uremia, Nephrol Dial Transplant 4:339–344, 1989.
136. El-Hajj Fuleihan G, Klerman E, Brown E, et al: The parathyroid hormone circadian rhythm is truly endogenous–a general clinical research center study, J Clin Endocrinol Metab 82:281–286, 1997.
137. Harms HM, Kaptaina U, Kulpmann WR, et al: Pulse amplitude and frequency modulation of parathyroid hormone in plasma, J Clin Endocrinol Metab 69:843–851, 1989.
138. Brown E: Biology of the extracellular Ca^{2+}-sensing receptor. In Bilezikian JP, Marcus R, and ML, editors: Principles of bone biology, ed 2, Elsevier, San Diego (in press).
139. Brown EM, Gamba G, Riccardi D, et al: Cloning and characterization of an extracellular Ca^{2+}-sensing receptor from bovine parathyroid, Nature 366:575–580, 1993.
140. Brown E, MacLeod R: Extracellular calcium sensing and extracellular calcium signaling, Physiol Rev 81:239–297, 2001.
141. Nemeth EF: Calcium receptors as novel drug targets. In Bilezikian JP, Raisz LG, Rodan RA, editors: Principles of bone biology, San Diego, 1996, Academic Press.
142. Brauner-Osborne H, Jensen AA, Sheppard PO, et al: The agonist-binding domain of the calcium-sensing receptor is located at the amino-terminal domain, J Biol Chem 274:18382–18386, 1999.
143. Hu J, Reyes-Cruz G, Chen W, et al: Identification of acidic residues in the extracellular loops of the seven-transmembrane domain of the human Ca^{2+} receptor critical for response to Ca^{2+} and a positive allosteric modulator, J Biol Chem 277:46622–46631, 2002.
144. Kifor O, Diaz R, Butters R, et al: The Ca^{2+}-sensing receptor (CAR) activates phospholipases C, A2, and D in bovine parathyroid and CAR-transfected, human embryonic kidney (HEK293) cells, J Bone Miner Res 12:715–725, 1997.
145. McNeil SE, Hobson SA, Nipper V, et al: Functional calcium-sensing receptors in rat fibroblasts are required for activation of src kinase and mitogen-activated protein kinase in response to extracellular calcium, J Biol Chem 273:1114–1120, 1998.
146. Chen CJ, Barnett JV, Congo DA, et al: Divalent cations suppress 3′,5′-adenosine monophosphate accumulation by stimulating a pertussis toxin-sensitive guanine nucleotide-binding protein in cultured bovine parathyroid cells, Endocrinology 124:233–240, 1989.
147. Wettschureck N, Lee E, Libutti SK, et al: Parathyroid-specific double knockout of gq and g11 alpha-subunits leads to a phenotype resembling germline knockout of the extracellular Ca^{2+} -sensing receptor, Mol Endocrinol 21:274–280, 2007.
148. Ritter CS, Pande S, Krits I, et al: Destabilization of parathyroid hormone mRNA by extracellular Ca^{2+} and the calcimimetic r-568 in parathyroid cells: role of cytosolic ca and requirement for gene transcription, J Mol Endocrinol 40:13–21, 2008.
149. Garrett JE, Tamir H, Kifor O, et al: Calcitonin-secreting cells of the thyroid express an extracellular calcium receptor gene, Endocrinology 136:5202–5211, 1995.
150. Riccardi D, Hall AE, Chattopadhyay N, et al: Localization of the extracellular Ca^{2+}/polyvalent cation-sensing protein in rat kidney, Am J Physiol 274:F611–622, 1998.
151. Hebert SC, Brown EM, Harris HW: Role of the $Ca^{(2+)}$-sensing receptor in divalent mineral ion homeostasis, J Exp Biol 200:295–302, 1997.
152. Quarles LD: Cation-sensing receptors in bone: a novel paradigm for regulating bone remodeling? J Bone Miner Res 12:1971–1974, 1997.
153. Chang W, Tu C, Chen TH, et al: The extracellular calcium-sensing receptor (CASR) is a critical modulator of skeletal development, Sci Signal 1, ra1, 2008.
154. Pollak MR, Brown EM, WuChou YH, et al: Mutations in the human Ca^{2+}-sensing receptor gene cause familial hypocalciuric hypercalcemia and neonatal severe hyperparathyroidism, Cell 75:1297–1303, 1993.
155. Pollak MR, Brown EM, Estep HL, et al: Autosomal dominant hypocalcaemia caused by a Ca^{2+}-sensing receptor gene mutation, Nat Genet 8:303–307, 1994.
156. Brown EM: Clinical lessons from the calcium-sensing receptor, Nat Clin Pract Endocrinol Metab 3:122–133, 2007.
157. Hauache OM: Extracellular calcium-sensing receptor: Structural and functional features and association with diseases, Braz J Med Biol Res 34:577–584, 2001.
158. Ho C, Conner DA, Pollak M, et al: A mouse model for familial hypocalciuric hypercalcemia and neonatal severe hyperparathyroidism, Nat Genet 11:389–394, 1995.
159. Cantley LK, Russell J, Lettieri D, et al: 1,25-dihydroxyvitamin D_3 suppresses parathyroid hormone secretion from bovine parathyroid cells in tissue culture Endocrinology 117:2114–2119, 1985.
160. Chan YL, McKay C, Dye E, et al: The effect of 1,25 dihydroxycholecalciferol on parathyroid hormone secretion by monolayer cultures of bovine parathyroid cells, Calcif Tissue Int 38:27–32, 1986.
161. Naveh-Many T, Rahaminov R, Livini N, et al: Parathyroid cell proliferation in normal and chronic renal failure in rats. The effects of calcium, phosphate, and vitamin D, J Clin Invest 96:1786–1793, 1995.
162. Almaden Y, Canalejo A, Hernandez A, et al: Direct effect of phosphorus on PTH secretion from whole rat parathyroid glands in vitro, J Bone Miner Res 11:970–976, 1996.
163. Slatopolsky E, Finch J, Denda M, et al: Phosphorus restriction prevents parathyroid gland growth. High phosphorus directly stimulates PTH secretion in vitro, J Clin Invest 97:2534–2540, 1996.
164. Habener JF, Potts JTJ: Relative effectiveness of magnesium and calcium on the secretion and biosynthesis of parathyroid in vitro, Endocrinology 98:197–202, 1976.

165. Strewler GJ: Familial benign hypocalciuric hypercalcemia: from the clinic to the calcium sensor, West J Med 160:579–580, 1994.
166. Brown EM: Physiology and pathophysiology of the extracellular calcium-sensing receptor, Am J Med 106:238–253, 1999.
167. Brown EM, Vassilev PM, Quinn S, et al: G-protein-coupled, extracellular $Ca^{(2+)}$-sensing receptor: a versatile regulator of diverse cellular functions, Vitam Horm 55:1–71, 1999.
168. Anast CS, Winnacker JL, Forte LF, et al: Impaired release of parathyroid hormone in magnesium deficiency, J Clin Endocrinol Metab 42:707–717, 1976.
169. Quitterer U, Hoffmann M, Freichel M, et al: Paradoxical block of parathormone secretion is mediated by increased activity of G alpha subunits, J Biol Chem 276:6763–6769, 2001.
170. Berson SA, Yalow RS: Immunochemical heterogeneity of parathyroid hormone in plasma, J Clin Endocrinol Metab 28:1037–1947, 1968.
171. Nguyen-Yamamoto L, Rousseau L, Brossard JH, et al: Synthetic carboxyl-terminal fragments of parathyroid hormone (PTH) decrease ionized calcium concentration in rats by acting on a receptor different from the PTH/PTH-related peptide receptor, Endocrinology 142:1386–1392, 2001.
172. D'Amour P, Brossard JH, Rousseau L, et al: Structure of non-(1–84) PTH fragments secreted by parathyroid glands in primary and secondary hyperparathyroidism, Kidney Int 68:998–1007, 2005.
173. Slatopolsky E, Finch J, Clay P, et al: A novel mechanism for skeletal resistance in uremia, Kidney Int 58:753–761, 2000.
174. Flueck JA, Dibella FB, Edis AJ, et al: Immunoheterogeneity of parathyroid hormone in venous effluent serum from hyperfunctioning parathyroid glands, J Clin Invest 60:1367–1375, 1977.
175. Brasier A, Wang C, Nussbaum S: Recovery of parathyroid hormone secretion after parathyroid adenomectomy, J Clin Endocrinol Metab 66:495–500, 1988.
176. Bringhurst FR, Stern AM, Yotts M: Peripheral metabolism of PTH: fate of the biologically active amino-terminus in vivo, Am J Physiol 255:E886–E893, 1988.
177. Bringhurst FR, Stern AM, Yotts M: Peripheral metabolism of [^{35}S]PTH in vivo: influence of alterations in calcium availability and parathyroid status, Endocrinology 122:237–245, 1989.
178. Martin KJ, Hruska KA, Freitag JJ, et al: The peripheral metabolism of parathyroid hormone, N Engl J Med 301:1092–1098, 1979.
179. Hilpert J, Nykjaer A, Jacobsen C, et al: Megalin antagonizes activation of the parathyroid hormone receptor, J Biol Chem 274:5620–5625, 1999.
180. Nussbaum SR, Zahradnik RJ, Lavigne JR, et al: Highly sensitive two-site immunoradiometric assay of parathyrin, and its clinical utility in evaluating patients with hypercalcemia, Clin Chem 33:1364–1367, 1987.
181. Blind E, Schmidt-Gayk H, Scharla S, et al: Two-site assay of intact parathyroid hormone in the investigation of primary hyperparathyroidism and other disorders of calcium metabolism compared with a midregion assay, J Clin Endocrinol Metab 67:353–360, 1988.
182. John M, Goodman W, Gao P, et al: A novel immunoradiometric assay detects full-length human PTH but not amino-terminally truncated fragments: implications for PTH measurements in renal failure, J Clin Endocrinol Metab 84:4287–4290, 1999.
183. Hercz G, Pei Y, Greenwood C, et al: Aplastic osteodystrophy without aluminum: the role of "suppressed" parathyroid function, Kidney Int 44:860–866, 1993.
184. Goodman WG, Ramirez JA, Belin TR, et al: Development of adynamic bone in patients with secondary hyperparathyroidism after intermittent calcitriol therapy, Kidney Int 46:1160–1166, 1994.
185. Wang M, Hercz G, Sherrard D, et al: Relationship between intact 1–84 parathyroid hormone and bone histomorphometric parameters in dialysis patients without aluminum toxicity, Am J Kidney Dis 26:836–844, 1995.
186. Goodman W, Veldhuis J, Belin T, et al: Suppressive effect of calcium on parathyroid hormone release in adynamic renal osteodystrophy and secondary hyperparathyroidism, Kidney Int 51:1590–1595, 1997.
187. Salusky IB, Goodman WG, Kuizon BD, et al: Similar predictive value of bone turnover using first- and second-generation immunometric PTH assays in pediatric patients treated with peritoneal dialysis, Kidney Int 63:1801–1808, 2003.
188. Kuizon BD, Goodman WG, Jüppner H, et al: Diminished linear growth during intermittent calcitriol therapy in children undergoing CCPD, Kidney Int 53:205–211, 1998.
189. Kuizon BD, Salusky IB: Intermittent calcitriol therapy and growth in children with chronic renal failure, Miner Electrolyte Metab 24:290–295, 1998.
190. Sanchez CP, Salusky IB, Kuizon BD, et al: Growth of long bones in renal failure: Roles of hyperparathyroidism, growth hormone and calcitriol, Kidney Int 54:1879–1887, 1998.
191. Rakel A, Brossard J, Patenaude J, et al: Overproduction of an amino-terminal form of PTH distinct from human pth(1–84) in a case of severe primary hyperparathyroidism: influence of medical treatment and surgery, Clin Endocrinol (Oxf) 62:721–727, 2005.
192. Rubin MR, Silverberg SJ, D'Amour P, et al: An n-terminal molecular form of parathyroid hormone (PTH) distinct from hpth(1–84) is overproduced in parathyroid carcinoma, Clin Chem 53:1470–1476, 2007.
193. Shimada T, Urakawa I, Isakova T, et al: Circulating FGF23 in dialysis patients is intact and biologically active, 2009. [Submitted].
194. Friedman PA, Gesek FA: Calcium transport in renal epithelial cells, Am J Physiol 264:F181–F198, 1993.
195. Bourdeau J: Mechanisms and regulation of calcium transport in the nephron, Semin Nephrol 13:191–201, 1993.
196. Suki WN: Calcium transport in the nephron, Am J Physiol 237:F1–F6, 1979.
197. Torikai S, Wang, M-S, Klein KL, et al: Adenylate cyclase and cell cyclic AMP of rat cortical thick ascending limb of Henle, Kidney Int 20:649–654, 1981.
198. Morel F, Imbert-Teboul M, Chabardes D: Distribution of hormone-dependent adenylate cyclase in the nephron and its physiological significance, Annu Rev Physiol 43:569–581, 1981.
199. van Abel M, Hoenderop JG, van der Kemp AW, et al: Coordinated control of renal $Ca^{(2+)}$ transport proteins by parathyroid hormone, Kidney Int 68:1708–1721, 2005.
200. Hoenderop JG, van der Kemp AW, Hartog A, et al: Molecular identification of the apical Ca^{2+} channel in 1,25-dihydroxyvitamin D_3-responsive epithelia, J Biol Chem 274:8375–8378, 1999.
201. Mensenkamp AR, Hoenderop JG, Bindels RJ: Trpv5, the gateway to Ca^{2+} homeostasis, Handb Exp Pharmacol, 207–220, 2007.
202. Bouhtiauy I, LaJeunesse D, Brunette MG: The mechanism of parathyroid hormone action on calcium reabsorption by the distal tubule, Endocrinology 128:251–258, 1991.
203. Bacskai BJ, Friedman PA: Activation of latent Ca^{2+} channels in renal epithelial cells by parathyroid hormone, Nature 347:388–391, 1990.
204. Takeyama K, Kitanaka S, Sato T, et al: 25-hydroxyvitamin D_3 1-alpha-hydroxylase and vitamin D synthesis, Science 277:1827–1830, 1997.
205. St. Arnaud R, Messerlian S, Moir JM, et al: The 25-hydroxyvitamin D 1-alpha-hydroxylase gene maps to the pseudovitamin D-deficiency rickets (PDDR) disease locus, J Bone Miner Res 12:1552–1559, 1997.
206. Fu GK, Lin D, Zhang MY, et al: Cloning of human 25-hydroxyvitamin D-1 alpha-hydroxylase and mutations causing vitamin D-dependent rickets type 1, Mol Endocrinol 11:1961–1970, 1997.
207. Henry H: Parathyroid hormone modulation of 25-hydroxyvitamin D3 metabolism by cultured chick kidney cells is mimicked and enhanced by forskolin, Endocrinology 116:503–510, 1985.
208. Murayama A, Takeyama K, Kitanaka S, et al: Positive and negative regulations of the renal 25-hydroxyvitamin D_3 1alpha-hydroxylase gene by parathyroid hormone, calcitonin, and 1-alpha,25$(OH)_2D_3$ in intact animals, Endocrinology 140:2224–2231, 1999.
209. Brenza HL, Kimmel-Jehan C, Jehan F, et al: Parathyroid hormone activation of the 25-hydroxyvitamin D_3-1α-hydroxylase gene promoter, Proc Natl Acad Sci U S A 95:1387–1391, 1998.
210. Kong XF, Zhu XH, Pei YL, et al: Molecular cloning, characterization, and promoter analysis of the human 25-hydroxyvitamin D_3-1alpha-hydroxylase gene, Proc Natl Acad Sci U S A 96:6988–6993, 1999.
211. Tanaka Y, Lorenc RS, Deluca HF: The role of 1,25-dihydroxyvitamin D_3 and parathyroid hormone in the regulation of chick renal 25-hydroxy-vitamin D_3-24-hydroxylase, Arch Biochem Biophys 171:521–526, 1975.
212. Shigematsu T, Horiuchi N, Ogura Y: Human parathyroid hormone inhibits renal 24-hydroxylase activity of 25-hydroxyvitamin d3 by a mechanism involving adenosine 3′,5′-monophosphate in rats, Endocrinology 118:1583–1589, 1986.
213. Econs M, Drezner M: Tumor-induced osteomalacia: unveiling a new hormone, N Engl J Med 330:1679–1681, 1994.
214. Kempson SA: Effect of metabolic acidosis on renal brush border membrane adaptation to low phosphorus diet, Kidney Int 22:225–233, 1982.
215. Pfister MF, Ruf I, Stange G, et al: Parathyroid hormone leads to the lysosomal degradation of the renal type II NA/P_i cotransporter, Proc Natl Acad Sci U S A 95:1909–1914, 1998.
216. Blaine J, Breusegem S, Giral H, et al: Differential regulation of renal NAPIIIA and NAPI-IIC trafficking by PTH, Renal Week ASN (San Francisco), 2007.
217. Forster IC, Hernando N, Biber J, et al: Proximal tubular handling of phosphate: a molecular perspective, Kidney Int 70:1548–1559, 2006.
218. Miyamoto K, Ito M, Tatsumi S, et al: New aspect of renal phosphate reabsorption: The type IIC sodium-dependent phosphate transporter, Am J Nephrol 27:503–515, 2007.
219. Virkki LV, Biber J, Murer H, et al: Phosphate transporters: a tale of two solute carrier families, Am J Physiol Renal Physiol 293:F643–654, 2007.
220. Tenenhouse HS: Phosphate transport: molecular basis, regulation and pathophysiology, J Steroid Biochem Mol Biol 103:572–577, 2007.
221. Riccardi D, Traebert M, Ward DT, et al: Dietary phosphate and parathyroid hormone alter the expression of the calcium-sensing receptor (car) and the Na^+-dependent P_i transporter (NaP_i-2) in the rat proximal tubule, Pflugers Arch 441:379–387, 2000.
222. Ba J, Brown D, Friedman PA: Calcium-sensing receptor regulation of PTH-inhibitable proximal tubule phosphate transport, Am J Physiol Renal Physiol 285:F1233–F1243, 2003.
223. Amizuka N, Lee HS, Khan MY, et al: Cell-specific expression of the parathyroid hormone (PTH)PTH-related peptide receptor gene in kidney from kidney-specific and ubiquitous promotors, Endocrinology 138:469–481, 1997.
224. Mohr H, Hesch RD: Different handling of parathyrin by basal-lateral and brush-border membranes of the bovine kidney cortex, Biochem J 188:649–656, 1980.
225. Kaufmann M, Muff R, Stieger B, et al: Apical and basolateral parathyroid hormone receptors in rat renal cortical membranes Endocrinology 134:1173–1178, 1994.
226. Traebert M, Volkl H, Biber J, et al: Luminal and contraluminal action of 1–34 and 3–34 PTH peptides on renal type IIa Na-P_i cotransporter, Am J Physiol Renal Physiol 278:F792–F798, 2000.
227. Segawa H, Yamanaka S, Onitsuka A, et al: Parathyroid hormone-dependent endocytosis of renal type IIC Na-P_i cotransporter, Am J Physiol Renal Physiol 292:F395–F403, 2007.
228. Capuano P, Bacic D, Stange G, et al: Expression and regulation of the renal na/phosphate cotransporter NAPI-IIA in a mouse model deficient for the PDZ protein PDZk1, Pflugers Arch 449:392–402, 2005.
229. Bell NH, Avery S, Sinha T, et al: Effects of dibutyryl cyclic adenosine 3′,5′-monophosphate and parathyroid extract on calcium and phosphorus metabolism in hypoparathyroidism and pseudohypoparathyroidism, J Clin Invest 51:816–823, 1972.
230. Neer RM, Tregear GW, Potts JT Jr: Renal effects of native parathyroid hormone and synthetic biologically active fragments in pseudohypoparathyroidism and hypoparathyroidism, J Clin Endocrinol Metab 44:420–423, 1977.
231. McElduff A, Lissner D, Wilkinson M, et al: A 6-hour human parathyroid hormone (1–34) infusion protocol: studies in normal and hypoparathyroid subjects, Calcif Tissue Int 41:267–273, 1987.
232. Segawa H, Kaneko I, Takahashi A, et al: Growth-related renal type II Na/P_i cotransporter, J Biol Chem 277:19665–19672, 2002.

233. Bergwitz C, Roslin NM, Tieder M, et al: Slc34a3 mutations in patients with hereditary hypophosphatemic rickets with hypercalciuria predict a key role for the sodium-phosphate cotransporter NaP$_i$-IIc in maintaining phosphate homeostasis, Am J Hum Genet 78:179–192, 2006.

234. Lorenz-Depiereux B, Benet-Pages A, Eckstein G, et al: Hereditary hypophosphatemic rickets with hypercalciuria is caused by mutations in the sodium-phosphate cotransporter gene slc34a3, Am J Hum Genet 78:193–201, 2006.

235. Ichikawa S, Sorenson AH, Imel EA, et al: Intronic deletions in the slc34a3 gene cause hereditary hypophosphatemic rickets with hypercalciuria, J Clin Endocrinol Metab 91:4022–4027, 2006.

236. Yamamoto T, Michigami T, Aranami F, et al: Hereditary hypophosphatemic rickets with hypercalciuria: a study for the phosphate transporter gene type IIc and osteoblastic function, J Bone Miner Metab 25:407–413, 2007.

237. Bezprozvanny I, Maximov A: Pdz domains: more than just a glue, Proc Natl Acad Sci U S A 98:787–789, 2001.

238. Shenolikar S, Voltz JW, Cunningham R, et al: Regulation of ion transport by the NHERF family of PDZ proteins, Physiology (Bethesda) 19:362–369, 2004.

239. Mahon M, Donowitz M, Yun C, et al: Na$^{(+)}$/H$^{(+)}$ exchanger regulatory factor 2 directs parathyroid hormone 1 receptor signalling, Nature 417:858–861, 2002.

240. Mahon M, Segre G: Stimulation by parathyroid hormone of a NHERF-1-assembled complex consisting of the parathyroid hormone i receptor, phospholipase Cbeta, and actin increases intracellular calcium in opossum kidney cells, J Biol Chem 279:23550–23558, 2004.

241. Gisler SM, Stagljar I, Traebert M, et al: Interaction of the type IIa Na/P$_i$ cotransporter with PDZ proteins, J Biol Chem 276:9206–9213, 2001.

242. Shenolikar S, Voltz JW, Minkoff CM, et al: Targeted disruption of the mouse NHERF-1 gene promotes internalization of proximal tubule sodium-phosphate cotransporter type IIa and renal phosphate wasting, Proc Natl Acad Sci U S A 99:11470–11475, 2002.

243. Mahon MJ: Ezrin promotes functional expression and parathyroid hormone-mediated regulation of the sodium-phosphate cotransporter 2a in llc-pk1 cells, Am J Physiol Renal Physiol 294:F667–675, 2008.

244. Jouishomme H, Whitfield JF, Chakravarthy B, et al: The protein kinase-C activation domain of the parathyroid hormone, Endocrinology 130:53–59, 1992.

245. Jouishomme H, Whitfield JF, Gagnon L, et al: Further definition of the protein kinase C activation domain of the parathyroid hormone, J Bone Miner Res 9:943–949, 1994.

246. Whitfield J, Isaacs R, Chakravarthy B, et al: Stimulation of protein kinase C activity in cells expressing human parathyroid hormone receptor by C- and N-terminally truncated fragments of parathyroid hormone 1–34, J Bone Miner Res 16:441–447, 2001.

247. Takasu H, Guo J, Bringhurst F: Dual signaling and ligand selectivity of the human PTH/PTHrP receptor, J Bone Miner Res 14:11–20, 1999.

248. Teitelbaum AP, Strewler GJ: Parathyroid hormone receptors coupled to cyclic adenosine monophosphate formation in an established renal cell line, Endocrinology 114:980–985, 1984.

249. Quamme G, Pfeilschifter J, Murer H: Parathyroid hormone inhibition of na+/phosphate cotransport in ok cells: generation of second messengers in the regulatory cascade, Biochem Biophys Res Commun 158:951–957, 1989.

250. Cole JA, Carnes DL, Forte LR, et al: Structure-activity relationships of parathyroid hormone analogs in the opossum kidney cell line, J Bone Miner Res 4:723–730, 1989.

251. Cole JA, Eber SL, Poelling RE, et al: A dual mechanism for regulation of kidney phosphate transport by parathyroid hormone, Am J Physiol 253:E221–E227, 1987.

252. Cole JA, Forte LR, Eber S, et al: Regulation of sodium-dependent phosphate transport by parathyroid hormone in opossum kidney cells: adenosine 3',5'-monophosphate-dependent and -independent mechanisms, Endocrinology 122:2981–2989, 1988.

253. Segre GV, Rosenblatt M, Tully GL III, et al: Evaluation of an in vitro parathyroid hormone antagonist in vivo in dogs, Endocrinology 116:1024–1029, 1985.

254. Arakawa T, D'Amour P, Rousseau L, et al: Overproduction and secretion of a novel amino-terminal form of parathyroid hormone from a severe type of parathyroid hyperplasia in uremia, Clin J Am Soc Nephrol 1:525–531, 2006.

255. D'Amour P, Brossard JH, Rakel A, et al: Evidence that the amino-terminal composition of non-(1–84) parathyroid hormone fragments starts before position 19, Clin Chem 51:169–176, 2005.

256. Martin KJ, McConkey CJ Jr, Caulfield MP: The role of protein kinase-A activity in the evaluation of agonist/antagonist properties of analogs of parathyroid hormone-related protein in opossum kidney cells, Endocrinology 131:2161–2164, 1992.

257. Martin KJ, McConkey CL, Garcia JC, et al: Protein kinase-A and the effects of parathyroid hormone on phosphate uptake in opossum kidney cells, Endocrinology 125:295–301, 1989.

258. Chambers TJ, Athanasou NA, Fuller K: Effect of parathyroid hormone and calcitonin on the cytoplasmic spreading of isolated osteoclasts, J Endocrinol 102:281–286, 1984.

259. Wong GL: Paracrine interactions in bone-secreted products of osteoblasts permit osteoclasts to respond to parathyroid hormone, J Biol Chem 259:4019–4022, 1984.

260. Perry HM III, Skogen W, Chappel J, et al: Partial characterization of a parathyroid hormone-stimulated resorption factor(s) from osteoblast-like cells, Endocrinology 125:2075–2082, 1989.

261. Parsons JA, Robinson CJ: Calcium shift into bone causing transient hypocalcaemia after injection of parathyroid hormone, Nature 230:581–582, 1971.

262. Talmage RV, Doppelt SH, Fondren FB: An interpretation of acute changes in plasma ^{45}Ca following parathyroid hormone administration to thyroparathyroidectomized rats, Calcif Tissue Res 22:117–128, 1976.

263. Bellido T, Ali AA, Plotkin LI, et al: Proteasomal degradation of Runx2 shortens parathyroid hormone-induced anti-apoptotic signaling in osteoblasts. A putative explanation for why intermittent administration is needed for bone anabolism, J Biol Chem 278:50259–50272, 2003.

264. Jilka RL: Molecular and cellular mechanisms of the anabolic effect of intermittent PTH, Bone 40:1434–1446, 2007.

265. Keller H, Kneissel M: Sost is a target gene for PTH in bone, Bone 37:148–158, 2005.

266. Leupin O, Kramer I, Collette NM, et al: Control of the Sost bone enhancer by PTH using mef2 transcription factors, J Bone Miner Res 22:1957–1967, 2007.

267. O'Brien CA, Plotkin LI, Galli C, et al: Control of bone mass and remodeling by PTH receptor signaling in osteocytes, PLoS ONE 3:e2942, 2008.

268. Bellido T, Ali AA, Gubrij I, et al: Chronic elevation of parathyroid hormone in mice reduces expression of sclerostin by osteocytes: a novel mechanism for hormonal control of osteoblastogenesis, Endocrinology 146:4577–4583, 2005.

269. Iida-Klein A, Guo J, Xie LY, et al: Truncation of the carboxyl-terminal region of the parathyroid hormone (PTH)/PTH-related peptide receptor enhances PTH stimulation of adenylate cyclase but not phospholipase C, J Biol Chem 270:8458–8465, 1995.

270. Habener JF, Potts JT Jr: Parathyroid physiology and primary hyperparathyroidism, In Avioli LV, Krane SM, editors: Metabolic bone disease, New York, 1978, Academic Press.

271. Finkelstein JS: Pharmacological mechanisms of therapeutics: parathyroid hormone. In Bilezikian JP, Raisz LG, Rodan RA, editors: Principles of bone biology, New York, 1996, Academic Press.

272. Noble BS: The osteocyte lineage, Arch Biochem Biophys 473:106–111, 2008.

273. You L, Temiyasathit S, Lee P, et al: Osteocytes as mechanosensors in the inhibition of bone resorption due to mechanical loading, Bone 42:172–179, 2008.

274. Kong Y, Yoshida H, Sarosi I, et al: Opgl is a key regulator of osteoclastogenesis, lymphocyte development and lymph-node organogenesis, Nature 397:315–323, 1999.

275. Li J, Sarosi I, Yan X, et al: RANK is the intrinsic hematopoietic cell surface receptor that controls osteoclastogenesis and regulation of bone mass and calcium metabolism, Proc Natl Acad Sci U S A 15:1566–1571, 2000.

276. Krishnan V, Moore TL, Ma YL, et al: Parathyroid hormone bone anabolic action requires cbfa1/runx2-dependent signaling, Mol Endocrinol 17:423–435, 2003.

277. Martin TJ, Sims NA, Ng KW: Regulatory pathways revealing new approaches to the development of anabolic drugs for osteoporosis, Osteoporos Int 19:1125–1138, 2008.

278. Wong BR, Rho J, Aaron J, et al: Trance is a novel ligand of the tumor necrosis factor receptor family that activates C-jun N-terminal kinase in T cells, J Biol Chem 272:25190–25194, 1997.

279. Anderson DA, Maraskovsky E, Billingsley WL, et al: A homologue of the TNF receptor and its ligand enhance T-cell growth and dendritic-cell function, Nature 390:175–179, 1997.

280. Yasuda H, Shima N, Nakagawa N, et al: Osteoclast differentiation factor is a ligand for osteoprotegerin/osteoclastogenesis-inhibitory factor and is identical to trance/rankl, Proc Natl Acad Sci U S A 95:3597–3602, 1998.

281. Quinn JM, Elliott J, Gillespie MT, et al: A combination of osteoclast differentiation factor and macrophage-colony stimulating factor is sufficient for both human and mouse osteoclast formation in vitro, Endocrinology 139:4424–4427, 1998.

282. Fuller K, Wong B, Fox S, et al: Oc activation by trance is necessary and sufficient for osteoblast-mediated activation of bone resorption in osteoclasts, J Exp Med 188:997–1001, 1998.

283. Lacey DL, Timms E, Tan HL, et al: Osteoprotegerin ligand is a cytokine that regulates osteoclast differentiation and activation, Cell 93:165–176, 1998.

284. Simonet SW, Lacey DL, Dunstan CR, et al: Osteoprotegerin: a novel secreted protein involved in the regulation of bone density, Cell 89:309–319, 1997.

285. Suda E, Goto M, Mochizuki S, et al: Isolation of a novel cytokine from human fibroblasts that specifically inhibits osteoclastogenesis, Biochem Biophys Res Comm 234:137–142, 1997.

286. Bucay N, Sarosi I, Dunstan DR, et al: Osteoprotegerin-deficient mice develop early onset osteoporosis and arterial calcification, Genes Dev 12:1260–1268, 1998.

287. Löwik CWGM, van der Pluijm G, Bloys H, et al: Parathyroid hormone (PTH) and PTH-like protein (PLP) stimulate interleukin-6 production by osteogenic cells: a possible role of interleukin-6 in osteoclastogenesis, Biochem Biophys Res Commun 162:1546–1552, 1989.

288. Paliwal I, Insogna K: Partial purification and characterization of the 9,000-dalton bone-resorbing activity from parathyroid hormone-related protein-treated saos2 cells (abstr #245), J Bone Miner Res 6(Supp 1):S144, 1991.

289. Felix R, Fleisch H, Elford PR: Bone-resorbing cytokines enhance release of macrophage colony-stimulating activity by the osteoblastic cell mc3t3-e1, Calcif Tissue Int 44:356–360, 1989.

290. Lee S, Lorenzo J: Parathyroid hormone stimulates trance and inhibits osteoprotegerin messenger ribonucleic acid expression in murine bone marrow cultures: correlation with osteoclast-like cell formation, Endocrinology 140:3552–3561, 1999.

291. Robling AG, Niziolek PJ, Baldridge LA, et al: Mechanical stimulation of bone in vivo reduces osteocyte expression of Sost/sclerostin J Biol Chem 283:5866–5875, 2008.

292. Martin A, David V, Laurence JS, et al: Degradation of MEPE, DMP1, and release of SIBLING ASARM-peptides (minhibins): ASARM-peptide(s) are directly responsible for defective mineralization in HYP, Endocrinology 149:1757–1772, 2008.

293. Martin JT, Moseley JM, Gillespie MT: Parathyroid hormone-related protein: biochemistry and molecular biology, Crit Rev Biochem Mol Biol 26:377–395, 1991.

294. Albright F: Case records of the Massachusetts General Hospital; case 27461, New Engl J Med 255:789–791, 1941.

295. Stewart AF, Horst R, Deftos LJ, et al: Biochemical evaluation of patients with cancer-associated hypercalcemia. Evidence for humoral and non-humoral groups, N Engl J Med 303:1377–1381, 1980.

296. Moseley JM, Kubota M, Diefenbach-Jagger H, et al: Parathyroid hormone-related protein purified from a human lung cancer cell line, Proc Natl Acad Sci U S A 84:5048–5052, 1987.

297. Strewler GJ, Stern PH, Jacobs JW, et al: Parathyroid hormone-like protein from human renal carcinoma cells. Structural and functional homology with parathyroid hormone, J Clin Invest 80:1803–1807, 1987.

298. Mangin M, Webb AC, Dreyer BE, et al: Identification of a cDNA encoding a parathyroid hormone-like peptide from a human tumor associated with humoral hypercalcemia of malignancy, Proc Natl Acad Sci U S A 85:597–601, 1988.

299. Burtis WJ, Brady TG, Orloff JJ, et al: Immunochemical characterization of circulating parathyroid hormone related protein in patients with humoral hypercalcemia of cancer, N Engl J Med 322:1106–1112, 1990.

300. Ikeda K, Weir EC, Mangin M, et al: Expression of messenger ribonucleic acids encoding a parathyroid hormone-like peptide in normal human and animal tissues with abnormal expression in human parathyroid adenomas and rat keratinocytes, Mol Endocrinol 2:1230–1236, 1988.

301. Thiede MA, Rodan GA: Expression of a calcium-mobilizing parathyroid hormone-like peptide in lactating mammary tissue, Science 242:278–280, 1988.

302. Burton, PBJ, Moniz C, Quirke P, et al: Parathyroid hormone-related peptide in the human fetal urogenital tract, Mol Cell Endocrinol 69:R13–R17, 1990.

303. Ferguson JE, Gorman JV, Bruns DE, et al: Abundant expression of parathyroid hormone-related protein in human amnion and its association with labor, Physiology 89:8384–8388, 1992.

304. van de Stolpe A, Karperien M, Löwik CWGM, et al: Parathyroid hormone-related peptide as an endogenous inducer of parietal endoderm differentiation, J Cell Biol 120:235–243, 1993.

305. Karaplis AC, Luz A, Glowacki J, et al: Lethal skeletal dysplasia from targeted disruption of the parathyroid hormone-related peptide gene, Genes Dev 8:277–289, 1994.

306. Weir EC, Philbrick WM, Amling M, et al: Targeted overexpression of parathyroid hormone-related peptide in chondrocytes causes skeletal dysplasia and delayed endochondral bone formation, Proc Natl Acad Sci U S A 93:10240–10245, 1996.

307. Mangin M, Ikeda K, Dreyer BE, et al: Isolation and characterization of the human parathyroid hormone-like peptide gene, Proc Natl Acad Sci U S A 86:2408–2412, 1989.

308. Pausova Z, Morgan K, Fujiwara TM, et al: Molecular characterization of an intragenic minisatellite (vntr) polymorphism in the human parathyroid hormone-related peptide gene in chromsome 12p12.1–11.2, Genomics 17:243–244, 1993.

309. Wu TL, Vasavada RC, Yang K, et al: Structural and physiological characterization of the mid-region secretory species of parathyroid hormone-related protein, J Biol Chem 271:24371–24381, 1996.

310. Yang KH, dePapp AE, Soifer NE, et al: Parathyroid hormone-related protein: evidence for isoform- and tissue-specific posttranslational processing, Biochemistry 33:7460–7469, 1994.

311. Jüppner H, Abou-Samra AB, Uneno S, et al: The parathyroid hormone-like peptide associated with humoral hypercalcemia of malignancy and parathyroid hormone bind to the same receptor on the plasma membrane of ros 17/2.8 cells, J Biol Chem 263:8557–8560, 1988.

312. Kemp BE, Moseley JM, Rodda CP, et al: Parathyroid hormone-related protein of malignancy: active synthetic fragments, Science 238:1568–1570, 1987.

313. Horiuchi N, Caulfield MP, Fisher JE, et al: Similarity of synthetic peptide from human tumor to parathyroid hormone in vivo and in vitro, Science 238:1566–1568, 1987.

314. Everhart-Caye M, Inzucchi SE, Guinness-Henry J, et al: Parathyroid hormone (PTH)-related protein(1–36) is equipotent to PTH(1–34) in humans, J Clin Endocrinol Metab 81:199–208, 1996.

315. Wu TL, Soifer NE, Burtis WJ, et al: Glycosylation of parathyroid hormone-related peptide secreted by human epidermal keratinocytes, J Clin Endocrinol Metab 73:1002–1007, 1991.

316. Orloff JJ, Soifer NE, Fodero JP, et al: Accumulation of carboxy-terminal fragments of parathyroid hormone-related protein in renal failure, Kidney Int 43:1371–1376, 1993.

317. Fenton AJ, Kemp BE, Hammonds RG Jr, et al: A potent inhibitor of osteoclastic bone resorption within a highly conserved pentapeptide region of parathyroid hormone-related protein; PTHrP(107–111), Endocrinology 129:3424–3426, 1991.

318. Fenton AJ, Kemp BE, Kent GN, et al: A carboxyl-terminal peptide from the parathyroid hormone-related protein inhibits bone resorption by osteoclasts, Endocrinology 129:1762–1768, 1991.

319. Cornish J, Callon K, Lin C, et al: Stimulation of osteoblast proliferation by C-terminal fragments of parathyroid hormone-related protein, J Bone Miner Res 14:915–922, 1999.

320. Sone T, Kohno H, Kikuchi H, et al: Human parathyroid hormone-related peptide-(107–111) does not inhibit bone resorption in neonatal mouse calvariae, Endocrinology 131:2742–2746, 1992.

321. Cornish J, Callon KE, Nicholson GC, et al: Parathyroid hormone-related protein-(107–139) inhibits bone resorption in vivo, Endocrinology 138:1299–1304, 1997.

322. Soifer NE, Dee K, Insogna KL, et al: Parathyroid hormone-related protein. Evidence for secretion of a novel mid-region fragment by three different cell types, J Biol Chem 267:18236–18243, 1992.

323. Burtis WJ, Dann P, Gaich GA, et al: A high abundance midregion species of parathyroid hormone-related protein: immunological and chromatographic characterization in plasma, J Clin Endocrinol Metab 78:317–322, 1994.

324. Orloff JJ, Ganz MB, Nathanson H, et al: A midregion parathyroid hormone-related peptide mobilizes cytosolic calcium and stimulates formation of inositol trisphosphate in a squamous carcinoma cell line, Endocrinology 137:5376–5385, 1996.

325. Kovacs CS, Lanske B, Hunzelman JL, et al: Parathyroid hormone-related peptide (pthrp) regulates fetal placental calcium transport through a receptor distinct from the PTH/PTHrP receptor, Proc Natl Acad Sci U S A 93:15233–15238, 1996.

326. Kovacs CS, Kronenberg HM: Maternal-fetal calcium and bone metabolism during pregnancy, puerperium, and lactation, Endocr Rev 18:832–872, 1997.

327. Rodda CP, Kubota M, Heath JA, et al: Evidence for a novel parathyroid hormone-related protein in fetal lamb parathyroid glands and sheep placenta: Comparison with a similar protein implicated in humoral hypercalcemia of malignancy, J Endocrinol 117:261–271, 1988.

328. Care A, Caple I, Abbas S, et al: The effect of fetal thyroparathyroidectomy on the transport of calcium across the ovine placenta to the fetus, Placenta 4:271–277, 1986.

329. Abbas SK, Pickard DW, Rodda CP, et al: Stimulation of ovine placental calcium transport by purified natural and recombinant parathyroid hormone-related protein (PTHrP) preparations, Q J Exp Physiol 74:549–552, 1989.

330. Garner S, Boass A, SU T: Parathyroid hormone is not required for normal milk composition or secretion or lactation-associated bone loss in normocalcemic rats, J Bone Miner Res 5, 1990.

331. Halloran B, DeLuca H: Calcium transport in small intestine during pregnancy and lactation, Am J Physiol 239:E64–E68, 1980.

332. Ratcliffe WA, Thompson GE, Care AD, et al: Production of parathyroid hormone-related protein by the mammary gland of the goat, J Endocrinol 133:87–93, 1980.

333. Yamamoto M, Duong LT, Fisher JE, et al: Suckling-mediated increases in urinary phosphate and 3′,5′-cyclic adenosine monophosphate excretion in lactating rats: possible systemic effect of parathyroid hormone-related protein, Endocrinology 129:2614–2622, 1991.

334. Grill V, Hillary J, Ho PMW, et al: Parathyroid hormone-related protein: a possible endocrine function in lactation, Clin Endocrinol 37:405–410, 1992.

335. Dobnig H, Kainer F, Stepan V, et al: Elevated parathyroid hormone-related peptide levels after human gestation: relationship to changes in bone and mineral metabolism, J Clin Endocrinol Metab 80:3699–3707, 1995.

336. Kovacs C, Chik C: Hyperprolactinemia caused by lactation and pituitary adenomas is associated with altered serum calcium, phosphate, parathyroid hormone (PTH), and PTH-related peptide levels, J Clin Endocrinol Metab 80:3036–3042, 1995.

337. Sowers M, Hollis B, Shapiro B, et al: Elevated parathyroid hormone-related peptide associated with lactation and bone density loss, J Am Med Assoc 276:549–554, 1996.

338. VanHouten JN, Dann P, Stewart AF, et al: Mammary-specific deletion of parathyroid hormone-related protein preserves bone mass during lactation, J Clin Invest 112:1429–1436, 2003.

339. Cross N, Hillman L, Allen S, et al: Calcium homeostasis and bone metabolism during pregnancy, lactation, and postweaning: a longitudinal study, Am J Clin Nutr 61:514–523, 1995.

340. Reid I, Wattie D, Evans M, et al: Post-pregnancy osteoporosis associated with hypercalcaemia, Clin Endocrinol (Oxf) 37:298–303, 1992.

341. Khosla S, van Heerden JA, Gharib H, et al: Parathyroid hormone-related protein and hypercalcemia secondary to massive mammary hyperplasia, N Engl J Med 322:1157, 1990.

342. Hens JR, Dann P, Zhang JP, et al: Bmp4 and pthrp interact to stimulate ductal outgrowth during embryonic mammary development and to inhibit hair follicle induction, Development 134:1221–1230, 2007.

343. Wysolmerski J, Philbrick W, Dunbar M, et al: Rescue of the parathyroid hormone-related protein knockout mouse demonstrates that parathyroid hormone-related protein is essential for mammary gland development, Development 125:1285–1294, 1998.

344. Guise TA, Yin JJ, Taylor SD, et al: Evidence for a causal role of parathyroid hormone-related protein in the pathogenesis of human breast cancer-mediated osteolysis, J Clin Invest 98:1544–1549, 1996.

345. Amizuka N, Warshawsky H, Henderson JE, et al: Parathyroid hormone-related peptide-depleted mice show abnormal epiphyseal cartilage development and altered endochondral bone formation, J Cell Biol 126:1611–1623, 1994.

346. Lee K, Lanske B, Karaplis AC, et al: Parathyroid hormone-related peptide delays terminal differentiation of chondrocytes during endochondral bone development, Endocrinology 137:5109–5118, 1996.

347. Schipani E, Lanske B, Hunzelman J, et al: Targeted expression of constitutively active PTH/PTHrP receptors delays endochondral bone formation and rescues PTHrP-less mice, Proc Natl Acad Sci U S A 94:13689–13694, 1997.

348. Philbrick WM, Dreyer BE, Nakchbandi IA, et al: Parathyroid hormone-related protein is required for tooth eruption, Proc Natl Acad Sci U S A 95:11846–11851, 1998.

349. Calvi LM, Shin HI, Knight MC, et al: Constitutively active PTH/PTHrP receptor in odontoblasts alters odontoblast and ameloblast function and maturation, Mech Dev 121:397–408, 2004.

350. Jobert AS, Zhang P, Couvineau A, et al: Absence of functional receptors parathyroid hormone and parathyroid hormone-related peptide in Blomstrand chondrodysplasia, J Clin Invest 102:34–40, 1998.

351. Zhang P, Jobert AS, Couvineau A, et al: A homozygous inactivating mutation in the parathyroid hormone/parathyroid hormone-related peptide receptor causing Blomstrand chondrodysplasia, J Clin Endocrinol Metab 83:3365–3368, 1998.

352. Karaplis AC, Bin He MT, Nguyen A, et al: Inactivating mutation in the human parathyroid hormone receptor type 1 gene in Blomstrand chondrodysplasia, Endocrinology 139:5255–5258, 1998.

353. Karperien MC, van der Harten HJ, van Schooten R, et al: A frame-shift mutation in the type I parathyroid hormone/parathyroid hormone-related peptide receptor causing Blomstrand lethal osteochondrodysplasia, J Clin Endocrinol Metab 84:3713–3720, 1999.

354. Schipani E, Kruse K, Jüppner H: A constitutively active mutant PTH-PTHrP receptor in Jansen-type metaphyseal chondrodysplasia, Science 268:98–100, 1995.

355. Schipani E, Langman CB, Parfitt AM, et al: Constitutively activated receptors for parathyroid hormone and parathyroid hormone-related peptide in Jansen's metaphyseal chondrodysplasia, New Engl J Med 335:708–714, 1996.

356. Minagawa M, Arakawa K, Minamitani K, et al: Jansen-type metaphyseal chondrodysplasia: analysis of PTH/PTH-related protein receptor messenger RNA by the

reverse transcription-polymerase chain method, Endocr J 44:493–499, 1997.
357. Schipani E, Langman CB, Hunzelman J, et al: A novel PTH/PTHrP receptor mutation in Jansen's metaphyseal chondrodysplasia, J Clin Endocrinol Metab 84:3052–3057, 1999.
358. Bitgood MJ, McMahon AP: Hedgehog and bmp genes are coexpressed at many diverse sites of cell-cell interaction in the mouse embryo, Dev Biol 172:126–138, 1995.
359. Stone DM, Hynes M, Armanini M, et al: The tumour-suppressor gene *Patched* encodes a candidate receptor for sonic hedgehog, Nature 384:129–134, 1996.
360. Marigo V, Davey RA, Zuo Y, et al: Biochemical evidence that Patched is the hedgehog receptor, Nature 384:176–179, 1996.
361. Suda N, Gillespie MT, Traianedes K, et al: Expression of parathyroid hormone-related protein in cells of osteoblast lineage, J Cell Physiol 166:94–104, 1996.
362. Amizuka N, Karaplis AC, Henderson JE, et al: Haplo-insufficiency of parathyroid hormone-related peptide (PTHrP) results in abnormal post-natal bone development, Dev Biol 175:166–176, 1996.
363. Philbrick WM, Wysolmerski JJ, Galbraith S, et al: Defining the roles of parathyroid hormone-related protein in normal physiology, Physiol Rev 76:127–173, 1996.
364. Wysolmerski JJ, Broadus AE, Zhou J, et al: Overexpression of parathyroid hormone-related protein in the skin of transgenic mice interferes with hair follicle development, Proc Natl Acad Sci U S A 91:1133–1137, 1994.
365. Qian J, Lorenz J, Maeda S, et al: Reduced blood pressure and increased sensitivity of the vasculature to parathyroid hormone-related protein (PTHrP) in transgenic mice overexpressing the PTH/PTHrP receptor in vascular smooth muscle, Endocrinology 140:1826–1833, 1999.
366. Maeda S, Sutliff R, Qian J, et al: Targeted overexpression of parathyroid hormone-related protein (PTHrP) to vascular smooth muscle in transgenic mice lowers blood pressure and alters vascular contractility, Endocrinology 140:1815–1825, 1999.
367. Thiede MA, Daifotis AG, Weir EC, et al: Intrauterine occupancy controls expression of the parathyroid hormone-related peptide gene in preterm rat myometrium Proc Natl Acad Sci U S A 87:6969–6973, 1990.
368. Jüppner H: Molecular cloning and characterization of a parathyroid hormone (PTH)/PTH-related peptide (PTHrP) receptor: a member of an ancient family of G protein-coupled receptors, Curr Opin Nephrol Hypertens 3:371–378, 1994.
369. Jüppner H, Schipani E: Receptors for parathyroid hormone and parathyroid hormone-related peptide: from molecular cloning to definition of diseases, Curr Opin Nephrol Hypertens 5:300–306, 1996.
370. Sneddon WB, Yang Y, Ba J, et al: Extracellular signal-regulated kinase activation by parathyroid hormone in distal tubule cells, Am J Physiol Renal Physiol 292:F1028–F1034, 2007.
371. Syme CA, Friedman PA, Bisello A: Parathyroid hormone receptor trafficking contributes to the activation of extracellular signal-regulated kinases but is not required for regulation of camp signaling, J Biol Chem 280:11281–11288, 2005.
372. Rey A, Manen D, Rizzoli R, et al: Proline-rich motifs in the parathyroid hormone (pth)/pth-related protein receptor c terminus mediate scaffolding of c-src with beta-arrestin2 for erk1/2 activation, J Biol Chem 281:38181–38188, 2006.
373. Singh AT, Gilchrist A, Voyno-Yasenetskaya T, et al: Gα12/gα13 subunits of heterotrimeric G proteins mediate parathyroid hormone activation of phospholipase d in umr-106 osteoblastic cells, Endocrinology 140:1826–1833, 2005.
374. Shigeno C, Yamamoto I, Kitamura N, et al: Interaction of human parathyroid hormone-related peptide with parathyroid hormone receptors in clonal rat osteosarcoma cells, J Biol Chem 34:18369–18377, 1988.
375. Nissenson RA, Diep D, Strewler GJ: Synthetic peptides comprising the amino-terminal sequence of a parathyroid hormone-like protein from human malignancies: binding to parathyroid hormone receptors and activation of adenylate cyclase in bone cells and kidney, J Biol Chem 263:12866–12871, 1988.
376. Orloff JJ, Wu TL, Heath HW, et al: Characterization of canine renal receptors for the parathyroid hormone-like protein associated with humoral hypercalcemia of malignancy, J Biol Chem 264:6097–6103, 1989.
377. Usdin TB, Gruber C, Bonner TI: Identification and functional expression of a receptor selectively recognizing parathyroid hormone, the pth2 receptor, J Biol Chem 270:15455–15458, 1995.
378. Hoare S, Usdin T: Molecular mechanisms of ligand-recognition by parathyroid hormone 1 (pth1) and pth2 receptors, Curr Pharm Des 7:689–713, 2001.
379. Behar V, Nakamoto C, Greenberg Z, et al: Histidine at position 5 is the specificity "switch" between two parathyroid hormone receptor subtypes, Endocrinology 137:4217–4224, 1996.
380. Gardella TJ, Luck MD, Jensen GS, et al: Converting parathyroid hormone-related peptide (PTHrP) into a potent PTH-2 receptor agonist, J Biol Chem 271:19888–19893, 1996.
381. Hoare SR, Bonner TI, Usdin TB: Comparison of rat and human parathyroid hormone 2 (pth2) receptor activation: PTH is a low potency partial agonist at the rat PTH2 receptor, Endocrinology 140:4419–4425, 1999.
382. Goold C, Usdin T, Hoare S: Regions in rat and human parathyroid hormone (pth) 2 receptors controlling receptor interaction with PTH and with antagonist ligands, J Pharmacol Exp Ther 299:678–690, 2001.
383. Usdin TB, Hoare SRJ, Wang T, et al: Tip39: a new neuropeptide and PTH2-receptor agonist from hypothalamus, Nature Neurosci 2:941–943, 1999.
384. Piserchio A, Usdin T, Mierke D: Structure of tuberoinfundibular peptide (tip39), J Biol Chem 275:27284–27290, 2000.
385. Hoare S, Usdin T: Tuberoinfundibular peptide (7 39) [tip(7 39)], a novel, selective, high affinity antagonist for the parathyroid hormone 1 receptor with no detectable agonist activity, J Pharmacol Exp Ther 295:761–770, 2000.
386. Jonsson K, John M, Gensure R, et al: Tuberoinfundibular peptide 39 binds to the parathyroid hormone (PTH)/PTH related peptide receptor, but functions as an antagonist, Endocrinology 142:704–709, 2001.
387. Hoare S, Usdin T: Specificity and stability of a new PTH1 receptor antagonist, mouse tip(7–39), Peptides 23:989–998, 2002.
388. Usdin T: The PTH2 receptor and tip39: a new peptide-receptor system, Trends Pharmacol Sci 4:128–130, 2000.
389. Usdin TB, Paciga M, Riordan T, et al: Tuberoinfundibular peptide of 39 residues is required for germ cell development, Endocrinology 149:4292–4300, 2008.
390. Rubin DA, Jüppner H: Zebrafish express the common parathyroid hormone/parathyroid hormone-related peptide (PTH1R) and a novel receptor (PTH3R) that is preferentially activated by mammalian and fugufish parathyroid hormone-related peptide, J Biol Chem 84:28185–28190, 1999.
391. Schneider H, Feyen JHM, Seuwen K, et al: Cloning and functional expression of a human parathyroid hormone (parathormone)/parathormone-related peptide receptor, Eur J Pharmacol 246:149–155, 1993.
392. Eggenberger M, Flühmann B, Muff R, et al: Structure of a parathyroid hormone/parathyroid hormone-related peptide receptor of the human cerebellum and functional expression in human neuroblastoma sk-n-mc cells, Brain Res Mol Brain Res 36:127–136, 1997.
393. Karperien M, van Dijk TB, Hoeijmakers T, et al: Expression pattern of parathyroid hormone/parathyroid hormone related peptide receptor mRNA in mouse postimplantation embryos indicates involvement in multiple developmental processes, Mech Dev 47:29–42, 1994.
394. Pausova Z, Bourdon J, Clayton D, et al: Cloning of a parathyroid hormone/parathyroid hormone-related peptide receptor (PTHR) cDNA from a rat osteosarcoma (umr106) cell line: chromosomal assignment of the gene in the human, mouse, and rat genomes, Genomics 20:20–26, 1994.
395. Smith DP, Zang XY, Frolik CA, et al: Structure and functional expression of a complementary DNA for porcine parathyroid hormone/parathyroid hormone-related peptide receptor, Biochim Biophys Acta 1307:339–347, 1996.
396. Smock S, Vogt G, Castleberry T, et al: Molecular cloning and functional characterization of the canine parathyroid hormone receptor 1 (PTH1), J Bone Miner Res 14(suppl. 1):S288, 1999.
397. Bergwitz C, Klein P, Kohno H, et al: Identification, functional characterization, and developmental expression of two nonallelic parathyroid hormone (PTH)/PTH-related peptide (PTHrP) receptor isoforms in *Xenopus laevis* (daudin) Endocrinology 139:723–732, 1998.
398. Rubin DA, Hellman P, Zon LI, et al: A G protein-coupled receptor from zebrafish is activated by human parathyroid hormone and not by human or teleost parathyroid hormone-related peptide: implications for the evolutionary conservation of calcium-regulating peptide hormones, J Biol Chem 274:23035–23042, 1999.
399. Tian J, Smorgorzewski M, Kedes L, et al: Parathyroid hormone-parathyroid hormone related protein receptor messenger RNA is present in many tissues besides the kidney, Am J Nephrol 13:210–213, 1993.
400. Urena P, Kong XF, Abou-Samra AB, et al: Parathyroid hormone (PTH)/PTH-related peptide (PTHrP) receptor mRNA are widely distributed in rat tissues, Endocrinology 133:617–623, 1993.
401. McKee RL, Goldman ME, Caulfield MP, et al: The 7–34 fragment of human hypercalcemia factor is a partial agonist/antagonist for parathyroid hormone-stimulated camp production Endocrinology 122:3008–3010, 1988.
402. Chorev M, Goodman ME, McKee RL, et al: Modifications of position 12 in parathyroid hormone and parathyroid hormone related protein: toward the design of highly potent antagonists, Biochemistry 29:1580–1586, 1990.
403. Chorev M, Roubini E, Goodman ME, et al: Effects of hydrophobic substitutions at position 18 on the potency of parathyroid hormone antagonists, Int J Pept Protein Res 36:465–470, 1990.
404. Yamaguchi DT, Hahn TJ, Iida-Klein A, et al: Parathyroid hormone-activated calcium channels in an osteoblast-like clonal osteosarcoma cell line. cAMP-dependent and cAMP-independent calcium channels, J Biol Chem 262:7711–7718, 1987.
405. Yamaguchi DT, Kleeman CR, Muallem S: Protein kinase C-activated calcium channel in the osteoblast-like clonal osteosarcoma cell line umr-106, J Biol Chem 262:14967–14973, 1987.
406. Schipani E, Weinstein LS, Bergwitz C, et al: Pseudohypoparathyroidism type IB is not caused by mutations in the coding exons of the human parathyroid hormone (PTH)/PTH-related peptide receptor gene, J Clin Endocrinol Metab 80:1611–1621, 1995.
407. Bettoun JD, Minagawa M, Kwan MY, et al: Cloning and characterization of the promoter regions of the human parathyroid hormone (PTH)/PTH-related peptide receptor gene: analysis of deoxyribonucleic acid from normal subjects and patients with pseudohypoparathyroidism type IB, J Clin Endocrinol Metab 82:1031–1040, 1997.
408. Manen D, Palmer G, Bonjour J, et al: Sequence and activity of parathyroid hormone/parathyroid hormone-related protein receptor promoter region in human osteoblast-like cells, Gene 218:49–56, 1998.
409. McCuaig KA, Clarke JC, White JH: Molecular cloning of the gene encoding the mouse parathyroid hormone/parathyroid hormone-related peptide receptor, Proc Natl Acad Sci U S A 91:5051–5055, 1994.
410. Kong XF, Schipani E, Lanske B, et al: The rat, mouse and human genes encoding the receptor for parathyroid hormone and parathyroid hormone-related peptide are highly homologous, Biochem Biophys Res Comm 200:1290–1299, 1994.
411. McCuaig KA, Lee H, Clarke JC, et al: Parathyoid hormone/parathyroid hormone related peptide receptor gene transcripts are expressed from tissue-specific and ubiquitous promoters, Nucleic Acids Res 23:1948–1955, 1995.
412. Joun H, Lanske B, Karperien M, et al: Tissue-specific transcription start sites and alternative splicing of the parathyroid hormone (PTH)/PTH-related peptide (PTHrP) receptor gene: a new PTH/PTHrP receptor splice variant that lacks the signal peptide, Endocrinology 138:1742–1749, 1997.
413. Bettoun JD, Minagawa M, Hendy GN, et al: Developmental upregulation of the human parathyroid hormone (PTH)/PTH-related peptide receptor gene

expression from conserved and human-specific promoters, J Clin Invest 102:958–967, 1998.
414. Giannoukos G, Williams L, Chilco P, et al: Characterization of an element within the rat parathyroid hormone/parathyroid hormone-related peptide receptor gene promoter that enhances expression in osteoblastic osteosarcoma 17/2.8 cells, Biochem Biophys Res Commun 258:336–340, 1999.
415. Qi LJ, Leung A, Xiong Y, et al: Extracellular cysteines of the corticotropin-releasing factor receptor are critical for ligand interaction, Biochemistry 36:12442–12448, 1997.
416. Lee C, Gardella TJ, Abou-Samra AB, et al: Role of the extracellular regions of the parathyroid hormone (PTH)/PTH-related peptide receptor in hormone binding, Endocrinology 135:1488–1495, 1994.
417. Jüppner H, Schipani E, Bringhurst FR, et al: The extracellular, amino-terminal region of the parathyroid hormone (PTH)/PTH-related peptide (PTHrP) receptor determines the binding affinity for carboxyl-terminal fragments of PTH(1–34), Endocrinology 134:879–884, 1994.
418. Castro M, Nikolaev VO, Palm D, et al: Turn-on switch in parathyroid hormone receptor by a two-step parathyroid hormone binding mechanism, Proc Natl Acad Sci U S A 102:16084–16089, 2005.
419. Cardoso JC, Pinto VC, Vieira FA, et al: Evolution of secretin family gpcr members in the metazoa, BMC Evol Biol 6:108, 2006.
420. Ishihara T, Nakamura S, Kaziro Y, et al: Molecular cloning and expression of a cDNA encoding the secretin receptor, EMBO J 10:1635–1641, 1991.
421. Lin HY, Harris TL, Flannery MS, et al: Expression cloning of an adenylate cyclase-coupled calcitonin receptor Science 254:1022–1024, 1991.
422. Fredriksson R, Schioth HB: The repertoire of g-protein-coupled receptors in fully sequenced genomes, Mol Pharmacol 67:1414–1425, 2005.
423. Kolakowski LFJ: Gcrdb: A G-protein-coupled receptor database, Receptors Channels 2:1–7, 1994.
424. Fredriksson R, Lagerstrom MC, Schioth HB: Expansion of the superfamily of G-protein-coupled receptors in chordates, Ann N Y Acad Sci 1040:89–94, 2005.
425. Kamesh N, Aradhyam GK, Manoj N: The repertoire of G protein-coupled receptors in the sea squirt *Ciona intestinalis*, BMC Evol Biol 8:129, 2008.
426. Pioszak AA, Parker NR, Suino-Powell K, et al: Molecular recognition of corticotropin-releasing factor by its G-protein-coupled receptor crfr1, J Biol Chem 283:32900–32912, 2008.
427. Grace CR, Perrin MH, Gulyas J, et al: Structure of the N-terminal domain of a type B1 G protein-coupled receptor in complex with a peptide ligand, Proc Natl Acad Sci U S A 104:4858–4863, 2007.
428. Sun C, Song D, Davis-Taber RA, et al: Solution structure and mutational analysis of pituitary adenylate cyclase-activating polypeptide binding to the extracellular domain of pac1-rs, Proc Natl Acad Sci U S A 104:7875–7880, 2007.
429. Carter P, Shimizu M, Luck M, et al: The hydrophobic residues phenylalanine 184 and leucine 187 in the type-1 parathyroid hormone (PTH) receptor functionally interact with the amino-terminal portion of PTH-(1–34), J Biol Chem 274:31955–31960, 1999.
430. Lee C, Luck MD, Jüppner H, et al: Kronenberg HM, Gardella TJ: Homolog-scanning mutagenesis of the parathyroid hormone (PTH) receptor reveals PTH-(1–34) binding determinants in the third extracellular loop, Mol Endocrinol 9:1269–1278, 1995.
431. Turner PR, Bambino T, Nissenson RA: A putative selectivity filter in the G-protein-coupled receptors for parathyroid hormone and secretin, J Biol Chem 271:9205–9208, 1996.
432. Turner PR, Bambino T, Nissenson RA: Mutations of neighboring polar residues on the second transmembrane helix disrupt signaling by the parathyroid hormone receptor, Mol Endocrinol 10:132–139, 1996.
433. Bergwitz C, Jusseaume SA, Luck MD, et al: Residues in the membrane-spanning and extracellular regions of the parathyroid hormone (PTH)-2 receptor determine signaling selectivity for PTH and PTH-related peptide, J Biol Chem 272:28861–28868, 1997.
434. Mannstadt M, Luck M, Gardella TJ, et al: Evidence for a ligand interaction site at the amino-terminus of the parathyroid hormone (PTH)/PTH-related protein receptor from cross-linking and mutational studies, J Biol Chem 273:16890–16896, 1998.
435. Bisello A, Adams AE, Mierke DF, et al: Parathyroid hormone-receptor interactions identified directly by photo cross-linking and molecular modeling studies, J Biol Chem 273:22498–22505, 1998.
436. Gensure R, Gardella T, Juppner H: Multiple sites of contact between the carboxyl terminal binding domain of PTHrP(1–36) analogs and the amino terminal extracellular domain of the PTH/PTHrP receptor identified by photoaffinity cross linking, J Biol Chem 276:28650–28658, 2001.
437. Greenberg Z, Bisello A, Mierke D, et al: Mapping the bimolecular interface of the parathyroid hormone (PTH) PTH1 receptor complex: spatial proximity between lys(27) (of the hormone principal binding domain) and leu(261) (of the first extracellular loop) of the human PTH1 receptor, Biochemistry 39:8142–8152, 2000.
438. Adams A, Bisello A, Chorev M, et al: Arginine 186 in the extracellular n-terminal region of the human parathyroid hormone 1 receptor is essential for contact with position 13 of the hormone, Mol Endocrinol 12:1673–1683, 1998.
439. Hoare S, Gardella T, Usdin T: Evaluating the signal transduction mechanism of the parathyroid hormone 1 receptor: effect of receptor-G-protein interaction on the ligand binding mechanism and receptor conformation, J Biol Chem 276:7741–7753, 2001.
440. Bergwitz C, Gardella TJ, Flannery MR, et al: Full activation of chimeric receptors by hybrids between parathyroid hormone and calcitonin, J Biol Chem 271: 26469–26472, 1996.
441. Gensure RC, Gardella TJ, Juppner H: Parathyroid hormone and parathyroid hormone-related peptide, and their receptors, Biochem Biophys Res Commun 328:666–678, 2005.
442. Wittelsberger A, Corich M, Thomas BE, et al: The mid-region of parathyroid hormone (1–34) serves as a functional docking domain in receptor activation, Biochemistry 45:2027–2034, 2006.
443. Nussbaum SR, Rosenblatt M, Potts JT Jr: Parathyroid hormone/renal receptor interactions: demonstration of two receptor-binding domains, J Biol Chem 255:10183–10187, 1980.
444. Rosenblatt M, Segre GV, Tyler GA, et al: Identification of a receptor-binding region in parathyroid hormone, Endocrinology 107:545–550, 1980.
445. Dong M, Lam PC, Pinon DI, et al: Spatial approximation between secretin residue five and the third extracellular loop of its receptor provides new insight into the molecular basis of natural agonist binding, Mol Pharmacol 74:413–422, 2008.
446. Fortin JP, Zhu Y, Choi C, et al: Membrane-tethered ligands are effective probes for exploring class b1 G protein-coupled receptor function, Proc Natl Acad Sci U S A 106:8049–8054, 2009.
447. Gardella TJ, Axelrod D, Rubin D, et al: Mutational analysis of the receptor-activating region of human parathyroid hormone, J Biol Chem 266:13141–13146, 1991.
448. Behar V, Bisello A, Bitan B, et al: Photoaffinity cross-linking identifies differences in the interactions of an agonist and an antagonist with the parathyroid hormone/parathyroid hormone-related protein receptor, J Biol Chem 275:9–17, 1999.
449. Gensure R, Carter P, Petroni B, et al: Identification of determinants of inverse agonism in a constitutively active parathyroid hormone/parathyroid hormone related peptide receptor by photoaffinity cross linking and mutational analysis, J Biol Chem 276:42692–42699, 2001.
450. Gardella TJ, Jüppner H, Wilson AK, et al: Determinants of [arg2]PTH-(1–34) binding and signaling in the transmembrane region of the parathyroid hormone receptor, Endocrinology 135:1186–1194, 1994.
451. Gensure R, Shimizu N, Tsang J, et al: Identification of a contact site for residue 19 ofparathyroid hormone (PTH) and PTH-related protein analogs in transmembrane domain two of the type 1 PTH receptor, Molecular Endocrinology, 2003. In Press.
452. Monticelli L, Mammi S, Mierke D: Molecular characterization of a ligand tethered parathyroid hormone receptor, Biophys Chem 95:165–172, 2002.
453. Vilardaga JP, Bunemann M, Krasel C, et al: Measurement of the millisecond activation switch of G protein-coupled receptors in living cells, Nat Biotechnol 21:807–812, 2003.
454. Piserchio A, Shimizu N, Gardella T, et al: Residue 19 of parathyroid hormone: structural consequences, Biochemistry 41:13217–13223, 2002.
455. Carter PH, Liu RQ, Foster WR, et al: Discovery of a small molecule antagonist of the parathyroid hormone receptor by using an N-terminal parathyroid hormone peptide probe, Proc Natl Acad Sci U S A 104:6846–6851, 2007.
456. Gardella TJ: Mimetic ligands for the pthr1: Approaches developments, and considerations IBMS BoneKEy on line. 6(2):71–85, 2009 February.
457. Dean T, Linglart A, Mahon MJ, et al: Mechanisms of ligand binding to the PTH/PTHrP receptor: selectivity of a modified pth(1–15) radioligand for gαs-coupled receptor conformations, Mol Endocrinol 20:931–942, 2006.
458. Hoare SR, Sullivan SK, Pahuja A, et al: Conformational states of the corticotropin releasing factor 1 (crf1) receptor: detection, and pharmacological evaluation by peptide ligands, Peptides 24:1881–1897, 2003.
459. Dean T, Vilardaga JP, Potts JT Jr, et al: Altered selectivity of parathyroid hormone (PTH) and PTH-related protein (PTHrP) for distinct conformations of the PTH/PTHrP receptor, Mol Endocrinol 22:156–166, 2008.
460. Horwitz MJ, Tedesco MB, Sereika SM, et al: Continuous PTH and PTHrP infusion causes suppression of bone formation and discordant effects on $1,25(OH)_2$ vitamin D, J Bone Miner Res 20:1792–1803, 2005.
461. Okazaki M, Ferrandon S, Vilardaga JP, et al: Prolonged signaling at the parathyroid hormone receptor by peptide ligands targeted to a specific receptor conformation, Proc Natl Acad Sci U S A 105:16525–16530, 2008.
462. Calvi L, Schipani E: The PTH/PTHrP receptor in Jansen's metaphyseal chondrodysplasia, J Endocrinol Invest 23:545–554, 2000.
463. Kenakin T: Functional selectivity through protean and biased agonism: who steers the ship? Mol Pharmacol 72:1393–1401, 2007.
464. Ferrandon S, Potts JT Jr, Gardella TJ, et al: Sustained cyclic amp production by parathyroid hormone receptor endocytosis, Nat Chem Biol 5:734–742, 2009.
465. Tawfeek HA, Abou-Samra AB: Important role for the V-type $H^{(+)}$-ATPase and the Golgi apparatus in the recycling of PTH/PTHrP receptor, Am J Physiol Endocrinol Metab 286:E704–E710, 2004.
466. Tawfeek HA, Qian F, Abou-Samra AB: Phosphorylation of the receptor for PTH and PTHrP is required for internalization and regulates receptor signaling, Mol Endocrinol 16:1–13, 2002.
467. Ferrari S, Bisello A: Cellular distribution of constitutively active mutant parathyroid hormone (PTH)/PTH related protein receptors and regulation of cyclic adenosine 3′,5′ monophosphate signaling by beta arrestin-2, Mol Endocrinol 15:149–163, 2001.
468. Vilardaga J, Frank M, Krasel C, et al: Differential conformational requirements for activation of g proteins and regulatory proteins, arrestin and grk in the G protein coupled receptor for parathyroid hormone (PTH)/PTH related protein, J Biol Chem 31:31, 2001.
469. Canalis E, Giustina A, Bilezikian JP: Mechanisms of anabolic therapies for osteoporosis, N Engl J Med 357:905–916, 2007.
470. Winer KK, Sinaii N, Peterson D, et al: Effects of once versus twice-daily parathyroid hormone 1–34 therapy in children with hypoparathyroidism, J Clin Endocrinol Metab 93:3389–3395, 2008.
471. Schlüter K-D, Hellstern H, Wingender E, et al: The central part of parathyroid hormone stimulates thymidine incorporation of chondrocytes, J Biol Chem 264:11087–11092, 1989.
472. Neugebauer W, Surewicz WK, Gordon HL, et al: Structural elements of human parathyroid hormone and their possible relation to biological activities, Biochemistry 31:2056–2063, 1992.
473. Rixon RH, Whitfield JF, Gagnon L, et al: Parathyroid hormone fragments may stimulate bone growth in ovariectomized rats by activating adenylyl cyclase, J Bone Miner Res 9:1179–1189, 1994.
474. Erdmann S, Muller W, Bahrami S, et al: Differential effects of parathyroid hormone fragments on collagen gene expression in chondrocytes, J Cell Biol 135:1179–1191, 1996.

475. Rao LG, Murray TM, Heersche JNM: Immunohistochemical demonstration of parathyroid hormone binding to specific cell types in fixed rat bone tissue, Endocrinology 113:805–810, 1983.

476. Demay M, Mitchell J, Goltzman D: Comparison of renal and osseous binding of parathyroid hormone and hormonal fragments, Am J Phyisol 249:E437–E446, 1985.

477. Rao LG, Murray TM: Binding of intact parathyroid hormone to rat osteosarcoma cells: major contribution of binding sites for the carboxyl-terminal region of the hormone, Endocrinology 117:1632–1638, 1985.

478. Murray TM, Rao LG, Rizzoli RE: Interaction of parathyroid hormone, parathyroid hormone-related peptide, and their fragments with conventional and nonconventional receptor sites. In Bilzikian JP, Levine MA, Marcus R, editors: The parathyroids. Basic and clinical concepts, New York, 1994, Raven Press.

479. Murray TM, Rao LG, Muzaffar SA, et al: Human parathyroid hormone carboxyterminal peptide (53–84) stimulates alkaline phosphatase activity in dexamethasone-treated rat osteosarcoma cells in vitro, Endocrinology 124:1097–1099, 1989.

480. Murray TM, Rao LG, Muzaffar SA: Dexamethasone-treated ros 17/2.8 rat osteosarcoma cells are responsive to human carboxylterminal parathyroid hormone peptide hpth(53–84): stimulation of alkaline phosphatase, Calcif Tissue Int 49:120–123, 1991.

481. Nakamoto C, Baba H, Fukase M, et al: Individual and combined effects of intact PTH, amino-terminal, and a series of truncated carboxyl-terminal PTH fragments on alkaline phosphatase activity in dexamethasone-treated rat osteoblastic osteosarcoma cells, ros 17/2.8, Acta Endocrinol 128:367–372, 1993.

482. Kaji H, Sugimoto T, Kanatani M, et al: Carboxyl-terminal PTH fragments stimulate osteoclast-like cell formation and osteoclastic activity, Endocrinology 134:1897–1904, 1994.

483. Fukayama S, Schipani E, Jüppner H, et al: Role of protein kinase-a in homologous down-regulation of parathyroid hormone (PTH)/PTH-related peptide receptor messenger ribonucleic acid in human osteoblast-like saos-2 cells, Endocrinology 134:1851–1858, 1994.

484. Guo J, Iida-Klein A, Huang X, et al: Parathyroid hormone (PTH)/PTH-related peptide receptor density modulates activation of phospholipase C and phosphate transport by PTH in llc-pk1 cells, Endocrinology 136:3884–3891, 1995.

485. Guo J, Lanske B, Liu B, et al: A functional carboxyl-terminal PTH receptor regulates growth of conditionally immortalized hypertrophic chondrocytes, J Bone Miner Res 11(suppl. 1):S305, 1996.

486. Sun BH, Mitnick M, Eielson C, et al: Parathyroid hormone increases circulating levels of fibronectin in vivo: modulating effect of overiectomy, Endocrinology 138:3918–3924, 1997.

487. Nasu M, Sugimoto T, Kaji H, et al: Carboxyl-terminal parathyroid hormone fragments stimulate type-1 procollagen and insulin-like growth factor-binding protein-5 mRNA expression in osteoblastic umr-106 cells, Endocr J 45:229–234, 1998.

488. Inomata N, Akiyama M, Kubota N, et al: Characterization of a novel PTH-receptor with specificity for the carboxyl-terminal region of PTH(1–84), Endocrinology 136:4732–4740, 1995.

489. Takasu H, Baba H, Inomata N, et al: The 69–84 amino acid region of the parathyroid hormone molecule is essential for the interaction of the hormone with the binding sites with carboxyl-terminal specificity, Endocrinology 137:5537–5543, 1996.

490. Usatii M, Rousseau L, Demers C, et al: Parathyroid hormone fragments inhibit active hormone and hypocalcemia-induced 1,25(OH)D$_2$ synthesis, Kidney Int 72:1330–1335, 2007.

491. Fukayama S, Tashjian AH, Davis JN: Signaling by N- and C-terminal sequences of parathyroid hormone-related protein in hippocampal neurons, Proc Natl Acad Sci U S A 92:10182–10186, 1995.

492. Orloff JJ, Ganz MB, Ribaudo AE, et al: Analysis of PTHrP binding and signal transduction mechanisms in benign and malignant squamous cells, Am J Physiol 262:E599–E607, 1992.

493. Gaich G, Orloff JJ, Atillasoy EJ, et al: Amino-terminal parathyroid hormone-related protein: specific binding and cytosolic calcium responses in rat insulinoma cells, Endocrinology 132:1402–1409, 1993.

494. Orloff JJ, Kats Y, Urena P, et al: Further evidence for a novel receptor for amino-terminal parathyroid hormone-related protein on keratinocytes and squamous carcinoma cell lines, Endocrinology 136:3016–3023, 1995.

495. Kaji H, Sugimoto T, Kanatani M, et al: Carboxyl-terminal peptides from parathyroid hormone-related protein stimulate osteoclast-like cell formation, Endocrinology 136:842–848, 1995.

496. Yamamoto S, Morimoto I, Yanagihara N, et al: Parathyroid hormone-related peptide-(1–34) [PTHrP-(1–34)] induces vasopressin release from the rat supraoptic nucleus in vitro through a novel receptor distinct from a type I or type II PTH/PTHrP receptor, Endocrinology 138:2066–2072, 1997.

497. Yamamoto S, Morimoto I, Zeki K, et al: Centrally administered parathyroid hormone (PTH)-related protein(1–34) but not PTH(1–34) stimulates arginine-vasopressin secretion and its messenger ribonucleic acid expression in supraoptic nucleus of the conscious rats, Endocrinology 139:383–388, 1998.

498. Zhou A, Assil I, Abou Samra A: Role of asparagine linked oligosaccharides in the function of the rat PTH/PTHrP receptor, Biochemistry 39:6514–6520, 2000.

499. Iida-Klein A, Guo J, Takamura M, et al: Mutations in the second cytoplasmic loop of the rat parathyroid hormone (PTH)/PTH-related peptide receptor result in selective loss of PTH-stimulated phospholipase c activity, J Biol Chem 272:6882–6889, 1997.

500. Huang Z, Chen Y, Pratt S, et al: The n-terminal region of the third intracellular loop of the parathyroid hormone (PTH)/PTH-related peptide receptor is critical for coupling to camp and inositol phosphate/Ca^{2+} signal transduction pathways, J Biol Chem 271:33382–33389, 1996.

501. Malecz N, Bambino T, Bencsik M, et al: Identification of phosphorylation sites in the G protein-coupled receptor for parathyroid hormone. Receptor phosphorylation is not required for agonist-induced internalization, Mol Endocrinol 12:1846–1856, 1998.

502. Qian F, Leung A, Abou-Samra A: Agonist-dependent phosphorylation of the parathyroid hormone/parathyroid hormone-related peptide receptor, Biochemistry 37:6240–6246, 1998.

503. Mahon MJ, Cole JA, Lederer ED, et al: Na$^+$/H$^+$ exchanger-regulatory factor 1 mediates inhibition of phosphate transport by parathyroid hormone and second messengers by acting at multiple sites in opossum kidney cells, Mol Endocrinol 17:2355–2364, 2003.

Chapter 2

CALCITONIN

T. JOHN MARTIN, DAVID M. FINDLAY, and PATRICK M. SEXTON

In the course of experiments seeking a factor that, in addition to parathyroid hormone (PTH), might contribute to the tight control of serum calcium in mammals, Copp and colleagues[1] discovered calcitonin. By perfusing the thyroparathyroid glands of dogs and sheep with high calcium concentrations, they obtained evidence for the secretion of a factor that rapidly lowered the blood calcium; they called this factor calcitonin and suggested that it was produced by the parathyroid gland. Subsequently, calcitonin was found by others to be produced by the thyroid in mammals. After it was noted that parathyroidectomy by cautery in the rat resulted in much greater calcium lowering than that resulting from surgery (Fig. 2-1),[2] it was found that acid extracts of rat thyroid injected into young rats caused a lowering of serum calcium, and the hypocalcemic factor was called *thyrocalcitonin*.[3] MacIntyre and co-workers,[4] using thyroparathyroid perfusions in dogs and goats, also established the thyroidal origin of the hypocalcemic agent. It was by then apparent that calcitonin and thyrocalcitonin were identical. The accepted nomenclature became calcitonin (CT), which described a new hormone of thyroid gland origin that was likely to be important in calcium homeostasis.

Synthesis, Secretion, and Cells of Origin

CT is produced by the C cells of the mammalian thyroid, with its secretion dependent on serum calcium levels.[5] Although the dominant site of production of CT in mammals is the thyroid C cell, the distribution of these cells throughout the thyroid gland varies considerably among mammalian species, and there is evidence that in some animals CT-producing cells might be found in other parts of the neck, including the thymus. In fish and in most birds, CT is produced by the ultimobranchial glands. Whereas in mammalian development the ultimobranchial bodies fuse with the posterior lobes of the developing thyroid to become the C cells, in submammalian vertebrates these bodies remain separate, and the ultimobranchial glands constitute a separate endocrine system. The CTs of ultimobranchial origin are highly potent in their actions upon mammalian targets. The physiologic significance of CT in fish and birds remains uncertain, although it is interesting to note that CT has been reported to suppress osteoclastic activity in the scales of freshwater and seawater teleosts.[6] Although there is little doubt that increased serum calcium is an important secretagogue for CT in normal and malignant C cells, the exact mechanisms by which calcium provokes exocytosis of CT have not been fully elucidated. The same extracellular calcium–sensing receptor that mediates decreased PTH secretion from parathyroid cells[7] is also found in C cells and is likely to represent the primary molecular entity through which C cells detect changes in extracellular calcium and control CT release.

Agents that elevate C cell cyclic adenosine monophosphate (cAMP) may stimulate CT secretion, since cAMP analogues have this effect both in vivo and in vitro. Probably the most important CT secretagogues, apart from calcium, are the gastrointestinal hormones. In the pig, gastrin appears to be an effective physiologic secretagogue, suggesting that CT may have a physiologic role postprandially as a hormone that assists uptake of calcium after a calcium-rich meal by preventing the efflux of calcium from bone into blood.[8] Although there is some evidence for this role in pigs and rats, studies in humans remain to be performed. Other gastrointestinal hormones, including glucagon, cholecystokinin, and secretin, are also capable of promoting CT secretion. The gastrin analogue, pentagastrin, has been used clinically as a provocative test for CT secretion in patients with medullary carcinoma of the thyroid. Other hormones that

influence calcium homeostasis may also directly or indirectly influence CT secretion. 1,25-Dihydroxyvitamin D_3 (1,25[OH]$_2$D$_3$) administration has been reported to increase plasma CT levels; this was suggested to occur via specific thyroid C cell receptors for 1,25(OH)$_2$D$_3$, which modify secretion of CT.[9] Both CT and 1,25(OH)$_2$D$_3$ levels are raised in pregnancy and lactation, leading to the suggestion that CT may act to protect the skeleton in the face of increased calcium demand by the fetus.

Serum and thyroid concentrations of CT increase markedly with age in the rat, in association with substantial increases in thyroid content of CT mRNA.[10] In normal rats subjected to acute calcium stimulation in vivo, thyroid CT mRNA is increased. On current evidence it seems that calcium can stimulate both synthesis and secretion of CT by thyroid C cells.

CT secretion has been studied extensively in patients with medullary carcinoma of the thyroid, who have elevated CT levels (see later). However, circulating CT levels in normal human subjects are very low and their measurement requires sensitive and specific assays. The level of CT in normal human blood appears to be less than 10 pg/mL (3 picomolar). Circulating levels of CT are increased in several pathologic states, such as CT-secreting tumors.[11,12] In addition to the CT monomer (≈3500 Daltons), high molecular weight forms circulate, and elevated levels of these molecules can be useful diagnostically in certain situations, such as acute pancreatitis[13,14] and infection/inflammatory conditions.[15] In fact, it has been reported that ProCT is toxic and that immunoneutralization with immunoglobulin (Ig)G that is reactive to this molecule significantly improves survival in animal models of sepsis.[16]

Chemistry

The CT sequence has been determined for many species, the common features being that it is a 32 amino acid peptide with a carboxyterminal proline amide and a disulfide bridge between cysteine residues at positions 1 and 7.[17] Based on their amino acid sequence homologies, the different CTs (Fig. 2-2) are classified into three groups: (1) *artiodactyl*, which includes porcine, bovine, and ovine; (2) *primate/rodent*, which includes human and rat CT; and (3) *teleost/avian*, which includes salmon, eel, goldfish, and chicken. The common structural features of the CT molecule contribute importantly to biological activity, with the standard assay that has been used since the discovery of CT being one that measures the hypocalcemic response in young rats. Subsequently, receptor-based assays have been used also, and structure/function relationships are largely shared in these

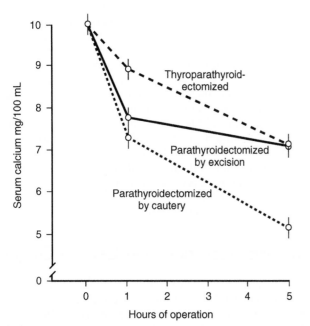

FIGURE 2-1. Comparison of the effects of surgical thyroparathyroidectomy with parathyroidectomy by cautery or surgery in the rat. (Data from Hirsch PF et al, Endocrinology 73:244–251, 1963.)

	1	2	3	4	5	6	7	8	9	10	11	12	13	14	15	16	17	18	19	20	21	22	23	24	25	26	27	28	29	30	31	32	
Salmon CT	C	S	N	L	S	T	C	V	L	G	K	L	S	Q	E	L	H	K	L	Q	T	Y	P	R	T	N	T	G	S	G	T	P	NH$_2$
Eel CT	C	S	N	L	S	T	C	V	L	G	K	L	S	Q	E	L	H	K	L	Q	T	Y	P	R	T	D	V	G	A	G	T	P	NH$_2$
Chicken CT	C	A	S	L	S	T	C	V	L	G	K	L	S	Q	E	L	H	K	L	Q	T	Y	P	R	T	D	V	G	A	G	T	P	NH$_2$
Goldfish CT	C	S	S	L	S	T	C	V	L	G	K	L	S	Q	E	L	H	K	L	Q	T	Y	P	R	T	N	V	G	A	G	T	P	NH$_2$
Stingray CT	C	T	S	L	S	T	C	V	V	G	K	L	S	Q	Q	L	H	K	L	Q	N	I	Q	R	T	D	V	G	A	A	T	P	NH$_2$
Porcine CT	C	S	N	L	S	T	C	V	L	S	A	Y	W	R	N	L	N	N	F	H	R	F	S	G	M	G	F	G	P	E	T	P	NH$_2$
Bovine CT	C	S	N	L	S	T	C	V	L	S	A	Y	W	K	D	L	N	N	Y	H	R	F	S	G	M	G	F	G	P	E	T	P	NH$_2$
Dog CT	C	S	N	L	S	T	C	V	L	G	T	Y	S	K	D	L	N	N	F	H	T	F	S	G	M	G	F	G	A	E	T	P	NH$_2$
Rabbit CT	C	G	N	L	S	T	C	M	L	G	T	Y	T	Q	D	L	N	K	F	H	T	F	P	Q	T	A	I	G	V	V	A	P	NH$_2$
Rat CT	C	G	N	L	S	T	C	M	L	G	T	Y	T	Q	D	L	N	K	F	H	T	F	P	Q	T	S	I	G	V	G	A	P	NH$_2$
Human CT	C	G	N	L	S	T	C	M	L	G	T	Y	T	Q	D	F	N	K	F	H	T	F	P	Q	T	A	I	G	V	G	A	P	NH$_2$

FIGURE 2-2. Alignment of CT sequences from different species. The shaded amino acids indicate identity with salmon CT. All CTs have a disulphide-bridged loop between cysteines (C) at position 1 and 7, a glycine at position 28, and a proline amide at position 32. Amino acids 4, 5, and 6 are also conserved across all species.

various assays. The order of biological potency of the CTs is, in general, teleost≥artiodactyl≥human, although absolute biological activities vary considerably among CT receptors of different species and receptor isoforms within species. Studies of substituted, deleted, and otherwise modified CTs have provided considerable information regarding structure/activity relationships of the CT molecule, showing, for example, that the ring structure serves to stabilize the molecule. The disulfide bridge of the ring can be chemically substituted by an N-N bond, as in aminosuberic eel CT, and this modification yields an extremely stable and fully potent CT variant.[18] The sequence differences among species are concentrated in the middle portion of the molecule, and these differences contribute to the wide variations in biological potencies. However, the outcomes of studies of structural requirements for biological activity have varied with the different biological assays used, and the type of receptor used is able to profoundly influence the results. For example, residues in the carboxyterminal half of salmon CT are more important for binding competition with the two rat receptor isoforms and the human receptor, whereas residues in the aminoterminus are more important for interaction with the porcine receptor.[5]

Calcitonin Gene

As with other hormonal peptides, CT is synthesized as a larger precursor molecule, which is processed by cleavage and amidation before secretion. CT is synthesized as a large molecular weight precursor (136 amino acids), with a leader sequence at the aminoterminus that is cleaved during transport of the molecule into the endoplasmic reticulum. A potentially important posttranslational modification of CT is that of glycosylation. It had been noted that the tripeptide sequence, Asn-Leu-Ser, found within the aminoterminal ring structure of CT is invariate among the CTs of different species. This sequence is an acceptor site for N-linked glycosylation. This, together with evidence for glycosylation of tumor CT, led to detailed studies showing that the CT precursor is indeed a glycoprotein, and that the only N-linked glycosylation site in the entire precursor was within the CT portion itself.[19] The biological significance of CT glycosylation has yet to be determined.

The complete sequences of the cDNA for human, rat, mouse, chicken, sheep, dog,[20] and various species of fish CTs and the DNA sequence of the full human CT gene have been determined.[21-23] These show that the hormone is flanked in the precursor by N- and C-terminal peptides, but the biological significance of these peptides is unknown. The human CT gene has been located in the p14-qter region of chromosome 11.[24]

ALTERNATIVE GENE PRODUCT—CGRP

The CT gene transcript actually encodes a second distinct peptide known as CT gene-related peptide (CGRP), which is produced by tissue-specific alternative splicing of the gene (Fig. 2-3). The mature CGRP and CT mRNAs predict proteins that share sequence identity in the aminoterminal regions, but in the carboxyterminal regions the nucleotide sequences are almost entirely different. The mature, secreted 32 and 37 amino acid CT and CGRP peptides, respectively, result from cleavage of both aminoterminal and carboxyterminal flanking sequences at specific cleavage sites, as depicted in Fig. 2-3.[24] CT mRNA is found largely in the thyroid, and CGRP mRNA is found primarily in the nervous system.[25] However, aberrant expression of CGRP may be seen in medullary thyroid carcinoma.[26] Two

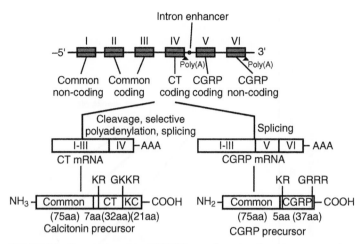

FIGURE 2-3. Organization of the CT/CGRP gene illustrating alternative patterns of processing of the primary transcript and subsequent protein processing. The exons are denoted I through VI in Roman numerals, introns are represented by a single line (not to scale).

different CT/CGRP genes, α and β, have been identified in man and rat.

Processing of the pre-mRNA to the CT mRNA transcript involves usage of exon 4 as a 3′-terminal exon with concomitant polyadenylation at the end of exon 4. Processing to produce the CGRP mRNA involves the exclusion of exon 4 and direct ligation of exon 3 to exon 5, with polyadenylation at the end of exon 6. The hCT/CGRP exon 4, like many differentially incorporated exons, has been characterized as having weak processing signals. Weak differential exons are frequently associated with special enhancer sequences that facilitate exon recognition in the presence of accessory factors that bind to the enhancer. Indeed, such an enhancer, located in the intron downstream of exon 4, has been described for the CT/CGRP gene. In addition, sequences within exon 4 are necessary for the inclusion of exon 4.[27]

Physiology—Bone and Kidney

The physiologic role of CT is not fully understood. It is currently viewed as an inhibitor of bone resorption, whose function is to prevent bone loss at times of stress on skeletal calcium conservation, particularly pregnancy, lactation, and growth. Earlier concepts of CT as a regulator of extracellular fluid calcium are probably relevant only in young and growing animals, in which rapid bone modeling and turnover are required for development of the skeleton. In the rat, for example, which is used for the in vivo assay of CT, the calcium-lowering effect of the hormone is less marked with increasing age of the animal (Fig. 2-4).[28] However, the ability of CT to counteract the effects of a calcium load was shown not to be impaired in older animals, at least in the rat[29]—an observation that has not been explained and that has not been extended to other species.

In normal adult human subjects, even quite large doses of CT have little effect on serum calcium levels. In those subjects in whom bone turnover is increased (e.g., in thyrotoxicosis, Paget's disease), CT treatment acutely inhibits bone resorption and lowers the serum calcium.[30] Given that the acute effect of CT on serum calcium is related to the prevailing rate of bone resorption, it is not surprising that CT has little or no effect on serum calcium in the mature animal or human subject, since the rate of bone resorption is slow in maturity. The physiologic function

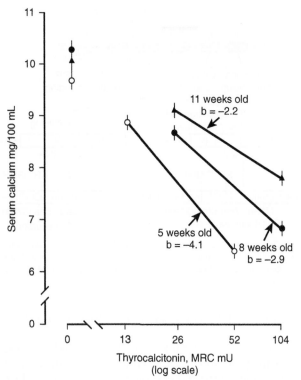

FIGURE 2-4. Decreasing hypocalcemic response to calcitonin with increasing age of the rat. (Data from Cooper CW et al, Endocrinology 81:610–617, 1967.)

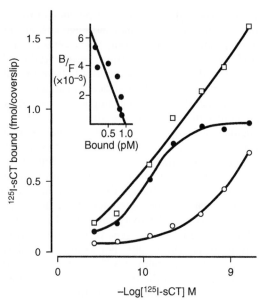

FIGURE 2-5. Saturation analysis of labeled calcitonin binding to rat osteoclasts. Scatchard analysis of specific binding (inset) shows receptor number of 4.8×10^6 per cell. (Data from Nicholson GC et al, J Clin Invest 78:355–360, 1986.)

of CT in maturity nevertheless may be to regulate the bone resorptive process in a continuous or intermittent manner. It follows that CT should not necessarily be regarded as a "calcium-regulating hormone" in maturity, but may yet be shown to be such in stages of rapid growth (e.g., in the young, in states of increased bone turnover). It is nevertheless important that bone resorption be regulated, and CT is the only hormone known to be capable of carrying out this function through a direct action on bone. Physiologic roles for other members of the CT family, such as amylin and CGRP, in the regulation of resorption have not yet been substantiated. An antiresorptive role for CT in maturity might become more important in circumstances in which skeletal integrity is at particular risk (e.g., in pregnancy and lactation). Evidence in support of such an important physiologic role for endogenous CT in protecting against bone loss is provided by experiments showing that cancellous bone loss in thyroparathyroidectomized rats treated with PTH was greater than that in similarly treated sham-operated controls.[31] In addition, mice in which the CT/CGRP gene was ablated showed a severe drop in bone mineral content during lactation, although the maternal skeleton recovered to baseline thereafter.[32,33]

CALCITONIN ACTIONS IN BONE

Osteoclasts

The first evidence of the mechanism of action of CT was obtained by showing in organ culture of bone that CT inhibited bone resorption.[34] Inhibition of resorption appeared to be explained by a direct action on osteoclasts. CT treatment of resorbing bone in vitro resulted in rapid loss of osteoclast ruffled borders and decreased release of lysosomal enzymes. In vivo evidence was also consistent with an inhibitory action upon bone resorption. Loss of ruffled borders in osteoclasts was seen in patients with

Paget's disease, in whom bone biopsies were taken before and 30 minutes after an injection of CT.[35] In the same clinical study, CT was noted to decrease the number of osteoclasts, in addition to altering their ultrastructure. CT infusion in rats led to an immediate reduction in the rate of excretion of hydroxyproline, consistent with inhibition of breakdown of bone collagen.[36] Other studies led to similar conclusions, with no evidence to suggest any increase in the active uptake of calcium by bone.[37]

Studies of the actions of hormones on isolated bone cell populations established that CT acts directly on osteoclasts, with receptor autoradiography showing osteoclasts as the only discernible bone cell targets.[38] Mammalian osteoclasts possess abundant, specific, high-affinity receptors for CT (Fig. 2-5), and CT stimulates cAMP formation in a sensitive and dose-dependent manner,[38] as well as increasing intracellular free calcium levels and protein kinase C activity.[39] As stated, the direct effect of CT upon the osteoclast was found to result in rapid inhibition of activity, reflected in cessation of motility and contraction of the cell. Although isolated osteoclasts remained quiescent in CT as long as the hormone was present, they regained activity when osteoblasts were added to the culture.[40] This escape of osteoclasts from inhibition by CT took place at a rate proportional to the number of osteoblasts with which they were in contact. CT reduced the cytoplasmic spreading of isolated osteoclasts in a dose-dependent manner. PTH had no effect unless osteoblasts were co-cultivated with the osteoclasts, in which case addition of PTH resulted in a marked increase in cytoplasmic spreading of osteoclasts. It cannot be assumed that these phenomena reflect the responses of cells in bone in vivo, but this work provided for the first time some useful direct observations of actions of hormones on isolated bone cell preparations containing osteoclasts. These observations though may be relevant to our interpretation of recent findings in mice rendered null for the CT/CGRP gene and in those haploinsufficient for the CT receptor (vide infra).

The molecular mechanisms by which CT decreases osteoclast function have yet to be fully defined. The rapid effects of the hormone may be brought about through actions on a cytoskeletal function of osteoclasts, after initial events involving generation of several intracellular second messengers. Early events in CT signal transduction have been studied in a variety of cell types and are described in greater detail later. The other means by which CT could inhibit resorption is through inhibition of osteoclast formation. In vivo data and results from CT inhibition of resorption in organ culture are suggestive of this. The development of methods of studying osteoclast formation in vitro from hemopoietic precursor cells has allowed this question to be addressed directly. Several reports have described CT inhibiting osteoclast-like cell formation in bone marrow cultures of human, baboon, and mouse origin.[41-44] However, these experiments were all conducted at relatively high CT concentrations, and the effects were small. In other studies, in which lower concentrations of CT were used, which nevertheless reduced CT receptor mRNA expression in developing mouse osteoclasts, no reduction in osteoclast formation was observed.[45-47] The multinucleated osteoclasts that formed in the continuous presence of exogenous CT had fewer nuclei though, and the osteoclasts generated under these conditions were deficient in CT receptor mRNA and protein but nevertheless capable of resorbing bone. In elegant studies of CT administration to mice, Ikegame et al[48] showed that the CT-induced drop in serum calcium was linked temporally to the loss of osteoclast ruffled borders. Further, frequent dosing of the animals resulted in insensitivity to CT in terms of recovery of osteoclast ruffled borders and return of serum calcium to control levels. It was significant that treatment of mice with CT initially rendered osteoclasts unable to bind ^{125}I-sCT, which recovered after a single treatment but not with repeated treatment.[48] These findings may be relevant to the mechanism of "escape" from CT that is observed clinically.

Osteoblasts

Although the best understood action of CT in bone is as an antiresorptive agent, numerous reports have described actions also on cells of the osteoblast lineage, as well as direct and indirect effects on bone formation. CT increased [^{3}H]thymidine incorporation in embryonic chicken calvariae, in the transformed murine calvarial cell lines MMB and MC-3T3-E1 and in primary cultures of cells prepared from newborn mouse calvaria.[49] CT was also shown to stimulate [^{3}H]thymidine incorporation in primary human osteoblasts[50] and to increase expression of insulin-like growth factors (IGFs) by human SaOS-2 cells.[51] None of these observations has been confirmed, and indeed data failing to show such effects of CT have been published.[52] In addition to the fact that relatively high concentrations of CT were used in these early experiments, results with primary osteoblasts should be interpreted with caution at present, because it is known that calvarial osteoblast preparations are contaminated with osteoclast precursors, and a recent report provides evidence that primary osteoblast preparations contain a substantial proportion of bone-specific macrophages, which have been termed "osteomacs."[53] This raises the possibility that the presumed osteoblast responses may actually be mediated by cells of the monocyte-macrophage lineage. Furthermore, no published evidence is convincing of specific, functional CT receptors in any cells of the osteoblast lineage. Inadequate criteria were used in a claim that ^{125}I-sCT was bound specifically to osteocyte-like cells, MLO-Y4.[54] In the same work, CT at high concentrations was associated with a small increase in cAMP and with protection of the cells from apoptosis induced by etoposide, tumor necrosis factor (TNF)-α or dexamethasone. It has been claimed that CT

can hasten and improve the process of fracture healing in normal[55] and osteoporotic rats.[56] If this proves to be the case, the mechanism could be similar to that of bisphosphonates, which have also been shown to enhance the strength of the healed fracture, apparently by modulating resorption during the remodeling phase of bone repair.[57] It could also relate to possible stimulation of angiogenesis by CT, which has been shown for human microvascular endothelial cells, albeit at supraphysiologic concentrations.[58]

NEW UNDERSTANDING OF THE ROLE OF CALCITONIN IN BONE: STUDIES IN GENETICALLY MANIPULATED MICE

The preceding discussion of the physiology of CT and its action on bone reflects views that have remained largely unaltered over many years, with few new data to change them. The data on which they are based, particularly since normal and low circulating CT levels cannot be measured with confidence (vide supra), do not provide a convincing argument for a specific physiologic role for calcitonin. Indeed, in a recent review, one of the co-discoverers of calcitonin[59] argued the case that calcitonin is not involved in calcium homeostasis or in any other important physiologic function, except possibly in protection of the skeleton under conditions of calcium stress. Some recent work has changed this situation. Ablation of the CT/CGRP gene in mice resulted in viable and fertile mice with no production of CT or CGRPα.[32] As expected, these mice were much less able than wild-type mice to overcome the hypercalcemia induced by a calcium load,[32] and they lost excessive bone during lactation.[33] The great surprise with these mice, however, was that they had increased bone mass, with histomorphometric parameters showing increased bone formation.[32] This suggested that a normal role for calcitonin might be that of an inhibitor of bone formation. The finding was unexpected and counterintuitive, and it was possible that the dual ablation of CT and CGRPα might explain it, although there was no obvious mechanism for this. Indeed, the increased bone formation phenotype was not found when CGRPα-deficient mice were examined,[60] thereby making calcitonin deficiency likely responsible for the increased bone formation. In reviewing the role of calcitonin, Hirsch[59] had considered the results obtained with the CT/CGRP−/− mice but regarded them as inconclusive; as information accumulates, the new physiology of calcitonin is becoming more apparent. The CT/CGRP-deficient mice were protected against ovariectomy-induced bone loss,[32,60] and, it was striking that after the age of 6 months these mice showed severe cortical porosity, even though indices of increased bone formation were maintained.[61,62] Taken together, the observations are indicative of an inhibitory effect of calcitonin on bone formation, most likely an indirect one, and a direct effect on bone resorption through action on the osteoclast.

The significance and importance of these findings were enhanced however with the outcome of the studies of Dacquin et al[63] in mice in which the CT receptor (CTR) was genetically manipulated. CTR−/− mice were embryologically lethal, and this was thought to be due to a placental effect. The CTR+/− mice, however, exhibited a bone phenotype virtually indistinguishable from the CT/CGRP−/− mice, with increased bone mass and increased bone formation on histomorphometry. Thus, the conclusion is that in mice the removal of calcitonin production or action results in an increased amount of bone, implying a physiologic role for calcitonin as a tonic inhibitor of bone formation. The same group prepared mice at least 94% deficient in the CTR and again found evidence of increased indices of bone formation.[64] How the effect on bone formation comes about remains to be determined. The lack of evidence for specific calcitonin receptors and responses in osteoblasts is compelling, so it is very likely that the physiologic roles of calcitonin in bone are brought about through two pathways: a direct effect on osteoclasts to inhibit resorption and an indirect one resulting in the elaboration of a critical, locally active factor that is necessary for bone formation. This could result from signals through receptors in the osteoclast or in the hypothalamus.[62,65] Resolution of this question will be a matter of very great interest, especially in light of ample recent evidence for central regulation of bone metabolism.[66]

RENAL ACTIONS OF CALCITONIN

When infused into thyroparathyroidectomized rats, CT caused a dose-dependent phosphaturia, but the effect on phosphate excretion was only a minor one in comparison with the phosphaturic effect of PTH.[67] Although this was demonstrated in human subjects also, in several species CT failed to have any effect on phosphate excretion. Thus, it seems unlikely that the phosphaturic effect is of any major physiologic significance.

A number of other renal effects of CT, including a transient increase in calcium excretion due probably to inhibition of renal tubular calcium reabsorption, have been noted.[68] Although this has not usually been regarded as an important effect of CT, it has been linked to the calcium-lowering effect of CT in hypercalcemic patients with metastatic bone disease. The use of CT in the treatment of hypercalcemia due to cancer has been based exclusively on the inhibition of osteolysis by CT. Some evidence has been produced that failure of the kidneys to excrete the calcium load derived from bone breakdown is a major contributor to the hypercalcemia. This has prompted careful study of the relative contributions to the hypocalcemic effect of CT of its renal and skeletal components. It was concluded that inhibition of renal tubular reabsorption by CT can induce a rapid fall in serum calcium, and that the magnitude of this effect depends upon the correction of volume depletion, which inevitably accompanies hypercalcemia.[69] Thus, the calciuretic action of CT may assume greater importance than was hitherto suspected.

CT receptors are present in rat kidney,[70] and the action of CT upon adenylate cyclase activity has been localized in the human nephron, predominantly to the medullary and cortical portions of the thick ascending limb and to the early portion of the distal convoluted tubule. The co-localization of the CT receptor mRNA expression and cell surface receptors with G protein–sensitive adenylate cyclase is consistent with cAMP being an important mediator of CT action in this organ. A possible role for CT in the kidney is to regulate $1,25(OH)_2D_3$ levels, with an original observation of enhanced 1-hydroxylation of 25(OH)D in the proximal straight tubule of the kidney by CT stimulation of the expression of 25(OH)D 1α-hydroxylase.[71] Subsequently, Shinki et al[72] showed that CT administration to rats induced renal CYP27B1 when serum calcium levels were normal or high, and this was supported by a report that CT treatment in rats increased renal production of *CYP27B1* mRNA.[73] CT stimulation of the expression of *CYP24* in CTR-transfected HEK-293 cells has also been reported.[74] The authors speculated that, since $1,25(OH)_2D_3$ and CT synergistically stimulate *CYP24* mRNA production in kidney cells, this latter action of CT could be part of the process by which it regulates serum calcium by controlling renal production of $1,25(OH)_2D_3$.

Peptides Related to Calcitonin

The CT peptides are homologous with the related peptides CGRP, amylin, and the adrenomedullins. Greatest identity is between the teleost CTs and amylin ($\approx 33\%$), with $\approx 22\%$ identity with the CGRPs and 16% with adrenomedullin. Less homology is observed between the mammalian CTs and the other peptides. Consistent with the homology between peptides, there is a limited degree of overlap in specificity among the binding sites for the peptide receptors, with CT-like actions seen with high concentrations of amylin and CGRP.

Amylin is a 37 amino acid peptide that is co-secreted with insulin from pancreatic β cells following nutrient ingestion. Amylin at physiologic concentrations is important in the integrated control of nutrient influx with potent actions, including inhibition of gastric emptying, gastric acid secretion, food intake, digestive enzyme secretion, and glucagon secretion.[75] Amylin at higher concentrations also acts to inhibit insulin secretion from the pancreas and to promote glycogen breakdown and to decrease insulin-stimulated incorporation of glucose into glycogen in skeletal muscle. Thus, amylin is thought to act as a partner to insulin in metabolic regulation, although this effect may not occur at normal circulating levels of the peptide.[76] In the kidney, amylin is proposed to have a diverse range of actions, including modulation of Ca^{2+} excretion and thiazide receptor levels, proliferative effects on tubule epithelium, and increasing renin activity.[77,78] Amylin–/– mice have been shown to have less bone as the result of increased bone resorption, and in vitro tests indicated that this may be due to release of an amylin-mediated attenuator of osteoclastogenesis.[63] These authors speculate that the receptor for this effect is independent of the CTR gene, which, with receptor activity modifying proteins (RAMPs), forms the basis of characterized amylin receptor phenotypes (see later). However, their conclusion is based on studies in animals with the amylin–/+, CTR–/+ genotype, and therefore RAMP/CTR-based amylin receptors cannot be excluded as the target for amylin action.

Amylin receptors are also widely expressed in brain, where administered peptide induces many potent effects. These include decreased appetite and gastric acid secretion, hyperthermia, adipsia, and reduction in growth hormone–releasing hormone. Central amylin injection may also modulate memory and the extrapyramidal motor system.[75,77] The molecular basis for amylin receptor phenotype is discussed later.

CGRP is a pleiotropic neuropeptide with a diverse range of actions including potent dilation of vascular beds, as well as relaxation of other smooth muscle, inotropy and chronotropy in the heart, and paracrine regulation of pituitary hormone release, and many central effects, such as suppression of appetite and gastric acid secretion, modulation of body temperature, and modulation of sympathetic outflow. CGRP also acts to modulate nicotinic acetylcholine receptor levels at neuromuscular junctions. CGRP weakly modulates calcium homeostasis, although this is likely to reflect its low affinity for interaction with CTRs. The actions of CGRP have been extensively reviewed elsewhere.[78,79] Specific CGRP receptors have been characterized in many tissues and it is likely that more than one subtype of receptor exists. CGRP receptors arise from hetero-oligomerization of RAMP1 with either the calcitonin receptor-like receptor (CLR) or CTR,[80,81] although weaker interactions are also seen with other RAMP/CLR- or RAMP/CTR-based receptors.[82]

Adrenomedullin was originally isolated from human pheochromocytoma and is abundant in the normal adrenal medulla,

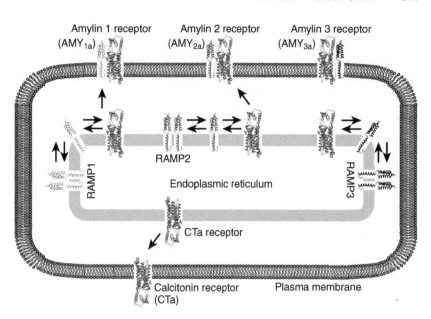

FIGURE 2-6. Representative illustration of complex formation between the calcitonin receptor (CT) and RAMPs 1, 2, and 3 in the endoplasmic reticulum (ER). All three RAMPs are postulated to exist as homodimers in the ER; however, in the presence of CTR an equilibrium is established in which hetero-oligomers between the receptor and each of the RAMPs are formed. To date, the stoichiometry of the oligomers remains unclear. AMY_{1a}, AMY_{2a}, and AMY_{3a} receptors are generated when the CTa receptor isoform is complexed with RAMP 1, 2, and 3, respectively. In addition, although the oligomers between the CT receptor and RAMPs can then be transported to the cell surface, the CT receptor is transported to the cell surface in the absence of RAMPs. The human CT receptor has two major splice variants, CTa and CTb, that arise from the absence or presence of a 16 amino acid insert in intracellular domain 1. The nomenclature for amylin receptors formed by the different receptor isoforms is denoted by (a) or (b) in the name (e.g., AMY_{1a} denotes an amylin receptor formed from the CTa receptor and RAMP 1). It has been hypothesized that RAMPs may reside in a homodimerized form in intracellular sorting compartments such as the endoplasmic reticulum.

hence its name. The full-length peptide of ≈50 amino acids shares approximately 25% homology with CGRP across its N-terminal 37 amino acids.[83] Adrenomedullin is a potent dilator of many vascular beds and is protective against conditions such as cardiac hypertrophy, perivascular fibrosis, renal damage, and pulmonary hypertension.[84,85] Adrenomedullin receptors arise from heterodimers of CLR and RAMP2 or RAMP3.[81] Both adrenomedullin and amylin can stimulate osteoblast proliferation at low concentration.[86] Fig. 2-6 illustrates complex formations between the CTR and RAMPs 1, 2, and 3.

Recently, new peptides related to the CT family of peptides have been identified. The calcitonin receptor–stimulating peptides (CRSPs) were originally isolated/cloned from porcine brain and, being localized principally to brain and pituitary, have been proposed as potential endogenous ligands for central CTRs.[87-89] However, not all CRSPs activate CTRs or related receptors, suggesting that they may also stimulate other receptors.[88] To date, homologous peptides have not been identified in humans or rodents, although bovine and canine homologues do exist.[89] In addition, a second adrenomedullin-like peptide (adrenomedullin 2; also known as intermedin) has been identified in multiple species, including human. This peptide has similar affinity for both CGRP and adrenomedullin receptors, although the physiologic significance of this peptide is still unclear.[82,90,91]

Low levels of hCTI occur in extracts of postmortem human brain. However, in addition to hCTI, low levels of material chromatographically and immunologically similar to sCT (sCTI) have been found, with concentrations in the brain ≈10 times greater than those in serum and cerebrospinal fluid. Similarly, extracts of rat brain diencephalon contain an sCT-like peptide.[93] Although hCTI has been detected in rat brain, only limited evidence has been found for the presence of rat CT (rCT) mRNA. Immunoreactive CT-like material also occurs in the pituitary of both mammals and lower vertebrates, although the identity of the pituitary CT remains to be established. The physiologic significance of CT-like immunoreactivity in the pituitary remains to be fully elucidated; however, CT receptors are present in the intermediate pituitary, and therefore the CT-like material may act as a paracrine regulator of these receptors. CT has been recently described as participating in a complex cross-talk between extracellular signaling molecules in the pituitary.[94] Treatment of pituitary cells with CT in culture modulates the secretion of prolactin,[95,96] and treatment of the cultures with an anticalcitonin antibody enhances it.[97] Targeted overexpression of calcitonin in gonadotrophs of mice leads to long-term hypoprolactinemia, decreased PRL gene expression, female subfertility, and a selective underdevelopment of lactotrophs.[98,99]

Calcitonin in the Central Nervous System

Intraventricular administration of CT generates potent effects that include analgesia and inhibition of appetite and gastric acid secretion, as well as modulation of hormone secretion and the extrapyramidal motor system.[77,79,81,92] Both immunoreactive CT-like peptide and CT receptors have been demonstrated in the brain and nervous system of rats, humans, and other species. Immunoreactive CT related antigenically to hCT (hCTI) has also been demonstrated in the nervous systems of protochordates, lizards, and pigeons, as well as at low levels in human and rat brain extracts. Furthermore, radioimmunoassay analyses point to the presence of sCT-like peptide material in human and rat brain.[93]

Calcitonin Receptors

RECEPTOR DISTRIBUTION

Direct evidence for binding of CT to osteoclasts was obtained from the work of Nicholson et al,[38] who used in vitro autoradiography to demonstrate ^{125}I-sCT binding specifically to osteoclasts and their precursor cells. The CT receptor became a required phenotypic feature to establish cells as osteoclasts.[100] Radioligand binding studies in tissue sections, membranes, and cultured cells have revealed an extensive extraskeletal distribution of CTRs. These sites include kidney, brain, pituitary, placenta, testis and spermatozoa, lung, and lymphocytes, as well as cancer-derived cells from lung, breast, pituitary, and embryonal carcinoma.[77]

The centrally mediated actions of CT correlate well with the locations of CT binding sites. Autoradiographic mapping revealed high binding densities associated with parts of the ventral striatum and amygdala, the hypothalamic and preoptic areas, as well as most of the circumventricular organs. High-density binding also occurs in parts of the periaqueductal gray, the reticular formation, most of the midline raphe nuclei, parabrachial nuclei, locus coeruleus, and solitary tract nucleus.[92,101,102] CTR mRNA has been confirmed in many of these sites, including kidney, brain, lung, placenta, and osteoclasts, along with many cancer cell lines. However, CTR mRNA studies have also provided evidence for previously uncharacterized sites of CTR expression, including prostate, normal and neoplastic breast, and thyroid.[77] As was discussed earlier, there is no evidence for CTR expression in osteoblasts.

As is discussed later, CT and amylin receptors derive from the same gene product, and consequently care needs to be taken in extrapolating the potential significance of CTR mRNA expression for CT biology. The same is also true for receptor localization studies where ^{125}I-sCT is used as the radioligand.

RECEPTOR CLONING

Our knowledge of the molecular basis of CT action, in terms of both ligand binding and postbinding events, was greatly augmented by the molecular cloning of CT receptors. The first cloned receptor was the porcine CTR, which was isolated by expression cloning from a cDNA library derived from the renal epithelial cell line, LLC-PK1.[103] Subsequently, the sequences of CTR genes from man, rat, mouse, rabbit, guinea pig, and several species of fish have been reported, and the phylogenetic relationships between CTRs of mammalian and nonmammalian species have been well summarized.[104] Analysis of the predicted protein translation product(s) revealed that these receptors comprise approximately 500 amino acids and belong to the class II (family B) subclass of G protein–coupled receptors, which include the receptors for other peptide hormones such as secretin, PTH, glucagon, glucagon-like peptide 1, vasoactive intestinal polypeptide, pituitary adenylate cyclase–activating peptide, and gastric inhibitory peptide.

RECEPTOR ISOFORMS

Receptor cloning also provided direct evidence for receptor heterogeneity and the existence of multiple receptor isoforms that arise from alternative splicing of the CTR mRNA primary transcript. The human receptor, of which there are at least 5 splice variants, is the most extensively studied. The most common hCTR splice variant occurs in intracellular domain 1, generating a 16 amino acid insert in this domain (I_{1+}).[105-107] These are now termed CTa (insert negative) and CTb (insert positive).[108] Additional splice variants have been identified in other species. In rodents, alternate splicing leads to two receptor isoforms (these have previously been termed C1a and C1b), which differ by the presence (C1b; E_{2+}) or absence (C1a) of an additional 37 amino acids in the second extracellular domain. However, it is unlikely that expression of the rodent C1b isoform occurs in humans. In rabbits, an additional splice variant, in which the exon encoding transmembrane domain 7 is spliced out (ΔTM7; delta e13), has been isolated.

Investigation of the significance of the splice variants revealed that inserts or deletions in the CTR structure lead to alterations in ligand binding (E_{2+}, Δamino47), signal transduction (I_{1+}), or both (ΔTM7). For the E_{2+} variants, there is a loss of affinity for peptides exhibiting weak α-helical secondary structure, such

as human CT, while peptides with strong helical secondary structure, such as salmon CT, maintain high affinity at this receptor.[109] In contrast, the CTb (I_{1+}) receptor isoform displays similar affinity to the CTa (I_{1-}) variant for CT-like peptides but has markedly altered G protein–coupling efficiency. The presence of the 16 amino acid insert leads to complete loss of intracellular calcium mobilization. Activation by calcitonin of its receptor can result in coupling to multiple different G proteins (see Fig. 2-6). The effect on signaling via Gs is cell type dependent but overall is maintained with decreased efficiency, leading to a 10- to 100-fold reduction in the potency of peptides for stimulation of cAMP production.[106] It is interesting to speculate about the functional significance of the different receptor isoforms, particularly those with apparently impaired signaling capacity. Accumulating evidence suggests that G protein–coupled receptors can form homodimers and heterodimers, and that these interactions can cross-modulate the activity of the partners. Indeed, in the case of the rabbit CTR (delta e13), Seck et al[110,111] reported that this isoform can complex with the CTa isoform and inhibit its cell surface expression and activity, thus exerting an endogenous dominant negative effect on CTR signaling.

RECEPTOR GENE

The *CTR* gene, like the genes for other class II G protein–coupled receptors, is complex, comprising at least 14 exons with introns ranging in size from 78 nucleotides to >20,000 nucleotides. The total receptor gene is estimated to exceed 70 kb in length.[112] The organization and size of the human gene are similar to the pig *CTR* gene, although with some interspecies differences in organization. For instance, in the pig the I1 insert is generated by selective use of alternate splice sites located in exon 8. However, in humans, the I1 insert occurs on a separate exon, with at least one additional exon proximal to exon 7 in the pig.[106] Isolation of the mouse *CTR* gene[113] revealed that the locations of introns within the coding region of the *mCTR* gene (exons E3-E14) are identical to those of the porcine and human *CTR* genes. The predicted structure of the mefugu fish gene is more complex than the human gene, with an additional nine exons.[104] It is interesting to note that both fish and mammalian genes code for micro-RNA (miR)-489 in intron 3, the function of which remains to be determined.

The regulatory portion of the gene contains three putative promoters (P1, P2, and P3), giving rise to multiple CTR isoforms, which differ in the 5′ region of the gene and generate 5′-untranslated regions of very different lengths, in a tissue specific manner.[113] Promoters P1 and P2 are utilized in osteoclasts, brain, and kidney, and the proximal promoter of the human CTR (hCTRP1) was transcriptionally active in all cell lines tested, with high-level activity dependent on an 11 bp Sp1/Sp3 binding site.[114] In contrast, promoter P3 appears to be osteoclast specific and is sensitive to the osteoclast-inducing cytokine, RANKL, as well as the RANKL-induced transcription factor, NFATc1, consistent with a role for the latter in regulating the *CTR* gene in osteoclasts.[115] The human *CTR* gene is located on chromosome 7 at 7q21.3. In the mouse it is in the proximal region of chromosome 6, while the pig gene is located in chromosomal band 9q11-12. These pig and mouse chromosomal regions are homologous to 7q in humans. It is interesting to note that the mouse *CTR* gene is expressed preferentially from the maternal allele in brain, with no allelic bias detected in other tissues, indicating that the mouse *CTR* gene is imprinted in a tissue-specific manner.[116]

RECEPTOR POLYMORPHISMS AND OSTEOPOROSIS

An interesting, but as yet unconfirmed, report describes an association between the expression of the CTa receptor mRNA in circulating monocytes of postmenopausal, but not premenopausal, women and their serum levels of bone alkaline phosphatase and urinary deoxypyridinolone.[117] The authors therefore suggested a link between CTR expression and increased bone resorption postmenopausally.

Restriction fragment length polymorphism (RFLP) studies have identified a polymorphism within the CTR gene coding sequence; Nakamura et al,[118] using the Alu I restriction enzyme, identified a polymorphism arising from a single nucleotide substitution, which leads to either a proline (CC genotype) or a leucine (TT genotype) at amino acid 447 in the human CTa receptor (amino acid 463 of the hCTb receptor), with heterozygotes designated TC. In this Japanese population, the proline heterozygote was the most prevalent (≈70%), with the leucine homozygote accounting for ≈10% of the population and the heterozygote for ≈20%. Additional analyses across different ethnic groups have revealed that the Leu homozygote is most prevalent in Caucasians, with decreased prevalence in African Americans and Hispanics and very low frequency in Asians (0% to 10%).[119-122]

The influence of the polymorphism on bone mineral density (BMD) has been studied by multiple investigators. Most studies have identified significant correlations between CTR genotype and osteoporotic markers (BMD, fracture risk); however there is considerable divergence among studies in regard to which genotype is more favorable. High incidence of the T allele (either Leu homozygotes or heterozygotes) has been correlated with both increased BMD[119,121,123] and decreased BMD.[119,124,125] The underlying basis for this divergence is unclear. It may be due to linkage disequilibrium of the CTR polymorphism with other genes involved in bone homeostasis. Alternatively, it may be related to the complex nature of action of CT and amylin (likely utilizing the same core receptor) alluded to above from gene knockout studies.[63] This work indicates that CT can affect both bone formation and resorption, while amylin may be important for osteoclastogenesis.

The CTR genotype has also been linked to body weight in premenopausal Japanese women,[87] and to incidence of kidney stones.[126] To date, in vitro studies have not identified significant functional differences in ligand binding or cAMP generation between the two polymorphic variants.[127] A large number of other, probably silent, polymorphisms in the hCTR, whose frequency varies among ethnic groups, have been identified.[127]

AMYLIN AND CALCITONIN GENE-RELATED PEPTIDE RECEPTORS

Recent work revealed that the CT receptor–like receptor (CLR), which has highest homology with the cloned CT receptor, is a CGRP receptor. Functionally, however, this receptor requires the coexpression of a novel protein, termed receptor activity modifying protein 1 (RAMP 1). RAMP 1 is a member of a family of three single transmembrane proteins and acts to modify the glycosylation of CLR, enhance the trafficking of the receptor protein to the cell surface and contributing to the cell surface ligand binding and specificity of the receptor. RAMP 2 and RAMP 3 also enhance the trafficking of CLR to the cell surface; association of CLR with RAMP 2 and RAMP 3 gives rise to adrenomedullin-like receptors.[128,129] It has been demonstrated[80,81] that the molecular identity of amylin receptors was also founded on RAMP-based hetero-oligomers. In this case, the RAMPs interacted with the CTR to form distinct amylin receptor phenotypes, depending on which RAMP was complexed with the receptor (see Fig. 2-6). It is intriguing that the CTR/RAMP 1 complex, in addition to being a high-affinity amylin receptor, potently interacts with CGRP.[80] This behavior may contribute to some of the heterogeneity seen in CGRP receptor analyses. Unlike CLR, CTRs do not require RAMPs to translocate to the cell surface and exhibit classic CTR phenotype under these conditions. Both RAMPs and receptors are subject to dynamic regulation, although in the case of CLR-based receptors, RAMPs often appear to be the major component regulated.[82,130]

SIGNALING

Usage of the cAMP pathway in mediating CT action in osteoclasts was discussed earlier. CT also stimulates adenylate cyclase activity in the kidney, with the pattern of CT responsiveness paralleling the distribution of CTRs in this tissue. CT induction of cAMP has now been documented in a large number of cultured CTR-bearing cells that include LLC-PK1 pig kidney cells, and cancers of lung, breast, and bone. Receptor cloning and expression studies have confirmed that cAMP production is an important component of CTR-mediated signaling.[103,105,106]

It is now apparent that G protein–coupled receptors can interact with and signal through multiple G proteins (Fig. 2-7). Thus, CT action in osteoclasts is probably regulated by alternate signaling pathways, in apparently species-specific ways. In mice, this response appears to be mediated predominantly by the protein kinase A pathway,[131,132] although inhibition of osteoclast-mediated bone resorption by CT can be mimicked by both dibutyryl cAMP and phorbol esters or blocked by protein kinase inhibitors.[133] Coupling of the CTR to G_q can also activate phospholipase C, leading to increased cytosolic calcium and triphosphate levels and activation of protein kinase C.[134] Thus, in human osteoclasts, activation of protein kinase C pathways appears to be the predominant mechanism of CT-mediated osteoclast inhibition,[39] although PKA may be more important in human odontoclasts.[135]

Calcitonin induction of interleukin (IL)-6 production in pituitary folliculo-stellate cells required both PKA and PKC signaling pathways.[136] In hepatocytes, even at very low concentrations, CT is capable of increasing cytosolic calcium.[137] CT-induced differentiation of early rat embryos is dependent upon intracellular calcium mobilization.[138] It is interesting to note that although CT inhibits proton extrusion from osteoclasts,[139] it can increase H^+ efflux from nonosteoclastic cells, in a PKC-dependent manner.[140] The significance of this activity is not clear. CT-induced changes mediated by cAMP or intracellular calcium in LLC-PK1 pig kidney cells are cell cycle dependent.[141] Expression of cloned receptors in a variety of cell types has now conclusively shown that CT receptors of human, rat, and porcine origin are capable of signaling through both cAMP and calcium-activated second messenger systems. It is important to note that comparison of the calcium response in cell lines expressing different CT receptor levels has suggested that the magnitude of the response is proportional to the receptor density, and it is therefore possible that relative receptor density in target tissues may influence the signaling pathway(s) activated.

CT treatment of CTR-bearing cells, in the presence of extracellular calcium, initiates a sustained rise in intracellular calcium, the extent of which is dependent on the concentration of the extracellular calcium and is proportional to the receptor

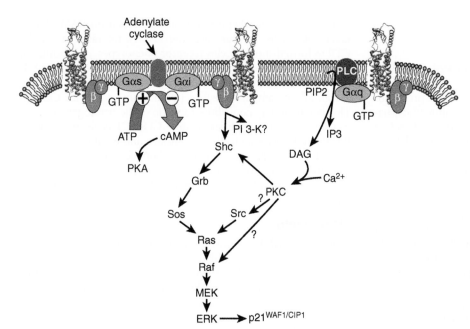

FIGURE 2-7. Calcitonin activation of the CTa receptor can lead to coupling to multiple different G proteins. Coupling to $G_{\alpha i}$ is seen less frequently and may be due, at least in part, to a PKC-dependent inhibition of G_i. The balance of activation of different G proteins and effectors is critical for the cell-specific actions of CT. Also illustrated is the current understanding of CT-induced MAPK activation, as delineated in stably transfected HEK-293 cells. ERK1/2 phosphorylation requires both PTX-sensitive G proteins (presumably Gi via $\beta\gamma$ subunits) and Gq. The latter leads to rises in intracellular calcium and activation of PKC, and both contribute to ERK phosphorylation. At least part of the activation occurs following phosphorylation of Shc and mobilization of its downstream effectors. Activation of ERK increases phosphorylation of p21[WAF/CIP1] and modulation of cell growth. Although strongly activated by CTa receptors, Gs is not involved in activation of MAPKs.

density.[142] Because osteoclasts, which express high levels of CTR, are reportedly exposed to calcium concentrations as high as 26 mM during bone resorption,[143] this phenomenon may have particular relevance for this cell type. CT and extracellular calcium both can cause intracellular calcium transients in isolated osteoclasts, and each agent greatly augments the signal produced by either agent alone.[144]

CTR-mediated activation of the MAPK pathway has been described,[145-147] with a role for both Gq and Gi/o proteins—the latter principally via $\beta\gamma$ G protein subunits, as is commonly the case for other G protein–coupled receptors. There is also evidence that CT can influence cell attachment by modulating components of focal adhesions and the cytoskeleton.[146] CT treatment of osteoclasts disrupts the F-actin ring that is thought to correspond to the sealing zone[64,148] and increases the tyrosine phosphorylation of paxillin and FAK. In rabbit osteoclasts, these actions were mediated by PKC.[146] These actions of CT, together with decreased osteoclast motility, cytosol retraction, and disassembly of podosomes, have been linked to modulation of the activity and intracellular localization of Pyk2 and Src in osteoclasts.[149] It has also been shown, in nonosteoclastic cells, that CT can cause cell death by aniokis, as the result of loss of cell attachment.[150]

It is interesting to note that recent work suggests that coexpression of RAMPs with the CTR leads to pathway-specific modulation of coupling, with strong augmentation of amylin-mediated Gs-coupling, but little effect on Gq- or Gi- mediated signaling, at least for RAMP 1– or RAMP 3–coupled receptors.[151]

RECEPTOR REGULATION

Regulation of the level and/or affinity of cell surface receptors is a key component in the physiologic and pathophysiologic responses to both endogenous and pharmacologically administered agents. The CTR is subject to both homologous (CT-induced) and heterologous regulation. CT-induced CTR downregulation was initially demonstrated in various transformed cell lines and subsequently in primary kidney cell cultures. The induction by CT of resistance to its own action in osteoclasts is such a specific process and correlates so closely in

dose dependence to CT efficacy as an agonist,[48] that it appears to be an important accompaniment of CT action. Proof of this might require genetic experiments, just as genetic manipulation has finally begun to cast light on the physiologic functions of CT.[32,63]

Receptor downregulation is mediated by specific loss of cell surface receptors, which occurs via an energy-dependent internalization of the ligand-receptor complex, in which the principal internalization pathway involves processing of the receptor-ligand complex into lysosomes and subsequent degradation of the receptor.[152] Receptor regulatory responses to CT are likely to be cell or tissue dependent. For example, in mouse or rat osteoclasts, a potent downregulation of CTR mRNA appears to be mediated by a cAMP-dependent mechanism, in addition to downregulation of the receptor by internalization.[153] Similar CT-mediated CTR regulation is also observed in human osteoclasts, but, as stated above, activation of protein kinase C pathways is suggested to be the predominant mechanism of CT-mediated osteoclast inhibition in human osteoclasts.[39] In contrast to these observations in osteoclasts, downregulation of CTRs in UMR106-06 cells and T47D cells is not accompanied by changes in CTR mRNA levels.[113] The CT-induced receptor mRNA loss in osteoclasts appears to be due principally to destabilization of receptor mRNA.[46] The 3′-untranslated region of the mouse and rat CTR mRNA contains four AUUUA motifs, as well as other A/U-rich domains, which can function as signals for rapid mRNA inactivation. Thus, addition of A/U-rich CTR 3′UTR sequences considerably shortens the mRNA half-life of a reporter gene, and evidence shows the involvement of AUF1 p40, HuR in the regulation of CTR mRNA.[154] It is also worth noting that the degree of internalization of human CTRs appears to be isoform specific, with the I_{1+} variant being resistant to internalization.[106] Thus, the regulation of receptors and consequently peptide responses may vary according to the levels of specific receptor isoforms present in each tissue.

Data on regulation of CTR by other agents are limited. In mouse osteoclast cultures, the glucocorticoid dexamethasone increased the level of cell surface CTR following upregulation of receptor mRNA levels, the latter mediated at the level of transcription.[46] Moreover, the CT-mediated decrease in cell surface receptor and mRNA was attenuated by dexamethasone. Increased production of CTR in response to glucocorticoid stimulation also occurs in the human T47D cell line, where cortisol is required for the expression of CTRs, suggesting that this may be a common regulatory mechanism for induction of CTR expression. It is worth noting the clinical evidence suggesting that glucocorticoids, given together with CT, might prevent to some extent the CT-induced resistance to its own action.[155]

Calcitonin and Its Receptors in Cancer

MEDULLARY CARCINOMA OF THE THYROID

The classic syndrome of CT excess is medullary carcinoma of the thyroid (MCT). This tumor clearly differs in origin from all other thyroid cancers, since it is a tumor of the C cells, derived from the ultimobranchial bodies. MCT may occur as a sporadic or a genetic (familial) tumor.[156-160] The only effective treatment for MCT is surgical. The earlier this can be performed in the course of this disease, the better is the likelihood of a cure. Once the tumor becomes palpable, any treatment is unlikely to be curative. Genetic testing for the locus of mutation in the responsible gene (the RET proto-oncogene) often has considerable clinical relevance in management, as early surgery is key to survival, especially in the syndrome known as multiple endocrine neoplasia type 2b (MEN-2b).

CALCITONIN RECEPTORS IN OTHER CANCERS

Specific high-affinity receptors for CT have been demonstrated in human lymphoid cell lines, in a human lung cancer cell line, in several human breast cancer cell lines, including MCF-7, T47D, and ZR-75, and in prostate cancer cells.[152,153,161,162] Indeed, CTR mRNA appears to be a frequent accompaniment of human tumors. The first clinical study of CT receptors in surgically obtained human breast cancers identified receptor mRNA production in all of 18 cancers by reverse transcription/polymerase chain reaction (PCR).[163]

In situ hybridization in the same study showed that CT receptor expression was confined to tumor cells in the sections. In contrast, a subsequent study, using laser capture microdissection and PCR, found that the CTR in breast cancer tissue was actually reduced compared with adjacent normal breast tissue.[164] The significance of the CTR in cancer cells is not known; however forced expression of human CT in LNCaP human prostate cancer cells was reported to dramatically enhance their oncogenic characteristics,[165] and CT is expressed endogenously in the prostate.[166] The same group also showed that CT increased hallmarks of invasiveness of prostate cancer cells, including the concentration and activity of MMP-2 and MMP-9.[167] Similar results have been reported for MDA-MB-231 human breast cancer cells.[168]

Calcitonin in Growth and Development

The presence of CT and its receptors in a large number of cell types and tissue sites suggests multiple physiologic roles. CTRs have been identified in bone, kidney, brain, pituitary, testis, prostate, spermatozoa, breast, lung, and lymphocytes, as well as in cancer-derived cells from lung, breast, prostate, pituitary, bone (osteoclastoma, osteogenic sarcoma), and embryonal carcinoma.[77] CT can potently modulate the growth of some CTR-bearing cells. Treatment with CT has been shown to stimulate the growth of human prostate cancer cells, in which the peptide increases both intracellular calcium and cAMP levels.[169] Conversely, knock-down of calcitonin receptor expression in these cells induced apoptosis and growth arrest.[162] The effects of CT on growth are clearly cell type dependent, since CT treatment repressed the growth of T47D human breast cancer cells, an action proposed to be mediated by the specific activation of the type II isoenzyme of the cAMP-dependent protein kinase.[161] In cells overexpressing the human CTR, CT inhibited cell growth and caused an accumulation of cells in the G2 phase of the cell cycle, associated with a prolonged increase in p21$^{WAF1/CIP1}$ expression[170] and sustained activation of the p42/44 MAP kinase proteins.[145]

Evidence has been found to be consistent with the involvement of CT in cell growth[161,169] and differentiation and in tissue development and remodeling.[171] CT may be involved in both blastocyst implantation and development[138,172] of the early blastocyst, and CT downregulates E-cadherin expression in rat uterine epithelium during implantation.[130] It was shown recently that CT promotes the outgrowth of trophoblast cells on endometrial epithelial cells, perhaps thereby facilitating embryo implantation.[173] Other reports indicate embryonic expression of the mouse CTR, suggesting that CTRs may play important roles in morphogenesis.[171] It has been reported that CT is expressed in the pregnant mouse mammary gland, exclusively in and secreted from the luminal epithelial cells, and that its expression is progesterone dependent.[174] It was found that CT induction spatiotemporally correlates with increases in progesterone-induced mammary gland proliferation and structural remodeling, suggesting that CT may be involved in one or both of these progesterone-dependent processes. As was discussed earlier, CT can inhibit cell proliferation[161] or can have mitogenic actions.[169] CT also may have a role in cell survival, and as discussed above has been claimed to be protective of drug-induced apoptosis in osteoblast-like and osteocyte-like cells[54] and prostate cancer cell lines,[175] and to promote the survival of osteoclasts.[134] On the other hand, CT has been found to potentiate neuronal death due to oxygen and glucose deprivation,[176] and to be pro-apoptotic in serum-deprived cells.[150]

Calcitonin as a Therapeutic

HYPERCALCEMIA

Calcitonin has been used in the treatment of hypercalcemia in many different conditions, especially malignancy, but its effective use is limited by rapid tachyphylaxis, often within 24 hours of use.[177] The mechanism of resistance seems to involve receptor downregulation, which to some extent is blocked by corticosteroid use (see Receptor Regulation earlier).[155]

OSTEOPOROSIS AND PAGET'S DISEASE OF BONE

The discussions in this chapter of the mechanism of action of CT provide some background for the use of CT in therapy. One of the most important unanswered questions concerning CT is whether its role as an inhibitor of bone resorption is such that CT deficiency can contribute to the development of osteoporosis. It is the antiresorptive action of CT that is the basis for its use clinically in osteoporosis, for which it is approved in several countries. Although its use remains somewhat controversial, CT administered by injection or by nasal spray has been found to decrease vertebral fracture risk in postmenopausal osteoporotic women.[178,179] A reported advantage of calcitonin is its analgesic effect on bone pain, which probably is mediated centrally[179]; CT treatment has modest effects on bone quantity (BMD) or bone turnover markers, but new evidence suggests improvement in bone quality parameters after administration of salmon CT nasal spray over 2 years. The results of the QUEST study, in which effects of CT on bone structure were assessed by high-resolution MRI, suggest therapeutic benefit of CT-NS compared with placebo in maintaining trabecular microarchitecture at multiple skeletal sites.[180] Similar protection by CT of bone structure was obtained in ovariectomized sheep, again with MRI used to assess bone changes.[181] A problem with CT use clinically is its bioavailability, and attempts are now being made to produce orally bioavailable CT, with promising results.[182,183]

CT given by subcutaneous injection was recognized as effective in the treatment of Paget's disease, with relief of pain, return of biochemical indices of disease activity toward normal, formation of normal lamellar bone, and filling in of osteolytic lesions. In long-term treatment of Paget's disease with CT, the number of osteoclasts declines progressively, either because of a direct effect on osteoclast precursors or as an indirect consequence of the acute inhibition of osteoclast function by CT. In Paget's disease, CT needs to be given by injection, since intranasal delivery is relatively ineffective, and its use generally has been supplanted by bisphosphonates, as is reviewed elsewhere in this book.

OSTEOARTHRITIS

A number of recent studies have suggested the potential benefit of CT in osteoarthritis. In both in vitro and in vivo animal models,[184,185] CT was found to attenuate the indices of progression of osteoarthritis, including degradation of collagen type II, a hallmark of articular cartilage damage. In humans, CT treatment reduced circulating CTX-II[186] and improved functional disability in patients, albeit in a small test group, selected for active disease.[187] The mechanism of action of CT in this putative chondroprotection is not clear. It has been claimed, on the one hand, that CT has direct effects on bovine articular chondrocytes via the CTR,[188] but a recent study was unable to find CTR expression or responsiveness to CT in human chondrocytes.[189] The findings are nonetheless intriguing and benefits could result from the effects of CT on subchondral bone, as have been described for bisphosphonate treatment of animal models of osteoarthritis.[190] Potential benefits of CT have also been suggested for inflammatory arthritis, since it was found to preserve bone morphology in a rat model of rheumatoid arthritis, particularly when used with prednisolone.[191]

Acknowledgments

Work from each of the authors' laboratories was supported by the National Health and Medical Research Council of Australia (NHMRC). PMS is a NHMRC Principal Research Fellow.

REFERENCES

1. Copp DH, Cameron EC, Cheney BA, et al: Evidence for calcitonin—a new hormone from the parathyroid that lowers blood calcium, Endocrinology 70:638–649, 1962.
2. Hirsch PF, Gauthier GF, Munson PL: Thyroid hypocalcemic principle and recurrent laryngeal nerve injury as factors affecting the response to parathyroidectomy in rats, Endocrinology 73:244–252, 1963.
3. Hirsch PF, Voelkel EF, Munson PL: Thyrocalcitonin: hypocalcemic hypophosphatemic principle of the thyroid gland, Science 146:412–413, 1964.
4. Foster GV, Baghdiantz A, Kumar MA, et al: Thyroid origin of calcitonin, Nature 202:1303–1305, 1964.
5. Pearse AG, Carvalheira AF: Cytochemical evidence for an ultimobranchial origin of rodent thyroid C cells, Nature 214(5091):929–930, 1967.
6. Suzuki N, Suzuki T, Kurokawa T: Suppression of osteoclastic activities by calcitonin in the scales of goldfish (freshwater teleost) and nibbler fish (seawater teleost), Peptides 21(1):115–124, 2000.
7. Brown EM, Gamba G, Riccardi D, et al: Cloning and characterization of an extracellular Ca(2+)-sensing receptor from bovine parathyroid, Nature 366(6455):575–580, 1993.
8. Care AD, Bates RF, Swaminathan R, et al: The role of gastrin as a calcitonin secretagogue, J Endocrinol 51(4):735–744, 1971.
9. Freake HC, MacIntyre I: Specific binding of 1,25-dihydroxycholecalciferol in human medullary thyroid carcinoma, Biochem J 206(1):181–184, 1982.
10. Jacobs JW, Simpson E, Penschow J, et al: Characterization and localization of calcitonin messenger ribonucleic acid in rat thyroid, Endocrinology 113(5):1616–1622, 1983.
11. Becker KL, Snider RH, Silva OL, et al: Calcitonin heterogeneity in lung cancer and medullary thyroid cancer, Acta Endocrinol (Copenh) 89(1):89–99, 1978.
12. Tobler PH, Dambacher MA, Born W, et al: A new bioactive form of human calcitonin, Cancer Res 43(8):3793–3799, 1983.
13. Canale DD, Donabedian RK: Hypercalcitoninemia in acute pancreatitis, J Clin Endocrinol Metab 40(4):738–741, 1975.

14. O'Neill WJ, Jordan MH, Lewis MS, et al: Serum calcitonin may be a marker for inhalation injury in burns, J Burn Care Rehabil 13(6):605–616, 1992.
15. Lind L, Bucht E, Ljunghall S: Pronounced elevation in circulating calcitonin in critical care patients is related to the severity of illness and survival, Intensive Care Med 21(1):63–66, 1995.
16. Becker KL, Nylen ES, Snider RH, et al: Immunoneutralization of procalcitonin as therapy of sepsis, J Endotoxin Res 9(6):367–374, 2003.
17. Martin TJ, Findlay DM, Moseley JM, et al: Calcitonin. In Avioli LV, Krane SM, editors: Metabolic Bone Disease and Clinically Related Disorders, ed 3, St. Louis, 1998, Academic Press, pp 95–121.
18. Yamauchi H, Shiraki M, Otani M, et al: Stability of [Asu1,7]-eel calcitonin and eel calcitonin in vitro and in vivo, Endocrinol Jpn 24(3):281–285, 1977.
19. Jacobs JW, Lund PK, Potts JT Jr, et al: Procalcitonin is a glycoprotein, J Biol Chem 256(6):2803–2807, 1981.
20. Mol JA, Kwant MM, Arnold IC, et al: Elucidation of the sequence of canine (pro)-calcitonin. A molecular biological and protein chemical approach, Regul Pept 35(3):189–195, 1991.
21. Jacobs JW, Goodman RH, Chin WW, et al: Calcitonin messenger RNA encodes multiple polypeptides in a single precursor, Science 213(4506):457–459, 1981.
22. Lasmoles F, Jullienne A, Day F, et al: Elucidation of the nucleotide sequence of chicken calcitonin mRNA: direct evidence for the expression of a lower vertebrate calcitonin-like gene in man and rat, Embo J 4(10):2603–2607, 1985.
23. Steenbergh PH, Hoppener JW, Zandberg J, et al: Calcitonin gene related peptide coding sequence is conserved in the human genome and is expressed in medullary thyroid carcinoma, J Clin Endocrinol Metab 59(2):358–360, 1984.
24. Rosenfeld MG, Amara SG, Evans RM: Alternative RNA processing: determining neuronal phenotype, Science 225(4668):1315–1320, 1984.
25. Zaidi M, Breimer LH, MacIntyre I: Biology of peptides from the calcitonin genes, Q J Exp Physiol 72(4):371–408, 1987.
26. Roos BA, Yoon MJ, Frelinger AL, et al: Tumor growth and calcitonin during serial transplantation of rat medullary thyroid carcinoma, Endocrinology 105(1):27–32, 1979.
27. Lou H, Gagel RF, Berget SM: An intron enhancer recognized by splicing factors activates polyadenylation, Genes Dev 10(2):208–219, 1996.
28. Cooper CW, Hirsch PF, Toverud SU, et al: An improved method for the biological assay of thyrocalcitonin, Endocrinology 81(3):610–616, 1967.
29. Harper C, Toverud SU: Ability of thyrocalcitonin to protect against hypercalcemia in adult rats, Endocrinology 93(6):1354–1359, 1973.
30. Martin TJ, Melick RA: The acute effects of porcine calcitonin in man, Australas Ann Med 18(3):258–263, 1969.
31. Yamamoto M, Seedor JG, Rodan GA, et al: Endogenous calcitonin attenuates parathyroid hormone-induced cancellous bone loss in the rat, Endocrinology 136(2):788–795, 1995.
32. Hoff AO, Catala-Lehnen P, Thomas PM, et al: Increased bone mass is an unexpected phenotype associated with deletion of the calcitonin gene, J Clin Invest 110(12):1849–1857, 2002.
33. Woodrow JP, Sharpe CJ, Fudge NJ, et al: Calcitonin plays a critical role in regulating skeletal mineral metabolism during lactation, Endocrinology 147(9):4010–4021, 2006.
34. Friedman J, Raisz LG: Thyrocalcitonin: inhibitor of bone resorption in tissue culture, Science 150(702):1465–1467, 1965.
35. Matthews JL, Martin JH: Immediate changes in the ultrastructure of bone cells following thyrocalcitonin administration. In Talmadge RV, Munson PL, editors: Calcium, Parathyroid Hormone and the Calcitonins, Amsterdam, 1972, Excerpta Medica, pp 375–382,.
36. Martin TJ, Robinson CJ, MacIntyre I: The mode of action of thyrocalcitonin, Lancet 1(7443):900–902, 1966.
37. Robinson CJ, Martin TJ, Matthews EW, et al: Mode of action of thyrocalcitonin, J Endocrinol 39(1):71–79, 1967.
38. Nicholson GC, Moseley JM, Sexton PM, et al: Abundant calcitonin receptors in isolated rat osteoclasts. Biochemical and autoradiographic characterization, J Clin Invest 78(2):355–360, 1986.

39. Samura A, Wada S, Suda S, et al: Calcitonin receptor regulation and responsiveness to calcitonin in human osteoclast-like cells prepared in vitro using receptor activator of nuclear factor-kappaB ligand and macrophage colony-stimulating factor, Endocrinology 141(10):3774–3782, 2000.

40. Chambers TJ, Athanasou NA, Fuller K: Effect of parathyroid hormone and calcitonin on the cytoplasmic spreading of isolated osteoclasts, J Endocrinol 102(3): 281–286, 1984.

41. MacDonald BR, Takahashi N, McManus LM, et al: Formation of multinucleated cells that respond to osteotropic hormones in long term human bone marrow cultures, Endocrinology 120(6):2326–2333, 1987.

42. Takahashi N, Mundy GR, Kuehl TJ, et al: Osteoclast-like cell formation in fetal and newborn long-term baboon marrow cultures is more sensitive to 1,25-dihydroxyvitamin D3 than adult long-term marrow cultures, J Bone Miner Res 2(4):311–317, 1987.

43. Linkhart TA, Linkhart SG, Kodama Y, et al: Osteoclast formation in bone marrow cultures from two inbred strains of mice with different bone densities, J Bone Miner Res 14(1):39–46, 1999.

44. Galvin RJ, Bryan P, Venugopalan M, et al: Calcitonin responsiveness and receptor expression in porcine and murine osteoclasts: a comparative study, Bone 23(3):233–240, 1998.

45. Ikegame M, Rakopoulos M, Martin TJ, et al: Effects of continuous calcitonin treatment on osteoclast-like cell development and calcitonin receptor expression in mouse bone marrow cultures, J Bone Miner Res 11(4):456–465, 1996.

46. Wada S, Udagawa N, Akatsu T, et al: Regulation by calcitonin and glucocorticoids of calcitonin receptor gene expression in mouse osteoclasts, Endocrinology 138(2):521–529, 1997.

47. Wada S, Udagawa N, Nagata N, et al: Calcitonin receptor down-regulation relates to calcitonin resistance in mature mouse osteoclasts, Endocrinology 137(3):1042–1048, 1996.

48. Ikegame M, Ejiri S, Ozawa H: Calcitonin-induced change in serum calcium levels and its relationship to osteoclast morphology and number of calcitonin receptors, Bone 35(1):27–33, 2004.

49. Farley JR, Tarbaux NM, Hall SL, et al: The anti-bone-resorptive agent calcitonin also acts in vitro to directly increase bone formation and bone cell proliferation, Endocrinology 123(1):159–167, 1988.

50. Farley J, Dimai HP, Stilt-Coffing B, et al: Calcitonin increases the concentration of insulin-like growth factors in serum-free cultures of human osteoblast-line cells, Calcif Tissue Int 67(3):247–254, 2000.

51. Villa I, Dal Fiume C, Maestroni A, et al: Human osteoblast-like cell proliferation induced by calcitonin-related peptides involves PKC activity, Am J Physiol Endocrinol Metab 284(3):E627–E633, 2003.

52. Naot D, Bava U, Matthews B, et al: Differential gene expression in cultured osteoblasts and bone marrow stromal cells from patients with Paget's disease of bone, J Bone Miner Res 22(2):298–309, 2007.

53. Chang MK, Raggatt LJ, Alexander KA, et al: Osteal tissue macrophages are intercalated throughout human and mouse bone lining tissues and regulate osteoblast function in vitro and in vivo, J Immunol 181(2):1232–1244, 2008.

54. Plotkin LI, Weinstein RS, Parfitt AM, et al: Prevention of osteocyte and osteoblast apoptosis by bisphosphonates and calcitonin, J Clin Invest 104(10):1363–1374, 1999.

55. Bulbul M, Esenyel CZ, Esenyel M, et al: Effects of calcitonin on the biomechanics, histopathology, and radiography of callus formation in rats, J Orthop Sci 13(2):136–144, 2008.

56. Li X, Luo X, Yu N, et al: Effects of salmon calcitonin on fracture healing in ovariectomized rats, Saudi Medical Journal 28(1):60–64, 2007.

57. Amanat N, McDonald M, Godfrey C, et al: Optimal timing of a single dose of zoledronic acid to increase strength in rat fracture repair, J Bone Miner Res 22(6):867–876, 2007.

58. Chigurupati S, Kulkarni T, Thomas S, et al: Calcitonin stimulates multiple stages of angiogenesis by directly acting on endothelial cells, Cancer Res 65(18):8519–8529, 2005.

59. Hirsch PF, Baruch H: Is calcitonin an important physiological substance? Endocrine 21(3):201–208, 2003.

60. Schinke T, Liese S, Priemel M, et al: Decreased bone formation and osteopenia in mice lacking alpha-calcitonin gene-related peptide, J Bone Miner Res 19(12):2049–2056, 2004.

61. Huebner AK, Schinke T, Priemel M, et al: Calcitonin deficiency in mice progressively results in high bone turnover, J Bone Miner Res 21(12):1924–1934, 2006.

62. Huebner AK, Keller J, Catala-Lehnen P, et al: The role of calcitonin and alpha-calcitonin gene-related peptide in bone formation, Arch Biochem Biophys 473(2):210–217, 2008.

63. Dacquin R, Davey RA, Laplace C, et al: Amylin inhibits bone resorption while the calcitonin receptor controls bone formation in vivo, J Cell Biol 164(4):509–514, 2004.

64. Davey RA, Turner A, McManus JF, et al: The calcitonin receptor plays a physiological role to protect against hypercalcemia in mice, J Bone Miner Res 2008 Mar 18 [Epub ahead of print].

65. Martin TJ, Sims NA: Osteoclast-derived activity in the coupling of bone formation to resorption, Trends Mol Med 11(2):76–81, 2005.

66. Takeda S, Elefteriou F, Levasseur R, et al: Leptin regulates bone formation via the sympathetic nervous system, Cell 111(3):305–317, 2002.

67. Robinson CJ, Martin TJ, MacIntyre I: Phosphaturic effect of thyrocalcitonin, Lancet 2(7454):83–84, 1966.

68. Williams CC, Matthews EW, Moseley JM, et al: The effects of synthetic human and salmon calcitonins on electrolyte excretion in the rat, Clin Sci 42(2):129–137, 1972.

69. Hosking DJ, Gilson D: Comparison of the renal and skeletal actions of calcitonin in the treatment of severe hypercalcaemia of malignancy, Q J Med 53(211):359–368, 1984.

70. Sexton PM, Adam WR, Moseley JM, et al: Localization and characterization of renal calcitonin receptors by in vitro autoradiography, Kidney Int 32(6):862–868, 1987.

71. Kawashima H, Torikai S, Kurokawa K: Calcitonin selectively stimulates 25-hydroxyvitamin D3–1 alpha-hydroxylase in proximal straight tubule of rat kidney, Nature 291(5813):327–329, 1981.

72. Shinki T, Ueno Y, DeLuca HF, et al: Calcitonin is a major regulator for the expression of renal 25-hydroxyvitamin D3–1alpha-hydroxylase gene in normocalcemic rats, Proc Natl Acad Sci U S A 96(14):8253–8258, 1999.

73. Murayama A, Takeyama K, Kitanaka S, et al: Positive and negative regulations of the renal 25-hydroxyvitamin D3 1alpha-hydroxylase gene by parathyroid hormone, calcitonin, and 1alpha,25(OH)2D3 in intact animals, Endocrinology 140(5):2224–2231, 1999.

74. Gao XH, Dwivedi PP, Omdahl JL, et al: Calcitonin stimulates expression of the rat 25-hydroxyvitamin D3–24-hydroxylase (CYP24) promoter in HEK-293 cells expressing calcitonin receptor: identification of signaling pathways, J Mol Endocrinol 32(1):87–98, 2004.

75. Young A: Amylin and the integrated control of nutrient influx, Adv Pharmacol 52:67–77, 2005.

76. Pittner RA, Albrandt K, Beaumont K, et al: Molecular physiology of amylin, J Cell Biochem 55(Suppl):19–28, 1994.

77. Sexton PM, Findlay DM, Martin TJ: Calcitonin, Curr Med Chem 6(11):1067–1093, 1999.

78. Poyner DR: Molecular pharmacology of receptors for calcitonin-gene-related peptide, amylin and adrenomedullin, Biochem Soc Trans 25(3):1032–1036, 1997.

79. Wimalawansa SJ: Calcitonin gene-related peptide and its receptors: molecular genetics, physiology, pathophysiology, and therapeutic potentials, Endocr Rev 17(5):533–585, 1996.

80. Christopoulos G, Perry KJ, Morfis M, et al: Multiple amylin receptors arise from receptor activity-modifying protein interaction with the calcitonin receptor gene product, Mol Pharmacol 56(1):235–242, 1999.

81. Morfis M, Christopoulos A, Sexton PM: RAMPs: 5 years on, where to now? Trends Pharmacol Sci 24(11):596–601, 2003.

82. Hay DL, Christopoulos G, Christopoulos A, et al: Pharmacological discrimination of calcitonin receptor: receptor activity-modifying protein complexes, Mol Pharmacol 67(5):1655–1665, 2005.

83. Wimalawansa SJ: Amylin, calcitonin gene-related peptide, calcitonin, and adrenomedullin: a peptide superfamily, Crit Rev Neurobiol 11(2–3):167–239, 1997.

84. Niu P, Shindo T, Iwata H, et al: Protective effects of endogenous adrenomedullin on cardiac hypertrophy, fibrosis, and renal damage, Circulation 109(14):1789–1794, 2004.

85. Kandler MA, Von Der Hardt K, Mahfoud S, et al: Pilot intervention: aerosolized adrenomedullin reduces pulmonary hypertension, J Pharmacol Exp Ther 306(3):1021–1026, 2003.

86. Cornish J, Reid IR: Effects of amylin and adrenomedullin on the skeleton, J Musculoskelet Neuronal Interact 2(1):15–24, 2001.

87. Katafuchi T, Hamano K, Kikumoto K, et al: Identification of second and third calcitonin receptor-stimulating peptides in porcine brain, Biochem Biophys Res Commun 308(3):445–451, 2003.

88. Katafuchi T, Hamano K, Minamino N: Identification, structural determination, and biological activity of bovine and canine calcitonin receptor-stimulating peptides, Biochem Biophys Res Commun 313(1):74–79, 2004.

89. Katafuchi T, Kikumoto K, Hamano K, et al: Calcitonin receptor-stimulating peptide, a new member of the calcitonin gene-related peptide family. Its isolation from porcine brain, structure, tissue distribution, and biological activity, J Biol Chem 278(14):12046–12054, 2003.

90. Roh J, Chang CL, Bhalla A, et al: Intermedin is a calcitonin/calcitonin gene-related peptide family peptide acting through the calcitonin receptor-like receptor/receptor activity-modifying protein receptor complexes, J Biol Chem 279(8):7264–7274, 2004.

91. Takei Y, Hyodo S, Katafuchi T, et al: Novel fish-derived adrenomedullin in mammals: structure and possible function, Peptides 25(10):1643–1656, 2004.

92. Sexton PM: Central nervous system binding sites for calcitonin and calcitonin gene-related peptide, Mol Neurobiol 5(2–4):251–273, 1991.

93. Hilton JM, Mitchelhill KI, Pozvek G, et al: Purification of calcitonin-like peptides from rat brain and pituitary, Endocrinology 139(3):982–992, 1998.

94. Denef C: Paracrinicity: the story of 30 years of cellular pituitary crosstalk, J Neuroendocrinol 20(1):1–70, 2008.

95. Shah GV, Wang W, Grosvenor CE, et al: Calcitonin inhibits basal and thyrotropin-releasing hormone-induced release of prolactin from anterior pituitary cells: evidence for a selective action exerted proximal to secretagogue-induced increases in cytosolic Ca2+. Endocrinology 127(2):621–628, 1990.

96. Judd AM, Kubota T, Kuan SI, et al: Calcitonin decreases thyrotropin-releasing hormone-stimulated prolactin release through a mechanism that involves inhibition of inositol phosphate production, Endocrinology 127(1):191–199, 1990.

97. Shah GV, Deftos LJ, Crowley WR: Synthesis and release of calcitonin-like immunoreactivity by anterior pituitary cells: evidence for a role in paracrine regulation of prolactin secretion, Endocrinology 132(3):1367–1372, 1993.

98. Yuan R, Kulkarni T, Wei F, et al: Targeted overexpression of calcitonin in gonadotrophs of transgenic mice leads to chronic hypoprolactinemia, Mol Cell Endocrinol 229(1–2):193–203, 2005.

99. Sarkar DK, Kim KH, Minami S: Transforming growth factor-beta 1 messenger RNA and protein expression in the pituitary gland: its action on prolactin secretion and lactotropic growth, Mol Endocrinol 6(11):1825–1833, 1992.

100. Takahashi N, Yamana H, Yoshiki S, et al: Osteoclast-like cell formation and its regulation by osteotropic hormones in mouse bone marrow cultures, Endocrinology 122(4):1373–1382, 1988.

101. Paxinos G, Chai SY, Christopoulos G, et al: In vitro autoradiographic localization of calcitonin and amylin binding sites in monkey brain, J Chem Neuroanat 27(4):217–236, 2004.

102. Hilton JM, Chai SY, Sexton PM: In vitro autoradiographic localization of the calcitonin receptor isoforms, C1a and C1b, in rat brain, Neuroscience 69(4):1223–1237, 1995.

103. Lin HY, Harris TL, Flannery MS, et al: Expression cloning of an adenylate cyclase-coupled calcitonin receptor, Science 254(5034):1022–1024, 1991.

104. Nag K, Kato A, Sultana N, et al: Fish receptor has novel features, General and Comparative Endocrinology 154:48–58, 2007.
105. Gorn AH, Lin HY, Yamin M, et al: Cloning, characterization, and expression of a human calcitonin receptor from an ovarian carcinoma cell line, J Clin Invest 90(5):1726–1735, 1992.
106. Moore EE, Kuestner RE, Stroop SD, et al: Functionally different isoforms of the human calcitonin receptor result from alternative splicing of the gene transcript, Mol Endocrinol 9(8):959–968, 1995.
107. Albrandt K, Brady EM, Moore CX, et al: Molecular cloning and functional expression of a third isoform of the human calcitonin receptor and partial characterization of the calcitonin receptor gene, Endocrinology 136(12):5377–5384, 1995.
108. Poyner DR, Sexton PM, Marshall I, et al: International Union of Pharmacology. XXXII. The mammalian calcitonin gene-related peptides, adrenomedullin, amylin, and calcitonin receptors, Pharmacol Rev 54(2):233–246, 2002.
109. Houssami S, Findlay DM, Brady CL, et al: Divergent structural requirements exist for calcitonin receptor binding specificity and adenylate cyclase activation, Mol Pharmacol 47(4):798–809, 1995.
110. Seck T, Baron R, Horne WC: Binding of filamin to the C-terminal tail of the calcitonin receptor controls recycling, J Biol Chem 278(12):10408–10416, 2003.
111. Seck T, Baron R, Horne WC: The alternatively spliced deltae13 transcript of the rabbit calcitonin receptor dimerizes with the C1a isoform and inhibits its surface expression, J Biol Chem 278(25):23085–23093, 2003.
112. Zolnierowicz S, Cron P, Solinas-Toldo S, et al: Isolation, characterization, and chromosomal localization of the porcine calcitonin receptor gene. Identification of two variants of the receptor generated by alternative splicing, J Biol Chem 269(30):19530–19538, 1994.
113. Anusaksathien O, Laplace C, Li X, et al: Tissue-specific and ubiquitous promoters direct the expression of alternatively spliced transcripts from the calcitonin receptor gene, J Biol Chem 276(25):22663–22674, 2001.
114. Pondel MD, Partington GA, Mould R: Tissue-specific activity of the proximal human calcitonin receptor promoter is mediated by Sp1 and an epigenetic phenomenon, FEBS Lett 554(3):433–438, 2003.
115. Shen Z, Crotti TN, Flannery MR, et al: A novel promoter regulates calcitonin receptor gene expression in human osteoclasts, Biochim Biophys Acta 1769(11–12):659–667, 2007.
116. Hoshiya H, Meguro M, Kashiwagi A, et al: Calcr, a brain-specific imprinted mouse calcitonin receptor gene in the imprinted cluster of the proximal region of chromosome 6, J Hum Genet 48(4):208–211, 2003.
117. Beaudreuil J, Taboulet J, Orcel P, et al: Calcitonin receptor mRNA in mononuclear leucocytes from postmenopausal women: decrease during osteoporosis and link to bone markers with specific isoform involvement, Bone 27(1):161–168, 2000.
118. Nakamura M, Zhang ZQ, Shan L, et al: Allelic variants of human calcitonin receptor in the Japanese population, Hum Genet 99(1):38–41, 1997.
119. Zofkova I, Zajickova K, Hill M, et al: Does polymorphism C1377T of the calcitonin receptor gene determine bone mineral density in postmenopausal women? Exp Clin Endocrinol Diabetes 111(7):447–449, 2003.
120. Tsai FJ, Chen WC, Chen HY, et al: The ALUI calcitonin receptor gene polymorphism (TT) is associated with low bone mineral density and susceptibility to osteoporosis in postmenopausal women, Gynecol Obstet Invest 55(2):82–87, 2003.
121. Braga V, Sangalli A, Malerba G, et al: Relationship among VDR (BsmI and FokI), COLIA1, and CTR polymorphisms with bone mass, bone turnover markers, and sex hormones in men, Calcif Tissue Int 70(6):457–462, 2002.
122. Nakamura M, Morimoto S, Zhang Z, et al: Calcitonin receptor gene polymorphism in Japanese women: correlation with body mass and bone mineral density, Calcif Tissue Int 68(4):211–215, 2001.
123. Braga V, Mottes M, Mirandola S, et al: Association of CTR and COLIA1 alleles with BMD values in peri- and postmenopausal women, Calcif Tissue Int 67(5):361–366, 2000.
124. Masi L, Becherini L, Gennari L, et al: Allelic variants of human calcitonin receptor: distribution and association with bone mass in postmenopausal Italian women, Biochem Biophys Res Commun 245(2):622–626, 1998.
125. Masi L, Cimaz R, Simonini G, et al: Association of low bone mass with vitamin D receptor gene and calcitonin receptor gene polymorphisms in juvenile idiopathic arthritis, J Rheumatol 29(10):2225–2231, 2002.
126. Chen WC, Wu HC, Lu HF, et al: Calcitonin receptor gene polymorphism: a possible genetic marker for patients with calcium oxalate stones, Eur Urol 39(6):716–719, 2001.
127. Wolfe LA 3rd, Fling ME, Xue Z, et al: In vitro characterization of a human calcitonin receptor gene polymorphism, Mutat Res 522(1–2):93–105, 2003.
128. McLatchie LM, Fraser NJ, Main MJ, et al: RAMPs regulate the transport and ligand specificity of the calcitonin-receptor-like receptor, Nature 393(6683):333–339, 1998.
129. Fraser NJ, Wise A, Brown J, et al: The amino terminus of receptor activity modifying proteins is a critical determinant of glycosylation state and ligand binding of calcitonin receptor-like receptor, Mol Pharmacol 55(6):1054–1059, 1999.
130. Udawela M, Hay DL, Sexton PM: The receptor activity modifying protein family of G protein coupled receptor accessory proteins, Semin Cell Dev Biol 15(3):299–308, 2004.
131. Suzuki H, Nakamura I, Takahashi N, et al: Calcitonin-induced changes in the cytoskeleton are mediated by a signal pathway associated with protein kinase A in osteoclasts, Endocrinology 137(11):4685–4690, 1996.
132. Granholm S, Lundberg P, Lerner UH: Calcitonin inhibits osteoclast formation in mouse haematopoietic cells independently of transcriptional regulation by receptor activator of NF-κB and c-Fms, J Endocrinol 195(3):415–427, 2007.
133. Zaidi M, Datta HK, Moonga BS, et al: Evidence that the action of calcitonin on rat osteoclasts is mediated by two G proteins acting via separate post-receptor pathways, J Endocrinol 126(3):473–481, 1990.
134. Offermanns S, Iida-Klein A, Segre GV, et al: G alpha q family members couple parathyroid hormone (PTH)/PTH-related peptide and calcitonin receptors to phospholipase C in COS-7 cells, Mol Endocrinol 10(5):566–574, 1996.
135. Takada K, Kajiya H, Fukushima H, et al: Calcitonin in human odontoclasts regulates root resorption activity via protein kinase A, J Bone Miner Metab 22(1):12–18, 2004.
136. Kiriyama Y, Tsuchiya H, Murakami T, et al: Calcitonin induces IL-6 production via both PKA and PKC pathways in the pituitary folliculo-stellate cell line, Endocrinology 142(8):3563–3569, 2001.
137. Yamaguchi M: Stimulatory effect of calcitonin on Ca2+ inflow in isolated rat hepatocytes, Mol Cell Endocrinol 75(1):65–70, 1991.
138. Wang J, Rout UK, Bagchi IC, et al: Expression of calcitonin receptors in mouse preimplantation embryos and their function in the regulation of blastocyst differentiation by calcitonin, Development 125(21):4293–4302, 1998.
139. Kajiya H, Okamoto F, Fukushima H, et al: Calcitonin inhibits proton extrusion in resorbing rat osteoclasts via protein kinase A, Pflugers Arch 445(6):651–658, 2003.
140. Santhanagopal A, Chidiac P, Horne WC, et al: Calcitonin (CT) rapidly increases NA(+)/H(+) exchange and metabolic acid production: effects mediated selectively by the C1A CT receptor isoform, Endocrinology 142(10):4401–4413, 2001.
141. Chakraborty M, Chatterjee D, Kellokumpu S, et al: Cell cycle-dependent coupling of the calcitonin receptor to different G proteins, Science 251(4997):1078–1082, 1991.
142. Stroop SD, Thompson DL, Kuestner RE, et al: A recombinant human calcitonin receptor functions as an extracellular calcium sensor, J Biol Chem 268(27):19927–19930, 1993.
143. Silver IA, Murrills RJ, Etherington DJ: Microelectrode studies on the acid microenvironment beneath adherent macrophages and osteoclasts, Exp Cell Res 175(2):266–276, 1988.
144. Malgaroli A, Meldolesi J, Zallone AZ, et al: Control of cytosolic free calcium in rat and chicken osteoclasts. The role of extracellular calcium and calcitonin, J Biol Chem 264(24):14342–14347, 1989.
145. Raggatt LJ, Evdokiou A, Findlay DM: Sustained activation of Erk1/2 MAPK and cell growth suppression by the insert-negative, but not the insert-positive isoform of the human calcitonin receptor, J Endocrinol 167(1):93–105, 2000.
146. Zhang Z, Baron R, Horne WC: Integrin engagement, the actin cytoskeleton, and c-Src are required for the calcitonin-induced tyrosine phosphorylation of paxillin and HEF1, but not for calcitonin-induced Erk1/2 phosphorylation, J Biol Chem 275(47):37219–37223, 2000.
147. Findlay DM, Sexton PM: Calcitonin, Growth Factors 22(4):217–224, 2004.
148. Okumura S, Mizoguchi T, Sato N, et al: Coordination of microtubules and the actin cytoskeleton is important in osteoclast function, but calcitonin disrupts sealing zones without affecting microtubule networks, Bone 39(4):684–693, 2006.
149. Shyu JF, Shih C, Tseng CY, et al: Calcitonin induces podosome disassembly and detachment of osteoclasts by modulating Pyk2 and Src activities, Bone 40(5):1329–1342, 2007.
150. Findlay DM, Raggatt LJ, Bouralexis S, et al: Calcitonin decreases the adherence and survival of HEK-293 cells by a caspase-independent mechanism, J Endocrinol 175(3):715–725, 2002.
151. Morfis M, Tilakaratne N, Furness SG, et al: Receptor activity modifying proteins differentially modulate the G protein-coupling efficiency of amylin receptors, Endocrinology 149:5423–5431, 2008.
152. Schneider HG, Raue F, Zink A, et al: Down-regulation of calcitonin receptors in T47D cells by internalization of calcitonin-receptor complexes, Mol Cell Endocrinol 58(1):9–15, 1988.
153. Wada S, Martin TJ, Findlay DM: Homologous regulation of the calcitonin receptor in mouse osteoclast-like cells and human breast cancer T47D cells, Endocrinology 136(6):2611–2621, 1995.
154. Yasuda S, Wada S, Arao Y, et al: Interaction between 3′ untranslated region of calcitonin receptor messenger ribonucleic acid (RNA) and adenylate/uridylate (AU)-rich element binding proteins (AU-rich RNA-binding factor 1 and Hu antigen R). Endocrinology 145(4):1730–1738, 2004.
155. Binstock ML, Mundy GR: Effect of calcitonin and glucocorticoids in combination on the hypercalcemia of malignancy, Ann Intern Med 93(2):269–272, 1980.
156. Hazard JB: The C cells (parafollicular cells) of the thyroid gland and medullary thyroid carcinoma. A review, Am J Pathol 88(1):213–250, 1977.
157. Sipple JH: Multiple endocrine neoplasia type 2 syndromes: historical perspectives, Henry Ford Hosp Med J 32(4):219–221, 1984.
158. Block MA, Jackson CE, Greenawald KA, et al: Clinical characteristics distinguishing hereditary from sporadic medullary thyroid carcinoma. Treatment implications, Arch Surg 115(2):142–148, 1980.
159. Wells SA Jr, Ontjes DA: Multiple endocrine neoplasia type II, Annu Rev Med 27:263–268, 1976.
160. Melvin KE, Tashjian AH Jr: The syndrome of excessive thyrocalcitonin produced by medullary carcinoma of the thyroid, Proc Natl Acad Sci U S A 59(4):1216–1222, 1968.
161. Ng KW, Livesey SA, Larkins RG, et al: Calcitonin effects on growth and on selective activation of type II isoenzyme of cyclic adenosine 3′:5′-monophosphate-dependent protein kinase in T 47D human breast cancer cells, Cancer Res 43(2):794–800, 1983.
162. Thomas S, Muralidharan A, Shah GV: Knock-down of calcitonin receptor expression induces apoptosis and growth arrest of prostate cancer cells, Int J Oncol 31(6):1425–1437, 2007.
163. Gillespie MT, Thomas RJ, Pu ZY, et al: Calcitonin receptors, bone sialoprotein and osteopontin are expressed in primary breast cancers, Int J Cancer 73(6):812–815, 1997.
164. Wang X, Nakamura M, Mori I, et al: Calcitonin receptor gene and breast cancer: quantitative analysis with laser capture microdissection, Breast Cancer Res Treat 83(2):109–117, 2004.
165. Thomas S, Chigurupati S, Anbalagan M, et al: Calcitonin increases tumorigenicity of prostate cancer cells: evidence for the role of protein kinase A and urokinase-type plasminogen receptor, Mol Endocrinol 20(8):1894–1911, 2006.

166. Chien J, Ren Y, Qing Wang Y, et al: Calcitonin is a prostate epithelium-derived growth stimulatory peptide, Mol Cell Endocrinol 181(1–2):69–79, 2001.

167. Sabbisetti V, Chigurupati S, Thomas S, et al: Calcitonin stimulates the secretion of urokinase-type plasminogen activator from prostate cancer cells: its possible implications on tumor cell invasion, Int J Cancer 118(11):2694–2702, 2006.

168. Han B, Nakamura M, Zhou G, et al: Calcitonin inhibits invasion of breast cancer cells: involvement of urokinase-type plasminogen activator (uPA) and uPA receptor, Int J Oncol 28(4):807–814, 2006.

169. Shah GV, Rayford W, Noble MJ, et al: Calcitonin stimulates growth of human prostate cancer cells through receptor-mediated increase in cyclic adenosine 3′,5′-monophosphates and cytoplasmic Ca2+ transients, Endocrinology 134(2):596–602, 1994.

170. Evdokiou A, Raggatt LJ, Atkins GJ, et al: Calcitonin receptor-mediated growth suppression of HEK-293 cells is accompanied by induction of p21WAF1/CIP1 and G2/M arrest, Mol Endocrinol 13(10):1738–1750, 1999.

171. Jagger C, Chambers T, Pondel M: Transgenic mice reveal novel sites of calcitonin receptor gene expression during development, Biochem Biophys Res Commun 274(1):124–129, 2000.

172. Zhu LJ, Cullinan-Bove K, Polihronis M, et al: Calcitonin is a progesterone-regulated marker that forecasts the receptive state of endometrium during implantation, Endocrinology 139(9):3923–3934, 1998.

173. Li HY, Shen JT, Chang SP, et al: Calcitonin promotes outgrowth of trophoblast cells on endometrial epithelial cells: involvement of calcium mobilization and protein kinase C activation, Placenta 29(1):20–29, 2008.

174. Ismail PM, DeMayo FJ, Amato P, et al: Progesterone induction of calcitonin expression in the murine mammary gland, J Endocrinol 180(2):287–295, 2004.

175. Salido M, Vilches J, Lopez A: Neuropeptides bombesin and calcitonin induce resistance to etoposide induced apoptosis in prostate cancer cell lines, Histol Histopathol 15(3):729–738, 2000.

176. Asrari M, Lobner D: Calcitonin potentiates oxygen-glucose deprivation-induced neuronal death, Exp Neurol 167(1):183–188, 2001.

177. Potts JT, Finkelstein J: Medical treatment of hypercalcemia. In DeGroot LJ, Jameson JL: Endocrinology, vol 2, ed 5, Philadelphia, 2006, WB Saunders.

178. Chesnut CH 3rd, Silverman S, Andriano K, et al: A randomized trial of nasal spray salmon calcitonin in postmenopausal women with established osteoporosis: the prevent recurrence of osteoporotic fractures study. PROOF Study Group, Am J Med 109(4):267–276, 2000.

179. Chesnut CH 3rd, Azria M, Silverman S, et al: Salmon calcitonin: a review of current and future therapeutic indications, Osteoporos Int 19(4):479–491, 2008.

180. Chesnut CH 3rd, Majumdar S, Newitt DC, et al: Effects of salmon calcitonin on trabecular microarchitecture as determined by magnetic resonance imaging: results from the QUEST study, J Bone Miner Res 20(9):1548–1561, 2005.

181. Jiang Y, Zhao J, Geusens P, et al: Femoral neck trabecular microstructure in ovariectomized ewes treated with calcitonin: MRI microscopic evaluation, J Bone Miner Res 20(1):125–130, 2005.

182. Lee YH, Sinko PJ: Oral delivery of salmon calcitonin, Adv Drug Deliv Rev 42(3):225–238, 2000.

183. Komarova SV, Shum JB, Paige LA, et al: Regulation of osteoclasts by calcitonin and amphiphilic calcitonin conjugates: role of cytosolic calcium, Calcif Tissue Int 73(3):265–273, 2003.

184. Behets C, Williams JM, Chappard D, et al: Effects of calcitonin on subchondral trabecular bone changes and on osteoarthritic cartilage lesions after acute anterior cruciate ligament deficiency, J Bone Miner Res 19(11):1821–1826, 2004.

185. Sondergaard BC, Oestergaard S, Christiansen C, et al: The effect of oral calcitonin on cartilage turnover and surface erosion in an ovariectomized rat model, Arthritis Rheum 56(8):2674–2678, 2007.

186. Bagger YZ, Tanko LB, Alexandersen P, et al: Oral salmon calcitonin induced suppression of urinary collagen type II degradation in postmenopausal women: a new potential treatment of osteoarthritis, Bone 37(3):425–430, 2005.

187. Manicourt DH, Azria M, Mindeholm L, et al: Oral salmon calcitonin reduces Lequesne's algofunctional index scores and decreases urinary and serum levels of biomarkers of joint metabolism in knee osteoarthritis, Arthritis Rheum 54(10):3205–3211, 2006.

188. Sondergaard BC, Wulf H, Henriksen K, et al: Calcitonin directly attenuates collagen type II degradation by inhibition of matrix metalloproteinase expression and activity in articular chondrocytes, Osteoarthritis Cartilage 14(8):759–768, 2006.

189. Lin Z, Pavlos NJ, Cake MA, et al: Evidence that human cartilage and chondrocytes do not express calcitonin receptor, Osteoarthritis Cartilage 16(4):450–457, 2008.

190. Hayami T, Pickarski M, Wesolowski GA, et al: The role of subchondral bone remodeling in osteoarthritis: reduction of cartilage degeneration and prevention of osteophyte formation by alendronate in the rat anterior cruciate ligament transection model, Arthritis Rheum 50(4):1193–1206, 2004.

191. Mancini L, Paul-Clark MJ, Rosignoli G, et al: Calcitonin and prednisolone display antagonistic actions on bone and have synergistic effects in experimental arthritis, Am J Pathol 170(3):1018–1027, 2007.

Chapter 3

VITAMIN D: From Photosynthesis, Metabolism, and Action to Clinical Applications

ROGER BOUILLON

Historic Overview

Rickets as a bone disease of young children was clearly described by Whistler in 1645[1] and Glisson in 1650.[2] The relationship of this disease with lack of exposure to sunlight was already suspected in the 19th century, since the incidence of rickets was higher in children living in large industrialized towns than in children living in rural districts (see Chapter 15).[3,4] Early in the 20th century, Huldshinsky,[5] Chick et al.,[6] and Hess and Weinstock[7] demonstrated that rachitic children were cured after exposure to sunlight. In the United Kingdom, following an independent line of research in search of essential nutritional factors, Mellanby and Cantag[8] raised dogs on a diet of oatmeal (the basic food in parts of the United Kingdom where rickets was endemic) and observed that they developed rickets, curable by cod liver oil.[9] However, McCollum et al.[10] could demonstrate that cod liver oil made vitamin A-deficient by aeration and heating was still able to cure rickets and thus contained a new essential nutrient called *vitamin D*.[10] The two discoveries of vitamin D were unified by the demonstration of Goldblatt and Soames[11] that irradiation of 7-dehydrocholesterol in the skin could produce the antirachitic vitamin D. Similar observations were made by Hess and Weinstock.[7] Windaus,[12] a German chemist, then identified the structure of vitamins D$_2$ and D$_3$ after irradiation of plant sterols (ergosterol) or 7-dehydrocholesterol,[12] which earned him the Nobel Prize in chemistry in 1928.

The elucidation of the mode of action of vitamin D can be separated in several phases: the discovery of (1) the endogenous activation of vitamin D by sequential hydroxylations at C_{25} and C_1; (2) the molecular mechanisms following the binding of 1,25-dihydroxyvitamin D [1,25(OH)$_2$D] to a specific and quite ubiquitous nuclear transcription factor, vitamin D receptor (VDR), a receptor now known to recruit a large number of proteins; and (3) the regulation of the expression of a very large number of genes (between 1% and 5% of the human genome) involved in either calcium homeostasis or related to cell proliferation or differentiation.

Table 3-1. Adequate Intake, Previous Recommended Dietary Allowance, Reasonable Daily Allowance, and Tolerable Upper Limit for Vitamin D

	Age (Years)	RDA* μg/d (IU)	AI† μg/d (IU)	Reasonable† Daily Allowance (IU)	UL‡ μg/d (IU)
Infants	0.0-1.0	7.5 μg (300 IU)	5 μg (200 IU)	200-400 IU	25 μg (1000 IU)
Children	1-10	10 μg (400 IU)	5 μg (200 IU)	200-400 IU	50 μg (2000 IU)
Adults	11-24	10 μg (400 IU)	5 μg (200 IU)	200-400 IU	50 μg (2000 IU)
	25-50	5 μg (200 IU)	5 μg (200 IU)	200-400 IU	50 μg (2000 IU)
	51-70	5 μg (200 IU)	10 μg (400 IU)	400-600 IU	50 μg (2000 IU)
	70+	5 μg (200 IU)	15 μg (600 IU)	600-800 IU	50 μg (2000 IU)
Pregnant or lactating women		10 μg (400 IU)	5 μg (200 IU)	200-400 IU	50 μg (2000 IU)

AI, Adequate intake; *RDA*, recommended dietary allowance; *UL*, upper limit.
*Data from the Food and Nutrition Board, National Research Council, NAS: Recommended Dietary Allowances, 10th ed. Washington, DC: National Academy Press, 1989.
†Data from the Food and Nutrition Board: Dietary Reference Intakes for Calcium, Phosphorus, Magnesium, Vitamin D and Fluoride. Washington, DC: National Academy Press, 1997. Fairly similar advice is given by the European Food Safety Authority.[23]
‡Similar upper levels for vitamin D intake were defined by the European Food Safety Authority,[23] defining 25 μg or 1000 IU/d as the upper limit for children 0 to 10 years of age and 50 μg or 2000 IU/d for children older than 11 years and adults.

Origin of Vitamin D: Nutrition and Photosynthesis

Vitamin D can be obtained from dietary sources of vegetal (vitamin D_2 or ergocalciferol) or animal origin (vitamin D_3 or cholecalciferol). About 50% of dietary vitamin D is absorbed by the enterocytes and transported to the blood circulation via chylomicrons. Part of this vitamin D is taken up by a variety of tissues (fat and muscle) before the chylomicron remnants and its vitamin D finally reaches the hepatocytes. The best food sources are fatty fish or its liver oils, but it is also found in small amounts in butter, cream, and egg yolk. Both human and cow's milk are poor sources of vitamin D, providing only 15 to 40 IU/L, and equally minimal concentrations of 25(OH)D or 1,25(OH)$_2$D.[13] Only an intake of pharmacologic amounts of vitamin D (6000 IU/d) can increase the vitamin D concentration of milk to a level equivalent to the daily requirements of an infant.[14] Vitamin D intake is a poor predictor of serum 25(OH)D concentrations in subjects with an intake between 2 and 20 μg/d.[15,16] It is very difficult to obtain adequate vitamin D from a natural diet. However, in North America, 98% of fluid and dried milk (≥400 IU/L), as well as some margarine, butter, and certain cereals, are fortified with vitamin D_2 (irradiated ergosterol) or D_3, but the real vitamin D content is frequently quite different from the labeling standard. Skim milk and even proprietary infant formula frequently do not have the stated vitamin D content.[17,18] Vitamin D is remarkably stable and does not deteriorate when food is heated or stored for long periods. The Second National Health and Nutrition Survey (NHANES II) reported a median intake of about 3 μg/d in adults (range 0 to 49 μg),[19] whereas a slightly lower median intake (2.3 μg) was recorded in older women.[20] In view of the low vitamin D content of a vegetarian diet (natural vitamin D intake is indeed related to intake of animal fat), vitamin D deficiency and rickets is a risk factor for strictly vegetarian children with insufficient sun exposure or vitamin D supplementation.[21]

Nature probably intended that most vitamin D would be generated by photosynthesis in the skin, with minor contribution from food sources. However, exposure to sunlight also increases the risk of dermal photodamage and several skin cancers, including melanoma. This was no real problem during human evolution, but with increasing life expectancy, the benefits of UV light for the photosynthesis of vitamin D should be compared with

Table 3-2. Symptoms of Vitamin D Toxicity

Hypercalciuria
Kidney stones
Hypercalcemia
Hyperphosphatemia
Polyuria
Polydipsia
Decalcification of bone
Ectopic calcification of soft tissues (kidney and lung)
Nausea and vomiting
Anorexia
Constipation
Headache
Hypertension

the lifetime risk of skin damage, especially since vitamin D supplementation can safely replace the skin synthesis. The recommended dietary allowances by the U.S. Food and Nutrition Board of the National Research Council and the 1998 updated recommendations are given in Table 3-1, and similar recommendations are still valid in Europe.[22,23] However, these recommendations were based on rudimentary knowledge of optimal vitamin D status and need to be revised upwards.

Hypervitaminosis can occur when pharmaceutical vitamin D is taken in excess, with a wide variety of symptoms and signs related to hypercalciuria, hypercalcemia, and metastatic calcifications (Table 3-2). The toxic dosage has not been established for all ages, but infants and children are more susceptible. Toxicity should always be monitored when daily doses markedly exceeding the present upper limit of more than 50 μg are given for a longer period. Overproduction of renal 1,25(OH)$_2$D by abnormal hormonal stimuli (as seen in fibroblast growth factor-23 [FGF-23] or Klotho-null mice) or absence of CYP24A1 (see later), the main catabolizing enzyme, causes the same calcemic side effects, with severe multiple-organ calcification (especially kidney, vascular wall, and heart valves) leading to premature death.[24]

Most vertebrates also accomplish their needs for vitamin D by photochemical synthesis in the skin; therefore, vitamin D is not a true vitamin. It is formed from 7-dehydrocholesterol (7DHC or provitamin D_3), which is present in large amounts in cell membranes of keratinocytes of the basal or spinous epidermal layers. By the action of ultraviolet B (UVB) light (290 to 315 mm), the B ring of 7DHC can be broken to form previtamin D_3. Previtamin D_3 is unstable, and in the lipid bilayer of membranes, it is rapidly isomerized to vitamin D_3 by thermal energy, followed by transport to the serum vitamin D–binding protein and uptake into the liver for further metabolization.

The production of previtamin D_3 is a nonenzymatic photochemical reaction which is not subject to regulation other than substrate (7DHC) availability and intensity of UVB irradiation. 7DHC is the last precursor in the de novo biosynthesis of cholesterol. The enzyme 7HDC-Δ7-reductase (or sterol Δ7-reductase) catalyses the production of cholesterol from 7DHC. Inactivating mutations of the 7DHC-Δ7-reductase gene[25] are the hallmark of the autosomal recessive Smith-Lemli-Opitz syndrome, characterized by high tissue and serum 7DHC levels and multiple anomalies, including craniofacial dysmorphism and mental retardation due to the lack of cholesterol synthesis.[26] These patients may exhibit sometimes increased serum vitamin D and 25(OH)D concentrations.[27] Likewise, animals pretreated with a specific sterol-Δ7-reductase inhibitor also exhibit an augmented vitamin D synthesis following UVB irradiation.[28] With increasing human age, cutaneous stores of provitamin D decrease, together with decreased photoproduction of vitamin D.[16] In cats and the feline species in general, the high cutaneous sterol-Δ7-reductase activity hampers photoproduction of vitamin D, making it a true vitamin.[29] Apart from substrate (7DHC) availability, the photochemical synthesis of vitamin D_3 in the skin largely depends on the amount of UVB photons that strike the basal epidermal layers. Glass, sunscreen, clothes, and skin pigment absorb UVB and blunt vitamin D_3 synthesis. Latitude, time of day, and season are factors that influence the intensity of solar radiation and the cutaneous production of vitamin D_3. Therefore, there is a risk for a shortage of vitamin D supply during winter and spring. In both the Northern and Southern hemispheres above 40 degrees latitude, vitamin D_3 synthesis of the skin decreases or disappears during winter months, owing to the low inclination of the sun and the atmospheric filtration of the shortest (but effective for vitamin D_3 synthesis) UV waves of sunlight. The importance of skin synthesis of vitamin D_3 to maintain normal vitamin D status is best reflected by the vitamin D deficiency observed in submarine personnel or inhabitants of Antarctica[30] during prolonged absence of sun exposure, and also by the extremely high prevalence of vitamin D deficiency in countries where exposure to sunlight is extremely low for cultural and religious reasons, as in several Arabian countries with strict adherence to Islamic rules for body covering.[31-34] Solar exposure of 2 hours per week of the face and hands is probably sufficient for maintaining normal 25(OH)D concentrations in children[35] and adults but should be further fine-tuned according to the climate and latitude.[36]

Nature has built in several feedback mechanisms to minimize the risk that prolonged sun exposure would cause vitamin D intoxication. Cutaneous vitamin D and especially previtamin D are photosensitive and will be degraded to inactive sterols (lumisterol, tachysterol) before they are translocated to the circulation (Fig. 3-1). Only a maximum of 10% to 15% of the provitamin D will be converted to vitamin D. Sunlight-induced melanin synthesis, acting as a natural sunscreen, provides an additional negative feedback.

Metabolism of Vitamin D

Vitamin D is biologically inert and requires two successive hydroxylations in the liver (on C_{25}) and kidney (on the α position of C_1), using cytochrome P450 enzymes[37,38] to form its hormonally active metabolite, $1\alpha,25$-dihydroxyvitamin D (see Fig. 3-1).

25-HYDROXYLATION

25(OH)D was the first metabolite identified after the availability of radiolabeled vitamin D_3.[39,40] Although the liver is probably the main tissue responsible for 25-hydroxylation of vitamin D, extrahepatic 25-hydroxylation has been observed in vitro in a large number of tissues. In vivo observations after hepatectomy in rats also revealed that the conversion rate of [^{3}H]-vitamin D was still about 10% when compared with intact rats.[40] The hepatic 25-hydroxylation step is probably performed by more than one enzyme, localized either in the inner mitochondrial membrane (CYP27A1 or sterol 27-hydroxylase) or in the microsomes (including CYP2D11, CYP2D25, CYP3A4, and especially CYP2R1).[37,41,42] CYP27A1 is a multifunctional enzyme with broad substrate specificity and is mainly involved in the 26- or 27-hydroxylation of cholesterol and bile-acid precursors.[37] The rather mild (if any) disturbance of vitamin D metabolism in animals or humans lacking this enzyme[43] indicates that the 25-hydroxylation of vitamin D does not rely exclusively on the activity of CYP27A1. It is therefore likely that a microsomal enzyme is the more physiologic enzyme, as initially suspected on the basis of hepatic enzyme activity being much higher and with lower K_m in the microsomal fraction when compared with mitochondrial 25-hydroxylase activity.[44] The microsomal enzyme activity is up-regulated by vitamin D deficiency or by prior exposure to phenobarbital. The most important 25-hydroxylase is probably CYP2R1, since a homozygous mutation was identified in a patient with classical rickets with low 25(OH)D levels.[42]

1α-HYDROXYLATION

25(OH)D is biologically inactive and requires further hydroxylation in the kidney[45,46] to the active hormone, $1,25(OH)_2D$, by 25-hydroxyvitamin D-1α-hydroxylase (CYP27B1). The production of $1,25(OH)_2D$ is regulated primarily at this final step by several factors (vide infra). The rat, mouse, and human 1α-hydroxylase have been cloned by several groups[47-51] and mapped on human chromosome 12q13.3 in close vicinity to the VDR gene. The proximal renal tubule is the principle site of 1α-hydroxylation, but high levels of 1α-hydroxylase mRNA have also been found in human keratinocytes,[48] and its gene expression is also observed in mouse macrophages[52] and about ten other tissues.[24] 1α-Hydroxylase activity is under tight control by $1,25(OH)_2D$ (negative but probably indirect feedback); parathyroid hormone (PTH), calcitonin, and insulin-like growth factor 1 (all positive feedback); and phosphate, calcium, and especially FGF-23 (negative regulation).[38,53,54] The promoters of the mouse and human 1α-hydroxylase genes have been characterized with a profound responsiveness to PTH and a negative regulation by $1,25(OH)_2D$[55,56] by complex chromatin and DNA modifications.[57]

Pseudovitamin D–deficiency rickets (PDDR), also known as *vitamin D-dependency rickets type I*, is an autosomal recessive disease characterized by failure to thrive, muscle weakness, skeletal deformities, hypocalcemia, secondary hyperparathyroidism, normal to high serum levels of 25(OH)D, and low serum $1,25(OH)_2D$ concentrations, all caused by impaired activity of the renal 1α-hydroxylase.[58] These patients recover with supplementation of physiologic doses of $1,25(OH)_2D$. The human CYP27B1 maps to the previously identified PDDR locus and mutations found in this gene in patients with PDDR provide the molecular genetic basis for the disease.[48,59]

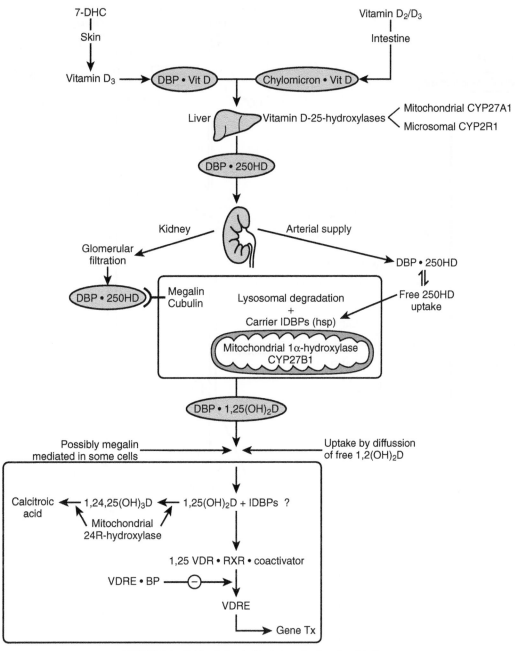

FIGURE 3-1. Origin of vitamin D: photosynthesis and metabolism.

24-HYDROXYLATION: CATABOLISM OR SPECIFIC FUNCTION?

An alternative hydroxylation of 25(OH)D occurs on carbon 24 by the multifunctional enzyme, 24-hydroxylase (CYP24A), mapped on human chromosome 20q13.[60] This enzyme not only initiates the catabolic cascade of 25(OH)D and 1,25(OH)$_2$D[61,62] by 24-hydroxylation but catalyzes also the dehydrogenation of the 24-OH group and performs 23-hydroxylation, resulting in 24-oxo-1,23,25(OH)$_3$D.[62] This C$_{24}$ oxidation pathway finally leads to calcitroic acid, which is the major end product of 1,25(OH)$_2$D (Fig. 3-2). In vivo evidence for this catabolic role of 24-hydroxylase was provided by the generation of mice deficient in the 24-hydroxylase gene, resulting in pathology consistent with systemic excess of 1,25(OH)$_2$D.[63] The expression of the 24-hydroxylase gene has been detected in virtually all nucleated cells. The induction of *CYP24A* belongs to the most sensitive biomarkers for responsiveness and is explained by the presence of several vitamin D responsive elements in its promoter.[64,65] As a consequence, *CYP24A* mRNA levels appear to fall under the detection limits in *VDR* knockout mice.[50,66] No human mutation in the 24-hydroxylase gene have yet been identified, but local overexpression of the enzyme may be involved in cancer.[67]

OTHER METABOLIC PATHWAYS FOR VITAMIN D AND ITS METABOLITES

Apart from the multifunctional 24-hydroxylation pathway, C$_{23}$ and C$_{26}$ hydroxylation of 1,25(OH)$_2$D is also possible in the absence of prior 24-hydroxylation. The 23-hydroxylation probably only becomes important in the case of vitamin D excess; its major locus is the kidney. In contrast, 26-hydroxylation is mainly performed outside the kidney. Both activities are necessary for

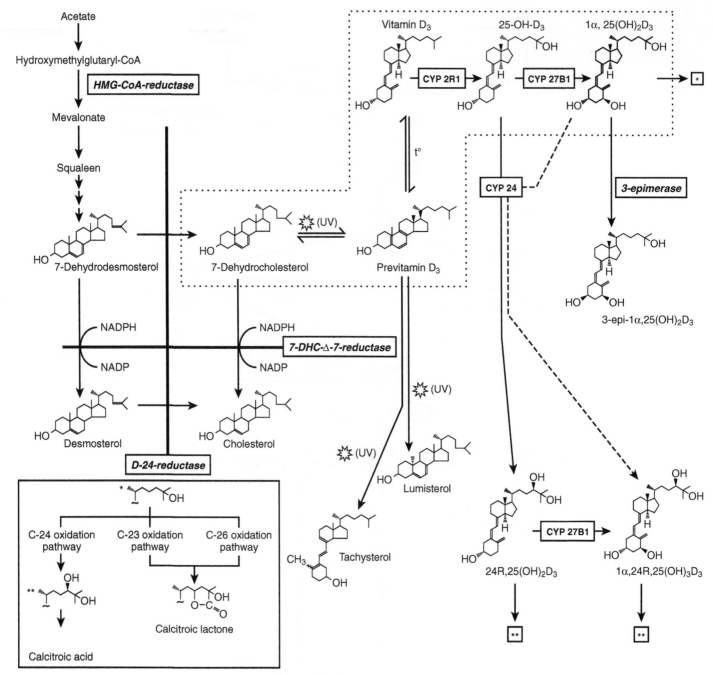

FIGURE 3-2. Catabolism of 1,25(OH)$_2$D.

the formation of 25(OH)D- or 1,25(OH)$_2$D-23,26-lactones (see Fig. 3-1). The A-ring metabolism involves the oxidation of C_{19} and the recently discovered 3-epimerisation. The latter, irreversible, reaction occurs only in a limited number of cells (e.g., keratinocytes, bone, and parathyroid cells) and is performed by hydroxysteroid dehydrogenases.[68]

The enzymes involved in the metabolic degradation of 1,25(OH)$_2$D do not recognize all vitamin D analogs in the same way. Indeed, analogs with either 20-epi or 20-methyl configuration or 16-ene structure show an impaired 23-hydroxylation. These or other analogs are then preferentially hydroxylated on C_{26} or on new terminal carbons of the side chain. Such alternative metabolism can certainly explain part of the specific selectivity profile of a number of analogs (vide infra).

Vitamin D is mainly excreted in the bile after esterification in the liver, but some of its more polar metabolites (e.g., calcitroic acid) are excreted via the urine. The enterohepatic recirculation of vitamin D esters is probably devoid of biological relevance.

Vitamin D Transport

Nutritional vitamin D is absorbed by the gut and then transported via the lymphatic system by chylomicrons[69] and stored in several tissues (e.g., fat and muscle). Skin-produced vitamin D probably binds directly to an α-globulin known as *vitamin D binding protein* (DBP) and is then transported to the liver, where it is hydroxylated and thereafter released as 25(OH)D.

Human DBP,[70] detected immunologically in 1959 as a group-specific component, or Gc-globulin,[71] is a 43-amino-acid glycoprotein synthesized by the liver. Long before DBP's functions had been characterized, its polymorphicity was already used in population genetics, parentage testing, and forensic medicine.[72] Worldwide, over 120 Gc alleles have been detected,[73] making the DBP locus one of the most polymorphic known. The Gc1F, Gc1S and Gc2 are the three most common alleles. Since in the many thousands of sera tested, none had been found of DBP deficiency, such a mutation was for a long time considered to be lethal; but this was contradicted by the generation of viable and fertile homozygous, DBP-deficient mice (DBP-null animals).[74] The existence of similarity among the genes and protein structure of DBP, albumin, and α-fetoprotein is long recognized.[75] The crystal structure, with or without actin, is now available and identified a surface cleft to bind 25(OH)D.[76]

ROLE OF VITAMIN D BINDING PROTEIN FOR VITAMIN D HOMEOSTASIS

DBP, the major plasma carrier of vitamin D_3, all its metabolites, and the vitamin D_3 analogs, has one vitamin D sterol-specific binding site.[75] The relative binding affinity is 25(OH)D-23,26-lactone > 25(OH)D = 24,25(OH)$_2$D = 25,26(OH)$_2$D (K_a = 5.10^8 mol/L at 4° C for human DBP) >> 1,25(OH)$_2$D (4.10^7 mol/L) >> vitamin D >> previtamin D.[77] The affinity for D_2 metabolites is slightly lower than for D_3 metabolites in mammals, but especially in birds. Since probably only non-DBP-bound vitamin D metabolites can readily cross the plasma membrane, and since the VDR has a much higher affinity for 1,25(OH)$_2$D than for 25(OH)D (100-fold difference), while the opposite is true for DBP, it is clear that 1,25(OH)$_2$D has substantially higher cellular uptake than 25(OH)D. This is also confirmed by the distribution space of (radiolabeled) metabolites: 25(OH)D has a distribution space similar to that of DBP and the plasma volume, whereas the distribution space of 1,25(OH)$_2$D is closer to that of intracellular water. The half-life of 25(OH)D and 1,25(OH)$_2$D in the human circulation is about 2 to 3 weeks and 4 to 6 hours, respectively.[78,79] DBP's function in the vitamin D endocrine system is assumed to reflect the "free hormone" hypothesis, which states that the unbound (free) rather than the protein-bound fraction of the active vitamin D hormone is responsible for the biological activity. The plasma concentration of DBP is increased by estrogens in most mammalian species and birds. In women, the DBP concentration therefore doubles at the end of pregnancy.[80] Recent studies with megalin knockout mice indicate that megalin, a lipoprotein-like receptor present at the surface of the proximal tubular cells in the kidney, is responsible for the reabsorption of DBP and of DBP complexed with vitamin D sterols. This megalin reabsorption mechanism may control the availability of the 25(OH)D/DBP complex for the 25(OH)D-1α-hydroxylation enzyme and explain the severe bone disease of megalin-deficient mice.[81]

OTHER FUNCTIONS OF VITAMIN D BINDING PROTEIN

DBP binds globular actin with a high affinity (K_a = 2 × 10^9 mmol/L).[82,83] Actin is the most abundant intracellular protein. The cell motility, shape, and size depend on the ability of globular actin to polymerize into filaments (F-actin). Upon cell injury or cell necrosis, actin is released into extracellular space. However, when actin is released from cells, it may rapidly form filaments with detrimental effects for the microcirculation. Two plasma proteins, DBP and gelsolin, bind actin avidly, thereby acting as "actin-scavenger" system.[84,85]

DBP-null (KO) mice, however, develop normally. They are nevertheless more sensitive to vitamin D deficiency and less sensitive to vitamin D excess, probably by an enhanced urinary loss of vitamin D metabolites.[74] The DBP and megalin KO mice, however, suggest that the main function of DBP is indeed to transport all vitamin D metabolites and preserve them from rapid clearance or urinary loss.

Action and Mode of Action

GENERAL CHARACTERISTICS OF THE VITAMIN D RECEPTOR

Protein

1,25(OH)$_2$D, the hormonally active form of vitamin D, exerts its effects mainly by activating the nuclear VDR, a member of the nuclear-receptor superfamily of ligand-activated transcription factors. Based on structure and function similarities between members of this family, different functional domains can be distinguished in these nuclear-receptor proteins. The short A/B domain at the N-terminus of VDR lacks the usual ligand-independent activation function (AF1). Two highly conserved zinc finger DNA binding motifs constitute the DNA-binding C domain, which also harbors the nuclear localization signal. The D domain or hinge region may regulate the receptor's flexibility between DNA-binding and ligand-binding domains and may be crucial to allowing the heterodimer complex of the ligand-binding domains to interact with two differently oriented response elements (direct repeat or palindrome orientation with variable number of spacer nucleotides). The large multifunctional E region contains the ligand-binding domain, as well as a dimerization surface and a ligand-dependent activation function (AF2) at the extreme C-terminus, represented by helix 12.[86]

Gene

The human *VDR* gene, consisting of 14 exons, spans more than 60 kb on chromosome 12.[87,88] The major *VDR* transcript is a 4.8 kb mRNA species, but multiple promoters and alternative splicing give rise to a multitude of less abundant transcripts that mostly vary in their 5′ untranslated region but encode the same 427-amino-acid protein.[88] However, two of these mRNAs are translated into VDR proteins that contain an additional 23 or 50 amino acids at the N-terminus.[88]

Genomic Actions

Binding of 1,25(OH)$_2$D to VDR generates conformational changes of VDR followed by heterodimerization with unliganded RXR and binding to vitamin D response elements (VDREs) in the promoter region of vitamin D target genes, with subsequent release of corepressors and recruitment of coactivators and general transcription factors for the assembly of an active transcriptional complex.[89] A putative crucial event in this respect is the mousetrap-like intramolecular folding of helix 12, closing off the ligand-binding pocket and exposing the AF2 domain for interaction with coactivators.[90] Corepressors bind and silence unliganded steroid receptors by recruitment of histone deacetylases, maintaining chromatin in a transcriptional repressive state.[91] Coactivators are a group of proteins that allow gene transcription in several waves of activities. First, coactivators of the CBP/p300 family and of the p160 protein family, including the steroid receptor coactivators (SRCs), are recruited.[92-94] These proteins possess intrinsic histone acetyltransferase (HAT) activity and by acetylating histone tails open up the chromatin structure, creating a chromatin environment permissive for gene transcription.[95] In a second wave, the vitamin D receptor interacting protein (DRIP) multimeric complex is recruited, followed by recruitment of basal transcription factors, as well as RNA polymerase II. Finally, target gene transcription is induced.[96] Gene expression can also be mediated by ATP-dependent chromatin remodeling complexes such as SWI/SNF-type and ISWI-type complexes and the multiprotein complex WINAC.[97-99] Distinct regulation of transcriptional coregulators may provide species-specific, tissue-specific, or developmental stage–specific regulation of nuclear receptor function.[100] Furthermore, the expression or the recruitment of these regulatory proteins is regulated by several intracellular signaling pathways[101] and by steroids themselves,[100] with receptor agonists or antagonists inducing preferential recruitment of coactivators or corepressors, respectively.[101]

A hexanucleotide direct repeat spaced by three nucleotides (DR3) is the cognate vitamin D response element (VDRE) to which RXR and VDR bind the 5′ and 3′ half-site, respectively, although alternative options appear to be possible, both with respect to dimer formation (VDR/VDR, VDR/RAR) and target-gene VDRE structure (DR4, DR6; IP9).[102]

Nongenomic Actions

Aside from the VDR transcriptional or genomic effects, several research groups have described rapid effects by 1,25(OH)$_2$D that are independent of transcription and would be mediated by a membrane receptor for 1,25(OH)$_2$D or by the localization of the nuclear VDR near the membrane.[103] These so-called nongenomic effects include the opening of calcium or chloride channels and the activation of second messenger signaling pathways (phosphoinositide turnover, activation of protein kinase C, and the Ras/Raf/ERK/MAPK pathway). A wide variety of rapid and transient modifications in the second messenger signaling system have also been observed for other steroid hormones.[104] At the tissue or cellular level, however, nongenomic activity of vitamin D and its analogs or metabolites have only been described for intestinal calcium absorption (transcaltachia) or cellular differentiation of leukemia cells.[105-107] This pathway seems to prefer 6-s-*cis* to the 6-s-*trans* configuration of vitamin D.[105] Moreover, the agonist/antagonist specificity differs for that of the genomic pathway.[108]

CLASSIC TARGET TISSUES

The action of 1,25(OH)$_2$D on bone, intestine, kidney, and parathyroid glands and its role in mineral metabolism is the result of a complex interplay between calcium and phosphate 1,25(OH)$_2$D, PTH, and phosphatonins. PTH induces calcium mobilization from bone and stimulates 1,25(OH)$_2$D production, but its secretion is inhibited by the action of 1,25(OH)$_2$D on the parathyroid glands (negative feedback). In a second negative feedback loop, 1,25(OH)$_2$D limits its own availability by inhibition of 1α-hydroxylase and stimulation of 24-hydroxylase, inducing 1,25(OH)$_2$D catabolism. In the last few years, considerable progress has been made in the understanding of phosphate homeostasis.[109] The phosphaturic hormone phosphatonin, or FGF-23, is produced by osteocytes and osteoblasts and inhibits the activity of the NPT2 protein. The *NPT2* gene encodes a renal sodium/phosphate cotransporter responsible for reabsorption of phosphate and represents a newly identified target gene for

1,25(OH)$_2$D.[110] Phosphatonin can be indirectly inactivated by a protease encoded by the *PEX* gene, which was identified as the gene that is defective in X-linked hypophosphatemic rickets. FGF-23 secretion is stimulated by 1,25(OH)$_2$D and impairs renal 1α-hydroxylase, creating an additional feedback system so that the production of 1,25(OH)$_2$D is tightly feedback regulated (Fig. 3-3).

Effects on Intestine

The absorption capacity of calcium along the gastrointestinal tract of the rat is dependent on the segment and follows the order ileum > jejunum > duodenum. The efficiency of the small intestine to absorb dietary calcium is increased by 1,25(OH)$_2$D,[111] and the abundance of the vitamin D receptor is highest in the duodenum, followed by jejunum and ileum. Although the exact mechanism by which 1,25(OH)$_2$D alters the flux of calcium

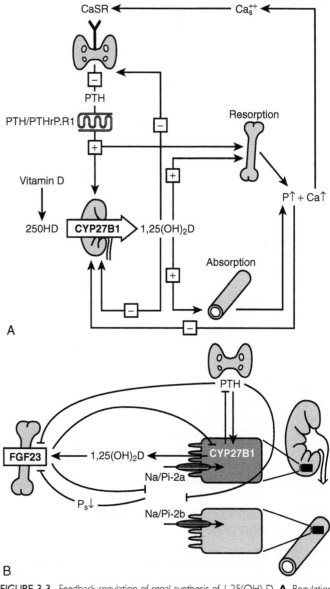

FIGURE 3-3. Feedback regulation of renal synthesis of 1,25(OH)$_2$D. **A,** Regulation of renal 1,25(OH)$_2$D synthesis by parathyroid hormone and calcium, with multiple feedback control mechanisms. *CaSR,* Calcium-sensing receptor. **B,** Regulation of renal 1,25(OH)$_2$D synthesis by FGF23 and phosphate, with several feedback control mechanisms.

across the intestinal absorptive cell is not known, $1,25(OH)_2D$ increases the production and activity of several proteins in the small intestine, including TRPV6 and V5, calbindin-D9K, alkaline phosphatase, and low-affinity Ca-ATPase (PMCA). The entry of Ca^{2+} from the intestinal lumen across the brush border membrane into the enterocyte is mainly regulated by the epithelial channels TRPV6 and V5.[112] The intracellular calcium transfer is considered to be dependent mainly on calbindin-D9K.[113] The transfer of Ca^{2+} from the cytoplasm to the extracellular space requires energy input because of an uphill concentration gradient and an unfavorable electrochemical gradient. Both the plasma membrane calcium pump and a sodium-calcium exchanger play important roles in this process. The stimulatory effect of $1,25(OH)_2D$ on the ATP-dependent uptake of Ca^{2+} at the basolateral membrane involves an increase in *PMCA* gene expression.[114] The essential role of the intestine for calcium and phosphate homeostasis was clearly demonstrated by the phenotype of *VDR* KO mice. Such *VDR*-null mice are phenotypically normal at birth, but after weaning, they develop hypocalcemia, secondary hyperparathyroidism, and hypophosphatemia despite very high levels of $1,25(OH)_2D$. They become growth retarded and develop severe rickets.[66,112,115,116] Mice deficient in 1α-hydroxylase display a similar phenotype.[117,118] This bone and calcium phenotype can be largely corrected by a high dietary calcium intake (especially in combination with high lactose intake) in both knockout models or $1,25(OH)_2D$ treatment of 1α hydroxylase–null mice.[112,119-125] These findings confirm previous observations in humans.[59,126,127] The data strongly suggest that the intestine is the primary target for $1,25(OH)_2D$'s action on calcium/bone homeostasis. This is largely confirmed by genetic mouse models of selective rescue or deletion of *VDR* in the intestine of transgenic mice.[128] The primary molecular targets, however, merit further exploration; ablation of *CaBP-9k* or *TRPV6* or even their combined deficiency have shown no major effects on basal intestinal calcium absorption or serum calcium levels when calcium intake is normal.[129] Paracellular intestinal calcium transport may also be part of the picture of vitamin D's action in that the expression of claudin 2 and claudin 12, both known to form paracellular calcium channels, are induced by $1,25(OH)_2D$ and decreased in the intestine of *VDR*-null mice.[130]

Effects on Kidney

The kidney is important both for the metabolism of $1,25(OH)_2D$ and the reabsorption of calcium and phosphate, processes regulated by $1,25(OH)_2D$. The kidney and more specifically the proximal tubule is the central tissue for 1α-hydroxylation of $25(OH)D$. Chronic renal failure reduces 1α-hydroxylase activity, which ultimately results in renal osteodystrophy or uremic bone disease. $1,25(OH)_2D$ also increased the distal tubular reabsorption of calcium; as in the intestine, TRP channels (now TRPV5), calbindin-D9K and 28K, and the plasma membrane calcium ATPase are involved. Whereas in the intestine, active calcium absorption in the duodenum takes place before the less-regulated diffusion process in the ileum, reabsorption of filtered calcium follows a more logical sequence of massive calcium-sodium reabsorption in the proximal convoluted tubuli, followed by specific, actively regulated calcium reabsorption in the distal parts of the nephron. The crucial role of $1,25(OH)_2D$-regulated renal calcium reabsorption was demonstrated by persistent hypercalciuria and reduction in bone mass in TRPV5-deficient mice.[131] The kidney is also the major component in phosphate homeostasis, as both PTH and FGF-23, in complex interplay with $1,25(OH)_2D$, are able to reduce renal phosphate reabsorption (see Fig. 3-3).

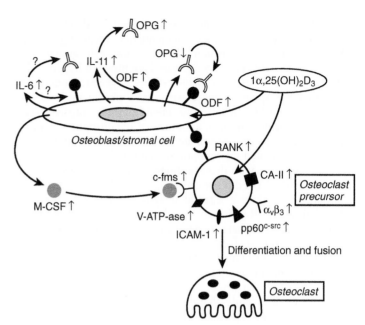

FIGURE 3-4. Effect of $1,25(OH)_2D$ on bone cells and osteoclastogenesis. In osteoblast/stromal cells, $1,25(OH)_2D$ induces ODF expression, down-regulates OPG, and stimulates M-CSF production. It also stimulates production of IL-6 and IL-11, which represent distinct signals in osteoclastogenesis. On osteoclast precursors, $1,25(OH)_2D$ induces the expression of RANK (or ODF receptor) and several osteoclast differentiation markers, such as the vitronectin receptor $\alpha v \beta 3$ and carbonic anhydrase-II. *CA-II,* Carbonic anhydrase-II; *c-fms,* M-CSF receptor; *M-CSF,* macrophage colony-stimulating factor; *ODF,* osteoclast differentiation factor; *OPG,* osteoprotegerin; *V-ATP-ase,* vacuolar adenosine triphosphatase.

Effects on Bone

$1,25(OH)_2D$ has dual effects on bone: it can stimulate osteoclastogenesis and bone resorption as well as modify osteoblast function and bone mineralization. The overall effects of vitamin D metabolites on bone are thus extremely complex. From observations in man and animals, it is clear that vitamin D deficiency or resistance impairs bone-matrix mineralization, whereas osteoblast activity and matrix synthesis are even stimulated. Excess $1,25(OH)_2D$ can clearly enhance osteoclastogenesis and bone resorption (Fig. 3-4). Because bone mineralization and bone structure can be largely normalized in vitamin D- or $1,25(OH)_2D$-deficient or resistant mice by sufficient supply of minerals via active or passive intestinal calcium absorption, it seems that direct effects of vitamin D metabolites on chondrocytes and bone cells are redundant if calcium and phosphate supply are guaranteed. However, most of the genes and proteins typically expressed in osteoblasts and osteoclasts are vitamin D regulated, so it is likely that $1,25(OH)_2D$ can fine-tune bone mineral homeostasis. Moreover, pharmacologic use of vitamin D metabolites or analogs might positively influence bone balance, as shown by human and animal experiments[132,133] and transgenic mice overexpressing osteoblast VDR.[134]

Effects on Growth Plate

The absence of VDR or 1α-hydroxylase creates no detectable phenotype in overall growth or growth plate of prenatal animals, but the longitudinal growth of long bones is impaired after weaning. X-ray analysis reveals advanced rickets, including widening of the epiphyseal growth plate, with an increased width and marked disorganization of the growth plate on histology, including impaired mineralization of hypertrophic chondrocytes.[66,115-118] This increased growth-plate width in VDR or 1α

hydroxylase–null mice cannot be explained by their (normal) chondrocyte proliferation and differentiation, including collagen X and osteopontin expression. The expansion of the growth plate can be largely explained by decreased apoptosis of hypertrophic chondrocytes.[135] Based on analysis of several genetic models with abnormal phosphate homeostasis, serum phosphate levels are probably crucial for hypertrophic chondrocyte apoptosis in vivo. This is confirmed in vitro: apoptosis of hypertrophic chondrocytes is regulated by phosphate levels via the activation of the caspase-9-mediated mitochondrial pathway.[136]

In accordance with these findings, chondrocyte-specific inactivation of the VDR did not cause a growth-plate phenotype and certainly not rickets.[137] Critical analysis of these mice, however, revealed that VDR action in chondrocytes regulates bone development and phosphate homeostasis by inducing expression of paracrine factors such as vascular endothelial growth factor and receptor activator of nuclear factor κB (NFκB) ligand expression, leading to impaired vascular invasion and decreased osteoclast number in the metaphysic, as well as increased bone mass of long bones of juvenile chondrocyte-specific VDR-null mice. In addition, FGF-23 expression in osteoblasts was decreased, probably linked to the increased gene expression profile of NPT2 and 1α-hydroxylase in the kidney and resulting in increased serum levels of phosphate and 1,25(OH)$_2$D.[137]

NONCALCEMIC OR NONCLASSIC ACTIONS OF VITAMIN D ENDOCRINE SYSTEM

The virtual ubiquitous expression of the VDR in all nucleated cells, the presence of a functional 1α-hydroxylase in at least 10 different tissues apart from the kidney, and the very large number of genes that are under direct or indirect control of 1,25(OH)$_2$D all point toward a more universal role for the vitamin D endocrine system than just regulation of calcium/phosphate/bone metabolism. This is not totally unexpected; most other ligands for nuclear receptors also have a very wide spectrum of activities such as androgens, estrogens, glucocorticoids, and retinoids.[24] Based on controlled observations in cells, tissues, and transgenic mice and on observational studies in humans, it seems that the functioning of nearly all major tissues or systems of the organism is modulated by vitamin D.

Skin

The combined presence of vitamin D production, 25-hydroxylase, 1α-hydroxylase, and VDR expression in the epidermis suggests the existence of a unique vitamin D intracrine system in which UVB-irradiated keratinocytes may supply their own needs for 1,25(OH)$_2$D. A role for vitamin D in epidermal homeostasis can also be expected from the prominent effects of vitamin D compounds on keratinocyte growth and differentiation.[138] The epidermal keratinocyte represents the major cell type in the epidermis and most likely the major cutaneous target cell for vitamin D, but many other cell types present in the epidermis are also vitamin D targets.

Based on studies of 1α hydroxylase–deficient mice, the repair of the essential barrier function of the skin is impaired in the absence of vitamin D action.[139] The major skin phenotype of both VDR-null mice and children with VDR mutations is, however, the development of total alopecia. Hair development at birth is normal, but hair loss starts after the first catagen and ultimately leads to alopecia totalis associated with large dermal cysts. The absence of alopecia in vitamin D–deficient WT mice or in mice with CYP27B1 mutations clearly suggests that the absence of

receptor and not its ligand is the cause of the skin phenotype. Mutations in the NR corepressor, hairless, or keratinocyte-specific loss of interaction of Lefl with β-catenin (part of the Wnt signaling pathway) produce a strikingly similar alopecia. There is therefore little doubt that ligand-independent effects of the VDR are required for normal keratinocyte stem cell function.

As expected from animal studies, no clear skin disorders are linked to vitamin D deficiency or insufficiency in humans. The very same photons that can generate the photoconversion of 7-dehydrocholesterol into previtamin D are also able to cause DNA damage and, ultimately, photoaging and increase the risk for skin cancer, so exposure to the UVB or sunlight needed to produce vitamin D always involves a small but cumulative risk of skin damage. This risk is especially relevant for humans with a fair skin type (phototypes 1 and 2).[140] Although 1,25(OH)$_2$D is able to generate a strong photoprotective effect against UVB-mediated events in cultured keratinocytes,[141,142] the overall effect is negative.

Cell Proliferation and Cancer

Exposure to 1,25(OH)$_2$D of virtually all normal cells and even most malignant cells results in an accumulation in the G0/G1 phase of the cell cycle.[143-145] This inhibition of cell proliferation involves a large number of mechanisms and genes, and the exact sequence of events between VDR-mediated transactivation of genes and the actual G0/G1 arrest is probably cell-type specific. A general downstream effect is the regulation of the E2F family of transcription factors, which act as master switch for a very large number of genes involved in cell-cycle progression. These EF factors are under the control of the retinoblastoma protein members (especially pocket proteins p107 and p130), and their phosphorylation state is regulated by cyclins and cyclin-dependent kinases (p18, p19, p21, or p27), many of which are regulated by 1,25(OH)$_2$D.[143,146] However, 1,25(OH)$_2$D may also inhibit cell growth by interfering with signaling pathways initiated by TGF-β, epidermal growth factor (IGF), prostaglandins,[147] and Wnt ligands,[148] as well as by intervening in other mitogenic signaling pathways (e.g., ERK/MAPK pathway and c-myc) (Fig. 3-5).[149-156] Moreover, 1,25(OH)$_2$D can regulate apoptosis and angiogenesis, mechanisms well known to be important for cancer cell expansion. In view of these well-established in vitro effects, one might expect a greater sensitivity for carcinogenesis in VDR-null mice. Epidermal, mammary, and intestinal cells of such animals do indeed show signs of hyperproliferation. Moreover, when exposed to chemocarcinogens or oncogens, VDR-null mice develop more mammary cancer–type lesions, skin tumors, and lymphomas.[157,158]

In humans, absolute VDR or CYP27B1 deficiencies are rare, but vitamin D deficiency is highly frequent. This obviously raises the question whether such vitamin D deficiency is associated with increased risk of cancer in humans. Such a hypothesis was originally reinforced by observations of higher cancer prevalence in areas of the United States and Japan with lower UVB exposure. Serum concentrations of 25(OH)D are, of course, a much better indication of the real vitamin D status, and a vast literature links lower levels of 25(OH)D with higher prevalence of the major cancers, especially colon and breast cancer, with more mixed results for prostate cancer. The inverse association between colorectal cancer or breast cancer and serum 25(OH)D levels was confirmed by the results of the Third National Health and Nutrition Examination Survey (NHANES III),[159] although 25(OH)D levels were not related to overall cancer mortality. In most of the

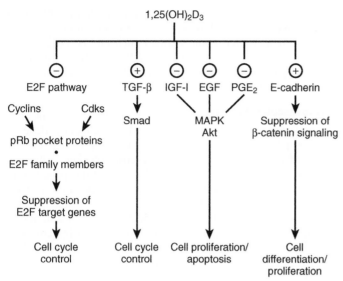

FIGURE 3-5. Effect of 1,25(OH)$_2$D on cell-cycle progression. 1,25(OH)$_2$D treatment leads to a cell cycle phase–specific effect characterized by an accumulation of cells in G$_1$ through modulation of different signaling pathways. (−), Inhibitory effect; (+), stimulatory effect; *EGF,* epidermal growth factor; *IGF-1,* insulin-like growth factor 1; *PGE2,* prostaglandin E2; *pRb,* retinoblastoma tumor-suppressor gene; *TGF-β,* transforming growth factor β.

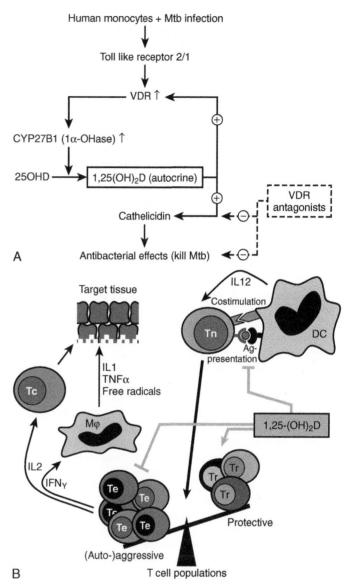

FIGURE 3-6. Immune effects of the vitamin D endocrine system. In the innate immune system, 1,25-(OH)$_2$D strengthens the antimicrobial function of monocytes/macrophages, for example, through enhanced expression of the cathelicidin antimicrobial peptide, eventually leading to better clearance of pathogenic microorganisms. In the acquired immune system, the immunomodulatory effects of 1,25(OH)$_2$D on players of the adaptive immune system can lead to the protection of target tissues in autoimmune diseases and transplantation. 1,25(OH)$_2$D inhibits the surface expression of MHC II–complexed antigen and of costimulatory molecules, as well as the production of the cytokine IL-12 in antigen-presenting cells (such as dendritic cells), thereby shifting the polarization of T cells from an (auto-)aggressive effector (Te) towards a protective or regulatory (Tr) phenotype. 1,25(OH)$_2$D also directly exerts its immunomodulatory effects at the level of T cells.

vast number of cross-sectional or observational studies, the higher cancer risk was found in subjects with serum 25(OH)D levels below 20 ng/mL, but most studies also revealed a significant trend across the different 25(OH)D subgroups and risk of cancer. Meta-analysis of studies addressing the association between 25(OH)D levels suggest that women with serum 25(OH)D of approximately 48 ng/mL (median of the top quintile) had a 50% lower risk of breast cancer than those with serum less than 13 ng/mL in the lowest quintile,[160] and that individuals with serum 25(OH)D levels greater than 32 ng/mL had a 50% lower incidence of colorectal cancer than those with relatively low levels (≤12 ng/mL).[161] However, a number of studies also link higher vitamin D nutritional status with a higher prevalence or more aggressive type of cancer.[24,162]

The final question is, of course, whether serum 25(OH)D is a predictor or has a causative relation with the overall cancer risk. Intervention studies should be able to provide the answer. In the Women's Health Initiative (WHI) study, a significant inverse relationship was found between baseline levels of serum 25(OH)D and subsequent colorectal cancer incidence, but postmenopausal women receiving calcium (1 g) plus vitamin D (400 IU) did not develop less colon cancer than control patients.[163] In a much smaller 4-yr study in postmenopausal women, higher doses of calcium (1.4 to 1.5 g) and vitamin D (1100 IU), which raised serum 25(OH)D to mean levels above 80 nmol/L, did significantly reduce overall cancer risk.[164] The small number of cancer deaths and a major confounding factor of calcium intake, however, limit the value of this study to hypothesis, and much larger prospective studies with substantial vitamin D supplementation are essential.

Immune Function and Vitamin D

All immune cells (antigen-presenting cells, T and B cells, natural killer [NK] cells, and even mast cells) express at certain stages of their differentiation a functional VDR. Antigen-presenting cells (dendritic cells and equivalent resident cells, as well as

monocytes/macrophages) can synthesize 1,25(OH)$_2$D using the same enzyme as in the kidney but controlled by immune stimuli instead of calciotropic hormones.[52,165-167] Finally, 1,25(OH)$_2$D regulates a wide range of genes that play crucial roles in the immune system. The overall effects are different for the innate immune system (largely mediated by monocytes/macrophages) than for the acquired immune system. The innate immune system, upon exposure to bacterial agents, is first stimulated to produce 1,25(OH)$_2$D (Fig. 3-6A) and thereafter activated by this paracrine 1,25(OH)$_2$D to become a more active macrophage, including the local production of a number of defensins (including cathelicidin). Defects in immune functions indispensable for antimicrobial activity have been observed in vitamin D–deficient mice.[168,169] The overall effects suggest that $1,25(OH)_2D$ enhances the natural defense against bacterial infection. In the human situation, low serum levels of 25(OH)D were repeatedly associated with increased susceptibility to and more rapid disease progression of tuberculosis.[170-174] This hypothesis is confirmed by the lower induction of cyclic adenosine monophosphate (cAMP) by monocytes incubated with 25(OH)D-deficient serum from sunlight-deprived African Americans.[175] Moreover, oral administration of vitamin D markedly improved tuberculosis outcome in small-scale studies.[176,177] Prospective clinical trials are ongoing to evaluate the effect of vitamin D supplementation on the evolution of various infections, including tuberculosis, to confirm the cause/effect relationship between vitamin D status and the native immune defense system.

The acquired immune system reacts in opposite ways to the native immune system (see Fig. 3-6B). Indeed, $1,25(OH)_2D$ inhibits dendritic cell maturation and generates a coordinated action on T cell gene expression of key cytokines (IL-1, IL-2, IL-12, IL-17, INF-γ) and genes needed for antigen presentation to T cells (MHC class II and cosignaling proteins). The global effect of these immune-modulating actions is thus a downregulation of the acquired immune system. This should have beneficial effects on the occurrence or evolution of autoimmune diseases. Vitamin D–deficient mice more easily develop a more severe type of such autoimmune diseases. For example, genetically predisposed NOD mice exposed to transient vitamin D deficiency early in life have a much higher incidence of type 1 diabetes than vitamin D–replete mice,[169,178] and 1α hydroxylase–deficient mice are more prone to several types of inflammatory bowel disease.[179] Moreover, $1,25(OH)_2D$ and more potent and selective analogs can significantly reduce spontaneous or experimental autoimmune diseases in rodents, such as type 1 diabetes in NOD mice, experimental allergic encephalitis, nephritis, or inflammatory bowel disease in rodents.[16,24,180]

Studies in human autoimmune diseases are, however, more complicated. VDR polymorphism is not clearly related to the risk for type 1 diabetes, according to a large meta-analysis.[181] However, polymorphism of the 1α-hydroxylase gene is associated with the risk of type 1 diabetes in cross-sectional as well as in family studies.[182] Consistent with data from NOD mice, several epidemiologic studies in humans report that vitamin D intake in early life may reduce later risk of type 1 diabetes. Risk reduction varied between 26% with cod liver oil to 78% with 2000 IU/d, with an overall effect of 30% reduction in five published reports.[180] Since 25(OH)D serum levels have not been measured in the cohorts of children, a threshold cannot be defined for optimal reduction of type 1 diabetes.

A low vitamin D status has also been repeatedly associated with a higher risk for multiple sclerosis. A large prospective, nested, case-control study among more than 7 million U.S. military personnel revealed that low 25(OH)D level was a strong risk factor for later occurrence of multiple sclerosis (odds ratio of about 2 for serum 25[OH]D <20 ng/mL, with possibly even greater "protection" by higher levels).[183] However, as for type 1 diabetes, no controlled, randomized intervention studies have yet proved a causal relation between vitamin D (deficiency or insufficiency) and later occurrence of autoimmune diseases, but randomized trials (especially in genetically at-risk groups) should receive high priority. All these observations, however, suggest that preventing vitamin D deficiency in the perinatal period,

early childhood, or adolescence may have long-lasting effects on autoimmune diseases. Moreover, there are several observations in mouse models that could explain such effects, such as the increased apoptosis of (autoreactive?) thymocytes or lymphocytes, the generation of regulatory T cells, and NKT cells after exposure to $1,25(OH)_2D$.[180,184]

Cardiovascular System

VDR-null mice, as well as 1α hydroxylase–null mice, develop high-renin hypertension and cardiac hypertrophy that can be prevented by treatment with an angiotensin blocker.[185] In vitro or in vivo exposure to $1,25(OH)_2D$ decreases renin production, probably by direct regulation of the gene expression via a VDRE in the promoter of renin. Observational studies in humans found an inverse association between $1,25(OH)_2D$ levels and blood pressure or plasma renin levels in normotensive or hypertensive individuals. Prospective cohort studies reported that incident hypertension over a 4-year follow-up is lowest when the serum 25(OH)D is 30 ng/mL or higher.[186] Also, in the NHANES III population, a significant negative relation between serum 25(OH)D concentrations and systolic, diastolic, and pulse pressure among the total adult population was observed.[187] The results of these observational studies are supported by two randomized controlled trials in which vitamin D treatment reduced blood pressure in hypertensive subjects and elderly community-dwelling women.

VDR-null mice display increased thrombogenicity and decreased fibrinolysis when exposed to inflammatory stimuli,[188] whereas $1,25(OH)_2D$ has beneficial effects on most cells of the vascular wall. In humans, a low vitamin D status is associated with a number of cardiovascular risk factors,[189] including the metabolic syndrome. The largest prospective intervention trial (WHI) with calcium (1g/d) and vitamin D (400 IU/d), however, revealed no increased nor decreased coronary or cerebrovascular risk after 7 years of follow-up.[190] Several large-scale observational studies demonstrated that survival and especially cardiovascular events were lower in patients on chronic renal replacement therapy treated with $1,25(OH)_2D$ analogs, compared with either untreated or $1,25(OH)_2D$-treated groups.[191] However, a large meta-analysis casts doubt on this conclusion.[192] In addition, vitamin D excess can have deleterious effects on all structures of the vascular wall, with ectopic calcification and organ failure of kidney, cardiac valves, myocardium, and most other soft tissues. These data suggest a beneficial effect of the vitamin endocrine system (within specific optimal limits) on cardiovascular targets but certainly need confirmation by a proper prospective, large-scale randomized trial.

Muscle and Muscle Function

VDR is expressed in myoblasts and is also present in low concentrations in mature striated muscle cells. *VDR*-null mice, even on a high calcium diet, show maturation problems of their muscle fibers, with smaller muscle fibers and expression of embryonic markers even after weaning.[193] Genes that are typically expressed early in life (e.g., *myf-5*) are under negative control by $1,25(OH)_2D$. Evaluation of muscle performance in VDR-resistant or vitamin D–deficient mice is difficult to interpret, because hypocalcemia may have major effects on calcium fluxes in muscle cells. Patients with chronic renal failure and vitamin D deficiency (thus combined deficiency of 25[OH]D and $1,25[OH]_2D$) can develop severe myopathy and inability to walk that can be promptly restored by appropriate vitamin D and/or analog treatment. Sarcopenia (progressive loss of muscle mass and strength) is highly prevalent in the elderly and frequently associated with vitamin D deficiency. Vitamin D supplementation can modestly and inconsistently improve muscle function and improve body sway. Meta-analysis of several prospective intervention studies revealed that vitamin D supplementation in vitamin D–deficient elderly subjects can modestly reduce the risk of falls;[194] this may explain, together with beneficial effects on bone, a reduced fracture risk.[195]

Glucose and Energy Metabolism

Several tissues which are important for energy and glucose metabolism, such as endocrine β cells, muscle, and fat cells, are also targets for vitamin D, so the obvious question is whether vitamin regulates or modulates overall metabolism apart from the effects of vitamin D on the immune system and autoimmune diabetes. Vitamin D deficiency in experimental animals (rodents and rabbits) impairs glucose tolerance.[180,196,197] VDR-null mice, however, did not have a consistently abnormal glucose tolerance; one strain differs from another strain.[24,180] This discrepancy between effects of ligand and receptor deficiency is not unique (see alopecia and immune effect) nor specific for vitamin D. Similar effects are known for thyroid hormone/thyroid receptor function. 1,25(OH)$_2$D has modest stimulatory effects on insulin production and secretion, probably mediated by the well-known effects of calcium on β-cell functions.

Most observational studies in humans link vitamin D insufficiency with nearly all aspects of the metabolic syndrome—including obesity, insulin resistance, fasting blood glucose or type 2 diabetes, hypertension, and hyperlipidemia.[24,180] This was confirmed in the NHANES study[198] and a Scandinavian cohort study,[199] as well as in a prospective British cohort study.[200] Baseline 25(OH)D levels were inversely associated with a 10-year risk of fasting hyperglycemia and insulin resistance, with the greatest risk in subjects with 25(OH)D levels below 20 ng/mL and the lowest risk in subjects with above 30 ng/mL.[200] Short-term interventional studies to correct severe vitamin D deficiency in a few subjects indicate improved glycemic control, but larger studies using 400 IU/d, such as in the WHI trial, could not demonstrate an effect on glucose levels.[201] A much smaller study was also negative, but post hoc analysis revealed a modest effect of a higher dose of vitamin D (700 IU/d) on subjects with fasting hyperglycemia at randomization.[202] In view of the high prevalence of vitamin D insufficiency and of metabolic syndrome and their association, it is highly desirable to demonstrate a causal link and then take appropriate actions.

Mortality

Because vitamin D status is associated with so many major diseases, it is worthwhile to explore whether vitamin D deficiency is associated with increased mortality. Indeed, in a prospective 8-year cohort study, all-cause and cardiovascular mortality was twofold higher when 25(OH)D levels were in the lower 2 quartiles (<17 ng/mL), compared with the upper quartile.[203] Similar results were obtained from the NHANES III study: mortality was about 1.5-fold higher when 25(OH)D levels were well below 20 ng/mL, and the lowest mortality was observed in subjects with 25(OH)D levels between 20 and 50 ng/mL.[204] Also, in patients on chronic hemodialysis, all-cause mortality was greater (significant 1.6-fold increase) when 25(OH)D levels fell below 10 ng/mL.[205] In addition, a meta-analysis of all studies using vitamin D supplementation for the prevention of fractures revealed a modest but significant (−8%) reduction in overall mortality in the vitamin D supplemented groups.[206]

Diagnostic and Therapeutic Aspects of Vitamin D

ASSAYS FOR VITAMIN D AND METABOLITES: METHODOLOGY AND APPLICATIONS

Vitamin D and about 30 of its metabolites are found in plasma. Measurements of their concentrations may be essential for clinical or research purposes.[207,208] Most techniques require a lipid extraction to free these compounds from their binding proteins (especially DBP). In view of the high molar extinction of vitamin D, UV absorptiometry can be used for measurement of vitamin D$_2$, vitamin D$_3$, or 25(OH)D after high-performance liquid chromatography (HPLC). However, competitive-binding assays or radioimmunoassay (RIA) are preferred for measurements of 25(OH)D, 1,25(OH)$_2$D, or 24,25(OH)$_2$D.[209] These assays remain difficult, as demonstrated by remarkably poor intralaboratory and especially interlaboratory quality-control studies.[210,211] Nonchromatographic assays using DBP overestimate the true 25(OH)D concentration by 10% to 20%, but nonspecific interferences (DBP, lipids?) in some assays can result in up to 100% higher values. The quality control of routine 25(OH)D assays revealed extreme problems with accuracy,[210] and since the definition of vitamin D deficiency or insufficiency is defined in absolute concentration (see later), there is urgent need for improved quality assurance.[210] The use of tandem mass spectrometry after liquid chromatography and serum extraction is now considered the gold standard, but this assay is not yet routinely available for purposes other than research.[212]

The measurement of serum concentrations of vitamin D$_2$ or D$_3$ is of little clinical value. Indeed, because of their short half-life in plasma, it reflects only recent exposure to UV light or nutritional intake. Serum 25(OH)D concentration is, however, an excellent reflection of the vitamin D status because of the rapid conversion of vitamin D into 25(OH)D and its long plasma half-life.[208,209] Its plasma concentration varies widely in normal subjects because of large variations in endogenous and exogenous supply of vitamin D (Table 3-3).

Plasma 25(OH)D concentration thus behaves as a true vitamin whose concentration depends on nutritional supply or synthesis in the skin after exposure to UVB light. Low exposure to UV light and low vitamin D intake is quite common in infants and elderly subjects if food sources are not supplemented with vitamin D. Plasma 25(OH)D concentrations are indeed low at birth (about half the maternal concentration because of the 2:1 ratio of maternal to fetal DBP concentration), and the natural vitamin D content of milk is low. Sun exposure was therefore evolution's solution to prevent rickets. However, in view of the relation between exposure to UVB light (especially in young children) and subsequent risk for skin malignancies, it is probably wise to advocate systematic vitamin D supplementation of all infants and young children. Whereas widespread vitamin D deficiency in infants was recognized and prevented in the beginning of the 20th century, a similar endemic deficiency in the elderly was only recognized and addressed at the end of the same century (see Treatment, later). Intestinal malabsorption of fat-soluble vitamins interrupts the absorption of exogenous (probably also endogenous) hepatobiliary excretion of vitamin D and therefore requires either substitution with large amounts of vitamin D or more physiologic doses (10 to 20 μg/d) of the more soluble 25(OH)D. A low calcium intake can markedly (twofold) increase the catabolism of 25(OH)D and will thus

Table 3-3. Plasma Concentration of 25(OH)D

Normal Fluctuation According to:

Dietary intake (+)*
Sun (UV light) exposure (+) influenced by seasonal life style and cultural
  habits
Age (−)
Skin pigmentation (−)
Latitude (−)
Sunscreen use (−)

Increased 25(OH)D Concentration

Exposure to pharmaceutical vitamin D[†]
Excess exposure to nutritional vitamin D
Excess exposure to UV light

Decreased 25(OH)D Concentration[‡]

Combined deficiency of access/exposure to nutritional vitamin D and UV light
  Major risk groups include:
    Infants, especially when born in late winter
    Women and children of immigrants with pigmented skin living in
      temperate climates
    Elderly population with limited mobility
    Subset of population with low exposure to sunshine because of
      socioeconomic, religious, or cultural reasons
Decreased intestinal absorption of vitamin D associated with fat malabsorption
  (e.g., associated with biliary cirrhosis)
Short bowel syndrome
Exocrine pancreas insufficiency
Gluten enteropathy
Increased loss or catabolism of vitamin D
Nephrotic syndrome
Chronic liver P450 activation by drugs (e.g., barbiturates or antiepileptic
  drugs)
Low calcium intake or absorption

*Positive or negative effects are indicated by + or −, respectively.
[†]Vitamin D toxicity with hypercalciuria, hypercalcemia, nephrocalcinosis, kidney
  stones, metastatic calcification, etc., are only observed if 25(OH)D
  concentrations exceed 100 ng/mL. Without access to pharmaceutical vitamin D,
  it is therefore unlikely to acquire clinical vitamin D toxicity.
[‡]For definition of vitamin D insufficiency or deficiency, see chapter-recommended
  daily intake and Table 3-5.

Table 3-4. Plasma Concentration of 1,25(OH)$_2$D

Decreased Concentrations	Increased Concentrations
Substrate Deficiency* (e.g., nutritional rickets, intestinal malabsorption)	**Substrate Excess[†]**
25(OH)D-1α-Hydroxylase Enzyme Deficiency	**25(OH)D-1α-Hydroxylase Enzyme Excess**
Inborn: Vitamin D-dependent rickets	Primary or tertiary
Organic: Renal insufficiency or anephric patients	hyperparathyroidism
Functional:	Hypothyroidism
Hypoparathyroidism	Glucocorticoid excess
Pseudohypoparathyroidism	Acromegaly
Hypomagnesemia	Granulomatous diseases
Tumoral osteomalacia	Idiopathic hypercalciuria
Hypercalcemia of malignancy	Hypophosphatemic rickets type 2
Hyperthyroidism	(+hypercalciuria)
Morbus Addison (acute)	Pregnancy
Severe insulin deficiency	Nutritional calcium deficiency
X-linked hypophosphatemia	Williams' syndrome
Rhabdomyolysis	
Tumoral calcinosis	
DBP Deficiency	**DBP Excess**
Fetus	Pregnancy
Nephrotic syndrome	Oral estrogen use
Liver cirrhosis	
	End-Organ Resistance
	True vitamin D resistance (so-called vitamin D–dependent rickets type 2)

DBP, Vitamin D-binding protein.
*In many cases of rickets or osteomalacia, 1,25(OH)$_2$D concentrations are still
  measurable or even nearly normal. This may be due to recent (and insufficient)
  access to vitamin D after long-term vitamin D deficiency. Nevertheless,
  such concentration is too low in comparison with the degree of secondary
  hyperparathyroidism. In any way, 25(OH)D is a better marker for vitamin D
  deficiency than 1,25(OH)$_2$D. A similar situation is observed in hypothyroidism
  when precursor hormone T$_4$ is a better marker for clinical hypothyroidism than
  the real hormone, T$_3$.
[†]Vitamin D excess only increases serum 1,25(OH)$_2$D when renal function remains
  normal and/or PTH secretion is elevated. Frequently, 1,25(OH)$_2$D levels are
  low or normal in vitamin D toxicity.
Monocyte activation can result in extrarenal synthesis of 1,25(OH)$_2$D, such as in
  sarcoidosis, tuberculosis, foreign body inflammation, lymphopenia, and some
  fungal infections.

facilitate substrate deficiency if the "nutritional" supply is marginal.[213]

The metabolism of 25(OH)D into 1,25(OH)$_2$D and 24,25(OH)$_2$D is tightly controlled by hormones, ions, and humoral factors. The plasma concentration of 1,25(OH)$_2$D is therefore regulated as a true hormone (Table 3-4), and measurements of its concentration can be useful for clinical exploration of unusual cases of rickets, osteopenia, and hypo- or hypercalcemia.

The serum concentration of 24,25(OH)$_2$D and 25,26(OH)$_2$D usually reflects the concentration of 25(OH)D and therefore does not contribute additional valuable clinical information. The 25(OH)D- and 1,25(OH)$_2$D-lactone concentrations are only increased in case of important substrate excess, but their measurement is not (yet) introduced in clinical practice.

All vitamin D metabolites are tightly bound to DBP. Since the hepatic 25-hydroxylase activity is not feedback regulated, the free (or total) 25(OH)D concentration is largely fluctuating according to substrate supply. In contrast, renal 25(OH)D-1α-hydroxylase is tightly controlled, and since the access to VDR in target tissues is dependent on the circulating free concentrations, free and not total 1,25(OH)$_2$D concentration is important.[80,214] The circulating DBP concentration is fairly stable, except when stimulated by estrogens (or pregnancy) or decreased by reduced synthesis (liver cirrhosis) or increased urinary loss (nephrotic

syndrome). The major arguments for the importance of free rather than total 1,25(OH)$_2$D are (1) in vitro experiments (biological activity of 1,25[OH]$_2$D on cultured cells)[215,216] and (2) in vivo observations such as increased steady-state concentration of 1,25(OH)$_2$D without signs of increased action during chronic estrogen use or in animals immunized against 1,25(OH)$_2$D-hapten-protein complex.[217]

Clinical Aspects of Vitamin D

RECOMMENDED DAILY INTAKE AND CLINICAL USE OF VITAMIN D

In contrast to some rare inborn diseases related to vitamin D production, metabolism, or action (see Chapter 11), vitamin D deficiency and insufficiency are extremely frequent worldwide, and the full scope of their prevalence has only recently been appreciated.[16,24,32] Vitamin D excess is also a serious disease but seems to occur rarely without the context of excess intake of vitamin D supplementation and is thus usually iatrogenic.

Before the discovery of the dual origin of vitamin D and the introduction of vitamin D supplementation of infants and children, rickets was highly prevalent among the poor in many European cities but also in children of wealthy families (see Chapter 15). The optimal dosage was determined over time, largely on a trial-and-error basis, since this happened well before even the concept of randomized clinical trials was conceived. The vitamin D content of 1 teaspoon of cod liver oil (later found to contain the equivalent of 400 IU of vitamin D_3) was found to be efficient and sufficient to prevent endemic rickets. Subsequently, a dose of 200 to 400 IU/d was considered protective. The recommended treatment dose for a child with established rickets was usually larger, partly because of the need for a loading dose. Most recommendations by various official nutritional boards around the world also suggested, up to recently, a daily intake of 5 or 10 μg of vitamin D for infants and children. Indeed, the standing committee on the scientific evaluation of dietary reference intakes (by the U.S. National Academy of Sciences Panel for vitamin D in partnership with the Institute of Medicine) carefully evaluated vitamin D requirements and recommendations in 1997 and suggested 5 μg as the daily supplement (see Table 3-1) ,[218] with similar recommendation by the European Food and Safety Authority.[23] Only one real randomized trial with regard to preventive action of vitamin D was ever published and found no cases of new rickets in young Turkish children treated with 400 IU/d for 18 months.[219,220] The recommended daily supplement for children, long set at 5 μg or 200 IU/d, was increased in 2008 to 10 μg or 400 IU of vitamin D_3/d by the American Academy of Pediatrics.[221] No well-designed prospective or randomized trials have ever used serum levels of 25(OH)D to define the minimal threshold for preventing or curing rickets. In clinical case studies, serum 25(OH)D levels found in simple vitamin D–deficiency rickets are well below 10 ng/mL and usually even below 5 ng/mL. Serum 25(OH)D levels are frequently low in newborn sera (cord sera); the mean level in newborns is usually only slightly above 50% of the 25(OH)D levels in the mother's serum.[80] Despite the cheap and effective strategies to prevent rickets, many countries or regions around the world are still facing endemic rickets affecting even a few percent of the infants or children,[222] especially in many Islamic countries, rural China, in children of immigrants in Western Europe, or in children born to mothers living in areas of high frequency of vitamin D insufficiency in general.[223] The disease prevalence or severity may be aggravated by simultaneous poor dietary calcium intake, such as in many African countries.[224] Poor vitamin D status in perinatal life or during childhood may also predispose to lower bone mass much later in life.[225]

Vitamin D is also known to be a major factor in maintaining bone integrity later in life, and most studies have dealt with the elderly or postmenopausal women. The idea for this role came from repeated and well-documented cross-sectional studies linking increasing PTH serum levels with increasing age and decreasing 25(OH)D levels. To define an optimal 25(OH)D level for optimal bone health, numerous studies have looked at surrogate endpoints (Table 3-5), but fortunately several intervention studies are now also available, including several meta-analyses of these data. Indeed, several surrogate endpoints have been evaluated to define a minimal or optimal threshold for 25(OH)D. Serum concentrations of 1,25(OH)₂D are not related to the substrate concentration if serum 25(OH)D exceeds 20 ng/mL in adults, but a positive relation with serum 25(OH)D has been observed when subjects with low 25(OH)D were included. Intervention studies reveal that 1,25(OH)₂D rapidly increases, even

Table 3-5. Strategies and Clinical Studies to Define Optimal Vitamin D Status for Bone Health

Hard Endpoints

Placebo-controlled intervention studies
Vitamin D/25(OH)D and fractures
Prospective/cross-sectional studies
25(OH)D and fractures

Surrogate Endpoints

Prospective/cross-sectional studies
25(OH)D and BMC/BMD
25(OH)D and bone turnover markers
Prospective/cross-sectional studies
25(OH)D and calcium absorption
Cross-sectional/intervention studies
25(OH)D and PTH
Cross-sectional/intervention studies
25(OH)D and 1,25(OH)₂D

BMC, Bone mineral content; *BMD,* bone mineral density; *PTH,* parathyroid hormone.

transiently above the normal level, when vitamin D supplementation is given to vitamin D–insufficient patients (25[OH]D levels < 12 to 20 ng/mL).[226] Thus, it seems that the plasma level of 1,25(OH)₂D is no longer substrate dependent once 25(OH)D levels exceed 20 ng/mL. PTH has been very extensively used as a surrogate marker for defining optimal vitamin D status. Undoubtedly PTH increases in groups of patients with low 25(OH)D levels; however, PTH concentrations increase only to levels above the normal range when 25(OH)D is very low, whereas in about a third of patients with low 25(OH)D levels, PTH remains normal. The threshold of 25(OH)D below which serum PTH starts to increase varies between 12 and 40 ng/mL in a large number of cross-sectional studies.[32] Such differences may partly be due to differences in accuracy of the 25(OH)D assay and differences in nutritional calcium intake and kidney function. Intervention studies are therefore more reliable. Serum PTH decreases after vitamin D supplementation when baseline levels are below 20 ng/mL.[32,227] Active intestinal calcium absorption is the primary target for vitamin D action and would thus represent an ideal surrogate endpoint for defining 25(OH)D levels. However, measuring intestinal calcium absorption is difficult because only dual-isotope techniques allow accurate estimations. Other methods, such as plasma concentrations of a calcium isotope after oral intake, provide a more crude estimation, whereas change in total serum calcium concentrations after a large oral calcium loading is a very poor estimation of active calcium absorption. Cross-sectional data suggested a minimal 25(OH)D level of 32 ng/mL for optimal calcium absorption but used a poor procedure to measure calcium absorption.[228,229] Other large cross-sectional studies could not identify a true 25(OH)D threshold but only a relation with serum 1,25(OH)₂D, either in adults[230] or adolescents.[231] Again, intervention studies with vitamin D supplementation revealed no[232] or only a minimal[233] increase in active intestinal calcium absorption in subjects with baseline 25(OH)D levels above 20 ng/mL. Cross-sectional data on 25(OH)D and bone mineral density (BMD) values could not demonstrate a strong correlation; this may be due to a long lag time between vitamin D intake and bone turnover or bone mass. Lower BMD levels, however, were observed in subjects with the lowest 25(OH)D levels (<12 ng/mL).[32,234] Fracture prevalence in cross-sectional or prospective studies according to 25(OH)D levels revealed that a higher fracture risk is associated with single point measurements of 25(OH)D levels below 20 ng/mL.[235] Finally, intervention studies with vitamin D and/or calcium supplements are most relevant to define the optimal vitamin D status. A very large number of studies have addressed this question, but only a limited number can be classified as well-designed randomized trials. Several meta-analyses came to slightly different conclusions. Vitamin D alone given to postmenopausal or elderly subjects cannot reliably reduce hip-fracture incidence,[219,236] and oral calcium supplementation alone also has no clear benefit on hip-fracture risk, with one study even revealing an increased risk.[194,237] Combined vitamin D and calcium supplementation, however, can reduce hip-fracture risk by about 20%, with a similar reduction on other nonvertebral fractures.[236,238] In these studies, a vitamin D dosage of 800 IU/d was more efficient than 400 IU/d.[195]

It thus seems that only combined high calcium intake (>1 g/d) and vitamin D supplementation (≥800 IU/d) has shown to be efficient for fracture reduction in target populations of elderly subjects, with the greatest effect in institutionalized patients. The corresponding 25(OH)D level is more disputed, mainly owing to lack of accuracy of 25(OH)D assays in older studies and the confusion about optimal (minimal) 25(OH)D in individual subjects and mean population levels. Because most intervention studies conclude that serum 25(OH)D levels increase by 1 ng/mL for each additional 100 IU of vitamin D supplement per day,[239] serum 25(OH)D levels (calculated from baseline population level and expected increase of 8 ng/mL for a 800 IU/d supplement) reached during the vitamin D intervention studies with positive fracture effects can be estimated as over 20 ng/mL in most adults, with mean levels closer to 30 ng/mL.[240] The amount of vitamin D needed to obtain a minimal 25(OH)D level above 20 ng/mL and a population mean closer to 30 ng/mL, of course, depends on the baseline 25(OH)D level and accesses to UVB and dietary vitamin D. Intervention studies, however, revealed that 400 IU/d is not sufficient to raise 25(OH)D above 20 ng/mL in more than 95% of the target population of postmenopausal or elderly Caucasians, whereas this can be better achieved by 800 IU/d.

Whereas a large body of literature and meta-analyses are available to define the relationship between vitamin D supplementation, 25(OH)D concentration, and future fracture risk, such data are far less available for defining optimal 25(OH)D levels and noncalcemic endpoints. For muscle function and falls, vitamin D supplements of 700 to 1100 IU/d were found to be modestly efficient, and serum 25(OH)D levels obtained by such interventions would be very similar to minimal 25(OH)D levels that seem to be effective for fracture reduction. For immune and cardiovascular effects, as well as for potential effects on cancer risks, no, very limited, or controversial intervention data are available. Observational data reveal that the greatest risks are observed in subjects with baseline 25(OH)D levels below 20 ng/mL. However, most cross-sectional studies also reveal that higher 25(OH)D levels (>30 to 40 ng/mL) are associated with the greatest risk reduction for cancer, autoimmune diseases, and metabolic endpoints. It is unlikely that these higher 25(OH)D levels increases serum 1,25(OH)$_2$D above the levels when substrate 25(OH)D exceeds 20 ng/mL, so the working hypothesis is that such higher 25(OH)D levels would be needed to allow local paracrine production of 1,25(OH)$_2$D. Although this is plausible, direct proof for this concept is still unresolved.

What are the options for vitamin D supplementation based on the available information? For infants and children, a daily intake of 400 IU/d should be assured from early life till adolescence, since this can prevent vitamin D–deficiency rickets. Real-life implementation is far from ideal in at-risk groups in Western countries and in many regions of the world where exposure to sunlight is minimal for geographic or sociocultural reasons. For elderly subjects and probably also for all adults, the minimal 25(OH)D level associated with the lowest risk for fractures, falls (based on intervention studies), and a number of major diseases (based on epidemiologic surveys) is above 20 ng/mL. This can be achieved by increasing vitamin D intake by 800 IU/d or equivalent per week or month.[241] In populations with better 25(OH)D baseline levels, 400 IU/d can be sufficient, and in some countries or regions of the world with mean 25(OH)D levels of 30 ng/mL, no vitamin D supplements may be needed. Alternative sources of vitamin D such as fatty fish are not a practical solution for many millions of mildly vitamin D–deficient subjects. Higher exposure to UVB light could certainly improve the vitamin D status but cannot be recommended to subjects with a fair-skin phototype (phototypes 1, 2) because of lifetime risk of photo-damage or skin cancer. Of course, for a number of patients with specific diseases (see Table 3-3) a higher dose of vitamin D or 25(OH)D or 1,25(OH)$_2$D is needed because of poor intestinal absorption, increased catabolism, or impaired metabolism.

There are a number of arguments that 25(OH)D levels over 30 to 40 ng/mL may provide additional benefits for bone, muscle, and noncalcemic endpoints. To reach such levels in over 97% of the population, daily supplements of at least 2000 IU/d (and usually more) would be needed, with or without substantially greater exposure to UVB.[229] Since severe vitamin D toxicity is usually observed only when 25(OH)D levels exceed 100 ng/mL, such levels of 30 to 40 ng/mL are probably safe. However, randomized, large-scale, long-term studies with supplements of 2000 IU/d or more do not exist; such doses were only evaluated in a few hundred subjects for a maximum of 6 months.[242] As a reminder of possible toxicity, it is worth remembering that a mild but significant increase in kidney stones was observed in the WHI trial when calcium supplements were combined with at least 400 IU/d of vitamin D for 7 years.[163] A causal relationship between vitamin D status and more major diseases has still to be proven, so it seems wise to defer recommendations for a generalized vitamin D intake above the present upper limits. However, in view of the solid hypotheses generated by observational studies, appropriate randomized controlled trials with multiple end points deserve a great priority.

WORLDWIDE VITAMIN D STATUS

Serum 25(OH)D levels, as the best marker for vitamin D status, vary widely in different populations around the world, and the frequency of vitamin D deficiency or insufficiency (Table 3-6) varies accordingly. In an extensive meta-analysis of cross-

Table 3-6. Vitamin D Nutritional Status as Described by Circulating Levels of 25(OH)D

Serum 25(OH)D		
Ng/mL	nmol/L	**Nutritional Status**
<10	<25	Vitamin D deficiency
10-20	25-50	Vitamin D insufficiency
>20*	>50*	Vitamin D sufficiency
>~100	>~250	Risk for toxicity

Optimal vitamin D status defined by serum 25(OH)D levels.
*Different opinions exist for defining the minimal threshold for optimal 25(OH)D levels; 30 ng/mL or 50 nmol/L is suggested by others.[272]

sectional studies on serum 25(OH)D levels in healthy subjects around the world (394 studies), average serum 25(OH)D levels were 21 ng/mL. Caucasians had slightly higher levels than non-Caucasians,[243] but this may be biased, since 25(OH)D levels are lower in subjects with darker skin when living in moderate climate zones. Older subjects (>75 yrs), as well as young children (<15 yr), had lower 25(OH)D levels. Latitude had only a minimal effect, demonstrating that apart from potential exposure to UVB light, many other factors—skin pigmentation, lifestyle, and nutritional factors—define vitamin D status. In more homogenous populations, the expected North-South gradient has been confirmed (e.g., in France),[244] whereas for all European populations, the North-South gradient was reversed, probably because of high fish intake in Scandinavian countries and differences in sun-seeking behavior.[34,245] In North America, NHANES data confirm that 25(OH)D levels remain relatively stable over time, with mean levels of 30 ng/mL[187] and thus substantially higher than in Europe, probably related to the widespread use of vitamin D–enriched food. Non-Hispanic U.S. blacks had mean levels of 20 ng/mL. In some countries, however, mean levels can be quite low.[246,247] Lower levels are usually observed in obese subjects or those with special risk factors (see Table 3-3). Low levels are also frequent in pregnant women and their infants, and this poses an additional risk in view of the potential late consequences of perinatal vitamin D deficiency.[248]

It is therefore obvious that mild vitamin D deficiency (see Table 3-6), even when defined conservatively as 25(OH)D levels under 20 ng/mL, is very widespread worldwide and can affect about one third to half of the world population. When insufficiency is defined by 25(OH)D levels below 30 ng/mL, then half of the healthy U.S. population (based on NHANES data) and about two thirds of the European population (and even more in most Muslim countries) would be vitamin D deficient.[16,249] It is therefore imperative that the health consequences of vitamin D status should be better evaluated and that the most severe forms of vitamin D deficiency or insufficiency (see Table 3-2) should be corrected by appropriate strategies.

Therapeutic Potential of 1,25(OH)₂D Analogs

The combined presence of 25(OH)D-1α-hydroxylase[48] and VDR in several tissues introduced the concept of a paracrine role for 1,25(OH)₂D.[250] These newly discovered functions of 1,25(OH)₂D create possible new therapeutic applications for immune modulation (e.g., for the treatment of autoimmune diseases or prevention of graft rejection), inhibition of cell proliferation (e.g., psoriasis), and induction of cell differentiation (cancer). To achieve growth inhibition or cell differentiation, supraphysiologic doses of 1,25(OH)₂D are needed, causing calcemic side effects. Therefore, new analogs of 1,25(OH)₂D have been developed to dissociate the antiproliferative and prodifferentiating effects from the calcemic and bone-metabolism effects.[251]

The secosteroid 1,25(OH)₂D, with its open B ring and side chain of 8 carbon atoms, is a very flexible molecule. Different modifications have already been introduced in the A, B, C, and D rings and in the side chain by addition or transposition of hydroxyl groups, introducing unsaturation, replacing a carbon atom with a hetero atom, inverting the stereochemistry, and/or shortening or lengthening the side chain.[251] During the last decade, over 500 analogs were synthesized and their biological potency reported in the non-patent literature.[251,252] Moreover, several thousands of analogs have been synthesized by pharmaceutical and academic research groups and reported briefly in patent literature. Some of these analogs demonstrate a clear dissociation between antiproliferative and calcemic effects. In the meantime, nonsteroidal analogs were synthesized with a totally new structure lacking the full CD region of 1,25(OH)₂D.[253,254]

No single or simple mechanism can explain the exact mechanism of superagonistic and selective activity profile (calcemic versus noncalcemic effects) of the new vitamin D analogs. Most of the biological effects of 1,25(OH)₂D are believed to be mediated via binding to the VDR, but surprisingly the binding affinity of the analogs to VDR does not always correlate with their potency. Some analogs extend the VDR half-life and induce different conformational changes to the VDR-ligand complex as assessed by limited proteolytic digestion and site-directed mutagenesis.[255-257] However, most analogs bind to the ligand-binding pocket of the VDR without major modifications of the surface of the ligand-binding domain of the receptor.[252,254,258] Nevertheless, the superagonists are able to enhance gene transcription at the level of coactivator recruitment or activity. The selective action of analogs, however, requires different mechanisms, such as different metabolism in different target cells or cell- or gene-specific regulation, depending on the VDR (e.g., homo-heterodimer configuration induced by specific analogs, presence or selective interaction with coactivators or repressor protein, etc).[251,259,260] Some analogs are selective agonists or antagonists for nongenomic rapid actions while being devoid of significant genomic activity.[105] Since for other steroid hormones (e.g., estrogens, androgens, glucocorticoids), it is now well established that analog-specific gene regulation can be generated by chemical modification of the parent ligand molecule, it is likely that among the many powerful selective vitamin D analogs, at least some will be found to be clinically useful for noncalcemic indications.

BONE DISORDERS

The role of vitamin D or its metabolites in the treatment of bone disorders characterized by defective mineralization, such as rickets and renal osteodystrophy, is well established. Presently only a few analogs are being evaluated in preclinical or human phase II trials for the prevention or cure of osteoporosis. The vitamin D analog, 2β-(3-hydroxypropoxy)-1,25(OH)₂D (ED-71), was found to be more potent than 1,25(OH)₂D in rodents and increased bone mineral mass and density in a phase III trial in Japanese postmenopausal women.[261] Another vitamin D analog, 2MD, was also very efficient for treatment of ovariectomy-induced bone loss in rats,[262] but clinical development was interrupted.

RENAL OSTEODYSTROPHY

Bone disease in patients with chronic renal failure is due to a complex set of mechanisms such as impaired 1,25(OH)₂D synthesis, vitamin D resistance, secondary hyperparathyroidism, increased FGF-23, and abnormal mineral handling (hyperphosphatemia, aluminum or fluoride excess, acidosis). While 1α(OH)D₃ and 1,25(OH)₂D are widely used for the prevention and cure of renal osteodystrophy, several analogs have been evaluated for this indication, with the aim of better PTH suppression with less risk for inducing hypercalcemia or hyperphosphatemia. Paracalcitol is widely used in the United States for control of secondary hyperparathyroidism. Its use was also associated with a lower rate of cardiovascular and overall mortality in comparison with patients receiving 1,25(OH)₂D or no vitamin D treatment.[191]

These results have been confirmed in a large number of similar nonrandomized studies, possibly biased by unequal patient selection, but prospective randomized clinical trials have not yet addressed this question.

CANCER

A large number of 1,25(OH)$_2$D analogs have been developed with potent antiproliferative and prodifferentiating effects on cancer cells in vitro[145] and reduced effects on calcium and bone metabolism.[251] Several potent analogs have already been tested in animal models for the treatment of different cancers.[158]

Although oral seocalcitol (EB 1089) was initially very promising in animal models and in early human studies, it did not provide clear benefits in later studies involving patients with advanced pancreatic and hepatocellular carcinoma. Large doses of oral 1,25(OH)$_2$D given in combination with taxol to patients with advanced prostate cancer was found to increase survival and decrease the risk of thrombosis,[263] but a phase III trial in similar patients was stopped early for as yet unknown reasons. Some other analogs are still in early clinical development for a variety of cancers, usually in combination with conventional chemotherapeutics.

SKIN

The epidermis is a unique tissue in that it can fully produce and activate the full vitamin D synthesis and metabolism pathways and is very sensitive to 1,25(OH)$_2$D. Calcitriol at pharmacologic concentrations potently induces growth arrest and differentiation of the epidermal keratinocyte.[138] The profound effects of calcitriol on keratinocyte proliferation and differentiation have led to the application of vitamin D analogs for skin diseases with disturbed keratinocyte proliferation and differentiation, primarily psoriasis.[264] Topical vitamin D analogs that display decreased calcemic activity (calcipotriol and tacalcitol) are now widely used for mild to moderate forms of psoriasis. Monotherapy with these vitamin D compounds achieves an equal effectiveness as topical medium-potency glucocorticoids, without a risk for skin atrophy. Mild irritation is the only frequently observed side effect.[264] During treatment with vitamin D analogs, the abnormal epidermal homeostasis is fully restored: keratinocyte proliferation is inhibited; the perturbed psoriatic differentiation profile is normalized, with a decrease of the premature expression of involucrin and type I transglutaminase and enhancement of filaggrin expression;[265] and the aberrant expression of cell adhesion molecules (integrins, ICAM1) also returns to normal.[266] The concomitant decrease of the inflammatory infiltrate is, however, incomplete,[265,266] which may account for the residual redness of the lesions after completion of therapy. This can, however, be further improved by combination with topical usage of corticosteroids.

IMMUNOLOGY

The detection of VDR in almost all cells of the immune system, especially antigen-presenting cells (macrophages and dendritic cells) and activated T lymphocytes, led to the investigation of a potential for 1,25(OH)$_2$D as an immunomodulator.[267-270] Vitamin D supplementation is now actively explored in several clinical trials for the stimulation of the natural immune defense and as adjuvant treatment of tuberculosis or other infectious diseases. Similar studies have started for the prevention of major autoimmune diseases. However, vitamin D analogs, though effective in animal models of autoimmunity, have not reached the stage of clinical trials in humans.

PROSTATE HYPERPLASIA

Since the prostate is both a VDR- and CYP27B1-expressing tissue, a vitamin D analog, elocalcitol, was evaluated in animal models of inflammatory prostate diseases and subsequently in patients with benign prostate hyperplasia, with modest beneficial effects requiring confirmation in large-scale clinical trials.[271]

Summary

Vitamin D is a flexible secosteroid that is normally produced in the skin from a cholesterol precursor, 7-dehydrocholesterol, during exposure to short-wave UVB sunlight. However, these UVB photons can also damage the skin and increase the risk for photoaging and skin cancer. Vitamin D can also be obtained from external sources such as fatty fish or vitamin D–enriched food. Two consecutive hydroxylations by two different P450 enzymes result in the production of 1,25(OH)$_2$D. This steroid hormone acts via a ligand-activated nuclear transcription factor present in almost all cells and regulates a large number of genes involved in calcium and bone homeostasis. However, numerous other genes (estimated as 3% of the human genome) involved in cell-cycle control, cell differentiation, or cell function (e.g., in the immune system) are also under the direct or indirect control of 1,25(OH)$_2$D. Moreover, 1,25(OH)$_2$D also induces several rapid and transient nongenomic biochemical reactions typically involved in second messenger signaling in a variety of cells.

Two essential vitamin D target tissues have been identified based on VDR knockout experiments: (1) the intestine for calcium and phosphorus absorption and secondarily for calcium and phosphate homeostasis and bone mineralization, because VDR or vitamin D deficiency results in rickets or osteomalacia; and (2) the skin, especially the hair follicle (for postnatal hair growth), since VDR-null mice and man develop total alopecia. Many other tissues involved in calcium transport (kidney, bone, growth plate) or serum calcium homeostasis (parathyroid gland) are targets of the vitamin D endocrine system. Moreover, 1,25(OH)$_2$D has noncalcemic effects in nearly all cells or tissues, and vitamin D deficiency is associated with a large number of major diseases such as (1) abnormal immune homeostasis (decreased native immune defense and increased risk of autoimmune diseases); (2) increased cell proliferation and increased risk of cancer; (3) cardiovascular risk factors (increased risk of hypertension by loss of vitamin D hormone or action) or metabolic diseases (all aspects of the metabolic syndrome); and (4) muscle dysfunction (increased risk of falls).

Vitamin D was discovered in the beginning of the 20th century, and vitamin D supplementation of 200 to 400 IU/d led to eradication of the widespread endemic disease, rickets. At the end of the same century, it became clear that vitamin D deficiency or insufficiency was widely present, especially so in the elderly and subjects with poor exposure to sunshine and nutritional vitamin D (immigrants with dark skin, people with poor skin exposure to sunlight because of sociocultural regions; see Chapter 15).

The definition of optimal vitamin D nutritional status is not finally settled, but all experts agree that at least a 25(OH)D level of 20 ng/mL (= 50 nmol/L) should be reached in all adults. Lower vitamin D status increases the risk for falls and osteoporotic fractures and is associated with a large number of human diseases. It is therefore imperative that a widespread supplementation program should be organized for all risk groups. Finally, future randomized clinical trials should generate the data to define the best vitamin D status for not only bone but also global health.

Chemical modifications of the parent 1,25(OH)$_2$D molecule, in line with ligands for other nuclear receptors, generated several thousands of analogs, some of which have a superagonistic and/or selective activity profile or are VDR antagonists. A few analogs are already in use for the treatment of hyperproliferative skin disorders, secondary hyperparathyroidism, and renal osteodystrophy. Vitamin D analogs are being explored for their potential use for a variety of other applications (cancer, immunology, inflammatory, or bone diseases).

Acknowledgments

The efficient help of my collaborators E. van Etten, A. Verstuyf, L. Verlinden, G. Eelen, G. Carmeliet, C. Mathieu, L. Lieben, R. Masuyama, and the financial support from the K.U. Leuven and Fonds voor Wetenschappelijk Onderzoek Vlaanderen is highly appreciated, as well as the secretarial assistance of D. De Graef.

REFERENCES

1. Whistler D: Morbo puerili Anglorum, quem patrio idiomate indigenae vocant. The Rickets. 1645, Lugduni Batavorum, pp 1–13.
2. Glisson F: De Rachitide sive morbo puerili, qui vulgo, London, 1650, The Rickets diciteur, pp 1–416.
3. Mozolowski W: Jedrzej Sniadecki (1768–1883) on the cure of rickets, Nature 143:121, 1939.
4. Palm TA: The geographic distribution and etiology of rickets, Practitioner 45:321–342, 1890.
5. Huldshinsky K: Heilung von Rachitis durch künstliche Höhensonne, Dtsch Med Wochenschr 45:712–713, 1919.
6. Chick HP, Dalyell EJ, Hume EM, et al: Studies of rickets in Vienna 1919–1922. Medical Research Council Special Report Series, No. 77, London, 1923, Medical Research Council.
7. Hess AF, Weinstock M: Antirachitic properties imparted to lettuce and to growing wheat by ultraviolet irradiation, Proc Soc Exp Biol Med 22:5–6, 1924.
8. Mellanby E, Cantag MD: Experimental investigation on rickets, Lancet 196:407–412, 1919.
9. McCollum EV, Simmonds N, Pitz W: The relation of unidentified dietary factors, the fat-soluble A and water-soluble B of the diet to the growth promoting properties of milk, J Biol Chem 27:33–38, 1916.
10. McCollum EV, Simmonds N, Becker JE, et al: Studies on experimental rickets. XXI. An experimental demonstration of the existence of a vitamin which promotes calcium deposition, J Biol Chem 53:293–312, 1922.
11. Goldblatt H, Soames KN: A study of rats on a normal diet irradiated daily by the mercury vapor quartz lamp or kept in darkness, Biochem J 17:294–297, 1923.
12. Windaus A, Linsert O: Vitamin D$_1$, Ann Chem 465:148, 1928.
13. Specker BL, Tsang RC, Hollis BW: Effect of race and diet on human-milk vitamin-D and 25-hydroxyvitamin D, Am J Dis Child 139:1134–1137, 1985.
14. Hollis BW: Vitamin D requirement during pregnancy and lactation, J Bone Miner Res 22:V39–V44, 2007.
15. Holick MF: Vitamin D and the kidney, Kidney Intl 32:912–929, 1987.
16. Holick MF: Vitamin D deficiency, N Engl J Med 357:266–281, 2007.
17. Chen TC, Shao Q, Heath H, et al: An update on the vitamin-D content of fortified milk from the United States and Canada, N Engl J Med 329:1507, 1993.
18. Holick MF, Shao Q, Liu WW, et al: The vitamin D content of fortified milk and infant formula, N Engl J Med 326:1178–1181, 1992.
19. Murphy SP, Calloway DH: Nutrient intakes of women in NHANES II, emphasizing trace minerals, fiber, and phytate, J Am Diet Assoc 86:1366–1372, 1986.
20. Krall EA, Sahyoun N, Tannenbaum S, et al: Effect of vitamin D intake on seasonal variations in parathyroid hormone secretion in postmenopausal women, N Engl J Med 321:1777–1783, 1989.
21. Lamberg-Allardt C, Karkkainen M, Seppanen R, et al: Low serum 25-hydroxyvitamin D concentrations and secondary hyperparathyroidism in middle-aged white strict vegetarians, Am J Clin Nutr 58:684–689, 1993.
22. Norman AW, Bouillon R, Whiting SJ, et al: 13th Workshop consensus for vitamin D nutritional guidelines, J Steroid Biochem Mol Biol 103:204–205, 2007.
23. European Food Safety Authority Scientific Committee on Food; Scientific Panel on Dietetic Products, Nutrition and Allergies: Tolerable upper intake levels for vitamin D and minerals. http://www.efsa.europa.eu/. 2006.
24. Bouillon R, Carmeliet G, Verlinden L, et al: Vitamin D and human health: lessons from vitamin D receptor null mice, Endocr Rev 29:726–776, 2008.
25. Kelley RI: RXH/Smith-Lemli-Opitz syndrome: mutations and metabolic morphogenesis, Am J Hum Genet 63:322–326, 1998.
26. Cunniff C, Kratz LE, Moser A, et al: Clinical and biochemical spectrum of patients with RSH/Smith-Lemli-Opitz syndrome and abnormal cholesterol metabolism, Am J Med Genet 68:263–269, 1997.
27. Rossi M, Federico G, Corso G, et al: Vitamin D status in patients affected by Smith-Lemli-Opitz syndrome, J Inherit Metab Dis 28:69–80, 2005.
28. Bonjour JP, Trechsel U, Granzer E, et al: The increase in skin 7-dehydrocholesterol induced by an hypocholesterolemic agent is associated with elevated 25-hydroxyvitamin D$_3$ plasma level, Pflügers Arch 410:165–168, 1987.
29. Morris JG: Ineffective synthesis of vitamin D in kittens exposed to sun or UV light is reversed by an inhibitor of 7-dehydrocholesterol-delta7-reductase. In Norman AW, Bouillon R, Thomasset M, editors: Vitamin D: Chemistry, Biology and Clinical Applications of the Steroid Hormone, Riverside, CA, 1997, University of California, pp 721–722.
30. Oliveri B, Zeni S, Lorenzetti MP, et al: Effect of one year residence in Antarctica on bone mineral metabolism and body composition, Eur J Clin Nutr 53:88–91, 1999.
31. Du X, Greenfield H, Fraser DR, et al: Vitamin D deficiency and associated factors in adolescent girls in Beijing, Am J Clin Nutr 74:494–500, 2001.
32. Lips P: Vitamin D deficiency and secondary hyperparathyroidism in the elderly: consequences for bone loss and fractures and therapeutic implications, Endocr Rev 22:477–501, 2001.
33. Lips P: Which circulating level of 25-hydroxyvitamin D is appropriate? J Steroid Biochem Mol Biol 89–90:611–614, 2004.
34. Lips P: Vitamin D status and nutrition in Europe and Asia, J Steroid Biochem Mol Biol 103:620–625, 2007.
35. Munns C, Zacharin MR, Rodda CP, et al: Prevention and treatment of infant and childhood vitamin D deficiency in Australia and New Zealand: a consensus statement, Med J Aust 185:268–272, 2006.
36. Working Group of the Australian and New Zealand Bone and Mineral Society ESoAoA: Vitamin D and adult bone health in Australia and New Zealand: a position statement, Med J Aust 182:281–285, 2005.
37. Gascon-Barré M: The vitamin D 25-hydroxylase. In Feldman D, Pike JW, Glorieux FH, editors: Vitamin D, San Diego, 2005, Academic Press, pp 47–67.
38. Henry HL: The 25-hydroxyvitamin D 1α-hydroxylase. In Feldman D, Pike JW, Glorieux FH, editors: Vitamin D, San Diego, 2005, Academic Press; 69–83.
39. Blunt JW, DeLuca HF, Schnoes HK: 25-Hydroxycholecalciferol. A biologically active metabolite of vitamin D$_3$, Biochemistry 7:3317–3322, 1968.
40. Ponchon G, Kennan AL, DeLuca HF: "Activation" of vitamin D by the liver, J Clin Invest 48:2032–2037, 1969.
41. Postlind H, Axen E, Bergman T, et al: Cloning, structure, and expression of a cDNA encoding vitamin D$_3$ 25-hydroxylase, Biochem Biophys Res Commun 241:491–497, 1997.
42. Cheng JB, Levine MA, Bell NH, et al: Genetic evidence that the human CYP2R1 enzyme is a key vitamin D 25-hydroxylase, Proc Natl Acad Sci U S A 101:7711–7715, 2004.
43. Maeda N, Reshef A, Lippoldt A, et al: Markedly reduced bile acid synthesis but maintained levels of cholesterol and vitamin D metabolites in mice with disrupted sterol 27-hydroxylase gene, J Biol Chem 273:14805–14812, 1998.
44. Bhattacharyya MH, DeLuca HF: The regulation of calciferol-25-hydroxylase in the chick, Biochem Biophys Res Commun 59:734–741, 1974.
45. Fraser DR, Kodicek E: Unique biosynthesis by kidney of a biologically active vitamin D metabolite, Nature 228:764–766, 1970.
46. Nicolaysen R, Eeglarsen N, Malm J: Physiology of calcium metabolism, Physiol Rev 33:424–444, 1953.
47. Monkawa T, Yoshida T, Wakino S, et al: Molecular cloning of cDNA and genomic DNA for human 25-hydroxyvitamin D$_3$ 1α-hydroxylase, Biochem Biophys Res Commun 239:527–533, 1997.
48. Fu GK, Lin D, Zhang MYH, et al: Cloning of human 25-hydroxyvitamin D-1α-hydroxylase and mutations causing vitamin D-dependent rickets type 1, Mol Endocrinol 11:1961–1970, 1997.
49. St-Arnaud R, Messerlian S, Moir JM, et al: The 25-hydroxyvitamin D 1-alpha-hydroxylase gene maps to the pseudovitamin D-deficiency rickets (PDDR) disease locus, J Bone Miner Res 12:1552–1559, 1997.
50. Takeyama K, Kitanaka S, Sato T, et al: 25-Hydroxyvitamin D$_3$ 1α-hydroxylase and vitamin D synthesis, Science 277:1827–1830, 1997.
51. Shinki T, Shimada H, Wakino S, et al: Cloning and expression of rat 25-hydroxyvitamin D$_3$-1α-hydroxylase cDNA, Proc Natl Acad Sci U S A 94:12920–12925, 1997.
52. Overbergh L, Decallonne B, Valckx D, et al: Identification and immune regulation of 25-hydroxyvitamin D-1-alpha-hydroxylase in murine macrophages, Clin Exp Immunol 120:139–146, 2000.
53. Bell NH: 25-Hydroxyvitamin D-1α-hydroxylases and their clinical significance, J Bone Miner Res 13:350–353, 1998.
54. Razzaque MS, Sitara D, Taguchi T, et al: Premature aging-like phenotype in fibroblast growth factor 23 null mice is a vitamin D-mediated process, FASEB J 20:720–722, 2006.
55. Brenza HL, Kimmel-Jehan C, Jehan F, et al: Parathyroid hormone activation of the 25-hydroxylation D$_3$–1α-hydroxylase gene promotor, Proc Natl Acad Sci U S A 95:1387–1391, 1998.
56. Murayama A, Takeyama K, Kitanaka S, et al: The promoter of the human 25-hydroxyvitamin D$_3$ 1α-hydroxylase gene confers positive and negative responsiveness to PTH, Calcitonin, and 1α,25(OH)$_2$D$_3$, Biochem Biophys Res Commun 249:11–16, 1998.
57. Kato S, Fujiki R, Kim MS, et al: Ligand-induced transrepressive function of VDR requires a chromatin remodeling complex, WINAC, J Steroid Biochem Mol Biol 103:372–380, 2007.
58. Fraser D, Kooh SW, Kind HP, et al: Pathogenesis of hereditary vitamin-D-dependent rickets, An inborn error of vitamin D metabolism involving defective conversion of 25-hydroxyvitamin D to 1α,25-dihydroxyvitamin D, N Engl J Med 289:817–822, 1973.
59. Kitanaka S, Takeyama K, Murayama A, et al: Inactivating mutations in the 25-hydroxyvitamin D$_3$ 1α-hydroxylase gene in patients with pseudovitamin D-deficient rickets, N Engl J Med 338:653–661, 1998.

60. Ohyama Y, Noshiro M, Eggertsen G, et al: Structural characterization of the gene encoding rat 25-hydroxyvitamin-D(3) 24-hydroxylase, Biochemistry 32:76–82, 1993.

61. Lohnes D, Jones G: Side chain metabolism of vitamin D₃ in osteosarcoma cell line UMR-106, J Biol Chem 262:14394–14401, 1987.

62. Akiyoshi-Shibata M, Sakaki T, Ohyama Y, et al: Further oxidation of hydroxycalcidiol by calcidiol 24-hydroxylase. A study with the mature enzyme expressed in Escherichia coli, Eur J Biochem 224:335–343, 1994.

63. St Arnaud R, Arabian A, Travers R, et al: Deficient mineralization of intramembranous bone in vitamin D-24-hydroxylase-ablated mice is due to elevated 1,25-dihydroxyvitamin D and not to the absence of 24,25-dihydroxyvitamin D, Endocrinology 141:2658–2666, 2000.

64. Meyer MB, Zella LA, Nerenz RD, et al: Characterizing early events associated with the activation of target genes by 1,25-dihydroxyvitamin D₃ in mouse kidney and intestine in vivo, J Biol Chem 282:22344–22352, 2007.

65. Omdahl J, May B: The 25-hydroxyvitamin D 24-hydroxylase. In Feldman D, Pike JW, Glorieux FH, editors: Vitamin D, San Diego, 2005, Academic Press, pp 85–104.

66. Yoshizawa T, Handa Y, Uematsu Y, et al: Mice lacking the vitamin D receptor exhibit impaired bone formation, uterine hypoplasia and growth retardation after weaning, Nat Genet 16:391–396, 1997.

67. Albertson DG, Ylstra B, Segraves R, et al: Quantitative mapping of amplicon structure by array CGH identifies CYP24 as a candidate oncogene, Nat Genet 25:144–146, 2000.

68. Reddy GS, Siucaldera ML, Schuster I, et al: Target tissue specific metabolism of 1,25(OH)₂D₃ through A-ring modification. In Norman AW, Bouillon R, Thomasset M, editors: Vitamin D: Chemistry, Biology and Clinical Applications of the Steroid Hormone, Riverside, CA, 1997, University of California, pp 139–146.

69. Dueland S, Pedersen JI, Helgerud P, et al: Absorption, distribution, and transport of vitamin-D₃ and 25-hydroxyvitamin-D₃ in the rat, Am J Physiol 245:E463–E467, 1983.

70. Bouillon R, Van Baelen H, Rombauts W, et al: The purification and characterisation of the human-serum binding protein for the 25-hydroxycholecalciferol (transcalciferin). Identity with group-specific component, Eur J Biochem 66:285–291, 1976.

71. Hirschfeld J: Immune-electrophoretic demonstration of qualitative differences in human sera and their relation to the haptoglobins, Acta Pathol Microbiol 47:160–168, 1959.

72. Westwood WAWDJ: Group-specific component: a review of the isoelectric focusing methods and auxiliary methods available for the separation of its phenotypes, Forensic Sci Int 32:135–150, 1986.

73. Cleve H, Constants J: The mutants of the vitamin-D-binding protein: more than 120 variants of the GC/DBP system, Vox Sang 54:215–225, 1988.

74. Cooke NE, Safadi FF, Magiera HM, et al: Biological consequences of vitamin D binding protein deficiency in a mouse model. In Norman AW, Bouillon R, Thomasset M, editors: Vitamin D: Chemistry, Biology and Clinical Applications of the Steroid Hormone, Riverside, CA, 1997, University of California, pp 105–111.

75. Laing CJ, Cooke NE: Vitamin D binding protein. In Feldman D, Pike JW, Glorieux FH, editors: Vitamin D, San Diego, 2005, Academic Press, pp 117–134.

76. Verboven C, Rabijns A, De MM, et al: A structural basis for the unique binding features of the human vitamin D-binding protein, Nat Struct Biol 9:131–136, 2002.

77. Bouillon R, Van Baelen H: The transport of vitamin D: significance of free and total concentrations of vitamin D metabolites. In Norman AW, Schaefer K, von Herrath K, et al: Vitamin D: Chemical, Biochemical and Clinical Endocrinology of Calcium Metabolism, Berlin, 1982, Walter de Gruyter, pp 1181–1186.

78. Vicchio D, Yergey A, Obrien K, et al: Quantification and kinetics of 25-hydroxyvitamin-D₃ by isotope dilution liquid chromatography/thermospray mass spectrometry, Biol Mass Spectrom 22:53–58, 1993.

79. Kumar R: The metabolism and mechanism of action of 1,25-dihydroxyvitamin-D₃, Kidney Intl 30:793–803, 1986.

80. Bouillon R, Van Assche FA, Van Baelen H, et al: Influence of the vitamin D-binding protein on the serum concentration of 1,25-dihydroxyvitamin D₃, J Clin Invest 67:589–596, 1981.

81. Nykjaer A, Dragun D, Walther D, et al: An endocytic pathway essential for renal uptake and activation of the steroid 25-(OH) vitamin D₃, Cell 96:507–515, 1999.

82. McLeod JF, Kowalski MA, Haddad JG: Interactions among serum vitamin D binding protein, monomeric actin, profilin, and profilactin, J Biol Chem 264:1260–1267, 1989.

83. Van Baelen H, Bouillon R, De Moor P: Vitamin D-binding protein (Gc-globulin) binds actin, J Biol Chem 255:2270–2272, 1980.

84. Goldschmidt-Clermont PJ, Van Baelen H, Bouillon R, et al: Role of group-specific component (vitamin D binding protein) in clearance of actin from the circulation in the rabbit, J Clin Invest 81:1519–1527, 1988.

85. Lee WM, Galbraith RM: The extracellular actin-scavenger system and actin toxicity, N Engl J Med 326:1335–1341, 1992.

86. Whitfield GK, Jurutka PW, Haussler CA, et al: Nuclear vitamin D receptor: structure-function, molecular control of gene transcription, and novel bioactions. In Feldman D, Pike JW, Glorieux FH, editors: Vitamin D, San Diego, 2005, Academic Press, pp 219–261.

87. Miyamoto K, Kesterson RA, Yamamoto H, et al: Structural organization of the human vitamin D receptor chromosomal gene and its promoter, Mol Endocrinol 11:1165–1179, 1997.

88. Crofts LA, Hancock MS, Morrison NA, et al: Multiple promoters direct the tissue-specific expression of novel N-terminal variant human vitamin D receptor gene transcripts, Proc Natl Acad Sci USA 95:10529–10534, 1998.

89. Haussler MR, Whitfield GK, Haussler CA, et al: The nuclear vitamin D receptor: biological and molecular regulatory properties revealed, J Bone Miner Res 13:325–349, 1998.

90. Masuyama H, Jefcoat SC Jr, MacDonald PN: The N-terminal domain of transcription factor IIB is required for direct interaction with the vitamin D receptor and participates in vitamin D-mediated transcription, Mol Endocrinol 11:218–228, 1997.

91. Nagy L, Kao J-YCD, Lin RJ, et al: Nuclear receptor repression mediated by a complex containing SMRT, mSin3A, and histone deacetylase, Cell 89:373–380, 1997.

92. Chakravarti D, LaMorte VJ, Nelson MC, et al: Role of CBP/P300 in nuclear receptor signalling, Nature 383:99–103, 1996.

93. Kamei Y, Xu L, Heinzel T, et al: A CBP integrator complex mediates transcriptional activation and AP-1 inhibition by nuclear receptors, Cell 85:403–414, 1996.

94. Rachez C, Freedman LP: Mechanisms of gene regulation by vitamin D(3) receptor: a network of coactivator interactions, Gene 246:9–21, 2000.

95. Spencer TE, Jenster G, Burcin MM, et al: Steroid receptor coactivator-1 is a histone acetyltransferase, Nature 389:194–198, 1997.

96. Rachez C, Gamble M, Chang CP, et al: The DRIP complex and SRC-1/p160 coactivators share similar nuclear receptor binding determinants but constitute functionally distinct complexes, Mol Cell Biol 20:2718–2726, 2000.

97. Kitagawa H, Fujiki R, Yoshimura K, et al: The chromatin-remodeling complex WINAC targets a nuclear receptor to promoters and is impaired in Williams syndrome, Cell 113:905–917, 2003.

98. Li B, Carey M, Workman JL: The role of chromatin during transcription, Cell 128:707–719, 2007.

99. Villagra A, Cruzat F, Carvallo L, et al: Chromatin remodeling and transcriptional activity of the bone-specific osteocalcin gene require CCAAT/enhancer-binding protein beta-dependent recruitment of SWI/SNF activity, J Biol Chem 281:22695–22706, 2006.

100. Li H, Chen JD: The receptor-associated coactivator 3 activates transcription through CREB-binding protein recruitment and autoregulation, J Biol Chem 273:5948–5954, 1998.

101. Lavinsky RM, Jepsen K, Heinzel T, et al: Diverse signaling pathways modulate nuclear receptor recruitment of N-CoR and SMRT complexes, Proc Natl Acad Sci U S A 95:2920–2925, 1998.

102. Carlberg C: The concept of multiple vitamin D signaling pathways, J Invest Dermatol Symp Proc 1:10–14, 1996.

103. Norman AW, Mizwicki MT, Norman DP: Steroid-hormone rapid actions, membrane receptors and a conformational ensemble model, Nat Rev Drug Discov 3:27–41, 2004.

104. Revelli A, Massobrio M, Tesarik J: Nongenomic effects of 1α,25-dihydroxyvitamin D₃, Trends Endocrinol Metab 9:419–422, 1998.

105. Norman AW, Zanello LP, De Song X, et al: Effectiveness of 1α,25(OH)₂-vitamin D₃-mediated signal transduction for genomic and rapid biological responses is dependent upon the conformation of the signaling ligand. In Norman AW, Bouillon R, Thomasset M, editors: Vitamin D: Chemistry, Biology and Clinical Applications of the Steroid Hormone, Riverside, CA, 1997, University of California, pp 331–333.

106. Norman AW, Bouillon R, Farach-Carson MC, et al: Demonstration that 1b,25-dihydroxyvitamin D₃ is an antagonist of the nongenomic but not genomic biological responses and biological profile of the three A-ring diastereomers of 1α,25-dihydroxyvitamin D₃, J Biol Chem 268:20022–20030, 1993.

107. Song X, Bishop JE, Okamura WH, et al: Stimulation of phosphorylation of mitogen-activated protein kinase by 1α,25-dihydroxyvitamin D₃ in promyelocytic NB4 leukemia cells: a structure-function study, Endocrinology 139:457–468, 1998.

108. Norman AW, Okamura WH, Farach-Carson MC, et al: Structure-function studies of 1,25-dihydroxyvitamin D₃ and the vitamin-D endocrine system. 1,25-Dihydroxy-pentadeuterio-previtamin D₃ (as a 6-s-cis analog) stimulates nongenomic but not genomic biological responses, J Biol Chem 268:13811–13819, 1993.

109. Strom TM, Juppner H: PHEX, FGF23, DMP1 and beyond, Curr Opin Nephrol Hypertens 17:357–362, 2008.

110. Taketani T, Miyamoto K-I, Tanaka K, et al: Gene structure and functional analysis of the human Na⁺/phosphate co-transporter, Biochem J 324:927–937, 1997.

111. Wasserman RH: Vitamin D and the intestinal absorption of calcium: a view and overview. In Feldman D, Pike JW, Glorieux FH, editors: Vitamin D, San Diego, 2005, Academic Press, pp 411–428.

112. Van Cromphaut SJ, Dewerchin M, Hoenderop JG, et al: Duodenal calcium absorption in vitamin D receptor-knockout mice: functional and molecular aspects, Proc Natl Acad Sci U S A 98:13324–13329, 2001.

113. Feher JJ: Facilitated calcium diffusion by intestinal calcium-binding protein, Cell Physiol 13:C303–C307, 1983.

114. Pannabecker TL, Chandler JS, Wasserman RH: Vitamin D-dependent transcriptional regulation of the intestinal plasma membrane calcium pump, Biochem Biophys Res Commun 213:499–505, 1995.

115. Li YC, Pirro AE, Amling M, et al: Targeted ablation of the vitamin D receptor: an animal model of vitamin D-dependent rickets type II with alopecia, Proc Natl Acad Sci U S A 94:9831–9835, 1997.

116. Erben RG, Soegiarto DW, Weber K, et al: Deletion of deoxyribonucleic acid binding domain of the vitamin D receptor abrogates genomic and nongenomic functions of vitamin D, Mol Endocrinol 16:1524–1537, 2002.

117. Dardenne O, Prud'homme J, Arabian A, et al: Targeted inactivation of the 25-hydroxyvitamin D(3)-1(alpha)-hydroxylase gene (CYP27B1) creates an animal model of pseudovitamin D-deficiency rickets, Endocrinology 142:3135–3141, 2001.

118. Panda DK, Miao D, Tremblay ML, et al: Targeted ablation of the 25-hydroxyvitamin-D 1-alpha-hydroxylase enzyme: evidence for skeletal, reproductive, and immune dysfunction, Proc Natl Acad Sci U S A 98:7498–7503, 2001.

119. Dardenne O, Prud'homme J, Hacking SA, et al: Correction of the abnormal mineral ion homeostasis with a high-calcium, high-phosphorus, high-lactose diet rescues the PDDR phenotype of mice deficient for the 25-hydroxyvitamin-D 1-alpha-hydroxylase (CYP27B1), Bone 32:332–340, 2003.

120. Amling M, Priemel M, Holzmann T, et al: Rescue of the skeletal phenotype of vitamin D receptor–ablated

mice in the setting of normal mineral ion homeostasis: formal histomorphometric and biomechanical analyses, Endocrinology 140:4982–4987, 1999.

121. Dardenne O, Prudhomme J, Hacking SA, et al: Rescue of the pseudo-vitamin D deficiency rickets phenotype of CYP27B1-deficient mice by treatment with 1,25-dihydroxyvitamin D_3: biochemical, histomorphometric, and biomechanical analyses, J Bone Miner Res 18:637–643, 2003.
122. Hoenderop JG, Dardenne O, Van AM, et al: Modulation of renal Ca^{2+} transport protein genes by dietary Ca^{2+} and 1,25-dihydroxyvitamin D_3 in 25-hydroxyvitamin D_3–1α-hydroxylase knockout mice, FASEB J 16:1398–1406, 2002.
123. Li YC, Amling M, Pirro AE, et al: Normalization of mineral ion homeostasis by dietary means prevents hyperparathyroidism, rickets, and osteomalacia, but not alopecia in vitamin D receptor-ablated mice, Endocrinology 139:4391–4396, 1998.
124. Rowling MJ, Gliniak C, Welsh J, et al: High dietary vitamin D prevents hypocalcemia and osteomalacia in CYP27B1 knockout mice, J Nutr 137:2608–2615, 2007.
125. Song Y, Kato S, Fleet JC: Vitamin D receptor (VDR) knockout mice reveal VDR-independent regulation of intestinal calcium absorption and ECaC2 and calbindin D9k mRNA, J Nutr 133:374–380, 2003.
126. Balsan S, Garabedian M, Larchet M, et al: Long-term nocturnal calcium infusions can cure rickets and promote normal mineralization in hereditary resistance to 1,25-dihydroxyvitamin D, J Clin Invest 77:1661–1667, 1986.
127. Hochberg Z, Tiosano D, Even L: Calcium therapy for calcitriol-resistant rickets, J Pediatr 121:803–808, 1992.
128. Lieben L, Masuyama R, Moermans K, et al: Intestinal-specific vitamin D receptor null mice maintain normal calcemia but display severe bone loss, J Bone Miner Res ASBMR Abstracts:SA238, 2008.
129. Benn BS, Ajibade D, Porta A, et al: Active intestinal calcium transport in the absence of transient receptor potential vanilloid type 6 and calbindin-D9k, Endocrinology 149:3196–3205, 2008.
130. Fujita H, Sugimoto K, Inatomi S, et al: Tight junction proteins claudin-2 and -12 are critical for vitamin D-dependent Ca^{2+} absorption between enterocytes, Mol Biol Cell 19:1912–1921, 2008.
131. Renkema KY, Nijenhuis T, van der Eerden BC, et al: Hypervitaminosis D mediates compensatory Ca^{2+} hyperabsorption in TRPV5 knockout mice, J Am Soc Nephrol 16:3188–3195, 2005.
132. Okano T, Tsugawa N, Masuda S, et al: Regulatory activities of 2b-(3-hydroxypropoxy)-1α,25-dihydroxyvitamin D_3, a novel synthetic vitamin D_3 derivative, on calcium metabolism, Biochem Biophys Res Commun 163:1444–1449, 1989.
133. Tilyard MW, Spears GFS, Thomson J, et al: Treatment of postmenopausal osteoporosis with calcitriol or calcium, N Engl J Med 326:357–362, 1992.
134. Gardiner EM, Sims NA, Thomas GP, et al: Elevated osteoblastic vitamin D receptor in transgenic mice yields stronger bones, Bone 23:S176, 1998.
135. Donohue MM, Demay MB: Rickets in VDR null mice is secondary to decreased apoptosis of hypertrophic chondrocytes, Endocrinology 143:3691–3694, 2002.
136. Sabbagh Y, Carpenter TO, Demay MB: Hypophosphatemia leads to rickets by impairing caspase-mediated apoptosis of hypertrophic chondrocytes, Proc Natl Acad Sci U S A 102:9637–9642, 2005.
137. Masuyama R, Stockmans I, Torrekens S, et al: Vitamin D receptor in chondrocytes promotes osteoclastogenesis and regulates FGF23 production in osteoblasts, J Clin Invest 116:3150–3159, 2006.
138. Bikle DD, Pillai S: Vitamin D, calcium, and epidermal differentiation, Endocr Rev 14:3–19, 1993.
139. Bikle DD, Chang S, Crumrine D, et al: 25 Hydroxyvitamin D 1 alpha-hydroxylase is required for optimal epidermal differentiation and permeability barrier homeostasis, J Invest Dermatol 122:984–992, 2004.
140. Gilchrest BA: Sun exposure and vitamin D sufficiency, Am J Clin Nutr 88:570S–577S, 2008.
141. De HP, Garmyn M, Verstuyf A, et al: 1,25-Dihydroxyvitamin D_3 and analogues protect primary human keratinocytes against UVB-induced DNA damage, J Photochem Photobiol B 78:141–148, 2005.
142. Gupta R, Dixon KM, Deo SS, et al: Photoprotection by 1,25 dihydroxyvitamin D_3 is associated with an increase in p53 and a decrease in nitric oxide products, J Invest Dermatol 127:707–715, 2007.
143. Jensen SS, Madsen MW, Lukas J, et al: Inhibitory effects of 1-alpha,25-dihydroxyvitamin D(3) on the G(1)-S phase-controlling machinery, Mol Endocrinol 15:1370–1380, 2001.
144. Colston K, Colston MJ, Feldman D: 1,25-dihydroxyvitamin D_3 and malignant melanoma: the presence of receptors and inhibition of cell growth in culture, Endocrinology 108:1083–1086, 1981.
145. Abe E, Miyaura C, Sakagami H, et al: Differentiation of mouse myeloid leukemia cells induced by 1 alpha,25-dihydroxyvitamin D_3, Proc Natl Acad Sci U S A 78:4990–4994, 1981.
146. Verlinden L, Eelen G, Beullens I, et al: Characterization of the condensin component Cnap1 and protein kinase Melk as novel E2F target genes down-regulated by 1,25-dihydroxyvitamin D_3, J Biol Chem 280:37319–37330, 2005.
147. Moreno J, Krishnan AV, Peehl DM, et al: Mechanisms of vitamin D-mediated growth inhibition in prostate cancer cells: inhibition of the prostaglandin pathway, Anticancer Res 26:2525–2530, 2006.
148. Aguilera O, Pena C, Garcia JM, et al: The Wnt antagonist DICKKOPF-1 gene is induced by 1-alpha,25-dihydroxyvitamin D_3 associated to the differentiation of human colon cancer cells, Carcinogenesis 28:1877–1884, 2007.
149. Tong WM, Kallay E, Hofer H, et al: Growth regulation of human colon cancer cells by epidermal growth factor and 1,25-dihydroxyvitamin D_3 is mediated by mutual modulation of receptor expression, Eur J Cancer 34:2119–2125, 1998.
150. Vink-van Wijngaarden T, Pols HA, Buurman CJ, et al: Inhibition of insulin- and insulin-like growth factor-I-stimulated growth of human breast cancer cells by 1,25-dihydroxyvitamin D_3 and the vitamin D_3 analogue EB1089, Eur J Cancer 32A:842–848, 1996.
151. Verlinden L, Verstuyf A, Convents R, et al: Action of $1,25(OH)2D_3$ on the cell cycle genes, cyclin D1, p21 and p27 in MCF-7 cells, Mol Cell Endocrinol 142:57–65, 1998.
152. Reitsma PH, Rothberg PG, Astrin SM, et al: Regulation of myc gene expression in HL-60 leukaemia cells by a vitamin D metabolite, Nature 306:492–494, 1983.
153. Matsumoto K, Hashimoto K, Nishida Y, et al: Growth-inhibitory effects of 1,25-dihydroxyvitamin D_3 on normal human keratinocytes cultured in serum-free medium, Biochem Biophys Res Commun 166:916–923, 1990.
154. Mercier T, Chaumontet C, Gaillard-Sanchez I, et al: Calcitriol and lexicalcitol (KH1060) inhibit the growth of human breast adenocarcinoma cells by enhancing transforming growth factor-beta production, Biochem Pharmacol 52:505–510, 1996.
155. Wu Y, Haugen JD, Zinsmeister AR, et al: 1 alpha,25-dihydroxyvitamin D_3 increases transforming growth factor and transforming growth factor receptor type I and II synthesis in human bone cells, Biochem Biophys Res Commun 239:734–739, 1997.
156. Rozen F, Pollak M: Inhibition of insulin-like growth factor I receptor signaling by the vitamin D analogue EB1089 in MCF-7 breast cancer cells: A role for insulin-like growth factor binding proteins, Int J Oncol 15:589–594, 1999.
157. Welsh J: Targets of vitamin D receptor signaling in the mammary gland, J Bone Miner Res 22:V86–V90, 2007.
158. Bouillon R, Eelen G, Verlinden L, et al: Vitamin D and cancer, J Steroid Biochem Mol Biol 102:156–162, 2006.
159. Freedman DM, Looker AC, Chang SC, et al: Prospective study of serum vitamin D and cancer mortality in the United States, J Natl Cancer Inst 99:1594–1602, 2007.
160. Garland CF, Gorham ED, Mohr SB, et al: Vitamin D and prevention of breast cancer: pooled analysis, J Steroid Biochem Mol Biol 103:708–711, 2007.
161. Giovannucci E: Strengths and limitations of current epidemiologic studies: vitamin D as a modifier of colon and prostate cancer risk, Nutr Rev 65:S77–S79, 2007.
162. Bouillon R, Bischoff-Ferrari H, Willett W: Vitamin D and health: perspectives from mice and man, J Bone Miner Res 23:974–979, 2008.
163. Wactawski-Wende J, Kotchen JM, Anderson GL, et al: Calcium plus vitamin D supplementation and the risk of colorectal cancer, N Engl J Med 354:684–696, 2006.
164. Lappe JM, Travers-Gustafson D, Davies KM, et al: Vitamin D and calcium supplementation reduces cancer risk: results of a randomized trial, Am J Clin Nutr 85:1586–1591, 2007.
165. Overbergh L, Stoffels K, Waer M, et al: Immune regulation of 25-hydroxyvitamin D-1-alpha-hydroxylase in human monocytic THP1 cells: mechanisms of interferon-gamma-mediated induction, J Clin Endocrinol Metab 91:3566–3574, 2006.
166. Stoffels K, Overbergh L, Giulietti A, et al: Immune regulation of 25-hydroxyvitamin-D_3–1α-hydroxylase in human monocytes, J Bone Miner Res 21:37–47, 2006.
167. Stoffels K, Overbergh L, Bouillon R, et al: Immune regulation of 1α-hydroxylase in murine peritoneal macrophages: unravelling the IFNgamma pathway, J Steroid Biochem Mol Biol 103:567–571, 2007.
168. Kankova M, Luini W, Pedrazzoni M, et al: Impairment of cytokine production in mice fed a vitamin D_3-deficient diet, Immunology 73:466–471, 1991.
169. Giulietti A, Gysemans C, Stoffels K, et al: Vitamin D deficiency in early life accelerates type 1 diabetes in non-obese diabetic mice, Diabetologia 47:451–462, 2004.
170. Chan TY: Vitamin D deficiency and susceptibility to tuberculosis, Calcif Tissue Int 66:476–478, 2000.
171. Davies PDO, Brown RC, Woodhead JS: Serum concentrations of vitamin D metabolites in untreated tuberculosis, Thorax 40:187–190, 1985.
172. Grange JM, Davies PDO, Brown RC, et al: A study of vitamin D levels in Indonesian patients with untreated pulmonary tuberculosis, Tubercle 66:187–191, 1985.
173. Waters WR, Palmer MV, Nonnecke BJ, et al: *Mycobacterium bovis* infection of vitamin D-deficient NOS2-/- mice, Microb Pathog 36:11–17, 2004.
174. Wilkinson RJ, Llewelyn M, Toossi Z, et al: Influence of vitamin D deficiency and vitamin D receptor polymorphisms on tuberculosis among Gujarati Asians in west London: a case-control study, Lancet 355:618–621, 2000.
175. Liu PT, Stenger S, Li H, et al: Toll-like receptor triggering of a vitamin D-mediated human antimicrobial response, Science 311:1770–1773, 2006.
176. Morcos MM, Gabr AA, Samuel S, et al: Vitamin D administration to tuberculous children and its value, Boll Chim Farm 137:157–164, 1998.
177. Nursyam EW, Amin Z, Rumende CM: The effect of vitamin D as supplementary treatment in patients with moderately advanced pulmonary tuberculous lesion, Acta Med Indones 38:3–5, 2006.
178. Zella JB, DeLuca HF: Vitamin D and autoimmune diabetes, J Cell Biochem 88:216–222, 2003.
179. Liu N, Nguyen L, Chun RF, et al: Altered endocrine and autocrine metabolism of vitamin D in a mouse model of gastrointestinal inflammation, Endocrinology 149:4799–4808, 2008.
180. Mathieu C, Gysemans C, Giulietti A, et al: Vitamin D and diabetes, Diabetologia 48:1247–1257, 2005.
181. Guo SW, Magnuson VL, Schiller JJ, et al: Meta-analysis of vitamin D receptor polymorphisms and type 1 diabetes: a HuGE review of genetic association studies, Am J Epidemiol 164:711–724, 2006.
182. Bailey R, Cooper JD, Zeitels L, et al: Association of the vitamin D metabolism gene *CYP27B1* with type 1 diabetes, Diabetes 56:2616–2621, 2007.
183. Munger KL, Levin LI, Hollis BW, et al: Serum 25-hydroxyvitamin D levels and risk of multiple sclerosis, JAMA 296:2832–2838, 2006.
184. Yu S, Cantorna MT: The vitamin D receptor is required for iNKT cell development, Proc Natl Acad Sci U S A 105:5207–5212, 2008.
185. Li YC, Kong J, Wei M, et al: 1,25-Dihydroxyvitamin D(3) is a negative endocrine regulator of the renin-angiotensin system, J Clin Invest 110:229–238, 2002.
186. Forman JP, Giovannucci E, Holmes MD, et al: Plasma 25-hydroxyvitamin D levels and risk of incident hypertension, Hypertension 49:1063–1069, 2007.
187. Scragg R, Sowers M, Bell C: Serum 25-hydroxyvitamin D, ethnicity, and blood pressure in the Third National Health and Nutrition Examination Survey, Am J Hypertens 20:713–719, 2007.
188. Aihara K, Azuma H, Akaike M, et al: Disruption of nuclear vitamin D receptor gene causes enhanced

thrombogenicity in mice, J Biol Chem 279:35798–35802, 2004.

189. Wang TJ, Pencina MJ, Booth SL, et al: Vitamin D deficiency and risk of cardiovascular disease, Circulation 117:503–511, 2008.

190. Hsia J, Heiss G, Ren H, et al: Calcium/vitamin D supplementation and cardiovascular events, Circulation 115:846–854, 2007.

191. Teng M, Wolf M, Lowrie E, et al: Survival of patients undergoing hemodialysis with paricalcitol or calcitriol therapy, N Engl J Med 349:446–456, 2003.

192. Palmer SC, McGregor DO, Macaskill P, et al: Meta-analysis: vitamin D compounds in chronic kidney disease, Ann Intern Med 147:840–853, 2007.

193. Endo I, Inoue D, Mitsui T, et al: Deletion of vitamin D receptor gene in mice results in abnormal skeletal muscle development with deregulated expression of myoregulatory transcription factors, Endocrinology 144:5138–5144, 2003.

194. Bischoff-Ferrari HA, wson-Hughes B, Baron JA, et al: Calcium intake and hip fracture risk in men and women: a meta-analysis of prospective cohort studies and randomized controlled trials, Am J Clin Nutr 86:1780–1790, 2007.

195. Bischoff-Ferrari HA, wson-Hughes B, Willett WC, et al: Effect of vitamin D on falls: a meta-analysis, JAMA 291:1999–2006, 2004.

196. Norman AW, Frankel BJ, Heldt AM, et al: Vitamin D deficiency inhibits pancreatic secretion of insulin, Science 209:823–825, 1980.

197. Nyomba BL, Bouillon R, De MP: Influence of vitamin D status on insulin secretion and glucose tolerance in the rabbit, Endocrinology 115:191–197, 1984.

198. Ford ES, Ajani UA, McGuire LC, et al: Concentrations of serum vitamin D and the metabolic syndrome among U.S. adults, Diabetes Care 28:1228–1230, 2005.

199. Hypponen E, Boucher BJ, Berry DJ, et al: 25-hydroxyvitamin D, IGF-1, and metabolic syndrome at 45 years of age: a cross-sectional study in the 1958 British Birth Cohort, Diabetes 57:298–305, 2008.

200. Forouhi NG, Luan J, Cooper A, et al: Baseline serum 25-hydroxy vitamin D is predictive of future glycemic status and insulin resistance: the Medical Research Council Ely Prospective Study 1990–2000, Diabetes 57:2619–2625, 2008.

201. de Boer IH, Tinker LF, Connelly S, et al: Calcium plus vitamin D supplementation and the risk of incident diabetes in the Women's Health Initiative, Diabetes Care 31:701–707, 2008.

202. Pittas AG, Harris SS, Stark PC, et al: The effects of calcium and vitamin D supplementation on blood glucose and markers of inflammation in nondiabetic adults, Diabetes Care 30:980–986, 2007.

203. Dobnig H, Pilz S, Scharnagl H, et al: Independent association of low serum 25-hydroxyvitamin D and 1,25-dihydroxyvitamin D levels with all-cause and cardiovascular mortality, Arch Intern Med 168:1340–1349, 2008.

204. Melamed ML, Michos ED, Post W, et al: 25-hydroxyvitamin D levels and the risk of mortality in the general population, Arch Intern Med 168:1629–1637, 2008.

205. Wolf M, Shah A, Gutierrez O, et al: Vitamin D levels and early mortality among incident hemodialysis patients, Kidney Int 72:1004–1013, 2007.

206. Autier P, Gandini S: Vitamin D supplementation and total mortality: a meta-analysis of randomized controlled trials, Arch Intern Med 167:1730–1737, 2007.

207. Porteous CE, Coldwell RD, Trafford DJH, et al: Recent developments in the measurement of vitamin D and its metabolites in human body fluids, J Steroid Biochem 28:785–801, 1987.

208. Bouillon R: Radiochemical assays for vitamin D metabolites: technical possibilities and clinical applications, J Steroid Biochem 19:921–927, 1983.

209. Schmidt-Gayk H, Bouillon R, Roth HJ: Measurement of vitamin D and its metabolites (calcidiol and calcitriol) and their clinical significance, Scand J Clin Lab Invest 57:35–45, 1997.

210. Binkley N, Krueger D, Gemar D, et al: Correlation among 25-hydroxy-vitamin D assays, J Clin Endocrinol Metab 93:1804–1808, 2008.

211. Lips P, Chapuy MC, Dawson-Hughes B, et al: An international comparison of serum 25-hydroxyvitamin D measurements, Osteoporos Int 9:394–397, 1999.

212. Maunsell Z, Wright DJ, Rainbow SJ: Routine isotope-dilution liquid chromatography-tandem mass spectrometry assay for simultaneous measurement of the 25-hydroxy metabolites of vitamins D_2 and D_3, Clin Chem 51:1683–1690, 2005.

213. Clements MR, Johnson L, Fraser DR: A new mechanism for induced vitamin-D deficiency in calcium deprivation, Nature 325:62–65, 1987.

214. Bouillon R, Van Baelen H: Transport of vitamin D: significance of free and total concentrations of the vitamin D metabolites, Calcif Tissue Int 33:451–453, 1981.

215. Bikle DD, Gee E: Free, and not total, 1,25-dihydroxyvitamin D regulates 25-hydroxyvitamin D metabolism by keratinocytes, Endocrinology 124:649–654, 1989.

216. Vanham G, Van Baelen H, Tan BK, et al: The effect of vitamin D analogs and of vitamin D-binding protein on lymphocyte proliferation, J Steroid Biochem 29:381–386, 1988.

217. Bouillon R, Van Baelen H: The transport of vitamin D. In Norman AW, Schaefer K, von Herrath D, et al, editors: Vitamin D: Basic Research and Its Clinical Application, Berlin, 1979, Walter de Gruyter, pp 137–143.

218. Dietary reference intakes for calcium, phosphorus, magnesium, vitamin D and fluoride. In: Food and Nutrition Board, Washington, 1997, National Academy Press, pp 1–30.

219. Lerch C, Meissner T: Interventions for the prevention of nutritional rickets in term born children, Cochrane Database Syst Rev CD00:61–64, 2007.

220. Beser E, Cakmakci T: Factors affecting the morbidity of vitamin D deficiency rickets and primary protection, East Afr Med J 71:358–362, 1994.

221. Wagner CL, Greer FR, the section on breastfeeding and committee on nutrition: Prevention of rickets and vitamin D deficiency in infants, children, and adolescents, Pediatrics 122:1142–1152, 2008.

222. Baroncelli GI, Bereket A, El KM, et al: Rickets in the Middle East: role of environment and genetic predisposition, J Clin Endocrinol Metab 93:1743–1750, 2008.

223. van der Meer I, Karamali NS, Boeke AJ, et al: High prevalence of vitamin D deficiency in pregnant non-Western women in The Hague, Netherlands, Am J Clin Nutr 84:350–353, 2006.

224. Pettifor JM: Rickets and vitamin D deficiency in children and adolescents, Endocrinol Metab Clin North Am 34:537–553, vii, 2005.

225. Javaid MK, Crozier SR, Harvey NC, et al: Maternal vitamin D status during pregnancy and childhood bone mass at age 9 years: a longitudinal study, Lancet 367:36–43, 2006.

226. Bouillon RA, Auwerx JH, Lissens WD, et al: Vitamin D status in the elderly: seasonal substrate deficiency causes 1,25-dihydroxycholecalciferol deficiency, Am J Clin Nutr 45:755–763, 1987.

227. Malabanan A, Veronikis IE, Holick MF: Redefining vitamin D insufficiency, Lancet 351:805–806, 1998.

228. Heaney RP, Dowell MS, Hale CA, et al: Calcium absorption varies within the reference range for serum 25-hydroxyvitamin D, J Am Coll Nutr 22:142–146, 2003.

229. Heaney RP: The case for improving vitamin D status, J Steroid Biochem Mol Biol 103:635–641, 2007.

230. Need AG, O'Loughlin PD, Morris HA, et al: Vitamin D metabolites and calcium absorption in severe vitamin D deficiency, J Bone Miner Res 23:1859–1863, 2008.

231. Abrams SA, Griffin IJ, Hawthorne KM, et al: Relationships among vitamin D levels, parathyroid hormone, and calcium absorption in young adolescents, J Clin Endocrinol Metab 90:5576–5581, 2005.

232. Zhu K, Bruce D, Austin N, et al: Randomized controlled trial of the effects of calcium with or without vitamin D on bone structure and bone-related chemistry in elderly women with vitamin D insufficiency, J Bone Miner Res 23:1343–1348, 2008.

233. Hansen KE, Jones AN, Lindstrom MJ, et al: Vitamin D insufficiency: disease or no disease? J Bone Miner Res 23:1052–1060, 2008.

234. Ooms ME, Lips P, Roos JC, et al: Vitamin D status and sex hormone binding globulin: determinants of bone turnover and bone mineral density in elderly women, J Bone Miner Res 10:1177–1184, 1995.

235. Cauley JA, LaCroix AZ, Wu L, et al: Serum 25-hydroxyvitamin D concentrations and risk for hip fractures, Ann Intern Med 149:242–250, 2008.

236. Boonen S, Lips P, Bouillon R, et al: Need for additional calcium to reduce the risk of hip fracture with vitamin D supplementation: evidence from a comparative meta-analysis of randomized controlled trials, J Clin Endocrinol Metab 92:1415–1423, 2007.

237. Reid IR, Bolland MJ, Grey A: Effect of calcium supplementation on hip fractures, Osteoporos Int 19:1119–1123, 2008.

238. Bischoff-Ferrari HA, Rees JR, Grau MV, et al: Effect of calcium supplementation on fracture risk: a double-blind randomized controlled trial, Am J Clin Nutr 87:1945–1951, 2008.

239. Heaney RP, Armas LA, Shary JR, et al: 25-Hydroxylation of vitamin D_3: relation to circulating vitamin D_3 under various input conditions, Am J Clin Nutr 87:1738–1742, 2008.

240. Roux C, Bischoff-Ferrari HA, Papapoulos SE, et al: New insights into the role of vitamin D and calcium in osteoporosis management: an expert roundtable discussion, Curr Med Res Opin 24:1363–1370, 2008.

241. Chel V, Wijnhoven HA, Smit JH, et al: Efficacy of different doses and time intervals of oral vitamin D supplementation with or without calcium in elderly nursing home residents, Osteoporos Int 19:663–671, 2008.

242. Vieth R: Vitamin D toxicity, policy, and science, J Bone Miner Res 22(Suppl 2):V64–V68, 2007.

243. Hagenau T, Vest R, Gissel TN, et al: Global vitamin D levels in relation to age, gender, skin pigmentation and latitude: an ecologic meta-regression analysis, Osteoporos Int 20:133–140, 2008.

244. Chapuy MC, Preziosi P, Maamer M, et al: Prevalence of vitamin D insufficiency in an adult normal population, Osteoporos Int 7:439–443, 1997.

245. van der Wielen RP, Lowik MR, van den BH, et al: Serum vitamin D concentrations among elderly people in Europe, Lancet 346:207–210, 1995.

246. Rahman SA, Chee WS, Yassin Z, et al: Vitamin D status among postmenopausal Malaysian women, Asia Pac J Clin Nutr 13:255–260, 2004.

247. Fraser DR: Vitamin D-deficiency in Asia, J Steroid Biochem Mol Biol 89–90:491–495, 2004.

248. van der Mei I, Ponsonby AL, Engelsen O, et al: The high prevalence of vitamin D insufficiency across Australian populations is only partly explained by season and latitude, Environ Health Perspect 115:1132–1139, 2007.

249. Bouillon R, Norman AW, Lips P: Vitamin D deficiency, N Engl J Med 357:1980–1981, 2007.

250. Bouillon R, Garmyn M, Verstuyf A, et al: Paracrine role for calcitriol in the immune system and skin creates new therapeutic possibilities for vitamin D analogs, Eur J Endocrinol 133:7–16, 1995.

251. Bouillon R, Okamura WH, Norman AW: Structure-function relationships in the vitamin D endocrine system, Endocr Rev 16:200–257, 1995.

252. Eelen G, Gysemans C, Verlinden L, et al: Mechanism and potential of the growth-inhibitory actions of vitamin D and analogs, Curr Med Chem 14:1893–1910, 2007.

253. Verstuyf A, Verlinden L, Van Baelen H, et al: The biological activity of nonsteroidal vitamin D hormone analogs lacking both the C- and D-rings, J Bone Miner Res 13:549–558, 1998.

254. Eelen G, Valle N, Sato Y, et al: Superagonistic fluorinated vitamin D(3) analogs stabilize helix 12 of the vitamin D receptor, Chem Biol 15:1029–1034, 2008.

255. Peleg S, Nguyen C, Woodard BT, et al: Differential use of transcription activation function 2 domain of the vitamin D receptor by 1,25-dihydroxyvitamin D_3 and its A ring-modified analogs, Mol Endocrinol 12:525–535, 1998.

256. Liu Y-Y, Collins ED, Norman AW, et al: Differential interaction of 1α,25-dihydroxyvitamin D_3 analogues and their 20-epi homologues with the vitamin D receptor, J Biol Chem 272:3336–3345, 1997.

257. van den Bemd GJCM, Pols HAP, Birkenhager JC, et al: Conformational change and enhanced stabilization of the vitamin D receptor by the 1,25-dihydroxyvitamin D_3 analog KH1060, Proc Natl Acad Sci U S A 93:10685–10690, 1996.

258. Rochel N, Wurtz JM, Mitschler A, et al: The crystal structure of the nuclear receptor for vitamin D bound to its natural ligand, Mol Cell 5:173–179, 2000.
259. Bouillon R, Allewaert K, Xiang DZ, et al: Vitamin D analogs with low affinity for the vitamin D binding protein: enhanced in vitro and decreased in vivo activity, J Bone Miner Res 6:1051–1057, 1991.
260. Dusso AS, Negrea L, Gunawardhana S, et al: On the mechanisms for the selective action of vitamin D analogs, Endocrinology 128:1687–1692, 1991.
261. Matsumoto T, Miki T, Hagino H, et al: A new active vitamin D, ED-71, increases bone mass in osteoporotic patients under vitamin D supplementation: a randomized, double-blind, placebo-controlled clinical trial, J Clin Endocrinol Metab 90:5031–5036, 2005.
262. Ke HZ, Qi H, Crawford DT, et al: A new vitamin D analog, 2MD, restores trabecular and cortical bone mass and strength in ovariectomized rats with established osteopenia, J Bone Miner Res 20:1742–1755, 2005.
263. Beer TM, Eilers KM, Garzotto M, et al: Weekly high-dose calcitriol and docetaxel in metastatic androgen-independent prostate cancer, J Clin Oncol 21:123–128, 2003.
264. Fogh K, Kragballe K: Vitamin D_3 analogues, Clin Dermatol 15:705–713, 1997.
265. Van de Kerkhof PCM: Reduction of epidermal abnormalities and inflammatory changes in psoriatic plaques during treatment with vitamin D_3 analogs, J Invest Dermatol Symp Proc 1:78–81, 1996.
266. Lu I, Gilleaudeau P, McLane JA, et al: Modulation of epidermal differentiation, tissue inflammation, and T-lymphocyte infiltration in psoriatic plaques by topical calcitriol, J Cutan Pathol 23:419–430, 1996.
267. Casteels K, Bouillon R, Waer M, et al: Immunomodulatory effects of 1,25-dihydroxyvitamin D_3, Curr Opin Nephrol Hypertens 4:313–318, 1995.
268. Baeke F, Van Etten E, Overbergh L, et al: Vitamin D_3 and the immune system: maintaining the balance in health and disease, Nutr Res Rev 20:106–118, 2007.
269. Van Etten E, Mathieu C: Immunoregulation by 1,25-dihydroxyvitamin D_3: basic concepts, J Steroid Biochem Mol Biol 97:93–101, 2005.
270. Mathieu C, Adorini L: The coming of age of 1,25-dihydroxyvitamin D(3) analogs as immunomodulatory agents, Trends Mol Med 8:174–179, 2002.
271. Adorini L, Penna G, Amuchastegui S, et al: Inhibition of prostate growth and inflammation by the vitamin D receptor agonist BXL-628 (elocalcitol), J Steroid Biochem Mol Biol 103:689–693, 2007.
272. Dawson-Hughes B, Heaney RP, Holick MF, et al: Estimates of optimal vitamin D status, Osteoporos Int 16:713–716, 2005.

Chapter 4

BONE DEVELOPMENT AND REMODELING

CHRISTA MAES and HENRY M. KRONENBERG

Despite its rigid and inert appearance, bone is an extremely dynamic tissue that develops and maintains the skeleton to fulfill at least five primary functions in the higher vertebrates: (1) The skeleton provides the crucial level arms that allow muscular activity to generate movement; (2) the skeleton provides rigid protection for internal organs, including the brain and spinal cord; (3) the skeleton is the site for storage and controlled systemic release of calcium and other ions, essential for electrolyte homeostasis of the extracellular fluid; (4) bones house the bone marrow and participate in the genesis of hematopoietic cells by providing the essential stromal/osteogenic niches that interact with hematopoietic precursors; and (5) evidence is accumulating that the skeleton may signal in a way that contributes to insulin-glucose homeostasis.

A series of distinct cell types control the development of bone and regulate its functions. Skeletal development and growth is driven to a large extent by the differentiation of chondrocytes that form and make up cartilage, and of osteoblasts that build mineralized bone. Postnatally, the skeleton is continuously turning over in a process called bone remodeling. In this process, packets of bone are constantly being removed and replaced in ways that meet mechanical demands by providing maximal strength for minimal material, while at the same time allowing the accretion and release of calcium and phosphate. The principal cellular players herein are the bone-forming osteoblasts and the osteoclasts, giant multinuclear cells derived from hematopoi-

etic precursors that break down (resorb) bone. The quantitatively dominant cell type in adult bone is the osteocyte, derived from osteoblasts and buried within the bone matrix. The roles of osteocytes are not fully understood but include the sensing of mechanical forces, the regulation of bone formation and resorption, and the regulation of phosphate homeostasis. Bone development and maintenance are closely associated with and dependent on angiogenesis, putting vascular endothelial cells in the picture as the fifth crucial cell type in bone. Over past decades, intensive research has focused on the cellular and molecular control of bone development and remodeling. In vitro cell systems have been extremely instructive, but recent advances have largely been driven by insights derived from genetically altered mice and lessons from human inherited disorders. This chapter reviews the main pathways that are currently known to govern the development of bone and the process of bone remodeling in the adult.

Skeletal Development

MECHANISMS OF BONE DEVELOPMENT

During embryonic development, the skeleton is established by the coordinated formation of well over 200 separate bones at sites distributed all over the body. Two distinct mechanisms are responsible for the development of bones—intramembranous and endochondral ossification—both of which depend on the coordinate growth, differentiation, function, and interaction of various cell types. Intramembranous ossification is responsible primarily for the formation of most of the craniofacial elements, as will be discussed briefly below. In contrast, all the long bones of the skeleton develop through endochondral ossification. This term connotes the formation of mineralized bone through the deposition of true bone matrix on top of scaffolding cartilaginous anlagen.

Intramembranous Ossification

The cranial and facial bones are derived largely from the neural crest through the process of intramembranous bone formation. In areas where bones are formed, mesenchymal precursor cells aggregate and form regions of high cell density, called condensations, that represent outlines of future skeletal elements. In intramembranous bones, the cells in these condensations then differentiate directly into osteoblasts that deposit "osteoid" or bone matrix rich in type I collagen, a process that occurs in close spatial interaction with vascular tissue. As the osteoblasts mature, the bone matrix becomes progressively mineralized. Terminally differentiated osteoblasts eventually become entrapped in the bone as osteocytes. Through modeling and remodeling (see later), the respective bones will reach their final shape and size. Membranous bones that derive as such from condensations that never form chondrocytes during development are restricted to the flat bones of the skull (calvarial bones and mandibles) and parts of the clavicles.[1-5] The subperiosteal bone collar or provisional cortex of long bones can be considered to form also by intramembranous bone formation, because the osteoblasts in this region differentiate directly from the perichondrial/periosteal mesenchyme and form bone adjacent to, instead of directly upon, a cartilage-derived matrix (see later). Unlike the formation of intramembranous bone directly from condensations, the formation of this intramembranous bone is regulated directly by signals from the adjacent chondrocytes, so can be thought of developmentally as part of endochondral bone formation. Intramembranous bone formation also occurs during bone repair after fracture, particularly when the bones are stabilized (fixed).[6-8]

Endochondral Ossification

Endochondral ossification is the mechanism responsible for the formation of all long bones of the axial skeleton (vertebrae and ribs) and the appendicular skeleton (limbs). Most of the axial skeleton is derived from cells of the paraxial mesoderm that condense early in embryogenesis on both sides of the neural tube and the notochord. Portions of this mesoderm form segmented structures called somites, portions of which later become the sclerotomes that will give rise to the vertebral bodies. The appendicular skeleton arises from the lateral plate mesoderm. The mechanisms underlying the early condensation, segmentation, differentiation, and patterning events define the precise arrangement of the individual anatomic elements and their patterning along the proximal-distal, dorsal-ventral, and posterior-anterior body axes. These mechanisms involve actions and cross-talk of several morphogens, including fibroblast growth factors (FGFs), sonic hedgehog (Shh), bone morphogenetic proteins (BMPs), and Wnts, as well as control by Notch signaling and by transcription factors encoded by *HOX*, *PAX1*, and *TBX* genes.[9]

As in intramembranous ossification, the development of the long bones proper starts with mesenchymal progenitor cells forming condensations at the sites where the bones will be formed.[10] Yet, in the mesenchymal condensations of endochondral bones, cells do not differentiate into osteoblasts but instead differentiate into chondrocytes that synthesize a characteristic extracellular matrix (ECM) rich in type II collagen and specific proteoglycans. As such, a cartilaginous model or anlage is established that prefigures the future bone. In mice, these differentiated cartilage structures appear around embryonic day 12, with the limb elements emerging in sequence along the proximodistal axis (i.e., hip to toes, shoulder to fingers). The sequential steps of the endochondral ossification process starting from this stage are illustrated in Fig. 4-1. Initially, the cartilage further enlarges through chondrocyte proliferation and matrix production. Chondrocytes in the midportion of the bone model then stop proliferating, undergo further maturation, and ultimately become hypertrophic. These large hypertrophic chondrocytes secrete a distinct matrix, containing type X collagen, which rapidly

becomes calcified. Concomitantly, cells in the connective tissues surrounding the cartilage element called the perichondrium differentiate into osteoblasts that deposit mineralized bone matrix—the "bone collar"—around the cartilage template. This bone collar forms the initiation site of the cortical bone, the dense outer envelope of compact, lamellar bone that provides the long bone with most of its strength and rigidity (see Fig. 4-1).

At this time in development (around embryonic day 14 to 15 in mice), the hypertrophic cartilage core becomes invaded by blood vessels. This process is accompanied by apoptosis of terminally differentiated hypertrophic chondrocytes, resorption of the calcified cartilage matrix by invading osteoclasts or related "chondroclasts," and deposition of mineralized bone matrix on the remnants of calcified cartilage by perichondrium/periosteum-derived osteoblasts. The net result is replacement of the cartilage model by bone, vascular, and marrow elements: the primary ossification center (see Fig. 4-1). With the disappearance of the diaphyseal cartilage, the remaining chondrocytes, restricted to the opposing ends of the long bone, provide the engine for subsequent bone lengthening. This process is typified by precise temporal and spatial regulation of chondrocyte proliferation and differentiation, with the chondrocytes first flattening out and forming longitudinal columns of rapidly proliferating cells, and next, as they reach the ends of the columns closest to the center of the bones, maturing further to hypertrophic chondrocytes (Fig. 4-2). Finally, at the border with the metaphysis, the terminally differentiated chondrocytes undergo apoptosis, and the calcified hypertrophic cartilage matrix is replaced with cancellous or trabecular bone (primary spongiosa) in a process requiring progressive neovascularization by metaphyseal capillaries (see Fig. 4-1 and cellular details in Fig. 4-2). Thus, similar to the initial formation of the primary ossification center, endochondral bone formation at the growth cartilage involves rigorous coupling of vascular invasion with maturation and activity of chondrocytes, osteoclasts, and osteoblasts.

At a certain time (around postnatal day 5 in mice), epiphyseal vessels, derived from the vascular network that overlays the cartilage tissue, invade the growth cartilage and initiate the formation of the secondary center of ossification. As a result, discrete layers of residual chondrocytes form true growth plates between the epiphyseal and metaphyseal bone centers, mediating further postnatal longitudinal bone growth. Ultimately, at least in humans, the growth plates completely disappear (close) at the end of adolescence in a process that actively requires the action of estrogen in both boys and girls, and growth stops. Remodeling of existing bone, replacing the primary spongiosa with lamellar bone in the secondary spongiosa and renewing the cortical bone, takes place throughout adult life, ensuring optimal mechanical properties of the skeleton and contributing to mineral ion homeostasis. This continual bone turnover is accomplished through the balanced action of osteoclasts and osteoblasts (see later) and results in a dynamic organization of honeycomb plate-like structures or trabeculae in the interior of the bone that are surrounded by blood vessels and bone marrow and housed within the cortical bone.

The mechanisms of embryonic bone development described here are largely recapitulated in the adult upon repair of bone defects. In contrast to soft tissues, which repair predominantly through the production of fibrous scar tissue at the site of injury, the skeleton possesses an astounding capacity to regenerate upon damage. As such, bone defects heal by forming new bone that is indistinguishable from adjacent, uninjured bone tissue. It has been appreciated for a long time that fracture repair in the adult

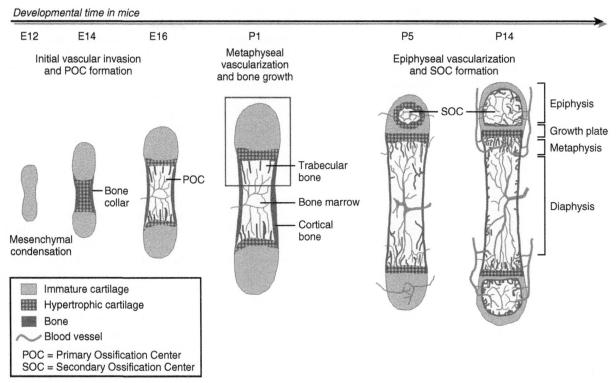

FIGURE 4-1. Stepwise schematic diagram of long bone development through endochondral ossification. Around embryonic day (E) 12 in mice, mesenchymal progenitor cells condense and differentiate into chondrocytes to form the cartilage anlagen that prefigure future long bones. Chondrocytes in the center become hypertrophic, while cells in the surrounding perichondrium differentiate into osteoblasts, forming a bone collar, the provisional cortical bone. The hypertrophic cartilage core subsequently is invaded by blood vessels and eroded and replaced by bone and marrow (primary ossification center [POC]). In the metaphysis, hypertrophic cartilage of the growth cartilage is continually replaced by trabecular bone, a process that relies on metaphyseal vascularization and mediates longitudinal bone growth. Around postnatal day (P) 5, epiphyseal vessels invade the avascular cartilage and initiate a secondary center of ossification (SOC). Discrete layers of residual chondrocytes form growth plates between the epiphyseal and metaphyseal bone centers to support further postnatal longitudinal bone growth. Ultimately (in humans), the growth plates close and growth stops. A detailed view of perinatal bone structure (boxed area) is provided in Fig. 4-2.

bears close resemblance to fetal skeletal tissue development, with both intramembranous and/or endochondral bone formation processes occurring depending on the type of fracture. In recent years, this close resemblance has been supported by genetic and molecular studies showing that similar signaling pathways (see later) are at work in both settings,[8,11-13] although additionally, some signaling molecules that are dispensable for development have been found to play essential roles in fracture repair.[14,15]

CELLULAR AND MOLECULAR CONTROL OF SKELETAL DEVELOPMENT

Our understanding of the regulatory mechanisms operating during skeletal development has grown tremendously over the past 20 years. Spontaneous mutations in humans and mice and experimental manipulation of genes by deletion or overexpression, causing loss- or gain-of-function, have identified many proteins involved in the differentiation of various cell types of bone and in the morphogenesis of individual bones. Here, we will review some of the principal growth and transcription factors and signaling cascades known to affect key aspects of bone development and maintenance, namely, chondrogenesis, vascular invasion of cartilage, resorption of cartilage and bone by chondroclasts/osteoclasts, and osteoblastogenesis.

Chondrogenesis

As outlined previously, a crucial step in endochondral bone development fundamentally entails the differentiation of cells in the mesenchymal condensations into chondrocytes. At least

some of the mesenchymal cells are probably osteochondroprogenitor cells with the potential to differentiate into chondrocytes or osteoblasts. The decision to follow a given differentiation pathway is determined by the expression of key transcription factors, likely under the influence of canonical Wnt signaling. As will be discussed in greater detail later, Wnt signaling results in the stabilization of β-catenin, which then can act as a transcription factor and regulate the expression of downstream target genes. Recent studies have provided evidence that in the perichondrium, where cells are destined to become osteoblasts, Wnt signaling is high (at least in part induced by Shh),[16] leading to high levels of β-catenin and inducing the expression of genes that mediate osteoblast differentiation (such as *Runx2*, a master regulator of osteoblastogenesis, see later), while inhibiting transcription of genes required for chondrocyte differentiation (such as *Sox9*). In the absence of β-catenin, these cells become chondrocytes instead of osteoblasts, as revealed via genetic modifications in mice. Conversely, in the inner region of the condensations, Wnt signaling must be low as these cells become chondrocytes.[17-19] The initial conversion of mesenchymal progenitor cells into chondrocytes is driven by the transcription factor Sox9, whereas the combined action of Sox9, 5 and 6, is required to direct the subsequent differentiation of chondrocytes throughout all phases of the chondrocyte lineage.[20-23]

In the growth cartilage, the most extensively studied cartilage, differentiation of committed cells along the chondrocyte lineage characteristically gives rise to a stratified organization of small, round periarticular chondrocytes (also previously termed resting

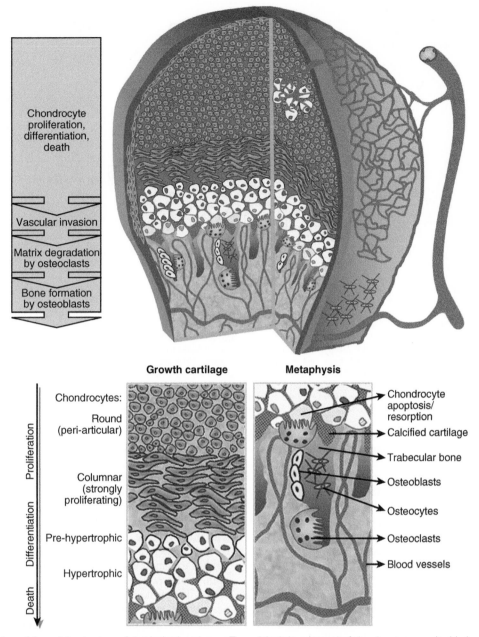

FIGURE 4-2. Schematic view of the cellular structure of developing long bones. The epiphysis is composed of chondrocytes, organized in layers of proliferation (round periarticular and flat columnar proliferating cells), progressive differentiation toward the metaphysis (pre-hypertrophic and hypertrophic chondrocytes), and cell death (apoptosis). The avascular cartilage is supplied by the epiphyseal blood vessel network that overlays its surface. In the metaphysis, blood vessels invading the terminal hypertrophic chondrocytes, osteoclasts resorbing the cartilage, and osteoblasts building bone on the cartilage remnants all act coordinately to replace the cartilage anlagen with bone and marrow.

or reserve chondrocytes, because these cells proliferate only slowly after birth and can become columnar chondrocytes), flattened, columnar proliferating chondrocytes, and pre-hypertrophic and hypertrophic chondrocytes (see Figs. 4-2 and 4-3). Because progression of the chondrocytes through these stages is the driving force of actual bone development and growth, it is not surprising that the process is tightly controlled by a myriad of local signaling molecules, the best characterized being BMPs and transforming growth factor-β (TGFβ), FGFs, parathyroid hormone (PTH)-related protein (PTHrP), and Indian hedgehog (Ihh). The importance of these molecules is reflected by the fact that mutations in their receptors have been found to cause severe human dwarfing conditions, such as constitutive activating mutations of FGF receptor (FGFR)3 in human achondropla-

sia and thanatophoric dysplasia[24-27] and PTH/PTHrP receptor mutations in Jansen and Blomstrand chondrodysplasia.[28-30] Here, we will briefly review the basic mechanisms by which these signaling systems control the pace of proliferation and differentiation of growth chondrocytes.[31-33]

BMPs, secreted proteins belonging to the TGFβ superfamily, transduce signals through serine/threonine kinase receptors, composed of type I and II subtypes, activating intracellular proteins of the Smad family that relay the BMP signal to target genes in the nucleus.[34] BMPs were first discovered as agents in bone matrix capable of inducing ectopic formation of cartilage and bone after injection into subcutaneous tissues.[35-38] Subsequent studies have shown that BMPs, some of which are also called growth and differentiation factors (GDFs) are, in fact, signaling

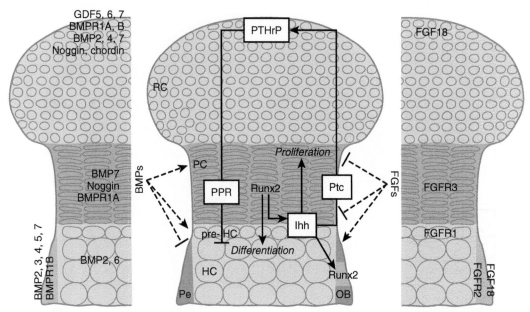

FIGURE 4-3. Regulation of chondrocyte proliferation and differentiation. Schematic representation of the epiphysis, with zones of periarticular round chondrocytes (*RC*), strongly proliferating columnar chondrocytes (*PC*), and (pre-)hypertrophic chondrocytes ([pre-]HC). Hypertrophic cartilage is surrounded by perichondrium (*Pe*), where osteoblasts (*OB*) develop. Centrally, the Indian hedgehog (*Ihh*)/parathyroid hormone-related protein (*PTHrP*)-negative feedback loop is indicated. Cells at the articular end of the bone secrete PTHrP, acting through the PTH/PTHrP receptor (PPR) on columnar chondrocytes to keep them in the proliferating pool and delay their differentiation. When the distance from the bone end becomes sufficiently large, cells escape the differentiation block and become Ihh-expressing pre-hypertrophic chondrocytes. In an as yet unknown manner, Ihh induces PTHrP expression. In addition, Ihh directly stimulates chondrocyte proliferation and converts perichondrial cells into OBs by inducing runt-related transcription factor 2 (Runx2), thereby determining the site of bone collar formation. Runx2 also favors Ihh expression and hypertrophic differentiation. Several bone morphogenetic protein (BMP) and fibroblast growth factor (FGF) family members are expressed at specific sites in the growth cartilage (left and right panels, respectively). BMPs and FGFs act antagonistically to modulate chondrocyte proliferation, Ihh expression, and terminal hypertrophic differentiation. *GDF*, Growth and differentiation factor; *Ptc*, patched; *BMPR*, BMP receptor; *FGFR*, FGF receptor.

proteins crucial for regulating development in almost all the principal organs and tissues.[39,40] In the morphogenesis of the skeleton, BMPs have been implicated in early limb patterning, as well as in the subsequent processes of chondrogenesis and osteogenesis. Initially, the role of BMPs in the correct formation of mesenchymal condensations was highlighted by the mutation of the *BMP5* gene in the mouse skeletal mutant short ear (se)[41] and by abnormalities observed in brachypodism (bp) mice that were attributed to mutations in the *GDF5* gene.[42] In both se and bp mice, the abnormalities were traced back to altered size or shape already apparent in the mesenchymal condensations of the respective skeletal elements that were affected. More recently, studies in which two BMP type I receptors were ablated at the condensation stage demonstrated that BMP signaling is essential for converting condensing mesenchyme into chondrocytes; the mutant cells expressed undetectable amounts of the essential Sox9, L-Sox5, and Sox6 transcription factors.[43] Similarly, when the potent BMP inhibitor noggin was introduced in early-stage mouse or chick limbs, mesenchymal condensation and chondrogenesis did not take place.[44,45] BMPs also play critical roles at later stages of cartilage development. These functions have been difficult to document in vivo because in some cases, inactivation of specific BMPs led to severe early defects and lethality (e.g., BMP-2, BMP-4), precluding investigation of the later stages; in other cases, removal of individual family members (such as BMP-7) displayed no defects in skeletogenesis, presumably because of functional redundancy between the various BMP ligands and receptors (around 20 BMP family members have been identified to date). Further, various models have yielded superficially contradictory results, presumably reflecting the multiple actions of BMPs and the interactions of BMP signaling with other pathways. Recent and ongoing studies therefore employ conditional (site-specific) and/or combined (multiple

targets) mutagenesis strategies. As such, it was shown in vivo that BMP signaling (through type I receptors on chondrocytes) positively regulates chondrocyte proliferation and survival, while concomitantly delaying the conversion to terminal hypertrophic differentiation,[46] confirming previous limb culture results.[47,48] These effects likely involve interactions between the BMP, FGF, and Ihh signaling pathways (see later); indeed BMP signaling seems to antagonize FGF actions and to promote Ihh expression. Studies in which BMP-2 and BMP-4 were ablated in limb development also revealed an essential role of BMP signaling in osteoblast differentiation (see later).[49] It is not surprising that perichondrium, chondrocytes, and osteoblasts express multiple BMPs, BMP receptors, and BMP antagonists to regulate this essential pathway (see Fig. 4-3).

The FGF pathway similarly involves multiple ligands and receptors in regulating skeletal development.[50] FGF18[51,52] and FGF9[53] appear to be the most important FGF ligands in regulating chondrogenesis identified so far. These ligands activate FGFR3 expressed on proliferating chondrocytes. Activating mutations in the *FGFR3* gene cause dominantly inherited human dwarfing chondrodystrophies due to impaired chondrocyte proliferation,[24] and FGFR3 inactivation in mice increases chondrocyte proliferation and prolongs growth.[54,55] This finding was surprising given that FGFs in most tissues act as potent mitogens; although this may pertain in early chondrogenesis, in which FGF18 stimulates proliferation,[56] later in development, signaling through FGFR3 constitutes a master block on chondrocyte proliferation through activation of STAT1, which activates the cell cycle inhibitor p21[Waf1/Cip1].[57-59] In addition, although previous in vitro experiments had indicated that FGF signaling accelerates the late steps of chondrocyte hypertrophy,[47] mouse models of achondroplasia and thanatophoric dysplasia have shown delayed hypertrophic differentiation of chondrocytes, strongly suggesting that FGFR3 signaling in vivo inhibits chondrocyte differentiation.[25,60-63] This effect is relayed by activation of the mitogen-activated protein kinase (MAPK) pathway in chondrocytes, which affects longitudinal growth by regulating hypertrophic chondrocyte differentiation and matrix deposition.[64-66] In vitro and in vivo experiments suggest that snail1 is required downstream of FGFR3 signaling for regulating its effects on chondrocyte proliferation and differentiation through activation of the Stat1/p21 and MAPK/Erks pathways, respectively.[67] Yet, the effects of FGFR3 are regulated only in part by direct signaling in chondrocytes, and in part indirectly by modulating the expression of the Ihh/PTHrP/BMP signaling pathways. Indeed, mice harboring an activating mutation in *FGFR3* have decreased expression of Ihh and its receptor and downstream target Patched (Ptc), and of BMP4, whereas in mice lacking FGFR3, Ihh, Ptc, and BMP4 expression are upregulated.[60,68,69] During chondrocyte differentiation, the FGF and BMP pathways generally appear to antagonize each other,[46] and both FGF signaling and BMP signaling regulate Ihh production (see Fig. 4-3). Thus, each of these pathways has multiple mechanisms for communicating with each other as they regulate chondrocyte and osteoblast differentiation.

A major regulatory system in growth chondrocytes is provided by Ihh, a member of the conserved family of hedgehog proteins, and PTHrP.[32] The Ihh/PTHrP pathway forms a negative-feedback loop that regulates the onset of hypertrophic differentiation (see Fig. 4-3). Ihh is produced by prehypertrophic and early hypertrophic chondrocytes and signals through its receptor Ptc to stimulate expression of PTHrP by chondrocytes located near the periarticular ends of bone. Increased production of Ihh or production of Ihh closer to the cells making PTHrP leads to increased PTHrP production. PTHrP in turn signals back to its receptor—the PTH/PTHrP receptor that also responds to PTH in osteoblasts and kidney—that is expressed at low levels by proliferating chondrocytes and strongly by prehypertrophic cells. This signaling slows down chondrocyte differentiation and keeps chondrocytes in the proliferative state (see Fig. 4-3). This slowed differentiation consequently delays the generation of cells that can produce Ihh; therefore, the production of PTHrP is lowered. Thus, a negative-feedback signaling pathway allows PTHrP and Ihh to regulate each other and, in turn, to control the pace of chondrocyte development in the growth plate.[32,70,71] It is important to note that the phenotype of the Ihh-/- mice[72] revealed that Ihh has additional functions in endochondral bone formation, independent of regulation of PTHrP production. Indeed, these mutant mice also displayed a marked decrease in chondrocyte proliferation and absence of mature osteoblasts and bone collar formation.[72] The regulation of chondrocyte proliferation represents a direct action of Ihh signaling to chondrocytes.[73,74] Ihh also accelerates the conversion of round periarticular chondrocytes to flat columnar chondrocytes.[75] Control of bone collar formation is mediated by Ihh-induced direct actions on perichondrial cells that are probably bipotential osteochondroprogenitors, and that are driven into the osteoblast lineage under the influence of Ihh stimulating the expression of Runx2. Runx2, an essential transcription factor in osteoblast development (see later), conversely also regulates Ihh expression and hypertrophic differentiation.[72,76-79] From this, it is evident that Ihh is a master regulator of endochondral bone development, coordinating chondrocyte proliferation, chondrocyte maturation, and osteoblast differentiation (see Fig. 4-3). Recently, a continued role for Ihh in the postnatal growth plate has been revealed by employing inducible mutagenesis in mice.[80]

Aside from the above mentioned factors, chondrogenesis is affected by several other growth factors, cytokines, and hormones, including growth hormone (GH) and insulin-like growth factors (IGFs), C-natriuretic peptide, retinoids, thyroid hormone, estrogen, androgen, 1,25-dihydroxyvitamin D_3 [1,25(OH)$_2$D$_3$], glucocorticoids, and others.[32,81]

Importantly, a main difference between mesenchymal condensations that differentiate toward the osteoblast lineage in and becoming intramembranous bones, and endochondral cartilaginous condensations is that the latter typically develop over a prolonged period in the absence of blood vessels. As an avascular tissue, cartilage consequently faces the challenge of hypoxia.[82,83] The main mediator of cellular responses to hypoxia is the transcription factor hypoxia-inducible factor (HIF).[84] Recently, HIF1α was shown to influence chondrocyte differentiation and to be required for survival of chondrocytes, because mice with conditional inactivation of HIF1α displayed aberrant apoptosis of chondrocytes located in the center of the growth cartilage, farthest from blood vessels.[85,86] The precise mechanisms by which HIF1 prevents chondrocyte apoptosis have yet to be fully explained. Part of the explanation may include an indirect survival effect of HIF1, mediated through induction of vascular endothelial growth factor (VEGF), as deletion of VEGF from cartilage also resulted in the apoptotic phenotype.[87,88] Alternatively, and not mutually exclusively, HIF1 may facilitate a vital switch in the metabolism of hypoxic chondrocytes by inducing the anaerobic glycolytic pathway,[86,89-91] and thereby allow their further differentiation up to the hypertrophic stage, when the chondrocytes induce vascular invasion (see next).

Vascular Invasion of Cartilage

Both temporally and spatially, chondrocyte differentiation is followed by vascular invasion of the terminally differentiated, hypertrophic cartilage. This step is an absolute requirement for endochondral bone development and growth to proceed, as physical blockage of blood vessel invasion into the hypertrophic cartilage of fetal skeletal explants completely halts their development,[92] and blocking the blood supply of bone in vivo results in reduced longitudinal growth.[93,94] The importance of skeletal vascularization goes beyond endochondral bone development. In fact, as a rule, any type of bone formation occurs in close spatial and temporal association with vascularization of the ossified tissue. The reasons that the vascular system is crucial for bone development, maintenance, and repair obviously include its intrinsic function to supply oxygen, nutrients, and growth factors/hormones to bone cells as required for their specified activities. In addition, the blood vessels serve to bring in (precursors of) osteoclasts that will degrade the cartilage or bone extracellular matrix, to remove end products of the resorption processes, and to bring in progenitors of osteoblasts that will deposit bone.[95-97]

During endochondral ossification, the initially avascular cartilage template is replaced by highly vascularized bone and marrow tissue through three consecutive vascularization events (see Fig. 4-1). First, initial vascular invasion of the cartilage anlagen during embryonic development (sometimes called quiescent angiogenesis) involves endothelial cells invading from the perichondrial tissues and organizing into immature blood vessels in the primary center of ossification. Second, capillary invasion at the metaphyseal border of the growth cartilage mediates rapid bone lengthening. Third, vascularization of the cartilage ends initiates the formation of secondary ossification centers (see Fig. 4-1). Although the vessel systems associated with the different stages of cartilage vascularization are believed to be substantially different,[98,99] a common feature is that invasion of cartilage at all times is preceded by chondrocyte hypertrophy. Immature chondrocytes are resistant to vascular invasion because of the production of angiogenic inhibitors, such as chondromodulin-I, troponin-I, and thrombospondins.[100-103] In contrast, when chondrocytes become hypertrophic, they switch to production of angiogenic stimulators, thereby becoming a target for capillary invasion and angiogenesis.[104,105] One exceptionally potent angiogenic stimulator, VEGF, has received much attention, as it is expressed at very high levels by hypertrophic cartilage, as well as by osteoblasts and osteoclasts. Although the regulation of VEGF expression is still largely unresolved and may vary depending on the developmental stage and specific location and cell type, several mechanisms have been implicated to date. Hypoxia seems to be a crucial trigger of VEGF expression in chondrocytes, osteoblasts, and possibly osteoclasts, through mechanisms that involve HIF both in vitro[106-109] and in vivo.[110] During early bone development, VEGF transcription may be induced by Runx2 (see later), given that expression of VEGF was impaired in Runx2-deficient mice and no blood vessel ingrowth into the cartilage occurred.[111] In addition, several hormones [including PTH, GH, and 1,25(OH)$_2$D$_3$] and locally produced growth factors (e.g., FGFs, TGFβ, BMPs, IGFs, platelet-derived growth factor [PDGF]) have been demonstrated to be involved, at least in vitro, in the regulation of VEGF expression.[112]

Important insight into the crucial physiologic function of VEGF-mediated angiogenesis in bone was first provided by Gerber et al.,[113] who inhibited VEGF action in juvenile mice through administration of a soluble VEGF receptor chimeric protein (sFlt-1). VEGF inhibition impaired vascular invasion of the growth plate, and concomitantly, trabecular bone formation and bone growth were reduced and the hypertrophic cartilage zone became enlarged, likely as the result of reduced osteoclast-mediated resorption (see later).[113] Additional mouse genetic studies performed over the past decade have univocally demonstrated that VEGF is an essential mediator of all three key vascularization stages of endochondral bone development. Although a mouse with the *VEGF* gene ablated in all cells could not be employed owing to early lethality of even heterozygous VEGF knockout embryos, several alternative mutagenesis approaches have been and are being exploited to investigate the role of VEGF in bone. These models include Cre/LoxP-mediated conditional inactivation of the *VEGF* gene (*VEGFa*) in type II collagen–expressing chondrocytes, and expression of only one of the three major VEGF isoforms by genetically engineered mice.[87,88,114-116] Altogether, these models have exposed multiple essential roles of VEGF and its isoforms in endochondral ossification, not only as a key inducer of vascularization but also as a direct modulator of bone development by affecting the various cell types involved. Perichondrial cells, osteoblasts, and osteoclasts are well documented to express several VEGF receptors and to respond to VEGF signaling through enhanced recruitment, differentiation, activity, and/or survival.[112,117,118] These pleiotrophic actions of VEGF on various cells in the bone environment may contribute to the tight coordination of vascularization, ossification, and matrix resorption that is characteristically seen in endochondral ossification. Indeed, the current model is that VEGF secretion in the bone environment will attract blood vessels and stimulate endothelial cells to form new blood vessels, which will be indirectly associated with increased potential delivery of osteoblast and osteoclast progenitors.[81] At the same time, VEGF signaling directly stimulates the recruitment and differen-

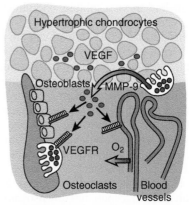

FIGURE 4-4. Vascular invasion and the role of vascular endothelial growth factor (VEGF). VEGF is produced at high levels by hypertrophic chondrocytes and is sequestered in part in the cartilage matrix upon its secretion. Trapped VEGF can be released from the matrix by proteases such as matrix metalloproteinase (MMP) 9 secreted by osteoclasts/chondroclasts during cartilage resorption. VEGF then can bind to its receptors (VEGFRs) on endothelial cells and stimulate the guided attraction of blood vessels to invade the terminal cartilage. Osteoblasts and osteoclasts also express VEGF receptors, and VEGF can affect their differentiation and function both directly and indirectly by enhancing metaphyseal vascularization, thus playing a coordinative role in the key events that mediate bone development and growth.

tiation of osteoblasts to form bone.[112,114,119,120] VEGF works as a chemoattractant stimulating osteoclast invasion of cartilage, and enhances osteoclast differentiation, survival, and resorptive activity.[121-127] A positive-feedback system is likely established, as chondroclast/osteoclast-derived matrix metalloproteinase (MMP) 9 may release more matrix-bound VEGF from the cartilage that is being resorbed (Fig. 4-4).[81,128]

Osteoclastogenesis and Skeletal Tissue Resorption

At the time of vascular invasion of hypertrophic cartilage, the chondrocytes undergo apoptosis, and remaining cellular debris and matrix components become degraded and are digested by co-invading osteoclasts (or related cells termed chondroclasts that have been postulated in the context of resorption of cartilage[128]) through their proteolytic enzyme products.[81] Beyond development, the osteoclast remains a key participant in the regulation of bone mass, as bone is constantly being remodeled throughout life (see later). Several pathologic conditions are due to an imbalance between bone formation and resorption, most frequently involving excessive osteoclast activity. Such skeletal diseases include osteoporosis, a common low bone mass disorder typically prevalent in postmenopausal women, as well as periodontal disease, rheumatoid arthritis, multiple myeloma, and metastatic cancer. On the other hand, osteopetrosis, a rare human disease characterized by increased bone mass and obliteration of the bone marrow cavity, is caused by impaired osteoclast differentiation and/or function. Many efforts have been made to dissect the regulatory pathways leading to functional osteoclasts.[129-134]

Osteoclastogenesis

Osteoclasts are giant multinucleated cells that have the unique capacity to efficiently degrade mineralized tissues. Osteoclasts are derived from hematopoietic precursor cells of the myelomonocytic lineage and share a common precursor with macrophages.[131] Recognition of the intertwining control and close interactions of the immune and skeletal systems has led recently to the emergence of the novel integrating field of osteoimmunol-

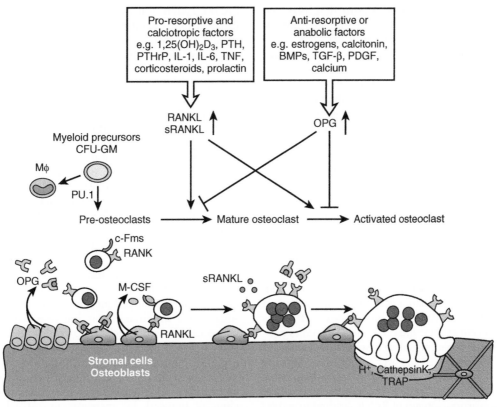

FIGURE 4-5. Osteoclastogenesis. The transcription factor PU.1 is indispensable for development of the osteoclast and macrophage (Mϕ) lineages from a common myeloid precursor. Macrophage-colony stimulating factor (M-CSF) acting upon the receptor c-Fms is required for the conversion of the progenitor to become a pre-osteoclast. Signaling through the membrane-bound receptor activator of nuclear factor-κB (RANK) promotes further differentiation of pre-osteoclasts to mature polykaryotic osteoclasts and their subsequent activation to bone-resorbing cells that secrete protons and lytic enzymes. RANK signaling is induced by receptor activator of nuclear factor-κB ligand (RANKL), present on osteoblasts and bone marrow stromal cells, as well as on lymphocytes and possibly in a soluble form in serum. The soluble antagonist osteoprotegerin (OPG) competes with RANK for RANKL binding, thereby functioning as a negative regulator of osteoclast differentiation, activation, and survival. RANKL expression is induced by pro-resorptive and calciotropic factors that stimulate osteoclastogenesis. Conversely, OPG is induced by factors that block bone catabolism and promote anabolic effects.

ogy.[131,132] Early differentiation of the bipotential macrophage/osteoclast precursor cells is regulated by PU.1, a versatile hematopoietic cell-specific transcriptional regulator of the ETS family of transcription factors. The commitment to macrophages/osteoclasts is dependent on a high level of activity of PU.1[131,135-137] (Fig. 4-5); PU.1 regulates the lineage fate decision of early progenitors by directly controlling expression of the *c-Fms* gene, which is a key determinant of differentiation into the macrophage/osteoclast lineage (see later).[138,139] Consequently, PU.1-null mice lack both macrophages and osteoclasts, and are osteopetrotic.[136,140,141] PU.1 also regulates the transcription of another key osteoclastogenesis control gene, encoding receptor activator of nuclear factor-κB (RANK) (see later) in myeloid progenitors.[142] Although mature macrophages and osteoclasts have some cell surface markers in common, the latter express high levels of tartrate-resistant acid phosphatase (TRAP), cathepsin K, vitronectin, calcitonin receptor, and $\alpha_v\beta_3$ integrin, which typify the osteoclast lineage (see later).[81]

After the precursor cells have committed to the osteoclast lineage, they are subjected to a complex multistep process that culminates in the generation of mature, multinuclear, activated osteoclasts; these steps include proliferation, maturation, and fusion of differentiating precursor cells, and finally activation of resorption (see Fig. 4-5).[81,130,132,134] Two critical cytokines are essential for osteoclastogenesis: macrophage-colony stimulating factor (M-CSF) and receptor activator of nuclear factor-κB ligand (RANKL) (also known previously as osteoprotegerin ligand

[OPGL], osteoclast differentiation factor [ODF], or tumor necrosis factor [TNF]-related activation-induced cytokine [TRANCE]). Both of these signaling molecules are strongly expressed by bone marrow stromal cells (i.e., osteoblast progenitors) and osteoblasts; M-CSF is produced in both a soluble and a membrane-bound form, and RANKL is made exclusively as a membrane protein by osteoblasts. The process of osteoclastogenesis requires direct cell-to-cell interaction between stromal/osteoblastic cells and osteoclast precursors, presumably because of these key membrane-bound ligands (see Fig. 4-5). Both PTH and 1,25(OH)$_2$D$_3$ and several other osteotropic factors stimulating resorption increase the expression of RANKL on stromal/osteoblastic cells[130,143,144] (see later). Moreover, before the identification of RANKL, in vitro investigation of osteoclastogenesis relied on contact-dependent co-culture of osteoclast progenitors with stromal/osteoblastic cells stimulated with PTH or 1,25(OH)$_2$D$_3$. Now we know that RANKL, together with M-CSF, is sufficient to induce in vitro osteoclast differentiation from spleen- or bone marrow–derived precursors in the complete absence of stromal/osteoblastic cells.[145] Furthermore, not only osteoblasts but also chondrocytes[146-148] and T cells[149,150] synthesize and secrete RANKL and are able to support osteoclastogenesis. This may be important physiologically during osteoclast differentiation and invasion at the hypertrophic cartilage during endochondral bone development and growth, and it definitely plays a major role pathologically. For instance, production of RANKL by T cells has been implicated as an activator of osteoclastic resorption in inflammatory mediated bone and cartilage destruction, as is seen in several autoimmune disorders, including rheumatoid arthritis,[81,130,151] likely working synergistically with TNFα.[152,153]

M-CSF and RANKL affect several steps of the osteoclastogenesis cascade by binding to their respective receptors, c-Fms and RANK, which are expressed by osteoclast progenitors and osteoclasts at all stages of differentiation. M-CSF signaling is essential early on in the lineage for proliferation, differentiation, and survival of osteoclast/macrophage precursors. The essential roles of M-CSF were illustrated through analysis of mice carrying the *op/op* mutation, an inactivating point mutation in the *M-CSF* gene; these mice have osteopetrosis with low numbers of macrophages and a complete lack of mature osteoclasts.[154-157]

RANKL is an essential inducer of multiple aspects of osteoclastogenesis, including osteoclast differentiation, fusion, activation of mature osteoclasts to resorb mineralized bone, and survival.[158-161] Through these actions, RANKL potently stimulates bone resorption. RANKL acts by binding to its signal transducing receptor, RANK, a member of the TNF receptor family present on pre-osteoclasts and mature osteoclasts. Consistent herewith, an activating mutation of the human *RANK* gene was found in patients with familial expansile osteolysis, a disease of excess bone resorption.[162] Recent genetic and cell biological studies have begun to elucidate the complex signaling cascade downstream of RANK/RANKL.[130,163] Briefly stated and oversimplified, the binding of RANKL to RANK on the surface of osteoclast precursors recruits the adaptor protein TNF receptor–associated factor (TRAF) 6 to the cytoplasmic domain of RANK, leading to activation of NF-κB and its translocation to the nucleus. NF-κB increases c-Fos expression, and c-Fos, as a component of the activator protein (AP)-1 complex, interacts with the master transcription factor for osteoclastogenesis, nuclear factor of activated T cells c1 (NFATc1), to induce osteoclast-specific genes (such as the genes encoding TRAP and calcitonin receptor; see later).[164-167]

The actions of RANKL are regulated negatively by a secreted soluble decoy receptor termed osteoprotegerin (OPG) (previously also known as osteoclastogenesis inhibitory factor [OCIF]), also a member of the TNF receptor superfamily. OPG sequesters RANKL molecules and thereby blocks their binding to RANK.[130,168] As such, OPG protects bone from excessive resorption; this conclusion is supported by the finding that certain homozygous deletions of OPG in humans can cause juvenile Paget's disease, a disorder characterized by increased bone remodeling, osteopenia, and fractures.[169] The relative concentrations of RANKL and OPG in bone thus are major determinants of bone mass and strength. OPG is widely expressed; it is not surprising that its expression by osteoblasts and stromal cells is positively regulated by bone anabolic or antiresorptive factors, such as estrogen and calcitonin.[130]

The essence of the RANK/RANKL/OPG cascade was further clarified by mouse genetic studies. Mice lacking RANKL[170] or RANK[171,172] and mice with increased circulating OPG by transgenic overexpression[173] were severely osteopetrotic owing to a block in osteoclastogenesis. Conversely, targeted mutagenesis of OPG,[174,175] overexpression of an *sRANKL* transgene,[176] and administration of RANKL[159,160] in mice all led to increased osteoclast formation, activation, and/or survival and resulted in an osteoporotic phenotype. In summary, RANKL and OPG act in an antagonistic fashion to regulate bone resorption, and their respective expression levels are under the control of proresorptive and antiresorptive factors, including several hormones, cytokines, and growth factors (see Fig. 4-5). Of note, RANK is broadly expressed, and these mouse studies indicate that the RANK/

RANKL system functions in tissues beyond bone. For instance, RANK/RANKL regulates lymph node formation and lactational mammary gland development in mice.[172,177] OPG has nonskeletal functions too, as it protects large arteries of mice from medial calcification.[174]

Other regulatory molecules have been implicated recently in the late stages of osteoclast differentiation, the fusion process, and activation of resorption. Co-stimulatory molecules acting in concert with M-CSF and RANKL to complete osteoclastogenesis include proteins containing an immunoreceptor tyrosine-based activation motif (ITAM) domain that is critical for the activation of calcium signaling and is found in adapter molecules like DNAX-activating protein (DAP)12 and the Fc receptor γ (FcRγ).[178] The resultant increase in intracellular calcium is required for activation of NFATc1. The fusion of mononuclear osteoclast precursor cells into mature multinucleated osteoclasts is regulated by a membrane protein called dendritic cell-specific transmembrane protein (DC-STAMP). DC-STAMP–deficient cells failed to fuse, and these mononuclear osteoclasts had reduced resorptive efficiency in vitro. Consequently, DC-STAMP–deficient mice exhibited increased bone mass.[179] These data may suggest that multinucleation and osteoclast enlargement could be associated with a higher degree of resorption efficiency.[180,181] Pathologically huge osteoclasts, containing substantially more nuclei than normal osteoclasts do, are seen for instance in Paget's disease of bone (up to 100 nuclei per cell; normal range is 3 to 20 nuclei per cell), in which localized excessive bone remodeling is initiated by increases in osteoclast-mediated bone resorption.[182]

Additional studies on the regulatory components of osteoclastogenesis not only will expand our basic understanding of the molecular mechanisms of osteoclast differentiation during bone development and remodeling but also offer opportunities to develop therapeutic means of intervention in osteoclast-related diseases. OPG and soluble recombinant RANK suppress osteoclastogenesis, while antibodies to RANK can stimulate osteoclast formation.[183] From the clinical point of view, the RANKL signaling pathway thus holds great promise as a strategy for suppressing excessive osteoclast formation in a variety of bone diseases, including osteoporosis, autoimmune arthritis, periodontitis, Paget's disease, and bone tumors/metastases.

Bone Resorption: Osteoclast Action and Proteolytic Enzymes

Bone resorption involves both dissolution of bone mineral and degradation of organic bone matrix. Osteoclasts are highly specialized to perform both of these functions. Upon activation of mature multinucleated osteoclasts, the cells attach themselves firmly to the bone surface, using specialized actin-rich podosomes (actin ring), through cytoskeleton reorganization and cellular polarization.[184-187] Within these tightly sealed zones of adhesion to the mineralized matrix, the osteoclasts form convoluted, villus-like membranes called "ruffled borders," which drastically increase the surface area of the cell membrane facing the resorption lacuna (Howship's lacuna). Via these ruffled membranes, the osteoclasts secrete abundant hydrochloric acid (involving the vacuolar H+-ATPase proton pump), mediating acidification of the compartment between the cell and the bone surface, as well as a myriad of enzymes such as lysosomal cathepsins, the phosphatase TRAP, and proteolytic MMPs (see later). The acidity of the environment leads to dissolution of the mineral phase (crystalline hydroxyapatite), activation of lytic enzymes, and digestion of organic matrix compounds (see Fig. 4-5). The sealing mechanism allows localized dissolving and degrading of the mineralized bone matrix, while simultaneously protecting neighboring cells from harm.[188,189] During the resorption process, dissolution of hydroxyapatite releases large amounts of soluble calcium, phosphate, and bicarbonate. Removal of these ions is needed (e.g., to maintain the acidic pH in the resorption lacuna) and apparently involves vesicular pathways and direct ion transport via different ion exchangers, channels, and pumps. The degradation products of the organic matrix after enzymatic digestion are transcytosed through the cell for secretion at the basolateral membrane.[188,189]

These complex processes of osteoclast recruitment, polarization on the bone surface, and export of acid and enzymes are orchestrated by many factors, including RANKL,[190-192] as well as by integrin-mediated signaling from the bone matrix itself.[193-195] The latter, which is particularly represented by the αvβ3 integrin in osteoclasts, was suggested to be important for osteoclast functioning based on the finding that inhibition of signaling through this αvβ3 integrin inhibited osteoclast-mediated bone resorption in vitro and in animal models of osteoporosis and malignant osteolysis (reviewed in refs. 196, 197). Integrins are heterodimeric cell-surface receptors, composed of an α and a β subunit, that mediate cell–matrix interactions and thus adhesion. The αvβ3 integrin, among various integrins the most highly expressed in osteoclasts, recognizes RGD(Arg-Gly-Asp)-containing matrix proteins such as vitronectin, osteopontin, and bone sialoprotein. Several components of the αvβ3 integrin signaling pathway localize to the sealing zone of actively resorbing osteoclasts, suggesting that they play a role in linking the matrix adhesion of osteoclasts to cytoskeletal organization, cell polarization, and activation for bone resorption. For these reasons, αvβ3 integrin appeared as a favorable candidate target for antiresorptive therapeutic interventions; in fact, small molecule inhibitors of the integrin are in clinical trial for the treatment of osteoporosis.[194,198]

Among the molecules that are important for the functional activity of osteoclasts per se, such as β3 integrin, but also c-Src, cathepsin K, carbonic anhydrase II, TRAP, and several ion channel proteins, many have been found to cause an osteopetrotic phenotype when deleted in mice or altered in humans. The absence of these genes does not affect the differentiation into morphologically normal osteoclasts; however, the osteoclasts are not functional, and they fail to resorb bone effectively.[81] For instance, cathepsin K, the key enzyme in the digestion of bone matrix by its activity in degrading type I collagen, is highly expressed by activated osteoclasts and secreted in the resorption lacuna.[199-201] Its deletion in mice led to osteopetrosis,[201-203] and mutations in the human cathepsin K gene cause pycnodysostosis.[204] Highly selective and potent cathepsin K inhibitors have been developed recently and have been shown to be useful antiresorptive agents for the treatment of osteoporosis, as well as promising therapeutic tools to reduce breast cancer–induced osteolysis and skeletal tumor burden.[205-208]

Besides cathepsin K, several proteolytic enzyme groups are involved in the degradation of organic components (collagens and proteoglycans) of bone and cartilage matrices after the mineral is dissolved.[209-211] One of these is the MMP family, which constitutes over 25 members, including secreted collagenases, stromelysins, gelatinases, and membrane-type (MT)-MMPs.[212,213] MMPs are synthesized as latent proenzymes that, upon proteolytic activation, can degrade numerous extracellular matrix components. As such, they are involved in the development, growth, and repair of tissues, but also in pathologic conditions associated with excessive matrix degradation, such as rheumatoid arthritis,

osteoarthritis, and tumor metastasis.[210,213-215] Several MMPs, including MMP9 and MMP14 (also known as MT1-MMP), are highly expressed in osteoclasts/chondroclasts,[128,216,217] but they are produced by many other cell types as well. Both of these molecules play a role in the cartilage resorption process associated with invasion by osteoclasts during endochondral ossification.[122,128,218-220] MMPs and proteolytic enzymes containing a disintegrin and metalloprotease domain (ADAMs) also possibly affect osteoclastogenesis per se, by modulating the bioavailability and presentation of RANKL through the proteolytic cleavage of its transmembrane form to soluble RANKL.[221,222]

Finally, after a limited period of resorptive activity, the osteoclast is thought to die via apoptosis (see later),[223,224] and the resorbed area of cartilage or bone is, in conditions of development, growth, and bone health, efficiently replaced by newly formed bone through the action of osteoblasts.

Osteoblastogenesis

The final step required to rebuild cartilage to bone during development consists of the differentiation of osteoblasts and the deposition of mineralized bone tissue by this specialized cell type. Osteoblasts are mesenchymal cells thought to descend from mesenchymal stem cells that are pluripotent and have the capacity to differentiate into a variety of cell types, including muscle cells (myoblasts), fat cells (adipocytes), chondrocytes, and osteoblasts (Fig. 4-6).[225-227] Differentiation of mesenchymal stem cells into distinct lineages is regulated by the expression of different transcription factors. MyoD transcription factors (MyoD, Myf5, and myogenin) regulate myogenic differentiation; C/EBP family (C/EBPβ, C/EBPδ, and C/EBPα) and PPARγ2 transcription factors regulate adipocyte differentiation (see Fig. 4-6).[228] In certain settings, osteoblasts and chondrocytes seem to share a common precursor, termed osteochondroprogenitor. Specific transcription factors direct the osteochondroprogenitors into the chondrocyte (the Sox family transcription factors Sox9, Sox5, and Sox6) or the osteoblast lineages (β-catenin, Runx2, and osterix; discussed later) (see Fig. 4-6).[31,229,230]

Committed pre-osteoblasts further differentiate into mature osteoblasts that secrete large amounts of type I collagen and other matrix components, which together are called osteoid. Subsequently, osteoblasts direct the mineralization of the osteoid in a process that requires active alkaline phosphatase (ALP), expressed on the osteoblast membrane. These mature osteoblasts express characteristic genes, including the gene encoding osteocalcin.[231] Ultimately, the cells die through apoptosis, or are converted to bone-lining cells, or become embedded within the bone matrix as osteocytes. Osteocytes are found dispersed throughout the bone matrix and have the potential to live as long as the organism itself. In fact, osteocytes are the most abundant cell type in bone, constituting over 90% of adult bone cells.[232,233] As osteoblasts become encased by the mineralized bone matrix that they themselves synthesized, they dramatically change their shape, sending out numerous dendritic processes that run inside lacunar cannaliculi.[234,235] These processes allow osteocytes to communicate with each other, with the vasculature, and with cells on the bone surface.[233,236-239] Osteocytes are well positioned to sense and respond to mechanical forces, and a growing body of evidence documents that osteocytes mediate the actions of mechanical forces to increase bone mass (see later). Osteocytes synthesize a series of proteins unique to this most differentiated member of the osteoblast lineage. These include dentin matrix protein (DMP)-1, matrix extracellular phosphoglycoprotein (MEPE) and FGF23, secreted proteins involved in systemic phosphate homeo-

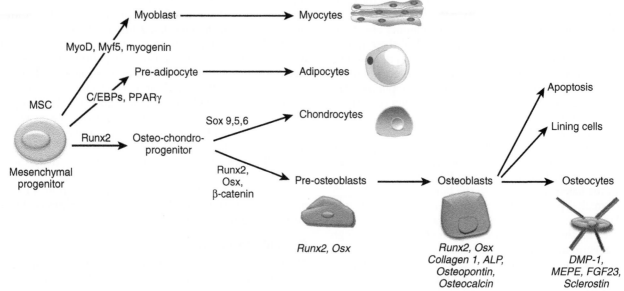

FIGURE 4-6. Osteoblast differentiation. Osteoblasts are derived from mesenchymal stem cells (MSCs) or progenitors that can become myocytes, adipocytes, or chondrocytes (driven by the indicated transcription factors) or can be directed into the osteoblast lineage, possibly through an osteochondroprogenitor intermediate. The transcription factors Runx2, Osx, and β-catenin mediate osteoblast differentiation and functioning. Progressive osteoblast differentiation is characterized by changes in gene expression typifying specific stages as indicated. See text for details.

stasis, and sclerostin (SOST), an inhibitor of Wnt action (see later).[237,240-244] Despite their relative inactivity compared with osteoblasts, osteocytes play a central role in the determination and maintenance of bone structure (see later).

A number of crucial transcription factors and signaling pathways determining osteoblastogenesis have been identified, and at least some of those are currently known to play a role in inherited human bone disease. Here, we will focus on discussing Wnt/β-catenin signaling and the transcription factors Runx2 and Osx, and we will briefly touch on other important signals, including BMPs, hedgehogs (Hh), and FGFs.

Wnt/β-Catenin Signaling

Wnts are a large family of secreted growth factors (19 different members in mouse and human genomes) that play essential roles in multiple developmental processes. Wnts are also required for adult tissue maintenance, and perturbations in Wnt signaling can lead to tumor formation and other diseases.[17,245-248] In the skeletal system, mutations in Wnt signaling components lead to skeletal malformations and diseases such as osteoporosis-pseudoglioma[249] and osteoarthritis.[250]

Wnts can transduce their signals through several different downstream signaling pathways. The best understood pathway is the canonical or Wnt/β-catenin pathway (Fig. 4-7).[251] Central to this pathway is the regulation of the protein stability of β-catenin, which acts as a transcription factor in the canonical Wnt pathway and is also involved in cell adhesion by binding to cadherins. In the absence of Wnts, cytoplasmic β-catenin is constitutively degraded through its phosphorylation by glycogen synthase kinase 3-β (GSK3-β) in a large protein complex brought together by axin and adenomatous polyposis coli (APC).[245,247,252,253] Phosphorylated β-catenin is recognized by a β-transducin repeat containing protein (β-TrCP) that targets it for proteasome-mediated degradation. Upon Wnt stimulation, the ligands bind to two synergistically acting families of Wnt (co)receptors, the Frizzled (Fz) receptor family members and low-density lipoprotein receptor-related proteins (LRP5 or LRP6), leading to the

recruitment of axin to LRP5/6 in the plasma membrane. The sequestering of axin at the plasma membrane likely leads to disassembly of the β-catenin destruction complex, thus inhibiting the phosphorylation/degradation of β-catenin.[254-259] Stabilized β-catenin protein then accumulates in the cytoplasm and translocates to the nucleus, where it interacts with members of the T cell factor/lymphoid enhancer factor (TCF/LEF) family of DNA-binding transcription factors to regulate the expression of downstream target genes (see Fig. 4-7).[260-262]

During the past decade, canonical Wnt signaling has been shown to play a significant role in the control of osteoblastogenesis and bone formation. Recent genetic studies analyzing conditional β-catenin loss- and gain-of-function mouse models provided compelling evidence that β-catenin is a crucial transcription factor determining the osteoblast lineage commitment of early osteochondroprogenitors, by inducing osteoblastic and suppressing chondrocytic differentiation.[17,263] Indeed, inactivation of β-catenin in mesenchymal progenitor cells blocked osteoblast differentiation, and mesenchymal cells in the perichondrium and calvarium differentiated into chondrocytes instead.[16,18,264] In addition, recent evidence showed that β-catenin plays an important role in the coupling between osteoblast and osteoclast activity by stimulating differentiated osteoblasts to produce OPG, an inhibitor of osteoclast formation (see earlier).[265,266]

In several clinical cases, mutations have been found in the Wnt receptor complexes that are associated with changes in bone mineral density and fractures. Loss-of-function mutations in LRP5 receptors cause osteoporosis-pseudoglioma syndrome,[249] whereas gain-of-function mutations in the same group that render LRP5 with reduced affinities for DKK1 and sclerostin (SOST), secreted antagonists of canonical Wnt signaling, result in high bone mass phenotypes.[267-271] These actions of LRP5 are indirect actions on bone: Activation of LRP5 in the duodenum suppresses serotonin secretion, and the lower blood levels of serotonin lead to an increase in bone mass through less activation of serotonin Htr1b receptors on osteoblasts.[272]

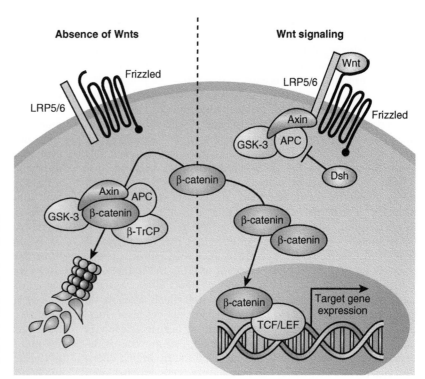

FIGURE 4-7. Canonical Wnt/β-catenin signaling pathway. In the absence of Wnt signals *(left),* β-catenin is associated with glycogen synthase kinase 3-β (GSK3-β) in a destruction complex that also contains Axin and adenomatous polyposis coli (APC). A hyperphosphorylated β-catenin is created by GSK3β and is bound by the β-transducin repeat containing protein (β-TrCP) component of the ubiquitin ligase complex, targeting β-catenin for proteasomal degradation. Wnt signaling through the Frizzled and LRP5/6 receptor complex *(right)* leads to inhibition of GSK3β through activation of Dishevelled (Dsh). Consequently, when Wnt signaling is active, β-catenin is stabilized, and the level of β-catenin in the cytoplasm becomes elevated. Accumulated β-catenin can translocate to the nucleus to interact with T cell factor/lymphoid enhancer factor (TCF/LEF) proteins and mediate transcription of target genes.

The protein inhibitors of Wnt signaling may have additional clinical relevance. For example, osteolytic bone lesions in patients with multiple myeloma are associated with the production of DKK1,[273,274] and homozygous loss-of-function mutations in SOST have been identified in patients diagnosed with sclerosteosis, a disfiguring disease associated with high bone mass.[275,276] Mutations affecting regulation of SOST transcription also cause van Buchem disease, a disease that resembles sclerosteosis.[241,277] These findings highlight the important role of canonical Wnt signaling in regulating human bone mass. Because osteocytes are the major producer of SOST, inhibition of this Wnt antagonist may offer a promising strategy for preventing bone loss.[17,278,279] Extensive research therefore is being conducted in this area based on the prospect that it may lead to the identification of targets of pharmacologic intervention useful in the management of osteoporosis.

Runx2 and Osx

Runx2, runt-related transcription factor 2 (previously known as core-binding factor a1 [Cbfa1], Osf2, or AML3), a transcription factor of the ancient runt family, has been demonstrated as absolutely essential for the induction of osteoblast differentiation and endochondral and intramembranous bone formation. Runx2-deficient mice completely lack osteoblasts and do not form bone at all; instead a completely cartilaginous skeleton develops without any true bone matrix.[280,281] In heterozygous (haploinsufficient) Runx2 mutant mice, the defect in osteoblast differentiation is limited to intramembranous bones.[280] The resulting phenotype in these mice closely resembles the cleidocranial dysplasia (CCD) syndrome in humans, a dominantly inherited developmental disorder of bone, and *RUNX2* was found to be mutated in most CCD patients.[282,283] Consistent with its function as an early transcriptional regulator of osteoblast differentiation, Runx2 is an early molecular marker of the osteoblast lineage, being highly expressed in perichondrial mesenchyme and in all osteoblasts.[280,284] Hypertrophic chondrocytes

also express Runx2, and Runx2 plays important roles in cartilage biology, as was mentioned earlier.

Runx2 can be sufficient to induce osteoblast differentiation in vitro.[285] Moreover, Runx2-null calvarial cells spontaneously differentiate into adipocytes and differentiate into chondrocytes in the presence of BMP-2 in vitro, but they do not differentiate into osteoblasts.[286] Thus, Runx2 is both sufficient and essential for differentiation of mesenchymal cells into osteoblasts, and it inhibits their differentiation into adipocytes and chondrocytes. Runx2 mediates osteoblast differentiation by inducing ALP activity, by regulating the expression of a variety of bone matrix protein genes, and by stimulating mineralization in immature mesenchymal cells and osteoblastic cells.[287] Furthermore, Runx2 regulates the expression of RANKL and OPG in osteoblasts, thus affecting osteoclast differentiation (see earlier).[288,289]

The DNA-binding sites of Runx2 have been identified in major osteoblast-specific genes, including the genes that encode type I collagen, (*Col1a1*), osteopontin, osteonectin, bone sialoprotein, osteocalcin, and *Runx2* itself, and Runx2 induced the expression of these genes or activated their promoters in vitro.[287] It is puzzling that although Runx2 strongly induced osteocalcin expression in vitro,[285,290] its overexpression in osteoblasts in vivo severely reduced osteocalcin expression.[291] Yet, expression of a dominant-negative form of Runx2 in osteoblasts also led to virtual absence of osteocalcin expression and caused impaired postnatal bone formation.[292] What is clear from these and other findings is that the regulation of different stages of osteoblast differentiation by Runx2 is very complex; Runx2 transcriptional regulation involves interactions with a myriad of transcriptional activators and repressors and other co-regulatory proteins that are under continued investigation. The current model is that Runx2 triggers the expression of major bone matrix protein genes and the acquisition of an osteoblastic phenotype at an early stage of osteoblast differentiation, while inhibiting the late osteoblast maturation stages and the transition into osteocytes. As such, Runx2 may play an important role in maintaining a supply of immature osteoblasts.[287]

Runx2 also regulates the expression of Osterix (encoded by the Osx or Sp7 gene), an SP family transcription factor with three zinc-finger motifs. Osterix is expressed in osteoblast progenitors, in osteoblasts, and at a lower level in (pre-)hypertrophic chondrocytes.[293] Similar to Runx2-deficient mice, mice lacking Osterix showed complete lack of osteoblasts and absence of both intramembranous and endochondral bone formation.[293] Thus, Osterix is a third transcription factor that is essential for osteoblast differentiation. Because Runx2 is expressed in the mesenchymal cells of Osx-null mice but Osterix is not expressed in Runx2-null mice, it can be concluded that Osterix acts downstream of Runx2.[293] Furthermore, the Osx gene contains a consensus Runx2-binding site in its promoter region, suggesting that Osterix might be a direct target of Runx2.[294] The transcriptional activity of Osterix involves its interaction with NFATc1, cooperatively forming a complex that binds to DNA and induces the expression of Col1a1.[295] The subtleties of how Osterix regulates osteoblast differentiation and function and which osteoblastic genes are directly regulated by Osterix have not yet been elucidated. Expression of genes characteristic of mature osteoblasts (such as those encoding bone sialoprotein, osteopontin, osteonectin, and osteocalcin) was absent in cells surrounding chondrocytes in Osx-null mice, and instead these cells express genes characteristic of chondrocytes (Sox9, Sox5, Col2a1).[293] Osterix has also been reported to inhibit chondrogenesis in vitro.[296,297] Thus, Osterix may be important for directing precursor cells away from the chondrocyte lineage and toward the osteoblast lineage. Overall, it is currently thought that Runx2 has a crucial role in the earliest determination stage of the osteoblast lineage, driving mesenchymal progenitors to become pre-osteoblasts, while Osterix regulates at a later stage the differentiation of pre-osteoblasts to functional, bone-forming osteoblasts expressing high levels of osteoblast markers (see Fig. 4-6).

Other Factors and Signaling Molecules Involved in Osteoblastogenesis

Besides β-catenin, Runx2, and Osterix, various other (non–bone-specific) transcription factors are involved in osteoblast differentiation and function, albeit not to a similar critical extent, as their inactivation does not completely abrogate bone formation. These include ATF4,[298-300] Msx1 and Msx2,[301-304] Dlx5, Dlx6, and Dlx3,[305-308] Twist,[309,310] activator protein-1 (AP1) and its related molecules (Fos/Jun),[311-315] and Schnurri-2 and -3.[230,316-322] A myriad of morphogens and signaling molecules control the activity of the transcription factors just described. These molecules include Wnts, as discussed before, as well as locally produced BMPs and TGFβ, Hedgehogs (particularly Ihh), FGFs, Notch ligands, IGFs, PDGF, and systemic factors like PTH, GH, prostaglandins, estrogens, androgens, $1,25(OH)_2D_3$ and glucocorticoids.[81,97,323]

Signaling pathways involving BMPs, Ihh, and FGFs have been mentioned previously in this chapter for their roles in chondrogenesis, but these signals also exert important functions in osteoblastogenesis and bone formation. Among BMP family members, BMP-2, BMP-4, and BMP-7 have been studied most extensively for their roles in osteogenesis during development, postnatal bone formation and remodeling, and fracture repair.[15,40,49] The double knockout of BMP-2 and BMP-4 in the limb completely disrupted osteoblast differentiation, demonstrating the crucial roles of these two BMPs in osteoblast differentiation.[49] Effects of BMP signaling in later stages of osteoblast differentiation are

suggested by studies using BMP antagonists. Targeting of noggin overexpression to differentiated osteoblasts by the osteocalcin promoter results in osteopenia by 8 months of age.[324] Likewise, overexpression of gremlin, another BMP antagonist, in differentiated osteoblasts results in reduced bone mineral density and fractures.[325]

BMP-2 has been shown to play a critical role in osteogenic differentiation: It promotes the commitment of pluripotent mesenchymal cells to the osteoblast lineage[326-329] and has been demonstrated to induce the expression of both Runx2 and Osx during osteoblastogenesis.[327,330-333] The precise mechanisms responsible for BMP-2-mediated gene regulation during osteoblast differentiation and bone formation are not well elucidated because of the considerable complexity and involvement of a myriad of interacting pathways. Nevertheless, the activity of BMP-2 as a potent inducer of bone formation is being applied to repair bone defects in humans.[323,334,335] A recent human genetic study indicated that polymorphisms in the BMP-2 gene are linked to a high risk for osteoporosis.[336]

The Hedgehog family member Ihh is required for endochondral but not for intramembranous bone formation, by controlling osteoblast differentiation in the perichondrium of long bones. Ihh-null mice completely lack endochondral ossification because of the lack of osteoblasts.[72,337] In these mice, Runx2 is expressed in chondrocytes but not in perichondrial cells. As well, nuclear β-catenin is absent in the perichondrial cells of Ihh-deficient mice.[16] Thus, Ihh is required for inducing the initial activity of Runx2 and β-catenin in perichondrial cells and triggering them to become endochondral osteoblasts, thereby coupling chondrocyte maturation with osteoblast differentiation during endochondral ossification. Chondrocyte-derived Ihh remains crucial for sustaining trabecular bone in the postnatal skeleton.[80] Skeletal abnormalities have been described in mutant mice lacking some of the intracellular mediators of Ihh signaling termed Gli proteins (three related transcription factors Gli1, Gli2, and Gli3)[338-341]; Gli2 mediates Ihh-induced osteoblast differentiation in mesenchymal cell lines by associating with Runx2 and stimulating its expression and function,[342] as well as by inducing BMP-2 expression.[343]

FGF signaling has been implicated in the proliferation of immature osteoblasts and the anabolic function of mature osteoblasts in vivo.[50-52,344-348] Whether and how osteoblast differentiation per se is affected by FGFs is currently elusive, but recent evidence indicates that FGF signaling induces BMP-2 expression and stimulates the expression and transcriptional activities of Runx2.[349-354] Conversely, Runx2 has been demonstrated to form a complex with Lef1 or TCF that binds to the promoter region of the gene encoding FGF18, inducing its expression.[355] These findings underscore once more how the various pathways that are essential for endochondral and intramembranous bone development physically and functionally converge. Moreover, the ultimate outcome relies on the complex integration of stimulatory and inhibitory signaling. For instance, Notch signaling suppresses osteoblast differentiation by diminishing Runx2 transcriptional activity via the Wnt/β-catenin pathway, actions that may be required to maintain a pool of undifferentiated mesenchymal progenitors in the bone marrow.[356-359]

Further characterization of the genetic pathways regulating osteoblastogenesis is under way and has been boosted by high hopes of finding effective therapeutic strategies to treat skeletal diseases and prevent pathologic bone loss, as in osteoporosis. Indeed, in this ever more widespread condition, current treatments as yet still most often target osteoclastic bone resorption, while compounds directed at the stimulation of osteoblastic bone formation are much sought after (see later).

Bone Remodeling and Skeletal Homeostasis

Throughout life, bone tissue maintains its integrity and responds to changes in functional demands by continuously turning over, a process termed bone remodeling.[360,361] Bone remodeling is needed to remove older matrix and cells and stress-induced microcracks to ensure biomechanical stability and to regulate mineral homeostasis of the whole organism. Osteoclasts initiate bone remodeling and perform the actual removal of old bone matrix, while osteoblasts subsequently become activated to lay down new bone. Disturbances in the delicate balance between bone resorption and bone formation lead to disorders such as osteopetrosis (reduced function of the osteoclasts), osteosclerosis (increased function of the osteoblasts), and osteoporosis (low bone mass caused by greater bone resorption than bone formation). The two first disease states are characterized by a high bone mass; osteoporosis, the more frequent condition, is typified by a decrease in bone density, severe trabecular and cortical porosity, and a high incidence of fractures. Here we will briefly review the principles and main regulatory determinants of the bone remodeling process, and will outline some of the current insights into how osteoclasts and particularly osteoblasts function to sustain additional skeletal functions in a broader physiologic perspective.

PRINCIPLES OF BONE REMODELING

Bone is constantly being renewed by undergoing a process of self-destruction followed by a regenerative process. Depending on mechanical and physiologic needs, osteoclasts resorb particular pockets or trenches of existing trabecular and cortical mineralized bone tissue, whereas osteoblasts lay down new bone at appropriate sites to replace the lost bone (Fig. 4-8). Packets of bone that are renewed during remodeling are called bone-remodeling units (BRUs) or bone multicellular units (BMUs).[360] It has been estimated that the adult human skeleton contains more than a million of these microscopic remodeling foci at any one time.[361] The bone in an activated BRU is first removed by osteoclastic bone resorption through a process that takes a few weeks (see Fig. 4-8). Lost bone is replaced by osteoblastic bone formation, lasting 3 to 4 months for one packet. This discrepancy in the kinetics of bone resorption and formation explains in part how increased resorption, even when accompanied by coupled increased formation, can cause bone loss, for example, in estrogen deficiency or hyperparathyroidism. Bone resorption that starts the remodeling cycle may be initiated by osteoblast lineage cells perceiving and responding to a remodeling signal (see later). The signal responsible for the completion of resorption in a remodeling cycle has not been determined in vivo, but several factors that reduce osteoclast formation or activity could play a role (see later). In healthy bones, cessation of resorption is followed by bone formation. During the time lag that occurs between the end of resorption and the beginning of formation, called the reversal phase, small cells are seen on the resorbed surface, perhaps osteoblast precursors that are attracted to the BRU. At this stage of the remodeling cycle, plump cuboidal osteoblastic cells differentiate on the bone surface and deposit the organized matrix that then becomes mineralized. The

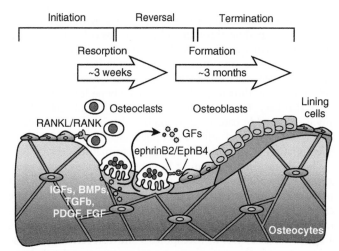

FIGURE 4-8. Three-phase model of bone remodeling. The skeleton is a metabolically active organ that undergoes continuous remodeling throughout life. Bone remodeling involves the removal of mineralized bone by osteoclasts, followed by the formation and subsequent mineralization of bone matrix by osteoblasts. Initiation starts with recruitment of hematopoietic precursors and their differentiation to osteoclasts, induced by osteoblast lineage cells that express osteoclastogenic ligands such as receptor activator of nuclear factor-κB ligand (RANKL). Osteoclasts become multinucleated and resorb bone. Transition is marked by switching from bone resorption to formation via coupling factors, possibly including diffusible growth factors (GFs) (e.g., hormones), membrane-bound molecules (e.g., ephrins), and factors embedded in bone matrix that become released upon osteoclastic bone resorption and can stimulate osteoblast recruitment, differentiation, and/or activity. During the termination phase, the resorbed lacuna is refilled through bone formation by osteoblasts that later flatten to form a layer of lining cells on the bone surface or become osteocytes connected by canaliculi within the bone.

bone formation period is completed after approximately 4 months, when the respective packet of bone, either on the surface of a trabecula or in the cortical haversian canal system, enters a quiescent period until the next remodeling cycle (see Fig. 4-8).[360]

Skeletal homeostasis remains intact as long as the activities of both osteoclasts and osteoblasts are balanced (coupled), and the net bone mass is maintained. This balance implies the existence of mechanisms that tightly coordinate the differentiation of osteoblasts and osteoclasts, as well as their migration to locations where they function. One prime aspect of the coupling principle is provided by the direct control of osteoclastogenesis by cells of the osteoblast lineage. Indeed, as was outlined previously in this chapter, osteoblasts and stromal cells control bone degradation by expressing M-CSF required for the proliferation of osteoclast precursors and RANKL, mediating the differentiation of hematopoietic osteoclast precursors toward mature multinucleated cells (osteoclastogenesis). Conversely, osteoclasts may reciprocally stimulate osteoblast differentiation and function to initiate the anabolic arm of the remodeling process. Osteoclastic bone resorption may well locally release the myriad of growth factors that are stored in the bone matrix, which can subsequently act as potent osteoblast stimuli. Growth factors like TGFβ, BMPs, IGFs, and PDGF are known to be incorporated into the bone matrix in high concentrations and to have the potency to attract osteoblastic cells and/or progenitors, and/or to stimulate proliferation and osteoblast differentiation and activity.[362-364] Direct signaling by osteoclasts to cells of the osteoblast lineage has been demonstrated recently and may participate in coupled osteoblastogenesis and bone formation. For instance, the ephrin/ Eph receptor system allows bidirectional signaling between osteoclasts and osteoblasts; osteoclasts express ephrin B2, and osteoblasts express its EphB4 receptor, both membrane-bound proteins.[365] Signaling through EphB4 into osteoblasts (forward signaling) enhances osteogenic differentiation, whereas signaling through ephrin B2 into osteoclast precursors (reverse signaling) suppresses osteoclast differentiation.[365] The overall outcome of such interaction thus is predicted to favor bone formation.[364,366] It has also been reported that the v-ATPase V0 subunit D2 not only is involved in osteoclast fusion but also regulates the secretion by osteoclasts of still unidentified factors that inhibit the differentiation of osteoblast precursors into mature cells.[367]

Thus, bone remodeling must be tightly controlled to maintain normal bone homeostasis, but the molecular mechanisms that control its initiation, progression, and cessation at any given site remain poorly understood. However, failure of this normal skeletal functioning is one of the most common early manifestations of aging, for example, in osteoporosis and osteoarthritis. These and a variety of other pathologic conditions affecting the skeleton (e.g., rheumatoid arthritis, periodontitis, Paget's disease, bone tumors) lead to perturbations in the bone remodeling process, predominantly shifting the balance toward increased degradation of bone owing to local and/or systemic alterations in the levels of hormones or proinflammatory cytokines that stimulate bone resorption (see next). Osteoporosis, characterized by low bone mass and high risk for debilitating fractures of the vertebrae and long bones, afflicts millions of people, particularly postmenopausal women (see later), and becomes increasingly prevalent with the aging of the general population. Estrogen deficiency increases both the number of sites at which remodeling is initiated and the extent of resorption at a given site (see next). Increased bone resorption is accompanied by increased bone formation as a result of coupling. However, the increase in bone formation is not sufficient to maintain bone balance and prevent

bone loss. The reason for this skeletal insufficiency in osteoporosis is not known; it could be due to lack of estrogen or other hormones, such as androgens, required for fully effective bone formation and is due in part to the above mentioned kinetic imbalance. In cancellous bone, the loss results in thinner trabeculae, which become rod-shaped rather than plate-like, and in trabecular discontinuity, which deprives them of mechanical function. In cortical bone, endosteal bone resorption causes thinning of the cortex and sometimes trabecularization of the endosteal surface. Enhanced resorption increases the size of haversian canals and the porosity of the cortical bone. The result of these changes is significant weakening of the respective bones and increased fracture risk.

CONTROL OF BONE REMODELING AND BONE MASS

Bone remodeling and the resultant net bone mass are influenced by a myriad of signals (Fig. 4-9); mechanical stimuli, endocrine molecules, and central regulatory systems profoundly affect bone resorption and bone formation and hence the balance between the two processes, in addition to local factors (discussed previously).

MECHANICAL LOADING

The skeletal system provides mechanical support and protection for the multiple organs of vertebrate organisms. To withstand loading in the most efficient way (maximal strength for minimal material), the skeleton constantly adjusts its bone mass and architecture in response to load through bone remodeling. In fact, adaptation and reshaping of the bone structure to mechanical forces require the replacement of existing bone packets or whole trabeculae with new ones appropriately oriented relative

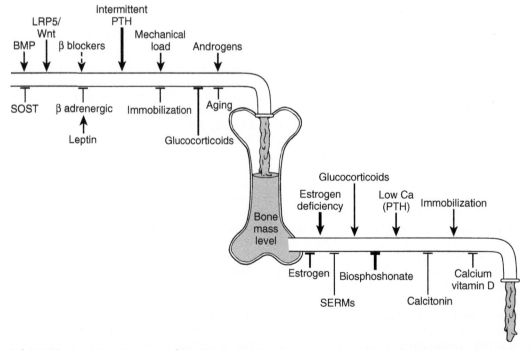

FIGURE 4-9. Control of skeletal homeostasis and bone mass. Schematic representation of the servo system that maintains bone mass at steady-state levels. Physiologic and pharmacologic stimulators and inhibitors of bone formation and resorption are listed. The relative impact, where known, is represented by the thickness of the *arrows*. *Solid lines* are current therapies, and *dotted lines*, putative ones. SERM, Selective estrogen receptor modulator. (Modified from Harada S, Rodan GA: Control of osteoblast function and regulation of bone mass, Nature 423:349–355, 2003.)

to prevailing mechanical loads. The close, dynamic relation between bone structure and the lines of force in bone may be maintained by responses to a mechanical strain threshold (force per unit area), below which osteoclastic removal of bone occurs, while a higher strain will stimulate the addition of bone. It has indeed long been recognized that mechanical stress induced by weight-bearing exercise increases osteoblast activity and induces bone formation. Conversely, the absence of mechanical stimulation resulting from prolonged immobilization or unloading causes severe bone loss. During immobilization, bone resorption increases and formation decreases, contributing to the bone loss seen to be associated with frailty and prolonged bed rest. Similarly, prolonged space flight, with the resulting lack of gravity forces on the skeleton, leads to marked loss of bone mass and increased bone fragility in astronauts.

Increasing evidence suggests that the main mechanosensing cell type of bone is the osteocyte (see earlier). The osteocyte is ideally situated within the lamellar bone to sense mechanical forces and may communicate signals to other osteocytes, osteoblasts, and osteoclasts on the bone surface through the connecting canalicular network.[233,368-370] Osteocytes have been demonstrated to have the potential to stimulate bone resorption in vitro and in vivo.[371,372] This modulation of bone remodeling has been suggested to be elicited by osteocyte apoptosis, which can be consequential to unloading.[373] Conversely, mechanical stimulation is capable of maintaining osteocyte viability.[374,375] Recent studies underscore the importance of osteocyte viability in maintenance of bone tissue health and the response to mechanical loading. Experimental destruction of osteocytes in murine bone, via targeted diphtheria toxin receptor expression under the control of the osteocyte-specific DMP-1 promoter, quickly led to a large-scale increase in bone resorption, decreased bone formation, and trabecular bone loss. Concomitantly, these mice were resistant to unloading-induced bone loss, indicating the requirement for osteocytes in the response to mechanical signals.[376]

The mechanisms by which a mechanical stimulus is transduced into biochemical signals in osteocytes and osteoblasts and the means whereby these cells then modulate bone remodeling activities have not been clearly identified. Influences that have been implicated in the process include shearing forces produced by fluid movement (e.g., in the canaliculi surrounding the osteocytic dendrites) and a variety of membrane proteins, including integrins, connexins, and stretch-sensitive ion channels.[233,236,239] For instance, mechanical stimulation increases expression of connexins, membrane-spanning proteins that form regulated channels; this allows the direct exchange of small molecules with adjacent cells, resulting in intercellular communication between cells.[239,377-379] Moreover, osteocytes respond in vitro and in vivo to increased load by altering their signaling. For example, in response to loading, osteocytes upregulate nitric oxide production, release prostaglandin (PG)E-2 and IGF-1, and decrease glutamate transporter expression.[233] DMP-1 expression is also robustly increased upon mechanical stimulation.[380] DMP-1 inactivation in mice is associated with a hypomineralized phenotype linked with elevated FGF-23 and defective osteocyte lacuna/canalicular network formation.[381] MEPE production in osteocytes is mechanosensitive as well, showing delayed production after mechanical stimulation, quite unlike that of DMP-1.[382] Targeted disruption of MEPE results in increased bone mass and confers a degree of resistance to age-related trabecular bone loss.[383] Because both DMP-1 and MEPE can regulate phosphate metabolism and bone mass, these findings suggest a potential

connection between exercise, local bone mineralization, phosphate homeostasis, and kidney function orchestrated via the osteocyte, which may be important toward an understanding of the full spectrum of consequences of the loss of osteocytes observed in aging bones.[233,237,243,384]

Of great interest also is the recent observation that mechanical loading changes the expression levels of *SOST* in osteocytes, resulting in a rapid decrease in sclerostin production.[385] As was mentioned, sclerostin inhibits Wnt signaling through binding to LRP5/6[240,241]; *SOST*-null mice have a very high bone mass,[386,387] whereas conversely transgenic mice overexpressing sclerostin in osteocytes suffer severe bone loss.[388] Osteocytes thus appear to use the Wnt/β-catenin pathway to transmit signals of mechanical loading to cells on the bone surface.[236,389]

SYSTEMIC FACTORS REGULATING CALCIUM HOMEOSTASIS

Bone remodeling also represents a major mechanism used by land vertebrates to regulate mineral homeostasis. The removal of calcium from bone, to maintain calcium homeostasis acutely, is facilitated by osteoclastic resorption of calcium-containing bone. The principal mediators in this process are PTH and its downstream effector 1,25(OH)$_2$D$_3$. Both these hormones act on osteoblastic cells to increase the production of RANKL and thereby potently activate osteoclastogenesis.[143,144,390]

The actions of PTH on bone are complex, with multiple direct actions on cells of the osteoblast lineage that vary, both with the state of differentiation of the cell and with its location in bone (periosteal vs. endosteal). The actions of PTH to increase osteoclast number and action dominate when levels of PTH are continuously elevated, but PTH also increases the rate of bone formation. In fact, when PTH is administered intermittently, this effect predominates and leads to a net increase in bone mass.[391-394] PTH enhances Runx2 expression and activity when administered intermittently; however, Runx2 is also involved in the catabolic effect of PTH through the induction of RANKL.[395,396] Intermittent PTH promotes osteoblast differentiation also in part by its ability to promote exit from the cell cycle, to activate Wnt signaling in osteoblasts, and to inhibit production of the Wnt antagonist sclerostin in osteocytes.[394,397-399] Furthermore, intermittent PTH prolongs osteoblast survival.[400] By controlling osteoblast function, PTH increases bone formation on cancellous, endocortical, and periosteal bone surfaces and has become a valuable clinical anabolic treatment strategy for osteoporotic conditions.[401,402]

Sex Steroids

Another significant endocrine input into bone remodeling and homeostasis is the pronounced influence of sex steroids, essential for maintenance of the adult skeleton (see Fig. 4-9). Skeletal preservation by estrogen in females may be related evolutionarily to the need for calcium stores for embryonic skeletal development. In mammalian adult males and females, including humans, estrogen has been identified as the major inhibitor of bone resorption by reducing osteoclast number. This explains the profound bone loss associated with estrogen deficiency, with postmenopausal osteoporosis being the most prominent type of bone pathology in humans.[223,403,404] Treatment of women with hormone replacement therapy (estrogen alone or estrogen plus progesterone) has been shown to prevent this bone loss.[405]

Recent studies have shed light on the mechanism of estrogen action on osteoclasts: Osteoclasts express estrogen receptors (ERα and ERβ) and estrogen acts directly on osteoclasts to increase apoptosis.[406,407] The regulation of osteoclast lifespan by estrogen involves induction of the Fas/FasL system causing apoptosis, a pathway that may be involved both in osteoclast cell-autonomous effects[407] and in indirect mechanisms mediated via the osteoblast.[408] Furthermore, estrogen can have nongenomic effects, or rapid signaling effects, thus inducing the phosphorylation of components of various signaling pathways (e.g., the MAPK pathway) or calcium regulation. Such effects may contribute to the induction of osteoclast apoptosis by estrogen without the need for direct binding of ERα to DNA.[403,409] Besides affecting osteoclast lifespan, estrogen was reported to decrease the responsiveness of osteoclast progenitor cells to RANKL, thereby reducing osteoclastogenesis.[410]

A variety of other mechanisms contribute to the beneficial effects of estrogen on bone. A prime role is played by cytokines regulated by estrogen that indirectly lead to changes in osteoclast number: Estrogen suppresses the production of osteoclastogenic cytokines such as interleukin (IL)-1, IL-6, IL-7, and TNFα in T cells and osteoblasts.[411-415] As well, a portion of the effects ascribed to estrogen deficiency were suggested recently to be in fact mediated by the resultant increase in pituitary gland–derived follicle-stimulating hormone (FSH) acting on osteoclasts.[416,417]

Androgens are important not only as a source of estrogen, through the action of aromatase, but also for their direct effect in stimulating bone formation.[418,419] Testosterone, responsible for the male phenotype characterized by a larger skeleton, has complex effects on bone metabolism. As an anabolic steroid, it stimulates bone formation in both males and females. In addition, testosterone can inhibit bone resorption directly, acting through the androgen receptor and through conversion by aromatase to estrogens. Androgens also increase periosteal bone formation, leading to larger and therefore stronger bones. Loss of androgens in males from chemical or surgical castration or an age-associated decline in androgen levels has the same adverse effect on the skeleton as estrogen loss in women, albeit the loss of testosterone in aging men is not as universal or as abrupt as the loss of estrogen at the time of menopause in women.[418-420]

Other Systemic Regulators of Bone Remodeling

In contrast to sex steroids, glucocorticoid excess is catabolic to bone, as is illustrated by glucocorticoid-induced osteoporosis, a devastating consequence of long-term use of glucocorticoids.[421] The mechanisms for glucocorticoid-induced bone loss are complex, including suppression of renal calcium reabsorption, reduction in intestinal calcium absorption, and hypogonadism, all of which lead to increased bone resorption and bone turnover. Perhaps more important, glucocorticoids have direct effects on the skeleton.[421] Glucocorticoids impair the replication, differentiation, and function of osteoblasts and induce the apoptosis of mature osteoblasts and osteocytes, leading to dramatic suppression of bone formation.[422-425] As well, glucocorticoids act directly on osteoclasts and prolong their lifespan; in addition, glucocorticoids may sensitize bone cells to regulators of bone remodeling and favor osteoclastogenesis, thus leading to overall increased bone resorption.[426-428]

Influences on bone remodeling by the GH/IGF axis,[429] thyroid hormones,[430] and prostaglandins[431] are reviewed in the indicated recent references.

CENTRAL CONTROL OF BONE REMODELING

The central nervous system (CNS) coordinates the activities of multiple organs throughout the body. Given the likely impor-

tance of coordinating skeletal responses to a variety of systemic challenges, perhaps it is not surprising that recent work shows that signals from the CNS and the sympathetic nervous system (SNS) profoundly influence bone remodeling and resultant bone mass (Fig. 4-10).

Leptin, an adipocyte-derived hormone mainly known for controlling appetite, energy metabolism, and reproduction, acts through the leptin receptor in the CNS (hypothalamus) and ultimately through the SNS to negatively regulate bone formation by osteoblasts.[432,433] Sympathetic signaling via β$_2$-adrenergic receptors (Adrβ$_2$) in osteoblasts inhibits proliferation through transcriptional factors such as Period (per), which also regulate the circadian clock,[434] and additionally favors bone resorption by increasing osteoblastic expression of RANKL[435] (see Fig. 4-10). These conclusions were drawn from a series of studies using mutant mice with deficiencies or lesions in portions of the leptin-hypothalamic-sympathetic pathways[432,433,435]; all of these models displayed a similar bone phenotype characterized by increased bone mass due to vastly increased osteoblast activity and bone formation accompanied by a mild increase in osteoclastic bone resorption. Part of this outcome is explained further by another action of leptin through hypothalamic receptors, which is to inhibit bone resorption by stimulating the expression of cocaine- and amphetamine-regulated transcript (CART), leading—through as yet unknown mechanisms—to reduced RANKL expression.[435,436] Evidence that leptin regulates bone turnover in part through a CNS/β-adrenergic system relay has driven attention toward the potential therapeutic benefits of β-adrenergic blockers in improving bone mass and strength in osteoporosis.[437-439] It is interesting to note that whereas the downstream effectors of leptin action on bone remodeling seem to be largely independent of its functions in energy metabolism and reproduction, a reciprocal regulatory function on energy metabolism and adiposity is exerted by osteoblasts (as outlined in the next section). In addition to CART, leptin interacts with the hypothalamic neuropeptides neuropeptide Y and neuromedin U, which themselves have been implicated in the central control of bone remodeling[440-442] (see Fig. 4-10). Furthermore, other neuroendocrine connections to bone remodeling have been made with the findings in mouse genetic and pharmacologic studies that both thyroid-stimulating hormone (TSH) and FSH act directly on bone cells to influence remodeling.[416,443,444] For additional readings on these subjects, see references 437 through 439, and 445 through 448.

ADDITIONAL ROLES OF OSTEOBLASTS AND OSTEOCLASTS IN INTEGRATING SKELETAL PHYSIOLOGIC FUNCTIONS

As was outlined earlier, bone remodeling is controlled by a myriad of mechanical, endocrine, local, and central signals, each aimed at fulfilling the functions of bone listed at the beginning of the chapter. A number of recent breakthroughs have shown that bone cells are not merely involved in bone remodeling and maintenance of bone mass, but have a number of critical functions that extend beyond the bone tissue proper. Among these newly described functions are the role of the skeleton in the regulation of immunity, hematopoiesis, and energy metabolism.

Interplay Between Bone Cells and the Immune and Hematopoietic Systems

With the growing elucidation of the molecular control of osteoclastogenesis, links with the immune system have increasingly emerged and given rise to a novel discipline of bone-related

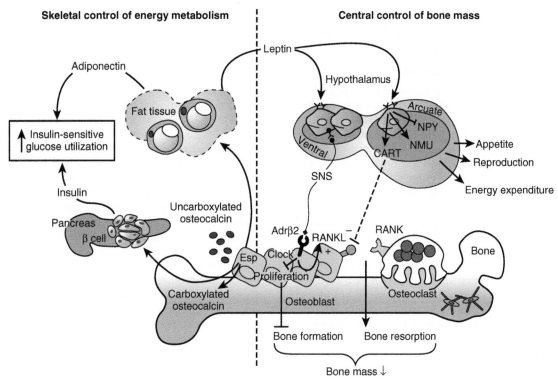

FIGURE 4-10. Interactions between bone, brain, and energy metabolism. The skeleton affects cells involved in metabolic control, such as pancreatic β cells and fat cells, which signal to brain centers and peripheral tissues to regulate energy and metabolic homeostasis *(left)*. Conversely, the central nervous system and brain neuropeptides regulate bone homeostasis *(right)*. Osteoblasts express osteotesticular protein tyrosine phosphatase (OT-PTP), a product of the *Esp* gene, which regulates γ-carboxylation of the osteoblast-specific protein osteocalcin. Whereas carboxylated osteocalcin has high affinity to bind the bone mineral, uncarboxylated osteocalcin is secreted into the serum and acts in a hormone-like manner to influence energy metabolism by increasing β cell proliferation and insulin secretion in the pancreas, and by increasing adipocyte secretion of adiponectin, an insulin-sensitizing adipokine. As a result, insulin sensitivity is enhanced. Thus, the skeleton functions as an endocrine regulator of energy metabolism *(left)*. Adipocytes also secrete the adipokine leptin, which binds to leptin receptors in the hypothalamus and regulates appetite, reproduction, and energy expenditure *(right)*. Leptin also regulates bone mass *(right)*. The leptin signal in the brain leads to stimulation of the sympathetic nervous system (SNS) and activation of the β₂-adrenergic receptor (Adrβ2) on osteoblasts, which decreases osteoblast proliferation (mediated by molecular clock genes) and bone formation, while increasing bone resorption through stimulation of receptor activator of nuclear factor-κB ligand (RANKL) expression. Yet, leptin also has inhibitory effects on bone resorption by binding to its receptor on neurons in the arcuate nucleus of the hypothalamus and increasing expression of the anorexigenic peptides cocaine- and amphetamine-related transcript (CART). Via an unknown mechanism, CART inhibits RANKL expression. Other neuropeptides, such as neuromedin U (NMU) and neuropeptide Y (NPY), also influence bone metabolism and thus play a role in the central control of bone mass.

studies termed osteoimmunology.[131] This field encompasses the complex interactions and molecular and functional overlap of the immune system and bone cells. For instance, not only osteoblasts and bone marrow stromal cells, but also immune cells, express M-CSF and RANKL, pivotal regulators of osteoclastogenesis. Particularly certain subsets of T cells rapidly upregulate surface expression of RANKL on activation, and therefore are capable of regulating osteoclast differentiation and activity. Additional cytokines, either produced by or regulating T cells, are responsible for the upregulation of osteoclast formation observed in a variety of conditions such as inflammation (e.g., arthritic joint disease), hyperparathyroidism, and estrogen deficiency causing osteoporosis.[411] These factors, which include TNFα, IL-1, and IL-6, function as co-stimulatory molecules for osteoclastogenesis. Another level of molecular overlap is provided by the fact that most osteoclastogenic cytokines, including M-CSF and RANKL, also regulate macrophages or dendritic cells that share myeloid precursor cells from the bone marrow during development.[131,133]

Although poorly understood at present, B cells also seem to modulate the bone remodeling balance.[449] Recently, it was shown that B cells constitute an important source of OPG in vivo, and that mice deficient in B cells or with arrested B cell differentiation

have reduced bone mass.[450,451] B cell progenitors themselves are capable of differentiating into osteoclasts in vitro.[452]

The close interaction between immune progenitors and the skeleton is facilitated by their proximity in the bone marrow. Moreover, bones do not merely house the bone marrow but also provide the appropriate environment for physiologic and pathologic blood cell development. Recent data have highlighted the importance of osteoblasts and osteogenic stromal cells as key regulators of hematopoietic cell development, hematopoietic stem cell maintenance, and blood cell mobilization, by providing the appropriate microenvironment for the hematopoietic system.[453-458] Accordingly, changes in bone that affect the bone marrow environment, in particular the osteoblast niche, can disrupt hematopoietic stem cells, leading to altered hematopoietic and immune cell development and/or potentially initiating myeloproliferative disease.[454,459-461] It remains to be determined whether and to what extent bone remodeling may dynamically respond to the changing demands of hematopoiesis. As a suggestive example, osteoclast resorptive activity on the endosteal bone surface, where hematopoietic cells reside,[456,462] was found to be capable of mediating the release of these hematopoietic cells to mobilize them into the circulation.[463,464] Furthermore, human hematologic diseases such as myelofibrotic disease often are associated with secondary bone pathology, suggesting that dysregulated hematopoietic differentiation may affect bone formation and/or resorption processes.

Skeletal Control of Energy Metabolism

The concept of an adipocyte-derived hormone regulating bone, as outlined earlier (leptin; see Fig. 4-10), led Karsenty to postulate the existence of reciprocal endocrine regulation from the skeleton. In search of bone-derived signals secreted into the circulation and able to modulate energy metabolism and adiposity, his research group discovered that a form of osteocalcin, one of the few osteoblast-specific gene products, acts as a hormone that increases insulin-sensitive glucose utilization and pancreatic β cell mass and reduces visceral fat (see Fig. 4-10).[465] Osteoblastic secretion of the hormone-like, undercarboxylated form of osteocalcin is controlled by a receptor-like protein tyrosine phosphatase, termed osteotesticular protein tyrosine phosphatase (OT-PTP), which is encoded by the *Esp* gene and expressed exclusively in osteoblasts. Mice lacking OT-PTP in osteoblasts have increased β cell activity that protects them from induced obesity and diabetes. These phenotypes are corrected by deleting one allele of osteocalcin. Osteocalcin deficiency in knockout mice leads to decreased insulin and adiponectin secretion, insulin resistance, higher serum glucose levels, and increased adiposity.[465,466] These findings indicate that the skeleton plays a previously unrecognized role in the regulation of energy metabolism and thereby may contribute to the onset and severity of metabolic disorders. The full significance of these novel findings established through elegant mouse genetics has yet to be fully defined in humans.

Conclusions

Bone formation during skeletal development involves a complex spatiotemporal coordination among multiple molecules, cell types, and tissues. A large number of morphogens, signaling molecules, and transcriptional regulators have been implicated in the regulation of bone development. Many of the developmental mechanisms are recapitulated or remain important later in bone homeostasis and/or pathology. The skeleton is a vital organ system essential to survival and well-being. Its major functions, including mechanical support and mineral homeostasis, are achieved by continuous remodeling throughout life. Osteoclasts and osteoblasts normally act in a coordinated manner to resorb and rebuild bone. Most bone disorders are due to bone loss resulting from an imbalance in the remodeling cycle, with bone resorption exceeding bone formation. A better understanding of the molecular mechanisms behind skeletal biology, largely derived from discoveries based on mouse and human genetics, has provided opportunities for developing therapies to treat diseases of bone. Additional advances in the molecular and genetic studies of bone, including integrative communication between pathways and cell types within and beyond the skeleton proper, may offer as yet unexplored targets for developing novel therapeutic options to treat various bone pathologies.

REFERENCES

1. Wilkie AO, Morriss-Kay GM: Genetics of craniofacial development and malformation, Nat Rev Genet 2:458–468, 2001.
2. Morriss-Kay GM, Wilkie AO: Growth of the normal skull vault and its alteration in craniosynostosis: insights from human genetics and experimental studies, J Anat 207:637–653, 2005.
3. Tapadia MD, Cordero DR, Helms JA: It's all in your head: new insights into craniofacial development and deformation, J Anat 207:461–477, 2005.
4. Huang LF, Fukai N, Selby PB, et al: Mouse clavicular development: analysis of wild-type and cleidocranial dysplasia mutant mice, Dev Dyn 210:33–40, 1997.
5. Matsuoka T, Ahlberg PE, Kessaris N, et al: Neural crest origins of the neck and shoulder, Nature 436:347–355, 2005.
6. Le AX, Miclau T, Hu D, et al: Molecular aspects of healing in stabilized and non-stabilized fractures, J Orthop Res 19:78–84, 2001.
7. Carter DR, Beaupre GS, Giori NJ, et al: Mechanobiology of skeletal regeneration, Clin Orthop Relat Res 355(suppl):S41–S55, 1998.
8. Behonick DJ, Xing Z, Lieu S, et al: Role of matrix metalloproteinase 13 in both endochondral and intramembranous ossification during skeletal regeneration, PLoS ONE 2:e1150, 2007.
9. Tabin C, Wolpert L: Rethinking the proximodistal axis of the vertebrate limb in the molecular era, Genes Dev 21:1433–1442, 2007.
10. Hall BK, Miyake T: All for one and one for all: condensations and the initiation of skeletal development, Bioessays 22:138–147, 2000.
11. Ferguson CM, Miclau T, Hu D, et al: Common molecular pathways in skeletal morphogenesis and repair, Ann N Y Acad Sci 857:33–42, 1998.
12. Thompson Z, Miclau T, Hu D, et al: A model for intramembranous ossification during fracture healing, J Orthop Res 20:1091–1098, 2002.
13. Gerstenfeld LC, Cullinane DM, Barnes GL, et al: Fracture healing as a post-natal developmental process: molecular, spatial, and temporal aspects of its regulation, J Cell Biochem 88:873–884, 2003.
14. Maes C, Coenegrachts L, Stockmans I, et al: Placental growth factor mediates mesenchymal cell development, cartilage turnover, and bone remodeling during fracture repair, J Clin Invest 116:1230–1242, 2006.
15. Tsuji K, Bandyopadhyay A, Harfe BD, et al: BMP2 activity, although dispensable for bone formation, is required for the initiation of fracture healing, Nat Genet 38:1424–1429, 2006.
16. Hu H, Hilton MJ, Tu X, et al: Sequential roles of Hedgehog and Wnt signaling in osteoblast development, Development 132:49–60, 2005.
17. Day TF, Yang Y: Wnt and hedgehog signaling pathways in bone development, J Bone Joint Surg Am 90(suppl 1):19–24, 2008.
18. Day TF, Guo X, Garrett-Beal L, et al: Wnt/beta-catenin signaling in mesenchymal progenitors controls osteoblast and chondrocyte differentiation during vertebrate skeletogenesis, Dev Cell 8:739–750, 2005.
19. Hill TP, Taketo MM, Birchmeier W, et al: Multiple roles of mesenchymal beta-catenin during murine limb patterning, Development 133:1219–1229, 2006.
20. Akiyama H, Chaboissier MC, Martin JF, et al: The transcription factor Sox9 has essential roles in successive steps of the chondrocyte differentiation pathway and is required for expression of Sox5 and Sox6, Genes Dev 16:2813–2828, 2002.
21. Akiyama H, Stadler HS, Martin JF, et al: Misexpression of Sox9 in mouse limb bud mesenchyme induces polydactyly and rescues hypodactyly mice, Matrix Biol 26:224–233, 2007.
22. Bi W, Deng JM, Zhang Z, et al: Sox9 is required for cartilage formation, Nat Genet 22:85–89, 1999.
23. Smits P, Li P, Mandel J, et al: The transcription factors L-Sox5 and Sox6 are essential for cartilage formation, Dev Cell 1:277–290, 2001.
24. Vajo Z, Francomano CA, Wilkin DJ: The molecular and genetic basis of fibroblast growth factor receptor 3 disorders: the achondroplasia family of skeletal dysplasias, Muenke craniosynostosis, and Crouzon syndrome with acanthosis nigricans, Endocr Rev 21:23–39, 2000.
25. Naski MC, Wang Q, Xu J, et al: Graded activation of fibroblast growth factor receptor 3 by mutations causing achondroplasia and thanatophoric dysplasia, Nat Genet 13:233–237, 1996.
26. Bellus GA, McIntosh I, Smith EA, et al: A recurrent mutation in the tyrosine kinase domain of fibroblast growth factor receptor 3 causes hypochondroplasia, Nat Genet 10:357–359, 1995.
27. Shiang R, Thompson LM, Zhu YZ, et al: Mutations in the transmembrane domain of FGFR3 cause the most common genetic form of dwarfism, achondroplasia, Cell 78:335–342, 1994.
28. Schipani E, Langman CB, Parfitt AM, et al: Constitutively activated receptors for parathyroid hormone and parathyroid hormone-related peptide in Jansen's metaphyseal chondrodysplasia, N Engl J Med 335:708–714, 1996.
29. Schipani E, Kruse K, Juppner H: A constitutively active mutant PTH-PTHrP receptor in Jansen-type metaphyseal chondrodysplasia, Science 268:98–100, 1995.
30. Karaplis AC, He B, Nguyen MT, et al: Inactivating mutation in the human parathyroid hormone receptor type 1 gene in Blomstrand chondrodysplasia, Endocrinology 139:5255–5258, 1998.
31. Goldring MB, Tsuchimochi K, Ijiri K: The control of chondrogenesis, J Cell Biochem 97:33–44, 2006.
32. Kronenberg HM: Developmental regulation of the growth plate, Nature 423:332–336, 2003.
33. Kappen C, Neubuser A, Balling R, et al: Molecular basis for skeletal variation: insights from developmental genetic studies in mice, Birth Defects Res B Dev Reprod Toxicol 80:425–450, 2007.
34. Shi Y, Massague J: Mechanisms of TGF-beta signaling from cell membrane to the nucleus, Cell 113:685–700, 2003.
35. Sampath TK, Reddi AH: Dissociative extraction and reconstitution of extracellular matrix components involved in local bone differentiation, Proc Natl Acad Sci U S A 78:7599–7603, 1981.
36. Urist MR: Bone: formation by autoinduction, Science 150:893–899, 1965.
37. Wozney JM, Rosen V, Celeste AJ, et al: Novel regulators of bone formation: molecular clones and activities, Science 242:1528–1534, 1988.
38. Luyten FP, Cunningham NS, Ma S, et al: Purification and partial amino acid sequence of osteogenin, a protein initiating bone differentiation, J Biol Chem 264:13377–13380, 1989.

39. Hogan BL: Bone morphogenetic proteins: multifunctional regulators of vertebrate development, Genes Dev 10:1580–1594, 1996.

40. Chen D, Zhao M, Mundy GR: Bone morphogenetic proteins, Growth Factors 22:233–241, 2004.

41. Kingsley DM: What do BMPs do in mammals? Clues from the mouse short-ear mutation, Trends Genet 10:16–21, 1994.

42. Storm EE, Huynh TV, Copeland NG, et al: Limb alterations in brachypodism mice due to mutations in a new member of the TGF beta-superfamily, Nature 368:639–643, 1994.

43. Yoon BS, Ovchinnikov DA, Yoshii I, et al: Bmpr1a and Bmpr1b have overlapping functions and are essential for chondrogenesis in vivo, Proc Natl Acad Sci U S A 102:5062–5067, 2005.

44. Pizette S, Niswander L: BMPs are required at two steps of limb chondrogenesis: formation of prechondrogenic condensations and their differentiation into chondrocytes, Dev Biol 219:237–249, 2000.

45. Tsumaki N, Nakase T, Miyaji T, et al: Bone morphogenetic protein signals are required for cartilage formation and differently regulate joint development during skeletogenesis, J Bone Miner Res 17:898–906, 2002.

46. Yoon BS, Pogue R, Ovchinnikov DA, et al: BMPs regulate multiple aspects of growth-plate chondrogenesis through opposing actions on FGF pathways, Development 133:4667–4678, 2006.

47. Minina E, Kreschel C, Naski MC, et al: Interaction of FGF, Ihh/Pthlh, and BMP signaling integrates chondrocyte proliferation and hypertrophic differentiation, Dev Cell 3:439–449, 2002.

48. Pathi S, Rutenberg JB, Johnson RL, et al: Interaction of Ihh and BMP/Noggin signaling during cartilage differentiation, Dev Biol 209:239–253, 1999.

49. Bandyopadhyay A, Tsuji K, Cox K, et al: Genetic analysis of the roles of BMP2, BMP4, and BMP7 in limb patterning and skeletogenesis, PLoS Genet 2:e216, 2006.

50. Ornitz DM: FGF signaling in the developing endochondral skeleton, Cytokine Growth Factor Rev 16:205–213, 2005.

51. Liu Z, Xu J, Colvin JS, et al: Coordination of chondrogenesis and osteogenesis by fibroblast growth factor 18, Genes Dev 16:859–869, 2002.

52. Ohbayashi N, Shibayama M, Kurotaki Y, et al: FGF18 is required for normal cell proliferation and differentiation during osteogenesis and chondrogenesis, Genes Dev 16:870–879, 2002.

53. Hung IH, Yu K, Lavine KJ, et al: FGF9 regulates early hypertrophic chondrocyte differentiation and skeletal vascularization in the developing stylopod, Dev Biol 307:300–313, 2007.

54. Colvin JS, Bohne BA, Harding GW, et al: Skeletal overgrowth and deafness in mice lacking fibroblast growth factor receptor 3, Nat Genet 12:390–397, 1996.

55. Deng C, Wynshaw-Boris A, Zhou F, et al: Fibroblast growth factor receptor 3 is a negative regulator of bone growth, Cell 84:911–921, 1996.

56. Liu Z, Lavine KJ, Hung IH, et al: FGF18 is required for early chondrocyte proliferation, hypertrophy and vascular invasion of the growth plate, Dev Biol 302:80–91, 2007.

57. Sahni M, Ambrosetti DC, Mansukhani A, et al: FGF signaling inhibits chondrocyte proliferation and regulates bone development through the STAT-1 pathway, Genes Dev 13:1361–1366, 1999.

58. Su WC, Kitagawa M, Xue N, et al: Activation of Stat1 by mutant fibroblast growth-factor receptor in thanatophoric dysplasia type II dwarfism, Nature 386:288–292, 1997.

59. Legeai-Mallet L, Benoist-Lasselin C, Munnich A, et al: Overexpression of FGFR3, Stat1, Stat5 and p21Cip1 correlates with phenotypic severity and defective chondrocyte differentiation in FGFR3-related chondrodysplasias, Bone 34:26–36, 2004.

60. Naski MC, Colvin JS, Coffin JD, et al: Repression of hedgehog signaling and BMP4 expression in growth plate cartilage by fibroblast growth factor receptor 3, Development 125:4977–4988, 1998.

61. Segev O, Chumakov I, Nevo Z, et al: Restrained chondrocyte proliferation and maturation with abnormal growth plate vascularization and ossification in human FGFR-3(G380R) transgenic mice, Hum Mol Genet 9:249–258, 2000.

62. Wang Y, Spatz MK, Kannan K, et al: A mouse model for achondroplasia produced by targeting fibroblast growth factor receptor 3, Proc Natl Acad Sci U S A 96:4455–4460, 1999.

63. Iwata T, Chen L, Li C, et al: A neonatal lethal mutation in FGFR3 uncouples proliferation and differentiation of growth plate chondrocytes in embryos, Hum Mol Genet 9:1603–1613, 2000.

64. Murakami S, Kan M, McKeehan WL, et al: Upregulation of the chondrogenic Sox9 gene by fibroblast growth factors is mediated by the mitogen-activated protein kinase pathway, Proc Natl Acad Sci U S A 97:1113–1118, 2000.

65. Murakami S, Balmes G, McKinney S, et al: Constitutive activation of MEK1 in chondrocytes causes Stat1-independent achondroplasia-like dwarfism and rescues the Fgfr3-deficient mouse phenotype, Genes Dev 18:290–305, 2004.

66. Yasoda A, Komatsu Y, Chusho H, et al: Overexpression of CNP in chondrocytes rescues achondroplasia through a MAPK-dependent pathway, Nat Med 10:80–86, 2004.

67. de Frutos CA, Vega S, Manzanares M, et al: Snail1 is a transcriptional effector of FGFR3 signaling during chondrogenesis and achondroplasias, Dev Cell 13:872–883, 2007.

68. Li C, Chen L, Iwata T, et al: A Lys644Glu substitution in fibroblast growth factor receptor 3 (FGFR3) causes dwarfism in mice by activation of STATs and ink4 cell cycle inhibitors, Hum Mol Genet 8:35–44, 1999.

69. Chen L, Li C, Qiao W, et al: A Ser(365)→Cys mutation of fibroblast growth factor receptor 3 in mouse downregulates Ihh/PTHrP signals and causes severe achondroplasia, Hum Mol Genet 10:457–465, 2001.

70. Lanske B, Karaplis AC, Lee K, et al: PTH/PTHrP receptor in early development and Indian hedgehog-regulated bone growth, Science 273:663–666, 1996.

71. Vortkamp A, Lee K, Lanske B, et al: Regulation of rate of cartilage differentiation by Indian hedgehog and PTH-related protein, Science 273:613–622, 1996.

72. St Jacques B, Hammerschmidt M, McMahon AP: Indian hedgehog signaling regulates proliferation and differentiation of chondrocytes and is essential for bone formation, Genes Dev 13:2072–2086, 1999.

73. Karp SJ, Schipani E, St Jacques B, et al: Indian hedgehog coordinates endochondral bone growth and morphogenesis via parathyroid hormone related protein dependent and independent pathways, Development 127:543–548, 2000.

74. Kobayashi T, Chung UI, Schipani E, et al: PTHrP and Indian hedgehog control differentiation of growth plate chondrocytes at multiple steps, Development 129:2977–2986, 2002.

75. Kobayashi T, Soegiarto DW, Yang Y, et al: Indian hedgehog stimulates periarticular chondrocyte differentiation to regulate growth plate length independently of PTHrP, J Clin Invest 115:1734–1742, 2005.

76. Inada M, Yasui T, Nomura S, et al: Maturational disturbance of chondrocytes in Cbfa1-deficient mice, Dev Dyn 214:279–290, 1999.

77. Kim IS, Otto F, Zabel B, et al: Regulation of chondrocyte differentiation by Cbfa1, Mech Dev 80:159–170, 1999.

78. Takeda S, Bonnamy JP, Owen MJ, et al: Continuous expression of Cbfa1 in nonhypertrophic chondrocytes uncovers its ability to induce hypertrophic chondrocyte differentiation and partially rescues Cbfa1-deficient mice, Genes Dev 15:467–481, 2001.

79. Ueta C, Iwamoto M, Kanatani N, et al: Skeletal malformations caused by overexpression of Cbfa1 or its dominant negative form in chondrocytes, J Cell Biol 153:87–100, 2001.

80. Maeda Y, Nakamura E, Nguyen MT, et al: Indian Hedgehog produced by postnatal chondrocytes is essential for maintaining a growth plate and trabecular bone, Proc Natl Acad Sci U S A 104:6382–6387, 2007.

81. Karsenty G, Wagner EF: Reaching a genetic and molecular understanding of skeletal development, Dev Cell 2:389–406, 2002.

82. Provot S, Schipani E: Fetal growth plate: a developmental model of cellular adaptation to hypoxia, Ann N Y Acad Sci 1117:26–39, 2007.

83. Schipani E: Hypoxia and HIF-1alpha in chondrogenesis, Ann N Y Acad Sci 1068:66–73, 2006.

84. Semenza GL: HIF-1, O(2), and the 3 PHDs: how animal cells signal hypoxia to the nucleus, Cell 107:1–3, 2001.

85. Provot S, Zinyk D, Gunes Y, et al: Hif-1alpha regulates differentiation of limb bud mesenchyme and joint development, J Cell Biol 177:451–464, 2007.

86. Schipani E, Ryan HE, Didrickson S, et al: Hypoxia in cartilage: HIF-1alpha is essential for chondrocyte growth arrest and survival, Genes Dev 15:2865–2876, 2001.

87. Maes C, Stockmans I, Moermans K, et al: Soluble VEGF isoforms are essential for establishing epiphyseal vascularization and regulating chondrocyte development and survival, J Clin Invest 113:188–199, 2004.

88. Zelzer E, Mamluk R, Ferrara N, et al: VEGFA is necessary for chondrocyte survival during bone development, Development 131:2161–2171, 2004.

89. Rajpurohit R, Koch CJ, Tao Z, et al: Adaptation of chondrocytes to low oxygen tension: relationship between hypoxia and cellular metabolism, J Cell Physiol 168:424–432, 1996.

90. Mobasheri A, Richardson S, Mobasheri R, et al: Hypoxia inducible factor-1 and facilitative glucose transporters GLUT1 and GLUT3: putative molecular components of the oxygen and glucose sensing apparatus in articular chondrocytes, Histol Histopathol 20:1327–1338, 2005.

91. Pfander D, Cramer T, Schipani E, et al: HIF-1alpha controls extracellular matrix synthesis by epiphyseal chondrocytes, J Cell Sci 116:1819–1826, 2003.

92. Colnot C, Lu C, Hu D, et al: Distinguishing the contributions of the perichondrium, cartilage, and vascular endothelium to skeletal development, Dev Biol 269:55–69, 2004.

93. Trueta J, Amato VP: The vascular contribution to osteogenesis. III. Changes in the growth cartilage caused by experimentally induced ischaemia, J Bone Joint Surg Br 42:571–587, 1960.

94. Brashear HR Jr: Epiphyseal avascular necrosis and its relation to longitudinal bone growth, J Bone Joint Surg Am 45:1423–1438, 1963.

95. Brandi ML, Collin-Osdoby P: Vascular biology and the skeleton, J Bone Miner Res 21:183–192, 2006.

96. Erlebacher A, Filvaroff EH, Gitelman SE, et al: Toward a molecular understanding of skeletal development, Cell 80:371–378, 1995.

97. Karsenty G: The complexities of skeletal biology, Nature 423:316–318, 2003.

98. Trueta J, Morgan JD: The vascular contribution to osteogenesis. I. Studies by the injection method, J Bone Joint Surg Br 42:97–109, 1960.

99. Brighton CT: Structure and function of the growth plate, Clin Orthop Relat Res (136):22–32, 1978.

100. Moses MA, Sudhalter J, Langer R: Identification of an inhibitor of neovascularization from cartilage, Science 248:1408–1410, 1990.

101. Hiraki Y, Inoue H, Iyama K, et al: Identification of chondromodulin I as a novel endothelial cell growth inhibitor: purification and its localization in the avascular zone of epiphyseal cartilage, J Biol Chem 272:32419–32426, 1997.

102. Shukunami C, Hiraki Y: Chondromodulin-I and tenomodulin: the negative control of angiogenesis in connective tissue, Curr Pharm Des 13:2101–2112, 2007.

103. Moses MA, Wiederschain D, Wu I, et al: Troponin I is present in human cartilage and inhibits angiogenesis, Proc Natl Acad Sci U S A 96:2645–2650, 1999.

104. Gerber HP, Ferrara N: Angiogenesis and bone growth, Trends Cardiovasc Med 10:223–228, 2000.

105. Descalzi CF, Melchiori A, Benelli R, et al: Production of angiogenesis inhibitors and stimulators is modulated by cultured growth plate chondrocytes during in vitro differentiation: dependence on extracellular matrix assembly, Eur J Cell Biol 66:60–68, 1995.

106. Cramer T, Schipani E, Johnson RS, et al: Expression of VEGF isoforms by epiphyseal chondrocytes during low-oxygen tension is HIF-1 alpha dependent, Osteoarthritis Cartilage 12:433–439, 2004.

107. Kim HH, Lee SE, Chung WJ, et al: Stabilization of hypoxia-inducible factor-1alpha is involved in the hypoxic stimuli-induced expression of vascular endothelial growth factor in osteoblastic cells, Cytokine 17:14–27, 2002.

108. Akeno N, Czyzyk-Krzeska MF, Gross TS, et al: Hypoxia induces vascular endothelial growth factor gene transcription in human osteoblast-like cells through

the hypoxia-inducible factor-2alpha, Endocrinology 142:959–962, 2001.

109. Knowles HJ, Athanasou NA: Hypoxia-inducible factor is expressed in giant cell tumour of bone and mediates paracrine effects of hypoxia on monocyte-osteoclast differentiation via induction of VEGF, J Pathol 215:56–66, 2008.

110. Wang Y, Wan C, Deng L, et al: The hypoxia-inducible factor alpha pathway couples angiogenesis to osteogenesis during skeletal development, J Clin Invest 117:1616–1626, 2007.

111. Zelzer E, Glotzer DJ, Hartmann C, et al: Tissue specific regulation of VEGF expression during bone development requires Cbfa1/Runx2, Mech Dev 106:97–106, 2001.

112. Dai J, Rabie AB: VEGF: an essential mediator of both angiogenesis and endochondral ossification, J Dent Res 86:937–950, 2007.

113. Gerber HP, Vu TH, Ryan AM, et al: VEGF couples hypertrophic cartilage remodeling, ossification and angiogenesis during endochondral bone formation, Nat Med 5:623–628, 1999.

114. Maes C, Carmeliet P, Moermans K, et al: Impaired angiogenesis and endochondral bone formation in mice lacking the vascular endothelial growth factor isoforms VEGF164 and VEGF188. Mech Dev 111:61–73, 2002.

115. Zelzer E, McLean W, Ng YS, et al: Skeletal defects in VEGF(120/120) mice reveal multiple roles for VEGF in skeletogenesis, Development 129:1893–1904, 2002.

116. Haigh JJ, Gerber HP, Ferrara N, et al: Conditional inactivation of VEGF-A in areas of collagen2a1 expression results in embryonic lethality in the heterozygous state, Development 127:1445–1453, 2000.

117. Maes C, Carmeliet G: Vascular and nonvascular roles of VEGF in bone development. In Ruhrberg C, editor: VEGF in Development, Austin, 2008, Springer, pp 79–90.

118. Zelzer E, Olsen BR: Multiple roles of vascular endothelial growth factor (VEGF) in skeletal development, growth, and repair, Curr Top Dev Biol 65:169–187, 2005.

119. Fiedler J, Leucht F, Waltenberger J, et al: VEGF-A and PlGF-1 stimulate chemotactic migration of human mesenchymal progenitor cells, Biochem Biophys Res Commun 334:561–568, 2005.

120. Mayr-Wohlfart U, Waltenberger J, Hausser H, et al: Vascular endothelial growth factor stimulates chemotactic migration of primary human osteoblasts, Bone 30:472–477, 2002.

121. Aldridge SE, Lennard TW, Williams JR, et al: Vascular endothelial growth factor receptors in osteoclast differentiation and function, Biochem Biophys Res Commun 335:793–798, 2005.

122. Engsig MT, Chen QJ, Vu TH, et al: Matrix metalloproteinase 9 and vascular endothelial growth factor are essential for osteoclast recruitment into developing long bones, J Cell Biol 151:879–889, 2000.

123. Henriksen K, Karsdal M, Delaisse JM, et al: RANKL and vascular endothelial growth factor (VEGF) induce osteoclast chemotaxis through an ERK1/2-dependent mechanism, J Biol Chem 278:48745–48753, 2003.

124. Nakagawa M, Kaneda T, Arakawa T, et al: Vascular endothelial growth factor (VEGF) directly enhances osteoclastic bone resorption and survival of mature osteoclasts, FEBS Lett 473:161–164, 2000.

125. Niida S, Kondo T, Hiratsuka S, et al: VEGF receptor 1 signaling is essential for osteoclast development and bone marrow formation in colony-stimulating factor 1-deficient mice, Proc Natl Acad Sci U S A 102:14016–14021, 2005.

126. Yang Q, McHugh KP, Patntirapong S, et al: VEGF enhancement of osteoclast survival and bone resorption involves VEGF receptor-2 signaling and beta(3)-integrin, Matrix Biol 27:589–599, 2008.

127. Yao S, Liu D, Pan F, et al: Effect of vascular endothelial growth factor on RANK gene expression in osteoclast precursors and on osteoclastogenesis, Arch Oral Biol 51:596–602, 2006.

128. Vu TH, Shipley JM, Bergers G, et al: MMP-9/gelatinase B is a key regulator of growth plate angiogenesis and apoptosis of hypertrophic chondrocytes, Cell 93:411–422, 1998.

129. Nakashima T, Takayanagi H: The dynamic interplay between osteoclasts and the immune system, Arch Biochem Biophys 473:166–171, 2008.

130. Boyle WJ, Simonet WS, Lacey DL: Osteoclast differentiation and activation, Nature 423:337–342, 2003.

131. Lorenzo J, Horowitz M, Choi Y: Osteoimmunology: interactions of the bone and immune system, Endocr Rev 29:403–440, 2008.

132. Takayanagi H: Osteoimmunology: shared mechanisms and crosstalk between the immune and bone systems, Nat Rev Immunol 7:292–304, 2007.

133. Boyce BF, Yao Z, Zhang Q, et al: New roles for osteoclasts in bone, Ann N Y Acad Sci 1116:245–254, 2007.

134. Xing L, Schwarz EM, Boyce BF: Osteoclast precursors, RANKL/RANK, and immunology, Immunol Rev 208:19–29, 2005.

135. Scott EW, Simon MC, Anastasi J, et al: Requirement of transcription factor PU.1 in the development of multiple hematopoietic lineages, Science 265:1573–1577, 1994.

136. DeKoter RP, Singh H: Regulation of B lymphocyte and macrophage development by graded expression of PU.1, Science 288:1439–1441, 2000.

137. Tondravi MM, McKercher SR, Anderson K, et al: Osteopetrosis in mice lacking haematopoietic transcription factor PU.1, Nature 386:81–84, 1997.

138. DeKoter RP, Walsh JC, Singh H: PU.1 regulates both cytokine-dependent proliferation and differentiation of granulocyte/macrophage progenitors, EMBO J 17:4456–4468, 1998.

139. Zhang DE, Hetherington CJ, Chen HM, et al: The macrophage transcription factor PU.1 directs tissue-specific expression of the macrophage colony-stimulating factor receptor, Mol Cell Biol 14:373–381, 1994.

140. Tondravi MM, McKercher SR, Anderson K, et al: Osteopetrosis in mice lacking haematopoietic transcription factor PU.1, Nature 386:81–84, 1997.

141. McKercher SR, Torbett BE, Anderson KL, et al: Targeted disruption of the PU.1 gene results in multiple hematopoietic abnormalities, EMBO J 15:5647–5658, 1996.

142. Kwon OH, Lee CK, Lee YI, et al: The hematopoietic transcription factor PU.1 regulates RANK gene expression in myeloid progenitors, Biochem Biophys Res Commun 335:437–446, 2005.

143. Huang JC, Sakata T, Pfleger LL, et al: PTH differentially regulates expression of RANKL and OPG, J Bone Miner Res 19:235–244, 2004.

144. Kitazawa S, Kajimoto K, Kondo T, et al: Vitamin D3 supports osteoclastogenesis via functional vitamin D response element of murine RANKL gene promoter, J Cell Biochem 89:771–777, 2003.

145. Quinn JM, Elliott J, Gillespie MT, et al: A combination of osteoclast differentiation factor and macrophage-colony stimulating factor is sufficient for both human and mouse osteoclast formation in vitro, Endocrinology 139:4424–4427, 1998.

146. Kishimoto K, Kitazawa R, Kurosaka M, et al: Expression profile of genes related to osteoclastogenesis in mouse growth plate and articular cartilage, Histochem Cell Biol 125:593–602, 2006.

147. Masuyama R, Stockmans I, Torrekens S, et al: Vitamin D receptor in chondrocytes promotes osteoclastogenesis and regulates FGF23 production in osteoblasts, J Clin Invest 116:3150–3159, 2006.

148. Usui M, Xing L, Drissi H, et al: Murine and chicken chondrocytes regulate osteoclastogenesis by producing RANKL in response to BMP2, J Bone Miner Res 23:314–325, 2008.

149. Horwood NJ, Kartsogiannis V, Quinn JM, et al: Activated T lymphocytes support osteoclast formation in vitro, Biochem Biophys Res Commun 265:144–150, 1999.

150. Weitzmann MN, Cenci S, Rifas L, et al: T cell activation induces human osteoclast formation via receptor activator of nuclear factor kappaB ligand-dependent and -independent mechanisms, J Bone Miner Res 16:328–337, 2001.

151. Kong YY, Feige U, Sarosi I, et al: Activated T cells regulate bone loss and joint destruction in adjuvant arthritis through osteoprotegerin ligand, Nature 402:304–309, 1999.

152. Lam J, Takeshita S, Barker JE, et al: TNF-alpha induces osteoclastogenesis by direct stimulation of macrophages exposed to permissive levels of RANK ligand, J Clin Invest 106:1481–1488, 2000.

153. Fuller K, Murphy C, Kirstein B, et al: TNFalpha potently activates osteoclasts, through a direct action independent of and strongly synergistic with RANKL, Endocrinology 143:1108–1118, 2002.

154. Felix R, Cecchini MG, Hofstetter W, et al: Impairment of macrophage colony-stimulating factor production and lack of resident bone marrow macrophages in the osteopetrotic op/op mouse, J Bone Miner Res 5:781–789, 1990.

155. Kodama H, Yamasaki A, Abe M, et al: Transient recruitment of osteoclasts and expression of their function in osteopetrotic (op/op) mice by a single injection of macrophage colony-stimulating factor, J Bone Miner Res 8:45–50, 1993.

156. Kodama H, Yamasaki A, Nose M, et al: Congenital osteoclast deficiency in osteopetrotic (op/op) mice is cured by injections of macrophage colony-stimulating factor, J Exp Med 173:269–272, 1991.

157. Yoshida H, Hayashi S, Kunisada T, et al: The murine mutation osteopetrosis is in the coding region of the macrophage colony stimulating factor gene, Nature 345:442–444, 1990.

158. Armstrong AP, Tometsko ME, Glaccum M, et al: A RANK/TRAF6-dependent signal transduction pathway is essential for osteoclast cytoskeletal organization and resorptive function, J Biol Chem 277:44347–44356, 2002.

159. Burgess TL, Qian Y, Kaufman S, et al: The ligand for osteoprotegerin (OPGL) directly activates mature osteoclasts, J Cell Biol 145:527–538, 1999.

160. Lacey DL, Timms E, Tan HL, et al: Osteoprotegerin ligand is a cytokine that regulates osteoclast differentiation and activation, Cell 93:165–176, 1998.

161. Lacey DL, Tan HL, Lu J, et al: Osteoprotegerin ligand modulates murine osteoclast survival in vitro and in vivo, Am J Pathol 157:435–448, 2000.

162. Hughes AE, Ralston SH, Marken J, et al: Mutations in TNFRSF11A, affecting the signal peptide of RANK, cause familial expansile osteolysis, Nat Genet 24:45–48, 2000.

163. Takayanagi H: Mechanistic insight into osteoclast differentiation in osteoimmunology, J Mol Med 83:170–179, 2005.

164. Takayanagi H, Kim S, Koga T, et al: Induction and activation of the transcription factor NFATc1 (NFAT2) integrate RANKL signaling in terminal differentiation of osteoclasts, Dev Cell 3:889–901, 2002.

165. Grigoriadis AE, Wang ZQ, Cecchini MG, et al: c-Fos: a key regulator of osteoclast-macrophage lineage determination and bone remodeling, Science 266:443–448, 1994.

166. Iotsova V, Caamano J, Loy J, et al: Osteopetrosis in mice lacking NF-kappaB1 and NF-kappaB2, Nat Med 3:1285–1289, 1997.

167. Lomaga MA, Yeh WC, Sarosi I, et al: TRAF6 deficiency results in osteopetrosis and defective interleukin-1, CD40, and LPS signaling, Genes Dev 13:1015–1024, 1999.

168. Boyce BF, Xing L: Functions of RANKL/RANK/OPG in bone modeling and remodeling, Arch Biochem Biophys 473:139–146, 2008.

169. Whyte MP, Obrecht SE, Finnegan PM, et al: Osteoprotegerin deficiency and juvenile Paget's disease, N Engl J Med 347:175–184, 2002.

170. Kong YY, Yoshida H, Sarosi I, et al: OPGL is a key regulator of osteoclastogenesis, lymphocyte development and lymph-node organogenesis, Nature 397:315–323, 1999.

171. Li J, Sarosi I, Yan XQ, et al: RANK is the intrinsic hematopoietic cell surface receptor that controls osteoclastogenesis and regulation of bone mass and calcium metabolism, Proc Natl Acad Sci U S A 97:1566–1571, 2000.

172. Dougall WC, Glaccum M, Charrier K, et al: RANK is essential for osteoclast and lymph node development, Genes Dev 13:2412–2424, 1999.

173. Simonet WS, Lacey DL, Dunstan CR, et al: Osteoprotegerin: a novel secreted protein involved in the regulation of bone density, Cell 89:309–319, 1997.

174. Bucay N, Sarosi I, Dunstan CR, et al: Osteoprotegerin-deficient mice develop early onset osteoporosis and arterial calcification, Genes Dev 12:1260–1268, 1998.

175. Mizuno A, Amizuka N, Irie K, et al: Severe osteoporosis in mice lacking osteoclastogenesis inhibitory factor/osteoprotegerin, Biochem Biophys Res Commun 247:610–615, 1998.

176. Mizuno A, Kanno T, Hoshi M, et al: Transgenic mice overexpressing soluble osteoclast differentiation factor

(sODF) exhibit severe osteoporosis, J Bone Miner Metab 20:337–344, 2002.

177. Fata JE, Kong YY, Li J, et al: The osteoclast differentiation factor osteoprotegerin-ligand is essential for mammary gland development, Cell 103:41–50, 2000.

178. Koga T, Inui M, Inoue K, et al: Costimulatory signals mediated by the ITAM motif cooperate with RANKL for bone homeostasis, Nature 428:758–763, 2004.

179. Yagi M, Miyamoto T, Sawatani Y, et al: DC-STAMP is essential for cell-cell fusion in osteoclasts and foreign body giant cells, J Exp Med 202:345–351, 2005.

180. Trebec DP, Chandra D, Gramoun A, et al: Increased expression of activating factors in large osteoclasts could explain their excessive activity in osteolytic diseases, J Cell Biochem 101:205–220, 2007.

181. Bar-Shavit Z: The osteoclast: a multinucleated, hematopoietic-origin, bone-resorbing osteoimmune cell, J Cell Biochem 102:1130–1139, 2007.

182. Roodman GD, Windle JJ: Paget disease of bone, J Clin Invest 115:200–208, 2005.

183. Hsu H, Lacey DL, Dunstan CR, et al: Tumor necrosis factor receptor family member RANK mediates osteoclast differentiation and activation induced by osteoprotegerin ligand, Proc Natl Acad Sci U S A 96:3540–3545, 1999.

184. Gil-Henn H, Destaing O, Sims NA, et al: Defective microtubule-dependent podosome organization in osteoclasts leads to increased bone density in Pyk2(-/-) mice, J Cell Biol 178:1053–1064, 2007.

185. Jurdic P, Saltel F, Chabadel A, et al: Podosome and sealing zone: specificity of the osteoclast model, Eur J Cell Biol 85:195–202, 2006.

186. Luxenburg C, Geblinger D, Klein E, et al: The architecture of the adhesive apparatus of cultured osteoclasts: from podosome formation to sealing zone assembly, PLoS ONE 2:e179, 2007.

187. Luxenburg C, Parsons JT, Addadi L, et al: Involvement of the Src-cortactin pathway in podosome formation and turnover during polarization of cultured osteoclasts, J Cell Sci 119:4878–4888, 2006.

188. Teitelbaum SL: Osteoclasts: what do they do and how do they do it? Am J Pathol 170:427–435, 2007.

189. Vaananen HK, Laitala-Leinonen T: Osteoclast lineage and function, Arch Biochem Biophys 473:132–138, 2008.

190. Wittrant Y, Theoleyre S, Couillaud S, et al: Regulation of osteoclast protease expression by RANKL, Biochem Biophys Res Commun 310:774–778, 2003.

191. Fujisaki K, Tanabe N, Suzuki N, et al: Receptor activator of NF-kappaB ligand induces the expression of carbonic anhydrase II, cathepsin K, and matrix metalloproteinase-9 in osteoclast precursor RAW264.7 cells, Life Sci 80:1311–1318, 2007.

192. Sundaram K, Nishimura R, Senn J, et al: RANK ligand signaling modulates the matrix metalloproteinase-9 gene expression during osteoclast differentiation, Exp Cell Res 313:168–178, 2007.

193. Nakamura I, Pilkington MF, Lakkakorpi PT, et al: Role of alpha(v)beta(3) integrin in osteoclast migration and formation of the sealing zone, J Cell Sci 112(Pt 22):3985–3993, 1999.

194. Nakamura I, Duong IT, Rodan SB, et al: Involvement of alpha(v)beta3 integrins in osteoclast function, J Bone Miner Metab 25:337–344, 2007.

195. Pfaff M, Jurdic P: Podosomes in osteoclast-like cells: structural analysis and cooperative roles of paxillin, proline-rich tyrosine kinase 2 (Pyk2) and integrin alphaVbeta3, J Cell Sci 114:2775–2786, 2001.

196. Nakamura I, Duong IT, Rodan SB, et al: Involvement of alpha(v)beta3 integrins in osteoclast function, J Bone Miner Metab 25:337–344, 2007.

197. Rodan SB, Rodan GA: Integrin function in osteoclasts, J Endocrinol 154(suppl):S47–S56, 1997.

198. Rodan SB, Rodan GA: Integrin function in osteoclasts, J Endocrinol 154(suppl):S47–S56, 1997.

199. Bossard MJ, Tomaszek TA, Thompson SK, et al: Proteolytic activity of human osteoclast cathepsin K: expression, purification, activation, and substrate identification, J Biol Chem 271:12517–12524, 1996.

200. Everts V, Korper W, Hoeben KA, et al: Osteoclastic bone degradation and the role of different cysteine proteinases and matrix metalloproteinases: differences between calvaria and long bone, J Bone Miner Res 21:1399–1408, 2006.

201. Kamiya T, Kobayashi Y, Kanaoka K, et al: Fluorescence microscopic demonstration of cathepsin K activity as the major lysosomal cysteine proteinase in osteoclasts, J Biochem 123:752–759, 1998.

202. Gowen M, Lazner F, Dodds R, et al: Cathepsin K knockout mice develop osteopetrosis due to a deficit in matrix degradation but not demineralization, J Bone Miner Res 14:1654–1663, 1999.

203. Saftig P, Hunziker E, Wehmeyer O, et al: Impaired osteoclastic bone resorption leads to osteopetrosis in cathepsin-K-deficient mice, Proc Natl Acad Sci U S A 95:13453–13458, 1998.

204. Johnson MR, Polymeropoulos MH, Vos HL, et al: A nonsense mutation in the cathepsin K gene observed in a family with pycnodysostosis, Genome Res 6:1050–1055, 1996.

205. Le Gall C, Bellahcene A, Bonnelye E, et al: A cathepsin K inhibitor reduces breast cancer induced osteolysis and skeletal tumor burden, Cancer Res 67:9894–9902, 2007.

206. Le Gall C, Bonnelye E, Clezardin P: Cathepsin K inhibitors as treatment of bone metastasis, Curr Opin Support Palliat Care 2:218–222, 2008.

207. Pearse RN: New strategies for the treatment of metastatic bone disease, Clin Breast Cancer 8(suppl 1):S35–S45, 2007.

208. Stoch SA, Wagner JA: Cathepsin K inhibitors: a novel target for osteoporosis therapy, Clin Pharmacol Ther 83:172–176, 2008.

209. Delaisse JM, Andersen TL, Engsig MT, et al: Matrix metalloproteinases (MMP) and cathepsin K contribute differently to osteoclastic bone activities, Microsc Res Tech 61:504–513, 2003.

210. Cawston TE, Wilson AJ: Understanding the role of tissue degrading enzymes and their inhibitors in development and disease, Best Pract Res Clin Rheumatol 20:983–1002, 2006.

211. Krane SM, Inada M: Matrix metalloproteinases and bone, Bone 43:7–18, 2008.

212. Ortega N, Behonick D, Stickens D, et al: How proteases regulate bone morphogenesis, Ann N Y Acad Sci 995:109–116, 2003.

213. Sternlicht MD, Werb Z: How matrix metalloproteinases regulate cell behavior, Annu Rev Cell Dev Biol 17:463–516, 2001.

214. Egeblad M, Werb Z: New functions for the matrix metalloproteinases in cancer progression, Nat Rev Cancer 2:161–174, 2002.

215. Martin TJ, Moseley JM: Mechanisms in the skeletal complications of breast cancer, Endocr Relat Cancer 7:271–284, 2000.

216. Sato T, del Carmen OM, Hou P, et al: Identification of the membrane-type matrix metalloproteinase MT1-MMP in osteoclasts, J Cell Sci 110(Pt 5):589–596, 1997.

217. Tezuka K, Nemoto K, Tezuka Y, et al: Identification of matrix metalloproteinase 9 in rabbit osteoclasts, J Biol Chem 269:15006–15009, 1994.

218. Colnot C, Thompson Z, Miclau T, et al: Altered fracture repair in the absence of MMP9, Development 130:4123–4133, 2003.

219. Holmbeck K, Bianco P, Chrysovergis K, et al: MT1-MMP-dependent, apoptotic remodeling of unmineralized cartilage: a critical process in skeletal growth, J Cell Biol 163:661–671, 2003.

220. Holmbeck K, Bianco P, Caterina J, et al: MT1-MMP-deficient mice develop dwarfism, osteopenia, arthritis, and connective tissue disease due to inadequate collagen turnover, Cell 99:81–92, 1999.

221. Hikita A, Yana I, Wakeyama H, et al: Negative regulation of osteoclastogenesis by ectodomain shedding of receptor activator of NF-kappaB ligand, J Biol Chem 281:36846–36855, 2006.

222. Lynch CC, Hikosaka A, Acuff HB, et al: MMP-7 promotes prostate cancer-induced osteolysis via the solubilization of RANKL, Cancer Cell 7:485–496, 2005.

223. Manolagas SC: Birth and death of bone cells: basic regulatory mechanisms and implications for the pathogenesis and treatment of osteoporosis, Endocr Rev 21:115–137, 2000.

224. Hughes DE, Dai A, Tiffee JC, et al: Estrogen promotes apoptosis of murine osteoclasts mediated by TGF-beta, Nat Med 2:1132–1136, 1996.

225. Caplan AI, Bruder SP: Mesenchymal stem cells: building blocks for molecular medicine in the 21st century, Trends Mol Med 7:259–264, 2001.

226. Chen Y, Shao JZ, Xiang LX, et al: Mesenchymal stem cells: a promising candidate in regenerative medicine, Int J Biochem Cell Biol 40:815–820, 2008.

227. Jiang Y, Jahagirdar BN, Reinhardt RL, et al: Pluripotency of mesenchymal stem cells derived from adult marrow, Nature 418:41–49, 2002.

228. Nishimura R, Hata K, Ikeda F, et al: Signal transduction and transcriptional regulation during mesenchymal cell differentiation, J Bone Miner Metab 26:203–212, 2008.

229. Harada S, Rodan GA: Control of osteoblast function and regulation of bone mass, Nature 423:349–355, 2003.

230. Karsenty G: Transcriptional control of skeletogenesis, Annu Rev Genomics Hum Genet 9:183–196, 2008.

231. Stein GS, Lian JB: Molecular mechanisms mediating proliferation/differentiation interrelationships during progressive development of the osteoblast phenotype, Endocr Rev 14:424–442, 1993.

232. Knothe Tate ML, Adamson JR, Tami AE, et al: The osteocyte, Int J Biochem Cell Biol 36:1–8, 2004.

233. Noble BS: The osteocyte lineage, Arch Biochem Biophys 473:106–111, 2008.

234. Kamioka H, Honjo T, Takano-Yamamoto T: A three-dimensional distribution of osteocyte processes revealed by the combination of confocal laser scanning microscopy and differential interference contrast microscopy, Bone 28:145–149, 2001.

235. Sugawara Y, Kamioka H, Honjo T, et al: Three-dimensional reconstruction of chick calvarial osteocytes and their cell processes using confocal microscopy, Bone 36:877–883, 2005.

236. Bonewald LF, Johnson ML: Osteocytes, mechanosensing and Wnt signaling, Bone 42:606–615, 2008.

237. Strom TM, Juppner H: PHEX, FGF23, DMP1 and beyond, Curr Opin Nephrol Hypertens 17:357–362, 2008.

238. Datta HK, Ng WF, Walker JA, et al: The cell biology of bone metabolism, J Clin Pathol 61:577–587, 2008.

239. Civitelli R: Cell-cell communication in the osteoblast/osteocyte lineage, Arch Biochem Biophys 473:188–192, 2008.

240. Poole KE, van Bezooijen RL, Loveridge N, et al: Sclerostin is a delayed secreted product of osteocytes that inhibits bone formation, FASEB J 19:1842–1844, 2005.

241. van Bezooijen RL, Ten Dijke P, Papapoulos SE, et al: SOST/sclerostin, an osteocyte-derived negative regulator of bone formation, Cytokine Growth Factor Rev 16:319–327, 2005.

242. Toyosawa S, Shintani S, Fujiwara T, et al: Dentin matrix protein 1 is predominantly expressed in chicken and rat osteocytes but not in osteoblasts, J Bone Miner Res 16:2017–2026, 2001.

243. Liu S, Gupta A, Quarles LD: Emerging role of fibroblast growth factor 23 in a bone-kidney axis regulating systemic phosphate homeostasis and extracellular matrix mineralization, Curr Opin Nephrol Hypertens 16:329–335, 2007.

244. Nampei A, Hashimoto J, Hayashida K, et al: Matrix extracellular phosphoglycoprotein (MEPE) is highly expressed in osteocytes in human bone, J Bone Miner Metab 22:176–184, 2004.

245. Clevers H: Wnt/beta-catenin signaling in development and disease, Cell 127:469–480, 2006.

246. Taipale J, Beachy PA: The Hedgehog and Wnt signalling pathways in cancer, Nature 411:349–354, 2001.

247. Logan CY, Nusse R: The Wnt signaling pathway in development and disease, Annu Rev Cell Dev Biol 20:781–810, 2004.

248. Klaus A, Birchmeier W: Wnt signalling and its impact on development and cancer, Nat Rev Cancer 8:387–398, 2008.

249. Gong Y, Slee RB, Fukai N, et al: LDL receptor-related protein 5 (LRP5) affects bone accrual and eye development, Cell 107:513–523, 2001.

250. Loughlin J, Dowling B, Chapman K, et al: Functional variants within the secreted frizzled-related protein 3 gene are associated with hip osteoarthritis in females, Proc Natl Acad Sci U S A 101:9757–9762, 2004.

251. Grigoryan T, Wend P, Klaus A, et al: Deciphering the function of canonical Wnt signals in development and disease: conditional loss- and gain-of-function mutations of beta-catenin in mice, Genes Dev 22:2308–2341, 2008.

252. Rubinfeld B, Albert I, Porfiri E, et al: Binding of GSK-3beta to the APC-beta-catenin complex and regulation

of complex assembly, Science 272:1023–1026, 1996.
253. Behrens J, Jerchow BA, Wurtele M, et al: Functional interaction of an axin homolog, conductin, with beta-catenin, APC, and GSK3beta, Science 280:596–599, 1998.
254. Mao J, Wang J, Liu B, et al: Low-density lipoprotein receptor-related protein-5 binds to Axin and regulates the canonical Wnt signaling pathway, Mol Cell 7:801–809, 2001.
255. Pinson KI, Brennan J, Monkley S, et al: An LDL-receptor-related protein mediates Wnt signalling in mice, Nature 407:535–538, 2000.
256. Tamai K, Semenov M, Kato Y, et al: LDL-receptor-related proteins in Wnt signal transduction, Nature 407:530–535, 2000.
257. Tamai K, Zeng X, Liu C, et al: A mechanism for Wnt coreceptor activation, Mol Cell 13:149–156, 2004.
258. Zeng X, Huang H, Tamai K, et al: Initiation of Wnt signaling: control of Wnt coreceptor Lrp6 phosphorylation/activation via frizzled, dishevelled and axin functions, Development 135:367–375, 2008.
259. Zeng X, Tamai K, Doble B, et al: A dual-kinase mechanism for Wnt co-receptor phosphorylation and activation, Nature 438:873–877, 2005.
260. Behrens J, von Kries JP, Kuhl M, et al: Functional interaction of beta-catenin with the transcription factor LEF-1, Nature 382:638–642, 1996.
261. Moon RT, Bowerman B, Boutros M, et al: The promise and perils of Wnt signaling through beta-catenin, Science 296:1644–1646, 2002.
262. Shitashige M, Hirohashi S, Yamada T: Wnt signaling inside the nucleus, Cancer Sci 99:631–637, 2008.
263. Kolpakova E, Olsen BR: Wnt/beta-catenin—a canonical tale of cell-fate choice in the vertebrate skeleton, Dev Cell 8:626–627, 2005.
264. Hill TP, Spater D, Taketo MM, et al: Canonical Wnt/beta-catenin signaling prevents osteoblasts from differentiating into chondrocytes, Dev Cell 8:727–738, 2005.
265. Glass DA, Bialek P, Ahn JD, et al: Canonical Wnt signaling in differentiated osteoblasts controls osteoclast differentiation, Dev Cell 8:751–764, 2005.
266. Glass DA, Karsenty G: In vivo analysis of Wnt signaling in bone, Endocrinology 148:2630–2634, 2007.
267. Ai M, Holmen SL, Van Hul W, et al: Reduced affinity to and inhibition by DKK1 form a common mechanism by which high bone mass-associated missense mutations in LRP5 affect canonical Wnt signaling, Mol Cell Biol 25:4946–4955, 2005.
268. Balemans W, Devogelaer JP, Cleiren E, et al: Novel LRP5 missense mutation in a patient with a high bone mass phenotype results in decreased DKK1-mediated inhibition of Wnt signaling, J Bone Miner Res 22:708–716, 2007.
269. Semenov MV, He X: LRP5 mutations linked to high bone mass diseases cause reduced LRP5 binding and inhibition by SOST, J Biol Chem 281:38276–38284, 2006.
270. Boyden LM, Mao J, Belsky J, et al: High bone density due to a mutation in LDL-receptor-related protein 5, N Engl J Med 346:1513–1521, 2002.
271. Little RD, Carulli JP, Del Mastro RG, et al: A mutation in the LDL receptor-related protein 5 gene results in the autosomal dominant high-bone-mass trait, Am J Hum Genet 70:11–19, 2002.
272. Yadav VK, Ryu JH, Suda N, et al: Lrp5 controls bone formation by inhibiting serotonin synthesis in the duodenum, Cell 135:825–837, 2008.
273. Qiang YW, Barlogie B, Rudikoff S, et al: Dkk1-induced inhibition of Wnt signaling in osteoblast differentiation is an underlying mechanism of bone loss in multiple myeloma, Bone 42:669–680, 2008.
274. Tian E, Zhan F, Walker R, et al: The role of the Wnt-signaling antagonist DKK1 in the development of osteolytic lesions in multiple myeloma, N Engl J Med 349:2483–2494, 2003.
275. Balemans W, Van Hul W: Identification of the disease-causing gene in sclerosteosis—discovery of a novel bone anabolic target? J Musculoskelet Neuronal Interact 4:139–142, 2004.
276. Balemans W, Cleiren E, Siebers U, et al: A generalized skeletal hyperostosis in two siblings caused by a novel mutation in the SOST gene, Bone 36:943–947, 2005.
277. Balemans W, Patel N, Ebeling M, et al: Identification of a 52 kb deletion downstream of the SOST gene in patients with van Buchem disease, J Med Genet 39:91–97, 2002.
278. Baron R, Rawadi G, Roman-Roman S: Wnt signaling: a key regulator of bone mass, Curr Top Dev Biol 76:103–127, 2006.
279. Krishnan V, Bryant HU, MacDougald OA: Regulation of bone mass by Wnt signaling, J Clin Invest 116:1202–1209, 2006.
280. Otto F, Thornell AP, Crompton T, et al: Cbfa1, a candidate gene for cleidocranial dysplasia syndrome, is essential for osteoblast differentiation and bone development, Cell 89:765–771, 1997.
281. Komori T, Yagi H, Nomura S, et al: Targeted disruption of Cbfa1 results in a complete lack of bone formation owing to maturational arrest of osteoblasts, Cell 89:755–764, 1997.
282. Lee B, Thirunavukkarasu K, Zhou L, et al: Missense mutations abolishing DNA binding of the osteoblast-specific transcription factor OSF2/CBFA1 in cleidocranial dysplasia, Nat Genet 16:307–310, 1997.
283. Mundlos S, Otto F, Mundlos C, et al: Mutations involving the transcription factor CBFA1 cause cleidocranial dysplasia, Cell 89:773–779, 1997.
284. Rabie AB, Tang GH, Hagg U: Cbfa1 couples chondrocytes maturation and endochondral ossification in rat mandibular condylar cartilage, Arch Oral Biol 49:109–118, 2004.
285. Ducy P, Zhang R, Geoffroy V, et al: Osf2/Cbfa1: a transcriptional activator of osteoblast differentiation, Cell 89:747–754, 1997.
286. Kobayashi H, Gao Y, Ueta C, et al: Multilineage differentiation of Cbfa1-deficient calvarial cells in vitro, Biochem Biophys Res Commun 273:630–636, 2000.
287. Komori T: Regulation of skeletal development by the Runx family of transcription factors, J Cell Biochem 95:445–453, 2005.
288. Enomoto H, Shiojiri S, Hoshi K, et al: Induction of osteoclast differentiation by Runx2 through receptor activator of nuclear factor-kappa B ligand (RANKL) and osteoprotegerin regulation and partial rescue of osteoclastogenesis in Runx2-/- mice by RANKL transgene, J Biol Chem 278:23971–23977, 2003.
289. Thirunavukkarasu K, Halladay DL, Miles RR, et al: The osteoblast-specific transcription factor Cbfa1 contributes to the expression of osteoprotegerin, a potent inhibitor of osteoclast differentiation and function, J Biol Chem 275:25163–25172, 2000.
290. Harada H, Tagashira S, Fujiwara M, et al: Cbfa1 isoforms exert functional differences in osteoblast differentiation, J Biol Chem 274:6972–6978, 1999.
291. Liu W, Toyosawa S, Furuichi T, et al: Overexpression of Cbfa1 in osteoblasts inhibits osteoblast maturation and causes osteopenia with multiple fractures, J Cell Biol 155:157–166, 2001.
292. Ducy P, Starbuck M, Priemel M, et al: A Cbfa1-dependent genetic pathway controls bone formation beyond embryonic development, Genes Dev 13:1025–1036, 1999.
293. Nakashima K, Zhou X, Kunkel G, et al: The novel zinc finger-containing transcription factor osterix is required for osteoblast differentiation and bone formation, Cell 108:17–29, 2002.
294. Nishio Y, Dong Y, Paris M, et al: Runx2-mediated regulation of the zinc finger Osterix/Sp7 gene, Gene 372:62–70, 2006.
295. Koga T, Matsui Y, Asagiri M, et al: NFAT and Osterix cooperatively regulate bone formation, Nat Med 11:880–885, 2005.
296. Kaback LA, Soung DY, Naik A, et al: Osterix/Sp7 regulates mesenchymal stem cell mediated endochondral ossification, J Cell Physiol 214:173–182, 2008.
297. Tominaga H, Maeda S, Miyoshi H, et al: Expression of osterix inhibits bone morphogenetic protein-induced chondrogenic differentiation of mesenchymal progenitor cells, J Bone Miner Metab 27:36–45, 2009.
298. Elefteriou F, Benson MD, Sowa H, et al: ATF4 mediation of NF1 functions in osteoblast reveals a nutritional basis for congenital skeletal dysplasia, Cell Metab 4:441–451, 2006.
299. Yang X, Karsenty G: ATF4, the osteoblast accumulation of which is determined post-translationally, can induce osteoblast-specific gene expression in non-osteoblastic cells, J Biol Chem 279:47109–47114, 2004.
300. Yang X, Matsuda K, Bialek P, et al: ATF4 is a substrate of RSK2 and an essential regulator of osteoblast biology: implication for Coffin-Lowry syndrome, Cell 117:387–398, 2004.
301. Liu YH, Tang Z, Kundu RK, et al: Msx2 gene dosage influences the number of proliferative osteogenic cells in growth centers of the developing murine skull: a possible mechanism for MSX2-mediated craniosynostosis in humans, Dev Biol 205:260–274, 1999.
302. Liu YH, Kundu R, Wu L, et al: Premature suture closure and ectopic cranial bone in mice expressing Msx2 transgenes in the developing skull, Proc Natl Acad Sci U S A 92:6137–6141, 1995.
303. Satokata I, Ma L, Ohshima H, et al: Msx2 deficiency in mice causes pleiotropic defects in bone growth and ectodermal organ formation, Nat Genet 24:391–395, 2000.
304. Satokata I, Maas R: Msx1 deficient mice exhibit cleft palate and abnormalities of craniofacial and tooth development, Nat Genet 6:348–356, 1994.
305. Acampora D, Merlo GR, Paleari L, et al: Craniofacial, vestibular and bone defects in mice lacking the Distal-less-related gene Dlx5, Development 126:3795–3809, 1999.
306. Holleville N, Mateos S, Bontoux M, et al: Dlx5 drives Runx2 expression and osteogenic differentiation in developing cranial suture mesenchyme, Dev Biol 304:860–874, 2007.
307. Li H, Marijanovic I, Kronenberg MS, et al: Expression and function of Dlx genes in the osteoblast lineage, Dev Biol 316:458–470, 2008.
308. Robledo RF, Rajan L, Li X, et al: The Dlx5 and Dlx6 homeobox genes are essential for craniofacial, axial, and appendicular skeletal development, Genes Dev 16:1089–1101, 2002.
309. Bialek P, Kern B, Yang X, et al: A twist code determines the onset of osteoblast differentiation, Dev Cell 6:423–435, 2004.
310. Lee MS, Lowe GN, Strong DD, et al: TWIST, a basic helix-loop-helix transcription factor, can regulate the human osteogenic lineage, J Cell Biochem 75:566–577, 1999.
311. Jochum W, David JP, Elliott C, et al: Increased bone formation and osteosclerosis in mice overexpressing the transcription factor Fra-1, Nat Med 6:980–984, 2000.
312. Sabatakos G, Sims NA, Chen J, et al: Overexpression of DeltaFosB transcription factor(s) increases bone formation and inhibits adipogenesis, Nat Med 6:985–990, 2000.
313. Wagner EF: Functions of AP1 (Fos/Jun) in bone development, Ann Rheum Dis 61(suppl 2):ii40–ii42, 2002.
314. Wagner EF, Eferl R: Fos/AP-1 proteins in bone and the immune system, Immunol Rev 208:126–140, 2005.
315. Kenner L, Hoebertz A, Beil T, et al: Mice lacking JunB are osteopenic due to cell-autonomous osteoblast and osteoclast defects, J Cell Biol 164:613–623, 2004.
316. Glimcher LH, Jones DC, Wein MN: Control of postnatal bone mass by the zinc finger adapter protein Schnurri-3, Ann N Y Acad Sci 1116:174–181, 2007.
317. Jones DC, Wein MN, Oukka M, et al: Regulation of adult bone mass by the zinc finger adapter protein Schnurri-3, Science 312:1223–1227, 2006.
318. Saita Y, Takagi T, Kitahara K, et al: Lack of Schnurri-2 expression associates with reduced bone remodeling and osteopenia, J Biol Chem 282:12907–12915, 2007.
319. Franceschi RT, Ge C, Xiao G, et al: Transcriptional regulation of osteoblasts, Cells Tissues Organs 189:144–152, 2009.
320. Komori T: Regulation of osteoblast differentiation by transcription factors, J Cell Biochem 99:1233–1239, 2006.
321. Marie PJ: Transcription factors controlling osteoblastogenesis, Arch Biochem Biophys 473:98–105, 2008.
322. Lian JB, Stein GS, Javed A, et al: Networks and hubs for the transcriptional control of osteoblastogenesis, Rev Endocr Metab Disord 7:1–16, 2006.
323. Yamaguchi A, Komori T, Suda T: Regulation of osteoblast differentiation mediated by bone morphogenetic proteins, hedgehogs, and Cbfa1, Endocr Rev 21:393–411, 2000.
324. Wu XB, Li Y, Schneider A, et al: Impaired osteoblastic differentiation, reduced bone formation, and severe osteoporosis in noggin-overexpressing mice, J Clin Invest 112:924–934, 2003.
325. Gazzerro E, Pereira RC, Jorgetti V, et al: Skeletal overexpression of gremlin impairs bone formation and causes osteopenia, Endocrinology 146:655–665, 2005.

326. Chen D, Ji X, Harris MA, et al: Differential roles for bone morphogenetic protein (BMP) receptor type IB and IA in differentiation and specification of mesenchymal precursor cells to osteoblast and adipocyte lineages, J Cell Biol 142:295–305, 1998.

327. Ryoo HM, Lee MH, Kim YJ: Critical molecular switches involved in BMP-2-induced osteogenic differentiation of mesenchymal cells, Gene 366:51–57, 2006.

328. Katagiri T, Yamaguchi A, Komaki M, et al: Bone morphogenetic protein-2 converts the differentiation pathway of C2C12 myoblasts into the osteoblast lineage, J Cell Biol 127:1755–1766, 1994.

329. Katagiri T, Yamaguchi A, Ikeda T, et al: The non-osteogenic mouse pluripotent cell line, C3H10T1/2, is induced to differentiate into osteoblastic cells by recombinant human bone morphogenetic protein-2, Biochem Biophys Res Commun 172:295–299, 1990.

330. Matsubara T, Kida K, Yamaguchi A, et al: BMP2 regulates Osterix through Msx2 and Runx2 during osteoblast differentiation, J Biol Chem 283:29119–29125, 2008.

331. Javed A, Bae JS, Afzal F, et al: Structural coupling of Smad and Runx2 for execution of the BMP2 osteogenic signal, J Biol Chem 283:8412–8422, 2008.

332. Lee KS, Kim HJ, Li QL, et al: Runx2 is a common target of transforming growth factor beta1 and bone morphogenetic protein 2, and cooperation between Runx2 and Smad5 induces osteoblast-specific gene expression in the pluripotent mesenchymal precursor cell line C2C12, Mol Cell Biol 20:8783–8792, 2000.

333. Celil AB, Campbell PG: BMP-2 and insulin-like growth factor-I mediate Osterix (Osx) expression in human mesenchymal stem cells via the MAPK and protein kinase D signaling pathways, J Biol Chem 280:31353–31359, 2005.

334. Govender S, Csimma C, Genant HK, et al: Recombinant human bone morphogenetic protein-2 for treatment of open tibial fractures: a prospective, controlled, randomized study of four hundred and fifty patients, J Bone Joint Surg Am 84:2123–2134, 2002.

335. Kirker-Head CA, Boudrieau RJ, Kraus KH: Use of bone morphogenetic proteins for augmentation of bone regeneration, J Am Vet Med Assoc 231:1039–1055, 2007.

336. Styrkarsdottir U, Cazier JB, Kong A, et al: Linkage of osteoporosis to chromosome 20p12 and association to BMP2, PLoS Biol 1:E69, 2003.

337. Long F, Chung UI, Ohba S, et al: Ihh signaling is directly required for the osteoblast lineage in the endochondral skeleton, Development 131:1309–1318, 2004.

338. Hilton MJ, Tu X, Cook J, et al: Ihh controls cartilage development by antagonizing Gli3, but requires additional effectors to regulate osteoblast and vascular development, Development 132:4339–4351, 2005.

339. Hui CC, Joyner AL: A mouse model of Greig cephalopolysyndactyly syndrome: the extra-toesJ mutation contains an intragenic deletion of the Gli3 gene, Nat Genet 3:241–246, 1993.

340. Miao D, Liu H, Plut P, et al: Impaired endochondral bone development and osteopenia in Gli2-deficient mice, Exp Cell Res 294:210–222, 2004.

341. Mo R, Freer AM, Zinyk DL, et al: Specific and redundant functions of Gli2 and Gli3 zinc finger genes in skeletal patterning and development, Development 124:113–123, 1997.

342. Shimoyama A, Wada M, Ikeda F, et al: Ihh/Gli2 signaling promotes osteoblast differentiation by regulating Runx2 expression and function, Mol Biol Cell 18:2411–2418, 2007.

343. Zhao M, Qiao M, Harris SE, et al: The zinc finger transcription factor Gli2 mediates bone morphogenetic protein 2 expression in osteoblasts in response to hedgehog signaling, Mol Cell Biol 26:6197–6208, 2006.

344. Jacob AL, Smith C, Partanen J, et al: Fibroblast growth factor receptor 1 signaling in the osteo-chondrogenic cell lineage regulates sequential steps of osteoblast maturation, Dev Biol 296:315–328, 2006.

345. Ornitz DM, Marie PJ: FGF signaling pathways in endochondral and intramembranous bone development and human genetic disease, Genes Dev 16:1446–1465, 2002.

346. Eswarakumar VP, Horowitz MC, Locklin R, et al: A gain-of-function mutation of Fgfr2c demonstrates the

roles of this receptor variant in osteogenesis, Proc Natl Acad Sci U S A 101:12555–12560, 2004.

347. Eswarakumar VP, Monsonego-Ornan E, Pines M, et al: The IIIc alternative of Fgfr2 is a positive regulator of bone formation, Development 129:3783–3793, 2002.

348. Yu K, Xu J, Liu Z, et al: Conditional inactivation of FGF receptor 2 reveals an essential role for FGF signaling in the regulation of osteoblast function and bone growth, Development 130:3063–3074, 2003.

349. Naganawa T, Xiao L, Coffin JD, et al: Reduced expression and function of bone morphogenetic protein-2 in bones of Fgf2 null mice, J Cell Biochem 103:1975–1988, 2008.

350. Choi KY, Kim HJ, Lee MH, et al: Runx2 regulates FGF2-induced Bmp2 expression during cranial bone development, Dev Dyn 233:115–121, 2005.

351. Franceschi RT, Xiao G: Regulation of the osteoblast-specific transcription factor, Runx2: responsiveness to multiple signal transduction pathways, J Cell Biochem 88:446–454, 2003.

352. Kim BG, Kim HJ, Park HJ, et al: Runx2 phosphorylation induced by fibroblast growth factor-2/protein kinase C pathways, Proteomics 6:1166–1174, 2006.

353. Kim HJ, Kim JH, Bae SC, et al: The protein kinase C pathway plays a central role in the fibroblast growth factor-stimulated expression and transactivation activity of Runx2, J Biol Chem 278:319–326, 2003.

354. Xiao G, Jiang D, Gopalakrishnan R, et al: Fibroblast growth factor 2 induction of the osteocalcin gene requires MAPK activity and phosphorylation of the osteoblast transcription factor, Cbfa1/Runx2, J Biol Chem 277:36181–36187, 2002.

355. Reinhold MI, Naski MC: Direct interactions of Runx2 and canonical Wnt signaling induce FGF18, J Biol Chem 282:3653–3663, 2007.

356. Engin F, Yao Z, Yang T, et al: Dimorphic effects of Notch signaling in bone homeostasis, Nat Med 14:299–305, 2008.

357. Zanotti S, Smerdel-Ramoya A, Stadmeyer L, et al: Notch inhibits osteoblast differentiation and causes osteopenia, Endocrinology 149:3890–3899, 2008.

358. Hilton MJ, Tu X, Wu X, et al: Notch signaling maintains bone marrow mesenchymal progenitors by suppressing osteoblast differentiation, Nat Med 14:306–314, 2008.

359. Sciaudone M, Gazzerro E, Priest L, et al: Notch 1 impairs osteoblastic cell differentiation, Endocrinology 144:5631–5639, 2003.

360. Martin TJ, Seeman E: Bone remodelling: its local regulation and the emergence of bone fragility, Best Pract Res Clin Endocrinol Metab 22:701–722, 2008.

361. Harada S, Rodan GA: Bone development and remodeling. In Degroot LJ, Jameson JL, editors: Endocrinology, St Louis, 2005, Elsevier.

362. Martin TJ, Sims NA: Osteoclast-derived activity in the coupling of bone formation to resorption, Trends Mol Med 11:76–81, 2005.

363. Sims NA, Gooi JH: Bone remodeling: multiple cellular interactions required for coupling of bone formation and resorption, Semin Cell Dev Biol 19:444–451, 2008.

364. Matsuo K, Irie N: Osteoclast-osteoblast communication, Arch Biochem Biophys 473:201–209, 2008.

365. Zhao C, Irie N, Takada Y, et al: Bidirectional ephrinB2-EphB4 signaling controls bone homeostasis, Cell Metab 4:111–121, 2006.

366. Edwards CM, Mundy GR: Eph receptors and ephrin signaling pathways: a role in bone homeostasis, Int J Med Sci 5:263–272, 2008.

367. Lee SH, Rho J, Jeong D, et al: v-ATPase V0 subunit d2-deficient mice exhibit impaired osteoclast fusion and increased bone formation, Nat Med 12:1403–1409, 2006.

368. Skerry TM: The response of bone to mechanical loading and disuse: fundamental principles and influences on osteoblast/osteocyte homeostasis, Arch Biochem Biophys 473:117–123, 2008.

369. You L, Temiyasathit S, Lee P, et al: Osteocytes as mechanosensors in the inhibition of bone resorption due to mechanical loading, Bone 42:172–179, 2008.

370. Han Y, Cowin SC, Schaffler MB, et al: Mechanotransduction and strain amplification in osteocyte cell processes, Proc Natl Acad Sci U S A 101:16689–16694, 2004.

371. Kogianni G, Mann V, Noble BS: Apoptotic bodies convey activity capable of initiating osteoclastogenesis

and localized bone destruction, J Bone Miner Res 23:915–927, 2008.

372. Zhao S, Zhang YK, Harris S, et al: MLO-Y4 osteocyte-like cells support osteoclast formation and activation, J Bone Miner Res 17:2068–2079, 2002.

373. Aguirre JI, Plotkin LI, Stewart SA, et al: Osteocyte apoptosis is induced by weightlessness in mice and precedes osteoclast recruitment and bone loss, J Bone Miner Res 21:605–615, 2006.

374. Mann V, Huber C, Kogianni G, et al: The influence of mechanical stimulation on osteocyte apoptosis and bone viability in human trabecular bone, J Musculoskelet Neuronal Interact 6:408–417, 2006.

375. Noble BS, Peet N, Stevens HY, et al: Mechanical loading: biphasic osteocyte survival and targeting of osteoclasts for bone destruction in rat cortical bone, Am J Physiol Cell Physiol 284:C934–C943, 2003.

376. Tatsumi S, Ishii K, Amizuka N, et al: Targeted ablation of osteocytes induces osteoporosis with defective mechanotransduction, Cell Metab 5:464–475, 2007.

377. Cherian PP, Siller-Jackson AJ, Gu S, et al: Mechanical strain opens connexin 43 hemichannels in osteocytes: a novel mechanism for the release of prostaglandin, Mol Biol Cell 16:3100–3106, 2005.

378. Civitelli R: Connexin43 modulation of osteoblast/osteocyte apoptosis: a potential therapeutic target? J Bone Miner Res 23:1709–1711, 2008.

379. Gluhak-Heinrich J, Gu S, Pavlin D, et al: Mechanical loading stimulates expression of connexin 43 in alveolar bone cells in the tooth movement model, Cell Commun Adhes 13:115–125, 2006.

380. Yang W, Lu Y, Kalajzic I, et al: Dentin matrix protein 1 gene cis-regulation: use in osteocytes to characterize local responses to mechanical loading in vitro and in vivo, J Biol Chem 280:20680–20690, 2005.

381. Feng JQ, Ward LM, Liu S, et al: Loss of DMP1 causes rickets and osteomalacia and identifies a role for osteocytes in mineral metabolism, Nat Genet 38:1310–1315, 2006.

382. Gluhak-Heinrich J, Pavlin D, Yang W, et al: MEPE expression in osteocytes during orthodontic tooth movement, Arch Oral Biol 52:684–690, 2007.

383. Gowen LC, Petersen DN, Mansolf AL, et al: Targeted disruption of the osteoblast/osteocyte factor 45 gene (OF45) results in increased bone formation and bone mass, J Biol Chem 278:1998–2007, 2003.

384. Quarles LD: Endocrine functions of bone in mineral metabolism regulation, J Clin Invest 118:3820–3828, 2008.

385. Robling AG, Niziolek PJ, Baldridge LA, et al: Mechanical stimulation of bone in vivo reduces osteocyte expression of Sost/sclerostin, J Biol Chem 283:5866–5875, 2008.

386. Loots GG, Kneissel M, Keller H, et al: Genomic deletion of a long-range bone enhancer misregulates sclerostin in Van Buchem disease, Genome Res 15:928–935, 2005.

387. Li X, Ominsky MS, Niu QT, et al: Targeted deletion of the sclerostin gene in mice results in increased bone formation and bone strength, J Bone Miner Res 23:860–869, 2008.

388. Winkler DG, Sutherland MK, Geoghegan JC, et al: Osteocyte control of bone formation via sclerostin, a novel BMP antagonist, EMBO J 22:6267–6276, 2003.

389. Robinson JA, Chatterjee-Kishore M, Yaworsky PJ, et al: Wnt/beta-catenin signaling is a normal physiological response to mechanical loading in bone, J Biol Chem 281:31720–31728, 2006.

390. Horwood NJ, Elliott J, Martin TJ, et al: Osteotropic agents regulate the expression of osteoclast differentiation factor and osteoprotegerin in osteoblastic stromal cells, Endocrinology 139:4743–4746, 1998.

391. Poole KE, Reeve J: Parathyroid hormone—a bone anabolic and catabolic agent, Curr Opin Pharmacol 5:612–617, 2005.

392. Martin TJ, Quinn JM, Gillespie MT, et al: Mechanisms involved in skeletal anabolic therapies, Ann N Y Acad Sci 1068:458–470, 2006.

393. Potts JT, Gardella TJ: Progress, paradox, and potential: parathyroid hormone research over five decades, Ann N Y Acad Sci 1117:196–208, 2007.

394. Jilka RL: Molecular and cellular mechanisms of the anabolic effect of intermittent PTH, Bone 40:1434–1446, 2007.

395. Krishnan V, Moore TL, Ma YL, et al: Parathyroid hormone bone anabolic action requires Cbfa1/Runx2-

dependent signaling, Mol Endocrinol 17:423–435, 2003.

396. Fu Q, Manolagas SC, O'Brien CA: Parathyroid hormone controls receptor activator of NF-kappaB ligand gene expression via a distant transcriptional enhancer, Mol Cell Biol 26:6453–6468, 2006.

397. Keller H, Kneissel M: SOST is a target gene for PTH in bone, Bone 37:148–158, 2005.

398. Leupin O, Kramer I, Collette NM, et al: Control of the SOST bone enhancer by PTH using MEF2 transcription factors, J Bone Miner Res 22:1957–1967, 2007.

399. O'Brien CA, Plotkin LI, Galli C, et al: Control of bone mass and remodeling by PTH receptor signaling in osteocytes, PLoS ONE 3:e2942, 2008.

400. Bellido T, Ali AA, Plotkin LI, et al: Proteasomal degradation of Runx2 shortens parathyroid hormone-induced anti-apoptotic signaling in osteoblasts: a putative explanation for why intermittent administration is needed for bone anabolism, J Biol Chem 278:50259–50272, 2003.

401. Girotra M, Rubin MR, Bilezikian JP: The use of parathyroid hormone in the treatment of osteoporosis, Rev Endocr Metab Disord 7:113–121, 2006.

402. Kousteni S, Bilezikian JP: The cell biology of parathyroid hormone in osteoblasts, Curr Osteoporos Rep 6:72–76, 2008.

403. Krum SA, Brown M: Unraveling estrogen action in osteoporosis, Cell Cycle 7:1348–1352, 2008.

404. Novack DV: Estrogen and bone: osteoclasts take center stage, Cell Metab 6:254–256, 2007.

405. Rossouw JE, Anderson GL, Prentice RL, et al: Risks and benefits of estrogen plus progestin in healthy postmenopausal women: principal results from the Women's Health Initiative randomized controlled trial, JAMA 288:321–333, 2002.

406. Kameda T, Mano H, Yuasa T, et al: Estrogen inhibits bone resorption by directly inducing apoptosis of the bone-resorbing osteoclasts, J Exp Med 186:489–495, 1997.

407. Nakamura T, Imai Y, Matsumoto T, et al: Estrogen prevents bone loss via estrogen receptor alpha and induction of Fas ligand in osteoclasts 1, Cell 130:811–823, 2007.

408. Krum SA, Miranda-Carboni GA, Hauschka PV, et al: Estrogen protects bone by inducing Fas ligand in osteoblasts to regulate osteoclast survival, EMBO J 27:535–545, 2008.

409. Kousteni S, Chen JR, Bellido T, et al: Reversal of bone loss in mice by nongenotropic signaling of sex steroids, Science 298:843–846, 2002.

410. Srivastava S, Toraldo G, Weitzmann MN, et al: Estrogen decreases osteoclast formation by down-regulating receptor activator of NF-kappa B ligand (RANKL)-induced JNK activation, J Biol Chem 276:8836–8840, 2001.

411. Pacifici R: Estrogen deficiency, T cells and bone loss, Cell Immunol 252:68–80, 2008.

412. Pacifici R, Brown C, Puscheck E, et al: Effect of surgical menopause and estrogen replacement on cytokine release from human blood mononuclear cells, Proc Natl Acad Sci U S A 88:5134–5138, 1991.

413. Weitzmann MN, Pacifici R: Estrogen deficiency and bone loss: an inflammatory tale, J Clin Invest 116:1186–1194, 2006.

414. Weitzmann MN, Roggia C, Toraldo G, et al: Increased production of IL-7 uncouples bone formation from bone resorption during estrogen deficiency, J Clin Invest 110:1643–1650, 2002.

415. Jilka RL, Hangoc G, Girasole G, et al: Increased osteoclast development after estrogen loss: mediation by interleukin-6, Science 257:88–91, 1992.

416. Sun L, Peng Y, Sharrow AC, et al: FSH directly regulates bone mass, Cell 125:247–260, 2006.

417. Martin TJ, Gaddy D: Bone loss goes beyond estrogen, Nat Med 12:612–613, 2006.

418. Vanderschueren D, Gaytant J, Boonen S, et al: Androgens and bone, Curr Opin Endocrinol Diabetes Obes 15:250–254, 2008.

419. Vanderschueren D, Vandenput L, Boonen S, et al: Androgens and bone, Endocr Rev 25:389–425, 2004.

420. Manolagas SC, Kousteni S, Jilka RL: Sex steroids and bone, Recent Prog Horm Res 57:385–409, 2002.

421. Canalis E, Mazziotti G, Giustina A, et al: Glucocorticoid-induced osteoporosis: pathophysiology and therapy, Osteoporos Int 18:1319–1328, 2007.

422. Migliaccio S, Brama M, Fornari R, et al: Glucocorticoid-induced osteoporosis: an osteoblastic disease, Aging Clin Exp Res 19:5–10, 2007.

423. O'Brien CA, Jia D, Plotkin LI, et al: Glucocorticoids act directly on osteoblasts and osteocytes to induce their apoptosis and reduce bone formation and strength, Endocrinology 145:1835–1841, 2004.

424. Weinstein RS, Jilka RL, Parfitt AM, et al: Inhibition of osteoblastogenesis and promotion of apoptosis of osteoblasts and osteocytes by glucocorticoids: potential mechanisms of their deleterious effects on bone, J Clin Invest 102:274–282, 1998.

425. Yun SI, Yoon HY, Jeong SY, et al: Glucocorticoid induces apoptosis of osteoblast cells through the activation of glycogen synthase kinase 3beta, J Bone Miner Metab 27:140–148, 2009.

426. Jia D, O'Brien CA, Stewart SA, et al: Glucocorticoids act directly on osteoclasts to increase their life span and reduce bone density, Endocrinology 147:5592–5599, 2006.

427. Kim HJ, Zhao H, Kitaura H, et al: Glucocorticoids suppress bone formation via the osteoclast, J Clin Invest 116:2152–2160, 2006.

428. Kim HJ, Zhao H, Kitaura H, et al: Glucocorticoids and the osteoclast, Ann N Y Acad Sci 1116:335–339, 2007.

429. Giustina A, Mazziotti G, Canalis E: Growth hormone, insulin-like growth factors, and the skeleton, Endocr Rev 29:535–559, 2008.

430. Bassett JH, Williams GR: Critical role of the hypothalamic-pituitary-thyroid axis in bone, Bone 43:418–426, 2008.

431. Miller SB: Prostaglandins in health and disease: an overview, Semin Arthritis Rheum 36:37–49, 2006.

432. Ducy P, Amling M, Takeda S, et al: Leptin inhibits bone formation through a hypothalamic relay: a central control of bone mass, Cell 100:197–207, 2000.

433. Takeda S, Elefteriou F, Levasseur R, et al: Leptin regulates bone formation via the sympathetic nervous system, Cell 111:305–317, 2002.

434. Fu L, Patel MS, Bradley A, et al: The molecular clock mediates leptin-regulated bone formation, Cell 122:803–815, 2005.

435. Elefteriou F, Ahn JD, Takeda S, et al: Leptin regulation of bone resorption by the sympathetic nervous system and CART, Nature 434:514–520, 2005.

436. Ahn JD, Dubern B, Lubrano-Berthelier C, et al: Cart overexpression is the only identifiable cause of high bone mass in melanocortin 4 receptor deficiency, Endocrinology 147:3196–3202, 2006.

437. Bonnet N, Pierroz DD, Ferrari SL: Adrenergic control of bone remodeling and its implications for the treatment of osteoporosis, J Musculoskelet Neuronal Interact 8:94–104, 2008.

438. Takeda S: Central control of bone remodelling, J Neuroendocrinol 20:802–807, 2008.

439. Karsenty G, Ducy P: The hypothalamic control of bone mass, implication for the treatment of osteoporosis, Ann Endocrinol (Paris) 67:123, 2006.

440. Sato S, Hanada R, Kimura A, et al: Central control of bone remodeling by neuromedin U, Nat Med 13:1234–1240, 2007.

441. Baldock PA, Sainsbury A, Couzens M, et al: Hypothalamic Y2 receptors regulate bone formation, J Clin Invest 109:915–921, 2002.

442. Baldock PA, Allison SJ, Lundberg P, et al: Novel role of Y1 receptors in the coordinated regulation of bone and energy homeostasis, J Biol Chem 282:19092–19102, 2007.

443. Abe E, Marians RC, Yu W, et al: TSH is a negative regulator of skeletal remodeling, Cell 115:151–162, 2003.

444. Sun L, Vukicevic S, Baliram R, et al: Intermittent recombinant TSH injections prevent ovariectomy-induced bone loss, Proc Natl Acad Sci U S A 105:4289–4294, 2008.

445. Wong IP, Zengin A, Herzog H, et al: Central regulation of bone mass, Semin Cell Dev Biol 19:452–458, 2008.

446. Karsenty G: Convergence between bone and energy homeostases: leptin regulation of bone mass, Cell Metab 4:341–348, 2006.

447. Cirmanova V, Bayer M, Starka L, et al: The effect of leptin on bone: an evolving concept of action, Physiol Res 57(suppl 1):S143-S151, 2008.

448. Patel MS, Elefteriou F: The new field of neuroskeletal biology, Calcif Tissue Int 80:337–347, 2007.

449. Horowitz MC, Bothwell AL, Hesslein DG, et al: B cells and osteoblast and osteoclast development, Immunol Rev 208:141–153, 2005.

450. Horowitz MC, Xi Y, Pflugh DL, et al: Pax5-deficient mice exhibit early onset osteopenia with increased osteoclast progenitors, J Immunol 173:6583–6591, 2004.

451. Li Y, Toraldo G, Li A, et al: B cells and T cells are critical for the preservation of bone homeostasis and attainment of peak bone mass in vivo, Blood 109:3839–3848, 2007.

452. Sato T, Shibata T, Ikeda K, et al: Generation of bone-resorbing osteoclasts from B220+ cells: its role in accelerated osteoclastogenesis due to estrogen deficiency, J Bone Miner Res 16:2215–2221, 2001.

453. Calvi LM, Adams GB, Weibrecht KW, et al: Osteoblastic cells regulate the haematopoietic stem cell niche, Nature 425:841–846, 2003.

454. Visnjic D, Kalajzic Z, Rowe DW, et al: Hematopoiesis is severely altered in mice with an induced osteoblast deficiency, Blood 103:3258–3264, 2004.

455. Porter RL, Calvi LM: Communications between bone cells and hematopoietic stem cells, Arch Biochem Biophys 473:193–200, 2008.

456. Zhang J, Niu C, Ye L, et al: Identification of the haematopoietic stem cell niche and control of the niche size, Nature 425:836–841, 2003.

457. Adams GB, Martin RP, Alley IR, et al: Therapeutic targeting of a stem cell niche, Nat Biotechnol 25:238–243, 2007.

458. Wu JY, Purton LE, Rodda SJ, et al: Osteoblastic regulation of B lymphopoiesis is mediated by Gsα-dependent signaling pathways, Proc Natl Acad Sci U S A 105:16976–16981, 2008.

459. Walkley CR, Olsen GH, Dworkin S, et al: A micro-environment-induced myeloproliferative syndrome caused by retinoic acid receptor gamma deficiency, Cell 129:1097–1110, 2007.

460. Walkley CR, Shea JM, Sims NA, et al: Rb regulates interactions between hematopoietic stem cells and their bone marrow microenvironment, Cell 129:1081–1095, 2007.

461. Larsson J, Ohishi M, Garrison B, et al: Nf2/merlin regulates hematopoietic stem cell behavior by altering microenvironmental architecture, Cell Stem Cell 3:221–227, 2008.

462. Gong JK: Endosteal marrow: a rich source of hematopoietic stem cells, Science 199:1443–1445, 1978.

463. Aicher A, Kollet O, Heeschen C, et al: The Wnt antagonist Dickkopf-1 mobilizes vasculogenic progenitor cells via activation of the bone marrow endosteal stem cell niche, Circ Res 103:796–803, 2008.

464. Kollet O, Dar A, Shivtiel S, et al: Osteoclasts degrade endosteal components and promote mobilization of hematopoietic progenitor cells, Nat Med 12:657–664, 2006.

465. Lee NK, Sowa H, Hinoi E, et al: Endocrine regulation of energy metabolism by the skeleton, Cell 130:456–469, 2007.

466. Lee NK, Karsenty G: Reciprocal regulation of bone and energy metabolism, Trends Endocrinol Metab 19:161–166, 2008.

Chapter 5

CALCIUM REGULATION, CALCIUM HOMEOSTASIS, AND GENETIC DISORDERS OF CALCIUM METABOLISM

RAJESH V. THAKKER, F. RICHARD BRINGHURST, and HARALD JÜPPNER

Calcium plays an important role in many physiologic pathways that include muscle contraction, the secretion of neurotransmitters and hormones, and the coagulation pathways, and it is an important component of the skeleton. Disturbances in extracellular calcium concentration may cause a variety of symptoms, the most common of which reflect abnormal neuromuscular activity. *Hypercalcemia* may lead to muscle weakness and areflexia, anorexia, constipation, vomiting, drowsiness, depression, confusion, other cognitive dysfunction, and coma. Hypercalcemia leads to hypercalciuria, which can result in medullary calcification, nephrocalcinosis, and renal failure. *Hypocalcemia*, conversely, may cause anxiety, seizures, muscle twitching, epilepsy, tetany, Chvostek's and Trousseau's signs, carpal or pedal spasm, stridor, bronchospasm, and intestinal cramps, as well as cataracts, skeletal malformations, and abnormal dentition. The control of body calcium involves a balance between the amounts that are absorbed from the gut, deposited into bone and cells, and excreted from the kidney (Fig. 5-1). This fine balance, involving three organs, is chiefly under the control of parathyroid hormone (PTH), which is synthesized and secreted by the parathyroid glands. Thus, hypocalcemia will lead to an increased secretion of PTH, whereas hypercalcemia will result in diminished PTH secretion. A number of clinical disorders characterized by derangements of calcium homeostasis are caused by

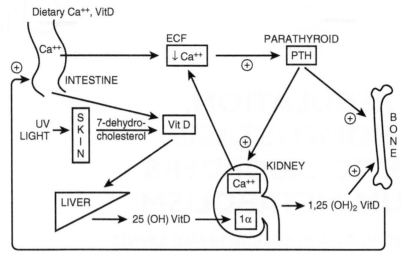

FIGURE 5-1. Regulation of extracellular fluid (ECF) calcium (Ca^{2+}) by parathyroid hormone (PTH) action on kidney, bone, and intestine. A decrease in ECF Ca^{2+} is sensed by the calcium-sensing receptor, leading to an increase in PTH secretion, which predominantly acts directly on kidney and bone that possess the PTH/PTHrP receptor (PTHR1; see Fig. 5-3). The skeletal effects of PTH are to increase (+) osteoclastic bone reabsorption, but because osteoclasts do not express the PTHR1, this action is mediated via the osteoblasts, which do have this receptor and in response release cytokines and factors that activate osteoclasts. In the kidney, PTH stimulates (+) the 1α-hydroxylase (1α) to increase the conversion of 25-hydroxy vitamin D [25(OH)D] to the active metabolite 1,25-dihydroxyvitamin D [1,25(OH)$_2$D]. In addition, PTH increases (+) reabsorption of Ca^{2+} from the renal distal tubule and inhibits reabsorption of phosphate from the proximal tubule, leading to hypercalcemia and hypophosphatemia. PTH also inhibits Na^+/H^+ antiporter activity and bicarbonate reabsorption, causing a mild hyperchloremic acidosis. Elevated 1,25(OH)$_2$D acts on the intestine to increase (+) absorption of dietary calcium and phosphate; it is important to note that PTH does not appear to have a direct action on the gut. In response to hypocalcemia and the increase in PTH secretion, all of these direct and indirect actions of PTH on the kidney, bone, and intestine will help to increase ECF Ca^{2+}, which in turn will act via the calcium-sensing receptor to decrease PTH secretion.

abnormalities of the parathyroid glands themselves. Thus, PTH oversecretion due to parathyroid tumors, which affect 3/1000 of the population, is a major cause of hypercalcemia, which may be associated with kidney stones, osteoporosis, and peptic ulcers. PTH deficiency as part of a syndrome occurs in 1/4000 live births, isolated hypoparathyroidism resulting in hypocalcemia appears to occur less frequently. This chapter will review (1) the physiologic and biochemical mechanisms underlying extracellular calcium homeostasis and (2) the genetic basis for disorders of calcium metabolism.

Regulation of Calcium Homeostasis

DISTRIBUTION AND METABOLIC ACTIONS OF CALCIUM

The total body content of calcium in a normal adult is approximately 1000 g, of which nearly all exists within the crystal structure of bone mineral; less than 1% is soluble in extracellular and intracellular fluid.[1,2] On average, bone mineral closely approximates the composition of hydroxyapatite [$Ca_{10}(PO4)_6(OH)_2$], which means that 6 mmol of phosphate are released with every 10 mmol of calcium mobilized during bone resorption (or about 1:2 on a mg/mg basis).[1,3]

In blood, calcium is partly bound to proteins. Albumin accounts for about 70% of the protein-bound fraction.[4] Another portion (about 6%) is associated with diffusible ion complexes.[1] Thus normally, only half of total plasma calcium is freely ionized, but it is this fraction that is most important physiologically and subject to stringent endocrine regulation. The normal ranges of total and ionized serum calcium in the adult are 8.5 to 10.5 mg/dL and 1.17 to 1.33 mmol, respectively.[5] The usual 2:1 ratio of total to ionized calcium may be disturbed by disorders such as metabolic acidosis (calcium binding to proteins is reduced at

acid pH) or by changes in serum protein concentrations, as in starvation, cirrhosis, dehydration, or multiple myeloma. When precise knowledge of the ionized calcium concentration is clinically important, direct measurement with calcium-selective electrodes should be performed.

Serum calcium is higher during infancy/childhood and adolescence than in the adult[6] but does not change at puberty or, in women, during the menstrual cycle. During pregnancy, total serum calcium and albumin decline progressively, but ionized calcium is minimally affected.[7,8] Fetal calcium content rises dramatically during the third trimester (to about 30 g at term),[9] and fetal serum total and ionized calcium concentrations both are higher than maternal levels, consistent with active placental transport of calcium.[10] Despite daily losses of 200 to 300 mg/d of calcium in breast milk, lactating women maintain normal levels of ionized calcium in blood by increasing intestinal calcium absorption in response to augmented production of 1,25(OH)$_2$D.[11,12]

Calcium entry into cells is strongly favored by a steep electrochemical gradient. Thus, the cell interior is electronegative, and cytosolic free calcium is in the range of 10^{-7} M, which is 10,000-fold lower than extracellular calcium concentrations. Calcium traverses the plasma membrane through various channels, including voltage-, receptor- and store-operated forms, the regulation of which is complex and tissue specific.[13,14] Intracellularly, nearly all (99%) calcium is sequestered in pools within mitochondria, endoplasmic reticula, or sarcoplasmic reticula or is tightly bound to the inner surface of the plasma membrane.[15] Sequestered calcium, especially that within the endoplasmic reticulum, may be released rapidly into the cytosol following activation of cell-surface receptors. In this way, it plays a critical role in signal transduction and in controlling calcium entry via store-operated channels. The extremely low cytosolic free calcium concentration is maintained by active calcium transport into intracellular pools or by extrusion out of the cell via high-affinity, low-capacity Ca^{2+}/H^+ adenosine triphosphatases (ATPases) and low-affinity, high-capacity Na^+/Ca^{2+} exchangers driven by the transmembrane sodium gradient.[16]

With the discovery of a G protein–coupled calcium-sensing receptor (CaSR) expressed in parathyroid, renal epithelial, and other cells, it has become clear that calcium can act as an extracellular ligand to directly control cellular function.[17] The principal actions of the CaSR with respect to calcium homeostasis include suppression of PTH secretion and, in the thick ascending loop of the renal tubule, inhibition of calcium, magnesium, and NaCl reabsorption. Extracellular calcium also is utilized directly for normal matrix mineralization in bone and cartilage and is required for activation of important circulating or extracellular enzymes and proteases. Intracellular calcium exerts a broad range of effects via interaction with key enzymes and effector molecules, including kinases, phosphatases, calmodulins, transcription factors, ion channels (including calcium channels), and troponins and other proteins involved in contraction, microtubule and microfilament assembly, and motility. The steep gradients between intracellular calcium and both extracellular and intracellularly sequestered calcium are crucial for normal neuromuscular activity and provide the potential required for rapid transients and waves of cytosolic free calcium that serve key second-messenger functions in both excitable and nonexcitable cells.[14,18]

CALCIUM ABSORPTION

Intestinal calcium absorptive efficiency in humans ranges broadly between 20% and 70%, declines steadily with age, and is strongly influenced by previous calcium intake, the presence of other nutrients, pregnancy, lactation, overall calcium balance, and the availability of vitamin D.[19-23] Fecal calcium includes the residual fraction of dietary calcium that is not absorbed, as well as a contribution from secreted calcium present in bile and other digestive juices ("endogenous fecal calcium"). Endogenous fecal calcium in humans normally amounts to 100 to 200 mg/d and is relatively unaffected by changes in dietary or serum calcium.[24,25]

Intestinal calcium absorption is adjusted physiologically in response to variations in calcium intake, as shown by radiocalcium kinetic and balance studies in normal subjects.[26,27] Obligate renal and intestinal excretion of calcium is such that calcium balance cannot be maintained if dietary calcium consistently falls below 200 to 400 mg/d, even though the percentage of calcium absorbed may be very high (i.e., 70%). As calcium intake increases, overall calcium absorption (in mg/d) rises, but the fractional absorption of ingested calcium declines progressively such that within the physiologic range of calcium intake, total net calcium absorption tends to plateau at approximately 400 mg/d. Consequently, urinary calcium excretion tends also to plateau at higher intakes. Additional buffering of changes in dietary calcium results from control of renal tubular calcium reabsorption and skeletal calcium release, but regulation of intestinal absorptive efficiency is critical for calcium balance.[26] The mechanisms of this inverse regulation of intestinal absorptive efficiency by changes in calcium availability are considered in the following discussion.

MECHANISMS AND SITES OF CALCIUM ABSORPTION

Calcium is absorbed throughout the intestine. In terms of rates of transport per unit length of mucosa, absorption is most efficient in the duodenum and proximal jejunum, which exhibit the highest levels of vitamin D–dependent calcium binding proteins and in which lower luminal pH (5 to 6) promotes dissociation of calcium from complexes with food constituents and other ions.[28,29] On the other hand, longer residence times in the more distal small bowel segments may allow absorption of a larger proportion of total calcium intake in the distal jejunum and ileum.[30,31] The ileum, for example, may become an important site of net calcium absorption during dietary restriction of calcium or when the residence time of luminal contents in more proximal bowel segments is reduced.[30,32]

Transcellular calcium absorption necessarily involves three steps: entry into the cell, diffusion across the cell, and extrusion from the cell (see Chapter 3). The first step, entry through the apical brush border, occurs via a member of the vanilloid (TRPV) superfamily of channels, namely TRPV6 (previously referred to as *CaT1* or *ECaC2*).[33,34] Another member of this family, TRPV5, appears to be dominantly involved in calcium reabsorption in the kidney (see later). The *TRPV6* and *TRPV5* genes are located on chromosome 7q33-35. Their structure includes six transmembrane regions, a short hydrophobic region between segments 5 and 6 that likely forms the calcium pore, and large intracellular domains at the N- and C-termini.[33] The pore region is highly selective for calcium,[35,36] and mutations in this region have been shown to abolish calcium permeability.[37] Posttranslational modification and glycosylation of TRPV6 occurs, but the functional effects of these modifications are not well defined. Similarly, the mechanisms regulating the activity of these molecules are not well understood. TRPV6 and TRPV5 expression varies significantly between species and in humans, and both genes are expressed in a variety of tissues.[38] Specifically, TRPV5 seems to be the major isoform expressed in the kidney, whereas TRPV6 is most highly expressed in the small intestine (restricted to the apical surface of epithelial cells).[39] Given the important role of $1,25(OH)_2D_3$ and other hormonal regulators in calcium absorption, the effects of these hormones on TRPV6 expression has recently been investigated. $1,25(OH)D_3$ clearly increases TRPV6 expression in vitro (see Chapter 3).[40] Furthermore, mice with targeted inactivation of the vitamin D receptor demonstrate a 90% reduction in TRPV6 expression and a threefold reduction in intestinal calcium absorption.[41] Additionally, calcium exposure appears to independently affect TRPV6 expression insofar as high calcium intake decreases TRPV6 expression, and low intake increases it.[41,42] Finally, TRPV6 expression is decreased in mice with targeted inactivation of their estrogen receptor-α gene and is increased in mice receiving exogenous estradiol administration.[43]

After calcium has entered the cell, it must be transported through the cytoplasm and extruded from the cell against a steep gradient. The mechanism by which calcium moves through the cell involves the small cytosolic protein calbindin D_{9k}. Calcium entering the cell via the apical TRPV6 channel becomes tightly associated with the calbindin, which buffers the relatively large mass of entering calcium and minimizes its impact upon cytosolic free-calcium concentrations. The calbindin/calcium complex then diffuses across the cytosol to the basolateral membrane. Free calcium then dissociates into the low-cytosolic calcium environment maintained immediately subjacent to the basolateral membrane by high-affinity membrane Ca^{2+}-ATPases located there. Finally, these calcium ATPases actively extrude calcium out of the cell.[29] The known cellular concentrations and kinetic properties of the calbindin D_{9k} molecule would support observed rates of duodenal calcium transport at submicromolar concentrations of cytosolic free calcium.[44] Indeed, the importance of this buffered diffusional process predicts that enterocyte calbindin D_{9k} content is likely to be a major determinant, along with TRPV6 activity, of the overall rate of enterocyte calcium transport.

RENAL CALCIUM EXCRETION

Regulation of renal calcium excretion is an important mechanism for homeostatic control of blood ionized calcium in the face of fluctuations in filtered load, as derived from intestinal calcium absorption and net bone resorption. When urinary calcium is viewed as a function of the amount of calcium actually absorbed by the gut (i.e., after regulation of intestinal absorptive efficiency has been factored out), the precision with which the kidney adjusts tubular calcium reabsorption to residual changes in filtered load becomes obvious. Ordinarily, the daily load of calcium filtered at the glomerulus (the product of the glomerular filtration rate[45] and ultrafilterable calcium[46]) is approximately 10,000 mg/d in adult humans, which means that the extracellular calcium pool is completely filtered several times a day. Since urinary calcium excretion (and net intestinal calcium absorption) is approximately 200 mg/d, only 2% of filtered calcium is excreted normally. This high ratio of filtered to excreted calcium affords ample opportunity for finely tuned hormonal control of calcium excretion, even though it may be difficult to measure the small changes involved.

SITES AND MECHANISMS OF RENAL CALCIUM REABSORPTION

Calcium is reabsorbed at multiple sites and by different mechanisms along the nephron. As in the intestine, the challenge of transporting calcium across the renal epithelium requires that adequate rates of transport be achieved without substantially increasing the concentration of calcium within the cytosol of the epithelial cell. This is accomplished mainly by use of paracellular diffusional mechanisms that are supplemented in some nephron segments by active transcellular transport, especially in response to hormonal stimulation.

Approximately 60% to 70% of tubular calcium reabsorption, like that of sodium, occurs in the proximal tubule.[46] Proximal tubular calcium reabsorption occurs mainly via passive diffusion along paracellular pathways, down the ambient (lumen-positive) electrochemical gradient.[47] Another 20% to 25% of the filtered calcium load is reabsorbed in Henle's loop.[46] This occurs mainly by paracellular diffusion in the cortical thick ascending limb (cTAL),[48-50] although active transcellular transport may play a minor role as well.[51,52] Calcium (and magnesium) reabsorption in this segment is severely impaired in patients with homozygous inactivating mutations in claudin 16 (CLDN16) (previously referred to as paracellin-1) or claudin 19 (CLDN19) protein, strongly expressed in tight junctions of the cTAL and presumably required for normal divalent cation conductance.[53-56] Hypercalcemia suppresses renal tubular calcium reabsorption even in the absence of PTH,[57] an effect likely due to direct activation of basolateral CaSRs in the cTAL (and possibly other nephron segments).[58] In the cTAL, activated CaSRs lower apical K^+ exit by inhibiting renal outer medullary K^+ channels (ROMKs), thereby blunting Na-K-2Cl cotransporter (NKCC2) activity and reducing the transepithelial voltage gradient that drives paracellular cation movement.[17,59-61] The critical importance of normal rates of Na-K-2Cl reabsorption for adequate calcium transport in the cTAL is highlighted clinically by the occurrence of dramatic hypercalciuria in patients with Bartter's syndromes, which involve defects in NKCC2, ROMK, or other transporters or channels required

for effective Na-K-2Cl reabsorption.[62] An analogous Bartter's-like phenotype may occur in some patients with activating CaSR mutations.[63] CaSR activation in the cTAL also antagonizes PTH-stimulated increases in calcium reabsorption, possibly by impairing cyclic adenosine monophosphate (cAMP) generation[61] (see later).

Only about 8% to 10% of filtered calcium is reabsorbed in more distal segments of the tubule, but calcium transport in the distal nephron is a key control point for hormonal regulation and involves predominantly transcellular reabsorption.[64-66] Cells in the late distal tubule exhibit striking co-localization of several unique proteins that are critical for effective transcellular calcium reabsorption. These include an apical epithelial calcium channel, TRPV5 (formerly ECaC1 or CaT2 and highly homologous to TRPV6, discussed earlier), the cytosolic calcium-binding protein, calbindin D_{28k}, basolateral plasma membrane calcium ATPase(s) (PMCAs), and basolateral NA^+/Ca^{2+} exchanger 1 (NCX1).[67-72] As in the intestinal epithelium, these cells admit calcium across their apical membranes via opening of TRPV5. Expression of this channel is up-regulated by PTH, thus enhancing calcium reabsorption (see later). In contrast, high intracellular calcium concentrations and increased calbindin D_{28k} levels reduce calcium reabsorption, possibly via enhanced buffering of subapical Ca^{2+} ions. Calcium bound to calbindin D_{28k} is ferried across the cell to the basolateral membrane, where it ultimately is extruded against a steep electrochemical gradient, predominantly via NCX1 (70% of Ca^{2+} flux),[73,74] but also by PMCA. As expected, mice lacking TRPV5[75] or calbindin D_{28k}[76] were found to manifest severe hypercalciuria.

Additional calcium absorption may occur in more distal nephron segments, such as cortical and medullary collecting ducts.[47] Proteins other than those described above may be involved in renal calcium reabsorption as well, including voltage-operated calcium channels[47,77] and Cl^- channels, as evidenced by the hypercalciuria seen in Dent's disease, an X-linked disorder due to inactivating mutations in the Cl^- channel ClC-5 that may be involved in endocytic vesicle function and protein trafficking.[78,79]

REGULATION OF RENAL CALCIUM REABSORPTION

Calcium excretion is affected by a variety of hormones, ions, nutrients, and drugs.[80,81] Among these, PTH is the principal physiologic regulator of renal tubular calcium transport, as appreciated clinically by the markedly abnormal overall relation of serum to urinary calcium in hyper- and hypoparathyroidism.[80,82,83] PTH acts to enhance tubular calcium reabsorption in the cTAL, distal convoluted tubules (DCT), and connecting tubules (CNT).[50,65,84,85] It augments DCT calbindin D_{28k} expression[86] and basolateral N^+/Ca^{2+} exchange,[87-91] increases the affinity for calcium of the basolateral Ca^{2+}-ATPase,[92] and hyperpolarizes the DCT cell,[93] which then activates the TRPV5 channel.[94] In immortalized murine distal tubular cells, PTH causes insertion into the apical membrane of new dihydropyridine-sensitive membrane calcium channels,[77] and it stimulates stretch-activated nonselective cation channels in rabbit CNT.[95] These are distinct from TRPV5 channels and may represent other mechanisms of apical calcium entry. PTH increases the surface expression or activity of TRPV5 epithelial calcium channels. In the cTAL, PTH also may increase some form of active transcellular transport,[51,52] and it may stimulate paracellular diffusional calcium transport by augmenting the transepithelial voltage gradient, at least in some segments and species.[96,97]

Studies in patients with inactivating vitamin D receptor mutations have demonstrated that $1,25(OH)_2D_3$ is required for the calcium-reabsorptive response to PTH.[98] It furthermore accelerates the increase in DCT cell calcium entry initiated by PTH,[99] and it directly increases DCT calcium reabsorption, apparently by driving higher expression of TRPV5, calbindin D_{28k}, and PMCA (see Chapter 3).[74,100-103] Another hormone affecting calcium reabsorption is calcitonin. When given in large doses, calcitonin acutely reduces proximal tubular calcium reabsorption by a mechanism independent of PTH;[104] however, an important role for calcitonin in the physiologic regulation of calcium reabsorption is thought to be unlikely. Hypercalciuria observed in states of excess growth hormone or cortisol seems likely to be secondary to an increased filtered load of calcium rather than to direct tubular actions of these hormones.[105-110] Estrogen treatment of normal postmenopausal women lowers urinary calcium excretion by increasing tubular calcium reabsorption.[111,112] In DCT of ovariectomized rats, 17β-estradiol acutely increases mRNA expression of all major components of the calcium transport pathway, including TRPV5, calbindin D_{28k}, NCX1, and PMCA1b.[113] Reported effects on tubular calcium reabsorption of insulin,[114] glucagon,[96] antidiuretic hormone,[96] and angiotensin II[115] are of uncertain physiologic or clinical significance.

Parathyroid Hormone Gene Structure and Function

The *PTH* gene is located on chromosome 11p15 and consists of 3 exons which are separated by 2 introns.[116] Exon 1 of the *PTH* gene is 85 bp in length and is untranslated (Fig. 5-2), whereas exons 2 and 3 encode the 115-amino-acid pre-proPTH peptide (see Chapter 1 for detailed discussion). Exon 2 is 90 bp in length and encodes the initiation (ATG) codon, the prehormone sequence, and part of the prohormone sequence. Exon 3 is 612 bp in size and encodes the remainder of the prohormone sequence, the 84 amino acids comprising the mature PTH peptide and the 3′ untranslated region.[117] The 5′ regulatory sequence of the human *PTH* gene contains a vitamin D response element 125 bp upstream of the transcription start site, which down-regulates PTH mRNA transcription in response to vitamin D receptor binding.[118,119] PTH gene transcription (as well as PTH peptide secretion) is also dependent upon the extracellular calcium and phosphate concentration,[120,121] although the presence of specific upstream "calcium or phosphate response element(s)" has not yet been demonstrated.[122,123] The secretion of mature PTH from the parathyroid chief cell is regulated through a G protein–coupled calcium-sensing receptor, which is also expressed in renal tubules and several other tissues, albeit at lower abundance. PTH mRNA is first translated into a pre-proPTH peptide. The "pre" sequence consists of a 25-amino-acid

signal peptide (leader sequence) which is responsible for directing the nascent peptide into the endoplasmic reticulum to be packaged for secretion from the cell.[124] The "pro" sequence is 6 amino acids in length, and although its function is less well defined than that of the "pre" sequence, it is also essential for correct PTH processing and secretion.[124] After the 84 amino acid–containing mature PTH peptide is secreted from the parathyroid cell, it is cleared from the circulation (with a short half-life of about 2 minutes) via nonsaturable hepatic and renal uptake (see Chapter 1).

PTH mediates its actions through a receptor it shares with PTH-related peptide (PTHrP also known as *PTHrH*, PTH-related hormone).[125,126] This PTH/PTHrP receptor (Fig. 5-3) is a member of a subgroup of G protein–coupled receptors, and its gene is located on chromosome 3p21.3.[127,128] The PTH/PTHrP receptor is highly expressed in kidney and bone, where it mediates the endocrine actions of PTH. However, during embryonic and postnatal development, the PTH/PTHrP receptor is most abundantly expressed in chondrocytes of the metaphyseal growth plate, where it mediates predominantly the autocrine/paracrine actions of PTHrP.[129,130] Mutations involving the genes that encode PTH, the calcium-sensing receptor, the PTH/PTHrP receptor, and $G_{s\alpha}$ all affect the regulation of calcium homeostasis and can thus be associated with genetic disorders characterized by hypercalcemia or hypocalcemia (Table 5-1).

Hypercalcemic Diseases

Similar to the findings in other tumor syndromes, the abnormal expression of an oncogene or the loss of a tumor-suppressor gene can result in abnormal proliferative activity of parathyroid cells. The molecular exploration of these genes has provided important novel insights into the pathogenesis of different forms of hyperparathyroidism. *Oncogenes* are genes whose abnormal expression may transform a normal cell into a tumor cell. The normal form of the gene is referred to as a *proto-oncogene*, and a single mutant allele may affect the phenotype of the cell; these genes may also be referred to as *dominant oncogenes* (Fig. 5-4A). The mutant versions (i.e., the oncogene), which are usually excessively or inappropriately active, may arise because of point mutations, gene amplifications, or chromosomal translocations. Tumor-suppressor genes, also referred to as *recessive oncogenes* or *anti-oncogenes*, normally inhibit cell proliferation, whereas their mutant versions in cancer cells have lost their normal function. In order to transform a normal cell into a tumor cell, both alleles of the tumor-suppressor gene must be inactivated. Inactivation arises by point mutations or, alternatively, by small or larger intragenic deletions that can involve substantial genomic portions or a whole chromosome. Larger deletions may be detected by cytogenetic methods, by Southern blot analysis, or by PCR-based analysis of polymorphic markers. Compared to genomic

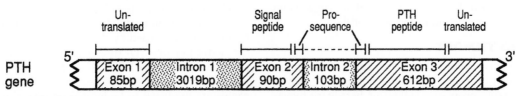

FIGURE 5-2. Schematic representation of the PTH gene, PTH mRNA, and PTH peptide. The PTH gene consists of 3 exons and 2 introns; the peptide is encoded by exons 2 and 3. The PTH peptide is synthesized as a precursor, which contains a presequence and a prosequence. The mature PTH peptide, which contains 84 amino acids, and larger carboxyl-terminal PTH fragments are secreted from the parathyroid cell. (From Parkinson D, Thakker R: A donor splice site mutation in the parathyroid hormone gene is associated with autosomal-recessive hypoparathyroidism, Nat Genet 1:149–153, 1992.)

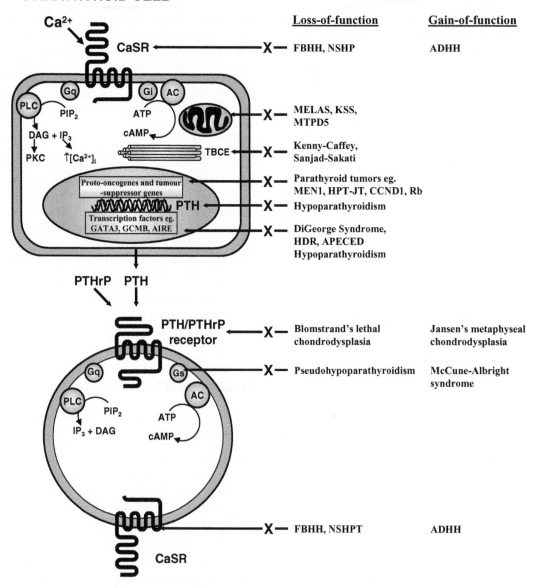

FIGURE 5-3. Schematic representation of some of the components involved in calcium homeostasis. Alterations in extracellular calcium are detected by the calcium-sensing receptor (CaSR), a 1078-amino-acid G protein–coupled receptor. The PTH/PTHrP receptor, which mediates the actions of PTH and PTHrP, is also a G protein–coupled receptor. Thus, Ca^{2+} and PTH and PTHrP involve G protein–coupled signaling pathways, and interaction with their specific receptors can lead to activation of G_s, G_i and G_q, respectively. G_s stimulates adenylcyclase (AC), which catalyses the formation of cAMP from ATP. G_i inhibits AC activity, and cAMP stimulates PKA, which phosphorylates cell-specific substrates. Activation of G_q stimulates PLC, which catalyses the hydrolysis of the phosphoinositide (PIP_2) to inositol triphosphate (IP_3), which increases intracellular calcium, and diacylglycerol (DAG), which activates PKC. These proximal signals modulate downstream pathways, resulting in specific physiologic effects. Abnormalities in several genes, which lead to mutations in proteins in these pathways, have been identified in specific disorders of calcium homeostasis (see Table 5-1).

DNA from other cells (e.g., leukocytes), genomic DNA from the patient's tumor cells typically lack certain chromosomal regions, and this finding is consequently referred to as *loss of heterozygosity* (LOH) (see Fig. 5-4B). Finding LOH, therefore, suggests an inactivating mutation or deletion in the other allele.

PARATHYROID TUMORS

Parathyroid tumors may occur as an isolated and sporadic endocrinopathy or as part of inherited tumor syndromes,[131] such as the multiple endocrine neoplasias (MEN) or hereditary hyperparathyroidism with jaw tumors (HPT-JT),[132] or in response to chronic overstimulation, as in uremic hyperparathyroidism.[133] Genetic analyses of kindreds with MEN1 and MEN2A and of tumor tissue from patients with single parathyroid adenomas have shown that some of the molecular mechanisms known to be involved in tumor genesis can also be responsible for the development of hyperparathyroidism.

Our current understanding indicates that sporadic parathyroid tumors are caused by single somatic mutations that lead to the activation or overexpression of proto-oncogenes such as parathyroid adenoma 1 (*PRAD1*) or *RET* (see Fig. 5-4A). Furthermore, different tumor-suppressor genes affecting the parathyroid glands are predicted to be located on several different chromosomes, and in a significant number of patients, LOH has been documented for one of these loci. For all these somatic mutations, a single point mutation or a deletion provides a growth

Table 5-1. Diseases of Calcium Homeostasis and Their Chromosomal Locations

Metabolic Abnormality	Disease	Inheritance	Gene Product	Chromosomal Location
Hypercalcemia	Multiple endocrine neoplasia type 1	Autosomal dominant	MENIN	11q13
	Multiple endocrine neoplasia type 2	Autosomal dominant	RET	10q11.2
	Hereditary hyperparathyroidism and jaw tumors (HPT-JT)	Autosomal dominant	PARAFIBROMIN	1q31-2 13q14
	Hyperparathyroidism	Sporadic	PRAD1/CCND1	11q13
			Retinoblastoma	13q14
			Unknown	1p32-pter
	Parathyroid carcinoma	Sporadic	PARAFIBROMIN	1q31.2
	Familial benign hypercalcemia (FBH)			
	FBH1	Autosomal dominant	CaSR	3q21.1
	FBH2	Autosomal dominant	Unknown	19p13
	FBH3 (FBH$_{OK}$)	Autosomal dominant	Unknown	19q13
	Neonatal hyperparathyroidism	Autosomal recessive	CaSR	3q21.1
		Autosomal dominant	CaSR	
	Jansen's disease	Autosomal dominant	PTHR/PTHrPR	3p21.3
	Williams syndrome	Autosomal dominant	Elastin, LIMK (and other genes)	7q11.23
	McCune-Albright syndrome	Somatic mutations during early embryonic development (?)	GNAS	20q13.3
Hypocalcemia	Isolated hypoparathyroidism	Autosomal dominant	PTH, GCNB	11p15*
		Autosomal recessive	PTH, GCMB	11p15*, 6p24.2
		X-linked recessive	Unknown (SOSC3)	Xq26-27
	Hypocalcemic hypercalciuria (ADHH)	Autosomal dominant	CaSR	3q21.1
	Hypoparathyroidism associated with polyglandular autoimmune syndrome (APECED)	Autosomal recessive	AIRE-1	21q22.3
	Hypoparathyroidism associated with KSS, MELAS, and MTPDS	Maternal	Mitochondrial genome	
	Hypoparathyroidism associated with complex congenital syndromes (DiGeorge)	Autosomal dominant	TBX1	22q11.2,10p
	HDR syndrome	Autosomal dominant	GATA3	10p14
	Blomstrand's lethal chondrodysplasia	Autosomal recessive	PTHR/PTHrPR	3p21.3
	Kenney-Caffey, Sanjad-Sakati	Autosomal dominant/recessive	TBCE	1q42.3
	Barakat	Autosomal recessive†	Unknown	?
	Lymphedema	Autosomal recessive	Unknown	?
	Nephropathy, nerve deafness	Autosomal dominant†	Unknown	?
	Nerve deafness without renal dysplasia	Autosomal dominant	Unknown	?
	Pseudohypoparathyroidism (type Ia)	Autosomal dominant paternally imprinted	GNAS exons 1–13	20q13.3
	Pseudohypoparathyroidism (type Ib)	Autosomal dominant paternally imprinted	Deletion upstream of or within GNAS locus	20q13.3

HDR, Hypoparathyroidism, deafness, renal dysplasia; *KSS*, Kearns-Sayre syndrome; *MELAS*, mitochondrial encephalopathy, stroke-like episodes, and lactic acidosis; *MTPDS*, mitochondrial trifunctional protein deficiency syndrome.
*Mutations of PTH gene identified only in some families.
†Most likely inheritance shown, location not known.
SOSC3 is shown in parenthesis at the genetic abnormality likely exerts a positive effect to alter SOSC3 expression.

advantage to a single parathyroid cell and its progeny, leading to their clonal expansion.

In hereditary forms of the disease, two distinct, sequentially occurring molecular defects are observed. The first "hit" (point mutation or deletion) is an inherited genetic defect, which affects only one allele that comprises a gene encoding an anti-oncogene (see Fig. 5-4B). Subsequently, a somatic mutation or deletion affecting the second allele occurs in a single parathyroid cell, and because of the resulting growth advantage, this mutation leads to its monoclonal expansion and thus the development of parathyroid tumors. Examples of this latter molecular mechanism in the development of hyperparathyroidism are the inactivation of tumor-suppressor genes such as the multiple endocrine neoplasia type 1 (*MEN1*) gene, the hyperparathyroidism–jaw tumor (*HPT–JT*) gene, and the retinoblastoma (*Rb*) gene (see Table 5-1).

PARATHYROID ADENOMA 1 AND *PTH* GENES

Investigations of the *PTH* gene in sporadic parathyroid adenomas detected abnormally sized restriction fragment length polymorphisms (RFLPs) with a DNA probe for the 5′ part of the PTH

gene in some adenomas,[134] indicating disruption of the gene. Further studies of the tumor DNA demonstrated that the first exon of the *PTH* gene (see Fig. 5-2) was separated from the fragments containing the second and third exons, and that a rearrangement had occurred, juxtaposing the 5′ PTH regulatory elements with "new" non-PTH DNA.[135] This rearrangement was not found in the DNA from the peripheral leukocytes of the patients, thereby indicating that it represented a somatic event and not an inherited germline mutation. Investigation of this rearranged DNA sequence localized it to chromosome 11q13, and detailed analysis revealed that it was highly conserved in different species and expressed in normal parathyroids and in parathyroid adenomas. The protein expressed as a result of this rearrangement, which was designated *PRAD1*, was demonstrated to encode a 295-amino-acid member of the cyclin-D family of cell-cycle regulatory proteins. Cyclins were initially characterized in the dividing cells of budding yeast, where they controlled the G_1 to S transition of the cell cycle, and in marine mollusks, where they regulated the mitotic phase (M-phase) of the cell cycle.[136] Cyclins have also been identified in man and have an important

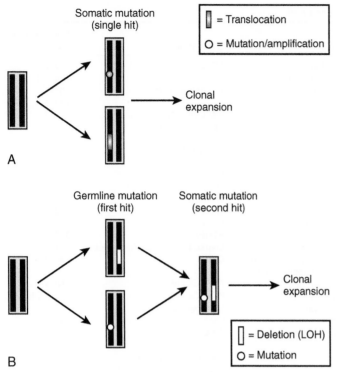

FIGURE 5-4. Schematic illustration of molecular defects that can lead to development of parathyroid tumors. **A,** Somatic mutation (point mutation or translocation) affecting a proto-oncogene (e.g., PRAD1 or RET) results in a growth advantage of single parathyroid cell and thus its clonal expansion. **B,** Inherited single point mutation or deletion affecting a tumor-suppressor gene (first hit) makes the parathyroid cell susceptible to a second, somatic "hit" (point mutation or deletion, i.e., LOH), which then leads to clonal expansion of a single cell.

Table 5-2. Multiple Endocrine Neoplasia Syndromes, Characteristic Tumors, and Associated Genetic Abnormalities*

Type (Chromosomal Location)	Tumors
MEN1 (11q13)	Parathyroids
	Pancreatic islets
	Gastrinoma
	Insulinoma
	Glucagonoma
	VIPoma
	Ppoma
	Pituitary (anterior)
	Prolactinoma
	Somatotrophinoma
	Corticotrophinoma
	Nonfunctioning
	Associated tumors
	Adrenal cortical
	Carcinoid
	Lipoma
	Angiofibromas
	Collagenomas
MEN2 (10 cen-10q 11.2)	
MEN2A	Medullary thyroid carcinoma
	Pheochromocytoma
	Parathyroid
MTC-only	Medullary thyroid carcinoma
MEN2B	Medullary thyroid carcinoma
	Pheochromocytoma
	Associated abnormalities
	Mucosal neuromas
	Marfanoid habitus
	Medullated corneal nerve fibers
	Megacolon

*Autosomal-dominant inheritance of the multiple endocrine neoplasia (MEN) syndromes has been established.

role in regulating many stages of cell-cycle progression. Thus PRAD1, which encoded a novel cyclin referred to as *cyclin D1* (CCND1), is an important cell-cycle regulator, and overexpression of PRAD1 may be an important event in the development of at least 15% of sporadic parathyroid adenomas.[137,138]

Interestingly, more than 66% of the transgenic mice overexpressing PRAD1 under the control of a mammary tissue-specific promoter were found to develop breast carcinoma in adult life,[139] and expression of this proto-oncogene under the control of the 5′ regulatory region of the *PTH* gene resulted in mild to moderate chronic hyperparathyroidism.[137,138] Taken together, these findings in transgenic animals provide further evidence for the conclusion that PRAD1 can be involved in the development of a significant number of parathyroid adenomas.

In addition to the rearrangement of the *PTH* gene in some parathyroid adenomas, a nonsense mutation of the *PTH* gene, Arg83Stop, that occurred in association with LOH of the *PTH* locus has been reported in a parathyroid adenoma.[140] The patient, who had presented with hypercalcemia and an undetectable serum PTH concentration, showed heterozygosity in the peripheral-blood leukocytes with wild-type and mutant alleles, but the parathyroid adenoma had a loss of the wild-type allele and retention of the mutant (Arg83Stop) allele, which predicts that the tumor secretes only a PTH peptide that is truncated after the 52nd amino acid. Following removal of the parathyroid adenoma, normocalcemia was restored.[140] These findings demonstrate that *PTH* nonsense mutations, which result in truncated forms of PTH not recognizable by standard hormone assays, may

be associated with parathyroid adenoma, and that endogenously produced N-terminal PTH fragments can be biologically active.[140]

MULTIPLE ENDOCRINE NEOPLASIA 1 GENE

MEN1 is characterized by the combined occurrence of tumors of the parathyroids, pancreatic islet cells, and anterior pituitary (Table 5-2).[141,142] Parathyroid tumors occur in 95% of MEN1 patients, and the resulting hypercalcemia is the first manifestation of MEN1 in about 90% of patients. Pancreatic islet cell tumors occur in 40% of MEN1 patients; gastrinomas, leading to the Zollinger-Ellison syndrome, are the most common type and also the important cause of morbidity and mortality in MEN1 patients. Anterior pituitary tumors occur in 30% of MEN1 patients, with prolactinomas representing the most common type. Associated tumors, which may also occur in MEN1, include adrenal cortical tumors, carcinoid tumors, lipomas, and cutaneous angiofibromas and collagenomas.[142,143] The gene causing MEN1 was localized to a less than 300-kb region on chromosome 11q13 by genetic mapping studies that investigated MEN1-associated tumors for LOH and by segregation studies in MEN1 families.[144] The results of these studies, which were consistent with Knudson's model for tumor development, indicated that the *MEN1* gene represented a putative tumor-suppressor gene (see Fig. 5-4B). Characterization of genes from this region led to the identification of the *MEN1* gene, which consists of 10 exons that encode a novel 610-amino-acid protein referred to as *menin*.[145,146] Over 1100 germline *MEN1* mutations have been identified, and the majority (>80%) are inactivating and are consistent with its role as a tumor-suppressor gene.[147,148] These mutations are diverse in their types, and in approximate percentages, 25% are nonsense, 45% are frameshift deletions or insertions, 9% are splice-site mutations, 20% are missense mutations, and 1% are whole or partial gene deletions.[144,147-149] In addition, the *MEN1* mutations are scattered throughout the 1830-bp coding region of the gene with no evidence for clustering. Correlations between the MEN1 germline mutations and the clinical manifestations of the disorder appear to be absent.[147-150] Tumors from MEN1 patients and non-MEN1 patients have been observed to harbor the germline mutation together with a somatic LOH involving chromosome 11q13, as expected from Knudson's model and the proposed role of the *MEN1* gene as a tumor suppressor.[148,151-161] The role of the *MEN1* gene in the etiology of familial isolated hyperparathyroidism (FIHP) has also been investigated, and germline *MEN1* mutations have been reported in 29 families with FIHP.[148,151,162-164] The sole occurrence of parathyroid tumors in these families is remarkable, and the mechanisms that determine the altered phenotypic expressions of these mutations remain to be elucidated.

The function of menin has been investigated by identifying its interactions with other proteins, and by under- or overexpression in in vitro studies. Menin has no homology to any known proteins or sequence motifs other than three nuclear localization signals (NLSs) in its C-terminal segment. Subcellular localization studies have shown that menin is predominantly a nuclear protein in nondividing cells, but in dividing cells, it is found in the cytoplasm. Menin has been shown to interact with a number of proteins that are involved in transcriptional regulation, genome stability, cell division, and proliferation.[148]

The functional role of menin as a tumor suppressor also has been investigated, and studies in human fibroblasts have revealed that menin acts as a repressor of telomerase activity via hTERT (a protein component of telomerase).[165] Furthermore, overexpression of menin in the human endocrine pancreatic tumor cell line (BON1) resulted in an inhibition of cell growth[166] that was accompanied by up-regulation of JunD expression but downregulation of delta-like protein 1/preadipocyte factor-1, proliferating cell nuclear antigen, and QM/Jif-1, which is a negative regulator of c-Jun.[166] These findings of growth suppression by menin were observed in other cell types. Thus, expression of menin in the RAS-transformed NIH3T3 cells partially suppressed the RAS-mediated tumor phenotype in vitro and in vivo.[167] Overexpression of menin in CHO-IR cells also suppressed insulin-induced AP-1 transactivation, and this was accompanied by an inhibition of c-Fos induction at the transcriptional level.[168] Furthermore, menin reexpression in *Men1*-deficient mouse Leydig tumor cell lines induced cell cycle arrest and apoptosis.[169] In contrast, depletion of menin in human fibroblasts resulted in their immortalization.[165] Thus, menin appears to have a large number of functions through interactions with proteins, and these mediate alterations in cell proliferation.

MULTIPLE ENDOCRINE NEOPLASIA 2 GENE (c-ret)

MEN2 describes the association (see Table 5-2) of medullary thyroid carcinoma (MTC), pheochromocytomas, and parathyroid tumors.[141,144] Three clinical variants of MEN2 are recognized: MEN2a, MEN2b, and MTC-only (see Table 5-2). MEN2a is the most common variant, and the development of MTC is associated with pheochromocytomas (50% of patients), which may be bilateral, and parathyroid tumors (20% of patients). MEN2b, which represents 5% of all MEN2 cases, is characterized

by the occurrence of MTC and pheochromocytoma in association with a Marfanoid habitus, mucosal neuromas, medullated corneal fibers, and intestinal autonomic ganglion dysfunction leading to multiple diverticula and megacolon. Parathyroid tumors do not usually occur in MEN2b. MTC-only is a variant in which medullary thyroid carcinoma is the sole manifestation of the syndrome. The gene causing all three MEN2 variants was mapped to chromosome 10cen-10q11.2, a region containing the *c-ret* proto-oncogene which encodes a tyrosine kinase receptor with cadherin-like and cysteine-rich extracellular domains, and a tyrosine kinase intracellular domain.[170,171] Specific mutations of *c-ret* have been identified for each of the three MEN2 variants. Thus in 95% of patients, MEN2a is associated with mutations of the cysteine-rich extracellular domain, and mutations in codon 634 (Cys→Arg) account for 85% of *MEN2A* mutations. However, a search for *c-ret* mutations in sporadic non-MEN2a parathyroid adenomas revealed no codon 634 mutations.[172,173] MTC-only is also associated with missense mutations in the cysteine-rich extracellular domain, and most mutations are in codon 618. However, MEN2b is associated with mutations in codon 918 (Met→Thr) of the intracellular tyrosine kinase domain in 95% of patients. Interestingly, the *c-ret* proto-oncogene is also involved in the etiology of papillary thyroid carcinomas and in Hirschsprung's disease. Mutational analysis of *c-ret* to detect mutations in codons 609, 611, 618, 634, 768, and 804 in MEN2a and MTC-only, and codon 918 in MEN2b, has been used in the diagnosis and management of patients and families with these disorders.[171,174]

HYPERPARATHYROIDISM–JAW TUMOR SYNDROME GENE

The HPT–JT syndrome is an autosomal-dominant disorder characterized by the development of parathyroid adenomas and carcinomas, and fibro-osseous jaw tumors.[175,176] In addition, some patients may also develop uterine tumors and renal abnormalities, which include Wilms' tumors, renal cysts, renal hamartomas, renal cortical adenomas, and papillary renal cell carcinomas.[177] Other tumors, including pancreatic adenocarcinomas, testicular mixed germ cell tumors with a major seminoma component, and Hurthle cell thyroid adenomas have also been reported in some patients.[132,177] It is important to note that the parathyroid tumors may occur in isolation and without any evidence of jaw tumors, and this may cause confusion with other hereditary hypercalcemic disorders such as MEN1, familial benign hypercalcemia (FBH) (which is also referred to as *familial hypocalciuric hypercalcemia* [FHH]), and FIHP.[178] HPT–JT can be distinguished from FBH, because in FBH, serum calcium levels are elevated during the early neonatal or infantile period, whereas in HPT–JT, such elevations are uncommon in the first decade. In addition, HPT–JT patients, unlike FBH patients, will have associated hypercalciuria. The distinction between HPT–JT patients and MEN1 patients, who have only developed the usual first manifestation of hypercalcemia (>90% of patients), is more difficult and is likely to be influenced by operative and histologic findings and by the occurrence of other characteristic lesions in each disorder. It is important to note that HPT–JT patients will usually have single adenomas or a carcinoma, but MEN1 patients will often have multiglandular parathyroid disease. The distinction between FIHP and HPT–JT in the absence of jaw tumors is difficult but important; HPT–JT patients may be at a higher risk of developing parathyroid carcinomas.[179-181] These distinctions may be helped by the identification of additional features, and a search for jaw tumors, renal, pancreatic, thyroid, and testicular abnormalities may help to identify HPT–JT patients. The jaw tumors in HPT–JT are different from the brown tumors observed in some patients with primary hyperparathyroidism and do not resolve after parathyroidectomy.[178] Indeed, ossifying fibromas of the jaw are an important distinguishing feature of HPT–JT from FIHP, and the occurrence of these may occasionally precede the development of hypercalcemia in HPT–JT patients by several decades. The gene causing HPT–JT is located on chromosome 1q31.2 and consists of 17 exons that encode a ubiquitously expressed and evolutionarily conserved 531-amino-acid protein, designated *parafibromin*.[132,182] This gene, *CDC73*, is also referred to as *HRPT2* (i.e., hyperparathyroidism type 2). *HRPT2* mutations associated with HPT–JT were found to be scattered throughout the 1593-bp coding region, with the majority (>80%) predicting a functional loss through premature truncation. A genotype-phenotype correlation was not apparent from these analyses.[177,182,184] The observation of LOH involving the chromosome 1q31.2 region in HPT–JT-associated tumors indicated that parafibromin may be acting as a tumor suppressor, consistent with Knudson's two-hit hypothesis.[177,178,182] This was supported by the observations of germline and somatic *HRPT2* mutations in HPT–JT-associated tumors.[177,182-185] Similar germline and somatic *HRPT2* mutations have also been found in sporadic parathyroid carcinomas, and the frequency of such mutations is high, ranging from 67% to 100%[183,186]; however, the frequency of *HRPT2* mutations in sporadic parathyroid adenomas is low at 0% to 4%, indicating that *HRPT2* mutations likely confer an aggressive growth potential to the parathyroid cells.[182-184,186,187] *HRPT2* mutations and allelic imbalances have also been identified in sporadic renal tumors,[188] and a loss or down-regulation of *HRPT2* expression has been reported in both breast and gastric cancers.[189,190] These studies indicate that *HRPT2* and its encoded protein, parafibromin, play a critical role in inherited and sporadic parathyroid cancers as well as other nonhereditary solid tumors. The role of parafibromin, which is predominantly a nuclear protein with a monopartite NLS,[191] was not readily apparent, inasmuch as it has no homologies to known proteins. However, the approximately 200 amino acids of the C-terminal domain shared over 25% sequence identity with the yeast Cdc73 protein which is a component of the yeast polymerase-associated factor 1 (PAF1) complex, a key transcriptional regulatory complex that interacts directly with RNA polymerase II.[182,192,193] Studies of the PAF1 complex in yeast and *Drosophila*, as well as in mammalian cells, have revealed that parafibromin, as part of the PAF1 complex, is a mediator of the key transcriptional events of histone modification, chromatin remodeling, initiation and elongation, and the wnt/β-catenin signaling pathway.[192-194] Studies of a mouse deleted for HRPTt2 have revealed that HRPT2 expression and the PARAFIBROMIN/PAF complex directly regulate genes (e.g., *H19*, *IgF1*, *Igf3*, *Igfbp4*, *Hmga1*, *Hmga2*, and *Hmga3*) that are involved in cell growth and apoptosis.[195]

LRP5 AND THE WNT/β-CATENIN PATHWAY

Aberrant Wnt/β-catenin signaling with an accumulation of β-catenin in the cytoplasm and nucleus is associated with several types of tumor development (e.g., adenomatous polyposis coli and colorectal cancer). Investigations of this pathway in parathyroid tumors have revealed that β-catenin accumulation occurs in parathyroid adenomas and in parathyroid tumors associated with chronic renal failure.[196] In addition, a protein-stabilizing mutation, Ser37Ala, in exon 3 of β-catenin was detected in over 7% of parathyroid adenomas but not parathyroid tumors of chronic renal failure, from Swedish patients[197,198] but

not North American[199] or Japanese[200] patients. The Ser37Ala β-catenin mutations were homozygous in the parathyroid adenomas, which had a higher expression of β-catenin and the non-phosphorylated active form of β-catenin.[198] In addition, MYC, which is a direct target of the Wnt/β-catenin signaling pathway in colorectal cancer cells and a critical mediator of the early stages of intestinal neoplasia, was also overexpressed, and the stable activity of endogenous β-catenin was found to be necessary for MYC and cyclin D1 expression.[196] Stability of β-catenin is regulated by Wnt ligands, which bind to the cell-surface frizzled receptors and LRP5 and LRP6 co-receptors that alter phosphorylation of several intracellular second messengers and consequently accumulation of nonphosphorylated β-catenin. Investigation of the Wnt signaling pathway in parathyroid tumors revealed that over 85% of adenomas and 100% of tumors from chronic renal failure patients have a shorter LRP5 transcript, which contained an in-frame deletion of 142 amino acids (residues 666 to 809) that encompassed the third YWTD beta propeller domain between the second and third epidermal growth factor repeats.[197] This internally truncated LRP5 receptor activated β-catenin signaling in parathyroid tumors by a mechanism that may involve an impaired inhibitory action of the WNT antagonist, DKK1.[197] The parathyroid tumors expressing the internally truncated LRP5 receptor did not harbor the β-catenin stabilizing mutation, Ser37Ala, and those that had the stabilizing β-catenin mutation did not express the truncated LRP5 receptor.[197] Thus, it seems that the presence of the stabilizing β-catenin mutation and the expression of the truncated LRP5 receptor are mutually exclusive. However, these studies demonstrate an important role for the WNT β-catenin signaling pathway in parathyroid tumorigenesis.

Rb GENE

The *Rb* gene, which is a tumor-suppressor gene[201] located on chromosome 13q14, is involved in the pathogenesis of retinoblastomas and a variety of common sporadic human malignancies including ductal breast, small cell lung carcinoma, and bladder carcinomas. Allelic deletion of the *Rb* gene has been demonstrated in all parathyroid carcinomas and in 10% of parathyroid adenomas[202,203] and was accompanied by abnormal staining patterns for the Rb protein in 50% of the parathyroid carcinomas but in none of the parathyroid adenomas.[202] These results demonstrate an important role for the *Rb* gene in the development of parathyroid carcinomas and may be of help in the histologic distinction of parathyroid adenoma from carcinoma.[202] The Rb protein may also be secondarily involved in parathyroid tumorigenesis by its interaction with the retinoblastoma-interacting zinc finger protein 1, RIZ1.[204] The findings of extensive deletions of the long arm of chromosome 13 (including the *Rb* locus) in some parathyroid adenomas and carcinomas,[203] and similar findings in pituitary carcinomas,[205] suggest that other tumor-suppressor genes on chromosome 13q may also have a role in the development of such tumors.

RETINOBLASTOMA-INTERACTING ZINC FINGER PROTEIN 1 GENE ON CHROMOSOME 1P

Loss of heterozygosity studies have revealed allelic loss of chromosome 1p32-pter in 40% of sporadic parathyroid adenomas.[206] This region is estimated to be about 110 cM, equivalent to about 110 million base pairs (Mbp) of DNA, but additional studies narrowed the interval containing this putative tumor-suppressor gene(s) to an approximately 4-cM (i.e., about 4-Mbp) region.[207] Investigations of one candidate gene, retinoblastoma-interacting zinc finger protein 1 (RIZ1), have revealed that over 25% of parathyroid tumors had LOH of the RIZ1 locus, and that over 35% of parathyroid tumors had hypermethylation of the RIZ1 promoter region.[204] Moreover, the RIZ1 promoter hypermethylation was related to LOH in these tumors, indicating that these two events may represent the "two hits" (see Fig. 5-4B) required for tumor development in Knudson's hypothesis for tumorigenesis.[204]

NONSYNDROMIC FAMILIAL ISOLATED HYPERPARATHYROIDISM

FIHP may represent an incomplete manifestation of a syndromic form such as MEN1, FHH, or HPT-JT.[163,164,182,208] Twenty-nine MEN1, nine HRPT2 and five CaSR germline mutations have been reported to date in FIHP kindreds.[164] However, it is important to note that the genetic etiology of nonsyndromic FIHP in the majority of families remains to be elucidated.[209,210] Thus, studies of 32 kindreds with nonsyndromic FIHP for mutations of the MEN1, CaSR, and HRPT2 genes have revealed that only one family harbored a germline mutation, and this involved the HRPT2 gene that encodes parafibromin.[209,210] However, studies of 10 other FIHP kindreds have indicated that another locus, referred to as HRPT3, on chromosome 2p13.3-p14, is likely to be involved in the etiology of nonsyndromic FIHP.[211] Thus, the genes and their underlying abnormalities that lead to nonsyndromic FIHP remain to be identified.

HYPERPARATHYROIDISM IN CHRONIC RENAL FAILURE

Chronic renal failure is often associated with a form of secondary hyperparathyroidism that may subsequently result in the hypercalcemic state of "tertiary" hyperparathyroidism. The parathyroid proliferative response in this condition led to the proposal that the autonomous parathyroid tissue might have undergone hyperplastic change and therefore be polyclonal in origin. However, studies of X-chromosome inactivation in parathyroids from patients on hemodialysis with refractory hyperparathyroidism have revealed at least one monoclonal parathyroid tumor in over 60% of patients.[133] In addition, LOH involving several loci on chromosome Xp11 was detected in one of these parathyroid tumors, thereby suggesting the involvement of a tumor-suppressor gene from this region in the pathogenesis of such tumors.[133] Interestingly, none of the parathyroid tumors from these patients with chronic renal failure had LOH involving loci from chromosome 11q13. This unexpected finding of monoclonal parathyroid tumors in the majority of patients with "tertiary" hyperparathyroidism suggests that an increased turnover of parathyroid cells in secondary hyperparathyroidism may possibly render the parathyroid glands more susceptible to mitotic nondisjunction or other mechanisms of somatic deletions, which may involve loci other than those—MEN1 and PRAD1—located on chromosome 11q13. In addition, as noted above, parathyroid tumors from patients with chronic renal failure have been shown to accumulate β-catenin and to have a truncated form of the LRP5 receptor, which lacks 142 amino acids.[196,197]

DISORDERS OF THE CALCIUM-SENSING RECEPTOR

Three hypercalcemic disorders due to mutations and/or reduced activity of CaSR have been reported,[208,212-217] which are FBH, also referred to as FHH, neonatal severe hyperparathyroidism (NSHPT), and autoimmune hypocalciuric hypercalcemia (AHH) (Table 5-3).

Table 5-3. Diseases Associated With Abnormalities of the Extracellular Calcium-Sensing Receptor (CaSR)

CaSR Abnormality and Disease	CaSR Genotype
Loss-of-function CaSR mutation	
Familial benign hypercalcemia	Heterozygous
Neonatal severe primary hyperparathyroidism	Heterozygous or homozygous (mutant)
Gain-of-function CaSR mutation	
Autosomal-dominant hypocalcemic hypercalciuria	Heterozygous
Bartter syndrome type V	Heterozygous
CaSR autoantibodies	
Autoimmune hypocalciuric hypercalcemia	Homozygous (normal)
Acquired hypoparathyroidism	Homozygous (normal)

FAMILIAL BENIGN HYPERCALCEMIA AND NEONATAL SEVERE HYPERPARATHYROIDISM

Mutational analyses of the human CaSR, which is a G protein–coupled receptor located on chromosome 3q21.1,[218] have revealed different mutations that result in a loss-of-function of the CaSR in patients with FBH and NSHPT.[212-217] Many of these mutations cluster around the aspartate- and glutamate-rich regions (codons 39-300) within the extracellular domain of the receptor, and this has been proposed to contain low-affinity calcium-binding sites, based on similarities to that of calsequestrin, in which the ligand-binding pockets also contain negatively charged amino acid residues.[208,219] Approximately two-thirds of the FBH kindreds investigated have been found to have unique heterozygous mutations of the CaSR, and expression studies of these mutations have demonstrated a loss of CaSR function whereby there is an increase in the calcium ion–dependent set-point for PTH release from the parathyroid cell.[212,217,220,221] NSHPT occurring in the offspring of consanguineous FBH families has been shown to be due to homozygous CaSR mutations.[212,213,215,222,223] However, some patients with sporadic neonatal hyperparathyroidism have been reported to be associated with de novo heterozygous CaSR mutations,[214] thereby suggesting that factors other than mutant gene dosage[222]—for example, the degree of set-point abnormality, the bony sensitivity to PTH, and the maternal extracellular calcium concentration—may also all play a role in the phenotypic expression of a CaSR mutation in the neonate. The remaining third of FBH families in whom a mutation within the coding region of the CaSR has not been demonstrated may either have an abnormality in the promoter of the gene or a mutation at one of the two other FBH loci that have been revealed by family linkage studies. One of these FBH loci is located on chromosome 19p and is referred to as FBH_{19p}.[224] Studies of another FBH kindred from Oklahoma that also suffered from progressive elevations in PTH, hypophosphatemia, and osteomalacia[225,226] demonstrated that this variant, designated FBH_{Ok}, was linked to chromosome 19q13.[227] These three FBH loci located on chromosomes 3q, 19p, and 19q have also been referred to as FBH (or FHH) types 1, 2, and 3, respectively.[227]

AUTOIMMUNE HYPOCALCIURIC HYPERCALCEMIA

Some patients who have the clinical features of FHH but not CaSR mutations may have AHH (see also Chapter 7). Four patients with AHH who all had other autoimmune manifestations have been reported[228]: three patients had antithyroid antibodies, and one had sprue with antigliadin and antiendomysial antibodies. These patients were shown to have circulating antibodies to the extracellular domain of the CaSR, and these antibodies stimulated PTH release from dispersed human parathyroid cells in vitro, probably by inhibiting the activation of the CaSR by extracellular calcium.[228] Thus, AHH is a condition of extracellular calcium sensing that should be considered in FHH patients who do not have *CaSR* mutations.

JANSEN'S DISEASE

Jansen's disease (Figs. 5-5 and 5-6) is an autosomal-dominant disease that is characterized by short-limbed dwarfism caused by an abnormal regulation of chondrocyte proliferation and differentiation in the metaphyseal growth plate and associated, usually severe, hypercalcemia and hypophosphatemia despite normal or undetectable serum levels of PTH or PTHrP.[229] These abnormalities are caused by mutations in the PTH/PTHrP receptor that lead to constitutive, PTH- and PTHrP-independent receptor activation.[230-232] Three different heterozygous mutations of the PTH/PTHrP receptor have been identified in the severe form of Jansen's disease, and these involve codon 223 (His→Arg), codon 410 (Thr→Pro), and codon 458 (Ile→Arg) (Fig. 5-7). Expression of the mutant receptors in COS-7 cells result in constitutive, ligand-independent accumulation of cAMP, while the basal accumulation of inositol phosphates is not measurably increased.[230-232] Since the PTH/PTHrP receptor is most abundantly expressed in kidney and bone and in the metaphyseal growth plate, these findings provide a likely explanation for the abnormalities observed in mineral homeostasis and growth plate development associated with this disorder. This conclusion is supported further by observations in mice which express the human PTH/PTHrP receptor, with the His223Arg mutation under the control of the rat α_1(II) promoter.[233] This promoter targeted expression of the mutant receptor to the layer of proliferative chondrocytes, delayed their differentiation into hypertrophic cells, and led, at least in animals with multiple copies of the transgene, to a mild impairment in growth of long bones. These observations are consistent with the conclusion that expression of a constitutively active human PTH/PTHrP receptor in growth plate chondrocytes

causes the characteristic metaphyseal changes in patients with Jansen's disease.

Another novel heterozygous PTH/PTHrP receptor mutation, T410R, was identified in several members of a small kindred with an apparently mild form of Jansen's disease.[234] Affected individuals had, compared to patients with the previously identified activating PTH/PTHrP receptor mutations,[230-232] less severe growth plate abnormalities, relatively normal stature, normal plasma calcium concentration, yet significant hypercalciuria and normal or suppressed plasma PTH levels. When tested in vitro, the PTH/PTHrP receptor with the T410R mutation showed less constitutive activity than that observed with the previously

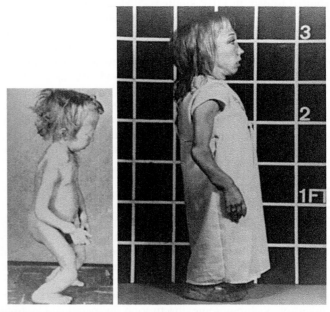

FIGURE 5-5. Patient with Jansen's metaphyseal chondrodysplasia at ages 5 *(left)* and 22 years *(right)*. (From Frame B, Poznanski AK: Conditions that may be confused with rickets. In DeLuca HF, Anast CS editors: Pediatric diseases related to calcium, New York, 1980, Elsevier, pp 269–289.[341])

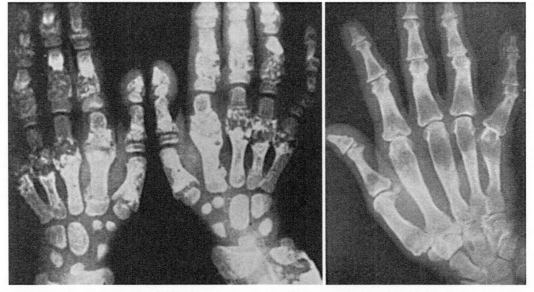

FIGURE 5-6. Hand radiographs at ages 10 *(left)* and 44 years *(right)* of the patient first described by Jansen. (From De Haas WHD, De Boer W, Griffioen F, et al: Metaphysial dysostosis: a late follow-up of the first reported case, J Bone Joint Surg Br 51:290–299, 1969.[342])

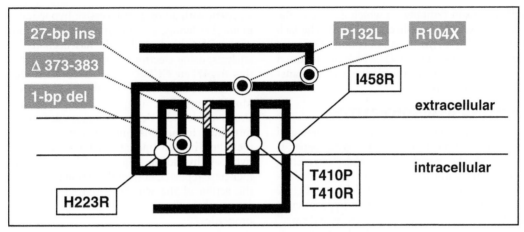

FIGURE 5-7. Schematic representation of the human PTH/PTHrP receptor. Approximate locations of heterozygous missense mutations that lead to constitutive receptor activation in patients with Jansen's disease are indicated by *open circles*. Homozygous loss-of-function mutations identified in patients with Blomstrand's disease are indicated by *striped boxes* or *grey circles*. The nucleotide exchange in exon M5 of the maternal PTH/PTHrP receptor allele introduces a novel splice acceptor site that leads to synthesis of an abnormal receptor protein which lacks portions of the fifth membrane-spanning domain (*stippled box*); for yet unknown reasons, the paternal allele is not expressed in this patient (see text for details).

described T410P mutant.[231,235] This less pronounced agonist-independent cAMP accumulation induced by the T410R mutation is consistent with the less severe skeletal and laboratory abnormalities observed in this milder form of Jansen's disease.

WILLIAMS SYNDROME

Williams syndrome is an autosomal-dominant disorder characterized by supravalvular aortic stenosis, elfin-like facies, psychomotor retardation, and infantile hypercalcemia. The underlying abnormality of calcium metabolism remains unknown, but abnormal $1,25(OH)_2D_3$ metabolism or decreased calcitonin production have been implicated, although none have been consistently demonstrated. Studies have demonstrated hemizygosity at the elastin locus on chromosome 7q11.23 in over 90% of patients with the classical Williams phenotype,[236-238] and only one patient had a cytogenetically identifiable deletion, thereby indicating that the syndrome is usually due to a microdeletion of 7q11.23.[238] Interestingly, ablation of the elastin gene in mice results in vascular abnormalities similar to those observed in patients with Williams syndrome.[239] However, the microdeletions that have been reported involve also another gene, designated LIM-kinase, that is expressed in the central nervous system.[240] The calcitonin receptor gene, which is located on chromosome 7q21, is not involved in the deletions found in Williams syndrome and is therefore unlikely to be implicated in the hypercalcemia of such children.[241] While deletion of the elastin and LIM-kinase genes can explain the respective cardiovascular and neurologic features of Williams syndrome, it seems likely that another, as yet uncharacterized, gene that is within this contiguously deleted region is involved in this disorder and could explain the abnormalities of calcium metabolism.

Hypocalcemic Disorders

HYPOPARATHYROIDISM

Hypoparathyroidism may occur as part of a pluriglandular autoimmune disorder or as a complex congenital defect, as for example in the DiGeorge syndrome. In addition, hypoparathyroidism may develop as a solitary endocrinopathy, and this has

been called *isolated* or *idiopathic hypoparathyroidism*. Familial occurrences of isolated hypoparathyroidism with autosomal-dominant, autosomal-recessive, and X-linked-recessive inheritances have been established.

PARATHYROID HORMONE GENE ABNORMALITIES

DNA sequence analysis of the *PTH* gene (see Fig. 5-2) from one patient with autosomal-dominant isolated hypoparathyroidism has revealed a single base substitution (T→C) in exon 2,[242] which resulted in the substitution of arginine (CGT) for cysteine (TGT) in the signal peptide. The presence of this charged amino acid in the midst of the hydrophobic core of the signal peptide impeded the processing of the mutant preproPTH, as demonstrated by in vitro studies. These revealed that the mutation impaired the interaction of the nascent protein with the translocation machinery and that cleavage of the mutant signal sequence by solubilized signal peptidase was ineffective.[242,243] Studies using transfected HEK293 cells showed that the mutant PTH is trapped intracellularly, predominantly in the endoplasmic reticulum (ER), which is toxic for the cells and leads to apoptosis.[244] In another family with autosomal-recessive hypoparathyroidism, a single base substitution (T→C) involving codon 23 of exon 2 was detected. This resulted in the substitution of proline (CCG) for the normal serine (TCG) in the signal peptide.[245] This mutation alters the −3 position of the pre-pro-PTH protein cleavage site. Indeed, amino acid residues at the −3 and −1 positions of the signal peptidase recognition site have to conform to certain criteria for correct processing through the rough endoplasmic reticulum (RER), and one of these is an absence of proline in the region −3 and +1 of the site. Thus, the presence of a proline, which is a strong helix-breaking residue, at the −3 position is likely to disrupt cleavage of the mutant pre-pro-PTH that would be subsequently degraded in the RER, and PTH would not be available.[245] Another abnormality of the *PTH* gene, involving a donor splice site at the exon 2/intron 2 boundary, has been identified in one family with autosomal-recessive isolated hypoparathyroidism.[246] This mutation involved a single base transition (g→c) at position 1 of intron 2, and an assessment of the effects of this alteration in the invariant gt dinucleotide of the 5′ donor splice site consensus on mRNA processing revealed that the mutation resulted in exon skipping, in which exon 2 of the *PTH* gene was lost, and exon 1 was spliced to exon 3. The lack of exon 2 would lead to a loss of the initiation codon (ATG) and the signal peptide sequence (see Fig. 5-2), which are required for the commencement of PTH mRNA translation and the translocation of the PTH peptide, respectively.

GLIAL CELLS MISSING B ABNORMALITIES

Glial cells missing B *(GCMB)*, which is the human homolog of the *Drosophila* gene, *Gcm*, and of the mouse *gcm2* gene, is expressed exclusively in the parathyroid glands, suggesting that it may be a specific regulator of parathyroid gland development.[247] Mice that were homozygous (–/–) for deletion of *gcm2* lacked parathyroid glands and developed the hypocalcemia and hyperphosphatemia observed in hypoparathyroidism.[247] However, despite their lack of parathyroid glands, Gcm2-deficient (–/–) mice did not have undetectable serum PTH levels, but instead had levels indistinguishable from those of eucalcemic normal (+/+, wild-type) and heterozygous (+/–) mice. This endogenous level of PTH in the Gcm2-deficient (–/–) mice was too low to correct the hypocalcemia, but exogenous continuous PTH infusion could correct the hypocalcemia.[247] Interestingly, there were no compensatory increases in PTHrP or 1,25(OH)$_2$D$_3$. These findings indicate that Gcm2 mice have a normal response (and not resistance) to PTH, and that the PTH in the serum of Gcm2-deficient mice was active. The auxiliary source of PTH was identified to be a cluster of PTH-expressing cells under the thymic capsule. These thymic PTH-producing cells also expressed the CaSR, and long-term treatment of the Gcm2-deficient mice with 1,25(OH)$_2$D$_3$ restored the serum calcium concentrations to normal and reduced the serum PTH levels, thereby indicating that the thymic production of PTH can be down-regulated.[247] However, it appears that this thymic production of PTH cannot be up-regulated, because serum PTH levels are not high despite the hypocalcaemia in the Gcm2-deficient mice. This absence of up-regulation would be consistent with the very small size of the thymic PTH-producing cell cluster when compared to the size of normal parathyroid glands. The development of the thymic PTH-producing cells likely involves Gcm1, which is the other mouse homolog of *Drosophila* Gcm.[248] Gcm1 expression, which could not be detected in parathyroid glands, colocalized with PTH expression in the thymus.[247] The specific role of Gcm2 in the development of the parathyroids from the third pharyngeal pouch has been further investigated by studying the expression of the Hoxa3-Pax1/9-Eya1 transcription factor and Sonic hedgehog–bone morphogenetic protein 4 (Shh-Bmp4) signaling networks.[249] These studies have revealed that Gcm2 (–/–) embryos that are 12 d.p.c. have a parathyroid-specific domain, but that this parathyroid domain undergoes coordinated programmed cell death (apoptosis) by 12.5 d.p.c. in the Gcm2-null mouse embryos.[249] Moreover, the expression of the transcription factors Hoxa3, Pax1, Pax9, Eya1, Tbx1, and of Shh and Bmp4 was normal in the third pharyngeal pouch of these Gcm2-null mouse embryos. These findings indicate that the Hoxa3-Pax1/9-Eya transcription factor cascade, the transcription factor Tbx1, and the Shh-Bmp4 signaling network all act upstream of Gcm2.[249] Moreover, these studies have revealed that Gcm2 has a role in promoting differentiation and survival of parathyroid cells in the developing embryo.[249]

Studies of patients with isolated hypoparathyroidism have shown that *GCMB* mutations are associated with autosomal-recessive and autosomal-dominant forms of the disease.[250-252] A homozygous intragenic deletion of *GCMB* has been identified in

a patient with autosomal-recessive hypoparathyroidism,[250] while in another family, a homozygous missense mutation (Arg47Leu) of the DNA binding domain has been reported.[251] Functional analysis, using electrophoretic mobility shift assays (EMSAs), of this Arg47Leu *GCMB* mutation revealed that it resulted in a loss of DNA binding to the GCM DNA binding site.[251] More recently, heterozygous *GCMB* mutations, which consist of single nucleotide deletions (c1389deT and c1399delC) that introduce frameshifts and premature truncations, have been identified in two unrelated families with autosomal-dominant hypoparathyroidism (Fig. 5-8).[252] By using a GCMB-associated luciferase reporter, both of these mutations were shown to inhibit the action of the wild-type transcription factor, thereby indicating that these GCMB mutants have dominant-negative properties.[252]

X-LINKED RECESSIVE HYPOPARATHYROIDISM

X-linked recessive hypoparathyroidism has been reported in two multigenerational kindreds from Missouri.[253,254] In this disorder, only males are affected, and they suffer from infantile onset of epilepsy and hypocalcemia due to an isolated defect in parathyroid gland development.[255] Relatedness of the two kindreds has been established by demonstrating an identical mitochondrial DNA sequence, inherited via the maternal lineage, in affected males from the two families.[256] Studies utilizing X-linked polymorphic markers in these families localized the mutant gene to chromosome Xq26-q27,[257] and a molecular deletion-insertion that involves chromosome 2p25 and Xq27 has been identified.[258] This deletion-insertion is located approximately 67 kb downstream of SOX3, and hence it is likely to exert a position effect on SOX3 expression. Moreover, SOX3 was shown to be expressed in the developing parathyroids of mouse embryos, and this indicates a likely role for SOX3 in the embryonic development of the parathyroid glands.[258] SOX3 belongs to a family of genes encoding high-mobility group (HMG) box transcription factors and is related to SRY, the sex-determining gene on the Y chromosome. The mouse homolog is expressed in the prestreak embryo and subsequently in the developing central nervous system (CNS) that includes the region of the ventral diencephalon, which induces development of the anterior pituitary and gives rise to the hypothalamus, olfactory placodes, and parathyroids.[258-261] The location of the deletion-insertion approximately 67 kb downstream of SOX3 in X-linked recessive hypoparathyroid patients is likely to result in altered SOX3 expression, since SOX3 expression has been reported to be sensitive to position effects caused by X-chromosome abnormalities.[262] Indeed, reporter construct studies of the mouse *Sox3* gene have demonstrated the presence of both 5′ and 3′ regulatory elements,[263] and thus it is possible that the deletion-insertion in the X-linked recessive hypoparathyroid patients may have a position effect on SOX3 expression and parathyroid development from the pharyngeal pouches. Indeed such position effects on SOX genes, which may be exerted over large distances, have been reported. For example, the very closely related *Sox2* gene has been shown to have regulatory regions spread over a long distance, both 5′ and 3′ to the coding region,[264] and disruption of sequences at some distance 3′ have been reported to lead to loss of expression in the developing inner ear and absence of sensory cells, whereas expression in other sites is unaffected.[265] Similarly for the *SRY* gene, which probably originated from SOX3,[266] both 5′ and 3′ deletions result in abnormalities of sexual development, and translocation breakpoints over 1 Mb upstream of the *SOX9* gene have been reported to result in Campomelic dysplasia due to

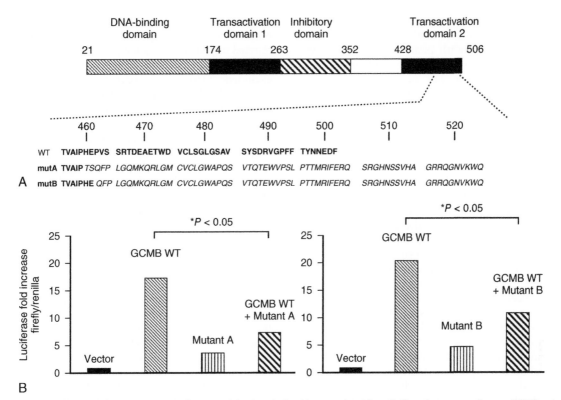

FIGURE 5-8. Heterozygous GCMB mutation can be a cause of autosomal-dominant isolated hypoparathyroidism. **A,** Domain structure of human GCMB and carboxyl-terminal amino acid sequence of wild-type human GCMB (WT) and of the mutants identified in families A (mutA) and B (mutB). Both single nucleotide deletions lead to a frameshift and translation of 65 novel amino acids after proline 464 and of 63 novel amino acids after glutamic acid 466, respectively. Novel amino acids are in *italics*. Numbering of amino acids above. **B,** Luciferase reporter assay using chicken fibroblast DF-1 cells. Cells were co-transfected with plasmids encoding wild-type human GCMB (GCMB WT), combined with either the c.1389delT mutant identified in family A *(left)*, the c.1399delC mutant identified in family B *(right)*, or empty vector; luciferase activity obtained with empty plasmid was defined as 1. (From Mannstadt M, Bertrand G, Muresan M, et al: Dominant-negative GCMB mutations cause an autosomal-dominant form of hypoparathyroidism, J Clin Endocrinol Metab 93:3568–3576, 2008.)

removal of elements that regulate SOX9 expression.[262] The molecular deletion-insertion identified in X-linked recessive hypoparathyroidism may similarly cause position effects on SOX3 expression, and this points to a potential role for the *SOX3* gene in the embryologic development of the parathyroid glands from the pharyngeal pouches.

PLURIGLANDULAR AUTOIMMUNE HYPOPARATHYROIDISM

Hypoparathyroidism may occur in association with candidiasis and autoimmune Addison's disease, and the disorder has been referred to as either the *autoimmune polyendocrinopathy-candidiasis-ectodermal dystrophy* (APECED) syndrome or the *autoimmune polyglandular syndrome type 1* (APS1).[267] This disorder has a high incidence in Finland, and a genetic analysis of Finnish families indicated autosomal-recessive inheritance of the disorder.[268] In addition, the disorder has been reported to have a high incidence among Iranian Jews, although the occurrence of candidiasis was less common in this population.[269] Linkage studies of Finnish families mapped the *APECED* gene to chromosome 21q22.3.[270] Further positional cloning approaches led to the isolation of a novel gene from chromosome 21q22.3. This gene, referred to as *AIRE* (autoimmune regulator), encodes a 545-amino-acid protein that contains motifs suggestive of a transcriptional factor and includes two zinc finger motifs, a proline-rich region, and three LXXLL motifs.[271] Four *AIRE1* mutations are commonly found in APECED families: (1) Arg257 Stop in Finnish, German, Swiss, British, and Northern Italian families; (2) Arg139 Stop in Sardin-

ian families; (3) Tyr85Cys in Iranian Jewish families; and (4) a 13-bp deletion in exon 8 in British, Dutch, German, and Finnish families.[271-275] AIRE1 has been shown to regulate the elimination of organ-specific T cells in the thymus, and thus APECED is likely to be caused by a failure of this specialized mechanism for deleting forbidden T cells and establishing immunologic tolerance.[276] Patients with APS1 may also develop other autoimmune disorders in association with organ-specific autoantibodies, which are similar to those in patients with non-APS1 forms of the disease. Examples of such autoantibodies and related diseases are GAD6S autoantibodies in diabetes mellitus type 1A and 21-hydroxylase autoantibodies in Addison's disease. Patients with APS1 may also develop autoantibodies that react with specific autoantigens that are not found in non-APS1 patients. Examples of this are autoantibodies to type 1 interferon omega (IFN-ω), which are present in all APS1 patients,[277] and to NACHT leucine-rich-repeat protein 5 (NALP5), which is a parathyroid-specific autoantibody present in 49% of patients with APS1 associated hypoparathyroidism.[278] NALP proteins are essential components of the inflammasome and activate the innate immune system in different inflammatory and autoimmune disorders such as vitiligo, which involves NALP1, and gout, which involves NALP3.[279] The precise role of NALP5 in APS1-associated hypoparathyroidism remains to be elucidated.

DIGEORGE SYNDROME

Patients with the DiGeorge syndrome (DGS) typically suffer from hypoparathyroidism; immunodeficiency; congenital heart defects; and deformities of the ear, nose, and mouth. The disorder arises from a congenital failure in the development of the derivatives of the third and fourth pharyngeal pouches, with resulting absence or hypoplasia of the parathyroids and thymus. Most cases of DGS are sporadic, but an autosomal-dominant inheritance of DGS has been observed. An association between the syndrome and an unbalanced translocation and deletions involving 22q11.2 have also been reported,[280] and this is referred to as *DGS type 1* (DGS1). In some patients, deletions of another locus on chromosome 10p have been observed in association with DGS,[281] and this is referred to as *DGS type 2* (DGS2). Mapping studies of the DGS1 deleted region on chromosome 22q11.2 have defined a 250-kb to 3000-kb critical region[282,283] that contained approximately 30 genes. Studies of DGS1 patients have reported deletions of several of the genes (e.g., *rnex40*, *nex2.2–nex3*, *UDF1L*, and *TBX1*) from the critical region,[280,284-286] and studies of transgenic mice deleted for such genes (e.g., *Udf1l*, *Hira*, and *Tbx1*) have revealed developmental abnormalities of the pharyngeal arches.[287-289] However, point mutations in DGS1 patients have only been detected in the *TBX1* gene,[290] and TBX1 is now considered to be the gene causing DGS1.[291] TBX1 is a DNA-binding transcriptional factor of the T-Box family and known to have an important role in vertebrate and invertebrate organogenesis and pattern formation. The *TBX1* gene is deleted in roughly 96% of all DGS1 patients. Moreover, DNA sequence analysis of unrelated DGS1 patients who did not have deletions of chromosome 22q11.2 revealed the occurrence of three heterozygous point mutations.[290] One of these mutations resulted in a frameshift with a premature truncation; the other two were missense mutations (Phe148Tyr and Gly310Ser). All of these patients had the complete pharyngeal phenotype but did not have mental retardation or learning difficulties. Interestingly, transgenic mice with deletion of Tbx1 have a phenotype that is similar to that of DGS1 patients.[289] Thus, Tbx1-null mutant mice (–/–) had all the developmental anomalies of DGS1 (i.e., thymic and parathyroid hypoplasia; abnormal facial structures and cleft palate; skeletal defects; and cardiac outflow tract abnormalities), whereas Tbx1 haploinsufficiency in mutant mice (+/–) was associated only with defects of the fourth branchial pouch (i.e., cardiac outflow tract abnormalities). The basis of the phenotypic differences between DGS1 patients, who are heterozygous, and the transgenic (+/–) mice remain to be elucidated. It is plausible that Tbx1 dosage, together with the downstream genes that are regulated by Tbx1 could provide an explanation, but the roles of these putative genes in DGS1 remains to be elucidated.

Some patients may have late-onset DGS1, and these develop symptomatic hypocalcemia in childhood or during adolescence, with only subtle phenotypic abnormalities.[292,293] These late-onset DGS1 patients have similar microdeletions in the 22q11 region. It is of interest to note that the age of diagnosis in the families of the three DGS1 patients with inactivating *TBX1* mutations ranged from 7 to 46 years, which is in keeping with late-onset DGS1.[290]

HYPOPARATHYROIDISM, DEAFNESS, AND RENAL ANOMALIES SYNDROME

The combined inheritance of hypoparathyroidism, deafness, and renal dysplasia (HDR) as an autosomal-dominant trait was reported in one family in 1992.[294] Patients had asymptomatic hypocalcemia, with undetectable or inappropriately normal serum concentrations of PTH and normal brisk increases in plasma cAMP in response to the infusion of PTH. The patients also had bilateral symmetrical sensorineural deafness involving all frequencies. The renal abnormalities consisted mainly of bilateral cysts that compressed the glomeruli and tubules and led to renal impairment in some patients. Cytogenetic abnormalities were not detected, and abnormalities of the *PTH* gene were excluded.[294] However, cytogenetic abnormalities involving chromosome 10p14-10pter were identified in two unrelated patients with features that were consistent with HDR. These two patients suffered from hypoparathyroidism, deafness, and growth and mental retardation. One patient also had a solitary dysplastic kidney with vesico-ureteric reflux and a uterus bicornis unicollis, and the other patient, who had a complex reciprocal insertional translocation of chromosomes 10p and 8q, had cartilaginous exostoses.[295] Neither of these patients had immunodeficiency or heart defects, which are key features of DGS2 (see earlier), and further studies defined two non-overlapping regions; thus, the DGS2 region was located on 10p13-14 and HDR on 10p14-10pter. Deletion mapping studies in two other HDR patients further defined a critical 200-kb region that contained GATA3,[295] which belongs to a family of zinc finger transcription factors that are involved in vertebrae embryonic development. DNA sequence analysis in other HDR patients identified mutations that resulted in a haploinsufficiency and loss of GATA3 function.[295-298] GATA3 has two zinc fingers; the C-terminal finger (ZnF2) binds DNA, and the N-terminal finger (2n-F1) stabilizes this DNA binding and interacts with other zinc finger proteins, such as the Friends of GATA (FOG).[299] HDR-associated mutations involving GATA3 ZnF2 or the adjacent basic amino acids were found to result in a loss of DNA binding, whereas those involving ZnF1 either lead to a loss of interaction with FOG2 ZnFs or altered DNA binding affinity.[297,298,300] These findings are consistent with the proposed three-dimensional model of GATA3 ZnF1, which has separate DNA-binding and protein-binding surfaces.[297,298,301]

Thus, the HDR-associated *GATA3* mutations can be subdivided into two broad classes that depend upon (1) whether they disrupt ZnF1 or ZnF2 and (2) their subsequent effects on interactions with FOG2 and altered DNA binding, respectively. The majority (>75%) of these HDR-associated mutations are predicted to result in truncated forms of the GATA3 protein. Each proband and family will generally have its own unique mutation, and there appears to be no correlation with the underlying genetic defect and the phenotypic variation (e.g., presence or absence of renal dysplasia). Over 90% of patients with two or three of the major clinical features of the HDR syndrome—hypoparathyroidism, deafness, or renal abnormalities—have a *GATA3* mutation.[298] The remaining 10% of HDR of patients who do not have a *GATA3* mutation of the coding region may harbor mutations in the regulatory sequences flanking the *GATA3* gene, or else they may represent heterogeneity. The phenotypes of HDR patients with *GATA3* mutations appear to be similar to those without *GATA3* mutations.[298]

The HDR phenotype is consistent with the expression pattern of GATA3 during human and mouse embryogenesis in the developing kidney, otic vesicle, and parathyroids. However, GATA3 is also expressed in the developing central nervous system (CNS) and the hematopoietic organs in man and mice, and this suggests that GATA3 may have a more complex role. Indeed, studies of mice that are deleted for a Gata3 allele (+/–), or both Gata3 alleles (–/–) have revealed important roles for Gata3 in the development of the brain, spinal cord, peripheral auditory system, T-cells, fetal liver hematopoiesis, and urogenital system.[302] Gata3[+/–] mice are viable, appear to be normal with a normal life span, and are fertile.[302] However, Gata3[+/–] mice have hearing loss that is associated with cochlear abnormalities which consist of a significant progressive morphologic degeneration that starts with the outer hair cells at the apex and eventually involves all the inner hair cells, pillar cells, and nerve fibers.[303,304] These studies have shown that hearing loss in Gata3 haploinsufficiency commences in the early postnatal period and is progressive through adulthood, and that it is peripheral in origin and is predominantly due to malfunctioning of the outer hair cells of the cochlea.[303,304] Gata 3[-/-] mice are embryonically lethal, and these null embryos die between 11 to 12 dpc.[302] Examination of these Gata3[-/-] embryos revealed a variety of abnormalities that included massive internal bleeding resulting in anemia, marked growth retardation, severe deformities of the brain and spinal cord, a hypopigmented retina, gross aberrations in fetal liver hematopoiesis, a total block of T-cell differentiation, and a retarded or missing lower jaw area.[302,305] These Gata3[-/-] mice had an anatomically normal sympathetic nervous system, yet the sympathetic ganglia lacked tyrosine hydroxylase and dopamine β-hydroxylase, which are key enzymes that convert tyrosine to L-dihydroxyphenylalanine (L-dopa), and dopamine to noradrenaline, respectively, in the catecholamine synthesis pathway. Thus, the Gata3[-/-] mice lacked noradrenaline in the sympathetic neurons, and this was contributing to the early embryonic lethality.[305] Feeding of catecholamine intermediates to the pregnant dams helped to partially rescue the Gata3[-/-] embryos to 12.5 to 16.5 dpc. These older, pharmacologically rescued Gata3[-/-] embryos showed abnormalities that could not be detected in the untreated mice.[305] These late embryonic defects included thymic hypoplasia, a thin-walled ventricular septum, a poorly developed mandible, other developmental defects in structures derived from the cephalic neural crest cells, renal hypoplasia, a failure to form the metanephros, and an aberrant elongation of the nephric duct along the antero-posterior axis of the embryo.[305,306] The defect of the nephric duct, which consisted of an abnormal morphogenesis and guidance in the developing kidney, was characterized by the loss of Ret expression that is an essential component of the glial-derived nerve factor (GDNF) signaling pathway involved in ureteric bud formation and nephric duct guidance.[306] Thus, Gata3 has a role in the differentiation of multiple cell lineages during embryogenesis, as well as key regulation of nephric duct morphogenesis and guidance of the nephric duct in its caudal extension in the pro/mesonephric kidney.[305,306]

It is important to note that HDR patients with *GATA3* haploinsufficiency do not have immune deficiency, and this suggests that the immune abnormalities observed in some patients with 10p deletions are most likely to be caused by other genes on 10p. Similarly, the facial dysmorphism and growth and developmental delay commonly seen in patients with larger 10p deletions were absent in the HDR patients with *GATA3* mutations, further indicating that these features were likely due to other genes on 10p.[295] These studies of HDR patients clearly indicate an important role for GATA3 in parathyroid development and in the etiology of hypoparathyroidism.

MITOCHONDRIAL DISORDERS ASSOCIATED WITH HYPOPARATHYROIDISM

Hypoparathyroidism has been reported to occur in three disorders associated with mitochondrial dysfunction: the Kearns-Sayre syndrome (KSS), the MELAS syndrome, and a mitochondrial trifunctional protein deficiency syndrome (MTPDS). KSS is characterized by progressive external ophthalmoplegia and pigmentary retinopathy before the age of 20 years and is often associated with heart block or cardiomyopathy. The MELAS syndrome

consists of a childhood onset of *m*itochondrial *e*ncephalopathy, *l*actic *a*cidosis and *s*troke-like episodes. In addition, varying degrees of proximal myopathy can be seen in both conditions. Both the KSS and MELAS syndromes have been reported to occur with insulin-dependent diabetes mellitus and hypoparathyroidism.[307,308] A point mutation in the mitochondrial gene tRNA leucine (UUR) has been reported in one patient with the MELAS syndrome who also suffered from hypoparathyroidism and diabetes mellitus.[219] Large deletions, consisting of 6741 and 6903 bp and involving more than 38% of the mitochondrial genome, have been reported in other patients who suffered from KSS, hypoparathyroidism, and sensorineural deafness.[309] Rearrangements and duplication of mitochondrial DNA have also been reported in KSS. Mitochondrial trifunctional protein deficiency (MTPDS) is a disorder of fatty acid oxidation that is associated with peripheral neuropathy, pigmentary retinopathy, and acute fatty liver degeneration in pregnant women who carry an affected fetus. Hypoparathyroidism has been observed in one patient with trifunctional protein deficiency.[310] The role of these mitochondrial mutations in the etiology of hypoparathyroidism remains to be further elucidated.

KENNEY-CAFFEY, SANJAD-SAKATI, AND KIRK-RICHARDSON SYNDROMES

Hypoparathyroidism has been reported to occur in over 50% of patients with the Kenney-Caffey syndrome, which is associated with short stature, osteosclerosis and cortical thickening of the long bones, delayed closure of the anterior fontanel, basal ganglia calcification, nanophthalmos, and hyperopia.[311] Parathyroid tissue could not be found in a detailed postmortem examination of one patient,[312] and this suggests that hypoparathyroidism may be due to an embryologic defect of parathyroid development. In the Kirk-Richardson and Sanjad-Sakati syndromes, which are similar, hypoparathyroidism is associated with severe growth failure and dysmorphic features.[313,314] This has been reported in patients of Middle Eastern origin.[313,314] Consanguinity was noted in the majority of the families, indicating that this syndrome is inherited as an autosomal-recessive disorder. Homozygosity and linkage disequilibrium studies located this gene to chromosome 1q42-q43.[315] Molecular genetic investigations have identified that mutations of the tubulin-specific chaperone (TBCE) are associated with the Kenney-Caffey and Sanjad-Sakati syndromes.[316] TBCE encodes one of several chaperone proteins required for the proper folding of α-tubulin subunits and the formation of α-β tubulin heterodimers (see Fig. 5-3).[316]

ADDITIONAL FAMILIAL SYNDROMES

Single familial syndromes in which hypoparathyroidism is a component have been reported (see Table 5-1). The inheritance of the disorder in some instances has been established, and molecular genetic analysis of the *PTH* gene has revealed no abnormalities. An association of hypoparathyroidism, renal insufficiency, and developmental delay has been reported in one Asian family in whom autosomal-recessive inheritance of the disorder was established; an analysis of the *PTH* gene in this family revealed no abnormalities.[317] The occurrence of hypoparathyroidism, nerve deafness, and a steroid-resistant nephrosis leading to renal failure, which has been referred to as the *Barakat syndrome*,[318] has been reported in four brothers from one family, and an association of hypoparathyroidism with congenital lymphedema, nephropathy, mitral valve prolapse, and brachytelephalangy has been observed in two brothers from another family.[319] Molecular genetic studies have not been reported from these two families.

CALCIUM-SENSING RECEPTOR ABNORMALITIES

CaSR abnormalities are associated with three hypocalcemic disorders: autosomal-dominant hypocalcemic hypercalciuria (ADHH), Bartter syndrome type V (i.e., ADHH with a Bartter-like syndrome), and a form of autoimmune hypoparathyroidism due to CaSR autoantibodies (see Table 5-3).

Autosomal-Dominant Hypocalcemic Hypercalciuria

CaSR mutations that result in loss-of-function abnormalities are associated with familial benign (hypocalciuric) hypercalcemia.[208,212-217] It was therefore postulated that gain-of-function mutations in *CaSR* lead to hypocalcemia with hypercalciuria, and the investigation of kindreds with autosomal-dominant forms of hypocalcemia have indeed identified such *CaSR* mutations.[208,320-324] The hypocalcemic individuals generally had normal serum intact PTH concentrations and hypomagnesemia, and treatment with vitamin D or its active metabolites to correct the hypocalcemia resulted in marked hypercalciuria, nephrocalcinosis, nephrolithiasis, and renal impairment. The majority (>80%) of *CaSR* mutations that result in a functional gain are located within the extracellular domain,[208,320-324] which is different from the findings in other disorders that are the result of activating mutations in G protein–coupled receptors.

Bartter Syndrome Type V

Bartter syndrome is a heterozygous group of autosomal-recessive disorders of electrolyte homeostasis characterized by hypokalemic alkalosis, renal salt wasting that may lead to hypotension, hyperreninemic hyperaldosteronism, increased urinary prostaglandin excretion, and hypercalciuria with nephrocalcinosis.[325,326] Mutations of several ion transporters and channels have been associated with Bartter syndrome, and five types are now recognized.[326] Type I is due to mutations involving the bumetanide-sensitive sodium-potassium-chloride co-transporter (NKCC2 or SLC12A2); type II is due to mutations of the outwardly rectifying renal potassium channel (ROMK); and type III is due to mutations of the voltage-gated chloride channel (CLC-Kb). Type IV is due to mutations of barttin, which is a beta subunit required for trafficking of CLC-Kb and CLC-Ka; this form is also associated with deafness, since barttin, CLC-Ka and CLC-Kb are also expressed in the marginal cells of the scala media of the inner ear that secrete potassium ion–rich endolymph. Type V is due to activating mutations of the CaSR. Patients with Bartter syndrome type V have the classic features of the syndrome: hypokalemic metabolic alkalosis, hyperreninemia, and hyperaldosteronism.[63,327] In addition, they develop hypocalcemia, which may be symptomatic and lead to carpopedal spasm and an elevated fractional excretion of calcium that may be associated with nephrocalcinosis.[63,327] Such patients have been reported to have heterozygous gain-of-function CaSR mutations, and in vitro functional expression of these mutations has revealed a more severe set-point abnormality for the receptor than that found in patients with ADHH.[63,224,327] This suggests that the additional features occurring in Bartter syndrome type V but not in ADHH are due to severe gain-of-function mutations of the CaSR.[326]

Autoimmune Acquired Hypoparathyroidism

Twenty percent of patients who had acquired hypoparathyroidism in association with autoimmune hypothyroidism were found to have autoantibodies to the extracellular domain of the CaSR.[228,328] The CaSR autoantibodies did not persist for long; 72% of patients who had acquired hypoparathyroidism for less than 5 years had detectable CaSR autoantibodies, whereas only 14% of patients with autoimmune hypoparathyroidism for more than 5 years had such autoantibodies.[328] The majority of the patients who had CaSR autoantibodies were females, a finding that is similar to that found in other autoantibody-mediated diseases. Indeed, a few autoimmune hypoparathyroidism patients have also had features of autoimmune polyglandular syndrome type 1 (APS1). These findings establish that the CaSR is an autoantigen in autoimmune hypoparathyroidism.[228,328]

BLOMSTRAND'S DISEASE

Blomstrand's chondrodysplasia is an autosomal-recessive human disorder characterized by early lethality, dramatically advanced bone maturation, and accelerated chondrocyte differentiation.[329] Affected infants are typically born to consanguineous healthy parents (only in one instance did unrelated healthy parents have two affected offspring),[330-334] show pronounced hyperdensity of the entire skeleton (Fig. 5-9) and markedly advanced ossification, and particularly the long bones are extremely short and poorly modeled. PTH/PTHrP receptor mutations that impair its functional properties were identified as the most likely cause of Blomstrand's disease (see Fig. 5-7). One of these defects is caused by a nucleotide exchange in exon M5 of the maternal PTH/PTHrP receptor allele, which introduces a novel splice acceptor site and thus leads to the synthesis of a receptor mutant that does not mediate, despite seemingly normal cell surface expression, the actions of PTH or PTHrP; the patient's paternal PTH/PTHrP receptor allele is, for yet unknown reasons, only poorly expressed.[335] In a second patient with Blomstrand's disease, the product of a consanguineous marriage, a nucleotide exchange was identified that changes proline at position 132 to leucine.[336,337] The resulting PTH/PTHrP receptor mutant showed, despite reasonable cell surface expression, severely impaired binding of radiolabeled PTH and PTHrP analogs, greatly reduced agonist-stimulated cAMP accumulation, and no measurable inositol phosphate response. Additional loss-of-function mutations of the PTH/PTHrP receptor have been identified in three unrelated patients with Blomstrand's disease. Two of these mutations led to a frameshift and a truncated protein due either to a homozygous single nucleotide deletion in exon EL2 [338] or a 27-bp insertion between exon M4 and EL2.[339] The other defect was a nonsense mutation at residue 104 and thus resulted in a truncated receptor protein.[339]

As in Jansen's disease, the identification of mutant PTH/PTHrP receptors provided a plausible explanation for the severe abnormalities in endochondral bone formation in patients with Blomstrand's disease. The disease is lethal, but it is likely that besides the striking skeletal defects, affected infants show abnormalities in other organs, including secondary hyperplasia of the parathyroid glands, presumably due to hypocalcemia. In addition, analysis of fetuses with Blomstrand's disease have revealed abnormal breast development and tooth impaction, highlighting the involvement of the PTH/PTHrP receptor in the normal development of breast and tooth.[340]

Concluding Remarks

Considerable advances have been made in identifying key proteins that are either directly or indirectly involved in the regula-

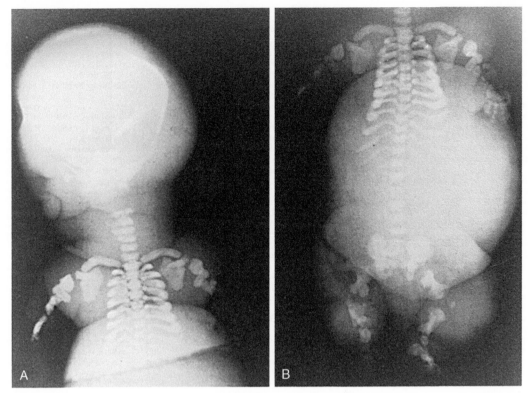

FIGURE 5-9. Radiologic findings in a patient with Blomstrand's disease. Note the markedly advanced ossification of all skeletal elements and the extremely short limbs, despite the comparatively normal size and shape of hands and feet. Furthermore, note that the clavicles are relatively long and abnormally shaped. (From Leroy JG, Keersmaeckers G, Coppens M, et al: Blomstrand lethal chondrodysplasia, Am J Med Genet 63:84–89, 1996.)

tion of PTH synthesis or secretion and in mediating its hormonal actions in the different target tissues. The subsequent identification of mutations in several of these proteins provided a plausible molecular explanation for a variety of familial and sporadic disorders of mineral ion homeostasis and/or bone development. In addition to these advances in further defining the biological role(s) of known proteins, genetic loci and/or candidate genes have been identified for multiple inherited disorders. It is likely that the molecular definition of these familial disorders, greatly aided by the rapid progress in the Human Genome Project, will provide further important insights into the regulation of body calcium and phosphate.

Acknowledgments

RVT is grateful to the Medical Research Council (UK) and Wellcome Trust for support and to Tracey Walker and Jennifer Accomando for their help in preparing the manuscript and expert secretarial assistance. HJ is supported by grants from the National Institutes of Health, National Institute of Diabetes and Digestive and Kidney Diseases (RO1-DK-46718 and PO1-DK-11794).

REFERENCES

1. Krane SM: Calcium, phosphate and magnesium. In Rasmussen H, editor: The International Encyclopedia of Pharmacology and Therapeutics, London, 1970, Pergamon Press, p 19.
2. Neer R, Berman M, Fisher L, et al: Multicompartmental analysis of calcium kinetics in normal adult males, J Clin Invest 46:1364–1379, 1967.
3. Glimcher MK, Krane SM: Organization and structure of bone and the mechanism of calcification. In Gould BS, Ramachandran GN, editors: Treatise on collagen, Part B, New York, 1968, Academic Press, pp 68–241.
4. Carr CW: Electrochemistry in biology and medicine, New York, 1955, John Wiley and Sons.
5. Bowers GN, Brassard C, Sena SF: Measurement of ionized calcium in serum with ion-selective electrodes: a mature technology that can meet the daily service needs, Clin Chem 32:1437–1447, 1986.
6. Krabbe S, Transbol I, Christiansen C: Bone mineral homeostasis, bone growth, and mineralization during years of pubertal growth: a unifying concept, Arch Dis Child 57:359–363, 1982.
7. Pitkin RM, Reynolds WA, Williams GA, et al: Calcium metabolism in normal pregnancy: a longitudinal study, Am J Obstet 133:781–790, 1979.
8. Gertner JM, Coustan OR, Kliger AS, et al: Pregnancy as a state of physiologic absorptive hypercalcemia, Am J Med 81:451–456, 1986.
9. Forbes GB: Calcium accumulation by the human fetus, Pediatrics 57:976–977, 1976.
10. Pitkin RM, Cruikshank DP, Schauberger CW, et al: Fetal calciotropic hormones and neonatal calcium homeostasis, Pediatrics 66:77–82, 1980.
11. Hillman L, Sateesha S, Haussler M, et al: Control of mineral homeostasis during lactation: interrelationships of 25-hydroxyvitamin D, 24,25-dihydroxyvitamin D, 1,25-dihydroxyvitamin, parathyroid hormone, calcitonin, prolactin, and estradiol, Am J Obstet Gynecol 139:471–476, 1981.
12. Greer FR, Tasang RC, Searcy JE, et al: Mineral homeostasis during lactation-relationship to serum 1,25-dihydroxyvitamin D, 25-hydroxyvitamin D, parathyroid hormone, and calcitonin, Am J Clin Nutr 36:431–437, 1982.
13. Barritt GJ: Receptor-activated Ca^{2+} inflow in animal cells: a variety of pathways tailored to meet different intracellular Ca^{2+} signalling requirements, Biochem J 337:153–169, 1999.
14. Berridge MJ: Elementary and global aspects of calcium signaling, J Physiol 499:291–306, 1997.
15. Carafoli E: Intracellular calcium homeostasis, Ann Rev Biochem 56:395–433, 1987.
16. Rasmussen H, Barrett PQ: Calcium messenger system: An integrated view, Physiol Rev 64:938–984, 1984.
17. Brown E, Pollack A, Hebert S: The extracellular calcium-sensing receptor: its role in health and disease, Annu Rev Med 49:15–29, 1998.
18. Rasmussen H: The calcium messenger system, N Engl J Med 314:1094–1101, 1986.
19. Heaney RP, Gallagher JC, Johnston CC, et al: Calcium nutrition and bone health in the elderly, Am J Clin Nutr 36:986–1013, 1982.
20. Allen LH: Calcium bioavailability and absorption: a review, Am J Clin Nutr 35:783–808, 1982.
21. Avioli LV, McDonald JE, Lee SW: Influence of aging on the intestinal absorption of 47-Ca in women and its relation to 47-Ca absorption in postmenopausal osteoporosis, J Clin Invest 44:1960–1967, 1965.
22. Ireland P, Fordtran JS: Effect of dietary calcium and age on jejunal calcium absorption in humans studied by intestinal perfusion, J Clin Invest 52:2672–2681, 1973.

23. Gallagher JC, Riggs BL, Eisman J, et al: Intestinal calcium absorption and serum vitamin D metabolites in normal subjects and osteoporotic patients, J Clin Invest 64:729–736, 1979.

24. Heaney RP, Skillman TG: Secretion and excretion of calcium by the human gastrointestinal tract, J Lab Clin Med 64:29–41, 1964.

25. Rose GA, Reed GW, Smith AH: Isotopic method for measurement of calcium absorption from the gastrointestinal tract, Br Med J 1:690–692, 1965.

26. Phang J, Berman M, Finerman G: Dietary perturbation of calcium metabolism in normal man: compartmental analysis, J Clin Invest 48:67–77, 1969.

27. Jung A, Bartholdi P, Mermillod B: Critical analysis of methods of analyzing human calcium kinetics, J Theor Biol 73:131–157, 1978.

28. Fordtran JS, Locklear TW: Ionic constituents and osmolality of gastric and small-intestinal fluids after eating, Am J Dig Dis 11:503–521, 1966.

29. Bronner F, Pansu D, Stein WD: An analysis of intestinal calcium transport across the rat intestine, Am J Physiol 250:G561–G569, 1986.

30. Marcus CS, Lengemann FW: Absorption of Ca^{45} and Sr^{85} from solid and liquid food at various levels of the alimentary tract of the rat, J Nutr 77:155–160, 1962.

31. Birge J, Peck WA, Berman M, et al: Study of calcium absorption in man: a kinetic analysis and physiologic model, J Clin Invest 48:1705–1713, 1969.

32. Dano P, Christiansen C: Calcium absorption and bone mineral content following intestinal shunt operations for obesity: a comparison of three types of procedures, Scand J Gastroenterol 9:775–779, 1974.

33. Hoenderop JG, van der Kemp AW, Hartog A, et al: Molecular identification of the apical Ca^{2+} channel in 1, 25-dihydroxyvitamin D3-responsive epithelia, J Biol Chem 274:8375–8378, 1999.

34. Peng JB, Chen XZ, Berger UV, et al: Molecular cloning and characterization of a channel-like transporter mediating intestinal calcium absorption, J Biol Chem 274:22739–22746, 1999.

35. Vennekens R, Prenen J, Hoenderop JG, et al: Pore properties and ionic block of the rabbit epithelial calcium channel expressed in HEK 293 cells, J Physiol 530:183–191, 2001.

36. Gunthorpe MJ, Benham CD, Randall A, et al: The diversity in the vanilloid (TRPV) receptor family of ion channels, Trends Pharmacol Sci 23:183–191, 2002.

37. Nilius B, Vennekens R, Prenen J, et al: The single pore residue Asp542 determines Ca^{2+} permeation and Mg^{2+} block of the epithelial Ca^{2+} channel, J Biol Chem 276:1020–1025, 2001.

38. den Dekker E, Hoenderop JG, Nilius B, et al: The epithelial calcium channels, TRPV5 & TRPV6: from identification towards regulation, Cell Calcium 33:497–507, 2003.

39. Zhuang L, Peng JB, Tou L, et al: Calcium-selective ion channel, CaT1, is apically localized in gastrointestinal tract epithelia and is aberrantly expressed in human malignancies, Lab Invest 82:1755–1764, 2002.

40. Wood RJ, Tchack L, Taparia S: 1,25-Dihydroxyvitamin D$_3$ increases the expression of the CaT1 epithelial calcium channel in the Caco-2 human intestinal cell line, BMC Physiol 1:11, 2001.

41. Van Cromphaut SJ, Dewerchin M, Hoenderop JG, et al: Duodenal calcium absorption in vitamin D receptor-knockout mice: functional and molecular aspects, Proc Natl Acad Sci U S A 98:13324–13329, 2001.

42. Song Y, Kato S, Fleet JC: Vitamin D receptor (VDR) knockout mice reveal VDR-independent regulation of intestinal calcium absorption and ECaC2 and calbindin D$_{9k}$ mRNA, J Nutr 133:374–380, 2003.

43. Van Cromphaut SJ, Rummens K, Stockmans I, et al: Intestinal calcium transporter genes are upregulated by estrogens and the reproductive cycle through vitamin D receptor-independent mechanisms, J Bone Miner Res 18:1725–1736, 2003.

44. Feher JJ, Fullmer CS, Wasserman RH: Role of facilitated diffusion of calcium by calbindin in intestinal calcium absorption, Am J Physiol 262:C517–C526, 1992.

45. Ruchon A, Tenenhouse H, Marcinkiewicz M, et al: Developmental expression and tissue distribution of Phex protein: effect of the Hyp mutation and relationship to bone markers, J Bone Miner Res 15:1440–1450, 2000.

46. Lassiter WE, Gottschalk CW, Mylle M: Micropuncture study of renal tubular reabsorption on calcium in normal rodents, Am J Physiol 204:771–775, 1963.

47. Friedman PA, Gesek FA: Cellular calcium transport in renal epithelia: measurement, mechanisms, and regulation, [Review] [418 refs]. Physiol Rev 75:429–471, 1995.

48. Bourdeau JE, Burg MB: Effects of PTH on calcium transport across the cortical thick ascending limb of Henle's loop, Am J Physiol 238:F350, 1979.

49. Suki WN, Rouse D, Ng RC, et al: Calcium transport in the thick ascending limb of Henle: heterogeneity of function in the medullary and cortical segments, J Clin Invest 66:1004–1009, 1980.

50. Shareghi GR, Agus ZS: Magnesium transport in the cortical thick ascending limb of Henle's loop of the rabbit, J Clin Invest 69:759, 1982.

51. Bourdeau JE, Burg MB: Effect of PTH on calcium transport across the cortical thick ascending limb of Henle's loop, Am J Physiol 239:F121–F126, 1980.

52. Friedman PA: Basal and hormone-activated calcium absorption in mouse renal thick ascending limbs, Am J Physiol 254:F62–F70, 1988.

53. Simon DB, Lu Y, Choate KA, et al: Paracellin-1, a renal tight junction protein required for paracellular Mg^{2+} resorption, Science 285:103–106, 1999.

54. Weber S, Hoffmann K, Jeck N, et al: Familial hypomagnesaemia with hypercalciuria and nephrocalcinosis maps to chromosome 3q27 and is associated with mutations in the PCLN-1 gene, Eur J Hum Genet 8:414–422, 2000.

55. Blanchard A, Jeunemaitre X, Coudol P, et al: Paracellin-1 is critical for magnesium and calcium reabsorption in the human thick ascending limb of Henle, Kidney Int 59:2206–2215, 2001.

56. Konrad M, Schaller A, Seelow D, et al: Mutations in the tight-junction gene claudin 19 (CLDN19) are associated with renal magnesium wasting, renal failure, and severe ocular involvement, Am J Hum Genet 79:949–957, 2006.

57. Quamme GA: Effect of hypercalcemia on renal tubular handling of calcium and magnesium, Can J Physiol Pharmacol 60:1275–1280, 1982.

58. Riccardi D, Hall AE, Chattopadhyay N, et al: Localization of the extracellular Ca^{2+}/polyvalent cation-sensing protein in rat kidney, Am J Physiol 274:F611–F622, 1998.

59. Wang WH, Lu M, Hebert SC: Cytochrome P-450 metabolites mediate extracellular Ca(2+)-induced inhibition of apical K$^+$ channels in the TAL, Am J Physiol 271:C103–C111, 1996.

60. Wang W, Lu M, Balazy M, et al: Phospholipase A2 is involved in mediating the effect of extracellular Ca^{2+} on apical K$^+$ channels in rat TAL, Am J Physiol 273:F421–F429, 1997.

61. Motoyama HI, Friedman PA: Calcium-sensing receptor regulation of PTH-dependent calcium absorption by mouse cortical ascending limbs, Am J Physiol Renal Physiol 283:F399–F406, 2002.

62. Barakat AJ, Rennert OM: Gitelman's syndrome (familial hypokalemia-hypomagnesemia), J Nephrol 14:43–47, 2001.

63. Vargas-Poussou R, Huang C, Hulin P, et al: Functional characterization of a calcium-sensing receptor mutation in severe autosomal dominant hypocalcemia with a Bartter-like syndrome, J Am Soc Nephrol 13:2259–2266, 2002.

64. Agus ZS, Chiu PJS, Goldberg M: Regulation of urinary calcium excretion in the rat, Am J Physiol 232:F545, 1977.

65. Costanzo LS, Windhager EE: Effect of PTH, ADH and cAMP on distal tubular Ca and Na reabsorption, Am J Physiol 239:F478–F485, 1980.

66. Costanzo LS: Comparison of calcium and sodium transport in early and late rat distal tubules: effect of amiloride, Am J Physiol 246:F937–F945, 1984.

67. Borke JL, Caride A, Verma AK, et al: Plasma membrane calcium pump and 28-kDa calcium binding protein in cells of rat kidney distal tubules, Am J Physiol 257:F842–F849, 1989.

68. Ramachandran C, Brunette MG: The renal Na$^+$/Ca^{++} exchange system is located exclusively in the distal tubule, Biochem J 257:259–264, 1989.

69. Reilly RF, Ellison DH: Mammalian distal tubule: physiology, pathophysiology, and molecular anatomy, [Review] [304 refs]. Physiol Rev 80:277–313, 2000.

70. Hoenderop JG, Hartog A, Stuiver M, et al: Localization of the epithelial Ca(2+) channel in rabbit kidney and intestine, J Am Soc Nephrol 11:1171–1178, 2000.

71. Kip SN, Strehler EE: Characterization of PMCA isoforms and their contribution to transcellular Ca^{2+} flux in MDCK cells, Am J Physiol Renal Physiol 284:F122–F132, 2003.

72. Loffing J, Kaissling B: Sodium and calcium transport pathways along the mammalian distal nephron: from rabbit to human, [Review] [142 refs]. Am J Physiol Renal Physiol 284:F628–F643, 2003.

73. Shimizu T, Yoshitomi K, Nakamura N, et al: Effects of PTH, calcitonin, and cAMP on calcium transport in rabbit distal nephron segments, Am J Physiol 259:F408–F414, 1990.

74. Bindels RJ, Hartog A, Timmermans J, et al: Active Ca^{2+} transport in primary cultures of rabbit kidney CCD: stimulation by 1,25-dihydroxyvitamin D3 and PTH, Am J Physiol 261:F799–F807, 1991.

75. Hoenderop JG, van Leeuwen JP, van der Eerden BC, et al: Renal Ca^{2+} wasting, hyperabsorption, and reduced bone thickness in mice lacking TRPV5, J Clin Invest 112:1906–1914, 2003.

76. Lee CT, Huynh VM, Lai LW, et al: Cyclosporine A-induced hypercalciuria in calbindin-D$_{28k}$ knockout and wild-type mice, Kidney Int 62:2055–2061, 2002.

77. Bacskai BJ, Friedman PA: Activation of latent Ca^{2+} channels in renal epithelial cells by parathyroid hormone, Nature 347:388–391, 1990.

78. Silva IV, Cebotaru V, Wang H, et al: The ClC-5 knockout mouse model of Dent's disease has renal hypercalciuria and increased bone turnover, J Bone Miner Res 18:615–623, 2003.

79. Christensen EI, Devuyst O, Dom G, et al: Loss of chloride channel ClC-5 impairs endocytosis by defective trafficking of megalin and cubilin in kidney proximal tubules, Proc Natl Acad Sci U S A 100:8472–8477, 2003.

80. Epstein FH: Calcium and the kidney, Am J Med 45:700–715, 1968.

81. Torikai S, Wang M-S, Klein KL, et al: Adenylate cyclase and cell cyclic AMP of rat cortical thick ascending limb of Henle, Kidney Int 20:649–654, 1981.

82. Bijvoet OLM: Kidney function in calcium and phosphate metabolism. In Avioli LV, Krane SM, editors: Metabolic Bone Disease, vol 1. New York, 1977, Academic Press, pp 49–140.

83. Peacock M, Robertson WG, Nordin BEC: Relation between serum and urinary calcium with particular reference to parathyroid activity, Lancet 1:384–386, 1969.

84. Shareghi GR, Stoner LC: Calcium transport across segments of the rabbit distal nephron in vitro, Am J Physiol 235:F367–F375, 1978.

85. Suki WN, Rouse D: Hormonal regulation of calcium transport in thick ascending limb renal tubules, Am J Physiol 241:F171, 1981.

86. Hemmingsen C: Regulation of renal calbindin-D$_{28k}$, [Review] [163 refs]. Pharmacol Toxicol 87:5–30, 2000.

87. Jayakumar A, Cheung L, Liang CT, et al: Sodium gradient-dependent calcium uptake in renal basolateral membrane vesicles, J Biol Chem 259:10827–10833, 1984.

88. Bomsztyk K, George JP, Wright FS: Effects of luminal fluid anions on calcium transport by proximal tubule, Am J Physiol 246:F600–F608, 1984.

89. Scoble JE, Mills S, Hruska KA: Calcium transport in canine renal basolateral membrane vesicles, effect of parathyroid hormones, J Clin Invest 75:1096–1105, 1985.

90. Bouhtiauy I, LaJeunesse D, Brunette MG: The mechanism of parathyroid hormone action on calcium reabsorption by the distal tubule, Endocrinology 128:251–258, 1991.

91. Shimizu T, Nakamura M, Yoshitomi K, et al: Interaction of trichlormethiazide or amiloride with PTH in stimulating Ca^{2+} absorption in rabbit CNT, Am J Physiol 261:F36–F43, 1991.

92. Tsukamoto Y, Saka S, Saitoh M: Parathyroid hormone stimulates ATP-dependent calcium pump activity by a different mode in proximal and distal tubules of the rat, Biochim Biophys Acta 1103:163–171, 1992.

93. Gesek FA, Friedman PA: On the mechanism of parathyroid hormone stimulation of calcium uptake by mouse distal convoluted tubule cells, J Clin Invest 90:749–758, 1992.

94. Hoenderop JG, Nilius B, Bindels RJ: Molecular mechanism of active Ca²⁺ reabsorption in the distal nephron, [Review] [85 refs]. Ann Rev Physiol 64:529–549, 2002.

95. Taniguchi J, Takeda M, Yoshitomi K, et al: Pressure- and parathyroid-hormone-dependent Ca²⁺ transport in rabbit connecting tubule: role of the stretch-activated nonselective cation channel, J Membr Biol 140:123–132, 1994.

96. de Rouffignac C, DiStefano A, Wittner M, et al: Consequences of differential effects of ADH and other peptide hormones on thick ascending limb of mammalian kidney, Am J Physiol 260:R1023–R1035, 1991.

97. Hebert SC: Extracellular calcium-sensing receptor: implications for calcium and magnesium handling in the kidney, Kidney Int 50:2129–2139, 1996.

98. Even L, Weisman Y, Goldray D, et al: Selective modulation by vitamin D of renal response to parathyroid hormone: a study in calcitriol-resistant rickets, J Clin Endocrinol Metab 81:2836–2840, 1996.

99. Friedman PA, Gesek FA: Calcium transport in renal epithelial cells, Am J Physiol 264:F181–F198, 1993.

100. Costanzo LS, Sheehe PR, Weiner IM: Renal actions of vitamin D in D-deficient rats, Am J Physiol 226:1490–1495, 1974.

101. Christakos S, Gabrielides C, Rhoten WB: Vitamin D-dependent calcium binding proteins: chemistry, distribution, functional considerations, and molecular biology, [Review] [251 refs]. Endocr Rev 10:3–26, 1989.

102. Van Baal J, Yu A, Hartog A, et al: Localization and regulation by vitamin D of calcium transport proteins in rabbit cortical collecting system, Am J Physiol 271: F985–F993, 1996.

103. Hoenderop JG, Muller D, Van Der Kemp AW, et al: Calcitriol controls the epithelial calcium channel in kidney, J Am Soc Nephrol 12:1342–1349, 2001.

104. Singer FR, Woodhouse NJ, Parkinson DK, et al: Some acute effects of administered porcine calcitonin in man, Clin Sci 37:181–190, 1969.

105. Chipman JJ, Zerwekh J, Nicar M, et al: Effect of growth hormone administration: reciprocal changes in serum 1a,25-dihydroxyvitamin D and intestinal calcium absorption, J Clin Endocrinol Metab 51:321–324, 1980.

106. Gertner JM, Tamborlane WV, Hintz RL, et al: The effects on mineral metabolism of overnight growth hormone infusion in growth hormone deficiency, J Clin Endocrinol Metab 53:818–822, 1981.

107. Wright NM, Papadea N, Wentz B, et al: Increased serum 1,25-dihydroxyvitamin D after growth hormone administration is not parathyroid hormone-mediated, Calcif Tissue Int 61:101–103, 1997.

108. Hahn TJ, Halstead LR, Baran DT: Effects of short-term glucocorticoid administration on intestinal calcium absorption and circulating vitamin D metabolite concentrations in man, J Clin Endocrinol Metab 52:111–114, 1981.

109. Lemann J, Jr, Piering WF, Lennon EJ: Studies of the acute effects of aldosterone and cortisol on the interrelationship between renal sodium, calcium and magnesium excretion in normal man, Nephron 7:117–130, 1970.

110. Findley JW, Adams ND, Lemann J, Jr, et al: Vitamin D metabolites and parathyroid hormone in Cushing's syndrome: relationship to calcium and phosphorus homeostasis, J Clin Endocrinol Metab 54:1039–1044, 1982.

111. Gallagher JC, Nordin BEC: Treatment with oestrogens of primary hyperparathyroidism in post-menopausal women, Lancet 1:503–507, 1972.

112. McKane W, Khosla S, Burritt M, et al: Mechanism of renal calcium conservation with estrogen replacement therapy in women in early menopause—a clinical research center study, J Clin Endocrinol Metab 80:3458–3464, 1995.

113. Van Abel M, Hoenderop JG, Dardenne O, et al: 1,25-dihydroxyvitamin D(3)-independent stimulatory effect of estrogen on the expression of ECaC1 in the kidney, J Am Soc Nephrol 13:2102–2109, 2002.

114. DeFronzo RA, Cooke CR, Andres R, et al: The effect of insulin on renal handling of sodium, potassium, calcium and phosphate in man, J Clin Invest 55:845–853, 1975.

115. Charbonneau A, Leclerc M, Brunette MG: Effect of angiotensin II on calcium reabsorption by the luminal membranes of the nephron, Am J Physiol Endocrinol Metab 280:E928–36, 2001.

116. Naylor SL, Sakaguchi AU, Szoka P, et al: Human parathyroid hormone gene (PTH) is on short arm of chromosome 11, Somat Cell Gene 9:609–616, 1983.

117. Vasicek T, McDevitt BE, Freeman MW, et al: Nucleotide sequence of genomic DNA encoding human parathyroid hormone, Proc Natl Acad Sci U S A 80:2127–2131, 1983.

118. Okazaki T, Igarashi T, Kronenberg HM: 5'-Flanking region of the parathyroid hormone gene mediates negative regulation by 1,25(OH)₂ vitamin D₃, J Biol Chem 263:2203–2208, 1989.

119. Demay MB, Kiernan MS, DeLuca HF, et al: Sequences in the human parathyroid hormone gene that bind the 1,25- dihydroxyvitamin D₃ receptor and mediate transcriptional repression in response to 1,25-dihydroxyvitamin D₃, Proc Natl Acad Sci U S A 89:8097–8101, 1992.

120. Naveh-Many T, Rahaminov R, Livini N, et al: Parathyroid cell proliferation in normal and chronic renal failure in rats, the effects of calcium, phosphate, and vitamin D, J Clin Invest 96:1786–1793, 1995.

121. Almaden Y, Canalejo A, Hernandez A, et al: Direct effect of phosphorus on PTH secretion from whole rat parathyroid glands in vitro, J Bone Miner Res 11:970–976, 1996.

122. Russell J, Lettieri D, Sherwood LM: Direct regulation by calcium of cytoplasmic messenger ribonucleic acid coding for pre-proparathyroid hormone in isolated bovine parathyroid cells, J Clin Invest 72:1851–1855, 1983.

123. Naveh-Many T, Friedlaender MM, Mayer H, et al: Calcium regulates parathyroid hormone messenger ribonucleic acid (mRNA), but not calcitonin mRNA in vivo in the rat, Dominant role of 1,25-dihydroxyvitamin D, Endocrinology 125:275–280, 1989.

124. Kemper B, Habener JF, Mulligan RC, et al: Preproparathyroid hormone: a direct translation product of parathyroid messenger RNA, Proc Natl Acad Sci U S A 71:3731–3735, 1974.

125. Jüppner H, Abou-Samra AB, Freeman MW, et al: A G protein-linked receptor for parathyroid hormone and parathyroid hormone-related peptide, Science 254:1024–1026, 1991.

126. Abou-Samra AB, Jüppner H, Force T, et al: Expression cloning of a common receptor for parathyroid hormone and parathyroid hormone-related peptide from rat osteoblast-like cells: a single receptor stimulates intracellular accumulation of both cAMP and inositol triphosphates and increases intracellular free calcium, Proc Natl Acad Sci U S A 89:2732–2736, 1992.

127. Gelbert L, Schipani E, Jüppner H, et al: Chromosomal location of the parathyroid hormone/parathyroid hormone-related protein receptor gene to human chromosome 3p21.2–p24.2, J Clin Endocrinol Metab 79:1046–1048, 1994.

128. Pausova Z, Bourdon J, Clayton D, et al: Cloning of a parathyroid hormone/parathyroid hormone-related peptide receptor (PTHR) cDNA from a rat osteosarcoma (UMR106) cell line: chromosomal assignment of the gene in the human, mouse, and rat genomes, Genomics 20:20–26, 1994.

129. Jüppner H, Gardella T, Brown E, et al: Parathyroid hormone and parathyroid hormone-related peptide in the regulation of calcium homeostasis and bone development. In DeGroot L, Jameson J, editors: Endocrinology, W.B. Saunders Company, 2000, Philadelphia, PA, pp 969–998.

130. Kronenberg H: Developmental regulation of the growth plate, Nature 423:332–336, 2003.

131. Thakker RV: Molecular genetics of parathyroid disease, Curr Opin Endocrinol Diabetes Obes 3:521–528, 1996.

132. Szabo J, Heath B, Hill VM, et al: Hereditary hyperparathyroidism-jaw tumor syndrome: the endocrine tumor gene HRPT2 maps to chromosome 1q21-q31, Am J Hum Genet 56:944–950, 1995.

133. Arnold A, Brown MF, Urena P, et al: Monoclonality of parathyroid tumors in chronic renal failure and in primary parathyroid hyperplasia, J Clin Invest 95:2047–2053, 1995.

134. Arnold A, Kim HG, Gaz RD, et al: Molecular cloning and chromosomal mapping of DNA rearranged with the parathyroid hormone gene in a parathyroid adenoma, J Clin Invest 83:2034–2040, 1989.

135. Motokura T, Bloom T, Kim HG, et al: A BCL1-linked candidate oncogene which is rearranged in parathyroid tumors encodes a novel cyclin, Nature 350:512–515, 1991.

136. Nurse P: Universal control mechanism regulating onset of M-phase, Nature 344:503–508, 1990.

137. Hosokawa Y, Yoshimoto K, Bronson R, et al: Chronic hyperparathyroidism in transgenic mice with parathyroid-targeted overexpression of cyclin D1/PRAD1, J Bone Miner Res 12(suppl 1):S110, 1997.

138. Imanishi Y, Hosokawa Y, Yoshimoto K, et al: Primary hyperparathyroidism caused by parathyroid-targeted overexpression of cyclin D1 in transgenic mice, J Clin Invest 107:1093–1102, 2001.

139. Wang TC, Cardiff RD, Zukerberg L, et al: Mammary hyperplasia and carcinoma in MMTV-cyclin D1 transgenic mice, Nature 369:669–671, 1994.

140. Au AY, McDonald K, Gill A, et al: PTH mutation with primary hyperparathyroidism and undetectable intact PTH, N Engl J Med 359:1184–1186, 2008.

141. Thakker RV: The molecular genetics of the multiple endocrine neoplasia syndromes, Clin Endocrinol (Oxf) 38:1–14, 1993.

142. Trump D, Farren B, Wooding C, et al: Clinical studies of multiple endocrine neoplasia type 1 (MEN1), QJM 89:653–669, 1996.

143. Marx S: Multiple endocrine neoplasia type 1. In Vogelstein B, Kinzler K, editors: The genetic basis of human cancer, New York, 1998, McGraw Hill, pp 489–506.

144. Thakker RV: Multiple endocrine neoplasia–syndromes of the twentieth century, J Clin Endocrinol Metab 83:2617–2620, 1998.

145. Chandrasekharappa SC, Guru SC, Manickam P, et al: Positional cloning of the gene for multiple endocrine neoplasia-type 1, Science 276:404–407, 1997.

146. Lemmens I, Van de Ven WJ, Kas K, et al: Identification of the multiple endocrine neoplasia type 1 (MEN1) gene, The European Consortium on MEN1, Hum Mol Genet 6:1177–1183, 1997.

147. Pannett AA, Thakker RV: Multiple endocrine neoplasia type 1, Endocr Relat Cancer 6:449–473, 1999.

148. Lemos MC, Thakker RV: Multiple endocrine neoplasia type 1 (MEN1): analysis of 1336 mutations reported in the first decade following identification of the gene, Hum Mutat 29:22–32, 2008.

149. Turner JJ, Leotlela PD, Pannett AA, et al: Frequent occurrence of an intron 4 mutation in multiple endocrine neoplasia type 1, J Clin Endocrinol Metab 87:2688–2693, 2002.

150. Bassett JH, Forbes SA, Pannett AA, et al: Characterization of mutations in patients with multiple endocrine neoplasia type 1, Am J Hum Genet 62:232–244, 1998.

151. Teh BT, Kytola S, Farnebo F, et al: Mutation analysis of the MEN1 gene in multiple endocrine neoplasia type 1, familial acromegaly and familial isolated hyperparathyroidism, J Clin Endocrinol Metab 83:2621–2626, 1998.

152. Heppner C, Kester MB, Agarwal SK, et al: Somatic mutation of the MEN1 gene in parathyroid tumours, Nat Genet 16:375–378, 1997.

153. Zhuang Z, Vortmeyer AO, Pack S, et al: Somatic mutations of the MEN1 tumor suppressor gene in sporadic gastrinomas and insulinomas, Cancer Res 57:4682–4686, 1997.

154. Zhuang Z, Ezzat SZ, Vortmeyer AO, et al: Mutations of the MEN1 tumor suppressor gene in pituitary tumors, Cancer Res 57:5446–5451, 1997.

155. Prezant TR, Levine J, Melmed S: Molecular characterization of the men1 tumor suppressor gene in sporadic pituitary tumors, J Clin Endocrinol Metab 83:1388–1391, 1998.

156. Debelenko LV, Brambilla E, Agarwal SK, et al: Identification of MEN1 gene mutations in sporadic carcinoid tumors of the lung, Hum Mol Genet 6:2285–2290, 1997.

157. Vortmeyer AO, Boni R, Pak E, et al: Multiple endocrine neoplasia 1 gene alterations in MEN1-associated and sporadic lipomas, J Natl Cancer Inst 90:398–399, 1998.

158. Farnebo F, Teh BT, Kytola S, et al: Alterations of the MEN1 gene in sporadic parathyroid tumors, J Clin Endocrinol Metab 83:2627–2630, 1998.

159. Carling T, Correa P, Hessman O, et al: Parathyroid MEN1 gene mutations in relation to clinical character-

istics of nonfamilial primary hyperparathyroidism, J Clin Endocrinol Metab 83:2960–2963, 1998.

160. Tanaka C, Kimura T, Yang P, et al: Analysis of loss of heterozygosity on chromosome 11 and infrequent inactivation of the MEN1 gene in sporadic pituitary adenomas, J Clin Endocrinol Metab 83:2631–2634, 1998.

161. Pannett AA, Thakker RV: Somatic mutations in MEN type 1 tumors, consistent with the Knudson "two-hit" hypothesis, J Clin Endocrinol Metab 86:4371–4374, 2001.

162. Teh BT, Esapa CT, Houlston R, et al: A family with isolated hyperparathyroidism segregating a missense MEN1 mutation and showing loss of the wild-type alleles in the parathyroid tumors, Am J Hum Genet 63:1544–1549, 1998.

163. Pannett AA, Kennedy AM, Turner JJ, et al: Multiple endocrine neoplasia type 1 (MEN1) germline mutations in familial isolated primary hyperparathyroidism, Clin Endocrinol (Oxf) 58:639–646, 2003.

164. Hannan FM, Nesbit MA, Christie PT, et al: Familial isolated primary hyperparathyroidism caused by mutations of the MEN1 gene, Nat Clin Pract Endocrinol Metab 4:53–58, 2008.

165. Lin SY, Elledge SJ: Multiple tumor suppressor pathways negatively regulate telomerase, Cell 113:881–889, 2003.

166. Stalberg P, Grimfjard P, Santesson M, et al: Transfection of the multiple endocrine neoplasia type 1 gene to a human endocrine pancreatic tumor cell line inhibits cell growth and affects expression of JunD, delta-like protein 1/preadipocyte factor-1, proliferating cell nuclear antigen, and QM/Jif-1, J Clin Endocrinol Metab 89:2326–2337, 2004.

167. Kim YS, Burns AL, Goldsmith PK, et al: Stable overexpression of MEN1 suppresses tumorigenicity of RAS, Oncogene 18:5936–5942, 1999.

168. Yumita W, Ikeo Y, Yamauchi K, et al: Suppression of insulin-induced AP-1 transactivation by menin accompanies inhibition of c-Fos induction, Int J Cancer 103:738–744, 2003.

169. Hussein N, Casse H, Fontaniere S, et al: Reconstituted expression of menin in Men1-deficient mouse Leydig tumour cells induces cell cycle arrest and apoptosis, Eur J Cancer 43:402–414, 2007.

170. Mulligan LM, Kwok JBJ, Healey CS, et al: Germ-line mutations of the RET proto-oncogene in multiple endocrine neoplasia type 2A, Nature 363:458–460, 1993.

171. Mulligan LM, Ponder BA: Genetic basis of endocrine disease: multiple endocrine neoplasia type 2, J Clin Endocrinol Metab 80:1989–1995, 1995.

172. Pausova Z, Janicic N, Konrad EM, et al: Analysis of the RET proto-oncogene in sporadic parathyroid tumors, J Bone Mineral Research 9:S151, 1994.

173. Padberg BC, Schroder S, Jochum W, et al: Absence of RET proto-oncogene point mutations in sporadic hyperplastic and neoplastic lesions of the parathyroid gland, Am J Pathol 147:1600–1607, 1995.

174. Heshmati HM, Gharib H, Khosla S, et al: Genetic testing in medullary thyroid carcinoma syndromes: mutation types and clinical significance, Mayo Clin Proc 72:430–436, 1997.

175. Kennett S, Pollick H: Jaw lesions in familial hyperparathyroidism, Oral Surg Oral Med Oral Pathol 31:502–510, 1971.

176. Jackson CE, Norum RA, Boyd SB, et al: Hereditary hyperparathyroidism and multiple ossifying jaw fibromas: a clinically and genetically distinct syndrome, Surgery 108:1006–1012; discussion 1012–3, 1990.

177. Bradley KJ, Hobbs MR, Buley ID, et al: Uterine tumours are a phenotypic manifestation of the hyperparathyroidism-jaw tumour syndrome, J Intern Med 257:18–26, 2005.

178. Cavaco BM, Barros L, Pannett AA, et al: The hyperparathyroidism-jaw tumour syndrome in a Portuguese kindred, QJM 94:213–222, 2001.

179. Wassif WS, Moniz CF, Friedman E, et al: Familial isolated hyperparathyroidism: a distinct genetic entity with an increased risk of parathyroid cancer, J Clin Endocrinol Metab 77:1485–1489, 1993.

180. Williamson C, Cavaco BM, Jauch A, et al: Mapping the gene causing hereditary primary hyperparathyroidism in a Portuguese kindred to chromosome 1q22-q31, J Bone Miner Res 14:230–239, 1999.

181. Weinstein LS, Simonds WF: HRPT2, a marker of parathyroid cancer, N Engl J Med 349:1691–1692, 2003.

182. Carpten JD, Robbins CM, Villablanca A, et al: HRPT2, encoding parafibromin, is mutated in hyperparathyroidism-jaw tumor syndrome, Nat Genet 32:676–680, 2002.

183. Shattuck TM, Valimaki S, Obara T, et al: Somatic and germ-line mutations of the HRPT2 gene in sporadic parathyroid carcinoma, N Engl J Med 349:1722–1729, 2003.

184. Howell VM, Haven CJ, Kahnoski K, et al: HRPT2 mutations are associated with malignancy in sporadic parathyroid tumours, J Med Genet 40:657–663, 2003.

185. Bradley KJ, Cavaco BM, Bowl MR, et al: Parafibromin mutations in hereditary hyperparathyroidism syndromes and parathyroid tumours, Clin Endocrinol (Oxf) 64:299–306, 2006.

186. Cetani F, Pardi E, Ambrogini E, et al: Genetic analyses in familial isolated hyperparathyroidism: implication for clinical assessment and surgical management, Clin Endocrinol (Oxf) 64:146–152, 2006.

187. Krebs LJ, Shattuck TM, Arnold A: HRPT2 mutational analysis of typical sporadic parathyroid adenomas, J Clin Endocrinol Metab 90:5015–5017, 2005.

188. Zhao J, Yart A, Frigerio S, et al: Sporadic human renal tumors display frequent allelic imbalances and novel mutations of the HRPT2 gene, Oncogene 26:3440–3449, 2007.

189. Zheng HC, Takahashi H, Li XH, et al: Downregulated parafibromin expression is a promising marker for pathogenesis, invasion, metastasis and prognosis of gastric carcinomas, Virchows Arch 452:147–155, 2008.

190. Selvarajan S, Sii LH, Lee A, et al: Parafibromin expression in breast cancer: a novel marker for prognostication? J Clin Pathol 61:64–67, 2008.

191. Bradley KJ, Bowl MR, Williams SE, et al: Parafibromin is a nuclear protein with a functional monopartite nuclear localization signal, Oncogene 26:1213–1221, 2007.

192. Rozenblatt-Rosen O, Hughes CM, Nannepaga SJ, et al: The parafibromin tumor suppressor protein is part of a human Paf1 complex, Mol Cell Biol 25:612–620, 2005.

193. Yart A, Gstaiger M, Wirbelauer C, et al: The HRPT2 tumor suppressor gene product parafibromin associates with human PAF1 and RNA polymerase II, Mol Cell Biol 25:5052–5060, 2005.

194. Mosimann C, Hausmann G, Basler K: Parafibromin/Hyrax activates Wnt/Wg target gene transcription by direct association with beta-catenin/Armadillo, Cell 125:327–341, 2006.

195. Wang P, Bowl MR, Bender S, et al: Parafibromin, a component of the human PAF complex, regulates growth factors and is required for embryonic development and survival in adult mice, Mol Cell Biol 28:2930–2940, 2008.

196. Bjorklund P, Akerstrom G, Westin G: Accumulation of nonphosphorylated beta-catenin and c-myc in primary and uremic secondary hyperparathyroid tumors, J Clin Endocrinol Metab 92:338–344, 2007.

197. Bjorklund P, Akerstrom G, Westin G: An LRP5 receptor with internal deletion in hyperparathyroid tumors with implications for deregulated WNT/beta-catenin signaling, PLoS Med 4:e328, 2007.

198. Bjorklund P, Lindberg D, Akerstrom G, et al: Stabilizing mutation of CTNNB1/beta-catenin and protein accumulation analyzed in a large series of parathyroid tumors of Swedish patients, Mol Cancer 7:53, 2008.

199. Costa-Guda J, Arnold A: Absence of stabilizing mutations of beta-catenin encoded by CTNNB1 exon 3 in a large series of sporadic parathyroid adenomas, J Clin Endocrinol Metab 92:1564–1566, 2007.

200. Ikeda S, Ishizaki Y, Shimizu Y, et al: Immunohistochemistry of cyclin D1 and beta-catenin, and mutational analysis of exon 3 of beta-catenin gene in parathyroid adenomas, Int J Oncol 20:463–466, 2002.

201. Weinberg RA: Tumor suppressor genes, Science 254:1138–1146, 1991.

202. Cryns VL, Thor A, Xu HJ, et al: Loss of the retinoblastoma tumor suppressor gene in parathyroid carcinoma, New Engl J Med 330:757–761, 1994.

203. Pearce SH, Trump D, Wooding C, et al: Loss of heterozygosity studies at the retinoblastoma and breast cancer susceptibility (BRCA2) loci in pituitary, parathyroid, pancreatic and carcinoid tumours, Clin Endocrinol (Oxf) 45:195–200, 1996.

204. Carling T, Du Y, Fang W, et al: Intragenic allelic loss and promoter hypermethylation of the RIZ1 tumor suppressor gene in parathyroid tumors and pheochromocytomas, Surgery 134:932–939; discussion 939–40, 2003.

205. Pei L, Melmed S, Scheithauer B, et al: Frequent loss of heterozygosity at the retinoblastoma susceptibility gene (RB) locus in aggressive pituitary tumors: evidence for a chromosome 13 tumor suppressor gene other than RB, Cancer Res 55:1613–1616, 1995.

206. Cryns VL, Yi SM, Tahara H, et al: Frequent loss of chromosomes arm 1p DNA in parathyroid adenomas, Genes Chromosomes & Cancer 13:9–17, 1995.

207. Williamson C, Pannett AA, Pang JT, et al: Localisation of a gene causing endocrine neoplasia to a 4 cM region on chromosome 1p35-p36, J Med Genet 34:617–619, 1997.

208. Brown EM, MacLeod RJ: Extracellular calcium sensing and extracellular calcium signaling, Physiol Rev 81:239–297, 2001.

209. Simonds WF, James-Newton LA, Agarwal SK, et al: Familial isolated hyperparathyroidism: clinical and genetic characteristics of 36 kindreds, Medicine (Baltimore) 81:1–26, 2002.

210. Simonds WF, Robbins CM, Agarwal SK, et al: Familial isolated hyperparathyroidism is rarely caused by germ-line mutation in HRPT2, the gene for the hyperparathyroidism-jaw tumor syndrome, J Clin Endocrinol Metab 89:96–102, 2004.

211. Warner JV, Nyholt DR, Busfield F, et al: Familial isolated hyperparathyroidism is linked to a 1.7 Mb region on chromosome 2p13.3–14, J Med Genet 43:e12, 2006.

212. Pollak MR, Brown EM, WuChou YH, et al: Mutations in the human Ca^{2+}-sensing receptor gene cause familial hypocalciuric hypercalcemia and neonatal severe hyperparathyroidism, Cell 75:1297–1303, 1993.

213. Chou YH, Pollak MR, Brandi ML, et al: Mutations in the human Ca(2+)-sensing-receptor gene that cause familial hypocalciuric hypercalcemia, Am J Hum Genet 56:1075–1079, 1995.

214. Pearce S, Trump D, Wooding C, et al: Calcium-sensing receptor mutations in familial benign hypercalcaemia and neonatal hyperparathyroidism, J Clin Invest 96:2683–2692, 1995.

215. Janicic N, Pausova Z, Cole DE, et al: Insertion of an Alu sequence in the Ca(2+)-sensing receptor gene in familial hypocalciuric hypercalcemia and neonatal severe hyperparathyroidism, Am J Hum Genet 56:880–886, 1995.

216. Aida K, Koishi S, Inoue M, et al: Familial hypocalciuric hypercalcemia associated with mutation in the human Ca(2+)-sensing receptor gene, J Clin Endocrinol Metab 80:2594–2598, 1995.

217. Heath H, III, Odelberg S, Jackson CE, et al: Clustered inactivating mutations and benign polymorphisms of the calcium receptor gene in familial benign hypocalciuric hypercalcemia suggest receptor functional domains, J Clin Endocrinol Metab 81:1312–1317, 1996.

218. Janicic N, Soliman E, Pausova Z, et al: Mapping of the calcium-sensing receptor gene (CASR) to human chromosome 3q13.3-21 by fluorescence in situ hybridization, and localization to rat chromosome 11 and mouse chromosome 16, Mamm Genome 6:798–801, 1995.

219. Morten KJ, Cooper JM, Brown GK, et al: A new point mutation associated with mitochondrial encephalomyopathy, Hum Mol Genet 2:2081–2087, 1993.

220. Pearce SH, Bai M, Quinn SJ, et al: Functional characterization of calcium-sensing receptor mutations expressed in human embryonic kidney cells, J Clin Invest 98:1860–1866, 1996.

221. Bai M, Quinn S, Trivedi S, et al: Expression and characterization of inactivating and activating mutations in the human Ca^{2+}-sensing receptor, J Biol Chem 271:19537–19545, 1996.

222. Pollak MR, Chou YH, Marx SJ, et al: Familial hypocalciuric hypercalcemia and neonatal severe hyperparathyroidism, Effects of mutant gene dosage on phenotype, J Clin Invest 93:1108–1112, 1994.

223. Bai M, Pearce SH, Kifor O, et al: In vivo and in vitro characterization of neonatal hyperparathyroidism resulting from a de novo, heterozygous mutation in the Ca^{2+}-sensing receptor gene: normal maternal calcium homeostasis as a cause of secondary hyperparathyroid-

ism in familial benign hypocalciuric hypercalcemia, J Clin Invest 99:88–96, 1997.

224. Heath H, III, Jackson CE, Otterrud B, et al: Genetic linkage analysis in familial benign (hypocalciuric) hypercalcemia: evidence for locus heterogeneity, Am J Hum Genet 53:193–200, 1993.

225. McMurtry CT, Schranck FW, Walkenhorst DA, et al: Significant developmental elevation in serum parathyroid hormone levels in a large kindred with familial benign (hypocalciuric) hypercalcemia, Am J Med 93:247–258, 1992.

226. Trump D, Whyte MP, Wooding C, et al: Linkage studies in a kindred from Oklahoma, with familial benign (hypocalciuric) hypercalcaemia (FBH) and developmental elevations in serum parathyroid hormone levels, indicate a third locus for FBH, Hum Genet 96:183–187, 1995.

227. Lloyd SE, Pannett AA, Dixon PH, et al: Localization of familial benign hypercalcemia, Oklahoma variant (FBHOk), to chromosome 19q13, Am J Hum Genet 64:189–195, 1999.

228. Kifor O, Moore FD, Jr, Delaney M, et al: A syndrome of hypocalciuric hypercalcemia caused by autoantibodies directed at the calcium-sensing receptor, J Clin Endocrinol Metab 88:60–72, 2003.

229. Jüppner H, Schipani E, Silve C: Jansen's metaphyseal chondrodysplasia and Blomstrand's lethal chondrodysplasia: two genetic disorders caused by PTH/PTHrP receptor mutations. In Bilezikian J, Raisz L, Rodan G, editors: Principles of bone biology, San Diego, CA, 2002, Academic Press, pp 1117–1135.

230. Schipani E, Kruse K, Jüppner H: A constitutively active mutant PTH-PTHrP receptor in Jansen-type metaphyseal chondrodysplasia, Science 268:98–100, 1995.

231. Schipani E, Langman CB, Parfitt AM, et al: Constitutively activated receptors for parathyroid hormone and parathyroid hormone-related peptide in Jansen's metaphyseal chondrodysplasia, New Engl, J Med 335: 708–714, 1996.

232. Schipani E, Langman CB, Hunzelman J, et al: A novel PTH/PTHrP receptor mutation in Jansen's metaphyseal chondrodysplasia, J Clin Endocrinol Metab 84:3052–3057, 1999.

233. Schipani E, Lanske B, Hunzelman J, et al: Targeted expression of constitutively active PTH/PTHrP receptors delays endochondral bone formation and rescues PTHrP-less mice, Proc Natl Acad Sci U S A 94:13689–13694, 1997.

234. Bastepe M, Raas-Rothschild A, Silver J, et al: A form of Jansen's metaphyseal chondrodysplasia with limited metabolic and skeletal abnormalities is caused by a novel activating PTH/PTHrP receptor mutation, J Clin Endocrinol Metab 89:3595–3600, 2004.

235. Schipani E, Jensen GS, Pincus J, et al: Constitutive activation of the cAMP signaling pathway by parathyroid hormone (PTH)/PTH-related peptide (PTHrP) receptors mutated at the two loci for Jansen's metaphyseal chondrodysplasia, Mol Endocrinol 11:851–858, 1997.

236. Ewart AK, Morris CA, Atkinson DL, et al: Hemizygosity at the elastin locus in a developmental disorder, Williams syndrome, Nature Genet 5:11–16, 1993.

237. Nickerson E, Greenberg F, Keating MT, et al: Deletions of the elastin gene at 7q11.23 occur in approximately 90% of patients with Williams syndrome, Am J Hum Genet 56:1156–1161, 1995.

238. Lowery MC, Morris CA, Ewart A, et al: Strong correlation of elastin deletions, detected by FISH, with Williams syndrome: evaluation of 235 patients, Am J Hum Genet 57:49–53, 1995.

239. Li D, Brooke B, Davis E, et al: Elastin is an essential determinant of arterial morphogenesis, Nature 393:276–280, 1998.

240. Tassabehji M, Metcalfe K, Fergusson WD, et al: LIM-kinase deleted in Williams syndrome, Nat Genet 13:272–273, 1996.

241. Perez Jurado LA, Li X, Francke U: The human calcitonin receptor gene (CALCR) at 7q21.3 is outside the deletion associated with the Williams syndrome, Cytogenet Cell Genet 70:246–249, 1995.

242. Arnold A, Horst SA, Gardella TJ, et al: Mutation of the signal peptide-encoding region of the preproparathyroid hormone gene in familial isolated hypoparathyroidism, J Clin Invest 86:1084–1087, 1990.

243. Karaplis AC, Lim SK, Baba H, et al: Inefficient membrane targeting, translocation, and proteolytic process-

ing by signal peptidase of a mutant preproparathyroid hormone protein, J Biol Chem 270:1629–1635, 1995.

244. Datta R, Waheed A, Shah GN, et al: Signal sequence mutation in autosomal dominant form of hypoparathyroidism induces apoptosis that is corrected by a chemical chaperone, Proc Natl Acad Sci U S A 104:19989–19994, 2007.

245. Sunthornthepvarakul T, Churesigaew S, Ngowngarmratana S: A novel mutation of the signal peptide of the preproparathyroid hormone gene associated with autosomal-recessive familial isolated hypoparathyroidism, J Clin Endocrinol Metab 84:3792–3796, 1999.

246. Parkinson D, Thakker R: A donor splice site mutation in the parathyroid hormone gene is associated with autosomal-recessive hypoparathyroidism, Nature Genet 1:149–153, 1992.

247. Günther T, Chen ZF, Kim J, et al: Genetic ablation of parathyroid glands reveals another source of parathyroid hormone, Nature 406:199–203, 2000.

248. Kim J, Jones B, Zock C, et al: Isolation and characterization of mammalian homologs of the Drosophila gene glial cells missing, Proc Natl Acad Sci U S A 95:12364–12369, 1998.

249. Liu Z, Yu S, Manley NR: Gcm2 is required for the differentiation and survival of parathyroid precursor cells in the parathyroid/thymus primordia, Dev Biol 305:333–346, 2007.

250. Ding C, Buckingham B, Levine MA: Familial isolated hypoparathyroidism caused by a mutation in the gene for the transcription factor GCMB, J Clin Invest 108:1215–1220, 2001.

251. Baumber L, Tufarelli C, Patel S, et al: Identification of a novel mutation disrupting the DNA binding activity of GCM2 in autosomal-recessive familial isolated hypoparathyroidism, J Med Genet 42:443–448, 2005.

252. Mannstadt M, Bertrand G, Muresan M, et al: Dominant-negative GCMB mutations cause an autosomal dominant form of hypoparathyroidism, J Clin Endocrinol Metab 93:3568–3576, 2008.

253. Peden V: True idiopathic hypoparathyroidism as a sex-linked recessive trait, Am J Human Genet 12:323–337, 1960.

254. Whyte M, Weldon V: Idiopathic hypoparathyroidism presenting with seizures during infancy: X-linked recessive inheritance in a large Missouri kindred, J Pediatr 99:628–611, 1981.

255. Whyte M, Kim G, Kosanovich M: Absence of parathyroid tissue in sex-linked recessive hypoparathyroidism, J Paediat 109:915, 1986.

256. Mumm S, Whyte MP, Thakker RV, et al: mtDNA Analysis shows common ancestry in two kindreds with X-linked recessive hypoparathyroidism and reveals a heteroplasmic silent mutation, Am J Hum Genet 60:153–159, 1997.

257. Thakker RV, Davies KE, Whyte MP, et al: Mapping the gene causing X-linked recessive idiopathic hypoparathyroidism to Xq26-Xq27 by linkage studies, J Clin Invest 86:40–45, 1990.

258. Bowl M, Nesbit M, Harding B, et al: An interstitial deletion-insertion involving chromosomes 2p25.3 and Xq27.1, near SOX3, causes X-linked recessive hypoparathyroidism, J Clin Invest 115:2822–2831, 2005.

259. Solomon NM, Ross SA, Morgan T, et al: Array comparative genomic hybridisation analysis of boys with X-linked hypopituitarism identifies a 3.9 Mb duplicated critical region at Xq27 containing SOX3, J Med Genet 41:669–678, 2004.

260. Rizzoti K, Brunelli S, Carmignac D, et al: SOX3 is required during the formation of the hypothalamo-pituitary axis, Nat Genet 36:247–255, 2004.

261. Collignon J, Sockanathan S, Hacker A, et al: A comparison of the properties of Sox-3 with Sry and two related genes, Sox-1 and Sox-2, Development 122:509–520, 1996.

262. Kleinjan DA, van Heyningen V: Long-range control of gene expression: emerging mechanisms and disruption in disease, Am J Hum Genet 76:8–32, 2005.

263. Brunelli S, Silva Casey E, Bell D, et al: Expression of Sox3 throughout the developing central nervous system is dependent on the combined action of discrete, evolutionarily conserved regulatory elements, Genesis 36:12–24, 2003.

264. Uchikawa M, Ishida Y, Takemoto T, et al: Functional analysis of chicken Sox2 enhancers highlights an array

of diverse regulatory elements that are conserved in mammals, Dev Cell 4:509–519, 2003.

265. Kiernan AE, Pelling AL, Leung KK, et al: Sox2 is required for sensory organ development in the mammalian inner ear, Nature 434:1031–1035, 2005.

266. Stevanovic M, Lovell-Badge R, Collignon J, et al: SOX3 is an X-linked gene related to SRY, Hum Mol Genet 2:2013–2018, 1993.

267. Ahonen P, Myllarniemi S, Sipila I, et al: Clinical variation of autoimmune polyendocrinopathy-candidiasis-ectodermal dystrophy (APECED) in a series of 68 patients, N Engl J Med 322:1829–1836, 1990.

268. Ahonen P: Autoimmune polyendocrinopathy–candidosis–ectodermal dystrophy (APECED): autosomal-recessive inheritance, Clin Genet 27:535–542, 1985.

269. Zlotogora J, Shapiro MS: Polyglandular autoimmune syndrome type I among Iranian Jews, J Med Genet 29:824–826, 1992.

270. Aaltonen J, Bjorses P, Sandkuijl L, et al: An autosomal locus causing autoimmune disease: autoimmune polyglandular disease type I assigned to chromosome 21, Nat Genet 8:83–87, 1994.

271. Nagamine K, Peterson P, Scott HS, et al: Positional cloning of the APECED gene, Nat Genet 17:393–398, 1997.

272. Pearce SH, Cheetham T, Imrie H, et al: A common and recurrent 13-bp deletion in the autoimmune regulator gene in British kindreds with autoimmune polyendocrinopathy type 1, Am J Hum Genet 63:1675–1684, 1998.

273. Scott HS, Heino M, Peterson P, et al: Common mutations in autoimmune polyendocrinopathy-candidiasis-ectodermal dystrophy patients of different origins, Mol Endocrinol 12:1112–1119, 1998.

274. Rosatelli MC, Meloni A, Devoto M, et al: A common mutation in Sardinian autoimmune polyendocrinopathy-candidiasis-ectodermal dystrophy patients, Hum Genet 103:428–434, 1998.

275. Bjorses P, Halonen M, Palvimo JJ, et al: Mutations in the AIRE gene: effects on subcellular location and transactivation function of the autoimmune polyendocrinopathy-candidiasis-ectodermal dystrophy protein, Am J Hum Genet 66:378–392, 2000.

276. Liston A, Lesage S, Wilson J, et al: AIRE regulates negative selection of organ-specific T cells, Nat Immunol 4:350–354, 2003.

277. Meager A, Visvalingam K, Peterson P, et al: Anti-interferon autoantibodies in autoimmune polyendocrinopathy syndrome type 1, PLoS Med 3:e289, 2006.

278. Alimohammadi M, Bjorklund P, Hallgren A, et al: Autoimmune polyendocrine syndrome type 1 and NALP5, a parathyroid autoantigen, N Engl J Med 358:1018–1028, 2008.

279. Eisenbarth SC, Colegio OR, O'Connor W, et al: Crucial role for the Nalp3 inflammasome in the immunostimulatory properties of aluminium adjuvants, Nature 453:1122–1126, 2008.

280. Scambler PJ, Carey AH, Wyse RK, et al: Microdeletions within 22q11 associated with sporadic and familial DiGeorge syndrome, Genomics 10:201–206, 1991.

281. Monaco G, Pignata C, Rossi E, et al: DiGeorge anomaly associated with 10p deletion, Am J Med Genet 39:215–216, 1991.

282. Gong W, Emanuel BS, Collins J, et al: A transcription map of the DiGeorge and velo-cardio-facial syndrome minimal critical region on 22q11, Hum Mol Genet 5:789–800, 1996.

283. Scambler PJ: The 22q11 deletion syndromes, Hum Mol Genet 9:2421–2426, 2000.

284. Augusseau S, Jouk S, Jalbert P, et al: DiGeorge syndrome and 22q11 rearrangements, Hum Genet 74:206, 1986.

285. Budarf ML, Collins J, Gong W, et al: Cloning a balanced translocation associated with DiGeorge syndrome and identification of a disrupted candidate gene, Nat Genet 10:269–278, 1995.

286. Yamagishi H, Garg V, Matsuoka R, et al: A molecular pathway revealing a genetic basis for human cardiac and craniofacial defects, Science 283:1158–1161, 1999.

287. Lindsay EA, Botta A, Jurecic V, Carattini-Rivera S, et al: Congenital heart disease in mice deficient for the DiGeorge syndrome region, Nature 401:379–383, 1999.

288. Magnaghi P, Roberts C, Lorain S, et al: HIRA, a mammalian homologue of Saccharomyces cerevisiae tran-

scriptional co-repressors, interacts with Pax3, Nat Genet 20:74–77, 1998.

289. Jerome LA, Papaioannou VE: DiGeorge syndrome phenotype in mice mutant for the T-box gene, Tbx1, Nat Genet 27:286–291, 2001.

290. Yagi H, Furutani Y, Hamada H, et al: Role of TBX1 in human del22q11.2 syndrome, Lancet 362:1366–1373, 2003.

291. Baldini A: DiGeorge's syndrome: a gene at last, Lancet 362:1342–1343, 2003.

292. Scire G, Dallapiccola B, Iannetti P, et al: Hypoparathyroidism as the major manifestation in two patients with 22q11 deletions, Am J Med Genet 52:478–482, 1994.

293. Sykes K, Bachrach L, Siegel-Bartelt J, et al: Velocardiofacial syndrome presenting as hypocalcemia in early adolescence, Arch Pediatr Adolesc Med 151:745–747, 1997.

294. Bilous R, Murty G, Parkinson D, et al: Autosomal dominant familial hypoparathyroidism, sensorineural deafness and renal dysplasia, N Engl J Med 327:1069–1084, 1992.

295. Van Esch H, Groenen P, Nesbit MA, et al: GATA3 haplo-insufficiency causes human HDR syndrome, Nature 406:419–422, 2000.

296. Muroya K, Hasegawa T, Ito Y, et al: GATA3 abnormalities and the phenotypic spectrum of HDR syndrome, J Med Genet 38:374–380, 2001.

297. Nesbit MA, Bowl MR, Harding B, et al: Characterization of GATA3 mutations in the hypoparathyroidism, deafness, and renal dysplasia (HDR) syndrome, J Biol Chem 279:22624–22634, 2004.

298. Ali A, Christie PT, Grigorieva IV, et al: Functional characterization of GATA3 mutations causing the hypoparathyroidism-deafness-renal (HDR) dysplasia syndrome: insight into mechanisms of DNA binding by the GATA3 transcription factor, Hum Mol Genet 16:265–275, 2007.

299. Tsang AP, Visvader JE, Turner CA, et al: FOG, a multitype zinc finger protein, acts as a cofactor for transcription factor GATA-1 in erythroid and megakaryocytic differentiation, Cell 90:109–119, 1997.

300. Zahirieh A, Nesbit MA, Ali A, et al: Functional analysis of a novel GATA3 mutation in a family with the hypoparathyroidism, deafness, and renal dysplasia syndrome, J Clin Endocrinol Metab 90:2445–2450, 2005.

301. Dai YS, Markham BE: p300 Functions as a coactivator of transcription factor GATA-4, J Biol Chem 276:37178–37185, 2001.

302. Pandolfi PP, Roth ME, Karis A, et al: Targeted disruption of the GATA3 gene causes severe abnormalities in the nervous system and in fetal liver haematopoiesis, Nat Genet 11:40–44, 1995.

303. van der Wees J, van Looij MA, de Ruiter MM, et al: Hearing loss following Gata3 haploinsufficiency is caused by cochlear disorder, Neurobiol Dis 16:169–178, 2004.

304. van Looij MA, van der Burg H, van der Giessen RS, et al: GATA3 haploinsufficiency causes a rapid deterioration of distortion product otoacoustic emissions (DPOAEs) in mice, Neurobiol Dis 20:890–897, 2005.

305. Lim KC, Lakshmanan G, Crawford SE, et al: Gata3 loss leads to embryonic lethality due to noradrenaline deficiency of the sympathetic nervous system, Nat Genet 25:209–212, 2000.

306. Grote D, Souabni A, Busslinger M, et al: Pax 2/8-regulated Gata 3 expression is necessary for morphogenesis and guidance of the nephric duct in the developing kidney, Development 133:53–61, 2006.

307. Moraes CT, DiMauro S, Zeviani M, et al: Mitochondrial DNA deletions in progressive external ophthalmoplegia and Kearns-Sayre syndrome, N Engl J Med 320:1293–1299, 1989.

308. Zupanc ML, Moraes CT, Shanske S, et al: Deletion of mitochondrial DNA in patients with combined features of Kearns-Sayre and MELAS syndromes, Ann Neurol 29:680–683, 1991.

309. Isotani H, Fukumoto Y, Kawamura H, et al: Hypoparathyroidism and insulin-dependent diabetes mellitus in a patient with Kearns-Sayre syndrome harbouring a mitochondrial DNA deletion, Clin Endocrinol (Oxf) 45:637–641, 1996.

310. Dionisi-Vici C, Garavaglia B, Burlina AB, et al: Hypoparathyroidism in mitochondrial trifunctional protein deficiency, J Pediatr 129:159–162, 1996.

311. Franceschini P, Testa A, Bogetti G, et al: Kenny-Caffey syndrome in two sibs born to consanguineous parents: evidence for an autosomal recessive variant, Am J Med Genet 42:112–116, 1992.

312. Boynton JR, Pheasant TR, Johnson BL, et al: Ocular findings in Kenny's syndrome, Arch Ophthalmol 97:896–900, 1979.

313. Richardson RJ, Kirk JM: Short stature, mental retardation, and hypoparathyroidism: a new syndrome, Arch Dis Child 65:1113–1117, 1990.

314. Sanjad SA, Sakati NA, Abu-Osba YK, et al: A new syndrome of congenital hypoparathyroidism, severe growth failure, and dysmorphic features, Arch Dis Child 66:193–196, 1991.

315. Parvari R, Hershkovitz E, Kanis A, et al: Homozygosity and linkage-disequilibrium mapping of the syndrome of congenital hypoparathyroidism, growth and mental retardation, and dysmorphism to a 1-cM interval on chromosome 1q42–43, Am J Hum Genet 63:163–169, 1998.

316. Parvari R, Hershkovitz E, Grossman N, et al: Mutation of TBCE causes hypoparathyroidism-retardation-dysmorphism and autosomal-recessive Kenny-Caffey syndrome, Nat Genet 32:448–452, 2002.

317. Parkinson D, Shaw N, Himsworth R, et al: Parathyroid hormone gene analysis in autosomal hypoparathyroidism using an intragenic tetranucleotide (AAAT)n polymorphism, Hum Genet 91:281–284, 1993.

318. Barakat AY, D'Albora JB, Martin MM, et al: Familial nephrosis, nerve deafness, and hypoparathyroidism, J Pediatr 91:61–64, 1977.

319. Dahlberg PJ, Borer WZ, Newcomer KL, et al: Autosomal or X-linked recessive syndrome of congenital lymphedema, hypoparathyroidism, nephropathy, prolapsing mitral valve, and brachytelephalangy, Am J Med Genet 16:99–104, 1983.

320. Pollak MR, Brown EM, Estep HL, et al: Autosomal dominant hypocalcaemia caused by a Ca²⁺-sensing receptor gene mutation, Nat Genet 8:303–307, 1994.

321. Finegold DN, Armitage MM, Galiani M, et al: Preliminary localization of a gene for autosomal-dominant hypoparathyroidism to chromosome 3q13, Pediatr Res 36:414–417, 1994.

322. Pearce SH, Williamson C, Kifor O, et al: A familial syndrome of hypocalcemia with hypercalciuria due to mutations in the calcium-sensing receptor, N Engl J Med 335:1115–1122, 1996.

323. Baron J, Winer K, Yanovski J, et al: Mutations in the Ca(2+)-sensing receptor gene cause autosomal dominant and sporadic hypoparathyroidism, Hum Mol Genet 5:601–606, 1996.

324. Okazaki R, Chikatsu N, Nakatsu M, et al: A novel activating mutation in calcium-sensing receptor gene associated with a family of autosomal dominant hypocalcemia, J Clin Endocrinol Metab 84:363–366, 1999.

325. Thakker RV: Molecular pathology of renal chloride channels in Dent's disease and Bartter's syndrome, Exp Nephrol 8:351–360, 2000.

326. Hebert SC: Bartter syndrome, Curr Opin Nephrol Hypertens 12:527–532, 2003.

327. Watanabe S, Fukumoto S, Chang H, et al: Association between activating mutations of calcium-sensing receptor and Bartter's syndrome, Lancet 360:692–694, 2002.

328. Li Y, Song YH, Rais N, et al: Autoantibodies to the extracellular domain of the calcium sensing receptor in patients with acquired hypoparathyroidism, J Clin Invest 97:910–914, 1996.

329. Blomstrand S, Claësson I, Såve-Söderbergh J: A case of lethal congenital dwarfism with accelerated skeletal maturation, Pediatr, Radiol 15:141–143, 1985.

330. Young ID, Zuccollo JM, Broderick NJ: A lethal skeletal dysplasia with generalised sclerosis and advanced skeletal maturation: Blomstrand chondrodysplasia, J Med Genet 30:155–157, 1993.

331. Leroy JG, Keersmaeckers G, Coppens M, et al: Blomstrand lethal chondrodysplasia, Am J Med Genet 63:84–89, 1996.

332. Loshkajian A, Roume J, Stanescu V, et al: Familial Blomstrand chondrodysplasia with advanced skeletal maturation: further delineation, Am J Med Genet 71:283–288, 1997.

333. den Hollander NS, van der Harten HJ, Vermeij-Keers C, et al: First-trimester diagnosis of Blomstrand lethal osteochondrodysplasia, Am J Med Genet 73:345–350, 1997.

334. Oostra RJ, Baljet B, Dijkstra PF, et al: Congenital anomalies in the teratological collection of museum Vrolik in Amsterdam, The Netherlands. II: skeletal dysplasia, Am J Med Genet 77:116–134, 1998.

335. Jobert AS, Zhang P, Couvineau A, et al: Absence of functional receptors parathyroid hormone and parathyroid hormone-related peptide in Blomstrand chondrodysplasia, J Clin Invest 102:34–40, 1998.

336. Zhang P, Jobert AS, Couvineau A, et al: A homozygous inactivating mutation in the parathyroid hormone/parathyroid hormone-related peptide receptor causing Blomstrand chondrodysplasia, J Clin Endocrinol Metab 83:3365–3368, 1998.

337. Karaplis AC, Bin He MT, Nguyen A, et al: Inactivating mutation in the human parathyroid hormone receptor type 1 gene in Blomstrand chondrodysplasia, Endocrinology 139:5255–5258, 1998.

338. Karperien MC, van der Harten HJ, van Schooten R, et al: A frame-shift mutation in the type I parathyroid hormone/parathyroid hormone-related peptide receptor causing Blomstrand lethal osteochondrodysplasia, J Clin Endocrinol Metab 84:3713–3720, 1999.

339. Karperien M, Sips H, Harten Hvd, et al: Novel mutations in the type I PTH/PTHrP receptor causing Blomstrand lethal osteochondrodysplasia (abstract), J Bone Mineral Res 16(Suppl 1):S549, 2001.

340. Wysolmerski JJ, Cormier S, Philbrick W, et al: Absence of functional type 1 PTH/PTHrP receptors in humans is associated with abnormal breast development and tooth impactation, J Clin Endocrinol Metab 86:1788–1794, 2001.

341. Frame B, Poznanski AK: Conditions that may be confused with rickets. In DeLuca HF, Anast CS, editors: Pediatric diseases related to calcium, New York, 1980, Elsevier, pp 269–289.

342. De Haas WHD, De Boer W, Griffioen F: Metaphysial dysostosis. A late follow-up of the first reported case, J Bone Joint Surg 51B:290–299, 1969.

Chapter 6

GENETIC DISORDERS OF PHOSPHATE HOMEOSTASIS

KENNETH E. WHITE, F. RICHARD BRINGHURST, and MICHAEL J. ECONS

The identification of genetic disorders associated with altered phosphate handling has been essential for providing new understanding of the mechanisms controlling phosphate homeostasis. Elevated fibroblast growth factor-23 (FGF23) is associated with syndromes manifested by hypophosphatemia with paradoxically low or normal $1,25(OH)_2$ vitamin D ($1,25(OH)_2D$) and include autosomal-dominant hypophosphatemic rickets (ADHR), X-linked hypophosphatemic rickets (XLH), tumor-induced osteomalacia (TIO), and autosomal-recessive hypophosphatemic rickets (ARHR). Heritable disorders of hyperphosphatemia and often elevated $1,25(OH)_2D$, such as tumoral calcinosis (TC) and hyperostosis-hyperphosphatemia syndrome (HHS), are associated with reduced FGF23 activity. Hereditary hypophosphatemia with hypercalciuria (HHRH) results from mutations in the phosphate transporter NPT2c, which directly results in impaired Pi reabsorption in the nephron. These collective findings have provided unique insight into the activity of FGF23 on renal Pi and vitamin D metabolism, as well as new insight into the pathophysiology of the various disorders. This chapter reviews the clinical manifestations of these disorders, their pathophysiology, current treatment, and strategies for developing new therapies.

Regulation of Phosphate Homeostasis

In contrast to calcium, phosphate is widely distributed in nonosseous tissues, both in inorganic form and as a component of numerous organic molecules ranging from nucleic acids and membrane phospholipids to small phosphoproteins and intermediates of carbohydrate metabolism. These soft-tissue phosphates nevertheless compose only about 15% of the total body content, the remainder of which is deposited as inorganic phosphate (Pi) in the mineral phase of bone.

Phosphate in serum exists almost exclusively as the free ion or in association with cations. Unlike calcium, only 12% of phosphate is protein bound.[1] Also in contrast to calcium, serum phosphate concentrations may vary substantially throughout the day. Carbohydrate ingestion may markedly reduce serum phosphate by moving serum phosphate from the extracellular to the intracellular space. Moreover, serum phosphate undergoes diurnal variation of as much as 1.5 mg/dL (0.5 mmol/L), with a nadir between 8 and 11 AM.[2] Interference with the measurement of phosphate in serum may occur during hypertriglyceridemia,[3] hypergammaglobulinemia,[4] or mannitol therapy,[5] depending on the method of analysis.

Fasting serum phosphate remains stable throughout the menstrual cycle and during pregnancy.[6-10] The placenta actively transports phosphate into the fetus, as reflected in the higher phosphate concentrations of newborn cord arterial and venous blood compared with maternal blood levels.[8] Lactating women, who may lose 100 to 500 mg of phosphorus daily in milk, nevertheless maintain normal levels of serum phosphate.[11,12] Serum phosphate concentrations are relatively high in the newborn (5 to 7 mg/dL),[8,13] decrease gradually thereafter, and then increase again briefly at puberty before reaching adult levels by age 18 to 20 years. Serum phosphate typically increases in women after menopause but decreases in the elderly.[14-16]

Phosphate is a ubiquitous constituent of a vast array of biomolecules. Of particular importance is the fundamental role of inorganic phosphate as a substrate for intracellular enzymes involved in glycolysis and respiration that synthesize high-energy phosphate bonds for storage of chemical energy in organophosphate compounds such as ATP, creatine phosphate, diphosphoglycerate (DPG), phosphoenolpyruvate, and others. Severe phosphate depletion leads to a concentration-dependent inhibition of glycolysis, accumulation of "triose phosphates" immediately proximal to glyceraldehyde 3-phosphate dehydrogenase, and decreased production of ATP. Adequate extracellular phosphate is required for normal mineralization of bone and cartilage,[17,18] and chronic hypophosphatemia of any cause may therefore lead to osteomalacia or, in children, rickets.

The average dietary intake of phosphate—derived largely from dairy products, cereals, and meats—is roughly twice the estimated minimum requirement of 400 mg/day.[19] Absorptive efficiency is high, averaging about 70%, and may increase further (=90%) if the intake of dietary phosphate decreases to less than 2 mg/kg/day.[20] Phosphate is avidly absorbed throughout the small intestine, but especially in the jejunum in animals and humans.[21-23]

In the jejunum, overall phosphate uptake consists of two components: a saturable, sodium-dependent process that is responsive to vitamin D (see later) and a nonsaturable, sodium-independent mechanism thought to represent paracellular diffusional transport.[21,24] The saturable mechanism reflects active transport via the transcellular route, the energy for which is derived from the transmembrane sodium gradient. In animal tissues and in human jejunal biopsies, the sodium phosphate cotransporter exhibits a K_m of approximately 0.05 mmol/L, half-maximal stimulation by 30 to 50 mmol/L sodium, and a ratio of two sodium molecules per molecule of phosphate transported.[21,25,26] Sodium-dependent active phosphate absorption is mediated by the NPT2b cotransporters present in the luminal brush-border membranes of enterocytes.[27,28] Sodium phosphate transporter NPT2b is the product of a different gene from that which encodes the predominant forms expressed in the renal proximal tubule (NPT2a and NPT2c).[27,28] For example, mice lacking the renal cotransporter manifest striking hyperphosphaturia because of continued intestinal phosphate absorption.[29] NPT2b is fully saturated at intraluminal phosphate concentrations of 1 to 2 mmol/L, which are easily achieved after most typical meals. Subsequent transport across the basolateral membrane does not require active transport and is thought to proceed via facilitated diffusion, although the transporter or channel involved has not been characterized.[30]

REGULATION OF PHOSPHATE ABSORPTION

The central role of vitamin D in the regulation of intestinal phosphate transport has been recognized for many years. Absorption of phosphate, like that of calcium, is strikingly augmented by 1,25(OH)$_2$D.[21,22,31-34] Basal fractional phosphate absorption in the absence of 1,25(OH)$_2$D is much higher than that of calcium, however. The action of 1,25(OH)$_2$D on phosphate transport has been studied in vitro by using intact intestinal segments, isolated enterocytes, and brush-border membrane vesicles (BBMVs).[24,35-39] In each case, stimulation by 1,25(OH)$_2$D was shown to result from activation of the sodium-dependent active transport mechanism and not the passive diffusional component. Specifically, 1,25(OH)$_2$D stimulates the maximal velocity of sodium-dependent phosphate cotransport by increasing expression of NPT2b, mainly or exclusively via a posttranscriptional mechanism.[30,40-43] Other studies have pointed to an additional, very rapid (minutes), nongenomic mechanism of 1,25(OH)$_2$D-dependent stimulation of intestinal phosphate transport, analogous to its nongenomic effect on duodenal calcium transport.[44,45]

Restriction of dietary phosphate increases intestinal NPT2b expression[41,43] and thus, like 1,25(OH)$_2$D, enhances the V_{max} of the saturable component of intestinal phosphate absorption.[46-48] This response also involves a posttranscriptional mechanism,[41,43] results in part from augmented renal synthesis of 1,25(OH)$_2$D,[30] but can be seen also in vitamin D–deficient or vitamin D receptor–null animals.[43,49-51]

PHOSPHATE EXCRETION

Renal tubular reabsorption is the overriding determinant of serum phosphate concentration and is subject to elaborate regulation by a wide variety of hormonal and metabolic factors. As noted earlier, the efficiency of intestinal phosphate absorption is high and not as closely regulated as is that of calcium. Consequently, urinary phosphate excretion is tightly correlated with phosphate intake.

Eighty percent of filtered phosphate is reabsorbed by the proximal tubule, and the capacity for phosphate transport appears to diminish between the early convoluted and the straight (pars recta) portions of the proximal tubule.[52-54] Additional phosphate may be reabsorbed in the distal tubule or cortical collecting tubule or both.[55-60] Phosphate must be actively transported across the luminal brush-border membrane against a steep electrochemical gradient. Consistent with this, renal phosphate transport requires luminal sodium ions and is blocked by inhibitors of Na$^+$/K$^+$-ATPase.[54,61-64] Dibasic phosphate is preferentially transported by the rat proximal tubule,[65-67] and studies with isolated perfused tubules have shown that increased intraluminal pH and decreased intracellular pH accelerate phosphate reabsorption by the intact cell.[68]

The two primary transport proteins responsible for Pi reabsorption in the kidney are the type II sodium-phosphate cotransporters NPT2a and NPT2c, expressed in the apical membrane of the proximal tubule. In the mouse, NPT2a is a critical phosphate cotransporter in the renal proximal tubule. Ablation of the NPT2a gene in the mouse results in a decrease in proximal tubular sodium phosphate cotransport, hypophosphatemia, and loss of regulation of phosphate reabsorption by both parathyroid hormone (PTH) and dietary phosphate.[29,69,70] Ablation of NPT2c in mice does not result in a phosphate phenotype,[71] thereby indicating that it may play a less central role in phosphate transport in the mouse. However, mutations in the gene coding NPT2c, *SLC34A3*, result in hereditary hypophosphatemic rickets with hypercalciuria (HHRH, see later), indicating that this transporter plays an important role in maintenance of phosphate homeostasis in humans.

Measurement of Renal Phosphate Transport

For clinical purposes, a relatively convenient way of measuring a patient's ability to reabsorb phosphate is to calculate the tubular maximum reabsorption of phosphate divided by the glomerular filtration rate (TMP/GFR). A simple nomogram has been developed by Walton and Bijvoet[72] that works well in most situations (Fig. 6-1).

REGULATION OF PHOSPHATE REABSORPTION

Parathyroid Hormone

PTH has a major effect on serum phosphate. The clinical relevance of this effect is demonstrated in patients with hyperparathyroidism, who develop phosphaturia and hypophosphatemia, as well as those with hypoparathyroidism, who have increased

NOMOGRAM FOR DERIVATION OF RENAL THRESHOLD PHOSPHATE CONCENTRATION

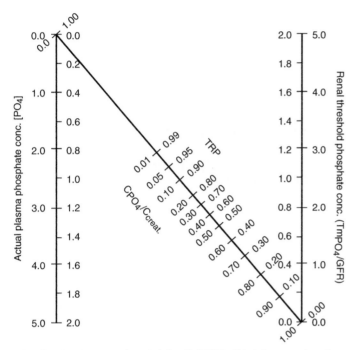

FIGURE 6-1. Nomogram for calculating TmP/GFR. Calculations are done from fasting samples obtained in the morning. The urine is collected for 1 to 2 hours (the time period is not critical). The $C_{PO4}/Ccreat = (U_{PO4} \times [Creat])/(U_{creat} \times [Pi])$. To use the nomogram to calculate TMP/GFR, a straight line is passed through the appropriate plasma phosphate concentration and the $C_{PO4}/Ccreat$. The line will intersect with the corresponding TMP/GFR value. For SI units, use the inside scales. For metric (mg/dL), use the outside scales. (From Walton RJ, Bijvoet OL: Nomogram for derivation of renal threshold phosphate concentration. Lancet 2:309–310, 1975.)

phosphate reabsorption and hyperphosphatemia. PTH rapidly (15 to 60 minutes) reduces the number of NPT2a cotransporters on the apical surface of the cells in the renal proximal tubule. The effect appears to result from microtubule-dependent internalization into endocytic vesicles and subsequent destruction of the transporters.[73,74] This acute down-regulation of NPT2a cotransporters does not involve reduction in NPT2a gene transcription,[75] although transcriptional suppression is seen after more prolonged PTH exposure.[76] After parathyroidectomy, rats manifest a two- to threefold increase in both protein and messenger RNA (mRNA) levels of NPT2a, which correlates with a striking increase in phosphate reabsorption.[75] Evidence exists for involvement of both PKA and protein kinase C (PKC), as well as MAPK signaling via PTH/PTHrP receptors in bringing about these responses.[77,78] Despite the fact that PTH clearly has a major effect on phosphate homeostasis, it should be kept in mind that the primary role of PTH is to regulate serum calcium level and not phosphate homeostasis. Recent studies of the role of FGF23 further illuminate this issue (see later).

Dietary Phosphate

Renal phosphate excretion is extremely sensitive to changes in dietary phosphate availability. Thus, dietary phosphate deprivation[79-86] or supplementation[80,82,87] rapidly evokes a compensatory increase or decrease, respectively, in renal phosphate reabsorption ($[Pi]_{Th}$). Compelling clinical and experimental evidence has established that these adaptations to dietary phosphate occur quite independently of PTH.[74,75,79-82,88]

Increased sodium-dependent phosphate transport by isolated brush-border membrane vesicles occurs within a few hours of phosphate deprivation[86,89] and reflects increased maximal velocity (rather than affinity) of the phosphate carrier,[89-91] consistent with an increased number of membrane transporters. This has been corroborated by direct immunohistologic demonstration that institution of a low-phosphate diet causes rapid (within 2 hours) insertion of NPT2a cotransporters into the apical plasma membrane of rat proximal tubular cells by a microtubule-dependent mechanism.[92-94] Up-regulation of NPT2a gene transcription occurs subsequently during more prolonged phosphate restriction (i.e., several days).[74] Similarly, high dietary phosphate rapidly reduces apical membrane NPT2a protein levels, with no change in NPT2a gene transcription for at least several hours.[74,95]

Fibroblast Growth Factor-23

Fibroblast growth factor-23 (FGF23), the gene identified as causative for autosomal dominant hypophosphatemic rickets (see later) and some forms of familial hyperphosphatemic tumoral calcinosis, does not appear to play a role in the rapid changes in phosphate reabsorption due to acute changes in intestinal phosphate.[96] However, there is substantial evidence that FGF23 plays a role in maintenance of normal phosphate homeostasis over the course of days.

FIBROBLAST GROWTH FACTOR-23 ACTIVITY

FGF23 has similar functions as PTH to reduce renal Pi reabsorption but has opposite effects on $1,25(OH)_2D$ production. FGF23 delivery leads to renal Pi wasting through the down-regulation of both NPT2a and NPT2c.[97] Under normal circumstances, hypophosphatemia is a strong positive stimulator for increasing serum $1,25(OH)_2D$ production. However, patients with ADHR, TIO, XLH, and ARHR manifest hypophosphatemia with paradoxically low or inappropriately normal serum $1,25(OH)_2D$ concentrations. In mice, the expression of the $1\alpha(OH)$ase enzyme and the catabolic $24(OH)$ase are reduced and elevated, respectively, when the animals are exposed to FGF23 by injection or by transgenic approaches.[98] Thus, the effects of FGF23 on the renal vitamin D metabolic enzymes is most likely responsible for the reductions in $1,25(OH)_2D$ in the setting of often marked hypophosphatemia in ADHR, XLH, TIO, and ARHR patients.

REGULATION OF FGF23 PRODUCTION

In humans, dietary Pi supplementation increased FGF23, whereas Pi restriction and the addition of Pi binders suppressed serum FGF23 (Fig. 6-2),[99] indicating that FGF23 plays a role in maintenance of Pi homeostasis. In animal studies, the FGF23 response to serum Pi appears to be much more dramatic than in the human studies. Mice given high and low Pi diets have increased and decreased serum FGF23 levels, respectively.[100]

Vitamin D has important regulatory effects on FGF23 in vivo. In mice, injections of 20 to 200 ng $1,25(OH)_2D$ led to dose-dependent increases in serum FGF23 concentrations.[98] These changes in FGF23 occurred before detectable changes in serum Pi, indicating that FGF23 may be directly regulated by vitamin D. Physiologically, this would be consistent with results examining the role of FGF23 in vitamin D metabolism, in that FGF23 has been shown to down-regulate the $1\alpha(OH)$ase mRNA.[97,98] Thus as $1,25(OH)_2D$ is elevated in the blood as a product of $1\alpha(OH)$ase activity, vitamin D would then increase FGF23

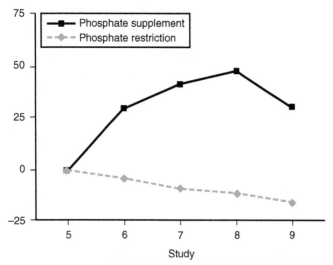

FIGURE 6-2. FGF23 levels in response to diet. Percent change in FGF23 during the intervention period (♦, phosphate depletion intervention as measured with the intact FGF23 assay; ■, phosphate loading intervention as measured with the intact FGF23 assay). The intervention, dietary phosphate depletion, or loading was started after the day 5 samples were collected. Values are presented as mean ± SE. (Data from Burnett SM, Gunawardene SC, Bringhurst FR et al: Regulation of C-terminal and intact FGF-23 by dietary phosphate in men and women, J Bone Miner Res 21:1187–1196, 2006.)

production, which would complete the negative-feedback loop and down-regulate 1α(OH)ase.

Serum Assays

FGF23 can be measured in the bloodstream via several assays. One widely used assay is a "C-terminal" FGF23 enzyme-linked immunosorbent assay (ELISA), with both the capture and detection antibodies binding C-terminal to the FGF23 $_{176}$RXXR$_{179}$/S cleavage site.[101] This assay thus recognizes full-length FGF23 as well as C-terminal fragments that could arise through proteolytic processing. The C-terminal assay is quantified relative to standards composed of FGF23-conditioned media produced from stable cell lines expressing the human protein, and it only recognizes the human FGF23 isoform. The normal mean for this assay is 55 ± 50 reference units (RU)/mL, and the upper limit of normal is 150 RU/mL. In a study with a large number of controls and TIO patients, this ELISA was used to examine FGF23 concentrations in TIO and XLH[101] and showed that serum FGF23 is detectable in normal individuals. The mean FGF23 was greater than 10-fold elevated in TIO patients, which rapidly fell after surgical removal of the tumor. Importantly, most XLH patients (13 out of 21) had elevated FGF23 compared to controls,[101] and in those with "normal" FGF23, these levels may be "inappropriately normal" in the setting of hypophosphatemia.

An "intact" FGF23 assay has been developed that uses conformation-specific monoclonal antibodies that span the $_{176}$RXXR$_{179}$/S$_{180}$ SPC cleavage site (see later) and thus recognize N-terminal and C-terminal regions of the FGF23 polypeptide.[102] In normal individuals, this assay has a mean circulating concentration of 29 pg/mL. The published upper limit of normal is 54 pg/mL.[102] The results of these two assays generally agree with regard to the relative ranges of FGF23 concentrations in XLH and in TIO patients, and that FGF23 is elevated in most XLH patients. Based upon limited data from two TIO patients undergoing resection, the intact assay was used to determine that the half-life of FGF23 is between 20 and 50 minutes.[103,104]

FGF23-Associated Syndromes

FGF23-associated syndromes, summarized in Table 6-1, can be divided into three groups:
1. Disorders associated with increased FGF23 bioactivity
2. Disorders associated with reduced FGF23 bioactivity
3. Genetic hypophosphatemia not associated with elevated FGF23

DISORDERS ASSOCIATED WITH INCREASED FGF23 BIOACTIVITY

Autosomal-Dominant Hypophosphatemic Rickets (OMIM No. 193100)

ADHR is a rare disorder characterized by low serum Pi concentrations due to decreased TmP/GFR and inappropriately low or normal circulating vitamin D concentrations.[105] ADHR was first described in a small family,[106] and subsequently, a large ADHR kindred with many affected individuals was evaluated.[105] This kindred provided an opportunity to test the phenotypic variability of ADHR in a large number of individuals with the same mutation. There was no evidence of genetic anticipation or imprinting. In contrast to the other genetic renal phosphate-wasting disorders, ADHR displays incomplete penetrance and variable age of onset. Important to the diagnosis and clinical management of ADHR, it was observed that this expanded ADHR family contains two subgroups of affected individuals. One subgroup consists of patients who presented during childhood with Pi wasting, rickets, and lower-extremity deformity in a pattern similar to the classic presentation of XLH. The second group consists of individuals who presented clinically during adolescence or adulthood. These individuals had bone pain, weakness, and insufficiency fractures but did not have lower extremity deformities.[105] The patients with adult-onset ADHR had clinical presentations essentially identical to patients who present with TIO (none of the ADHR patients developed tumors). The molecular mechanisms for early-onset ADHR resembling XLH and late-onset ADHR resembling TIO are currently unknown. To date, all patients that have been described with delayed onset of clinically evident disease are female. In addition to these two groups, we found unaffected individuals who are carriers for the ADHR mutation and two patients who were treated for hypophosphatemia and rickets but later lost the Pi wasting defect.[105] Thus, the clinical manifestations of ADHR are more variable than those observed in XLH.

To identify the gene for ADHR, the ADHR Consortium undertook a family-based positional cloning approach. A genomewide linkage scan in the large ADHR kindred described earlier demonstrated linkage to chromosome 12p13.3 (homologous to mouse chromosome 6).[107] FGF23 was identified using exon prediction programs on genomic DNA sequence from the Human Genome Project.[108] The FGF23 gene is composed of three coding exons and contains an open reading frame of 251 residues.[108] The tissue with the highest FGF23 expression is bone, where FGF23 mRNA is observed in osteoblasts, osteocytes, flattened bone-lining cells, and osteoprogenitor cells.[109] Quantitative RT-PCR showed that FGF23 mRNA was most highly expressed in long bone, followed by thymus, brain, and heart.[110]

Western blot analysis has demonstrated that wild-type FGF23 is secreted as a full-length 32-kD protein, as well as cleavage products of 20 kD (N-terminal) and 12 kD (C-terminal).[110-112]

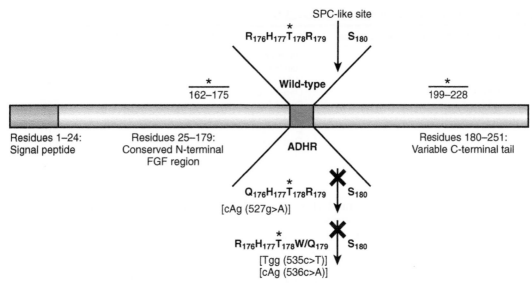

FIGURE 6-3. Model of FGF23 protein domains and effect of the ADHR mutations. FGF23 has a 24-residue signal peptide followed by residues 25 to 179 that comprise the conserved N-terminal FGF-like domain. The SPC-like site is interrupted by the ADHR mutations at R_{176} and R_{179} and divides the FGF-like domain from the variable C-terminal tail region. FGF23 undergoes glycosylation at three regions (denoted *), with the T_{178} most likely being the glycosylated residue that protects the mature protein from SPC degradation between R_{179} and S_{180} and is therefore critical for maintaining intact, active FGF23.

Table 6-1. Primary Heritable and Acquired Disorders Involving Fibroblast Growth Factor-23

Disorder	Gene Mutated	Mutation Consequence	Relationship to FGF23	Effect on Serum Pi	Effect on Serum 1,25D	Intact ELISA [FGF23]	C-Terminal ELISA [FGF23]	Animal Models
ADHR	FGF23	Gain of function	Stabilize full-length, active FGF23	↓	↔	↔ or ↑	↔ or ↑	—
XLH	PHEX	Loss of function	Increased FGF23 production in osteocytes	↓	↔	↔ or ↑	↔ or ↑	Hyp mouse (Phex-null)
ARHR	DMP1	Loss of function	Increased FGF23 production in osteocytes	↓	↔	↔ or ↑	↔ or ↑	Dmp1-null mouse
TIO	—	—	FGF23 highly produced by tumor	↓	↔	↔ or ↑	↔ or ↑	FGF23 general and bone-specific transgenics
TC	FGF23	Loss of function	Destabilize full-length, active FGF23	↑	↔ or ↑	↓	↑	Fgf23-null mice
TC	GALNT3	Loss of function	Destabilize full-length, active FGF23	↑	↔ or ↑	↓	↑	Galnt3-null mouse
HHS	GALNT3	Loss of function	Destabilize full-length, active FGF23	↑	↔ or ↑	↓	↑	Some HHS mutations are the same as in GALNT3-TC
TC	KL	Loss of function	Decreased FGF23-dependent signaling	↑	↔ or ↑	↑	↑	KL-knockdown, and KL-null mice

Cleavage of FGF23 occurs within a subtilisin-like proprotein convertase (SPC) proteolytic site ($_{176}$RXXR$_{179}$/S$_{180}$) that separates the conserved FGF-like N-terminal domain from the variable C-terminal tail (Fig. 6-3).

The ADHR mutations replace arginine (R) residues at FGF23 positions 176 or 179 with glutamine (Q) or tryptophan (W) within the SPC cleavage site, $_{176}$RXXR$_{179}$/S$_{180}$ (Table 6-2 and see Fig. 6-3).[108,111,112] The SPCs are a family of serine proteases that process a wide variety of proteins including neuropeptides, peptide hormones, growth factors, membrane-bound receptors, blood coagulation factors, and plasma proteins.[113] SPC substrates are cleaved C-terminal to the basic motif K/R-X$_n$-K/R, where X$_n$ = 2, 4, or 6 residues of any amino acid.[114,115] The SPCs, such as the furin protease, are largely expressed in the trans-Golgi network and possess similar but not exact substrate specificities.

Following insertion of these mutations into wild-type FGF23, FGF23 secreted from mammalian cells was primarily produced as the full-length protein (32 kD) active polypeptide, as opposed to the 32-kD cleavage products typically observed for wild-type FGF23 expression.[111] Peptide sequencing demonstrated that the 32-kD FGF23 form corresponded to full-length FGF23 after cleavage of the signal peptide (residues 25 to 251) and that the 12-kD isoform was the C-terminal portion of FGF23 downstream from the SPC cleavage site after R179 (residues 180 to 251) (see Fig. 6-3).[112] As further evidence that FGF23 is processed intracellularly, the cleavage of wild-type FGF23 between R179/S180 is inhibited by a nonspecific SPC competitive inhibitor, Dec-RVKR-CMK, at concentrations between 25 and 50 μM.[110,116] These studies show that the RXXR motif in FGF23 is central to its intracellular processing.

Table 6-2. Mutations in the Human Fibroblast Growth Factor-23 Gene

FGF23 Mutation	Predicted Amino Acid Substitution	Demonstrated or Predicted Effect on FGF23	Disorder	Reference
527G>A	R176Q	Stabilized	ADHR	108
535C>T	R179W	Stabilized	ADHR	108
536G>A	R179Q	Stabilized	ADHR	108, 251, 252
123C>T	H41Q	Destabilized	FTC	253
160C>A	Q54K	Destabilized	FTC	190
211A>G	S71G	Destabilized	FTC	187, 188
287C>T	M96T	Destabilized	FTC	191
386C>T	S129F	Destabilized	FTC	189

The SPC family is usually associated with the production of the active form of their substrate polypeptides. However, cleavage of FGF23 at the RXXR motif appears to be inactivating. In this regard, when full-length FGF23 or N-terminal (residues 25 to 179) and C-terminal (residues 180 to 251) fragments were injected into rodents, only the full-length protein lowered circulating phosphate concentrations.[112] Since the full-length form of FGF23 induces hypophosphatemia, it is likely that the ADHR mutations increase the biological activity of FGF23 by stabilizing the full-length form and increasing its concentrations in the serum. Indeed, severely affected ADHR patients have increased circulating levels of FGF23.[117]

Tumor-Induced Osteomalacia

TIO is an acquired disorder of renal Pi wasting that is associated with tumors. Patients with TIO present with hypophosphatemia with inappropriately suppressed 1,25(OH)$_2$D concentrations and elevated alkaline phosphatase levels.[118] Osteomalacia is observed in bone biopsies. Clinical symptoms include gradual onset of muscle weakness, fatigue, and bone pain, especially from ankles, legs, hips, and back.[118,119] Insufficiency fractures are common, and proximal muscle weakness can become severe enough for patients to require a wheelchair or become bed bound.[118]

The study of TIO introduced the idea for the existence of possible tumor-produced circulating factors, referred to as *phosphatonins*, that act upon the kidney to decrease Pi reabsorption.[120,121] Support for these factors primarily comes from the knowledge that if the responsible tumor is surgically removed, the abnormalities in Pi wasting and vitamin D metabolism are rapidly corrected, as well as the fact that PTH, which decreases renal Pi reabsorption, is usually within normal ranges in TIO patients. Other studies have supported this hypothesis by showing that implantation of tumor tissue into nude mice resulted in increased urinary Pi excretion.[122] To determine whether FGF23 could be involved in TIO as phosphatonin, five TIO tumors and several control tissues were tested by Northern blot for the presence of FGF23 transcripts, and it was determined that FGF23 mRNA was highly expressed in all of these tumors.[123] Furthermore, FGF23 was present in a tumor lysate by Western blot analysis, with an anti–human FGF23 antibody.[123]

FGF23 was also independently identified in RNA from TIO tumors. Transcripts from tumors were isolated by differential selection using comparisons to mRNAs present in normal bone.[124] The highly expressed transcripts were then subcloned, and the individual mRNAs were stably expressed in Chinese hamster ovary (CHO) cells, then injected into nude mice to form tumor masses.[124] The cells that produced FGF23 recapitulated the TIO phenotype in vivo by causing hypophosphatemia, elevated alkaline phosphatase, and inappropriately low 1,25(OH)$_2$D concentrations.[124] In addition, the mice that received implanted cells also showed growth retardation, kyphosis, and osteomalacia. Further, there was marked decrease in the renal 1α(OH)ase. Both the biochemical and metabolic bone profiles were remarkably similar to those observed in TIO and ADHR patients. These experiments provided evidence that FGF23 was a phosphaturic substance and had dramatic effects on enzymes involved in vitamin D metabolism, and increased circulating FGF23 concentrations were consistent with the idea that FGF23 was at least in part responsible for the TIO phenotype. Serum FGF23 is elevated in patients with TIO,[101,102] and tumors that cause TIO have a dramatic overexpression of FGF23 mRNA.[123] Surgical resection of the tumor results in rapid decreases in serum FGF23.[101]

X-Linked Hypophosphatemic Rickets (OMIM No. 307800)

XLH is an X-linked dominant disorder and the most common form of heritable rickets.[125] XLH is fully penetrant with variable severity. XLH patients present with laboratory findings that include hypophosphatemia with normocalcemia and inappropriately normal or low 1,25(OH)$_2$D concentrations.[125] Skeletal defects include lower-extremity deformities from rickets, bone pain, osteomalacia, fracture, and enthesopathy (calcification of the tendons and ligaments).[125] It was determined by the Hyp Consortium that XLH is caused by inactivating mutations in PHEX (phosphate-regulating gene with homologies to endopeptidases on the X chromosome).[126] Based upon sequence homology, PHEX encodes a protein that is a member of the M13 family of membrane-bound metalloproteases. Other members of this enzyme class include neutral endopeptidase (NEP) and endothelin-converting enzymes 1 and 2 (ECE-1 and ECE-2).[126,127] This protease family is known to cleave small peptide hormones, therefore it is likely that PHEX has similar activity. Over 160 inactivating PHEX mutations have been described in XLH patients, including genomic variations that cause missense, nonsense, frameshift, and splicing changes (see PHEX Locus database: *www.phexdb.mcgill.ca*). Of note, although XLH is a renal Pi wasting disorder, PHEX shows the highest expression in bone cells such as osteoblasts, osteocytes, and odontoblasts in teeth, as well as lower expression in the parathyroid glands, lung, brain, and skeletal muscle but no expression in kidney.[128] Taken together with the biochemical phenotype of XLH, PHEX protein homology and tissue expression are consistent with the hypothesis that PHEX interacts with small circulating factors outside of the kidney.

A valuable tool for the study of the pathophysiology of XLH has been the *Hyp* mouse, which has 3′ deletion in the *Phex* gene from intron 15 through the 3′ UTR[129] and does not make a stable Phex transcript.[128] This rodent model parallels the XLH phenotype, characterized by hypophosphatemia with inappropriately normal 1,25(OH)$_2$D levels and normal serum calcium, as well as growth retardation and bone mineralization defects.[130] Parabiosis studies between the *Hyp* mouse and a normal mouse pointed to the presence of a humoral factor, a phosphatonin, being transferred through the circulation of the *Hyp* mouse to the normal mouse to cause isolated renal Pi wasting.[131] After the identification of *PHEX/Phex*, it was logically postulated that the enzyme may directly degrade a phosphaturic substance; however, recent studies suggest a more complex pathophysiology.

X-Linked Hypophosphatemic Rickets and Fibroblast Growth Factor-23

As described earlier, patients with XLH have overlapping phenotypes with ADHR patients. Because XLH results from a mutation in PHEX, which shares homology to a family of extracellular proteases, and ADHR arises from mutations in a protease cleavage site, it was logically hypothesized that circulating FGF23 would be cleaved and inactivated by PHEX. Thus, by mutational inactivation of PHEX in XLH, serum FGF23 concentrations would then elevate and cause renal Pi wasting. As described earlier, lending further support to this hypothesis were parabiosis studies between *Hyp* and normal mice, which pointed to the presence of a humoral phosphaturic factor in the *Hyp* mouse being transferred to the normal mouse. However, evidence to date has not supported a direct enzyme-substrate relationship between FGF23 and PHEX. In this regard, it was shown that recombinant PHEX did not cleave FGF23 but did cleave a positive control substrate.[110] Furthermore, another report provided evidence that recombinant FGF23 was not cleaved by PHEX in cultured HEK293 cells coexpressing the proteins.[116] This latter study expressed native FGF23 that was not epitope tagged to ensure that the additional residues did not cause conformational changes within FGF23 and interfere with potential PHEX activity.[116]

Several reports have established that FGF23 is elevated in many XLH patients.[101,102,132] To understand the possible relationship between PHEX and FGF23, quantitative real-time RT-PCR was used to test *Hyp* bone for FGF23 mRNA concentrations versus wild-type bone. Interestingly, FGF23 mRNA in bone tissue from *Hyp* mice was elevated compared to levels present in control mice,[110] and serum concentrations of FGF23 have been reported to be 10-fold higher in *Hyp* mice when compared to normal mice (our unpublished results and Ref. 133). This finding provides support for the idea that there is a cellular connection between inactive PHEX mutants (or lack of Phex expression in *Hyp* mice) and the up-regulation of FGF23 mRNA in bone cells. The elevated FGF23 mRNA levels may indicate that the increase in serum FGF23 in XLH patients is due to overproduction and secretion of FGF23 by skeletal cells, as opposed to the alternative hypothesis of a decreased rate of FGF23 degradation by cell surface proteases after secretion into the circulation. Although the interactions between FGF23 and PHEX are most likely indirect, the encoded proteins are coexpressed in osteoblasts and osteocytes.[109,110,128] At present, the PHEX substrate and the mechanisms for phosphate sensing are unknown.

The current therapy for XLH, ADHR, and TIO includes oral replacement of phosphorus in combination with high-dose $1,25(OH)_2D$. This regimen "treats" XLH by increasing serum Pi concentrations and ameliorates much of the metabolic bone disease, but it does not directly "cure" the disorder by reversing the underlying molecular defects in kidney and in bone. In this regard, several studies have attempted to reverse the XLH phenotype. Transgenic expression of wild-type PHEX under the control of the bone-specific mouse pro-alpha(I) collagen gene[134]

and the osteocalcin (OG2)[135] promoters on the *Hyp* background was undertaken. Interestingly, the defective mineralization of bone and teeth in the *Hyp* mice was partially resolved with PHEX under the regulation of the collagen promoter, and dry ash weight increased with the OG2 PHEX, indicating improved mineralization. However, the hypophosphatemia was not normalized in either study, indicating that expression of PHEX under the temporal regulation of an osteoblast-specific promoter is not sufficient to rescue the *Hyp* phenotype. Furthermore, expression of PHEX to levels observed in wild-type animals was not obtained in all studies. Importantly, a recent report of a transgenic model overexpressing PHEX in the *Hyp* mouse—using the human beta-actin promoter for directing expression in a wider tissue distribution (bone, skin, lung, muscle, heart)—resulted in similar results as the bone-specific promoter studies,[136] further demonstrating that proper spatial-temporal expression of Phex is critical for normal mineral metabolism.

Treatment of X-Linked Hypophosphatemic Rickets

The current standard of care is combination therapy with phosphate and $1,25(OH)_2D$ (calcitriol) or 1-hydroxyvitamin D_3.[137-139] Therapy is labor intensive, and patients and caregivers should understand this before initiating treatment. As in any medical encounter, patients should be fully informed about potential side effects of therapy.

The objectives of therapy in children are to correct or prevent deformity from rickets, promote growth, and lessen bone pain. In some cases, marked improvement in lower-extremity deformity is noted with medical therapy. In this regard, we frequently give a course of medical therapy before performing osteotomies to correct lower-extremity deformities. Most affected children probably should be treated if a system exists to administer and monitor therapy. However, in some instances, it may be acceptable not to treat but rather to follow mildly affected children carefully (no less than twice a year).

The indications for treatment of adult patients are more controversial. There are no data to suggest that current treatment regimens prevent enthesopathy (calcifications of tendons and ligaments). Pseudofractures are common in moderately to severely affected adult XLH patients. Since pseudofractures are often painful, may lead to fracture, and generally respond well to treatment, we generally recommend medical therapy for patients with pseudofractures. XLH patients frequently complain of bone pain,[121] presumably due to osteomalacia. Treatment lessens osteomalacia and bone pain, and it is therefore reasonable to treat patients with this complaint. Additionally, it is advisable to treat patients who have nonunion after fractures or osteotomies, because treatment may improve fracture healing. In light of the complexity of therapy, potential side effects (see later), and lack of increased risk of fracture in patients without pseudofractures,[121] therapy is not recommended in asymptomatic patients who do not have pseudofractures.

Once the decision is made to initiate therapy, it is best to start at a low dose of calcitriol and phosphate (to avoid diarrhea from phosphate) and gradually increase therapy over several months. Some clinicians maintain a "high dose" phase for up to 1 year. During this phase of therapy, the calcitriol dose may be as high as 50 ng/kg per day in two divided doses, but not more than 3.0 mcg/day. However, not all experienced clinicians use this high-dose phase and some will use a maximum of 25 ng/kg. Also, 20 to 40 mg/kg of phosphate is administered in four divided doses (up to a maximum of 2 g per day). Serum calcium, phosphorus, and creatinine levels, as well as urine calcium and creatinine concentrations, are routinely monitored on a monthly basis during the high-dose phase. The doses of calcitriol and phosphate are adjusted based on the laboratory results. Hypercalciuria may be the first sign of healing of osteomalacia (theoretically, osteomalacic bone is capable of taking up more calcium and phosphate than bone that is histologically normal). Although some clinicians recommend administering phosphate over five doses per day initially, we do not ask patients to wake up to take medication at night for the following reasons: (1) serum phosphate concentrations tend to rise at night in XLH patients,[140] (2) there is an exaggerated nocturnal rise in PTH concentrations in XLH patients, and (3) it is very difficult for patients to wake up to take medication every night for a chronic condition. After approximately 1 year on high-dose therapy, patients are switched to a long-term "maintenance" phase with approximately 10 to 20 ng/kg per day of calcitriol and no change in the dose of phosphate. While patients are on maintenance therapy, we continue to see them and monitor serum and urine biochemistries at least every 3 to 4 months.

Preliminary data indicate that standard therapy may have the undesirable affect of increasing FGF23 concentrations. It is possible that calcitriol, phosphate, or both stimulate the production of FGF23 in XLH patients despite the fact that they are still hypophosphatemic.[141] This is currently an active area of research; however, physicians may want to consider not using a high-dose phase.

Careful follow-up is required when employing combined therapy, because the two agents balance each other's effects. Administration of phosphate alone will lead to secondary hyperparathyroidism, and administration of 1,25(OH)$_2$D alone commonly leads to hypercalciuria and hypercalcemia. Hence a patient on combined therapy can develop hypercalciuria as a consequence of either too much 1,25(OH)$_2$D or too little phosphate. Because of this balance, any time it becomes necessary to interrupt phosphate administration, it is necessary to discontinue 1,25(OH)$_2$D therapy as well.

Diarrhea and gastrointestinal upset frequently develop from phosphate administration. To minimize diarrhea, the phosphate dose should be increased gradually. If diarrhea develops, it is best to decrease (or stop) the dose of phosphate (and calcitriol; see earlier) and slowly increase therapy as tolerated. Since hypercalcemia may develop from calcitriol therapy, patients should be given instructions on the symptoms of hypercalcemia, such as depression, confusion, anorexia, nausea, vomiting, polyuria, and dehydration. Serum biochemistries should be measured if a patient experiences any symptoms of hypercalcemia. It should not be assumed that patients on high-dose calcitriol who develop nausea, vomiting, and lethargy have food poisoning or another benign etiology of their symptoms until proven otherwise.

The most common and potentially serious complication of therapy is the development of nephrocalcinosis.[142-147] With the widespread use of renal ultrasound, nephrocalcinosis has been noted with increasing frequency. In most cases, the nephrocalcinosis is observed without evident changes in glomerular filtration rate (GFR). Its occurrence may be related to phosphate dosage, and some authors assert that phosphate administration leads to hyperabsorption of oxalate, which results in nephrocalcinosis.[148] However, this assertion remains unproven, and patients who received vitamin D$_2$ but no phosphate can develop nephrocalcinosis.[149] Thus hypercalciuria and hypercalcemia may contribute to (or at least aggravate) this problem. Kidney biopsy specimens from three treated patients with nephrocalcinosis showed that renal calcifications are located mainly intratubularly

and are composed exclusively of calcium phosphate.[150] Of note, a report of two patients with nephrocalcinosis for 2 decades indicates that it was not associated with impaired renal function.[149] Although these data are somewhat reassuring, the available data are not strong enough to completely allay concerns about renal complications of even carefully monitored therapy, and we are aware of at least one XLH patient with end-stage renal failure after long-term therapy.

A second, less common complication is the development of tertiary hyperparathyroidism.[151-154] Presumably, tertiary hyperparathyroidism results from chronic stimulation of the parathyroid glands by phosphate therapy. Although this complication is more likely in patients who are getting too much phosphate, it also can occur in optimally treated individuals. In tertiary hyperparathyroidism, renal function may decline, necessitating a reduction in the dose of phosphate and calcitriol or cessation of therapy. This will lead to the redevelopment or worsening of the bone disease. A small number of such patients have undergone total parathyroidectomy with autotransplant to the forearm. In a number of these patients, the transplanted tissue has shown a propensity to proliferate and lead to the redevelopment of tertiary hyperparathyroidism. Removal of this hyperplastic tissue from the forearm site leads to a reduction in serum PTH levels. Theoretically, total parathyroidectomy followed by treatment with 1,25(OH)$_2$D and phosphate is a potential option. However, this approach is not recommended, because it results in lifelong hypoparathyroidism.

Although treatment complications cannot be prevented entirely, careful monitoring may minimize treatment-related problems. Serum calcium, phosphorus, and creatinine levels and urine calcium and creatinine concentrations should be monitored monthly while patients are on high-dose therapy and every 3 to 4 months while on maintenance therapy. A 24-hour urine phosphorus measurement is often useful to gauge compliance with therapy. Serum PTH concentration should be measured at yearly intervals as appropriate. We have not seen patients with elevated urinary oxalate caused by therapy. A renal ultrasound should be obtained as a baseline at the start of therapy and periodically thereafter.

In light of the difficulty with combined therapy and the complications attributable at least in part to therapy, additional therapeutic options are being explored. These include the use of human GH,[155] 24,25(OH)$_2$D,[156] and diuretics.[157] None of these are alternatives to combined therapy, but each has been employed as adjuvant therapy.

A continued search for better therapeutic agents is needed because it is increasingly clear that the present-day combined therapy is not curative and is accompanied by a high complication rate. However, if therapy with combined phosphate and 1,25(OH)$_2$D is monitored carefully, growth rates increase, rickets is corrected, and bowing of the lower extremities is significantly reduced.[137,139,147,158-161]

Autosomal Recessive Hypophosphatemic Rickets (OMIM No. 241520)

Dentin matrix protein-1 (DMP1) is a member of the small integrin-binding ligand, N-linked glycoprotein (SIBLING) family and is highly and specifically expressed in osteocytes. Both *Dmp1*-null mice and patients with ARHR manifest rickets and osteomalacia with isolated renal Pi wasting associated with elevated FGF23. Mutational analyses revealed that one ARHR family carried a mutation that ablated the DMP1 start codon (Met1Val), and a second family exhibited a deletion in the DMP1 C-terminus (1484-1490del).[162] Mutations have also been identified in DMP1 splicing sites, which likely result in nonfunctional protein.[163]

Mechanistic studies using the *Dmp1*-null mouse have demonstrated that loss of Dmp1 impairs osteocyte maturation, leading to markedly elevated FGF23 mRNA and protein expression. The hypophosphatemia results in pathological changes in bone mineralization,[162] which can be largely but not completely abrogated by high-phosphate diet in *Dmp1*-null mice. Importantly, *Dmp1*-null mice are biochemical phenocopies of the *Hyp* mouse, and patients with ARHR and XLH (as well as the *Dmp1*-null and *Hyp* mice) share a distinctive bone histology characterized by periosteocytic lesions of nonmineralized bone.[162] Thus, these findings suggest that PHEX (mutated in XLH) may also have a role in osteocyte maturation in a parallel pathway to DMP1 that leads to overexpression of FGF23.

Other Disorders Involving FGF23

Fibrous Dysplasia

Fibrous dysplasia (FD) is a disorder caused by activating somatic mutations in the *GNAS1* gene, encoding the α subunit of the stimulatory G protein, G_s.[164,165] The skeletal defects in FD are characterized by fibrous lesions and co-localized mineralization defects, which contribute to the morbidity in these patients.[166] A significant proportion of FD patients also manifest various degrees of renal Pi wasting and subsequent hypophosphatemia,[167] which can lead to hypophosphatemic rickets and osteomalacia. Extraskeletal clinical manifestations of FD can occur, such as abnormal skin pigmentation, premature puberty, and hyperthyroidism; the disease is then referred to as *McCune-Albright syndrome* (MAS). In one study of FD patients, increased FGF23 serum levels correlated negatively to serum Pi and $1,25(OH)_2D_3$ but positively to skeletal disease burden.[109] FGF23 mRNA and protein were localized to fibrous cells in the fibrous bone lesions of FD, as well as osteogenic and endothelial cells associated with microvascular walls in bone.[109] Therefore, it is likely that FGF23 plays an important role in the pathogenesis of the phosphate wasting that is often seen in FD/MAS.

FD patients are often treated with bisphosphonates, which can lead to improvement of symptoms. It was reported that several MAS patients significantly reduced their elevated FGF23 levels after pamidronate therapy, further supporting a central role of FGF23 in FD/MAS.[168] The mechanisms of action for this reduction of serum FGF23 levels is unclear, but one plausible explanation is that osteogenic cells overproducing FGF23 in FD/MAS may undergo apoptosis, thus leading to decreased production of FGF23.

The reason why the bone cells associated with lesions in FD overexpress FGF23 is not understood. Normally, FGF23 is expressed in osteogenic cells,[109,110] but it is possible that improperly differentiated cells of FD lesions may have lost regulatory mechanisms required to suppress FGF23 production. Speculatively, this is analogous to FGF23 overexpression in TIO tumors, which are not subject to normal regulatory mechanisms.[169]

Osteoglophonic Dysplasia (OMIM No. 166250)

Activating mutations in fibroblast growth factor receptors 1-3 (FGFR1-3) are responsible for a diverse group of skeletal disorders. In general, mutations in FGFR1-2 cause syndromes involving craniosynostosis, whereas the dwarfing syndromes are associated with FGFR3 mutations. Osteoglophonic dysplasia (OGD) is a "crossover" disorder that has skeletal phenotypes

associated with FGFR1-2 mutations as well as with FGFR3 mutations. In this regard, OGD patients present with craniosynostosis, prominent supraorbital ridge, and depressed nasal bridge, as well as with rhizomelic dwarfism and nonossifying bone lesions that show some similarity on x-ray to FD lesions.[170] OGD is an autosomal dominant disorder that is caused by missense mutations in highly conserved residues comprising the ligand-binding and transmembrane domain of FGFR1, thus defining novel roles for this receptor as a negative regulator of long-bone growth. Of significance, three out of the four OGD patients studied had isolated renal Pi wasting with inappropriately low $1,25(OH)_2D$ concentrations.[171] In one of these patients, a sample was available for analysis of plasma FGF23 concentrations, which were significantly elevated above control levels.[171] It was hypothesized that the associated metaphyseal lesions, which may be similar to FD lesions, produce FGF23 which causes renal Pi wasting. Although only a few patients have been assessed, owing to the rarity of the disorder, OGD may have parallels with FD whereby the lesional burden of a patient is proportional to the FGF23 production and the extent of Pi wasting.[108]

Linear Nevus Sebaceous Syndrome

Linear nevus sebaceous syndrome (LNSS) is a rare congenital disorder involving cutaneous lesions characterized by papillomatous epidermal hyperplasia and excess sebaceous glands.[172,173] Additional aberrations are often present in LNSS patients, including developmental defects of the brain which are associated with seizures, as well as eye complications.[174]

Another rare association with LNSS is hypophosphatemic rickets, which usually presents within the first years of life, often as skeletal pain and insufficiency fractures.[175] The primary cause of LNSS in currently unknown, but a report described elevated serum FGF23 in a patient with simultaneous therapy-resistant hypophosphatemic rickets.[176] Treatment with octreotide and excision of the nevus were followed by normalization of serum FGF23 and regression of symptoms, implying a role of FGF23 in the development of hypophosphatemic rickets in this disorder.[176]

DISORDERS ASSOCIATED WITH REDUCED FGF23 BIOACTIVITY

Tumoral Calcinosis (OMIM No. 211900)

Familial TC is an heritable autosomal recessive disorder characterized by ectopic calcified tumoral masses, dental abnormalities, and soft-tissue ectopic and vascular calcification.[177-179] Biochemical abnormalities include hyperphosphatemia, increased TmP/GFR, and inappropriately normal or elevated $1,25(OH)_2D$ concentrations. Calcium and PTH are typically within the normal reference range, although suppressed PTH levels also occur.[178] Biochemically, TC is the mirror image of the Pi-wasting disorder ADHR.[105,106] Hyperostosis-hyperphosphatemia syndrome (HHS) is a rare disorder in which patients present with a similar biochemical profile to TC and have localized hyperostosis.[180,181]

Tumoral Calcinosis/HHS Due to GALNT3 Mutations

The gene first identified for the heritable form of TC was UDP-N-acetyl-alpha-D-galactosamine: polypeptide N-acetylgalactosaminyl transferase-3 (*GALNT3*), in which potentially inactivating mutations in GALNT3 were detected.[182] GALNT3 is expressed in the trans-Golgi network and initiates O-linked glycosylation of nascent proteins. In another family with a reported autosomal dominant TC, the clinical symptoms in this family were in fact caused by two different bi-allelic GALNT3 mutations, further supporting an autosomal recessive inheritance of this disorder.[183] The patients with TC due to GALNT3 mutations were originally reported to have serum FGF23 levels approximately 30-fold above the normal mean when assessed with the C-terminal FGF23 ELISA.[182] Importantly, it was demonstrated that the TC patients did indeed have elevated C-terminal FGF23, but the same individuals had low circulating FGF23 when measured with the intact FGF23 ELISA.[184,185] These findings were then confirmed by demonstrating that loss of GALNT3 resulted in the production of nonfunctional FGF23 protein due to intracellular degradation.[186] FGF23 is O-glycosylated on residues within the $_{176}RH\underline{T}R_{179}/S_{180}$ site (specifically at threonine 178), thus the lack of glycosylation at this residue is thought to expose the SPC site and lead to degradation and destabilization of intact, active FGF23.[186]

HHS is due to inactivating mutations in GALNT3,[180] and these patients also manifest inappropriate ELISA ratios of C-terminal to intact FGF23.[180,181] It has been shown that some of the HHS mutations are the same as those that result in TC,[181] indicating that genetic background may influence disease phenotype and/ or that TC and HHS may represent ranges of severity within the same disease.

Tumoral Calcinosis Due to FGF23 Mutations

It was also discovered that the TC syndrome is caused by recessive mutations in the FGF23 gene. Groups reported mutations giving rise to an amino acid change from a serine to a glycine at residue 71 (S71G),[187,188] or from a serine to a phenylalanine at residue 129 (S129F).[189] Other missense mutations have also been identified, including Q54K[190] and M96T.[191] These FGF23 TC mutations (summarized in Table 6-2) occur within the FGF23 N-terminal FGF-like domain (residues 25 to 180).[190] The TC alterations apparently destabilize intact FGF23, as supported by the findings that the TC patients with FGF23 mutations have the same FGF23 ELISA pattern as GALNT3-TC patients, that is, markedly elevated C-terminal concentrations in concert with low intact values[187,188] and the fact that these mutants are proteolytically cleaved prior to cellular secretion.[187-189] This cleavage is in part mediated by SPC proteases, inasmuch as addition of the ADHR mutations in tandem with the S71G TC mutations in the FGF23 cDNA resulted in rescue of full-length FGF23 production.[192] Thus the common element in GALNT3-TC and FGF23-TC is the lack of secretion of intact FGF23. This lack of active FGF23 then results in elevation of serum Pi through increased renal reabsorption, which in turn most likely results in elevated secretion of nonfunctional FGF23 fragments through a positive-feedback cycle.

Tumoral Calcinosis Due to Klotho Mutations

FGF23 is a member of class of FGFs including FGF19 and FGF21 that are endocrine, as opposed to paracrine/autocrine, factors. FGF23 requires the coreceptor alpha-Klotho (KL) for bioactivity, whereas FGF19 and FGF21 require beta-Klotho.[193-195] KL-null mice have severe calcifications as well as markedly elevated serum Pi,[196] which parallels Fgf23-null mice[197] and that of TC patients. Both the KL-null and Fgf23-null mice, however, have more severe phenotypes than that observed in TC patients. Importantly, the defects in the KL-null and Fgf23-null mice can largely be ameliorated with a low Pi diet to reduce serum Pi.[198,199] In parallel with Fgf23-null mice, KL-null mice have increased NPT2a in the proximal tubule,[200] indicating that the hyperphos-

phatemia in these animals is secondary to increased renal reabsorption of Pi.

KL is produced as two isoforms due to alternative splicing of the same gene. Membrane-bound KL (mKL) is a 130-kD single-pass transmembrane protein characterized by a large extracellular domain and a very short (10-residue) intracellular domain that does not possess signaling capabilities.[201] The secreted form of KL (sKL) is approximately 80 kD and is spliced within exon 3 to result in a KL protein that does not contain the transmembrane domain and is thus secreted into the circulation.[201]

The most likely mechanism for FGF23 signaling through KL is the recruitment of canonical FGF receptors (FGFRs) to form active signaling complexes. One group has identified a specific complex between FGFR1c and KL.[193] In contrast, others demonstrated that multiple FGFRs (FGFR1c, FGFR3c, and FGFR4) can interact with KL and FGF23 and signal through mitogen-activated protein kinase (MAPK) cascades.[202] Importantly, within the kidney, KL localizes to the distal tubule,[200] but FGF23 is known to mediate its effects on NPT2a, NPT2c, and the vitamin D metabolizing enzymes within the proximal tubule.[97,124] It has been shown that p-ERK1/2 signaling occurs in the DCT within minutes of FGF23 delivery, indicating that a potential intrarenal signaling axis occurs for FGF23.[203] However, the mechanisms underlying this local DCT-PT axis in the kidney following FGF23 delivery remain largely unclear.

Since Klotho (KL) is a coreceptor for FGF23, this gene was tested as a candidate for TC in a 13-year-old female with hypothesized end-organ resistance to renal FGF23 activity. This patient presented with hyperphosphatemia, hypercalcemia, elevated PTH, elevated intact and C-terminal FGF23 over 100- to 550-fold elevation of the normal means[204] (in contrast to the differential C-terminal to intact ELISA ratios in GALNT3- and FGF23-TC), as well as ectopic calcifications in the heel and brain. She had normal pubertal development, and her disease paralleled KL-null mice with regard to ectopic calcifications and dramatic elevation of circulating FGF23.[193] This patient was shown to have a recessive mutation in a highly conserved residue (Histidine193Arginine, or H193R) in the extracellular domain of KL (the "KL1" domain). Mutant KL expression was markedly reduced in vitro compared to that of wild-type KL, which resulted in a striking reduction in the ability of KL to mediate FGF23-dependent signaling.[204] Thus, an inactivating H193R KL mutation results in a TC phenotype and demonstrates that KL is required for FGF23 bioactivity. Interestingly, recent findings in a rickets patient indicated that overexpression of KL (through a genomic rearrangement) resulted in hypophosphatemia and hyperparathyroidism.[205]

In sum, it is clear that in human disorders of phosphate handling and the corresponding mouse models, increased FGF23 bioactivity is associated with renal phosphate wasting and inappropriately normal 1,25(OH)$_2$ vitamin D concentrations, and that the converse biochemical relationships exist with loss of FGF23 bioactivity in the hormone itself or in its receptor complex (summarized in Fig. 6-4).

GENETIC HYPOPHOSPHATEMIA NOT ASSOCIATED WITH ELEVATED FGF23

Hereditary Hypophosphatemic Rickets with Hypercalciuria

HHRH was first described in a consanguineous Bedouin tribe.[206] Similar to the disease entities described earlier, HHRH is characterized by hypophosphatemia; however, HHRH is distinguished

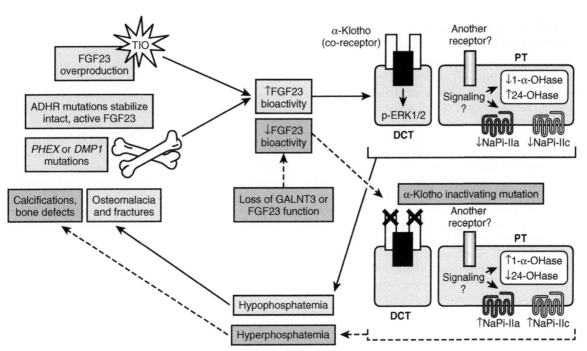

FIGURE 6-4. Genes involved in FGF23 activity. Summary of genes involved in gain of FGF23 bioactivity through intrinsic stabilization (*FGF23* gene [ADHR]) or overproduction (TIO; *PHEX* gene [XLH]; *DMP1* gene [ARHR]) *(solid pathways)* and involved in loss of FGF23 bioactivity through mutations that compromise intact FGF23 production (*FGF23* and *GALNT3* genes) or its signaling complex (*KL* gene) *(dashed pathways)*.

by elevated 1,25(OH)D concentrations and suppressed PTH. The distinguishing biochemical characteristic of this disorder when compared to the FGF23-related diseases such as ADHR and XLH is the notable increase in serum 1,25(OH)D as a compensatory response to the prevailing hypophosphatemia.[206] Affected individuals also have markedly elevated urine calcium excretion, with increased intestinal absorption of phosphorus and calcium that can lead to nephrolithiasis. Clinically, patients with HHRH have rickets and short stature. Additional analysis of this kindred revealed 21 members with "intermediate" phenotypes, which led to an initial hypothesis that HHRH was inherited through an autosomal codominant mode. This group of patients manifested hypercalciuria, mild hypophosphatemia, and elevated calcitriol levels but no apparent bony abnormalities.[207]

To identify the genetic defect responsible for HHRH, a genome wide linkage scan was performed in combination with homozygosity mapping in the large Bedouin kindred in which HHRH was first described. Using this approach, the disorder was mapped to a 1.6-Mb region on chromosome 9q34, which contains the *SLC34A3* gene that encodes NPT2c.[208,209] A recessive, single-nucleotide deletion was then identified in this gene (228delC). Subsequently, in three unrelated HHRH families, a compound heterozygous deletion and missense mutations were found,[208] and additional mutations have more recently been identified.[210-212] These are loss-of-function changes and most likely result in impaired Pi reabsorption in the kidney nephron through reduced plasma membrane expression of NPT2c or the uncoupling of Na-Pi cotransport in the proximal tubule.[211,212] One of the key physiologic implications of identifying disease-causing mutations in NPT2c was the fact that this transporter now appears to have a significant role in renal Pi reabsorption throughout life and is not limited to perinatal Pi homeostasis as previously hypothesized. The fact that NPT2c mutations lead to disease in humans but not in mice[71] may indicate that this transporter plays a more important role in humans than in mice.

HHRH is clinically managed somewhat differently from the hypophosphatemia associated with XLH or ADHR. Phosphate supplementation is an effective treatment, but oral calcitriol is contraindicated; calcitriol levels in this disease are already elevated.

Clinical Consequences and Treatment of Hypophosphatemia

Chronic hypophosphatemia reflects ongoing renal phosphate wasting, either from one of the genetic disorders described or from diseases associated with primary or secondary hyperparathyroidism, vitamin D deficiency or resistance, elevated PTHrP, or more generalized proximal tubular dysfunction (i.e., Fanconi's syndrome). Sustained phosphate wasting may occur also in Dent's disease[213]; in neurofibromatosis[214]; with various metabolic, hormonal, or electrolyte disturbances (poorly controlled diabetes,[215] hypokalemia,[216] or hypomagnesemia[217]); or following exposure to certain drugs or toxins (ethanol,[218] toluene,[219] heavy metals, cisplatin, or foscarnet[220]). The major clinical manifestations of sustained hypophosphatemia relate to the skeletal complications of rickets and osteomalacia noted earlier. Chronic phosphate depletion also may predispose to the development of acute, severe hypophosphatemia in certain clinical settings associated with rapid phosphate translocation into cells, such as intravenous glucose administration, insulin therapy of diabetic ketoacidosis, acute respiratory alkalosis, treatment of pernicious anemia, uncontrolled hematologic malignancy, or use of hematopoietic cytokines.[221,222] Management of chronic hypophosphatemia involves correction of the underlying disorder (where possible) or measures directed at improving the skeletal disease, as described above for XLH.

CLINICAL FEATURES OF ACUTE HYPOPHOSPHATEMIA

The clinical manifestations of acute severe hypophosphatemia reflect a generalized impairment of cellular energy metabolism, reduced generation of ATP and other intracellular high-energy organophosphates, and associated global tissue or organ dysfunction. Neuromuscular signs and symptoms are particularly common, with muscle weakness (with or without rhabdomyolysis[223]) and any of a number of other findings, including lethargy, confusion, disorientation, hallucinations, dysarthria, dysphagia, oculomotor palsies, anisocoria, nystagmus, ataxia, cerebellar tremor, ballismus, hyporeflexia, impaired sphincter control, distal sensory deficits, paresthesia, hyperesthesia, generalized or Guillain Barré-like ascending paralysis, central pontine myelinolysis, seizures, coma, and death.[224-228] Confusion, flaccid paralysis, areflexia, seizures, and other major sequelae generally are observed only when serum phosphate falls below 0.8 mg/dL, although abnormalities in muscle electrolyte content and membrane potential were demonstrable in animals with experimental phosphate depletion and much less severe hypophosphatemia (1.5 to 2 mg/dL).[229]

Reversible respiratory failure due to respiratory muscle weakness may occur at serum phosphate levels below 2 mg/dL,[230-232] and reversible left ventricular dysfunction has been described with both acute and chronic severe hypophosphatemia.[227,233] In patients with septic shock and severe hypophosphatemia (less than 2 mg/dL, average of 1 mg/dL), correction of hypophosphatemia acutely improved left ventricular stroke work index and systolic blood pressure.[234] Various abnormalities in renal tubular function have been detected in phosphate-depleted animals, including tubular acidosis and impaired reabsorption of glucose, sodium, and calcium.[82,235-237] Erythrocyte concentrations of ATP and 2,3-DPG are directly linked to that of extracellular inorganic phosphate, and severe hypophosphatemia may cause increased erythrocyte fragility, abnormal membrane composition, and excessive oxyhemoglobin affinity. Hemolysis, with membrane rigidity and microspherocytosis, may occur when serum phosphate is below 0.5 mg/dL,[238-240] whereas oxyhemoglobin dissociation may be sufficiently impaired when serum phosphate is less than 1 mg/dL to provoke a substantial increase in the cardiac output required for maintenance of adequate oxygen delivery to peripheral tissues.[239,241-243] Studies in animals have disclosed significant impairment of critical leukocyte functions (chemotaxis, phagocytosis, bacterial killing), platelet and hemostatic dysfunction, and spontaneous gastrointestinal bleeding during severe hypophosphatemia (less than 1 mg/dL). The appearance of these abnormalities correlates with reductions in leukocyte and platelet ATP content.[244]

TREATMENT OF ACUTE HYPOPHOSPHATEMIA

The accumulated evidence suggests that acute, severe hypophosphatemia (<1.5 mg/dL), particularly in the setting of underlying phosphate depletion or when associated with infection or neurologic, cardiopulmonary, or hematologic dysfunction, constitutes a dangerous electrolyte abnormality that should be corrected promptly with intravenous sodium or potassium phosphate, as appropriate. Although the cumulative deficit in body phosphate in such patients cannot be accurately predicted from knowledge of the serum phosphate alone,[245] available data indicate that phosphate may be safely administered intravenously at initial doses of 0.2 to 0.8 mmol/kg in elemental phosphorous equivalents over 6 hours (i.e., 10 to 50 mmol over 6 hours), with doses greater than 4 mmol/hr reserved for those with serum phosphate less than 1.5 mg/dL and normal renal function.[231,232,234,246,247] Higher doses (1.5 to 3 mmol/kg/12 hr) can cause significant hyperphosphatemia, particularly when renal function is diminished, are not necessary for prevention of severe hypophosphatemia, and thus should be avoided.[248,249] One large study conducted in a surgical intensive care unit employed a weight-based algorithm (approximately 0.5 mmol phosphate/kg for severe hypophosphatemia (<1.5 mg/dL) and 0.25 mmol/kg for moderate hypophosphatemia (up to 2.2 mg/dL)) to empirically treat all patients with hypophosphatemia and successfully restored normal serum phosphate in 76% of cases.[250] Patients were appropriately excluded for GFR < 25 mL/min, oliguria (<30 mL/hr), hypocalcemia or hypercalcemia, concurrent phosphate-containing parenteral nutrition, or extremes of body weight. The argument for empirical treatment of moderate or severe hypophosphatemia may be more compelling in an intensive care unit setting than for patients less acutely ill on general care units. In the latter case, oral repletion often may suffice, and the threshold for intravenous phosphate therapy and the dose administered should reflect consideration of the risk of hypophosphatemic sequelae, the likely severity and duration of the underlying phosphate depletion, and the presence and severity of symptoms consistent with those of hypophosphatemia. Renal function must be considered and serum phosphate and calcium monitored closely. Recommended protocols (as noted earlier) rarely engender hyperphosphatemia and more often are insufficient, requiring additional infusions on successive days for normalization of serum phosphate.

Possible Future Therapeutic Avenues

As evidence accumulates supporting the role of FGF23 in rare as well as more common disorders of phosphate homeostasis, this molecule is becoming an attractive therapeutic target. Using a novel approach to understanding the mechanisms underlying XLH, neutralizing antibodies targeting FGF23 were administered to *Hyp* mice.[133] After 4 weeks of treatment, injection of the monoclonal antibodies resulted in complete normalization of the serum Pi and 1,25(OH)$_2$D concentrations. Additionally, the *Hyp* rachitic lesions were ameliorated, and bone and tail length increased.[133] Exploring the mechanisms for these physiologic changes indicated that the inactivation of FGF23 in the mice led to increases in NPT2a protein and in 1α(OH)ase mRNA in the renal proximal tubule.[133] These studies reinforce the concept that FGF23 has a central role in XLH.

As described, serum FGF23 concentrations are elevated in ADHR, XLH, TIO, and FD. TIO tumors can be difficult to locate, and all of these disorders can be debilitating. Certainly, the inactivation of circulating FGF23 in the *Hyp* mouse, which causes the dramatic reversal in disease phenotype, leads to the exciting possibility of the use of FGF23 antibodies to treat these disorders of renal Pi handling. Ameliorating the symptoms of TIO by using the FGF23 antibodies until the tumor is found, or treating XLH early in life, could alleviate potentially harmful effects of long-term Pi and vitamin D therapy, such as hyperparathyroidism and nephrocalcinosis with resulting renal insufficiency.

The most direct potential application for recombinant FGF23 could be in familial tumoral calcinosis. Several groups have demonstrated that inactivating mutations in *FGF23* lead to FTC,[187-189] thus delivering recombinant FGF23 may completely resolve the disorder by directly treating the molecular defect through replacement of missing or mutant FGF23. Additional data are required to determine if FGF23 would be a potential treatment for GALNT3-mediated TC. Whether ADHR-mutant FGF23 (mutant at positions 176 and/or 179) would provide a "longer-acting" form of therapy as a result of stabilization of the full-length polypeptide compared to the labile wild-type form remains to be determined.

Acknowledgments

The authors would like to acknowledge the funding support of the National Institutes of Health through grants DK063934 (KEW), DK11794 (FRB), and AR42228 (MJE), as well as the Indiana Genomic Initiative (INGEN) of Indiana University, supported in part by Lilly Endowment, Inc.

REFERENCES

1. Walser M: Ion association. VI. Interactions between calcium, magnesium, inorganic phosphate, citrate and protein in normal human plasma, J Clin Invest 40:723–730, 1961.
2. Somell A, Alveryd A: Diurnal variations in the urinary excretion of calcium and phosphate in hyperparathyroidism, Acta Chir Scand 142:357–359, 1976.
3. Adam A, Boulanger J, Azzouzi M, et al: Colorimetric vs enzymatic determination of serum phosphorus, Clin Chem 30:1724–1725, 1984.
4. Landowne RA: Immunoglobulin interference with phosphorus and chloride determinations with the Coulter chemistry, Clin Chem 25:1189–1190, 1979.
5. Donhowe JM, Freier EF, Wong ET, et al: Factitious hypophosphatemia related to mannitol therapy, Clin Chem 27:1765–1769, 1981.
6. Pitkin RM, Reynolds WA, Williams GA, et al: Calcium metabolism in normal pregnancy: a longitudinal study, Am J Obstet Gynecol 133:781–790, 1979.
7. MacDonald RG, MacDonald HN: Erythrocyte 2,3-diphosphoglycerate and associated haematological parameters during the menstrual cycle and pregnancy, Br J Obstet Gynaecol 84:427–433, 1977.
8. Reitz RE, Daane TA, Woods JR, et al: Calcium, magnesium, phosphorus, and parathyroid hormone interrelationships in pregnancy and newborn infants, Obstet Gynecol 50:701–705, 1977.
9. Cruikshank DP, Pitkin RM, Reynolds WA, et al: Altered maternal calcium homeostasis in diabetic pregnancy, J Clin Endocrinol Metab 50:264–267, 1980.
10. Baran DT, Whyte MP, Haussler MR, et al: Effect of the menstrual cycle on calcium-regulating hormones in the normal young woman, J Clin Endocrinol Metab 50:377–379, 1980.
11. Hillman L, Sateesha S, Haussler M, et al: Control of mineral homeostasis during lactation: interrelationships of 25-hydroxyvitamin D, 24,25-dihydroxyvitamin D, 1,25-dihydroxyvitamin D, parathyroid hormone, calcitonin, prolactin, and estradiol, Am J Obstet Gynecol 139:471–476, 1981.
12. Greer FR, Tsang RC, Searcy JE, et al: Mineral homeostasis during lactation: relationship to serum 1,25-dihydroxyvitamin D, 25-hydroxyvitamin D, parathyroid hormone and calcitonin, Am J Clin Nutr 36:431–437, 1982.
13. Pitkin RM, Cruikshank DP, Schauberger CW, et al: Fetal calcitropic hormones and neonatal calcium homeostasis, Pediatrics 66:77–82, 1980.
14. Aitken JM, Gallagher MJ, Hart DM, et al: Plasma growth hormone and serum phosphorus concentrations in relation to the menopause and to oestrogen therapy, J Endocrinol 59:593–598, 1973.
15. Halloran BP, Lonergan ET, Portale AA: Aging and renal responsiveness to parathyroid hormone in healthy men, J Clin Endocrinol Metab 81:2192–2197, 1996.
16. Cirillo M, Ciacci C, De Santo NG: Age, renal tubular phosphate reabsorption, and serum phosphate levels in adults, N Engl J Med 359:864–866, 2008.
17. Boskey AL, Posner AS: The role of synthetic and bone extracted Ca-phospholipid-PO₄ complexes in hydroxyapatite formation, Calcif Tissue Res 23:251–258, 1977.
18. Lian JB, Cohen-Solal L, Kossiva D, et al: Changes in phosphoproteins of chicken bone matrix in vitamin D-deficient rickets, FEBS Lett 149:123–125, 1982.
19. Marxhall DH, Nordin BE, Speed R: Calcium, phosphorus and magnesium requirement, Proc Nutr Soc 35:163–173, 1976.
20. Wilz DR, Gray RW, Dominguez JH, et al: Plasma 1,25-(OH)2-vitamin D concentrations and net intestinal calcium, phosphate, and magnesium absorption in humans, Am J Clin Nutr 32:2052–2060, 1979.

21. Wasserman RH, Taylor AN: Intestinal absorption of phosphate in the chick: effect of vitamin D and other parameters, J Nutr 103:586–599, 1973.
22. Kowarski S, Schachter D: Effects of vitamin D on phosphate transport and incorporation into mucosal constituents of rat intestinal mucosa, J Biol Chem 244:211–217, 1969.
23. Hurwitz S, Bar A: Absorption of calcium and phosphorus along the gastrointestinal tract of the laying fowl as influenced by dietary calcium and egg shell formation, J Nutr 86:433–438, 1965.
24. Lee DB, Walling MW, Corry DB, et al: 1,25-Dihydroxyvitamin D₃ stimulates calcium and phosphate absorption by different mechanisms: contrasting requirements for sodium, Adv Exp Med Biol 178:189–193, 1984.
25. Danisi G, Murer H, Straub RW: Effects of pH and sodium on phosphate transport across brush border membrane vesicles of small intestine, Adv Exp Med Biol 178:173–180, 1984.
26. Borowitz SM, Ghishan FK: Phosphate transport in human jejunal brush-border membrane vesicles, Gastroenterology 96:4–10, 1989.
27. Hilfiker H, Hattenhauer O, Traebert M, et al: Characterization of a murine type II sodium-phosphate cotransporter expressed in mammalian small intestine, Proc Natl Acad Sci U S A 95:14564–14569, 1998.
28. Feild JA, Zhang L, Brun KA, et al: Cloning and functional characterization of a sodium-dependent phosphate transporter expressed in human lung and small intestine, Biochem Biophys Res Commun 258:578–582, 1999.
29. Beck L, Karaplis AC, Amizuka N, et al: Targeted inactivation of Npt2 in mice leads to severe renal phosphate wasting, hypercalciuria, and skeletal abnormalities, Proc Natl Acad Sci U S A 95:5372–5377, 1998.
30. Peterlik M, Wasserman RH: Effect of vitamin D on transepithelial phosphate transport in chick intestine, Am J Physiol 234:E379–E388, 1978.
31. Murer H, Hildmann B: Transcellular transport of calcium and inorganic phosphate in the small intestinal epithelium, Am J Physiol 240:G409–G416, 1981.
32. Chen TC, Castillo L, Korycka-Dahl M, et al: Role of vitamin D metabolites in phosphate transport of rat intestine, J Nutr 104:1056–1060, 1974.
33. Corradino RA: Embryonic chick intestine in organ culture. A unique system for the study of the intestinal calcium absorptive mechanism, J Cell Biol 58:64–78, 1973.
34. Brickman AS, Hartenbower DL, Norman AW, et al: Actions of 1 alpha-hydroxyvitamin D₃ and 1,25-dihydroxyvitamin D₃ on mineral metabolism in man. I. Effects on net absorption of phosphorus, Am J Clin Nutr 30:1064–1069, 1977.
35. Walling MW: Intestinal Ca and phosphate transport: differential responses to vitamin D₃ metabolites, Am J Physiol 233:E488–E494, 1977.
36. Birge SJ, Miller R: The role of phosphate in the action of vitamin D on the intestine, J Clin Invest 60:980–988, 1977.
37. Danisi G, Straub RW: Unidirectional influx of phosphate across the mucosal membrane of rabbit small intestine, Pflugers Arch 385:117–122, 1980.
38. Cross HS, Peterlik M: Vitamin D activates (Na⁺-K⁺) ATPase: a possible regulation of phosphate and calcium uptake by cultured embryonic chick small intestine, Adv Exp Med Biol 178:163–171, 1984.
39. Karsenty G, Lacour B, Ulmann A, et al: Early effects of vitamin D metabolites on phosphate fluxes in isolated rat enterocytes, Am J Physiol 248:G40–G45, 1985.
40. Fuchs R, Peterlik M: Vitamin D-induced transepithelial phosphate and calcium transport by chick jejunum.

Effect of microfilamentous and microtubular inhibitors, FEBS Lett 100:357–359, 1979.
41. Hattenhauer O, Traebert M, Murer H, et al: Regulation of small intestinal Na-P(i) type IIb cotransporter by dietary phosphate intake, Am J Physiol 277:G756–G762, 1999.
42. Xu H, Bai L, Collins JF, et al: Age-dependent regulation of rat intestinal type IIb sodium-phosphate cotransporter by 1,25-(OH)(2) vitamin D(3), Am J Physiol Cell Physiol 282:C487–493, 2002.
43. Segawa H, Kaneko I, Yamanaka S, et al: Intestinal Na-P(i) cotransporter adaptation to dietary P(i) content in vitamin D receptor null mice, Am J Physiol Renal Physiol 287:F39–F47, 2004.
44. Nemere I, Yoshimoto Y, Norman AW: Calcium transport in perfused duodena from normal chicks: enhancement within fourteen minutes of exposure to 1,25-dihydroxyvitamin D₃, Endocrinology 115:1476–1483, 1984.
45. Nemere I: Apparent nonnuclear regulation of intestinal phosphate transport: effects of 1,25-dihydroxyvitamin D₃,24,25-dihydroxyvitamin D₃, and 25-hydroxyvitamin D₃, Endocrinology 137:2254–2261, 1996.
46. Quamme GA: Phosphate transport in intestinal brush-border membrane vesicles: effect of pH and dietary phosphate, Am J Physiol 249:G168–G176, 1985.
47. Caverzasio J, Danisi G, Straub RW, et al: Adaptation of phosphate transport to low phosphate diet in renal and intestinal brush border membrane vesicles: influence of sodium and pH, Pflugers Arch 409:333–336, 1987.
48. Danisi G, Caverzasio J, Trechsel U, et al: Phosphate transport adaptation in rat jejunum and plasma level of 1,25-dihydroxyvitamin D₃, Scand J Gastroenterol 25:210–215, 1990.
49. Armbrecht HJ: Age-related changes in calcium and phosphorus uptake by rat small intestine, Biochim Biophys Acta 882:281–286, 1986.
50. Lee DB, Walling MW, Brautbar N: Intestinal phosphate absorption: influence of vitamin D and non-vitamin D factors, Am J Physiol 250:G369–G373, 1986.
51. Cramer CF, McMillan J: Phosphorus adaptation in rats in absence of vitamin D or parathyroid glands, Am J Physiol 239:G261–G265, 1980.
52. Knox FG, Osswald H, Marchand GR, et al: Phosphate transport along the nephron, Am J Physiol 233:F261–F268, 1977.
53. Dennis VW, Stead WW, Myers JL: Renal handling of phosphate and calcium, Annu Rev Physiol 41:257–271, 1979.
54. Dennis VW, Brazy PC: Divalent anion transport in isolated renal tubules, Kidney Int 22:498–506, 1982.
55. Amiel C, Kuntziger H, Richet G: Micropuncture study of handling of phosphate by proximal and distal nephron in normal and parathyroidectomized rat. Evidence for distal reabsorption, Pflugers Arch 317:93–109, 1970.
56. Haas JA, Berndt T, Knox FG: Nephron heterogeneity of phosphate reabsorption, Am J Physiol 234:F287–F290, 1978.
57. Le Grimellec C, Roinel N, Morel F: Simultaneous Mg, Ca, P, K and Cl analysis in rat tubular fluid. IV. During acute phosphate plasma loading, Pflugers Arch 346:189–204, 1974.
58. Pastoriza-Munoz E, Colindres RE, Lassiter WE, et al: Effect of parathyroid hormone on phosphate reabsorption in rat distal convolution, Am J Physiol 235:F321–F330, 1978.
59. Peraino RA, Suki WN: Phosphate transport by isolated rabbit cortical collecting tubule, Am J Physiol 238:F358–F362, 1980.
60. Shareghi GR, Agus ZS: Phosphate transport in the light segment of the rabbit cortical collecting tubule, Am J Physiol 242:F379–F384, 1982.

61. Schneider EG, McLane LA: Evidence for a peritubular-to-luminal flux phosphate in the dog kidney, Am J Physiol 232:F159–F166, 1977.
62. Ullrich KJ: Mechanisms of cellular phosphate transport in rat kidney proximal tubule, Adv Exp Med Biol 103:21–35, 1978.
63. Ullrich KJ, Capasso G, Rumrich G, et al: Coupling between proximal tubular transport processes. Studies with ouabain, SITS and HCO3-free solutions, Pflugers Arch 368:245–252, 1977.
64. Ullrich KJ, Murer H: Sulphate and phosphate transport in the renal proximal tubule, Philos Trans R Soc Lond B Biol Sci 299:549–558, 1982.
65. Hoffmann N, Thees M, Kinne R: Phosphate transport by isolated renal brush border vesicles, Pflugers Arch 362:147–156, 1976.
66. Burckhardt G, Stern H, Murer H: The influence of pH on phosphate transport into rat renal brush border membrane vesicles, Pflugers Arch 390:191–197, 1981.
67. Cheng L, Sacktor B: Sodium gradient-dependent phosphate transport in renal brush border membrane vesicles, J Biol Chem 256:1556–1564, 1981.
68. Ullrich KJ, Rumrich G, Kloss S: Phosphate transport in the proximal convolution of the rat kidney. III. Effect of extracellular and intracellular pH, Pflugers Arch 377:33–42, 1978.
69. Hoag HM, Martel J, Gauthier C, et al: Effects of Npt2 gene ablation and low-phosphate diet on renal Na(+)/phosphate cotransport and cotransporter gene expression, J Clin Invest 104:679–686, 1999.
70. Zhao N, Tenenhouse HS: Npt2 gene disruption confers resistance to the inhibitory action of parathyroid hormone on renal sodium-phosphate cotransport, Endocrinology 141:2159–2165, 2000.
71. Segawa H, Onitsuka A, Kuwahata M, et al: Type IIc sodium-dependent phosphate transporter regulates calcium metabolism, J Am Soc Nephrol 20:104–113, 2008.
72. Walton RJ, Bijvoet OL: Nomogram for derivation of renal threshold phosphate concentration, Lancet 2:309–310, 1975.
73. Pfister MF, Lederer E, Forgo J, et al: Parathyroid hormone-dependent degradation of type II Na+/Pi cotransporters, J Biol Chem 272:20125–20130, 1997.
74. Lotscher M, Wilson P, Nguyen S, et al: New aspects of adaptation of rat renal Na-Pi cotransporter to alterations in dietary phosphate, Kidney Int 49:1012–1018, 1996.
75. Takahashi F, Morita K, Katai K, et al: Effects of dietary Pi on the renal Na+-dependent Pi transporter NaPi-2 in thyroparathyroidectomized rats, Biochem J 333(Pt 1):175–181, 1998.
76. Kempson SA, Lotscher M, Kaissling B, et al: Parathyroid hormone action on phosphate transporter mRNA and protein in rat renal proximal tubules, Am J Physiol 268:F784–F791, 1995.
77. Traebert M, Volkl H, Biber J, et al: Luminal and contraluminal action of 1-34 and 3-34 PTH peptides on renal type IIa Na-P(i) cotransporter, Am J Physiol Renal Physiol 278:F792–F798, 2000.
78. Bacic D, Schulz N, Biber J, et al: Involvement of the MAPK-kinase pathway in the PTH-mediated regulation of the proximal tubule type IIa Na+/Pi cotransporter in mouse kidney, Pflugers Arch 446:52–60, 2003.
79. Wen SF: Micropuncture studies of phosphate transport in the proximal tubule of the dog. The relationship to sodium reabsorption, J Clin Invest 53:143–153, 1974.
80. Trohler U, Bonjour JP, Fleisch H: Inorganic phosphate homeostasis. Renal adaptation to the dietary intake in intact and thyroparathyroidectomized rats, J Clin Invest 57:264–273, 1976.
81. Goldfarb S, Westby GR, Goldberg M, et al: Renal tubular effects of chronic phosphate depletion, J Clin Invest 59:770–779, 1977.
82. Steele TH, DeLuca HF: Influence of dietary phosphorus on renal phosphate reabsorption in the parathyroidectomized rat, J Clin Invest 57:867–874, 1976.
83. Crawford JD, Osborne MM Jr, Talbot NB, et al: The parathyroid glands and phosphorus homeostasis, J Clin Invest 29:1448–1461, 1950.
84. Chambers EL Jr, Goldman L, Gordan GS, et al: Tests for hyperparathyroidism: tubular reabsorption of phosphate, phosphate deprivation, and calcium infusion, J Clin Endocrinol Metab 16:1507–1521, 1956.

85. McCrory WW, Forman CW, Mc NH, et al: Renal excretion of inorganic phosphate in newborn infants, J Clin Invest 31:357–366, 1952.
86. Caverzasio J, Bonjour JP: Mechanism of rapid phosphate (Pi) transport adaptation to a single low Pi meal in rat renal brush border membrane, Pflugers Arch 404:227–231, 1985.
87. Thompson DD, Hiatt HH: Effects of phosphate loading and depletion on the renal excretion and reabsorption of inorganic phosphate, J Clin Invest 36:566–572, 1957.
88. Hruska KA, Klahr S, Hammerman MR: Decreased luminal membrane transport of phosphate in chronic renal failure, Am J Physiol 242:F17–F22, 1982.
89. Levine BS, Ho K, Hodsman A, et al: Early renal brush border membrane adaptation to dietary phosphorus, Miner Electrolyte Metab 10:222–227, 1984.
90. Brunette MG, Chan M, Maag U, et al: Phosphate uptake by superficial and deep nephron brush border membranes. Effect of the dietary phosphate and parathyroid hormone, Pflugers Arch 400:356–362, 1984.
91. Murer H, Stern H, Burckhardt G, et al: Sodium-dependent transport of inorganic phosphate across the renal brush border membrane, Adv Exp Med Biol 128:11–23, 1980.
92. Boyer CJ, Xiao Y, Dugre A, et al: Phosphate deprivation induces overexpression of two proteins related to the rat renal phosphate cotransporter NaPi-2, Biochim Biophys Acta 1281:117–123, 1996.
93. Lotscher M, Kaissling B, Biber J, et al: Role of microtubules in the rapid regulation of renal phosphate transport in response to acute alterations in dietary phosphate content, J Clin Invest 99:1302–1312, 1997.
94. Ritthaler T, Traebert M, Lotscher M, et al: Effects of phosphate intake on distribution of type II Na/Pi cotransporter mRNA in rat kidney, Kidney Int 55:976–983, 1999.
95. Levi M, Lotscher M, Sorribas V, et al: Cellular mechanisms of acute and chronic adaptation of rat renal P(i) transporter to alterations in dietary P(i), Am J Physiol 267:F900–F908, 1994.
96. Berndt T, Thomas LF, Craig TA, et al: Evidence for a signaling axis by which intestinal phosphate rapidly modulates renal phosphate reabsorption, Proc Natl Acad Sci U S A 104:11085–11090, 2007.
97. Larsson T, Marsell R, Schipani E, et al: Transgenic mice expressing fibroblast growth factor 23 under the control of the alpha1(I) collagen promoter exhibit growth retardation, osteomalacia, and disturbed phosphate homeostasis, Endocrinology 145:3087–3094, 2004.
98. Shimada T, Hasegawa H, Yamazaki Y, et al: FGF-23 is a potent regulator of vitamin D metabolism and phosphate homeostasis, J Bone Miner Res 19:429–435, 2004.
99. Burnett SM, Gunawardene SC, Bringhurst FR, et al: Regulation of C-terminal and intact FGF-23 by dietary phosphate in men and women, J Bone Miner Res 21:1187–1196, 2006.
100. Perwad F, Azam N, Zhang MY, et al: Dietary and serum phosphorus regulate fibroblast growth factor 23 expression and 1,25-dihydroxyvitamin D metabolism in mice, Endocrinology 146:5358–5364, 2005.
101. Jonsson KB, Zahradnik R, Larsson T, et al: Fibroblast growth factor 23 in oncogenic osteomalacia and X-linked hypophosphatemia, N Engl J Med 348:1656–1663, 2003.
102. Yamazaki Y, Okazaki R, Shibata M, et al: Increased circulatory level of biologically active full-length FGF-23 in patients with hypophosphatemic rickets/osteomalacia, J Clin Endocrinol Metab 87:4957–4960, 2002.
103. Khosravi A, Cutler CM, Kelly MH, et al: Determination of the elimination half-life of fibroblast growth factor-23, J Clin Endocrinol Metab 92:2374–2377, 2007.
104. Takeuchi Y, Suzuki H, Ogura S, et al: Venous sampling for fibroblast growth factor-23 confirms preoperative diagnosis of tumor-induced osteomalacia, J Clin Endocrinol Metab 89:3979–3982, 2004.
105. Econs MJ, McEnery PT: Autosomal dominant hypophosphatemic rickets/osteomalacia: clinical characterization of a novel renal phosphate-wasting disorder, J Clin Endocrinol Metab 82:674–681, 1997.
106. Bianchine JW, Stambler AA, Harrison HE: Familial hypophosphatemic rickets showing autosomal domi-

nant inheritance, Birth Defects Orig Artic Ser 7:287–295, 1971.
107. Econs MJ, McEnery PT, Lennon F, et al: Autosomal dominant hypophosphatemic rickets is linked to chromosome 12p13, J Clin Invest 100:2653–2657, 1997.
108. ADHR Consortium: Autosomal dominant hypophosphataemic rickets is associated with mutations in FGF23, Nat Genet 26:345–348, 2000.
109. Riminucci M, Collins MT, Fedarko NS, et al: FGF-23 in fibrous dysplasia of bone and its relationship to renal phosphate wasting, J Clin Invest 112:683–692, 2003.
110. Liu S, Guo R, Simpson LG, et al: Regulation of fibroblastic growth factor 23 expression but not degradation by PHEX, J Biol Chem 278:37419–37426, 2003.
111. White KE, Carn G, Lorenz-Depiereux B, et al: Autosomal-dominant hypophosphatemic rickets (ADHR) mutations stabilize FGF-23, Kidney Int 60:2079–2086, 2001.
112. Shimada T, Muto T, Urakawa I, et al: Mutant FGF-23 responsible for autosomal dominant hypophosphatemic rickets is resistant to proteolytic cleavage and causes hypophosphatemia in vivo, Endocrinology 143:3179–3182, 2002.
113. Seidah NG, Chretien M: Proprotein and prohormone convertases: a family of subtilases generating diverse bioactive polypeptides, Brain Res 848:45–62, 1999.
114. Molloy SS, Bresnahan PA, Leppla SH, et al: Human furin is a calcium-dependent serine endoprotease that recognizes the sequence Arg-X-X-Arg and efficiently cleaves anthrax toxin protective antigen, J Biol Chem 267:16396–16402, 1992.
115. Nakayama K: Furin: a mammalian subtilisin/Kex2p-like endoprotease involved in processing of a wide variety of precursor proteins, Biochem J 327(Pt 3):625–635, 1997.
116. Benet-Pages A, Lorenz-Depiereux B, Zischka H, et al: FGF23 is processed by proprotein convertases but not by PHEX, Bone 35:455–462, 2004.
117. Imel EA, Hui SL, Econs MJ: FGF23 concentrations vary with disease status in autosomal dominant hypophosphatemic rickets, J Bone Miner Res 22:520–526, 2007.
118. Ryan EA, Reiss E: Oncogenous osteomalacia. Review of the world literature of 42 cases and report of two new cases, Am J Med 77:501–512, 1984.
119. Schapira D, Ben Izhak O, Nachtigal A, et al: Tumor-induced osteomalacia, Semin Arthritis Rheum 25:35–46, 1995.
120. Cai Q, Hodgson SF, Kao PC, et al: Brief report: inhibition of renal phosphate transport by a tumor product in a patient with oncogenic osteomalacia, N Engl J Med 330:1645–1649, 1994.
121. Econs MJ, Samsa GP, Monger M, et al: X-Linked hypophosphatemic rickets: a disease often unknown to affected patients, Bone Miner 24:17–24, 1994.
122. Chalew SA, Lovchik JC, Brown CM, et al: Hypophosphatemia induced in mice by transplantation of a tumor-derived cell line from a patient with oncogenic rickets, J Pediatr Endocrinol Metab 9:593–597, 1996.
123. White KE, Jonsson KB, Carn G, et al: The autosomal dominant hypophosphatemic rickets (ADHR) gene is a secreted polypeptide overexpressed by tumors that cause phosphate wasting, J Clin Endocrinol Metab 86:497–500, 2001.
124. Shimada T, Mizutani S, Muto T, et al: Cloning and characterization of FGF23 as a causative factor of tumor-induced osteomalacia, Proc Natl Acad Sci U S A 98:6500–6505, 2001.
125. Tenenhouse HS, Econs MJ: Mendelian hypophosphatemias. In Scriver CR, editor: The metabolic and molecular basis of inherited disease, 1998, pp 5039–5068.
126. PEXConsortium: A gene (PEX) with homologies to endopeptidases is mutated in patients with X-linked hypophosphatemic rickets. The HYP Consortium, Nat Genet 11:130–136, 1995.
127. Francis F, Strom TM, Hennig S, et al: Genomic organization of the human PEX gene mutated in X-linked dominant hypophosphatemic rickets, Genome Res 7:573–585, 1997.
128. Beck L, Soumounou Y, Martel J, et al: Pex/PEX tissue distribution and evidence for a deletion in the 3′ region of the Phex gene in X-linked hypophosphatemic mice, J Clin Invest 99:1200–1209, 1997.
129. Wang Y, Spatz MK, Kannan K, et al: A mouse model for achondroplasia produced by targeting fibroblast growth factor receptor 3, Proc Natl Acad Sci U S A 96:4455–4460, 1999.

130. Eicher EM, Southard JL, Scriver CR, et al: Hypophosphatemia: mouse model for human familial hypophosphatemic (vitamin D-resistant) rickets, Proc Natl Acad Sci U S A 73:4667–4671, 1976.

131. Meyer RA Jr, Meyer MH, Gray RW: Parabiosis suggests a humoral factor is involved in X-linked hypophosphatemia in mice, J Bone Miner Res 4:493–500, 1989.

132. Weber TJ, Liu S, Indridason OS, et al: Serum FGF23 levels in normal and disordered phosphorus homeostasis, J Bone Miner Res 18:1227–1234, 2003.

133. Aono Y, Yamazaki Y, Yasutake J, et al: Therapeutic effects of anti-FGF23 antibodies in hypophosphatemic rickets/ssteomalacia, J Bone Miner Res 2009 May 6 [Epub ahead of print].

134. Bai X, Miao D, Panda D, et al: Partial rescue of the Hyp phenotype by osteoblast-targeted PHEX (phosphate-regulating gene with homologies to endopeptidases on the X chromosome) expression, Mol Endocrinol 16:2913–2925, 2002.

135. Liu S, Guo R, Tu Q, et al: Overexpression of Phex in osteoblasts fails to rescue the Hyp mouse phenotype, J Biol Chem 277:3686–3697, 2002.

136. Erben RG, Mayer D, Weber K, et al: Overexpression of human PHEX under the human beta-actin promoter does not fully rescue the Hyp mouse phenotype, J Bone Miner Res 20:1149–1160, 2005.

137. Glorieux FH, Marie PJ, Pettifor JM, et al: Bone response to phosphate salts, ergocalciferol, and calcitriol in hypophosphatemic vitamin D-resistant rickets, N Engl J Med 303:1023–1031, 1980.

138. Glorieux FH, Scriver CR, Reade TM, et al: Use of phosphate and vitamin D to prevent dwarfism and rickets in X-linked hypophosphatemia, N Engl J Med 287:481–487, 1972.

139. Costa T, Marie PJ, Scriver CR, et al: X-linked hypophosphatemia: effect of calcitriol on renal handling of phosphate, serum phosphate, and bone mineralization, J Clin Endocrinol Metab 52:463–472, 1981.

140. Carpenter TO, Mitnick MA, Ellison A, et al: Nocturnal hyperparathyroidism: a frequent feature of X-linked hypophosphatemia, J Clin Endocrinol Metab 78:1378–1383, 1994.

141. Imel EA, DiMeglio LA, Hui SL, et al: Treatment of XLH with calcitriol and phosphate increases FGF23 concentration, J Bone Miner Res 22(Suppl 1):W123.S123, 2007.

142. Reid IR, Hardy DC, Murphy WA, et al: X-linked hypophosphatemia: a clinical, biochemical, and histopathologic assessment of morbidity in adults, Medicine (Baltimore) 68:336–352, 1989.

143. Goodyer PR, Kronick JB, Jequier S, et al: Nephrocalcinosis and its relationship to treatment of hereditary rickets, J Pediatr 111:700–704, 1987.

144. Stickler GB, Morgenstern BZ: Hypophosphataemic rickets: final height and clinical symptoms in adults, Lancet 2:902–905, 1989.

145. Balsan S, Tieder M: Linear growth in patients with hypophosphatemic vitamin D-resistant rickets: influence of treatment regimen and parental height, J Pediatr 116:365–371, 1990.

146. Bettinelli A, Bianchi ML, Mazzucchi E, et al: Acute effects of calcitriol and phosphate salts on mineral metabolism in children with hypophosphatemic rickets, J Pediatr 118:372–376, 1991.

147. Verge CF, Lam A, Simpson JM, et al: Effects of therapy in X-linked hypophosphatemic rickets, N Engl J Med 325:1843–1848, 1991.

148. Reusz GS, Latta K, Hoyer PF, et al: Evidence suggesting hyperoxaluria as a cause of nephrocalcinosis in phosphate-treated hypophosphataemic rickets, Lancet 335:1240–1243, 1990.

149. Eddy MC, McAlister WH, Whyte MP: X-linked hypophosphatemia: normal renal function despite medullary nephrocalcinosis 25 years after transient vitamin D$_2$-induced renal azotemia, Bone 21:515–520, 1997.

150. Alon U, Donaldson DL, Hellerstein S, et al: Metabolic and histologic investigation of the nature of nephrocalcinosis in children with hypophosphatemic rickets and in the Hyp mouse, J Pediatr 120:899–905, 1992.

151. Rasmussen H, Anast C: Familial hypophosphatemic rickets and vitamin D-dependent rickets. In Stanbury JB, Wyngaarden JB, Fredrickson DS et al, editors: The metabolic basis of inherited disease, ed 5, New York, 1983, McGraw-Hill, p 1743.

152. Rasmussen H, Tenenhouse HS: Hypophosphatemias. In Scriver CR, Beaudet AL, Sly WS, Valle D, editors: The metabolic basis of inherited disease, ed 6, New York, 1989, McGraw Hill, p 2581.

153. Blydt-Hansen TD, Tenenhouse HS, Goodyer P: PHEX expression in parathyroid gland and parathyroid hormone dysregulation in X-linked hypophosphatemia, Pediatr Nephrol 13:607–611, 1999.

154. Firth RG, Grant CS, Riggs BL: Development of hypercalcemic hyperparathyroidism after long-term phosphate supplementation in hypophosphatemic osteomalacia. Report of two cases, Am J Med 78:669–673, 1985.

155. Wilson DM, Lee PD, Morris AH, et al: Growth hormone therapy in hypophosphatemic rickets, Am J Dis Child 145:1165–1170, 1991.

156. Carpenter TO, Keller M, Schwartz D, et al: 24,25 Dihydroxyvitamin D supplementation corrects hyperparathyroidism and improves skeletal abnormalities in X-linked hypophosphatemic rickets: a clinical research center study, J Clin Endocrinol Metab 81:2381–2388, 1996.

157. Hanna JD, Niimi K, Chan JC: X-linked hypophosphatemia. Genetic and clinical correlates, Am J Dis Child 145:865–870, 1991.

158. Drezner MK, Lyles KW, Haussler MR, et al: Evaluation of a role for 1,25-dihydroxyvitamin D$_3$ in the pathogenesis and treatment of X-linked hypophosphatemic rickets and osteomalacia, J Clin Invest 66:1020–1032, 1980.

159. Rasmussen H, Pechet M, Anast C, et al: Long-term treatment of familial hypophosphatemic rickets with oral phosphate and 1 alpha-hydroxyvitamin D$_3$, J Pediatr 99:16–25, 1981.

160. Harrell RM, Lyles KW, Harrelson JM, et al: Healing of bone disease in X-linked hypophosphatemic rickets/osteomalacia. Induction and maintenance with phosphorus and calcitriol, J Clin Invest 75:1858–1868, 1985.

161. Chesney RW, Mazess RB, Rose P, et al: Long-term influence of calcitriol (1,25-dihydroxyvitamin D) and supplemental phosphate in X-linked hypophosphatemic rickets, Pediatrics 71:559–567, 1983.

162. Feng JQ, Ward LM, Liu S, et al: Loss of DMP1 causes rickets and osteomalacia and identifies a role for osteocytes in mineral metabolism, Nat Genet 38:1310–1315, 2006.

163. Lorenz-Depiereux B, Bastepe M, Benet-Pages A, et al: DMP1 mutations in autosomal recessive hypophosphatemia implicate a bone matrix protein in the regulation of phosphate homeostasis, Nat Genet 38:1248–1250, 2006.

164. Schwindinger WF, Francomano CA, Levine MA: Identification of a mutation in the gene encoding the alpha subunit of the stimulatory G protein of adenylyl cyclase in McCune-Albright syndrome, Proc Natl Acad Sci U S A 89:5152–5156, 1992.

165. Weinstein LS, Shenker A, Gejman PV, et al: Activating mutations of the stimulatory G protein in the McCune-Albright syndrome, N Engl J Med 325:1688–1695, 1991.

166. Albright F, Butler A, Bloomberg E: Rickets resistant to vitamin D therapy, Am J Dis Child 54:529–547, 1937.

167. Collins MT, Chebli C, Jones J, et al: Renal phosphate wasting in fibrous dysplasia of bone is part of a generalized renal tubular dysfunction similar to that seen in tumor-induced osteomalacia, J Bone Miner Res 16:806–813, 2001.

168. Yamamoto T, Imanishi Y, Kinoshita E, et al: The role of fibroblast growth factor 23 for hypophosphatemia and abnormal regulation of vitamin D metabolism in patients with McCune-Albright syndrome, J Bone Miner Metab 23:231–237, 2005.

169. Folpe AL, Fanburg-Smith JC, Billings SD, et al: Most osteomalacia-associated mesenchymal tumors are a single histopathologic entity: an analysis of 32 cases and a comprehensive review of the literature, Am J Surg Pathol 28:1–30, 2004.

170. Beighton P, Cremin BJ, Kozlowski K: Osteoglophonic dwarfism, Pediatr Radiol 10:46–50, 1980.

171. White KE, Cabral JM, Davis SI, et al: Mutations that cause osteoglophonic dysplasia define novel roles for FGFR1 in bone elongation, Am J Hum Genet 76:361–367, 2005.

172. Lovejoy FH Jr, Boyle WE Jr: Linear nevus sebaceous syndrome: report of two cases and a review of the literature, Pediatrics 52:382–387, 1973.

173. Mehregan AH, Hardin I: Generalized follicular hamartoma. Complicated by multiple proliferating trichilemmal cysts and palmar pits, Arch Dermatol 107:435–438, 1973.

174. Brodsky MC, Kincannon JM, Nelson-Adesokan P, et al: Oculocerebral dysgenesis in the linear nevus sebaceous syndrome, Ophthalmology 104:497–503, 1997.

175. Carey DE, Drezner MK, Hamdan JA, et al: Hypophosphatemic rickets/osteomalacia in linear sebaceous nevus syndrome: a variant of tumor-induced osteomalacia, J Pediatr 109:994–1000, 1986.

176. Hoffman WH, Jueppner HW, Deyoung BR, et al: Elevated fibroblast growth factor-23 in hypophosphatemic linear nevus sebaceous syndrome, Am J Med Genet A 134:233–236, 2005.

177. Inclan A, Leon P, Camjeo M: Tumoral calcinosis, JAMA 121:490–495, 1943.

178. Mitnick PD, Goldfarb S, Slatopolsky E, et al: Calcium and phosphate metabolism in tumoral calcinosis, Ann Intern Med 92:482–487, 1980.

179. Prince MJ, Schaeffer PC, Goldsmith RS, et al: Hyperphosphatemic tumoral calcinosis: association with elevation of serum 1,25-dihydroxycholecalciferol concentrations, Ann Intern Med 96:586–591, 1982.

180. Frishberg Y, Topaz O, Bergman R, et al: Identification of a recurrent mutation in GALNT3 demonstrates that hyperostosis-hyperphosphatemia syndrome and familial tumoral calcinosis are allelic disorders, J Mol Med 83:33–38, 2005.

181. Ichikawa S, Guigonis V, Imel EA, et al: Novel GALNT3 mutations causing hyperostosis-hyperphosphatemia syndrome result in low intact fibroblast growth factor 23 concentrations, J Clin Endocrinol Metab 92:1943–1947, 2007.

182. Topaz O, Shurman DL, Bergman R, et al: Mutations in GALNT3, encoding a protein involved in O-linked glycosylation, cause familial tumoral calcinosis, Nat Genet 36:579–581, 2004.

183. Ichikawa S, Lyles KW, Econs MJ: A novel GALNT3 mutation in a pseudoautosomal dominant form of tumoral calcinosis: evidence that the disorder is autosomal recessive, J Clin Endocrinol Metab 90:2420–2423, 2005.

184. Garringer HJ, Fisher C, Larsson TE, et al: The role of mutant UDP-N-acetyl-alpha-D-galactosamine-polypeptide N-acetylgalactosaminyltransferase 3 in regulating serum intact fibroblast growth factor 23 and matrix extracellular phosphoglycoprotein in heritable tumoral calcinosis, J Clin Endocrinol Metab 91:4037–4042, 2006.

185. Ichikawa S, Imel EA, Sorenson AH, et al: Tumoral calcinosis presenting with eyelid calcifications due to novel missense mutations in the glycosyl transferase domain of the GALNT3 gene, J Clin Endocrinol Metab 91:4472–4475, 2006.

186. Frishberg Y, Ito N, Rinat C, et al: Hyperostosis-hyperphosphatemia syndrome: a congenital disorder of O-glycosylation associated with augmented processing of fibroblast growth factor 23, J Bone Miner Res 22:235–242, 2007.

187. Benet-Pages A, Orlik P, Strom TM, et al: An FGF23 missense mutation causes familial tumoral calcinosis with hyperphosphatemia, Hum Mol Genet 14:385–390, 2005.

188. Larsson T, Yu X, Davis SI, et al: A novel recessive mutation in fibroblast growth factor-23 causes familial tumoral calcinosis, J Clin Endocrinol Metab 90:2424–2427, 2005.

189. Araya K, Fukumoto S, Backenroth R, et al: A novel mutation in fibroblast growth factor 23 gene as a cause of tumoral calcinosis, J Clin Endocrinol Metab 90:5523–5527, 2005.

190. Garringer HJ, Malekpour M, Esteghamat F, et al: Molecular genetic and biochemical analyses of FGF23 mutations in familial tumoral calcinosis, Am J Physiol Endocrinol Metab 295:E929–937, 2008.

191. Chefetz I, Heller R, Galli-Tsinopoulou A, et al: A novel homozygous missense mutation in FGF23 causes familial tumoral calcinosis associated with disseminated visceral calcification, Hum Genet 118:261–266, 2005.

192. Larsson T, Davis SI, Garringer HJ, et al: Fibroblast growth factor-23 mutants causing familial tumoral calcinosis are differentially processed, Endocrinology 146:3883–3891, 2005.

193. Urakawa I, Yamazaki Y, Shimada T, et al: Klotho converts canonical FGF receptor into a specific receptor for FGF23, Nature 444:770–774, 2006.

194. Lin BC, Wang M, Blackmore C, et al: Liver-specific activities of FGF19 require Klotho beta, J Biol Chem 282:27277–27284, 2007.

195. Kurosu H, Choi M, Ogawa Y, et al: Tissue-specific expression of betaKlotho and fibroblast growth factor (FGF) receptor isoforms determines metabolic activity of FGF19 and FGF21, J Biol Chem 282:26687–26695, 2007.

196. Tsujikawa H, Kurotaki Y, Fujimori T, et al: Klotho, a gene related to a syndrome resembling human premature aging, functions in a negative regulatory circuit of vitamin D endocrine system, Mol Endocrinol 17:2393–2403, 2003.

197. Shimada T, Kakitani M, Yamazaki Y, et al: Targeted ablation of Fgf23 demonstrates an essential physiological role of FGF23 in phosphate and vitamin D metabolism, J Clin Invest 113:561–568, 2004.

198. Segawa H, Yamanaka S, Ohno Y, et al: Correlation between hyperphosphatemia and type II Na-Pi cotransporter in klotho mice, Am J Physiol Renal Physiol 292:F769–F779, 2007.

199. Sitara D, Razzaque MS, Hesse M, et al: Homozygous ablation of fibroblast growth factor-23 results in hyperphosphatemia and impaired skeletogenesis, and reverses hypophosphatemia in Phex-deficient mice, Matrix Biol 23:421–432, 2004.

200. Li SA, Watanabe M, Yamada H, et al: Immunohistochemical localization of Klotho protein in brain, kidney, and reproductive organs of mice, Cell Struct Funct 29:91–99, 2004.

201. Matsumura Y, Aizawa H, Shiraki-Iida T, et al: Identification of the human klotho gene and its two transcripts encoding membrane and secreted klotho protein, Biochem Biophys Res Commun 242:626–630, 1998.

202. Kurosu H, Ogawa Y, Miyoshi M, et al: Regulation of fibroblast growth factor-23 signaling by klotho, J Biol Chem 281:6120–6123, 2006.

203. Farrow EG, Davis SI, Summers LJ, et al: Initial FGF23-mediated signaling occurs in the distal convoluted tubule, J Am Soc Nephrol 20:955–960, 2009.

204. Ichikawa S, Imel EA, Kreiter ML, et al: A homozygous missense mutation in human KLOTHO causes severe tumoral calcinosis, J Clin Invest 117:2684–2691, 2007.

205. Brownstein CA, Adler F, Nelson-Williams C, et al: A translocation causing increased alpha-klotho level results in hypophosphatemic rickets and hyperparathyroidism, Proc Natl Acad Sci U S A 105:3455–3460, 2008.

206. Tieder M, Modai D, Samuel R, et al: Hereditary hypophosphatemic rickets with hypercalciuria, N Engl J Med 312:611–617, 1985.

207. Tieder M, Modai D, Shaked U, et al: "Idiopathic" hypercalciuria and hereditary hypophosphatemic rickets. Two phenotypical expressions of a common genetic defect, N Engl J Med 316:125–129. 1987.

208. Bergwitz C, Roslin NM, Tieder M, et al: SLC34A3 mutations in patients with hereditary hypophosphatemic rickets with hypercalciuria predict a key role for the sodium-phosphate cotransporter NaPi-IIc in maintaining phosphate homeostasis, Am J Hum Genet 78:179–192, 2006.

209. Lorenz-Depiereux B, Benet-Pages A, Eckstein G, et al: Hereditary hypophosphatemic rickets with hypercalciuria is caused by mutations in the sodium-phosphate cotransporter gene SLC34A3, Am J Hum Genet 78:193–201, 2006.

210. Ichikawa S, Sorenson AH, Imel EA, et al: Intronic deletions in the SLC34A3 gene cause hereditary hypophosphatemic rickets with hypercalciuria, J Clin Endocrinol Metab 91:4022–4027, 2006.

211. Levi M: Novel NaPi-2c mutations that cause mistargeting of NaPi-2c protein and uncoupling of Na-Pi cotransport cause HHRH, Am J Physiol Renal Physiol 295:F369–F370, 2008.

212. Jaureguiberry G, Carpenter TO, Forman S, et al: A novel missense mutation in SLC34A3 that causes hereditary hypophosphatemic rickets with hypercalciuria in humans identifies threonine 137 as an important determinant of sodium-phosphate cotransport in NaPi-IIc, Am J Physiol Renal Physiol 295:F371–F379, 2008.

213. Lloyd SE, Gunther W, Pearce SH, et al: Characterisation of renal chloride channel, CLCN5, mutations in hypercalciuric nephrolithiasis (kidney stones) disorders, Hum Mol Genet 6:1233–1239, 1997.

214. Konishi K, Nakamura M, Yamakawa H, et al: Case report: hypophosphatemic osteomalacia in von Recklinghausen neurofibromatosis, Am J Med Sci 301:322–328, 1991.

215. Raskin P, Pak CYC: The effect of chronic insulin therapy on phosphate metabolism in diabetes mellitus, Diabetologia 21:50–53, 1981.

216. Dillon MJ, Shah V, Mitchell MD: Bartter's syndrome: 10 cases in childhood, Q J Med 48:429–446, 1979.

217. Jubiz W, Canterbury JM, Reiss E, et al: Circadian rhythm in serum parathyroid hormone concentration in human subjects: correlation with serum calcium, phosphate, albumin and growth hormone levels, J Clin Invest 51:2040–2046, 1972.

218. Larsson L, Rebel K, Sorbo B: Severe hypophosphatemia: a hospital survey, Acta Med Scand 214:221–223, 1983.

219. Weinstein S, Scottolini AG, Bhagavan NV: Low neutrophl alkaline phosphatase in renal tubular acidosis with hypophosphatemia after toluene sniffing, Clin Chem 31:330–331, 1985.

220. Aschan J, Ringden O, Ljungman P, et al: Foscarnet for treatment of cytomegalovirus infections in bone marrow transplant recipients, Scand J Infect Dis 24:143–150, 1992.

221. Perek J, Mettelman M, Gafter U, et al: Hypophosphatemia accompanying blastic crisis in a patient with malignant lymphoma, J Cancer Res Clin Oncol 108:351–353, 1984.

222. Clark R, Lee E: Severe hypophosphatemia during stem cell harvesting in chronic myeloid leukaemia, Br J Haematol 90:450–452, 1995.

223. Knochel JP: Neuromuscular manifestations of electrolyte disorders, Am J Med 72:521–535, 1982.

224. Silvis SE, DiBartolomeo AG, Aaker HM: Hypophosphatemia and neurological changes secondary to oral caloric intake, Am J Gastroenterol 73:215–222, 1980.

225. Silvis SE, Paragas PU Jr: Paresthesias, weakness, seizures and hypophosphatemia in patients receiving hyperalimentation, Gastroenterology 62:513, 1972.

226. Furlan AJ, Hanson M, Cooperman A, et al: Acute areflexic paralysis. Association with hyperalimentation and hypophosphatemia, Arch Neurol 32:706–707, 1975.

227. O'Connor LR, Klein KL, Bethune JE: Hyperphosphatemia in lactic acidosis, N Engl J Med 297:707–709, 1977.

228. Michell AW, Burn DJ, Reading PJ: Central pontine myelinolysis temporally related to hypophosphataemia, J Neurol Neurosurg Psychiatry 74:820, 2003.

229. Fuller TJ, Carter NW, Barcenas C, et al: Reversible changes of the muscle cell in experimental phosphorus deficiency, J Clin Invest 57:1019–1024, 1976.

230. Newman JH, Neff TA, Ziporin P: Acute respiratory failure associated with hypophosphatemia, N Engl J Med 296:1101, 1977.

231. Aubier M, Murciano D, Lecocguic Y, et al: Effect of hypophosphatemia on diaphragmatic contractility in patients with acute respiratory failure, N Engl J Med 313:420–424, 1985.

232. Gravelyn T, Brophy N, Siegert C, et al: Hypophosphatemia-associated respiratory muscle weakness in a general inpatient population, Am J Med 84:870–876, 1988.

233. Rasmussen A, Buus S, Hessov I: Postoperative myocardial performance during glucose-induced hypophosphatemia, Acta Chir Scand 151:13–15, 1985.

234. Bollaert P-E, Levy B, Nace L, et al: Hemodynamic and metabolic effects of rapid correction of hypophosphatemia in patients with septic shock, Chest 107:1698–1701, 1995.

235. Coburn JW, Massry SG: Changes in serum and urinary calcium during phosphate depletion: studies on mechanisms, J Clin Invest 49:1073–1087, 1970.

236. Agus ZS, Gardner LB, Beck LH, et al: Effects of parathyroid hornone on renal tubular reabsorption of calcium, sodium, and phosphate, Am J Physiol 224:1143–1148, 1973.

237. Emmett M, Goldfarb S, Agus ZS, et al: The pathophysiology of acid-base changes in chronically phosphate-depleted rats, J Clin Invest 59:291, 1977.

238. Lichtman MA, Miller DR, Cohen J, et al: Reduced red cell glycolysis, 2,3-diphosphoglycerate and adenosine triphosphate concentration and increased hemoglobin oxygen affinity caused by hypophosphatemia, Ann Intern Med 74:562–568, 1971.

239. Klock JC, Williams HE, Mentzer WC: Hemolytic anemia and somatic cell dysfunction in severe hypophosphatemia, Arch Intern 134:360–364, 1974.

240. Jacob JS, Amsden P: Acute hemolytic anemia with rigid red cells in hypophosphatemia, N Engl J Med 285:1446, 1971.

241. Marshall DH, Nordin BEC, Speed R: Calcium, phosphorus and magnesium requirements, Proc Nutr Soc 35:163–173, 1976.

242. Garner GB, et al: Dietary phosphorus and salmonellosis in guinea pigs, Fed Proc 26:799, 1967.

243. Rajan K: Hepatic hypoxia secondary to hypophosphatemia, Clin Res 23:521, 1973.

244. Craddock PR, Yawata Y, VanSanten L, et al: Acquired phagocyte dysfunction. A complication of the hypophosphatemia of parenteral hyperalimentation, N Engl J Med 290:1403–1407, 1974.

245. Lentz RD, Brown DM, Kjellstrand CM: Treatment of severe hypophosphatemia, Ann Intern Med 89:941–944, 1978.

246. Rosen G, Boullata J, O'Rangers E, et al: Intravenous phosphate repletion regimen for critically ill patients with moderate hypophosphatemia, Crit Care Med 23:1204–1210, 1995.

247. Clark C, Sacks G, Dickerson R, et al: Treatment of hypophosphatemia in patients receiving specialized nutrition support using a graduated dosing scheme: results from a prospective clinical trial, Crit Care Med 23:1504–1511, 1995.

248. Winter RJ, Harris CJ, Phillips LS, et al: Diabetic ketoacidosis. Induction of hypocalcemia and hypomagnesemia by phosphate therapy, Am J Med 67:897–900, 1979.

249. Zipp NB, Bacon GE, Spencer ML, et al: Hypocalcemia, hypomagnesemia and transient hypoparathyroidism during therapy with potassium phosphate in diabetic ketoacidosis, Diabetes Care 2:265, 1979.

250. Taylor BE, Huey WY, Buchman TG, et al: Treatment of hypophosphatemia using a protocol based on patient weight and serum phosphorus level in a surgical intensive care unit, J Am Coll Surg 198:198–204, 2004.

251. Kruse K, Woelfel D, Strom TM: Loss of renal phosphate wasting in a child with autosomal dominant hypophosphatemic rickets caused by a FGF23 mutation, Horm Res 55:305–308, 2001.

252. Negri AL, Negrotti T, Alonso G, et al: [Different forms of clinical presentation of an autosomal dominant hypophosphatemic rickets caused by a FGF23 mutation in one family], Medicina (B Aires) 64:103–106, 2004.

253. Masi L, Gozzini A, Franchi A, et al: A novel recessive mutation of fibroblast growth factor-23 in tumoral calcinosis, J Bone Joint Surg Am 91:1190–1198, 2009.

Chapter 7

PRIMARY HYPERPARATHYROIDISM

SHONNI J. SILVERBERG and JOHN P. BILEZIKIAN

Primary hyperparathyroidism (PHPT) is characterized by hypercalcemia and elevated parathyroid hormone (PTH) levels. The disease today bears little resemblance to the severe disorder of "stones, bones, and groans" described by Fuller Albright and others in the 1930s.[1-6] Osteitis fibrosa cystica was the hallmark of classic PHPT. Radiography of the skeleton showed brown tumors of the long bones, subperiosteal bone resorption, distal tapering of the clavicles and phalanges, and "salt-and-pepper"–appearing erosions of the skull on radiograph (Fig. 7-1).[7] Nephrocalcinosis was present in 80% of patients, and neuromuscular dysfunction with muscle weakness was also common. With the advent of the automated serum chemistry autoanalyzer in the 1970s, the diagnosis of PHPT became much more common, with a four- to fivefold increase in incidence.[8-10] Classic symptomatology, concomitantly, became much less common. In the United States and elsewhere in the developed world, symptomatic PHPT is now the exception rather than the rule, with more than three-fourths of patients having no symptoms attributable to their disease, making PHPT a disease which has "evolved" from its classic presentation (Table 7-1).[11-14] Nephrolithiasis is still seen, although much less frequently than in the past. Now, radiologically evident bone disease is rare, but bone involvement is readily detected by bone mass measurement. This chapter describes the clinical picture of PHPT as it presents today, how it can be differentiated from other causes of hypercalcemia, and its clinical course. Issues in management, many of which are still unresolved, are also addressed. A detailed discussion of our current understanding of the etiology of this disease can be found in Chapter 8.

Pathology

PARATHYROID ADENOMAS

By far the most common lesion found in patients with PHPT is the solitary parathyroid adenoma, occurring in 80% of patients.[7,14] Several risk factors have been identified in the development of

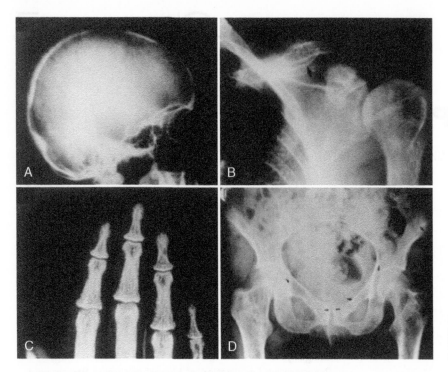

FIGURE 7-1. Radiologic representation of osteitis fibrosa cystica in classic primary hyperparathyroidism. **A,** Salt-and-pepper skull. **B,** Cystic bone disease of the clavicle. **C,** Subperiosteal bone resorption of the digits. **D,** Cortical erosions.

Table 7-1. Changing Profile of Primary Hyperparathyroidism

	Cope (1930–1965)	Heath et al. (1965–1974)	Mallette et al. (1965–1972)	Silverberg et al. (1984–2009)
Nephrolithiasis (%)	57	51	37	17
Skeletal disease (%)	23	10	14	1.4
Hypercalciuria (%)	NR	36	40	39
Asymptomatic (%)	0.6	18	22	80

NR, Not reported.

PHPT. These include a history of neck irradiation[16] and prolonged use of lithium therapy for affective disorders.[17-18] While in most cases a single adenoma is found, multiple parathyroid adenomas have been reported in 2% to 4% of cases.[19] These may be familial or sporadic. Parathyroid adenomas can be discovered in many unexpected anatomic locations (see Chapter 5). Embryonal migration patterns of parathyroid tissue account for a plethora of possible sites of ectopic parathyroid adenomas. The most common sites are within the thyroid gland, the superior mediastinum, and within the thymus.[20] Occasionally, the adenoma may ultimately be identified in the retroesophageal space, the pharynx, the lateral neck, and even the alimentary submucosa of the esophagus.[21-23] On histologic examination, most parathyroid adenomas are encapsulated and composed of parathyroid chief cells. Adenomas containing mainly oxyphilic or oncocytic cells are rare but can give rise to clinical PHPT.

MULTIGLANDULAR PARATHYROID DISEASE

In approximately 15% of patients with PHPT, all four parathyroid glands are involved. There are no clinical features that differentiate single versus multiglandular disease. The etiology of four-gland parathyroid hyperplasia is multifactorial. In nearly half of cases, it is associated with a familial hereditary syndrome such as multiple endocrine neoplasia (MEN) type 1 or type 2a.

Clinical Presentation

INCIDENCE

The incidence of PHPT has changed dramatically.[8,9,24,25] Prior to the advent of the multichannel autoanalyzer in the early 1970s, Heath et al.[8] reported an incidence of 7.8 cases per 100,000 persons in Rochester, Minnesota. With the introduction of routine calcium measurements in the mid-1970s, this rate rose precipitously to 51.1 cases per 100,000 in the same community. Once prevalent cases were diagnosed (the "sweeping" effect), the incidence declined to approximately 27 per 100,000 persons per year. A report from Rochester, Minnesota, suggested that newly diagnosed cases of PHPT have been declining continuously since the mid-1970s.[24] The decline in incidence is not explained by a change in the use of multichannel chemical screening because, in the United States, it is only in the very late 1990s that use of this technique became limited. Moreover, such declines in incidence are not apparent at other medical centers. It is possible that the special demographics of Rochester, Minnesota, combined with the rather complete discovery of PHPT in a population that receives virtually all of its care in one system (ideal epidemiologic surveillance) would naturally be associated with declining numbers for years thereafter. The analogy here might be to overfishing a small pond. Unrelated to the Rochester, Minnesota, experience, the United States may soon experience a decline in new cases of PHPT because multichannel screening is now more limited. On the other hand, greater appreciation of the potential of parathyroid hormone to be a catabolic force in postmenopausal women with osteoporosis has led to measurement of PTH even in subjects who do not have hypercalcemia. This trend has led to the emergence of a new entity, normocalcemic PHPT. A number of factors and forces are thus likely to influence the incidence of PHPT in the future (see later discussion).

CLINICAL FEATURES

PHPT occurs predominantly in individuals in their middle years, with a peak incidence between ages 50 and 60 years. However, the disease is seen at all ages. Women are affected more frequently than men, in a ratio of approximately 3:1. At the time of diagnosis, most patients with PHPT do not have classic symptoms or signs associated with disease. Kidney stones are uncommon, and fractures are rare.[14] Diseases associated epidemiologically with PHPT have included hypertension,[26-28] peptic ulcer disease, gout, or pseudogout.[29,30] Some concomitant disorders such as hypertension are commonly seen, but it is not established that any of these associated disorders are etiologically linked to the disease. The only exception is the MEN syndromes, in which MEN1 is often seen with peptic ulcer disease, and MEN2 may be associated with a pheochromocytoma. Constitutional complaints such as weakness, easy fatigability, depression, and intellectual weariness are seen with some regularity (see later discussion).[31]

The physical examination is generally unremarkable. Band keratopathy, a hallmark of classic PHPT, occurs because of deposition of calcium phosphate crystals in the cornea but is virtually never seen grossly. Even by slit-lamp examination, this finding is rare. The neck shows no masses. The neuromuscular system is normal.

DIFFERENTIAL DIAGNOSIS

The diagnosis of PHPT is made when hypercalcemia and elevated PTH levels are present. The other major cause of hypercalcemia, malignancy, is readily distinguished from PHPT. Patients with hypercalcemia of malignancy typically have advanced disease that has already been diagnosed. An exception is multiple myeloma, in which hypercalcemia can be the initial manifestation. These diseases can be easily distinguished; PTH levels are suppressed in multiple myeloma. The differential diagnosis of hypercalcemia, however, includes a number of other etiologies, including rare ones.[32]

Improved testing for PTH, especially immunoradiometric (IRMA) and immunochemiluminometric (ICMA) assay, has facilitated the distinction between PHPT and hypercalcemia of malignancy. In recent years, it has become clear that the "intact" immunoradiometric assay for PTH ("intact" IRMA) may significantly overestimate the concentration of biologically active parathyroid hormone. In 1998, Lepage et al.[33] demonstrated a large non-(1–84) PTH fragment that comigrated with a large aminoterminally truncated fragment (PTH[7–84]) and had substantial cross-reactivity in commercially available IRMAs. This large, inactive moiety constituted as much as 50% (20% to 90%) of immunoreactivity by IRMA for PTH in individuals with chronic renal failure.[34] Recognition of this molecule led to the development of a new IRMA utilizing affinity purified polyclonal antibodies to PTH(39–84) and to the extreme N-terminal amino acid regions, PTH(1–4).[35,36] This assay detects only the full-length PTH molecule, PTH(1–84). It does not detect the large inactive

fragment the normally circulates This assay has clear utility in uremic patients, in whom the "intact" IRMA has been shown to considerably overestimate elevations in biologically active hormone concentration.[33,37,38] In PHPT, it is less clear that this assay will aid in the diagnostic evaluation.

A small percentage of patients with PHPT have PTH levels that are within the normal reference range as measured either by the classic IRMA or the newer PTH(1–84) assay. In these patients, levels tend to be in the upper range of normal. In PHPT, such values, although within the normal range, are clearly abnormal in a hypercalcemic setting. This is even more evident in patients younger than 45 years of age. Because PTH levels normally rise with age, the broad normal range for the older IRMA (10 to 65 pg/mL) reflects values for the entire population. In the younger-than-45 individual, one expects a narrower, lower normal range (10 to 45 pg/mL), so hypercalcemia and a PTH level of 50 pg/mL is distinctly abnormal. Occasionally, in either a younger or older patient, the PTH level as measured by the established IRMA will not even be in the upper end of the normal range but as low as 30 pg/mL. Such unusual examples generally require a more careful consideration of other causes of hypercalcemia. But in the end, these individuals are likely to have PHPT also because non–PTH dependent hypercalcemia should suppress the PTH concentration to levels that are either undetectable or at the lower limits of the reference range. Souberbielle et al.[39] have illustrated that the normal range is very much a function of whether or not the reference population is or is not vitamin D deficient. When vitamin D deficient individuals were excluded, the upper limit of the PTH reference interval decreased from 65 to 46 pg/mL. When vitamin D–deficient individuals were excluded from the subjects used to establish a reference interval for "whole PTH," the upper limit decreased from 44 to 34 ng/L.

Ninety percent of patients with hypercalcemia will be shown either to have PHPT or malignancy. Although there are many other causes of hypercalcemia (Table 7-2), they constitute only approximately 10% of the hypercalcemic population. Here also, the PTH assay is useful. With the exception of lithium and thiazide use and familial hypocalciuric hypercalcemia (FHH), virtually all other causes of hypercalcemia are associated with suppressed levels of PTH. If the patient can be safely withdrawn

Table 7-2. Differential Diagnosis of Hypercalcemia

Primary hyperparathyroidism
Benign
Parathyroid carcinoma
Hypercalcemia of malignancy
Nonparathyroid endocrine causes
  Thyrotoxicosis
  Pheochromocytoma
  Addison's disease
  Islet cell tumors
Drug-related hypercalcemia
  Vitamin D
  Vitamin A
  Thiazide diuretics
  Lithium
  Estrogen and antiestrogens
Familial hypocalciuric hypercalcemia
Miscellaneous
Immobilization
Milk-alkali syndrome
Parenteral nutrition

from lithium or thiazide, this should be attempted. Serum calcium and PTH levels are then reassessed 3 months later. If the serum calcium and PTH levels continue to be elevated, the diagnosis of PHPT is made. While patients can generally be readily withdrawn from a thiazide diuretic, patient safety must be the first consideration in any decision to withdraw lithium therapy. The recent emergence of a number of alternative therapeutic approaches may make this option realistic. FHH is differentiated from PHPT by (1) family history, (2) markedly lowered urinary calcium excretion, and (3) the specific gene abnormality (see Chapter 8).

Rarely, a patient with malignancy will be shown to have elevated PTH levels due to ectopic secretion of native PTH from the tumor itself.[32] Much more commonly, the malignancy is associated with the secretion of parathyroid hormone–related protein (PTHrP), a molecule that does not cross-react in the IRMA and ICMA assay. Finally, it is possible that a malignancy is present in association with PHPT. When the PTH level is elevated in someone with a malignancy, this is more likely to be the case than a true ectopic PTH syndrome.

Using the third-generation assay for PTH(1–84), a second molecular form of PTH(1–84) that is immunologically intact at both extremes has been identified. This molecule reacts only poorly in second-generation PTH assays. This molecular species represents less than 10% of the immunoreactivity in normal individuals and up to 15% in renal failure patients. It has been shown to be overexpressed, however, in a limited number of patients with a severe form of PHPT or with parathyroid cancer.[41]

Occasionally a patient with PHPT has normal calcium levels. Although the term "normocalcemic PHPT" has been in use for decades, there has been considerable controversy concerning the accuracy of this designation. In many cases, the increases in PTH levels were more apparent than real and attributable to the limitations of available assay technology. The midmolecule radioimmunoassay for PTH, previously in common use, measured hormone fragments in addition to the intact molecule. The latter are retained, leading to spuriously elevated PTH levels, particularly in those with renal insufficiency, in whom clearance of hormone fragments is impaired. Alternative explanations for hyperparathyroidism in so-called normocalcemic PHPT patients have been discovered, including hypercalciuria, renal insufficiency, and certain forms of liver and gastrointestinal disease. In recent years, it has become clear that many patients designated as having normocalcemic PHPT in fact were vitamin D deficient. Vitamin D deficiency with coexisting PHPT can give the semblance of normal calcium levels when in fact they would have been hypercalcemic if the vitamin D levels were normal. Furthermore, we now appreciate that the normal circulating physiologic range of 25-hydroxyvitamin D (25[OH]D) may be significantly higher than the levels once used to diagnose vitamin D deficiency. The diagnosis of normocalcemic PHPT requires that the patient have levels of 25(OH)D within the normal minimum physiologic range of 30 ng/mL.

With these points in mind, patients with elevated PTH levels and normal calcium levels have been reported. These subjects do not have serum calcium levels that extend occasionally into the abnormal range nor do they have any of the known secondary causes for an elevated PTH level. An explanation for why this entity is being seen today may reside in the fact that endocrinologists and other osteoporosis specialists currently evaluate the skeletal status of women at risk for osteoporosis not only with determination of bone density but also with calciotropic hormone measurements. These patients may represent the earliest manifestations of PHPT, a "forme fruste" of the disease. That these patients should exist is not surprising, insofar as clinical manifestations of PHPT are already present when the disorder is commonly diagnosed with hypercalcemia.[42,43] One would expect the earliest phase of this disease to be characterized by elevated PTH levels in the absence of hypercalcemia. During this clinically silent period, the patient would not come to medical attention because the serum calcium is normal. However, if these patients were to have PTH levels measured, one might expect to discover them. Several reports describing these individuals have recently been reported, with several patients progressing to overt hypercalcemia while under observation.[44-46] Frankly low or low-normal serum calcium concentrations suggest an adaptive response to hypocalcemia with high PTH levels. Secondary hyperparathyroidism can be seen in patients with renal insufficiency, malabsorption, or any of the other vitamin D–deficiency states. Rarely, patients with PHPT and coexisting vitamin D deficiency will present with low calcium concentration. PTH levels are high. In such patients, correction of the vitamin D deficiency is associated with a rise in serum calcium concentration into the hypercalcemic range.[47]

OTHER BIOCHEMICAL FEATURES

In PHPT, serum phosphorus tends to be in the lower range of normal, but frank hypophosphatemia is present in less than a fourth of patients. The hypophosphatemia, when present, represents the phosphaturic actions of PTH. Average total urinary calcium excretion is at the upper end of the normal range, with about 40% of all patients having hypercalciuria. Serum 25(OH)D levels tend to be in the lower end of the normal range. While mean values of $1,25(OH)_2D_3$ are in the high-normal range, approximately a third of patients have frankly elevated levels of $1,25(OH)_2D_3$.[48] This pattern is due to the actions of PTH to facilitate the conversion of 25(OH)D to $1,25(OH)_2D$. A mild hyperchloremia is seen occasionally, due to the effect of PTH on renal acid-base balance. A typical biochemical profile is shown in Table 7-3.

The Skeleton

The classic radiologic bone disease of PHPT, osteitis fibrosa cystica, is rarely seen today in the United States. Most series place the incidence of osteitis fibrosa cystica at less than 2% of patients with PHPT. The absence of classic radiographic features (salt-

Table 7-3. Biochemical Profile in Primary Hyperparathyroidism ($n = 137$)

	Patients (Mean ± SEM)	Normal Range
Serum calcium	10.7 ± 0.1 mg/dL	8.2–10.2 mg/dL
Serum phosphorus	2.8 ± 0.1 mg/dL	2.5–4.5 mg/dL
Total alkaline phosphatase	114 ± 5 IU/L	<100 IU/L
Serum magnesium	2.0 ± 0.1 mg/dL	1.8–2.4 mg/dL
PTH (IRMA)	119 ± 7 pg/mL	10–65 pg/mL
25(OH)D	19 ± 1 ng/mL	30–100 ng/mL
$1,25(OH)_2D$	54 ± 2 pg/mL	15–60 pg/mL
Urinary calcium	240 ± 11 mg/g creatinine	
Urine DPD	17.6 ± 1.3 nmol/mmol creatinine	<14.6 nmol/mmol creatinine
Urine PYD	46.8 ± 2.7 nmol/mmol creatinine	<51.8 nmol/mmol creatinine

DPD, Deoxypyridinoline; *PTH (IRMA)*, parathyroid hormone (immunoradiometric assay); *PYD*, pyridinoline.

and-pepper skull, tapering of the distal third of the clavicle, brown tumors) does not mean that the skeleton is not involved in the metabolic processes associated with hyperparathyroid bone disease. With more sensitive techniques, it has become clear that skeletal involvement in the hyperparathyroid process is actually quite common. This section reviews the profile of the skeleton in PHPT as it is reflected in assays for bone markers, bone densitometry, and bone histomorphometry.

BONE MARKERS

Both bone resorption and bone formation are stimulated by PTH. Markers of bone turnover, which reflect those dynamics, provide clues to the extent of skeletal involvement in PHPT.[12] The study of bone markers in PHPT has been of considerable interest for several reasons. First, this inquiry sheds light on which markers accurately reflect skeletal activity in the patient with PHPT. Second, the evaluation of markers of bone turnover in PHPT has provided insight into the hyperparathyroid process in bone. Finally, clues to the extent of postoperative improvements in bone mineral density (BMD) might be provided by markers of bone turnover.

Bone Formation Markers

Bone formation is reflected by osteoblast products, including bone-specific alkaline phosphatase activity, osteocalcin, and type 1 procollagen peptide.[12] Despite the availability of these sensitive measurements of bone formation, the total alkaline phosphatase activity—part of the multichannel biochemical screening profile—is still widely assessed in PHPT. In PHPT, levels can be mildly elevated, but in many patients, total alkaline phosphatase values are within normal limits.[49,50] In a small study from our group,[51] bone-specific alkaline phosphatase activity correlated with PTH levels and BMD at the lumbar spine and femoral neck. Osteocalcin is also generally increased in patients with PHPT.[51-53] Osteocalcin correlates with other indices of bone formation. Assays for procollagen extension peptides reflect osteoblast activation and bone formation but have not been shown to have significant predictive or clinical utility in PHPT.[53] In a small study of patients with PHPT, C-terminal propeptide of human type 1 procollagen (PICP) levels were higher than in control subjects,[54] but distinct elevations were much less impressive than those seen for alkaline phosphatase, osteocalcin, or even hydroxyproline (see later).

Bone Resorption Markers

Markers of bone resorption include the osteoclast product, tartrate-resistant acid phosphatase (TRAP), and collagen breakdown products such as hydroxyproline, hydroxypyridinium cross-links of collagen, and N- and C-telopeptides of type 1 collagen.[12] Urinary hydroxyproline, once the only available marker of bone resorption, no longer offers sufficient sensitivity or specificity to make it a useful tool in the assessment of patients with PHPT. Although urinary hydroxyproline was frankly elevated in patients with osteitis fibrosa cystica, in mild asymptomatic PHPT, it is now generally normal. Hydroxypyridinium cross-links of collagen, pyridinoline (PYD) and deoxypyridinoline (DPD), on the other hand, are often elevated in PHPT. They return to normal after parathyroidectomy.[55] DPD and PYD both correlate positively with PTH concentrations. N- and C-terminal peptides of type I collagen (NTX and CTX) are likely to have utility, but they have not been studied extensively in PHPT. Other markers of bone resorption have also been limited in their application to bone turnover in PHPT. For example, studies of TRAP are

limited, although levels have been shown to be elevated.[47] In the case of the PYD cross-linked telopeptide domain of type I collagen (ICTP), pooled data from patients with high turnover diseases (i.e., PHPT as well as hyperthyroidism) suggest that this marker may reflect calcium kinetics and histomorphometric indices.[12] Data specifically relevant to PHPT are not yet available. Bone sialoprotein, a phosphorylated glycoprotein which makes up approximately 5% to 10% of the noncollagenous bone protein, appears to reflect processes associated with both bone formation and bone resorption. In PHPT, bone sialoprotein levels are elevated and correlate with urinary PYD and DPD.[55] Thus, sensitive assays of bone formation and bone resorption are both elevated in mild PHPT.

Longitudinal Bone Marker Studies

Studies of bone markers in the longitudinal follow-up of patients with PHPT are limited but indicate a reduction in these turnover markers following parathyroidectomy. Information from our group,[55,56] Guo et al.,[57] and Tanaka et al.[58] all report declining levels of bone markers following surgery, although the choice of markers in the individual studies differed. Data are also emerging concerning the kinetics of change in bone resorption versus bone formation following parathyroidectomy. We have found that markers of bone resorption decline rapidly following cure of PHPT, while indices of bone formation follow a more gradual decrease.[55] Urinary PYD and DPD decreased significantly as early as 2 weeks following parathyroidectomy, preceding reductions in alkaline phosphatase. Similar data were reported from Tanaka et al.,[58] who demonstrated a discrepancy between changes in NTX (reflecting bone resorption) and osteocalcin (reflecting bone formation) following parathyroidectomy, and Minisola et al.,[54] who reported a drop in bone resorptive markers and no significant change in alkaline phosphatase or osteocalcin. Short-term studies reported a brief increase in PICP immediately following parathyroidectomy, while bone resorptive markers fell promptly. The persistence of elevated bone formation markers coupled with rapid declines in bone resorption markers indicates a shift in the coupling between bone formation and bone resorption toward an anabolic buildup of bone mineral postoperatively. Increases in bone density postoperatively provide support for this idea.

CYTOKINES

Although studies of bone markers shed light on the skeletal manifestations of PHPT, other molecules have been studied to elucidate the mechanism underlying the effects of PTH excess on bone. These factors, or cytokines, released in response to PTH, lead to important direct and indirect effects on bone cells. Some, such as interleukins (ILs)-1, -6, and -11, transforming growth factor β (TGF-β), epidermal growth factor (EGF), and tumor necrosis factor (TNF), stimulate bone resorption. Others, including IL-4, insulin-like growth factor 1 (IGF-1), TGF-β, and interferons, may be anabolic for bone. Alterations in the levels of some or all of these cytokines may account for the mechanism of accelerated bone turnover and selective bone loss in PHPT.

IL-6 and TNF-α have been studied as possible mediators of bone resorption in PHPT. In vitro and in vivo data support an effect of PTH in stimulating production of IL-6, which in turn leads to increased osteoclastogenesis.[59,60] Furthermore, antibodies to IL-6 prevent PTH-mediated bone resorption. In PHPT, serum levels of TNF-α and IL-6 are increased and fall following parathyroidectomy.[61] Importantly, TNF and IL-6 concentrations correlate with the level of PTH in patients with PHPT. Bone turnover markers correlate with levels of these cytokines as well, supporting an important role of the cytokines in mediating the skeletal effects of PTH excess in PHPT.[62,63] Furthermore, IL-6 soluble receptor has recently been reported to predict rates of bone loss in mild PHPT. Although cytokine levels did not correlate significantly with bone density measurements in the report of Grey et al.,[61] it should be noted that bone density was not assessed at the site containing mostly cortical bone (the radius) where the catabolic effects of excess PTH would be expected to be seen most clearly. More information is needed to confirm these observations, especially with appropriate control subjects, and to test for potential involvement of other bone-resorptive cytokines in PHPT.

The involvement of other factors in the anabolic effect of PHPT on bone is also being studied. Levels of IGF-1, which is well documented to be a direct mediator of PTH action in bone, and insulin-like growth factor–binding protein 3 (IGFBP-3), the major binding protein for IGF-1, change following parathyroidectomy in PHPT.[64] The alteration in the ratio of IGF-1 to IGFBP-3 supports enhanced delivery of IGF-1 to tissues following surgery, an increase inversely proportional to the observed rise in lumbar spine and femoral neck bone density. It is not known whether the anabolic properties of PTH at cancellous sites (e.g., lumbar spine) can be explained by IGF-1 prior to surgery.

BONE DENSOMETRY

The advent of bone mineral densitometry as a major diagnostic tool for osteoporosis occurred at a time when the clinical profile of PHPT was changing from a symptomatic to an asymptomatic disease. This fortuitous timing allowed questions about skeletal involvement in PHPT to be addressed when specific radiologic features of PHPT had all but disappeared. Bone mass measurements could provide information about the actual state of bone mineral with great accuracy and precision. The known physiologic proclivity of PTH to be catabolic at sites of cortical bone make a cortical site essential to any complete densitometric study of PHPT. By convention, the distal third of the radius is the site used. The early densitometric studies in PHPT also revealed another physiologic property of PTH, namely, to be anabolic at cancellous sites. The lumbar spine became an important site to measure not only because it is predominantly cancellous bone, but also because postmenopausal women are at risk for cancellous bone loss. In PHPT, bone density at the distal third of the radius is diminished.[65,66] Bone density at the lumbar spine is only minimally reduced. The hip region, containing a relatively equal mixture of cortical and cancellous elements, shows bone density intermediate between the cortical and cancellous sites (Fig. 7-2). The results support not only the notion that PTH is catabolic for cortical bone but also the view that PTH is anabolic in cancellous bone.[67-69] In postmenopausal women, the same pattern was observed.[66] Postmenopausal women with PHPT, therefore, show a reversal of the pattern typically associated with postmenopausal bone loss: preferential loss of cancellous bone. The reduced bone density at the distal radius (cortical bone) and preserved density at the lumbar spine (cancellous bone) suggest that PHPT helps protect postmenopausal women from bone loss due to estrogen deficiency.

Observations of skeletal health in PHPT made by bone densitometry have established the importance of this technology in the evaluation of all patients with PHPT. Without this information, the data set leading to surgical recommendations is incomplete. The Consensus Development Conference on Asymptomatic Primary Hyperparathyroidism in 1990 implicitly acknowledged

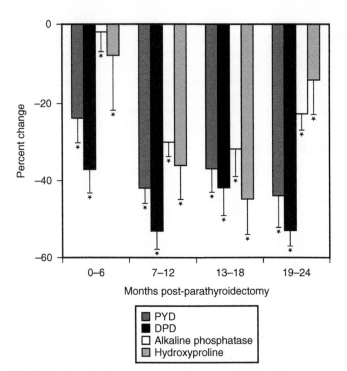

FIGURE 7-2. Bone densitometry in primary hyperparathyroidism. Data are shown in comparison to age- and sex-matched normal subjects. Divergence from expected values is different at each site ($P < 0.0001$). (Data from Silverberg SJ, Shane E, de la Cruz L et al: Skeletal disease in primary hyperparathyroidism, J Bone Miner Res 4:283–291, 1989.)

this point when bone mineral densitometry was included as a separate criterion for clinical decision making.[70] Since that time, bone densitometry has become an indispensable component of both evaluating the patient and establishing clinical guidelines for management and monitoring.

The bone density profile in which there is relative preservation of skeletal mass at the vertebrae and diminution at the more cortical distal radius is not always seen in PHPT. While this pattern is evident in the vast majority of patients, a small group of patients have evidence of vertebral osteopenia at the time of presentation. In our natural history study, approximately 15% of patients had a lumbar spine Z score of less than −1.5 at the time of diagnosis.[72] Only half of these patients were postmenopausal women, so not all vetebral bone loss could be attributed entirely to estrogen deficiency. These patients are of interest with regard to changes in bone density following parathyroidectomy and are discussed in further detail later. The extent of vertebral bone involvement will vary as a function of disease severity. In the typical mild form of the disease, the pattern described earlier is seen. When PHPT is more advanced, there will be more generalized involvement, and the lumbar spine will not appear to be protected. When PHPT is severe or more symptomatic, all bones can be extensively involved.

BONE HISTOMORPHOMETRY

Analyses of percutaneous bone biopsies from patients with PHPT have provided direct information that could only be indirectly surmised by bone densitometry and by bone markers. Both static and dynamic parameters present a picture of cortical thinning, maintenance of cancellous bone volume (Fig. 7-3), and a very dynamic process associated with high turnover and accelerated bone remodeling.

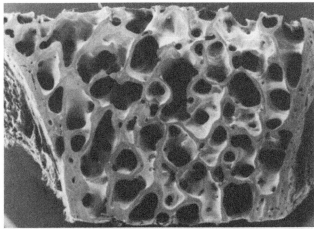

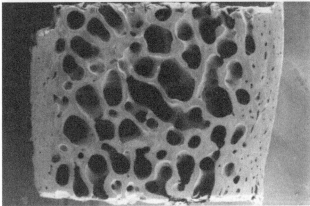

FIGURE 7-3. Scanning electron micrograph of bone biopsy specimens in a normal subject *(top)* and an age- and sex-matched patient with primary hyperparathyroidism *(bottom)*. The cortices of the hyperparathyroid sample are markedly thinned, but cancellous bone and trabecular connectivity appear to be well preserved. (Magnification ×31.25.) (From Parisien MV, Silverberg SJ, Shane E et al: Bone disease in primary hyperparathyroidism, Endocrinol Metab Clin North Am 19:19–34, 1990.)

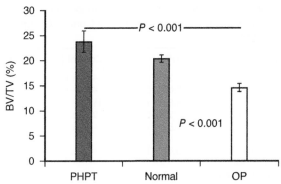

FIGURE 7-4. Cancellous bone volume in primary hyperparathyroidism. Cancellous bone volume was analyzed from bone biopsy specimens of the iliac crest. Comparisons are between 16 women with primary hyperparathyroidism, 17 women with postmenopausal osteoporosis, and 31 women with no known disorder of bone metabolism. Subjects were matched for age and other indices. (Data from Parisien M, Cosman F, Mellish RW et al: Bone structure in postmenopausal hyperparathyroid, osteoporotic and normal women, J Bone Miner Res 10:1393–1399, 1995.)

Cortical thinning, inferred by bone mineral densitometry, is clearly documented in a quantitative manner by iliac crest bone biopsy.[72-74] Van Doorn et al.[75] demonstrated a positive correlation between PTH levels and cortical porosity. These findings are consistent with the known effect of PTH to be catabolic at endocortical surfaces of bone. Osteoclasts are thought to erode more deeply along the corticomedullary junction under the influence of PTH.

Histomorphometric studies have contributed most by elucidating the nature of cancellous bone preservation in PHPT.[75] Again, as suggested by bone densitometry, cancellous bone volume is clearly well preserved in PHPT. This is seen as well among postmenopausal women with PHPT. Several studies have shown that cancellous bone is actually increased in PHPT as compared to normal subjects.[76,77] When cancellous bone volume is compared among age- and sex-matched subjects with PHPT or postmenopausal osteoporosis, a dramatic difference is evident (Fig. 7-4). Whereas postmenopausal women with osteoporosis have reduced cancellous bone volume, women with PHPT have higher cancellous bone volume.[77] This observation suggests that while PHPT is said to be a risk factor for postmenopausal osteoporosis, it is a syndrome of bone loss. The region(s) of bone loss in PHPT is directed toward the cortical bone compartment, with good maintenance of cancellous bone volume unless the PHPT is unusually active.

Preservation of cancellous bone volume even extends to comparisons with the expected losses associated with the effects of aging on cancellous bone physiology. In a study of 27 patients with PHPT (10 men and 17 women), static parameters of bone turnover (osteoid surface, osteoid volume, and eroded surface) were increased, as expected, in patients relative to control subjects.[78] However, in control subjects, trabecular number varied inversely with age, while trabecular separation increased with advancing age. Both of these observations are expected concomitants of aging. In marked contrast, in the patients with PHPT, no such age dependency was seen. There was no relationship between trabecular number or separation and age in PHPT, suggesting that the actual plates and their connections were being maintained over time more effectively than one would have expected through the aging process. Thus, PHPT seems to retard the normal age-related processes associated with trabecular loss.

In PHPT, indices of trabecular connectivity are greater than expected, while indices of disconnectivity are decreased. When three matched groups of postmenopausal women were assessed (a normal group, a group with postmenopausal osteoporosis, and a group with PHPT), women with PHPT were shown to have trabeculae with less evidence of disconnectivity compared with normals, despite increased levels of bone turnover,[76,78] so cancellous bone is preserved in PHPT through the maintenance of well-connected trabecular plates. In order to determine the mechanism of cancellous bone preservation in PHPT, static and dynamic histomorphometric indices were compared between normal and hyperparathyroid postmenopausal women. In normal postmenopausal women, there is an imbalance in bone formation and resorption which favors excess bone resorption. In postmenopausal women with PHPT, on the other hand, the adjusted apposition rate is increased. Bone formation, thus favored, may explain the efficacy of PTH at cancellous sites in patients with osteoporosis.[67,79-81] Assessment of bone remodeling variables in patients with PHPT shows increases in the active bone-formation period[77] (Table 7-4). The increased bone formation rate and total formation period may explain the preservation of cancellous bone seen in this disease.

Recently, further analysis of trabecular microarchitecture has taken advantage of newer technologies that have largely been confirmatory. In a three-dimensional analysis of transiliac bone biopsies using microCT technology, a highly significant correla-

Table 7-4. Wall Width and Remodeling Variables in Primary Hyperparathyroidism (PHPT) and Control Groups (Mean ± SEM)

Variable	PHPT (n = 19)	Control (n = 34)	P
Wall width (μm)	40.26 ± 0.36	34.58 ± 0.45	<0.0001
Eroded perimeter (%)	9.00 ± 0.86	4.76 ± 0.39	<0.0001
Osteoid perimeter (%)	26.84 ± 2.79	15.04 ± 1.09	<0.0001
Osteoid width (μm)	13.39 ± 0.54	9.92 ± 0.36	<0.0001
Single-labeled perimeter (%)	11.56 ± 1.63	4.47 ± 0.48	<0.0001
Double-labeled perimeter (%)	10.41 ± 1.28	4.45 ± 0.65	<0.0001
Mineralizing perimeter (%)	16.19 ± 1.75	6.68 ± 0.83	<0.0001
Mineralizing perimeter/ osteoid perimeter (%)	63.0 ± 5.0	44.04 ± 4.0	<0.01
Mineral apposition rate (μm/day)	0.63 ± 0.03	0.63 ± 0.02	NS
Bone formation rate (μm²/μm/day)	0.10 ± 0.01	0.042 ± 0.006	<0.0001
Adjusted apposition rate (μm/day)	0.40 ± 0.04	0.29 ± 0.03	<0.015
Activation frequency/year	0.95 ± 0.12	0.45 ± 0.06	<0.0002
Mineralization lag time (days)	44.0 ± 6.5	57.0 ± 8.9	NS
Osteoid maturation time (days)	22.5 ± 1.8	16.6 ± 0.9	<0.003
Total formation period (days)	129.2 ± 21.0	208.8 ± 32.5	NS
Active formation period (days)	67.8 ± 5.1	57.3 ± 2.3	<0.05
Resorption period (days)	48.4 ± 7.3	84.8 ± 25.0	NS
Remodeling period (days)	172.5 ± 25.2	299.9 ± 55.1	NS

Modified from Dempster DW, Parisien M, Silverberg SJ et al: On the mechanism of cancellous bone preservation in postmenopausal women with mild primary hyperparathyroidism, J Clin Endocrinol Metab 84:1562–1566, 1999.
NS, Not significant.

tion was observed with the conventional histomorphometry[82] described earlier. In comparison to age-matched control subjects without PHPT, postmenopausal women with PHPT had higher bone volume (BV/TV), higher bone surface area (BS/TV), higher connectivity density (Conn.D), and lower trabecular separation (Tb.Sp.). There were also less marked age-related declines in BV/TV and Conn.D as compared to controls, with no decline in BS/TV. Using the technique of backscattered electron imaging (qBEI) to evaluate trabecular BMD distribution (BMDD) in iliac crest bone biopsies, Roschger et al.[83] showed reduced average mineralization density and increase in the heterogeneity of the degree of mineralization, consistent with reduced mean age of bone tissue. Studies of collagen maturity using Fourier Transform Infrared Spectroscopy provide further support for these observations.[84] Bone strength, therefore, in PHPT has to take into account a number of factors related to skeletal properties of bone besides BMD.[85]

FRACTURES

Fractures were an integral element of classic PHPT, but their importance in modern-day disease is unclear. In a case-control study published in 1975, Dauphine et al.[86] suggested that back pain and vertebral crush fractures might be part of the presenting clinical profile of PHPT. Since that time, reports on fracture incidence have been conflicting. A retrospective review of lateral chest radiographs of patients who underwent parathyroidectomy showed an increased incidence of vertebral fractures in one study,[87] while Wilson et al.[88] found no increase in such fractures

in a cohort of 174 consecutive patients who had mild asymptomatic PHPT.

In a study that focused on hip fracture, a population-based prospective analysis (mean of 17 years' duration; 23,341 person years) showed women with PHPT in Sweden not to be at increased risk.[89] In a much smaller study (46 patients, 44 controls), fractures at any site were increased in hyperparathyroidism.[90] This study is flawed not only by its small sample size but also by the unusually high fracture incidence in both patients (48%) and control subjects (28%) and by the use of thyroid medication in a significantly greater number of patients (28%) relative to control subjects.

The Mayo Clinic experience with PHPT and risk of fracture reviewed 407 cases of PHPT recognized during the 28-year period between 1965 and 1992.[91] Fracture risk was assessed by comparing fractures at a number of sites with numbers of fractures expected on the basis of sex and age from the general population. The clinical presentation of these patients with PHPT was typical of the mild form of the disease, with the serum calcium being only modestly elevated at 10.9 ± 0.6 mg/dL. The data from this retrospective epidemiologic study indicate that overall fracture risk was significantly increased at many sites such as the vertebral spine, the distal forearm, the ribs, and the pelvis. There was no increase in hip fractures. After multivariate analysis, age and female sex remained significant independent predictors of fracture risk. These data, however, are subject to potential ascertainment bias. Patients with PHPT are typically followed more conscientiously, and thus fractures at some of these sites may have been recognized by greater surveillance. This may certainly be true of the vertebral spine and the ribs but unlikely in the case of fractures of the forearm. One might expect to see an increased incidence of distal forearm fractures, since the hyperparathyroid process tends to lead to reduction of cortical bone (distal forearm) in preference to cancellous bone (vertebral spine). Unfortunately, there were no densitometric data provided in this study, so one could not relate bone density to fracture incidence. It is difficult to know whether this study in fact confirms an expectation of preferential distal forearm fractures in PHPT or whether some other process is at work conferring universally greater fracture risk in these patients. In a more recent study, Vignali et al.[92] studied the incidence of vertebral fractures in PHPT as determined by DXA-based vertebral fracture assessment (VFA). In this case control study, 150 consecutive patients and 300 healthy women matched for age and menopausal age were studied. Vertebral fractures were detected in more subjects with PHPT (24.6%) than the control subjects (4.0%; P < 0.001). Among asymptomatic PHPT patients, only those who met surgical guidelines showed a higher incidence of vertebral fractures compared with controls. We still lack prospective, controlled studies to determine fracture incidence in PHPT.

Even the expectation of an increased fracture risk at a cortical site, like the forearm, in PHPT is fraught with uncertainties. The expectation is based upon bone-density data and the presumption that in this disease, it is as predictive of fracture as it is in postmenopausal women who do not have PHPT. By analogy with osteoporosis, it is reasonable to consider bone density as a risk factor for fracture in PHPT, but other issues could lead to a different relationship between bone density and fracture risk in PHPT. It is now known that bone density is only one of several important qualities of bone. These other qualities are influential in the overall assessment of fracture risk. Bone size, for example, influences fracture risk. From the clinical trials of parathyroid hormone in the treatment of osteoporosis, as well as in observations of PHPT per se, it is likely that bone size is affected by PTH. Cortical thinning through PTH-mediated endosteal resorption is compensated for by PTH-mediated periosteal apposition, leading to bone that may be increased in cross-sectional diameter. This increase in bone size provides biomechanical protection for the skeleton. In PHPT, an interesting paradigm is set up: cortical thinning tends to increase fracture risk, whereas increased bone size tends to reduce fracture risk. In addition, as noted, micro-architecture of bone does not show the same kind of deterioration that is commonly seen in postmenopausal osteoporosis. The relative preservation of microarchitecture in PHPT is another factor that may protect bone. More recent studies in which hyperparathyroid bone has been studied with regard to bone mineralization density[83] and collagen quality[84] may also be relevant to this discussion (see earlier). These considerations emphasize the need for prospective studies of site-specific fracture incidence in PHPT.[85,92-94]

Nephrolithiasis

In the past, classic clinical descriptions of PHPT emphasized skeletal involvement and kidney stones as principal complications of the disease.[95] The cause of nephrolithiasis in PHPT is probably multifactorial. An increase in the amount of calcium filtered at the glomerulus due to the hypercalcemia of hyperparathyroidism may lead to hypercalciuria despite the physiologic actions of PTH to facilitate calcium reabsorption. A component of absorptive hypercalciuria exists in this disorder. The enhanced intestinal calcium absorption is believed to be due to increased production of $1,25(OH)_2D$, a consequence of another physiologic action of PTH, namely to increase the synthesis of this active metabolite.[96,97] Urinary calcium excretion is correlated with $1,25(OH)_2D$ levels.[97,98] In addition, increased intestinal calcium absorption seen in nephrolithiasis[99] may also occur in PHPT. The skeleton provides yet another possible source for the increased levels of calcium in the glomerular filtrate. Hyperparathyroid bone resorption might contribute to hypercalciuria, and subsequently to nephrolithiasis, even though there is no convincing evidence to support this hypothesis.[100] Finally, alteration in local urinary factors, such as a reduction in inhibitor activity or an increase in stone-promoting factors, may predispose some patients with PHPT to nephrolithiasis.[100,101] It remains unclear whether the urine of patients with hyperparathyroid stone disease is different in this regard from that of other stone formers.

Studies in the 1970s and 1980s documented a higher incidence of renal stone disease than do reports of more recent experience. With the decreased incidence of osteitis fibrosa cystica, studies in the modern era have tended to focus on patients with kidney stones. Conflicting results have emerged, with one group providing evidence that $1,25(OH)_2D_3$ plays an etiologic role in the development of nephrolithiasis in PHPT and other groups unable to document differences in $1,25(OH)_2D_3$ levels between those with and without renal stone disease.[95,100-102]

Although the incidence of nephrolithiasis is much less common than the incidence in the classic, older presentation of PHPT, kidney stones remain the most common manifestation of symptomatic PHPT (see Table 7-1). Estimates in recent studies place the incidence of kidney stones at 15% to 20% of all patients.[103] Other renal manifestations of PHPT include hypercalciuria, which is seen in approximately 40% of patients, and

nephrocalcinosis, the frequency of which is unknown. It is important to note that in patients with PHPT who do not have renal stone disease, there is no relationship between extent of hypercalciuria and the development of kidney stones.[104]

In the 1930s, it was generally accepted that bone and stone disease did not coexist in the same patient with classic PHPT.[1,6] Albright and Reifenstein[1] postulated that low dietary calcium intake would lead to bone disease, while adequate or high dietary calcium levels would be associated with stone disease. Dent et al.,[105] who provided convincing evidence against this construct, proposed the existence of two forms of circulating PTH, one causing renal stones and the other causing bone disease. A host of mechanisms, including differences in dietary calcium, calcium absorption, forms of circulating PTH, and levels of $1,25(OH)_2D_3$, were proposed to account for the clinical distinction between bone and stone disease in PHPT.[100,105] Today, there is no clear evidence for two distinct subtypes of PHPT. In our patients with PHPT, we could not identify a distinctive set of biochemical data for patients with stone disease.[95] Furthermore, although our population did not include patients with classic hyperparathyroid bone disease, we found no evidence to support the notion that the processes affecting the skeleton and kidneys in hyperparathyroidism occur in different subsets of patients. Urinary calcium excretion per gram of creatinine, levels of $1,25(OH)_2D$, and BMD at all sites were indistinguishable among patients with and without nephrolithiasis. Cortical bone demineralization is as common and as extensive in those with and without nephrolithiasis.[95,100]

Other Organ Involvement

NEUROCOGNITIVE AND NEUROPSYCHOLOGICAL FEATURES

Over the years, PHPT has been associated with complaints referable to many different organ systems. Perhaps the most common complaints have been those of weakness and easy fatigability.[31] Classic PHPT used to be associated with a distinct neuromuscular syndrome characterized by type II muscle cell atrophy.[106,107] Originally described by Vicale in 1949,[108] the syndrome consisted of easy fatigability, symmetric proximal muscle weakness, and muscle atrophy. Both the clinical and electromyographic features of this disorder were reversible after parathyroid surgery.[109,110] In the milder, less symptomatic form of the disease that is common today, this disorder is rarely seen.[111] In a group of 42 patients with mild disease, none had complaints consistent with the classic neuromuscular dysfunction described above. Although over half of all patients had nonspecific complaints of paresthesias and muscle cramps, electromyographic studies did not confirm the picture of past observations.

The "psychic groans" described by early observers of patients with classic PHPT remain a source of controversy today. Patients with PHPT often report some degree of behavioral and/or psychiatric symptomatology. A retrospective look at patients with more severe disease revealed a 23% incidence of psychiatric symptomatology ($n = 441$).[112] More recent studies have shown some abnormalities on psychological tests preoperatively, with no improvement after surgery.[113,114] The study of Solomon et al.[115] studied psychiatric rather than neuropsychological symptoms.[115] Using the SCL-90-R rating scale, they observed a constellation of abnormalities, most of which improved after successful surgery. The control group, who underwent neck surgery for nodular thyroid disease, had similar postoperative improvement. This study documented psychiatric symptoms in the patients with PHPT but could not distinguish the improvement in symptomatology to cure of hyperparathyroidism or to the effects of a successful surgical procedure.

The surgical literature provides further data supporting postoperative improvements. Data from Clark et al.[116] on 152 patients (thyroid surgery control subjects) found 40% of patients reporting less fatigue after cure. Similar findings were reported by Pasieka and Parsons[117] and Burney et al.[118]

The subject of neurocognitive and neuropsychological impairment was reviewed in detail by Silverberg et al.[119] The more recent literature continues to be unclear on whether the symptomatology is specific to PHPT and whether it is improved following successful parathyroid surgery.[119-124] Silverberg et al.[119] have pointed out key limitations in experimental design in many of the published studies. The lack of adequate controls and the value of some of the quantitative instruments have been problematic. There are now three randomized, prospective trials in which this issue has been addressed.[125-127] Despite the rigorous experimental design, with control built into these more recent studies, there was great variability in which features of PHPT if any were improved or not following successful parathyroid surgery. Some of the randomized clinical trials are not yet complete. It is clear that the issue remains unsettled.

CARDIOVASCULAR SYSTEM

Interest in the effect of PHPT on cardiovascular function is rooted in pathophysiologic observations of the hypercalcemic state. Hypercalcemia has been associated with increases in blood pressure, left ventricular hypertrophy, heart muscle hypercontractility, and arrhythmias.[128-130] Furthermore, evidence of calcium deposition has been documented in the form of calcifications in the myocardium, heart valves, and coronary arteries. The association of overt cardiovascular symptomatology with modern-day PHPT is unclear. Hypertension, a common feature of PHPT when it is part of a MEN syndrome with pheochromocytoma or hyperaldosteronism, has also been reported to be more prevalent in sporadic, asymptomatic PHPT than in appropriately matched control groups. The mechanism of this association is unknown, and the condition does not clearly remit following cure of the hyperparathyroid state.[131,132]

An explanation for the inconsistent results reported in the literature on the cardiovascular manifestations of PHPT relates to the fact that the clinical profile of the disease has changed. As a result, the cohorts that have been studied have varied greatly in the severity of their underlying disease. This is particularly true in terms of the serum calcium and parathyroid hormone concentrations, with data from cohorts with marked hypercalcemia and hyperparathyroidism showing the most cardiovascular involvement. Since it is known that both calcium and PTH can independently affect the cardiovascular system, such variability among cohorts can give rise to the inconsistent results that have been reported in the literature. Nevertheless, one can consider this topic usefully in the following terms: mortality, hypertension, cardiac, and noncardiac vascular abnormalities, as well as more subtle functional changes in the cardiovascular system.

Cardiovascular Mortality

There is little doubt that in very active PHPT, cardiovascular mortality is increased.[133-136] Of some interest are the postoperative observations in which the higher cardiovascular mortality rate persists for years after cure.[137] These observations differ markedly from those in which asymptomatic PHPT have been studied. Although limited, the studies have not shown any increase in mortality.[138-139] The Mayo Clinic studies help to bring these observations together. In the mildly hypercalcemic individuals, overall and cardiovascular mortality was reduced, but in those whose serum calcium was in the highest quartile, cardiovascular mortality was increased.[139] The idea that the more common asymptomatic form of PHPT is not associated with increased mortality is supported by data from Nilsson et al.[140] and by other studies[141-142] in which more recently enrolled subjects had better survival than those who had been entered earlier and presumably had more active disease.

Hypertension

This discussion excludes subjects with MEN syndromes in whom a pheochromocytoma may be causative. But hypertension is also a frequent observation among those with mild disease. Most but not all studies have not shown that hypertension is reversed or ameliorated after successful parathyroid surgery for PHPT.[143-146]

Cardiac Manifestations of Primary Hyperparathyroidism

Coronary Artery Disease

Both calcium and PTH have independently been shown to be associated with coronary heart disease.[147-148] Aside from autopsy studies such as those of Roberts and Waller,[149] in which coronary atherosclerosis was seen in hyperparathyroid subjects with levels of calcium that would these days be occasioned with alarm (16.8 to 27.4 mg/dL), the more recent literature has been controversial. Even more recent studies, however, have tended to agree with the idea that the incidence of coronary artery disease in PHPT is more likely to be present as a function of the serum calcium level.[142] Some studies have actually found that in mild PHPT, there is better exercise tolerance as determined by the electrocardiogram.[150] If valvular and myocardial calcifications are regarded separately, the level of the serum calcium again seems to be the determinant.[151-152] Given these differing views, it is also noteworthy that the risk of cardiovascular death in PHPT seems to be related more to traditional risk factors for cardiovascular disease than to the hyperparathyroidism per se.

Left Ventricular Hypertrophy

Left ventricular hypertrophy (LVH) is considered separately because it is itself a strong predictor of cardiovascular disease and mortality. Moreover, different from the parameters described above, in which involvement seems to be a function of the serum calcium level, LVH has been seen across a wide range of calcium levels.[153-154] The idea has been advanced that LVH is more a function of the PTH level than it is the serum calcium.[152,155-156] If it could be shown that when PTH is returned to normal after successful parathyroidectomy LVH is reversible, this observation could have important management implications. Unfortunately, the literature does not give a clear view on this point, with a few but by no means all studies suggesting regression of LVH following parathyroidectomy.[152-153,155-157]

Electrocardiographic Manifestations

Classically, marked hypercalcemia is associated with a reduced QT interval.[158] In most patients with mild hypercalcemia, however, abnormalities on the electrocardiogram are not seen. Moreover, no other conduction abnormalities or arrhythmogenic potential are observed.[159-160]

Vascular Manifestations of Primary Hyperparathyroidism

Carotid Plaque

Calcium has been reported in a recent population-based study of Rubin et al.[161] to be associated with carotid plaque thickness. Consistent abnormalities in carotid intima-medial thickness (IMT), a strong predictor of systemic atherosclerosis and cerebrovascular events, have not been confirmed in mild hyperparathyroidism.[162-165]

Vascular Function

The evidence implicating vascular dysfunction in PHPT has been focused upon those with more severe disease than we see now.[162,166,167] However, in those with lower calcium levels, Baykan et al.[168] also found impaired flow-mediated (endothelial) dilation that negatively correlated with calcium levels. There is a preliminary report on endothelial dysfunction in PHPT[169] and two studies that have reported increased vascular stiffness.[169-170]

GASTROINTESTINAL MANIFESTATIONS

Primary hyperparathyroidism has long been thought to be associated with an increased incidence of peptic ulcer disease. Most recent studies suggest that the incidence of peptic ulcer disease in PHPT is approximately 10%, a figure similar to its percentage in the general population. An increased incidence of peptic ulcer disease is seen in patients with PHPT due to MEN1, in which approximately 40% of patients have clinically apparent gastrinomas (Zollinger-Ellison syndrome). In those patients, PHPT is associated with increased clinical severity of gastrinoma, and treatment of the associated PHPT has been reported to benefit patients with Zollinger-Ellison syndrome.[171] Despite this, current recommendations (Consensus Conference Guidelines for Therapy of MEN1) state that the coexistence of Zollinger-Ellison syndrome does not represent sufficient indication for parathyroidectomy, since medical therapy is so successful.[172]

Although hypercalcemia can underlie pancreatitis, most large series have not reported an increased incidence of pancreatitis in patients with PHPT with serum calcium levels under 12 mg/dL. The Mayo Clinic experience from 1950 to 1975 found that only 1.5% of those with PHPT had coexisting pancreatitis, and alternative explanations for pancreatitis were found for several patients. Regarding pancreatitis in pregnancy in patients with PHPT, these conditions may coexist, but there is no evidence for a causal relationship between the disorders.[173]

OTHER SYSTEMIC INVOLVEMENT

Many organ systems were affected by the hyperparathyroid state in the past. Anemia, band keratopathy, and loose teeth are no longer part of the clinical syndrome of PHPT. Gout and pseudogout are seen infrequently, and their etiologic relationship to PHPT is not clear.

Vitamin D Deficiency and Symptomatic Primary Hyperparathyroidism

Much of this chapter has focused on asymptomatic PHPT as the predominating clinical profile in the modern era. Certainly in countries where biochemical screening tests are routinely employed, this description is accurate. However, reports from other countries have revisited the older, more classic descriptions of PHPT as a disease of "stones, bones, and groans."[174-176] The lack of routine screening tests does not explain completely this older form of the disease in the 1990s in these other countries.

Rather, patients who have been described from China, Brazil, India, and Saudi Arabia have a common underlying vitamin D deficiency. Years ago, PHPT and vitamin D deficiency were described as a potent negative combination by Lumb and Stanbury.[177] Even in mild, asymptomatic PHPT, we have shown that indices of disease activity are generally higher among those whose 25(OH)D levels are low.[47] Mechanisms to explain this clinical observation are speculative, but it is intriguing to consider vitamin D–*PTH* gene interactions. An endogenous regulator of *PTH* gene function is 1,25(OH)$_2$D.[178] When vitamin D deficiency is present in PHPT, it is possible that the abnormal PTH cells are stimulated further to produce PTH.

Evaluation

The diagnosis of PHPT is confirmed by demonstrating an elevated PTH level in the face of hypercalcemia. Further biochemical assessment should include serum phosphorus, alkaline phosphatase, vitamin D metabolites, albumin, and creatinine. A morning 2-hour or 24-hour urine collection should be obtained for calcium and creatinine. A urinary bone resorption marker such as serum CTX or urinary N-telopeptide can be helpful. Radiographs of the skeleton are no longer recommended in view of the rarity of radiologically evident bone disease. Bone densitometry, on the other hand, is performed in all patients. It is important to obtain densitometry at three sites: the lumbar spine, hip, and distal third of the radius. Because of the differing amounts of cortical and cancellous bone at the three sites and the different effects of PTH on cortical and cancellous bone, measurement at all three sites allows a picture of the total effect of the hyperparathyroid process on the skeleton. Bone biopsy is not part of the routine evaluation of PHPT. Although kidney stones are present in 15% to 20% of patients by history, clinicians who see many patients with asymptomatic PHPT do not routinely search for occult nephrolithiasis or nephrocalcinosis. In the view of many experts, the yield of discovering calcifications in the kidney by x-ray or ultrasound is so low as to make it not useful.

Natural History

Over the past 25 years, new knowledge of the natural history of PHPT with or without surgery has been very helpful in guiding decisions regarding surgery in patients with asymptomatic PHPT. The longest prospective observational trial has been conducted by the authors and their colleagues.[179-180] This project began in 1984 in an effort to define the natural history of asymptomatic PHPT. The study included detailed analyses of pathophysiologic, densitometric, histomorphometric, and other skeletal features of PHPT.[179-180] Much of the information gleaned from that study have been summarized already in earlier sections of this chapter. The 15-year follow-up of this study constitutes the longest natural history study of this disorder and was recently reported.[180]

Recommendations for surgery or observation were made on the basis of the 1990 set of NIH guidelines, but both groups included patients who did or did not meet surgical guidelines. This is because some patients opted for surgery even if they didn't meet the guidelines, while others opted for a conservative approach even if they did meet guidelines for surgery. As will be described in the following, this imperfect design was followed

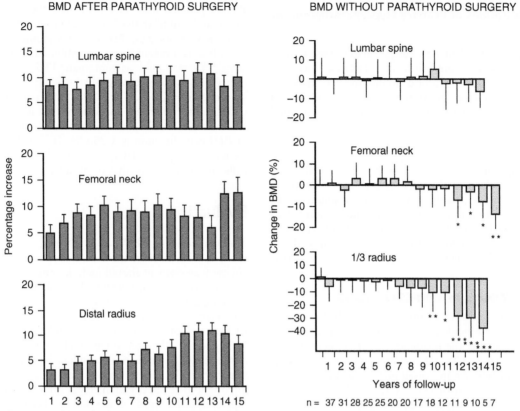

FIGURE 7-5. Longitudinal course of bone density in primary hyperparathyroidism. Data are presented as percentage change from preoperative baseline bone density measurement by site following parathyroidectomy (*left*) or in patients followed with no intervention (*right*). (Data from Rubin MR, Bilezikian JP, McMahon DJ et al: The natural history of primary hyperparathyroidism with or without parathyroid surgery after 15 years, J Clin Endocrinol Metab 93:3462–3470, 2008.)

by three studies that were truly randomized but were of much shorter duration.[125-127] The results with regard to natural history from all studies are remarkably concordant.

NATURAL HISTORY WITH SURGERY

Parathyroidectomy resulted in normalization of the serum calcium and PTH levels permanently. Postoperatively, there was a marked improvement in BMD at all sites (lumbar spine, femoral neck, and distal one-third radius) amounting to gains above 10%. The improvement was most rapid at the lumbar spine, but all sites showed persistent gains for the 15 years of follow-up (Fig. 7-5). The improvements were seen in those who met and did not meet surgical criteria at study entry, confirming the salutary effect of parathyroidectomy in this regard on all patients.

NATURAL HISTORY WITHOUT SURGERY

In subjects who did not undergo parathyroid surgery, serum calcium remained stable for about 12 years, with a tendency for the serum calcium level to rise in years 13 to 15. Other biochemical indices such as PTH, vitamin D metabolites, and urinary calcium did not change for the entire 15 years of follow-up in the group as a whole. Bone density at all three sites remained stable for the first 8 to 10 years. However, after this period of stability, declining cortical BMD was seen at the hip and the distal one-third radius sites. Although the numbers became limiting after 10 years of follow-up, it is noteworthy that a small majority of the subjects lost more than 10% of their BMD over the 15 years of observation. Even though this decline was

observed in the majority of subjects, only 37% of subjects met one or more guidelines for surgery after the 15 years of follow-up.

RANDOMIZED STUDIES OF THE NATURAL HISTORY OF ASYMPTOMATIC PRIMARY HYPERPARATHYROIDISM

Although the long natural history study of asymptomatic PHPT has added much to our knowledge about this disease over time, randomized clinical trials have added data with a more rigorous design that have confirmed the observational data. The three trials are limited by their short duration. In 2004, Rao et al.[125] reported on their randomized controlled trial of parathyroidectomy versus no surgery. The study was not completely enrolled and thus included only 53 subjects, assigned either to parathyroid surgery (*n* = 25) or to no surgery (*n* = 28). The follow-up was for at least 2 years. BMD significantly increased at the femoral neck and total hip, along with normalization of the serum calcium and PTH. In those who did not undergo parathyroid surgery, there were no changes in the lumbar spine or femoral neck bone density, but total hip density significantly declined. Forearm BMD declined, an oddity considering the vulnerability of this site to the catabolic actions of PTH. Biochemical indices were all stable.

In 2007, Bollerslev et al.[126] reported interim results of their randomized trial of parathyroidectomy versus no surgery. This study from three Scandinavian countries was larger, with 191 patients who were randomized to medical observation or to surgery. After surgery, biochemical indices normalized and BMD

Table 7-5. Comparison of New and Old Guidelines for Surgery in Asymptomatic Primary Hyperparathyroidism

Measurement	Guidelines, 1990	Guidelines, 2002	Guidelines, 2008
Serum calcium (above normal)	1–1.6 mg/dL	1.0 mg/dL	1.0 mg/dL
24-hour urinary calcium	>400 mg	>400 mg	
Creatinine clearance	Reduced by 30%	Reduced by 30%	<60 mL/min
Bone mineral density	Z-score < −2.0 (forearm)	T-score < −2.5 (any site)	T-score < −2.5; fragility fracture
Age	<50	<50	<50

increased. In the group that did not undergo parathyroid surgery, BMD did not change.

Also in 2007, Ambrogini et al.[127] reported the results of their randomized controlled trial of parathyroidectomy versus observation. Surgery was associated with a significant increase in BMD of the lumbar spine and hip after 1 year.

GUIDELINES TO THERAPY

Parathyroidectomy remains the only currently available option for cure of PHPT. As the disease profile has changed, questions have been raised concerning the advisability of surgery in asymptomatic patients. If asymptomatic patients have a benign natural history, the surgical alternative is not an attractive one. On the other hand, asymptomatic patients may display levels of hypercalcemia or hypercalciuria that cause concern for the future. Similarly, bone-mass measurements can be frankly low at cortical or (less commonly) cancellous sites. In an effort to address such issues, two consensus development conferences (in 1991 and 2002) on the management of asymptomatic PHPT[70,181] were followed in 2009 by the Third International Workshop on the Management of Asymptomatic Primary Hyperthyroidism, the proceedings of which have been published.[182-187] The 2009 Workshop convened a panel of international experts who reviewed the evidence on aspects of the clinical profile of asymptomatic PHPT with a few towards revising the guidelines for surgery. The most recent guidelines that emerged from that conference should be helpful to the clinician faced with the asymptomatic hyperparathyroid patient: *All* symptomatic patients are advised to undergo parathyroidectomy. Surgery is advised in asymptomatic patients with (1) serum calcium greater than 1 mg/dL above the upper limits of normal; (2) reduction in creatinine clearance to less than 60 mL/min; (3) reduced bone density (T-score < −2.5 at any site or the presence of a fragility fracture); and (4) age younger than 50 years. The most recent guidelines are shown in Table 7-5. It is noteworthy that urinary calcium excretion is no longer regarded as a guideline for surgery, because urinary calcium excretion in subjects with PHPT who have not had a kidney stone is not predictive of the risk for subsequent nephrolithiasis (see earlier discussion). A second change in the guidelines reflects the fact that a fragility fracture is now included as a guideline for surgery. Since two-thirds of vertebral compression fractures are asymptomatic, this brings up the question of whether all patients with asymptomatic PHPT should have a vertebral x-ray or other imaging study (i.e., vertebral fracture assessment) to rule out this possibility. The 2009 Workshop did not address this question.

A number of points were discussed which did not lead to specific recommendations, including the issues of the putative neurocognitive and cardiovascular aspects of PHPT. The Workshop panel also acknowledged a potential role of vitamin D deficiency in fueling processes associated with abnormal parathyroid glandular activity. Finally, the panel also recognized, for the first time, the entity of normocalcemic PHPT.

Surgery

A large percentage of those patients who meet the surgical guidelines listed in Table 7-5 are asymptomatic. Some asymptomatic patients who meet surgical guidelines elect not to have surgery. Among the reasons why surgery is not sought are personal choice, intercurrent medical conditions, and previous unsuccessful parathyroid surgery. Conversely, there are patients who meet none of the NIH guidelines for parathyroidectomy but opt for surgery nevertheless. Physician and patient input remain very important factors in the decision regarding parathyroid surgery.

PREOPERATIVE LOCALIZATION OF HYPERFUNCTIONING PARATHYROID TISSUE

A number of imaging tests have been developed and applied singly or in combination to the challenge of preoperative localization. The rationale for locating abnormal parathyroid tissue prior to surgery is that the glands can be notoriously unpredictable in their location. Although the majority of parathyroid adenomas are identified in regions proximate to their embryologically intended position (the four poles of the thyroid gland), many are not. In such situations, previous surgical experience and skill are needed to locate the ectopic parathyroid gland. In such hands, 95% of abnormal parathyroid glands will be discovered and removed at the time of initial parathyroid surgery. However, in the patient with previous neck surgery, such high success rates are not generally achieved, even by expert parathyroid surgeons. Preoperative localization of the abnormal parathyroid tissue can be extremely helpful under these circumstances. Since imaging technology has become more sophisticated and has captured the attention of patients with PHPT who are attracted to the idea of the gland being definitively localized prior to surgery, preoperative parathyroid imaging is being performed routinely prior to surgery.

Noninvasive Imaging

Noninvasive parathyroid imaging studies include technetium (Tc)-99m sestamibi scintigraphy, ultrasound, computed tomography (CT) scanning, magnetic resonance imaging (MRI), and positron emission tomography (PET) scanning (see also Chapter 9). Tc-99m sestamibi is generally regarded to be the most sensitive and specific imaging modality, especially when it is combined with single-photon emission CT (SPECT). For the single parathyroid adenoma, sensitivity has ranged from 80% to 100%, with a 5% to 10% false-positive rate. On the other hand, sestamibi scintigraphy and the other localization tests have a relatively poor record in the context of multiglandular disease.[188] The success of ultrasonography is highly operator dependent.[189] In centers where there is great expertise, this noninvasive approach is most attractive. Abnormalities identified by ultrasound as possible parathyroid tissue may prove to be a thyroid nodule or lymph node, which underscores the importance of the skill and experience of the ultrasonographer. Rapid spiral thin-slice CT scanning of the neck and mediastinum with evaluation of axial, coronal, and sagittal views can add much to the search for elusive parathyroid tissue.[190] MRI can also identify abnormal parathyroid tissue, but it is time consuming and expensive. It is also less sensitive than the other noninvasive modalities. It can nonetheless be useful when the search with these other noninvasive approaches has been unsuccessful. PET with or without simultaneous CT scan (PET/CT) can be used, but like MRI, it is expensive and does not have the kind of experiential basis that make it attractive. There are also specificity issues because FDG, the scanning agent, accumulates in the thyroid, making differentiation between parathyroid adenoma and thyroid nodules difficult.

Invasive Imaging

Parathyroid Fine-Needle Aspiration

Fine-needle aspiration (FNA) of a parathyroid gland, identified by any of the aforementioned modalities, can be performed and the aspirate analyzed for PTH. This technique is not recommended for routine de novo cases.[191] A theoretic concern with this approach is the possibility that parathyroid cells could be deposited outside the parathyroid gland in the course of the aspiration. Autoseeding of parathyroid tissue would be an unwanted consequence of this procedure if it were to occur.

Arteriography and Selective Venous Sampling for Parathyroid Hormone

In situations where the gland has not been identified by any of the techniques described, the combination of arteriography and selective venous sampling can provide both anatomic and functional localization of abnormal parathyroid tissue. This approach, however, is costly and requires an experienced interventional radiologist. It is also performed in only a few centers in the United States. This approach is reserved now only for those individuals who have had previous unsuccessful parathyroid surgery in whom all other localization techniques have failed.[192]

SURGICAL APPROACH

In the hands of an expert parathyroid surgeon, parathyroidectomy is a highly successful procedure with infrequent complications. A standard surgical approach is the four-gland parathyroid gland exploration under general or local anesthesia, with or without preoperative localization. This approach has been reported to lead to surgical cure in over 95% of cases (see Chapter 9).[193]

Several alternative approaches have emerged that focus upon the single gland and not the total four-gland neck exploration that used to be routinely employed. Unilateral approaches are appealing in a disease in which only a single gland is involved in approximately 85% of cases. These procedures include a unilateral operation in which the gland on the same side that harbors the adenoma is ascertained to be normal. Since multiple parathyroid adenomas are unusual, a normal parathyroid gland is considered by some to be sufficient evidence for single-gland disease. Another limited surgical approach that has emerged in many centers as the approach of choice is the minimally invasive parathyroidectomy (MIP).[194-195] Preoperative parathyroid imaging is necessary, and the procedure is directed only to the site where the abnormal parathyroid gland has been visualized.[196] Preoperative blood is obtained for comparison of the PTH concentration

with an intraoperative sample obtained after removal of the "abnormal" parathyroid gland. The availability of a rapid PTH assay in or near the operating room is necessary for this procedure. If the level falls by more than 50% following resection, into the normal range, the gland that has been removed is considered to be the sole source of overactive parathyroid tissue, and the operation is terminated. If the PTH level does not fall by more than 50%, into the normal range, the operation is extended to a more traditional one in a search for other overactive parathyroid tissue. There is a risk (albeit small) that the minimally invasive procedure may miss other overactive gland(s) that are suppressed in the presence of a dominant gland.

In Europe, MIP is being performed with an endoscopic camera.[197-198] Yet another variation on this theme is the use of preoperative sestamibi scanning with an intraoperative gamma probe to help locate enlarged parathyroid glands. The MIP procedure seems to be as successful as more standard approaches, in the range of 95% to 98%.[199-200]

IMMEDIATE POSTOPERATIVE COURSE

After surgery, biochemical indices return rapidly to normal.[201,202] Serum calcium and PTH levels normalize, and urinary calcium excretion falls by as much as 50%. The serum calcium no longer tends to become abnormally low, a situation characteristic of an earlier time when PHPT was a symptomatic disease with overt skeletal involvement. The acute reversal of hyperparathyroidism was associated with a robust deposition of calcium into the skeleton at a pace that could not be compensated for by supplemental calcium. Thus, postoperative hypocalcemia was routine and sometimes a serious short-term complication ("hungry bone syndrome"). Occasionally, postoperative hypocalcemia still occurs, especially if preoperative bone turnover markers are elevated. More typically, however, the early postoperative course is not complicated by symptomatic hypocalcemia.

Postoperative course after successful parathyroid surgery leads to normalization of the biochemical indices of the disease and improvements in BMD, as mentioned (Fig. 7-6). The capacity of the skeleton to restore itself is seen dramatically in young patients with severe PHPT. Kulak et al.[203] reported two patients with osteitis fibrosa cystica who experienced increases in bone density that ranged from 260% to 430% 3 to 4 years following surgery. Similar observations have been made by Tritos and Hartzband[204] and by DiGregorio.[205]

Medical Management

Surgery is generally not recommended in patients who do not meet any surgical guidelines. Among typical cohorts in the United States, about 50% of patients with PHPT will fit into this category. The most recent guidelines for management of asymptomatic PHPT restated the position that it is reasonable to pursue a nonsurgical course of management in those who do not meet criteria for surgery. In those patients who are not going to have parathyroid surgery, the Workshop[183] suggested a set of monitoring steps which are summarized in Table 7-6. This includes annual measurements of the serum calcium concentration, a calculated creatinine clearance, and regular monitoring of BMD.

GENERAL MEASURES

Patients should be instructed to remain well hydrated and to avoid thiazide diuretics. Prolonged immobilization, which

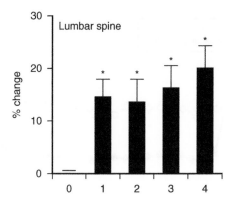

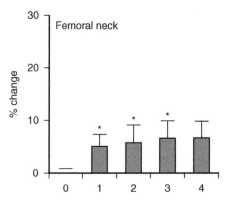

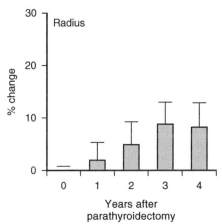

FIGURE 7-6. Bone mineral density following parathyroidectomy in 14 primary hyperparathyroid patients with vertebral osteopenia. The cumulative percentage change from preoperative baseline (year 0) is shown for each site. *Asterisk* denotes change from baseline at $P < 0.05$. (Data from Silverberg SJ, Locke FG, Bilezikian JP: Vertebral osteopenia: A new indication for surgery in primary hyperparathyroidism, J Clin Endocrinol Metab 81:4007–4012, 1996.)

can increase hypercalcemia and hypercalciuria, should also be avoided.

DIET

Dietary management of PHPT has long been an area of controversy. Many patients are advised to limit their dietary calcium intake because of the hypercalcemia. However, it is well known that low dietary calcium can lead to increased PTH levels in normal individuals.[206-208] In patients with PHPT, even though the abnormal PTH tissue is not as sensitive to slight perturbations in the circulating calcium concentration, it is still possible that PTH levels will rise when dietary calcium is tightly restricted. Conversely, diets enriched in calcium could suppress PTH levels in

Table 7-6. Comparison of New and Old Management Guidelines for Patients With Asymptomatic Primary Hyperparathyroidism Who Do Not Undergo Parathyroid Surgery

Measurement	Older Guidelines	Newer Guidelines
Serum calcium	Semiannually	Annually
24-hour urinary calcium	Annually	Not recommended
Creatinine clearance	Annually	Not recommended
Serum creatinine	Annually	Annually
Bone density	Annually	Annually or biannually
Abdominal x-ray	Annually	Not recommended

From Bilezikian JP, Khan AA, Potts JT Jr on behalf of the Third International Workshop on the Management of Asymptomatic Primary Hyperthyroidism: Guidelines for the management of asymptomatic primary hyperparathyroidism: Summary statement from the Third International Workshop, J Clin Endocrinol Metab 94:335–339, 2009.

PHPT, as shown by Insogna et al.[209] Dietary calcium could also be variably influenced by ambient levels of $1,25(OH)_2D$. In patients with normal levels of $1,25(OH)_2D_3$, Locker et al.[210] noted no difference in urinary calcium excretion between those on high (1000 mg/day) and low (500 mg/day) calcium intake diets. On the other hand, in those with elevated levels of $1,25(OH)_2D_3$, high calcium diets were associated with worsening hypercalciuria. This observation suggests that dietary calcium intake in patients can be liberalized to 1000 mg/day if $1,25(OH)_2D_3$ levels are not increased but should be more tightly controlled if $1,25(OH)_2D_3$ levels are elevated.

PHARMACEUTICALS

Phosphate

Oral phosphate can lower the serum calcium by up to 1 mg/dL.[211-212] A complex interplay of mechanisms leads to this moderating effect of oral phosphate. First, calcium absorption falls in the presence of intestinal phosphorus. Second, concomitant increases in serum phosphorus will tend to reduce circulating $1,25(OH)_2D_3$ levels. Third, phosphate can be an antiresorptive agent. Finally, increased serum phosphorus reciprocally lowers serum calcium. Problems with oral phosphate include limited gastrointestinal tolerance, possible further increase in PTH levels, and the possibility of soft-tissue calcifications after long-term use. It is essentially not used anymore in the management of PHPT.

Bisphosphonates

Bisphosphonates are conceptually attractive in PHPT because they are antiresorptive agents with an overall effect to reduce bone turnover. Although they do not affect PTH secretion directly, bisphosphonates could reduce serum and urinary calcium levels. Early studies with the first-generation bisphosphonates were disappointing. Etidronate has no effect.[213] Clodronate use was associated in several studies with a reduction in serum and urinary calcium,[214] but the effect was transient.

Alendronate has been studied most extensively in PHPT. Studies by Rossini et al.[215] and Hassani et al.[216] were followed by those of Chow et al.,[217] Parker et al.,[218] and Kahn et al.[219] These studies were all characterized by a randomized, controlled design. Typically, BMD of the lumbar spine and hip regions increases along with reductions in bone turnover markers. Except for the study of Chow et al.,[217] serum calcium was unchanged. These results suggest that a bisphosphonate-like alendronate might be useful in patients with low bone density in whom parathyroid surgery is not to be performed.

Estrogens and Selective Estrogen-Receptor Modulators

The earliest studies on the use of estrogen replacement therapy in PHPT date back to the early 1970s. A 0.5 to 1.0 mg/dL reduction in total serum calcium levels in postmenopausal women with PHPT who receive estrogen replacement therapy is generally seen. Gallagher and Nordin[220] first reported a calcium-lowering effect in 10 postmenopausal women given ethinyl estradiol. A prompt lowering of both serum and urinary calcium excretion was noted after 1 week of therapy, with continued reductions at 4 weeks (mean serum calcium [normal range, 8.9 to 10.2 mg/dL]: 12.0 to 11.6 to 11.3 mg/dL; $P < 0.0025$; and mean urinary calcium, 402 to 291 to 283 mg/g creatinine; $P < 0.0005$). Subsequent studies have reported similar declines in serum and urinary calcium in response to both ethinyl estradiol and conjugated equine estrogens.[221] Although levels of PTH were not measured in the earlier studies, Marcus et al.[221] and Selby and Peacock[222] reported no change in PTH as measured by a C-terminal radioimmunoassay. Grey et al.[223] also found no changes in intact PTH levels.

Various approaches to skeletal dynamics have been used in studies of metabolic and skeletal responses to estrogen replacement therapy in women with PHPT. Gallagher and Wilkinson[224] demonstrated normalization of calcium balance, with a decrease in output relative to intake. Studies of BMD in estrogen-treated patients with PHPT have documented a salutary effect of treatment on BMD at the femoral neck and lumbar spine.[223]

The role of cytokines in the skeletal response to estrogen therapy in PHPT is unknown. While the local anabolic actions of PTH may be mediated in part by IGF-1, estrogens play an important independent role in regulating the synthesis of this cytokine. Moreover, postmenopausal women have lower levels of IGF-1 than their premenopausal counterparts. A further decrease is found in osteoporotic postmenopausal women, arguing against a simple age-related effect. The precise role of IGF-1 in mediating the response to estrogen replacement in PHPT remains unclear, with decreased (oral administration of ethinyl estradiol, conjugated equine estrogen, or estradiol valerate) or slightly increased (transdermal estrogen) levels reported. In view of the recent concerns expressed about chronic estrogen use in the Women's Health Study, estrogen use is no longer recommended for medical management of hyperparathyroidism.

Raloxifene, a selective estrogen-receptor modulator, has been studied in PHPT, but the data are sparse. In a short-term (8-week) trial of 18 postmenopausal women, raloxifene (60 mg/day) was associated with a statistically significant although small (0.5 mg/dL) reduction in the serum calcium concentration and in markers of bone turnover.[225] No long-term data or data on bone density are available.

Inhibition of Parathyroid Hormone

The most specific pharmacologic approach to primary PHPT is to inhibit the synthesis and secretion of PTH from the parathyroid glands. Interest is now focused upon compounds that act on the parathyroid cell calcium-sensing receptor. This G protein–coupled receptor recognizes calcium as its cognate ligand.[226-228] When activated by increased extracellular calcium, the calcium-sensing receptor signals the cell via a G protein–transducing pathway to raise the intracellular calcium concentration, which inhibits PTH secretion. Molecules that mimic the effect of extracellular calcium by altering the affinity of calcium for the receptor could activate this receptor and inhibit parathy-

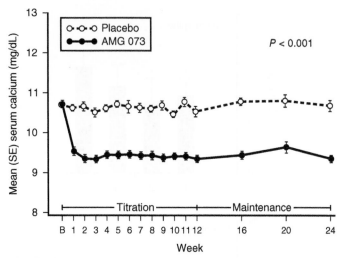

FIGURE 7-7. Changes in serum calcium concentrations with administration of the calcimimetic cinacalcet (solid line) or placebo (broken line) in patients with primary hyperparathyroidism. (Data from Shoback DM, Bilezikian JP, Turner SA et al: The calcimimetic cinacalcet normalizes serum calcium in subjects with primary hyperparathyroidism, J Clin Endocrinol Metab 88:5644–5649, 2003.)

roid cell function. The phenylalkylamine (R)-N(3-methoxy-α-phenylethyl)-3-(2-chlorophenyl)-1-propylamine (R-568) is one such calcimimetic compound. R-568 was found to increase cytoplasmic calcium and reduce PTH secretion in vitro, as well as in normal postmenopausal women.[229-230] This drug also was shown to inhibit PTH secretion in postmenopausal women with PHPT.[231] A second-generation ligand, cinacalcet, has been the subject of recent more extensive investigation in PHPT. Studies conducted by the authors and their colleagues[232-234] indicate that this drug can reduce the serum calcium concentration to normal in PHPT (Fig. 7-7), but despite normalization of the serum calcium concentration, PTH levels do not return to normal; they do fall by 35% to 50% after administration of drug. Urinary calcium excretion does not change; serum phosphorus levels increase but are maintained in the lower range of normal; and 1,25(OH)$_2$D$_3$ levels do not change. The average BMD does not change, even after 3 years of administration of cinacalcet. Marcocci[235] has recently shown that cinacalcet is effective in subjects with intractable PHPT, Silverberg et al.[236] have shown that cinacalcet reduces calcium levels effectively in inoperable parathyroid carcinoma.

Unusual Presentations

NEONATAL PRIMARY HYPERPARATHYROIDISM

Neonatal PHPT is a rare form of the disorder caused by homozygous inactivation of the calcium-sensing receptor.[237] When present in a heterozygous form, it is a benign hypercalcemic state known as familial hypercalciuric hypercalcemia (FHH). However, in the homozygous neonatal form, hypercalcemia is severe and the outcome fatal unless recognized early. The treatment of choice is early subtotal parathyroidectomy to remove the majority of hyperplastic parathyroid tissue.

PRIMARY HYPERPARATHYROIDISM IN PREGNANCY

Primary hyperparathyroidism in pregnancy is primarily of concern for its potential effect on the fetus and neonate.[238-239]

Complications of PHPT in pregnancy include spontaneous abortion, low birth weight, supravalvular aortic stenosis, and neonatal tetany. The last condition is a result of fetal parathyroid gland suppression by high levels of maternal calcium, which readily crosses the placenta during pregnancy. These infants, used to hypercalcemia in utero, have functional hypoparathyroidism after birth, and can develop hypocalcemia and tetany in the first few days of life. Today, with most patients (pregnant or not) presenting with a mild form of PHPT, an individualized approach to the management of the pregnant patient with PHPT is advised. Many of those with very mild disease can be followed safely, with successful neonatal outcomes without surgery. However, parathyroidectomy during the second trimester remains the traditional recommendation for this condition.

ACUTE PRIMARY HYPERPARATHYROIDISM

Acute PHPT is known variously as *parathyroid crisis, parathyroid poisoning, parathyroid intoxication,* and *parathyroid storm.* Acute PHPT describes an episode of life-threatening hypercalcemia of sudden onset in a patient with PHPT.[240-243] Clinical manifestations of acute PHPT are mainly those associated with severe hypercalcemia. Nephrocalcinosis or nephrolithiasis is frequently seen. Radiologic evidence of subperiosteal bone resorption is also commonly present. Laboratory evaluation is remarkable not only for very high serum calcium levels but for extreme elevations in PTH to approximately 20 times normal.[242] In this way, acute PHPT resembles parathyroid carcinoma. A history of persistent mild hypercalcemia has been reported in 25% of patients. However, given the rarity of this condition, the risk of developing acute PHPT in a patient with mild asymptomatic PHPT is very low. Intercurrent medical illness with immobilization may precipitate acute PHPT. Early diagnosis, with aggressive medical management followed by surgical cure, is essential for a successful outcome.

PARATHYROID CANCER

An indolent yet potentially fatal disease, parathyroid carcinoma accounts for less than 0.5% of cases of PHPT.[244] The cause of the disease is unknown, and no clear risk factors have been identified. There is no evidence to support the malignant degeneration of previously benign parathyroid adenomas. Manifestations of hypercalcemia are the primary effects of parathyroid cancer. The disease tends not to have a bulk tumor effect, spreading slowly in the neck. Metastatic disease is a late finding, with lung (40%), liver (10%), and lymph node (30%) involvement seen most commonly.

The clinical profile of parathyroid cancer differs from that of benign PHPT in several important ways.[244-245] First, no female predominance is seen among patients with carcinoma. Second, elevations in serum calcium and PTH are far greater. As a consequence, the hyperparathyroid disease tends to be much more severe, with the classic targets of PTH excess involved in most cases. Nephrolithiasis or nephrocalcinosis is seen in up to 60% of patients; overt radiologic evidence of skeletal involvement is seen in 35% to 90% of patients. A palpable neck mass, distinctly unusual in benign PHPT, has been reported in 30% to 76% of patients with parathyroid cancer.[246]

Grossly, malignant glands are large, often exceeding 12 g. They tend to be adherent to adjacent structures. Microscopically, the trabecular arrangement of the tumor cells is divided by thick, fibrous bands. Capsular and blood vessel invasion is common by these cells that often contain mitotic figures.[246]

Parathyroid carcinoma has also been reported in hereditary syndromes of hyperparathyroidism,[247-250] particularly in hyperparathyroidism-jaw tumor (HPT-JT) syndrome,[251] a rare autosomal disorder in which as many as 15% of patients will have malignant parathyroid disease. Because cystic changes are common, this disorder has also been referred to as *cystic parathyroid adenomatosis.*[252] In HPT-JT, ossifying fibromas of the maxilla and mandible are seen in 30% of cases. Less commonly, kidney lesions, including cysts, polycystic disease, hamartomas, or Wilms tumors can be present.[253] Parathyroid carcinoma has also been reported in familial isolated hyperparathyroidism.[248,254] Recently, parathyroid carcinoma, as defined pathologically, has been reported in MEN1 syndrome and with somatic *MEN1* mutations.[255-257] However, recurrent parathyroid disease in MEN1 may mimic but not actually be due to malignancy. Only one case of parathyroid carcinoma has been reported in the MEN2A syndrome.[258]

Loss of the retinoblastoma tumor suppressor gene used to be considered a marker for parathyroid cancer,[210] but more recent studies do not unequivocally support this impression.[259] Work by Shattuck et al.[260-261] have provided new insights into the molecular pathogenesis of parathyroid cancer. Parathyroid carcinomas from 10 of 15 patients with sporadic parathyroid cancer carried a mutation in the HRPT2 gene. The HRPT2 gene that encodes for the parafibromin protein has been shown to be mutated in a substantial number of patients with parathyroid cancer. Marcocci et al.[244] have recently reviewed this topic, pointing out a potential role for parafibromin in parathyroid cancer. In 3 of 15 patients with parathyroid cancer, Shattuck et al.[261] showed that the mutation was in the germline. The presence of the mutation in the germline suggests that this disease might be related in some way to the HPT-JT syndrome, in which this gene has been implicated.[261] In addition, there is an increased risk of parathyroid cancer in the HPT-JT syndrome. In fact, in patients with a germline mutation, certain clinical features in them and their relatives are indicative of the HPT-JT syndrome or phenotypic variants.[262-264]

Surgery is the only effective therapy currently available for this disease. The greatest chance for cure occurs with the first operation. Once the disease recurs, cure is unlikely, although the disease may smolder for many years thereafter. The tumor is not radiosensitive, although there are isolated reports of tumor regression with localized radiation therapy. Traditional chemotherapeutic agents have not been useful. When metastasis occurs, isolated removal is an option, especially if only one or two nodules are found in the lung. Such isolated metastasectomies are never curative but they can lead to prolonged remissions, sometimes lasting for several years. Similarly, local debulking of tumor tissue in the neck can be palliative, although malignant tissue is invariably left behind.

Chemotherapy has had a very limited role in this disease. Bradwell and Harvey[265] have attempted an immunotherapeutic approach by injecting a patient who had severe hypercalcemia due to parathyroid cancer with immunogenic PTH. Coincident with a rise in antibody titer to PTH, previous refractory hypercalcemia fell impressively. A more recent report[266] provided evidence of antitumor effect in a single case of PTH immunization in metastatic parathyroid cancer. Recent attention has been focused instead on control of hypercalcemia in this devastating disease. The intravenous bisphosphonates have been used in their capacity as agents that treat severe hypercalcemia. Although efficacious in that regard, they do not have an enduring effect. The calcimimetic agents hold promise for offering calcium-lowering effects on an outpatient basis. Our group[267] reported on a single patient treated with the calcimimetic, R-568; despite widely metastatic disease, the patient had serum calcium levels maintained in a range that allowed him to return to normal functioning for nearly 2 years. A wider experience by Silverberg et al.[236] gives even more evidence that cinacalcet has utility in the management of parathyroid cancer. The U.S. Food and Drug Administration approved this calcimimetic for the treatment of hypercalcemia in patients with parathyroid cancer. Based upon extensive studies,[268] cinacalcet has also been approved for use in patients with secondary hyperparathyroidism on hemodialysis. Use of this agent in parathyroid cancer led to improvement in serum calcium levels and a decrease in symptoms of nausea, vomiting, and mental lethargy, which are common concomitants of marked hypercalcemia. There are no data on the effect of cinacalcet on tumor growth in parathyroid cancer. Although many questions remain, this agent offers an option for control of intractable hypercalcemia when surgical removal of cancerous tissue is no longer an option.

Summary

This chapter has presented a comprehensive summary of the modern-day presentation of PHPT. As an asymptomatic disorder in economically more developed countries, its presentation has raised issues regarding the extent to which patients who are asymptomatic may nevertheless show involvement in target organs; who should be recommended for parathyroid surgery; who can be safely followed without surgical intervention; as well as newer pharmacologic approaches to management. Questions about the natural history and pathophysiology of the disorder continue to be of great interest. Inasmuch as this disorder appears to be evolving in several different ways, it is clear that additional careful studies are required to continue to gain new insights into this disease.

Acknowledgment

Supported in part by National Institutes of Health grants NIDDK 32333, DK066329, and RR 00645.

REFERENCES

1. Albright F, Reifenstein EC: The Parathyroid Glands and Metabolic Bone Disease, Baltimore, 1948, Williams & Wilkins.
2. Cope O: The story of hyperparathyroidism at the Massachusetts General Hospital, N Engl J Med 21:1174–1182, 1966.
3. Bauer W: Hyperparathyroidism: Distinct disease entity, J Bone Joint Surg 15:135–141, 1933.
4. Bauer W, Federman DD: Hyperparathyroidism epitomized: Case of Captain Charles E. Martell, Metabolism 11:21–22, 1962.
5. Mandl F: Therapeutische Versuch bei Ostitis fibrosa generalisata mittels Extirpation eines Epithelkörperchentumors, Wien Klin Wochenschr 50:1343–1344, 1925.
6. Albright F, Aub JC, Bauer W: Hyperparathyroidism: A common and polymorphic condition as illustrated by seventeen proven cases from one clinic, JAMA 102:1276–1287, 1934.
7. Silverberg SJ, Bilezikian JP: Clinical presentation of primary hyperparathyroidism in the United States. In Marcus R, Levine MA, editors: The Parathyroids, New York, 2001, Academic Press, pp 349–360.
8. Heath H, Hodgson SF, Kennedy MA: Primary hyperparathyroidism: Incidence, morbidity, and economic impact in a community, N Engl J Med 302:189–193, 1980.
9. Mundy GR, Cove DH, Fisken R: Primary hyperparathyroidism: Changes in the pattern of clinical presentation, Lancet 1:1317–1320, 1980.
10. Scholz DA, Purnell DC: Asymptomatic primary hyperparathyroidism, Mayo Clin Proc 56:473–478, 1981.
11. Bilezikian JP: Primary hyperparathyroidism. In DeGroot L, editor, Arnold A (section ed): www.ENDOTEXT.org (April 2009 version). Dartmouth, 2009, MDTEXT.COM Inc.
12. Silverberg SJ, Bilezikian JP: Primary hyperparathyroidism. In Seibel MJ, Robins SP, Bilezikian JP, editors: Dynamics of Bone and Cartilage Metabolism, San Diego, 2006, Elsevier, pp 767–778.
13. Silverberg SJ, Bilezikian JP: The diagnosis and management of asymptomatic primary hyperparathyroidism, Nat Clin Pract Endocrinol Metab 2:494–503, 2006.
14. Bilezikian JP, Silverberg SJ: Primary hyperparathyroidism. In Rosen C, editor: Primer on the Metabolic Bone Diseases and Disorders of Mineral Metabolism, ed 7, Washington, DC, 2008, American Society for Bone and Mineral Research, pp 302–306.
15. Golden SH, Robinson KA, Saldanha I, Anton B, Ladenson PW: Prevalence and incidence of endocrine and metabolic disorders in the United States: A comprehensive review, J Clin Endocrinol Metab 94:1853–1878, 2009.

16. Rao SD, Frame B, Miller MJ, et al: Hyperparathyroidism following head and neck irradiation, Arch Intern Med 140:205–207, 1980.
17. Nordenstrom J, Strigard K, Perbeck L, et al: Hyperparathyroidism associated with treatment of manic-depressive disorders by lithium, Eur J Surg 158:207–211, 1992.
18. McHenry CR, Rosen IB, Rotstein LE, et al: Lithiumogenic disorders of the thyroid and parathyroid glands as surgical disease, Surgery 108:1001–1005, 1992.
19. Attie JN, Bock G, Auguste L: Multiple parathyroid adenomas: Report of 33 cases, Surgery 108:1014–1019, 1990.
20. Nudelman IL, Deutsch AA, Reiss R: Primary hyperparathyroidism due to mediastinal parathyroid adenoma, Int Surg 72:104–108, 1987.
21. Sloane JA: Parathyroid adenoma in submucosa of esophagus, Arch Pathol Lab Med 102:242–243, 1978.
22. Joseph MP, Nadol JB, Pilch BZ, Goodman ML: Ectopic parathyroid tissue in the hypopharyngeal mucosa (pyriform sinus), Head Neck Surg 5:70–74, 1982.
23. Gilmour JR: Some developmental abnormalities of the thymus and parathyroids, J Pathol Bacteriol 52:213–218, 1941.
24. Wermers RA, Khosla S, Atkinson EJ, et al: The rise and fall of primary hyperparathyroidism, Ann Intern Med 126:433–440, 1997.
25. Melton LJ III: The epidemiology of primary hyperparathyroidism in North America, J Bone Miner Res 17(Suppl 2):N12–N17, 2002.
26. Ringe JD: Reversible hypertension in primary hyperparathyroidism: Pre- and postoperative blood pressure in 75 cases, Klin Wochenschr 62:465–469, 1984.
27. Broulik PD, Horky K, Pacovsky V: Blood pressure in patients with primary hyperparathyroidism before and after parathyroidectomy, Exp Clin Endocrinol 86:346–352, 1985.
28. Rapado A: Arterial hypertension and primary hyperparathyroidism, Am J Nephrol 6(suppl 1):49–50, 1986.
29. Bilezikian JP, Aurbach GD, Connor TB, et al: Pseudogout following parathyroidectomy, Lancet 1:445–447, 1973.
30. Geelhoed GW, Kelly TR: Pseudogout as a clue and complication in primary hyperparathyroidism, Surgery 106:1036–1041, 1989.
31. Silverberg SJ: Non-classical target organs in primary hyperparathyroidism, J Bone Min Res 17(Suppl 2):N117–N125, 2003.
32. Jacobs TP, Bilezikian JP: Rare causes of hypercalcemia, J Clin Endocrinol Metab 90:6316–6322, 2005.
33. Lepage R, Roy L, Brossard JH, et al: A non-(1–84) circulating parathyroid hormone (PTH) fragment interferes significantly with intact PTH commercial assay

measurements in uremic samples, Clin Chem 44:805–809, 1998.
34. Quarles LD, Lobough B, Murphy G: Intact parathyroid hormone over-estimates the presence and severity of parathyroid-mediated osseous abnormalities in uremia, J Clin Endocrinol Metab 75:145–150, 1992.
35. John MR, Goodman WG, Gao P, Cantor T, Salusky IB, Jueppner H: A novel immunoradiometric assay detects full-length human PTH but not amino-terminally truncated fragments: Implications for PTH measurement in renal failure, J Clin Endocrinol Metab 84:4287–4290, 1999.
36. Gao P, Scheibel S, D'Amour P, et al: Development of a novel immunoradiometric assay exclusively for biologically active whole parathyroid hormone 1–84. Implications for improvement of accurate assessment of parathyroid function, J Bone Miner Res, 16:4:605–614, 2001.
37. Slatopolsky E, Finch JL, Clay P, et al: A novel mechanism for skeletal resistance in uremia, Kidney Int 58:753–761, 2000.
38. Silverberg SJ, Brown I, LoGerfo P, Gao P, Cantor T, Bilezikian JP: Clinical utility of an immunoradiometric assay for whole PTH (1–84) in primary hyperparathyroidism, J Clin Endocrinol Metab 88:4725–4730, 2003.
39. Souberbielle JC, Cormier C, Kindermans C, et al: Vitamin D status and redefining serum parathyroid hormone reference range in the elderly, J Clin Endocrinol Metab 86:3086–3090, 2001.
40. D'Amour P, Brossard JH, Rousseau L, et al: Amino-terminal form of parathyroid hormone (PTH) with immunologic similarities to hPTH(1–84) is overproduced in primary and secondary hyperparathyroidism, Clin Chem 49:2037–2044, 2003.
41. Rubin MR, Silverberg SJ, D'Amour P, et al: An N-terminal molecular form of parathyroid hormone (PTH) distinct from hPTH(1–84) is overproduced in parathyroid carcinoma, Clin Chem 53:1470–1476, 2007.
42. Rao DS, Wilson RJ, Kleerekoper M, Parfitt AM: Lack of biochemical progression or continuation of accelerated bone loss in mild asymptomatic primary hyperparathyroidism, J Clin Endocrinol Metab 67:1294–1298, 1988.
43. Silverberg SJ, Gartenberg F, Jacobs TP, et al: Longitudinal measurements of bone density and biochemical indices in untreated primary hyperparathyroidism, J Clin Endocrinol Metab 80:723–728, 1995.
44. Hagag P, Revet-Zak I, Hod N, Horne T, Rapoport MJ, Weiss M: Diagnosis of normocalcemic hyperparathyroidism by oral calcium loading test, J Endocrinol Invest 26:327–332, 2003.
45. Silverberg SJ, Bilezikian JP: "Incipient" primary hyperparathyroidism: a "forme fruste" of an old disease, J Clin Endocrinol Metab 88:5348–5352, 2003.

46. Lowe H, McMahon DJ, Rubin MR, Bilezikian JP, Silverberg SJ: Normocalcemic primary hyperparathyroidism: further characterization of a new clinical phenotype, J Clin Endocrinol Metab 92:3001–3005, 2007.

47. Silverberg SJ, Shane E, Dempster DW, Bilezikian JP: Vitamin D deficiency in primary hyperparathyroidism, Am J Med 107:561–567, 1999.

48. Vieth R, Bayley TA, Walfish PG, et al: Relevance of vitamin D metabolite concentrations in supporting the diagnosis of primary hyperparathyroidism, Surgery 110:1043–1046, 1991.

49. Silverberg SJ, Gartenberg F, Jacobs TP, et al: Longitudinal measurements of bone density and biochemical indices in untreated primary hyperparathyroidism, J Clin Endocrinol Metab 80:723–728, 1995.

50. Seibel MJ: Molecular Markers of bone metabolism in primary hyperparathyroidism. In Bilezikian JP, editor: The Parathyroids: Basic and Clinical Concepts, New York, 2001, Academic Press, pp 399–410.

51. Price PA, Parthemore JG, Deftos LJ: New biochemical marker for bone metabolism. Measurement by radioimmunoassay of bone Gla-protein in the plasma of normal subjects and patients with bone disease, J Clin Invest 66:878–883, 1980.

52. Deftos LJ, Parthemore JG, Price PA: Changes in plasma bone Gla-protein during treatment of bone disease, Calcif Tissue Int 34:121–124, 1982.

53. Ebeling PR, Peterson JM, Riggs BL: Utility of type 1 procollagen propeptide assays for assessing abnormalities in metabolic bone diseases, J Bone Miner Res 7:1243–1250, 1992.

54. Minisola S, Romagnoli E, Scarnecchia L, et al: Serum CITP in patients with primary hyperparathyroidism: Studies in basal conditions and after parathyroid surgery, Eur J Endocrinol 130:587–591, 1994.

55. Seibel MJ, Gartenberg F, Silverberg SJ, et al: Urinary hydroxypyridinium cross-links of collagen in primary hyperparathyroidism, J Clin Endocrinol Metab 74:481–486, 1992.

56. Seibel MJ, Woitge HW, Pecherstorfer M, et al: Serum immunoreactive bone sialoprotein as a new marker of bone turnover in metabolic and malignant bone disease, J Clin Endocrinol Metab 81:3289–3294, 1996.

57. Guo CY, Thomas WER, Al-Dehaimi AW, et al: Longitudinal changes in bone mineral density and bone turnover in women with primary hyperparathyroidism, J Clin Endocrinol Metab 81:3487–3491, 1996.

58. Tanaka Y, Funahashi H, Imai T, et al: Parathyroid function and bone metabolic markers in primary and secondary hyperparathyroidism, Semin Surg Oncol 13:125–133, 1997.

59. Greenfield EM, Shaw SM, Gornik SA, Banks MA: Adenyl cyclase and interleukin 6 are downstream effectors of PTH resulting in stimulation of bone resorption, J Clin Invest 96:1238–1244, 1995.

60. Pollock JH, Blaha MJ, Lavish SA, et al: In vivo demonstration that PTH and PTHrP stimulate expression by osteoblasts of IL-6 and LIF, J Bone Miner Res 11:754–759, 1996.

61. Grey A, Mitnick M, Shapses S, et al: Circulating levels of IL-6 and TNF-alpha are elevated in primary hyperparathyroidism and correlate with markers of bone resorption, J Clin Endocrinol Metab 81:3450–3454, 1996.

62. Insogna K, Mitnick M, Pascarella J, et al: Role of the interleukin-6 soluble receptor cytokine system in mediating increased skeletal sensitivity to parathyroid hormone in perimenopausal women, J Bone Miner Res 17:N108–N116, 2002.

63. Grey A, Mitnick MA, Shapses S, Ellison A, Gundberg C, Insogna K: Circulating levels of interleukin-6 and tumor necrosis factor-alpha are elevated in PHPT and correlate with markers of bone resorption: A clinical research center study, J Clin Endocrinol Metab 81:3450–3454, 1996.

64. Rosen CJ, Bing-you R, Silverberg SJ, Bilezikian JP: Enhancement of cancellous bone mass after parathyroidectomy is associated with changes in circulating insulin-like growth factor binding proteins, J Bone Miner Res 9(suppl I):C424, 1994.

65. Silverberg SJ, Shane E, DeLaCruz L, et al: Skeletal disease in primary hyperparathyroidism, J Bone Miner Res 4:283–291, 1989.

66. Bilezikian JP, Silverberg SJ, Shane E, et al: Characterization and evaluation of asymptomatic primary hyperparathyroidism, J Bone Miner Res 6(suppl I):585–589, 1991.

67. Dempster DW, Cosman F, Parisien M, et al: Anabolic actions of parathyroid hormone on bone, Endocr Rev 14:690–709, 1993.

68. Bilezikian JP, Rubin MR, Finkelstein J: Parathyroid hormone as an anabolic therapy for women and men, J Endocrinol Invest 28(Suppl 7):41–49, 2005.

69. Canalis E, Giustina A, Bilezikian JP: Mechanisms of anabolic therapies for osteoporosis, N Engl J Med 357:905–916, 2007.

70. National Institutes of Health: Consensus development conference statement on primary hyperparathyroidism, J Bone Miner Res 6:s9–s13, 1991.

71. Silverberg SJ, Locker FG, Bilezikian JP: Vertebral osteopenia: A new indication for surgery in primary hyperparathyroidism, J Clin Endocrinol Metab 81:4007–4012, 1996.

72. Parisien M, Silverberg SJ, Shane E, et al: The histomorphometry of bone in primary hyperparathyroidism: Preservation of cancellous bone structure, J Clin Endocrinol Metab 70:930–938, 1990.

73. Parfitt AM: Accelerated cortical bone loss: Primary and secondary hyperparathyroidism. In Uhthoff H, Stahl E, editors: Current Concepts of Bone Fragility, Berlin, 1986, Springer-Verlag, pp 279–285.

74. Parfitt AM: Surface specific bone remodeling in health and disease. In Kleerekoper M, editor: Clinical Disorders of Bone and Mineral Metabolism, New York, 1989, Mary Ann Liebert, pp 7–14.

75. Van Doorn L, Lips P, Netelenbos JC, Hackengt WHL: Bone histomorphometry and serum intact PTH (I-84) in hyperparathyroid patients, Calcif Tissue Int 44S:N36, 1989.

76. Parisien M, Cosman F, Mellish RWE, et al: Bone structure in postmenopausal hyperparathyroid, osteoporotic and normal women, J Bone Miner Res 10:1393–1399, 1995.

77. Dempster DW, Parisien M, Silverberg SJ, et al: On the mechanism of cancellous bone preservation in postmenopausal women with mild primary hyperparathyroidism, J Clin Endocrinol Metab 84:1562–1566, 1999.

78. Parisien M, Mellish RWE, Silverberg SJ, et al: Maintenance of cancellous bone connectivity in primary hyperparathyroidism: Trabecular and strut analysis, J Bone Miner Res 7:913–920, 1992.

79. Lindsay R, Nieves J, Formica C, et al: Randomised controlled study of effect of parathyroid hormone on vertebral-bone mass and fracture incidence among postmenopausal women on oestrogen with osteoporosis, Lancet 350:550–555, 1997.

80. Dempster DW, Cosman F, Kurland ES, et al: Effects of daily treatment with parathyroid hormone on bone microarchitecture and turnover in patients with osteoporosis: A paired biopsy study, J Bone Miner Res 16:1846–1853, 2001.

81. Neer RM, Arnaud CD, Zanchetta JR, et al: Effect of parathyroid hormone (1–34) on fractures and bone mineral density in postmenopausal women with osteoporosis, N Engl J Med 344:1434–1441, 2001.

82. Dempster DW, Müller R, Zhou H, et al: Preserved three-dimensional cancellous bone structure in mild primary hyperparathyroidism, Bone 41:19–24, 2007.

83. Roschger P, Dempster DW, Zhou H, et al: New observations on bone quality in mild primary hyperparathyroidism as determined by quantitative backscattered electron imaging, J Bone Miner Res 22:717–723, 2007.

84. Zoehrer R, Dempster DW, Bilezikian JP, et al: Bone quality determined by Fourier transform infrared imaging analysis in mild primary hyperparathyroidism, J Clin Endocrinol Metab 93:3484–3489, 2008.

85. Bilezikian JP: Bone strength in primary hyperparathyroidism, Osteoporos Int 14(Suppl 5):S113–S117, 2003.

86. Dauphine RT, Riggs BL, Scholz DA: Back pain and vertebral crush fractures: An unemphasized mode of presentation for primary hyperparathyroidism, Ann Intern Med 83:365–367, 1975.

87. Kochesberger G, Buckley NJ, Leight GS, et al: What is the clinical significance of bone loss in primary hyperparathyroidism, Arch Intern Med 147:1951–1953, 1987.

88. Wilson RJ, Rao S, Ellis B, et al: Mild asymptomatic primary hyperparathyroidism is not a risk factor for vertebral fractures, Ann Intern Med 109:959–962, 1988.

89. Larsson K, Ljunghall S, Krusemo UB, et al: The risk of hip fractures in patients with primary hyperparathyroidism: A population-based cohort study with a follow-up of 19 years, J Intern Med 234:585–593, 1993.

90. Kenny AM, MacGillivray DC, Pilbeam CC, et al: Fracture incidence in postmenopausal women with primary hyperparathyroidism, Surgery 118:109–114, 1995.

91. Khosla S, Melton LJ, Wermers RA, et al: Primary hyperparathyroidism and the risk of fracture: A population-based study, J Bone Miner Res 14:1700–1707, 1999.

92. Vignali E, Viccica C, Diacinti D, et al: Morphometric vertebral fractures in postmenopausal women with primary hyperparathyroidism, J Clin Endocrinol Metab April 28, 2009 [Epub ahead of print].

93. Parfitt AM: Parathyroid hormone and periosteal bone expansion, J Bone Min Res 17:1741–1743, 2002.

94. Mosekilde L: Primary hyperparathyroidism and the skeleton, Clin Endocrinol (Oxf) 69:1–19, 2008.

95. Silverberg SJ, Shane E, Jacobs TP, et al: Nephrolithiasis and bone involvement in primary hyperparathyroidism, 1985–1990, Am J Med 89:327–334, 1990.

96. Pak CYC, Ohata M, Lawrence EC, Snyder W: The hypercalciurias: Causes, parathyroid functions and diagnostic criteria, J Clin Invest 54:387–391, 1974.

97. Kaplan RA, Haussler MR, Deftos LJ, et al: The role of 1,25(OH)2D in the mediation of intestinal hyperabsorption of calcium in primary hyperparathyroidism and absorptive hypercalciuria, J Clin Invest 59:756–760, 1977.

98. Broadus AE, Horst RL, Lang R, et al: The importance of circulating 1,25(OH)2D in the pathogenesis of hypercalciuria and renal stone formation in primary hyperparathyroidism, N Engl J Med 302:421–426, 1980.

99. Pak CYC, Holt K: Nucleation and growth of brushite and calcium oxalate in urine of stone formers, Metabolism 25:665–673, 1976.

100. Pak CYC, Nicar MJ, Peterson R, et al: Lack of unique pathophysiologic background for nephrolithiasis in primary hyperparathyroidism, J Clin Endocrinol Metab 53:536–542, 1981.

101. Pak CYC: Effect of parathyroidectomy on crystallization of calcium salts in urine of patients with primary hyperparathyroidism, Invest Urol 17:146–151, 1979.

102. Berger AD, Wu W, Eisner BH, Cooperberg MR, Duh QY, Stoller ML: Patients with primary hyperparathyroidism-why do some form stones? J Urol 181:2141–2145, 2009.

103. Klugman VA, Favus M, Pak CYC: Nephrolithiasis in primary hyperparathyroidism. In Bilezikian JP, editor: The Parathyroids: Basic and Clinical Concepts, New York, 2001, Academic Press, pp 437–450.

104. Peacock M: Primary hyperparathyroidism and the kidney: Biochemical and clinical spectrum, J Bone Miner Res 17(Suppl 2): N87–N94, 2002.

105. Dent CE, Hartland BV, Hicks J, Sykes ED: Calcium intake in patients with primary hyperparathyroidism, Lancet 2:336–342, 1961.

106. Auerbach GD, Mallette LE, Patten BM, et al: Hyperparathyroidism: Recent studies, Ann Intern Med 79:566–581, 1973.

107. Patten BM, Bilezikian JP, Mallette LE, et al: The neuromuscular disease of hyperparathyroidism, Ann Intern Med 80:182–194, 1974.

108. Vicale CT: Diagnostic features of muscular syndrome resulting from hyperparathyroidism, osteomalacia owing to renal tubular acidosis and perhaps to related disorders of calcium metabolism, Trans Am Neurol Assoc 74:143–147, 1949.

109. Frame B, Heinze EG, Block MA, Manson AGA: Myopathy in primary hyperparathyroidism: Observations in three patients, Ann Intern Med 68:1022–1027, 1968.

110. Rollinson RD, Gilligan BS: Primary hyperparathyroidism presenting as a proximal myopathy, Aust N Z J Med 7:420–421, 1977.

111. Turken SA, Cafferty M, Silverberg SJ, et al: Neuromuscular involvement in mild, asymptomatic primary hyperparathyroidism, Am J Med 87:553–557, 1989.

112. Joborn C, Hetta J, Johansson H, et al: Psychiatric morbidity in primary hyperparathyroidism, World J Surg 2:476–481, 1998.

113. Brown GG, Preisman RC, Kleerekoper MD: Neurobehavioral symptoms in mild hyperparathyroidism:

related to hypercalcemia but not improved by parathyroidectomy, Henry Ford Med J 35:211–215, 1987.
114. Cogan MG, Covey CM, Arieff AI, Clark OH: Central nervous system manifestations of hyperparathyroidism, Am J Med 65:963–970, 1978.
115. Solomon BL, Schaaf M, Smallridge RC: Psychologic symptoms before and after parathyroid surgery, Am J Med 96:101–106, 1994.
116. Clark OH: Presidential address: Asymptomatic primary hyperparathyroidism: Is parathyroidectomy indicated? Surgery 116:947, 1994.
117. Pasieka JL, Parsons L: Prospective surgical outcome study of relief of symptoms following surgery in patients with primary hyperparathyroidism, World J Surg 22:513–519, 1998.
118. Burney RE, Jones KR, Christy B, Thompson NW: Health status improvement after surgical correction of primary hyperparathyroidism in patients with high and low preoperative calcium levels, Surgery 125: 608–614, 1999.
119. Silverberg SJ, Lewiecki EM, Mosekilde L, Peacock M, Rubin MR: Presentation of asymptomatic primary hyperparathyroidism: Proceedings of the Third International Workshop, J Clin Endocrinol Metab 94:351–365, 2009.
120. Caillard C, Sebag F, Mathonnet M, et al: Prospective evaluation of quality of life (SF-36v2) and nonspecific symptoms before and after cure of primary hyperparathyroidism (1-year follow-up), Surgery 141:153–159; discussion 159–160, 2007.
121. Dotzenrath CM, Kaetsch AK, Pfingsten H: Neuropsychiatric and cognitive changes after surgery for primary hyperparathyroidism, World J Surg 5:680–685, 2006.
122. Eigelberger MS, Cheah WK, Ituarte PH, et al: The NIH criteria for parathyroidectomy in asymptomatic primary hyperparathyroidism: Are they too limited? Ann Surg 239:528–535, 2004.
123. Roman SA, Sosa JA, Mayes L, et al: Parathyroidectomy improves neurocognitive deficits in patients with primary hyperparathyroidism, Surgery 138:1121–1128; discussion 1128–1129, 2005.
124. Walker MD, McMahon DJ, Inabnet WB, et al: Neuropsychological features of primary hyperparathyroidism: A prospective study, J Clin Endocrinol Metab 94:1951–1959, 2009.
125. Rao DS, Phillips ER, Divine GW, Talpos GB: Randomized, controlled clinical trial of surgery vs no surgery in mild asymptomatic primary hyperparathyroidism, J Clin Endocrinol Metab 89:5415–5422, 2004.
126. Bollerslev J, Jansson S, Mollerup CL, et al: Medical observation compared with parathyroidectomy, for asymptomatic primary hyperparathyroidism: A prospective, randomized trial, J Clin Endocrinol Metab 92:1687–1692, 2007.
127. Ambrogini E, Cetani F, Cianferotti L, et al: Surgery or no surgery for mild asymptomatic primary hyperparathyroidism: A prospective, randomized clinical trial, J Clin Endocrinol Metab 92:3114–3121, 2007.
128. Symons C, Fortune F, Greenbaum RA, Dandona P: Cardiac hypertrophy, hypertrophic cardiomyopathy and hyperparathyroidism—an association, Br Heart J 54:539–542, 1985.
129. Diamond TH, Kawalski DL, van der Merwe TL, Myburgh DP: Hypercalcemia due to parathyroid adenoma and hypertrophic cardiomyopathy, S Afr Med J 71:448–449, 1987.
130. Stefenelli T, Mayr H, Bergler-Klein J, et al: Primary hyperparathyroidism: Incidence of cardiac abnormalities and partial reversibility after successful parathyroidectomy, Am J Med 95:197–202, 1993.
131. Bradley EL III, Wells JO: Primary hyperparathyroidism and hypertension, Am Surg 49:569–570, 1983.
132. Dominiczak AF, Lyall F, Morton JJ: Blood pressure, left ventricular mass and intracellular calcium in primary hyperparathyroidism, Clin Sci 78:127–132, 1990.
133. Palmer M, Adami HO, Bergstrom R, et al: Mortality after surgery for primary hyperparathyroidism: A follow-up of 441 patients operated on from 1956 to 1979, Surgery 102:1–7, 1987.
134. Ronni-Sivula H: Causes of death in patients previously operated on for primary hyperparathyroidism, Ann Chir Gynaecol 74:13–18, 1985.
135. Hedback G, Tisell LE, Bengtsson BA, et al: Premature death in patients operated on for primary hyperparathyroidism, World J Surg 14:829–835; discussion 36, 1990.
136. Ljunghall S, Jakobsson S, Joborn C, Palmer M, Rastad J, Akerstrom G: Longitudinal studies of mild primary hyperparathyroidism, J Bone Miner Res 6(Suppl 2):S111–S116; discussion S21–24, 1991.
137. Hedback G, Oden A, Tisell LE: The influence of surgery on the risk of death in patients with primary hyperparathyroidism, World J Surg 15:399–405; discussion 6–7, 1991.
138. Soreide JA, van Heerden JA, Grant CS, Yau Lo C, Schleck C, Ilstrup DM: Survival after surgical treatment for primary hyperparathyroidism, Surgery 122:1117–1123, 1997.
139. Wermers RA, Khosla S, Atkinson EJ, et al: Survival after the diagnosis of hyperparathyroidism: a population-based study, Am J Med 104:115–122, 1998.
140. Nilsson IL, Yin L, Lundgren E, Rastad J, Ekbom A: Clinical presentation of primary hyperparathyroidism in Europe: nationwide cohort analysis on mortality from nonmalignant causes, J Bone Miner Res 17(Suppl 2):N68–74, 2002.
141. Hedbäck G, Odén A: Increased risk of death from primary hyperparathyroidism: an update, Eur J Clin Invest 28:271–276, 1998.
142. Vestergaard P, Mollerup CL, Frokjaer VG, et al: Cardiovascular events before and after surgery for primary hyperparathyroidism, World J Surg 27:216–222, 2003.
143. Nainby-Luxmoore JC, Langford HG, Nelson NC, et al: A case-comparison study of hypertension and hyperparathyroidism, J Clin Endocrinol Metab 55:303–306, 1982.
144. Ringe JD: Reversible hypertension in primary hyperparathyroidism: pre- and postoperative blood pressure in 75 cases, Klin Wochenschr 62:465–469, 1984.
145. Rapado A: Arterial hypertension and primary hyperparathyroidism. Incidence and follow-up after parathyroidectomy, Am J Nephrol 6(Suppl 1):49–50, 1986.
146. Lind L, Jacobsson S, Palmer M, Lithell H, Wengle B, Ljunghall S: Cardiovascular risk factors in primary hyperparathyroidism: a 15-year follow-up of operated and unoperated cases, J Intern Med 230:29–35, 1991.
147. Lind L, Skarfors E, Berglund L, et al: Serum calcium: A new, independent, prospective risk factor for myocardial infarction in middle-aged men followed for 18 years, J Clin Epidemiol 50:967–973, 1997.
148. Kamycheva E, Sundsfjord J, Jorde R: Serum parathyroid hormone levels predict coronary heart disease: The Tromso Study, Eur J Cardiovasc Prev Rehabil 11:69–74, 2004.
149. Roberts WC, Waller BF: Effect of chronic hypercalcemia on the heart. An analysis of 18 necropsy patients, Am J Med 71:371–384, 1981.
150. Nilsson IL, Aberg J, Rastad J, Lind L: Maintained normalization of cardiovascular dysfunction 5 years after parathyroidectomy in primary hyperparathyroidism, Surgery 137:632–638, 2005.
151. Stefenelli T, Mayr H, Bergler-Klein J, et al: Primary hyperparathyroidism: incidence of cardiac abnormalities and partial reversibility after successful parathyroidectomy, Am J Med 95:197–202, 1993.
152. Dalberg K, Brodin LA, Juhlin-Dannfelt A, Farnebo LO: Cardiac function in primary hyperparathyroidism before and after operation. An echocardiographic study, Eur J Surg 162:171–176, 1996.
153. Nuzzo V, Tauchmanova L, Fonderico F, et al: Increased intima-media thickness of the carotid artery wall, normal blood pressure profile and normal left ventricular mass in subjects with primary hyperparathyroidism, Eur J Endocrinol 147:453–459, 2002.
154. Nilsson IL, Aberg J, Rastad J, Lind L: Left ventricular systolic and diastolic function and exercise testing in primary hyperparathyroidism-effects of parathyroidectomy, Surgery 128:895–902, 2000.
155. Piovesan A, Molineri N, Casasso F, et al: Left ventricular hypertrophy in primary hyperparathyroidism. Effects of successful parathyroidectomy, Clin Endocrinol (Oxf) 50:321–328, 1999.
156. Almqvist EG, Bondeson AG, Bondeson L, et al: Cardiac dysfunction in mild primary hyperparathyroidism assessed by radionuclide angiography and echocardiography before and after parathyroidectomy, Surgery 132:1126–1132; discussion 32, 2002.
157. Stefenelli T, Abela C, Frank H, et al: Cardiac abnormalities in patients with primary hyperparathyroidism: implications for follow-up, J Clin Endocrinol Metab 82(1):106–112, 1997.
158. Lind L, Ridefelt P, Rastad J, Akerstrom G, Ljunghall S: Cytoplasmic calcium regulation and the electrocardiogram in patients with primary hyperparathyroidism, Clin Physiol 14(1):103–110, 1994.
159. Rosenqvist M, Nordenstrom J, Andersson M, Edhag OK: Cardiac conduction in patients with hypercalcaemia due to primary hyperparathyroidism, Clin Endocrinol (Oxf) 37(1):29–33, 1992.
160. Barletta G, De Feo ML, Del Bene R, et al: Cardiovascular effects of parathyroid hormone: a study in healthy subjects and normotensive patients with mild primary hyperparathyroidism, J Clin Endocrinol Metab 85(5):1815–1821, 2000.
161. Baykan M, Erem C, Erdogan T, et al: Assessment of left ventricular diastolic function and the Tei index by tissue Doppler imaging in patients with primary hyperparathyroidism, Clin Endocrinol (Oxf) 66(4):483–488, 2007.
162. Nilsson IL, Aberg J, Rastad J, Lind L: Endothelial vasodilatory dysfunction in primary hyperparathyroidism is reversed after parathyroidectomy, Surgery 126(6):1049–1055, 1999.
163. Kosch M, Hausberg M, Vormbrock K, Kisters K, Rahn KH, Barenbrock M: Studies on flow-mediated vasodilation and intima-media thickness of the brachial artery in patients with primary hyperparathyroidism, Am J Hypertens 13(7):759–764, 2000.
164. Lumachi F, Ermani M, Frego M, et al: Intima-media thickness measurement of the carotid artery in patients with primary hyperparathyroidism. A prospective case-control study and long-term follow-up, In Vivo 20(6B):887–890, 2006.
165. Fallo F, Camporese G, Capitelli E, Andreozzi GM, Mantero F, Lumachi F: Ultrasound evaluation of carotid artery in primary hyperparathyroidism, J Clin Endocrinol Metab 88(5):2096–2099, 2003.
166. Neunteufl T, Katzenschlager R, Abela C, et al: Impairment of endothelium-independent vasodilation in patients with hypercalcemia, Cardiovasc Res 40(2):396–401, 1998.
167. Kosch M, Hausberg M, Vormbrock K, et al: Impaired flow-mediated vasodilation of the brachial artery in patients with primary hyperparathyroidism improves after parathyroidectomy, Cardiovasc Res 47(4):813–818, 2000.
168. Baykan M, Erem C, Erdogan T, et al: Impairment of flow mediated vasodilatation of brachial artery in patients with primary hyperparathyroidism, Int J Cardiovasc Imaging 23(3):323–328, 2007.
169. Smith JC, Page MD, John R, et al: Augmentation of central arterial pressure in mild primary hyperparathyroidism, J Clin Endocrinol Metab 85(10):3515–3519, 2000.
170. Rubin MR, Maurer MS, McMahon DJ, Bilezikian JP, Silverberg SJ: Arterial stiffness in mild primary hyperparathyroidism, J Clin Endocrinol Metab 90(6):3326–3330, 2005.
171. Marx S: Multiple endocrine neoplasia type 1. In Bilezikian JP, editor: The Parathyroids, New York, 2001, Academic Press, pp 535–584.
172. Brandi ML, Gagel RF, Angeli A: Consensus Guidelines for diagnosis and therapy of MEN type 1 and type 2, J Clin Endocrinol Metab 86:5658–5671, 2001.
173. Khoo TK, Vege SS, Abu-Lebdeh HS, et al: Acute pancreatitis in primary hyperparathyroidism: a population-based study, J Clin Endocrinol Metab 94:2115–2118, 2009.
174. Harinarayan DV, Gupta N, Kochupillai N: Vitamin D status in primary hyperparathyroidism in India, Clin Endocrinol 43:351–358, 1995.
175. Meng XW, Xing XP, Liu SQ, Shan ZW: The diagnosis of primary hyperparathyroidism—analysis of 134 cases, Ann Acad Med Singapore 16:116–122, 1994.
176. Luong KVQ, Nguyen LTH: Coexisting hyperthyroidism and hyperparathyroidism with vitamin D deficient osteomalacia in a Vietnamese immigrant, Endocr Pract 2:250–254, 1996.
177. Lumb GA, Stanbury SW: Parathyroid function in vitamin D deficiency in primary hyperparathyroidism, Am J Med 54:833–839, 1974.
178. Feldman D: Vitamin D, parathyroid hormone and calcium: A complex regulatory network, Am J Med 107:637–639, 1999.
179. Silverberg SJ, Shane E, Jacobs TP, Siris E, Bilezikian JP: A 10-year prospective study of primary hyperparathy-

roidism with or without parathyroid surgery, New Engl J Med 341:1249–1255, 1999.

180. Rubin MR, Bilezikian JP, McMahon DJ, et al: The natural history of primary hyperparathyroidism with or without parathyroid surgery after 15 years, J Clin Endocrinol Metab 93:3462–3470, 2008.

181. Bilezikian JP, Potts JT Jr, El-Hajj Fuleihan G, et al: Summary statement from a workshop on asymptomatic primary hyperparathyroidism: a perspective for the 21st century, J Clin Endocrinol Metab 87:5353–5361, 2002.

182. Khan AA, Bilezikian JP, Potts JT Jr on behalf of the Third International Workshop on Asymptomatic Primary Hyperparathyroidism: the diagnosis and management of asymptomatic primary hyperparathyroidism revisited, J Clin Endocrinol Metab 94:333–334, 2009.

183. Bilezikian JP, Khan AA, Potts JT Jr on behalf of the Third International Workshop on Asymptomatic Primary Hyperthyroidism: guidelines for the management of asymptomatic primary hyperparathyroidism: Summary statement from the Third International Workshop, J Clin Endocrinol Metab 94:335–339, 2009.

184. Eastell R, Arnold A, Brandi ML, et al: Diagnosis of Asymptomatic Primary Hyperparathyroidism: proceedings of the Third International Workshop, J Clin Endocrinol Metab 94:340–350, 2009.

185. Silverberg SJ, Lewiecki EM, Mosekilde L, Peacock M, Rubin MR: Presentation of Asymptomatic Primary Hyperparathyroidism: proceedings of the Third International Workshop, J Clin Endocrinol Metab 94:351–365, 2009.

186. Udelsman R, Pasieka JL, Sturgeon C, Young JEM, Clark OH: Surgery for asymptomatic primary yyperparathyroidism: proceedings of the Third International Workshop, J Clin Endocrinol Metab 94:366–372, 2009.

187. Khan A, Grey A, Shoback D: Medical management of asymptomatic primary hyperparathyroidism: proceedings of the Third International Workshop, J Clin Endocrinol Metab 94:373–381, 2009.

188. Civelek A, Ozalp E, Donovan P, Udelsman R: Prospective evaluation of delayed technetium-99M sestamibi SPECT scintigraphy for preoperative localization of primary hyperparathyroidism, Surgery 131:149–157, 2002.

189. Van Husen R, Kim LT: Accuracy of surgeon-performed ultrasound in parathyroid localization, World J Surg 1122–1126, 2004.

190. Mortenson ME, Evans DB, Hunter GJ, et al: Parathyroid exploration in the reoperative neck: improved preoperative localization with 4D-computer tomography, J Am Coll Surg 206:888–895, 2008.

191. Maser C, Donovan P, Satos F, et al: Sonographically guided fine needle aspiration with rapid parathyroid hormone assay, Ann Surg Oncol 13:1690–1695, 2006.

192. Udelsman R, Donovan PI: Remedial parathyroid surgery: changing trends in 130 consecutive cases, Ann Surg 244:471–479, 2006.

193. Clark OH: How should patients with primary hyperparathyroidism be treated? J Clin Endocrinol Metab 88:3011–3014, 2003.

194. Udelsman R: Six hundred fifty-six consecutive explorations for primary hyperparathyroidism, Ann Surgery 235(5):665–672, 2002.

195. Irvin CL, Solorzano CC, Carneiro DM: Quick intraoperative parathyroid hormone assay: Surgical adjunct to allow limited parathyroidectomy, improved success rate and predict outcome, World J Surg 28:1287–1292, 2004.

196. Udelsman R, Donovan POI, Sokoll LT: One hundred consecutive minimally invasive parathyroid explorations, Ann Surg 232:331–339, 2000.

197. Miccoli P, Berti P, Materazzi G, Ambrosini CE, Fregoli L, Donatini G: Endoscopic bilateral neck exploration versus quick intraoperative parathormone assay (qPTHa) during endoscopic parathyroidectomy: A prospective randomized trial, Surg Endosc 22:398–400, 2008.

198. Henry JF, Sebag F, Tamagnini P, Forman C, Silaghi H: Endoscopic parathyroid surgery: results of 365 consecutive procedures, World J Surg 28:1219–1223, 2004.

199. Westerdahl J, Bergenfelz A: Unilateral versus bilateral neck exploration for primary hyperparathyroidism:

200. Russell CF, Dolan SJ, Laird JD: Randomized clinical trial comparing scan-directed unilateral versus bilateral cervical exploration for primary hyperparathyroidism due to solitary adenoma, Br J Surg 93(4):418–421, 2006.

201. Silverberg SJ, Gartenberg F, Jacobs TP, et al: Increased bone mineral density following parathyroidectomy in primary hyperparathyroidism, J Clin Endocrinol Metab 80:729–734, 1995.

202. Silverberg SJ, Shane E, Jacobs TP, et al: Primary hyperparathyroidism: 10-year course with or without parathyroid surgery, N Engl J Med 341:1249–1255, 1999.

203. Kulak CAM, Bandeira C, Voss D, et al: Marked improvement in bone mass after parathyroidectomy in osteitis fibrosa cystica, J Clin Endocrinol Metab 83:732–735, 1998.

204. Tritos NA, Hartzband P: Rapid improvement of osteoporosis following parathyroidectomy in a premenopausal woman with acute primary hyperparathyroidism, Arch Intern Med 139:1498, 1999.

205. DiGregorio S: Hiperparatiroidismo primario: Dramatico incremento de la masa ostea post paratiroidectomia, Diagn Osteol 1:11–15, 1999.

206. Dawson-Hughes B, Stern DT, Shipp CC, Rasmussen HM: Effect of lowering dietary calcium intake on fractional whole body calcium retention, J Clin Endocrinol Metab 67:62–68, 1998.

207. Barger-Lux MJ, Heaney RP: Effects of calcium restriction on metabolic characteristics of premenopausal women, J Clin Endocrinol Metab 76:103–107, 1993.

208. Calvo MS, Kumar R, Heath H: Persistently elevated parathyroid hormone secretion and action in young women after four weeks of ingesting high phosphorus, low calcium diets, J Clin Endocrinol Metab 70:1334–1340, 1990.

209. Insogna KL, Mitnick ME, Stewart AF, et al: Sensitivity of the parathyroid hormone-1, 25-dihydroxyvitamin D axis to variations in calcium intake in patients with primary hyperparathyroidism, N Engl J Med 313:1126–1130, 1985.

210. Locker FG, Silverberg SJ, Bilezikian JP: Optimal dietary calcium intake in primary hyperparathyroidism, Am J Med 102:543–550, 1997.

211. Purnell DC, Scholz DA, Smith LM, et al: Treatment of primary hyperparathyroidism, Am J Med 56:800–809, 1984.

212. Broadus AE, Magee JS, Mallette LE, et al: A detailed evaluation of oral phosphate therapy in selected patients with primary hyperparathyroidism, J Clin Endocrinol Metab 56:953–961, 1983.

213. Kaplan RA, Geho WB, Poindexter C, et al: Metabolic effects of diphosphonate in primary hyperparathyroidism, J Clin Pharmacol 17:410–419, 1977.

214. Shane E, Baquiran DC, Bilezikian JP: Effects of dichloromethylene diphosphonate on serum and urinary calcium in primary hyperparathyroidism, Ann Intern Med 95:23–27, 1981.

215. Rossini M, Gatti D, Isaia G, Sartori L, Braga V, Adami S: Effects of oral alendronate in elderly patients with osteoporosis and mild primary hyperparathyroidism, J Bone Miner Res 16:113–119, 2001.

216. Hassani S, Braunstein GD, Seibel MJ, et al: Alendronate therapy of primary hyperparathyroidism, Endocrinologist 11:459–464, 2001.

217. Chow CC, Chan WB, Li JKY, et al: Oral alendronate increases bone mineral density in postmenopausal women with primary hyperparathyroidism, J Clin Endocrinol Metab 88:581–587, 2003.

218. Parker CR, Blackwell PJ, Fairbairn KJ, Hosking DJ: Hyperparathyroid-related osteoporosis: A 2-year study, J Clin Endocrinol Metab 87:4482–4489, 2002.

219. Kahn AA, Bilezikian JP, Kung AW, et al: Alendronate in primary hyperparathyroidism: A double-blind, randomized, placebo-controlled trial, J Clin Endocrinol Metab 89:3319–3325, 2004.

220. Gallagher JC, Nordin BEC: Treatment with oestrogens of primary hyperparathyroidism in post-menopausal women, Lancet 1:503–507, 1972.

221. Marcus R, Madvig P, Crim M, et al: Conjugated estrogens in the treatment of postmenopausal women with hyperparathyroidism, Ann Intern Med 100:633–640, 1984.

222. Selby PL, Peacock M: Ethinyl estradiol and norethindrone in the treatment of primary hyperparathyroidism

in postmenopausal women, N Engl J Med 314:1481–1485, 1986.

223. Grey AB, Stapleton JP, Evans MC, et al: Effect of hormone replacement therapy on BMD in post-menopausal women with primary hyperparathyroidism, Ann Intern Med 125:360–368, 1996.

224. Gallagher JC, Wilkinson R: The effect of ethinyl estradiol on calcium and phosphorus metabolism of postmenopausal women with primary hyperparathyroidism, Clin Sci Mol Med 45:785–802, 1973.

225. Rubin MA, Lee KH, McMahon DJ, Silverberg SJ: Raloxifene lowers serum calcium and markers of bone turnover in postmenopausal women with primary hyperparathyroidism, J Clin Endocrinol Metab 88:1174–1178, 2003.

226. Nemeth EF, Scarpa A: Rapid mobilization of cellular calcium in bovine parathyroid cells evoked by extracellular divalent cations. Evidence for a cell surface calcium receptor, J Biol Chem 262:5188–5196, 1987.

227. Brown EM, Gamba G, Riccardi D, et al: Cloning and characterization of an extracellular Ca^2-sensing receptor from bovine parathyroid, Nature 366:575–580, 1993.

228. Brown EM, Pollak M, Seidman CE: Calcium ion sensing cell surface receptors, N Engl J Med 333:234–240, 1995.

229. Fox J, Hadfield S, Petty BA, Nemeth EF: A first generation calcimimetic compound (NPS R-568) that acts on the parathyroid cell calcium receptor: A novel therapeutic approach for hyperparathyroidism, J Bone Miner Res 8:S181, 1993.

230. Heath H III, Sanguinetti EL, Oglseby S, Marriott TB: Inhibition of human parathyroid hormone secretion in vivo by NPS R-568, a calcimimetic drug that targets the parathyroid cell surface calcium receptor, Bone 16:85S, 1995.

231. Silverberg SJ, Marriott TB, Bone HG III, et al: Short term inhibition of parathyroid hormone secretion by a calcium receptor agonist in primary hyperparathyroidism, N Engl J Med 307:1506–1510, 1997.

232. Shoback DM, Bilezikian JP, Turner SA, McCary LC, Guo MD, Peacock M: The calcimimetic AMG 073 normalizes serum calcium in patients with primary hyperparathyroidism, J Clin Endocrinol Metab 88:5644–5649, 2003.

233. Peacock M, Bilezikian JP, Klassen PS, Guo MD, Turner SA, Shoback DM: Cinacalcet hydrochloride maintains long-term normocalcemia in patients with primary hyperparathyroidism, J Clin Endocrinol Metab 90:135–141, 2005.

234. Wüthrich RP, Martin D, Bilezikian JP: The role of calcimimetics in the treatment of hyperparathyroidism, Eur J Clin Invest 37:915–922, 2007.

235. Marcocci C, Chanson P, Shoback D, et al: Cinacalcet reduces serum calcium concentrations in patients with intractable primary hyperparathyroidism, J Clin Endocrinol Metab 2009 June 2 [Epub ahead of print]

236. Silverberg SJ, Rubin MR, Faiman C, et al: Cinacalcet HCl reduces the serum calcium concentration in inoperable parathyroid carcinoma, J Clin Endocrinol Metab 92:3803–3808, 2007.

237. Marx SJ, Fraser D, Rapoport A: Familial hypocalciuric hypercalcemia: Mild expression of the gene in heterozygotes and severe expression in homozygotes, Am J Med 78:15–22, 1985.

238. Kristoffersson A, Dahlgren S, Lithner F, Jarhult J: Primary hyperparathyroidism in pregnancy, Surgery 97:326–330, 1985.

239. Lowe DK, Orwoll ES, McClung MR, et al: Hyperparathyroidism and pregnancy, Am J Surg 145:611–619, 1983.

240. Fitzpatrick LA, Bilezikian JP: Acute primary hyperparathyroidism, Am J Med 82:275–282, 1987.

241. Bayat-Mokhtari F, Palmieri GMA, Moinuddin M, et al: Parathyroid storm, Arch Intern Med 140:1092–1095, 1980.

242. Fitzpatrick LA: Acute primary hyperparathyroidism. In Bilezikian JP, editor: The Parathyroids: Basic and Clinical Concepts, New York, 2001, Academic Press, pp 527–534.

243. Shane E, Bilezikian JP: Parathyroid carcinoma: A review of 62 patients, Endocr Rev 3:218–226, 1982.

244. Marcocci C, Cetani F, Rubin MR, Silverberg SJ, Pinchera A, Bilezikian JP: Parathyroid carcinoma, J Bone Min Res 23:1869–1880, 2008.

245. Shane E: Parathyroid carcinoma, J Clin Endocrinol Metab 86:485–493, 2001.
246. LiVolsi V: Morphology of the parathyroid glands. In Becker KL, editor: Principles and Practice of Endocrinology and Metabolism, ed 3, Philadelphia, 2000, Lippincott Williams & Wilkins.
247. Streeten EA, Weinstein LS, Norton JA, et al: Studies in a kindred with parathyroid carcinoma, J Clin Endocrinol Metab 75:362–366, 1992.
248. Wassif WS, Moniz CF, Friedman E, et al: Familial isolated hyperparathyroidism: a distinct genetic entity with an increased risk of parathyroid cancer, J Clin Endocrinol Metab 77:1485–1489, 1993.
249. Yoshimoto K, Endo H, Tsuyuguchi M, et al: Itakura Familial isolated primary hyperparathyroidism with parathyroid carcinomas: clinical and molecular features, Clin Endocrinol (Oxf) 48:67–72, 1998.
250. Marx SJ, Simonds WF, Agarwal SK, et al: Hyperparathyroidism in hereditary syndromes: special expressions and special managements, J Bone Miner Res 17(Suppl 2):N37–43, 2002.
251. Chen JD, Morrison C, Zhang C, Kahnoski K, Carpten JD, Teh BT: Hyperparathyroidism-jaw tumour syndrome, J Intern Med 253:634–642, 2003.
252. Mallette LE, Malini S, Rappaport MP, Kirkland JL: Familial cystic parathyroid adenomatosis, Ann Intern Med 107:54–60, 1987.
253. Carpten JD, Robbins CM, Villablanca A, et al: HRPT2, encoding parafibromin, is mutated in hyperparathyroidism-jaw tumors syndrome, Nat Genet 32:676–680, 2002.
254. Simonds WF, James-Newton LA, Agarwal SK, et al: Familial isolated hyperparathyroidism: clinical and genetic characteristics of 36 kindreds, Medicine (Baltimore) 81:1–26, 2002.
255. Dionisi S, Minisola S, Pepe J, et al: Concurrent parathyroid adenomas and carcinoma in the setting of multiple endocrine neoplasia type 1: presentation as hypercalcemic crisis, Mayo Clin Proc 77:866–869, 2002.
256. Agha A, Carpenter R, Bhattacharya S, Edmonson SJ, Carlsen E, Monson JP: Parathyroid carcinoma in multiple endocrine neoplasia type 1 (MEN1) syndrome: Two case reports of an unrecognized entity, J Endocrinol Invest 30:145–149, 2007.
257. Haven CJ, van Puijenbroek M, Tan MH, et al: Identification of MEN1 and HRPT2 somatic mutations in paraffin-embedded (sporadic) parathyroid carcinomas, Clin Endocrinol (Oxf) 67:370–376, 2007.
258. Jenkins PJ, Satta MA, Simmgen M, et al: Metastatic parathyroid carcinoma in the MEN2A syndrome, Clin Endocrinol (Oxf) 47:747–751, 1997.
259. Dotzenrath C, Teh BT, Farnebo F, et al: Allelic loss of the retinoblastoma tumor suppressor gene: A marker for aggressive parathyroid tumors? J Clin Endocrinol Metab 81:3194, 1996.
260. Shattuck TM, Valimaki S, Abara T, et al: Somatic and germ-line mutations of the HRPT2 gene in sporadic parathyroid carcinoma, N Eng J Med 349:1722–1929, 2003.
261. Weinstein LS, Simonds WF: HRPT2, a marker of parathyroid cancer, N Eng J Med 349:1691–1692, 2003.
262. Carpten JD, Robbins CM, Villablanca A, et al: HRPT2, encoding parafibromin is mutated in hyperparathyroidism-jw tumor sydrome, Nat Genet 32:676–680, 2002.
263. Marx SJ, Simonds WF, Agarwal SK, et al: Hyperparathyroidism in hereditary syndromes: special expressions and special managements, J Bone Miner Res 17(Suppl 2):N37–N43, 2002.
264. Simonds WF, James-Newton LA, Agarwal SK, et al: Familial isolated hyperparathyroidism: clinical and genetic characteristics of 36 kindreds, Medicine (Baltimore) 81:1–26, 2002.
265. Bradwell AR, Harvey TC: Control of hypercalcemia of parathyroid carcinoma by immunisation, Lancet 353:370–373, 1999.
266. Betea D, Bradwell AR, Harvey TC, et al: Hormonal and biochemical normalization and tumor shrinkage induced by anti-parathyroid hormone immunotherapy in a patient with metastatic parathyroid carcinoma, J Clin Endocrinol Metab 89:3413–3420, 2004.
267. Collins MT, Skarulis MC, Bilezikian JP, et al: Treatment of hypercalcemia secondary to parathyroid carcinoma with a novel calcimimetic agent, J Clin Endocrinol Metab 83:1083–1088, 1998.
268. Block GA, Martin KJ, deFrancisco ALM, et al: Cinacalcet for secondary hyperparathyroidism in patients receiving hemodialysis, N Engl J Med 350:1516–1525, 2004.

Chapter 8

MALIGNANCY-ASSOCIATED HYPERCALCEMIA AND MEDICAL MANAGEMENT

MARA J. HORWITZ and ANDREW F. STEWART

The History of Malignancy-Associated Hypercalcemia

Malignancy is the second most common cause of hypercalcemia in the general population and by far the most common cause among inpatients. Hypercalcemia was first reported in patients with cancer in the 1920s.[1] The first large series of patients with malignancy-associated hypercalcemia (MAHC) was reported in 1936 by Gutman and colleagues.[2] This group of patients primarily had multiple myeloma and breast cancer; skeletal invasion by tumor was extensive radiologically. The authors inferred that the cause of hypercalcemia in these patients was skeletal invasion by the malignancy.

This mechanism was assumed to be operative in all instances of MAHC until 1941, when Albright[3] described a hypercalcemic patient with renal carcinoma and a solitary skeletal metastasis. He reasoned that a single bone metastasis was inadequate to cause hypercalcemia. Furthermore, he noted that the patient was hypophosphatemic, not hyperphosphatemic, as would be expected from the combination of rapid dissolution of skeletal phosphate-containing hydroxyapatite and parathyroid suppression induced by the hypercalcemia. Albright suggested that the hypercalcemia in this patient was etiologically distinct from that in the previously described patients with breast cancer and multiple myeloma and proposed that hypercalcemia resulted from secretion by the renal carcinoma of parathyroid hormone (PTH) or another humoral factor that resembled PTH. Support for Albright's humoral hypothesis was presented in 1956, when two groups reported that surgical or other eradication of tumor reversed hypercalcemia in patients with carcinoma unaccompanied by skeletal involvement.[4,5] After additional reports supporting the "humoral hypothesis," Lafferty[6] in 1966 reviewed 50 patients with humorally mediated hypercalcemia. By definition, these patients had no detectable skeletal metastases on radiographs or manifested disappearance of the hypercalcemia with tumor ablation or both. Histologically, the patients proved to have predominantly squamous (particularly lung), renal, bladder, and gynecologic malignancies.

Thus, by the end of the 1960s, two broad mechanistic categories of MAHC had clearly been demonstrated.[7-9] In one group of patients, hypercalcemia develops through skeletal invasion and destruction by tumor, a condition we have referred to as local osteolytic hypercalcemia (LOH)[2,7-10] (Table 8-1). In the other group of patients, hypercalcemia develops predominantly through a humoral mechanism, a condition we have referred to as humoral hypercalcemia of malignancy (HHM).[11-13] Subsequently, two additional mechanistic subtypes were well described. These include authentic ectopic hyperparathyroidism and $1,25(OH)_2$-vitamin D–induced hypercalcemia in patients with lymphomas. These four types are summarized in Table 8-1 and are discussed in detail later.

Clinical Features of Malignancy-Associated Hypercalcemia

Hypercalcemia occurring in a patient with cancer indicates that the overall prognosis for the patient in question is very poor. For example, in a study by Ralson and collaborators,[14] the onset

Table 8-1. Tumor Histology in Malignancy-Associated Hypercalcemia

Tumors COMMONLY Associated With Local Osteolytic Hypercalcemia

Multiple myeloma
Lymphoma
Breast cancer

Tumors COMMONLY Associated With Humoral Hypercalcemia of Malignancy

Squamous carcinoma (lung, head and neck, esophagus, cervix, vulva, skin)
Renal carcinoma
Bladder carcinoma
Ovarian carcinoma
Breast carcinoma
HTLV-1 lymphoma
Endocrine tumors (pheochromocytoma, adrenocortical carcinoma, islet carcinoma, carcinoids)

Tumors Associated With 1,25(OH)$_2$D Overproduction

Lymphoma*
Ovarian dysgerminoma

Tumors Associated With Authentic Ectopic PTH Secretion

Common Tumors Rarely Associated With Hypercalcemia

Colon adenocarcinoma
Stomach adenocarcinoma
Prostate adenocarcinoma
Small cell carcinoma
Thyroid carcinoma
CNS malignancies

CNS, Central nervous system; HTLV-1, human T cell lymphoma/leukemia virus 1; PTH, parathyroid hormone.
*Has been reported with many different histologic types of lymphoma.

of hypercalcemia was associated with a 30-day survival rate of only 50%.

The clinical manifestations of the hypercalcemia that accompanies cancer are no different from those that accompany other hypercalcemic disorders. Polyuria, polydipsia, dehydration, renal compromise, constipation, and varying degrees of neurologic dysfunction ranging from lethargy or confusion to coma are common. The electrocardiogram may show shortening of the QTc interval.[15,16] The correlation between the degree of hypercalcemia and a given patient's neurologic function is poor. Other factors (such as the rate of development of hypercalcemia, the presence of underlying central nervous system dysfunction, the presence of other metabolic disorders, and the use of a variety of medications) may profoundly influence the effects of a given degree of hypercalcemia. Patients with skeletal metastases may report skeletal pain or pathologic fractures or both. Sometimes the onset of hypercalcemia can be ascribed to factors other than tumor progression (e.g., recent immobilization, addition of a thiazide diuretic, prerenal or renal azotemia leading to inadequate renal calcium clearance, hypophosphatemia resulting from inadequate oral intake, gastrointestinal fluid losses, medications, parenteral calcium administration in the form of hyperalimentation). These events should be specifically sought because their correction may reverse a given patient's hypercalcemia.

No study has precisely defined the relation of tumor size to the presence or absence of hypercalcemia. Nonetheless, to the extent that tumor size has been studied, it would seem clear that small, occult tumors rarely cause MAHC.[2-12,17,18] A corollary of this statement is that when a patient has MAHC, the tumor that is responsible usually is readily apparent after only a modestly rigorous search; conversely, if a tumor has not been found after 2 or 3 days of evaluation in a hospitalized, hypercalcemic patient, it is unlikely that a malignancy is the cause of the hypercalcemia.

Thus, a careful history and physical examination with attention to the skin, oropharynx, esophagus, pulmonary system, liver, genitourinary tract, hematopoietic system, and breasts and a limited laboratory and radiologic investigation focused on the hematologic system, esophagus, kidneys, bladder, gynecologic structures, and skeleton will almost invariably lead to rapid definition of the responsible tumor. Occasionally, retroperitoneal tumors (renal carcinomas, lymphomas, pancreatic tumors) may be difficult to demonstrate. Finally, endocrine tumors (e.g., islet carcinomas, pheochromocytomas, ovarian carcinoids) may lead to hypercalcemia and yet may be small and difficult or impossible to localize.

In approaching the evaluation and treatment of a patient with hypercalcemia and cancer, it is important to bear in mind that hypercalcemia may occur in patients with cancer for all the same reasons that it occurs in patients without cancer. For example, in a series of 133 patients with cancer and hypercalcemia encountered between 1978 and 1984, we identified 8 patients with cancer in whom hypercalcemia ultimately proved to result not from cancer but from coexisting primary hyperparathyroidism.[12] Similarly, we have observed hypercalcemia resulting from tuberculosis, sarcoidosis, immobilization, vitamin D intoxication, hyperthyroidism, thiazide use, Addison's disease, and other causes in patients initially perceived as having MAHC. Thus, the entire differential diagnosis of hypercalcemia should be entertained in every patient in whom hypercalcemia is identified, even if it appears at the outset that cancer will prove to be the ultimate cause. This approach is particularly important for the following reasons: (1) in contrast to the poor ultimate prognosis in MAHC, most causes of hypercalcemia other than cancer are readily treatable; (2) identifying a treatable, nonmalignant cause of hypercalcemia in a patient with cancer may dramatically change the overall perception of a case by the patient's physicians; and (3) treatment approaches may vary.

It is important to say a word about the tumor histologies associated with hypercalcemia (see Table 8-1). Virtually all tumor types have been reported to cause hypercalcemia, but, as will be described in the sections on LOH and HHM, certain tumor types are particularly common causes of hypercalcemia. Conversely, certain other common tumor types (prostate, colon, oat cell, thyroid, and gastric carcinomas, and primary central nervous system malignancies are examples) almost never cause hypercalcemia[2-12,17,18] (see Table 8-1). When these tumors are identified in a patient with hypercalcemia, other tumors or other nonmalignant causes of hypercalcemia should be sought.

Major advances have been made over the past three decades in our understanding of the precise pathophysiologic mechanisms responsible for the various subtypes of MAHC. The sections that follow are divided into four subcategories: LOH, HHM, authentic ectopic hyperparathyroidism, and unusual causes of HHM.

Local Osteolytic Hypercalcemia

Hypercalcemia can result from direct skeletal involvement by a primary hematologic neoplasm or by skeletal metastases from a nonhematologic neoplasm. Patients with LOH account for approximately 20% of patients in a series of patients with MAHC.[2-12,17-22] The malignancies that most commonly lead to LOH are multiple myeloma, leukemia, lymphoma, and breast cancer[2-12,17-22] (see Table 8-1). This list is not exhaustive, for many other tumor types occasionally have been reported to cause hypercalcemia through skeletal metastasis.[2-12,17-22]

Hypercalcemia that occurs in patients with multiple myeloma and breast cancer was initially attributed to the direct physical destruction of bone by malignant cells. This concept is now seen as naive, for it is clear that simply having malignant tumor cells in the bone marrow compartment is insufficient to cause hypercalcemia. First, bone resorption surrounding malignant cells in bone marrow is always accomplished by osteoclasts, not tumor cells, indicating that osteoclast recruitment and activation by tumors are required. Second, although some tumor metastases in bone are commonly associated with LOH (breast cancer and myeloma are examples), certain other tumor types typically associated with destructive skeletal metastases (e.g., small cell and prostate carcinomas)[23,24] only rarely cause hypercalcemia. Moreover, one large study reported an inverse correlation between the number of bone metastases and the serum calcium concentration in a series of hypercalcemic patients with breast cancer.[25] Thus, the pathophysiology of the hypercalcemia in LOH is based on paracrine factors or cytokines that are capable of activating osteoclasts, and these are produced by only certain types of malignant cells in the bone marrow. It is these factors that produce hypercalcemia in LOH.

A search for these so-called osteoclast-activating factors, or OAFs, began in the 1970s with reports by Mundy and others[26,27] that short-term cultures of bone marrow aspirates from patients with myeloma or lymphoma contain a bone-resorbing factor or family of bone-resorbing factors that are capable of stimulating osteoclasts in vitro. Despite work over the past four decades, the precise array of cytokines that compose OAFs remains incompletely resolved. At the time of this writing, the most attractive candidates include receptor activator of nuclear factor (NF)-κB ligand (RANK-L), macrophage inflammatory protein-1α (MIP-1α), interleukin-1α, interleukin-6, parathyroid hormone–related protein (PTHrP, see later), and tumor necrosis factor-α (TNF-α).[28-31] In patients with lymphoma, studies by Dewhirst and others[30] have suggested a role for interleukin-1. Thus, it seems likely that the generic term, OAF, actually constitutes a group of such factors that can mediate hypercalcemia in a tumor-specific fashion.

The discovery and elucidation of the RANK-RANK-L system in the late 1990s provided a particularly exciting advance and recently has been reviewed in detail as it relates to bone metastasis and myeloma.[31,32] In brief, osteoclast precursors (macrophages) and mature osteoclasts express the receptor, RANK. Osteoblasts and marrow stromal cells normally express the ligand (RANK-L) and upregulate RANK-L in response to agents that recruit osteoclast precursors and induce them to form osteoclasts and initiate and enhance bone resorption. Thus, for example, PTH and PTHrP act via the PTH receptor on marrow stromal cells and osteoblasts and induce them to produce more RANK-L. This then stimulates osteoclast precursors to form more osteoclasts and induces mature osteoclasts to become more active as well. It is interesting to note that osteoblasts and marrow stromal cells also produce a soluble or secreted decoy RANK receptor called osteoprotegerin (OPG). OPG serves to balance the bone resorption induced by the RANK-RANK-L pathway. Increases in OPG production by marrow stromal cells and osteoblasts can completely prevent osteoclast recruitment and bone resorption. Thus, osteoclast number and activity ultimately depend on the balance between OPG and RANK-L in the marrow microenvironment. This, in turn, depends on how much OPG and RANK-L are produced by marrow stromal cells and osteoblasts, and, in the case of skeletal metastases or myeloma cells, whether they activate or serve as surrogates for the native RANK-L system. To be more specific, credible evidence now suggests that myeloma cells themselves may produce large amounts of RANK-L, and, through direct interaction with RANK on osteoclast precursors, may activate osteoclast recruitment and further activate bone resorption, leading to the massive osteolysis characteristic of multiple myeloma.[28,31] These observations have not only pathophysiologic implications but potentially therapeutic ones as well, as is discussed later.

Another characteristic feature of myeloma bone disease is that bone formation by osteoblasts is absent. Thus, the skeletal demineralization of myeloma can be seen as being due in part to dramatic increases in bone resorption, as described earlier, acting in concert with dramatic reductions in osteoblastic bone formation. This marked uncoupling of bone formation from resorption is not well understood, but it is believed that cytokines or other paracrine factors produced by malignant plasma cells may be responsible for this suppression of bone formation in myeloma. In support of this possibility, Tian and colleagues[33] recently reported that myeloma cells greatly overproduce DKK-1, an antagonist of the wnt signaling pathway that is known to be critical for osteoblast function. More recently, the Roodman group[34] has reported that interleukin-3 (IL-3) secreted by malignant plasma cells can also act to suppress bone formation. DKK and IL-3 findings also suggest novel therapeutic strategies for inducing bone formation in patients with myeloma. It is possible that the marked infiltration of malignant plasma cells characteristic of myeloma replaces marrow stromal cells that might otherwise serve as a source of osteoblast precursors, and this lack of osteoblast precursors thus results in inadequate bone formation.

Progress also has been made in our understanding of the cellular mechanisms responsible for bone resorption by skeletal metastasis in breast cancer. An increasing number of reports suggest a role for PTHrP as a local or intraskeletal mediator of osteoclast activation in women with breast cancer bone metastases.[29,35-38] Immunohistochemical analysis by Southby and associates[37] demonstrated that 12 (92%) of 13 breast cancer skeletal metastases contained PTHrP, whereas only 3 (17%) of 18 nonskeletal breast cancer metastases contained PTHrP. These findings have been confirmed at the in situ hybridization level for PTHrP messenger RNA (mRNA) in breast cancers metastatic to bone or soft tissue.[38] In addition to suggesting a role for PTHrP as a local bone-resorbing factor, these studies suggest that PTHrP somehow may serve to favor metastasis to the skeleton, as well as tumor growth, in patients with breast cancer. Guise and collaborators[36] showed this concept to be true: In human breast cancer cell lines bioengineered to express PTHrP at high or low levels, those producing large quantities of PTHrP were more likely to lead to bone metastasis than were those expressing low levels. Moreover, after the development of bone metastases, a local skeletal vicious cycle appeared to develop in which PTHrP induces osteoclastic bone resorption, which in turn leads to the local release of TGF-β from resorbed bone. This locally released TGF-β further induces tumor-derived PTHrP production and accelerated bone resorption.[36]

Hypercalcemia will develop in approximately one third of women with breast cancer and bone metastases treated with estrogen or antiestrogens such as tamoxifen.[39,40] The mechanisms responsible for this "estrogen flare" in breast cancer remain undefined. Frequently, the hypercalcemia will resolve spontaneously if hypercalcemia can be controlled over the short term and endocrine therapy can be continued.[40] It has been suggested that the tamoxifen-induced hypercalcemic flare predicts a favorable tumor response. Valentin-Opran and colleagues[41] suggested, after work with cultured breast cancer cell lines, that estrogen exposure enhances the production of undefined bone-resorbing factors.

From a clinical and biochemical standpoint, LOH is associated with accelerated bone resorption[11-13,35,42] (Fig. 8-1), hypercalcemia, and appropriate suppression of PTH[11,12] (Fig. 8-2), nephrogenous cyclic adenosine monophosphate (cAMP) (Fig. 8-3), and 1,25(OH)$_2$-vitamin D (1,25[OH]$_2$D) (Fig. 8-4).[11,12] PTHrP is not detectable in the circulation[19-22] (Fig. 8-5). As a

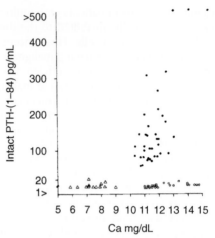

FIGURE 8-2. Immunoreactive parathyroid hormone in the serum of patients with primary hyperparathyroidism *(solid circles)*, hypoparathyroidism *(triangles)*, and hypercalcemia of malignancy *(open circles)* as measured with a two-site immunoradiometric assay for parathyroid hormone (1-84). Note the clear separation of patients with hyperparathyroidism from those with malignancy-associated hypercalcemia. (Data from Nussbaum SR, Zahradnik RJ, Lavigne JR, et al: Highly sensitive two-site immunoradiometric assay of parathyrin and its clinical utility in evaluating patients with hypercalcemia, Clin Chem 33:1364–1366, 1987.)

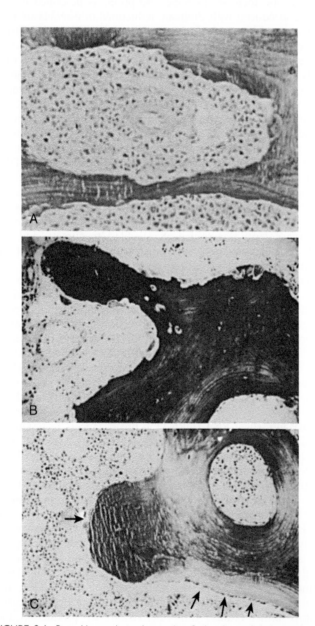

FIGURE 8-1. Bone biopsy photomicrographs. **A,** Local osteolytic hypercalcemia secondary to leukemia. Note the presence of leukemic cells in the marrow space and numerous osteoclasts lining the trabecular surface. **B,** Humoral hypercalcemia of malignancy caused by squamous carcinoma. Note the absence of tumor in the marrow space but the presence of numerous active osteoclasts on the trabecular surface. Also note the absence of osteoblasts and osteoid. **C,** Hyperparathyroidism. Note the abundant osteoclasts, osteoblasts, and osteoid. Osteoclasts are indicated by small arrows, and osteoblasts by large arrows. (**B** and **C** from Stewart AF, Vignery A, Silverate A, et al: Quantitative bone histomorphometry in humoral hypercalcemia of malignancy: uncoupling of bone cell activity, J Clin Endocrinol Metab 55:219–227, 1982.)

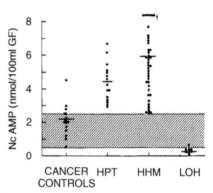

FIGURE 8-3. Nephrogenous cyclic adenosine monophosphate excretion in patients with normocalcemia and cancer (cancer controls), primary hyperparathyroidism (HPT), humoral hypercalcemia of malignancy (HHM), and local osteolytic hypercalcemia (LOH). (Data from Stewart AF, Horst R, Deftos LJ, et al: Biochemical evaluation of patients with cancer-associated hypercalcemia: evidence for humoral and nonhumoral groups, N Engl J Med 303:1377–1383, 1980.)

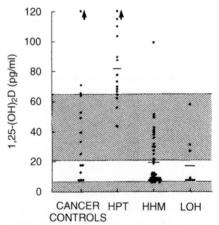

FIGURE 8-4. Plasma 1,25-dihydroxyvitamin D concentration in the four groups described in Figure 8-3. (Data from Stewart AF, Horst R, Deftos LJ, et al: Biochemical evaluation of patients with cancer-associated hypercalcemia: evidence for humoral and non-humoral groups, N Engl J Med 303:1377–1383, 1980.)

result of hypercalcemia and suppressed PTH, fractional calcium excretion is increased[11] (Fig. 8-6). With the presence of bone resorption, which delivers a phosphorus load into the extracellular fluid, together with suppression of PTH (limiting phosphorus excretion), one might expect the serum phosphorus concentration to be elevated in patients with LOH. Conversely, one might expect the serum phosphorus concentration to be low as a reflection of poor dietary intake and the phosphaturic effects of hypercalcemia. In fact, it is usually normal[11,12] (Fig. 8-7), as is the tubular maximum for phosphorus (TmP/glomerular filtration rate [GFR])[11,12] (see Fig. 8-7), which presumably reflects a balance between these opposing forces. Bone radionuclide scans typically display widespread metastases in breast cancer associated with LOH. In contrast, bone scans may be entirely negative in patients with multiple myeloma. This difference reflects the uptake of radionuclide in areas of bone formation (e.g., blastic metastases in breast cancer) but not in areas of osteoclastic activity. Scans may be positive in patients with myeloma in whom fractures and fracture callous formation have developed. As noted earlier, bone biopsy discloses markedly increased osteoclastic bone resorption in both breast cancer and myeloma associated with LOH (see Fig. 8-1), a finding reflected by increases in biochemical markers of bone resorption such as deoxypyridinoline and N-telopeptide excretion.[42]

Humoral Hypercalcemia of Malignancy

Humoral hypercalcemia of malignancy (HHM) accounts for approximately 80% of patients in unselected series of individuals with MAHC.[2-12,17-22] Approximately 50% of patients with HHM have an underlying squamous carcinoma of the lung, cervix, esophagus, larynx, oropharynx, vulva, skin, or other site[2-12,17-22] (see Table 8-1). Carcinomas of the kidney, ovary, and bladder also are very common.[2-14,19-22] It is interesting to note that breast cancer not only may cause MAHC through LOH and skeletal metastases but also may cause hypercalcemia in the absence of skeletal metastases in a classic HHM scenario[43,44] (see Table 8-1). Human T cell lymphoma/leukemia virus-I lymphomas, 90% of which are associated with hypercalcemia, also operate through this mechanism.[45,46] Finally, hypercalcemia resulting from endocrine tumors such as pheochromocytomas[47,48] and islet cell carcinomas[49,50] may cause hypercalcemia through this mechanism. As is the case with LOH, virtually every tumor type has been reported on occasion to cause HHM. It is interesting to note that not every tumor that causes hypercalcemia is malignant. Examples of systemic secretion of PTHrP by benign neoplasms (mammary hypertrophy and uterine leiomyomas are examples) have been reported to cause "humoral hypercalcemia of benignancy."[51]

Since the advent of Albright's humoral theory of hypercalcemia of malignancy in the 1940s,[3] several substances have been proposed as candidates for the humoral mediator responsible for HHM. In the 1960s, Gordan and coworkers[52] suggested that elevated circulating levels of four phytosterols (plant-derived vitamin D analogues) were present in patients with breast carcinoma. Subsequent studies showed, however, that these same phytosterols were present in equivalent concentrations in

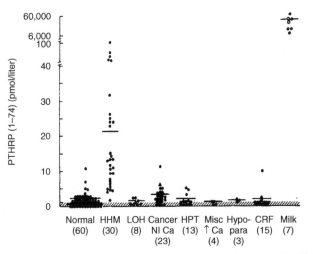

FIGURE 8-5. Immunoreactive parathyroid hormone–related protein (PTHrP) in plasma from patients with the clinical syndromes listed below the x-axis. Note that patients with humoral hypercalcemia of malignancy (HHM) have elevated circulating PTHrP concentrations. (Data from Burtis WJ, Brady TG, Orloff JJ, et al: Immunochemical characterization of circulating parathyroid hormone-related protein in patients with humoral hypercalcemia of malignancy, N Engl J Med 322:1106–1112, 1990.)

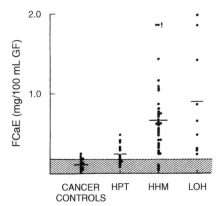

FIGURE 8-6. Fasting calcium excretion in the four groups described in Figure 8-3. Note that on average, patients with humoral hypercalcemia of malignancy (HHM) and local osteolytic hypercalcemia (LOH) appear to be more calciuric than do patients with primary hyperparathyroidism (HPT). Compare these findings with those in Figure 8-8. (Data from Stewart AF, Horst R, Deftos LJ, et al: Biochemical evaluation of patients with cancer-associated hypercalcemia: evidence for humoral and non-humoral groups, N Engl J Med 303:1377–1383, 1980.)

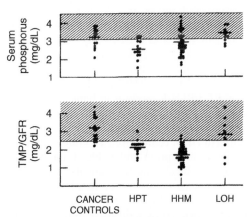

FIGURE 8-7. Serum phosphorus and renal phosphorus threshold in the four groups described in Figure 8-3. (Data from Stewart AF, Horst R, Deftos LJ, et al: Biochemical evaluation of patients with cancer-associated hypercalcemia: evidence for humoral and non-humoral groups, N Engl J Med 303:1377–1383, 1980.)

normal and lactating women, and that the potency of these analogues was inadequate to cause hypercalcemia.[53] The phytosterol theory thus lost support.

With the discovery in the 1970s that prostaglandin E2 (PGE2) was a potent stimulator of bone resorption both in tissue culture[54] and in experimental animals in vivo,[55] the possibility arose that the hypercalcemia associated with HHM was due to systemic PGE2 secretion by tumors. Seyberth and colleagues[56] and others reported that urinary metabolites of PGE2 were elevated in patients with MAHC, and that therapy with prostaglandin synthesis inhibitors (aspirin, indomethacin) reversed the hypercalcemia in several patients. However, subsequent, more extensive studies have not shown frequent responses to indomethacin.[57] It is the current view of most investigators that PGE2 does not act as a systemic mediator of bone resorption in most cases of HHM, and that therapy with prostaglandin synthesis inhibitors is usually ineffective. It should be clear, however, that these observations do not exclude a role for PGE2 or other arachidonate metabolites in HHM at the local level within the skeleton.

As was noted earlier, Albright[3] initially had suggested that PTH was the responsible humoral factor. This concept subsequently gained wide acceptance, as evidenced by the entrance into common usage in the 1960s and 1970s of the terms "ectopic hyperparathyroidism" and "pseudohyperparathyroidism."[6] Evidence in support of the "ectopic PTH" thesis included (1) the humoral nature of the syndrome[4,5,10]; (2) the hypophosphatemia and renal phosphate–wasting characteristic of the syndrome; and (3) the apparent failure of suppression of PTH observed in the early generations of PTH radioimmunoassays.[58,59] It is now clear, as is described later, that although bona fide ectopic hyperparathyroidism does indeed exist (see later), it is extremely rare and fails to account for most instances of HHM.

Today, it is widely accepted that the vast majority of cases of HHM are due to the secretion of PTHrP by tumors. Evidence for this statement can be summarized as follows: (1) tumors associated with HHM produce and secrete PTHrP, which leads to elevated circulating concentrations of PTHrP[19-22] (see Fig. 8-5); (2) PTHrP infusion into laboratory animals and humans reproduces the key features of the HHM syndrome in vivo[60-65]; and (3) infusion of neutralizing antisera against PTHrP reverses the HHM syndrome in laboratory animal models.[66,67]

The pathophysiology of HHM is now quite clear. Under normal circumstances, PTHrP is widely expressed among essentially all tissues and serves as a local paracrine or autocrine factor, but it does not enter the systemic circulation.[68,69] However, in malignant and occasionally benign tumors, *PTHrP* gene expression may be significantly upregulated, and PTHrP now enters the circulation. Because of the structural homology between PTHrP and PTH, PTHrP is able to bind to and activate the common PTH/PTHrP receptor in bone and kidney, with the result that patients with HHM mimic many of the cardinal features of primary hyperparathyroidism. As is summarized later, hypercalcemia in HHM results from a combination of accelerated osteoclastic bone resorption and reduced ability of the kidney to clear calcium. Biochemically, patients with HHM display increases in circulating concentrations of PTHrP[19-22] (see Fig. 8-5), and bone biopsies display a marked increase in osteoclastic resorption, accompanied by a decrease in osteoblastic bone formation[13] (see Fig. 8-1). These histologic results have been corroborated more recently by the use of biochemical markers of bone turnover such as bone-specific alkaline phosphatase, osteo-

calcin, N-telopeptide of collagen, and deoxypyridinoline cross-links.[42] This quantitatively striking uncoupling of bone resorption from formation leads to a large calcium flux from the skeleton into the extracellular fluid and accounts primarily for the hypercalcemia observed in HHM. The cellular basis for this dramatic uncoupling is not known. Circulating PTH concentrations are reduced in patients with HHM[19-22,70] (see Fig. 8-2), but nephrogenous cyclic adenosine monophosphate (NcAMP) excretion is increased (see Fig. 8-3),[11,12] a reflection of the increases in circulating PTHrP. Although the increase in NcAMP excretion is of little diagnostic importance today, the elevation in NcAMP and the ability of PTHrP to stimulate adenylyl cyclase in the kidney in vitro led to the identification and purification of PTHrP.[69]

HHM is associated with suppression of plasma $1,25(OH)_2D$[11,12] (see Fig. 8-4). The mechanisms responsible for the reduction in $1,25(OH)_2D$ in HHM as compared with primary hyperparathyroidism have recently begun to be elucidated. First, Horwitz et al.[64] have demonstrated that chronic infusion of PTHrP in humans serves as a poor agonist of $1,25(OH)_2D$ production, in contrast to infusion of PTH, which leads to robust, dose-related increases in $1,25(OH)_2D$. Second, Dean et al[71] have recently demonstrated that whereas PTH and PTHrP may *associate* with the common human PTH-PTHrP receptor equivalently, their *dissociation* rates differ markedly, with PTH remaining bound to the receptor and activating signal transduction, while PTHrP dissociates rapidly, inactivating downstream signaling. Because of the low $1,25(OH)_2D$ concentrations in patients with HHM, one might predict that intestinal calcium absorption does not contribute to their hypercalcemia, in contrast to those with primary hyperparathyroidism, in whom dietary calcium intake increases serum calcium. This inability to absorb dietary calcium in humans with malignancy-associated hypercalcemia has been directly documented using intestinal ^{45}Ca absorption.[72]

Fractional calcium excretion by the kidney has been reported to be elevated[10,11] (see Fig. 8-5) or reduced[73,74] in patients with HHM. These conflicting reports result from the fact that accurate measurements of the GFR, on which calcium excretion measurement is based, are not possible in patients with advanced cancer, rapidly declining renal function, and markedly reduced muscle mass (and therefore creatinine release) who are undergoing aggressive hydration and diuretic therapy. To address this issue more directly, Horwitz and others[62-64] recently demonstrated in normal healthy volunteers infused with PTH or PTHrP that both peptides have potent and equivalent effects in stimulating renal tubular (presumably distal) reabsorption of calcium (Fig. 8-8). Thus, in addition to the bone-resorbing effects of PTHrP, the anticalciuric effects of PTHrP contribute to hypercalcemia in HHM.

Finally, similar to PTH, PTHrP inhibits proximal tubular phosphorus reabsorption.[60-64] Thus, in HHM, the serum phosphorus concentration is characteristically reduced[11,12] (see Fig. 8-7) as long as renal function remains normal, a phenomenon that is reflected in a reduction in the TmP/GFR[11,12] (see Fig. 8-7).

Bone radionuclide scans characteristically display a complete absence of skeletal metastases or the presence of only a few skeletal metastases,[2-12,17-22] which is a reflection of the primarily humoral nature of the syndrome. It is important to note that the syndrome reverses with successful eradication of the tumor in question, thus underscoring the humoral nature of the syndrome.[2-12,17,18] Unfortunately, this outcome is not common.

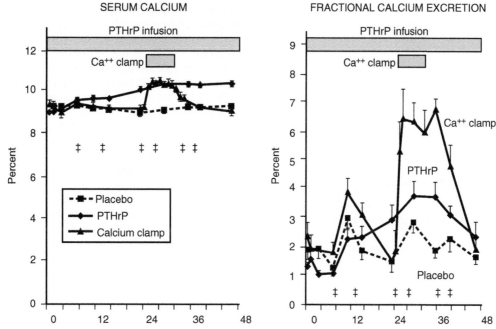

FIGURE 8-8. Fractional calcium excretion in normal subjects infused with calcium chloride or parathyroid hormone–related protein (PTHrP). *Left,* Serum calcium concentrations are shown in three groups of normal healthy volunteers infused with vehicle alone, with PTHrP to achieve a serum calcium of 10.3 mg/dL, or with calcium chloride (calcium clamp) to achieve an identical serum calcium of 10.3 mg/dL. *Right,* Response in fractional calcium excretion in the three groups. In the control (vehicle) group, fractional calcium excretion remains stable at approximately 2%. In the calcium clamp group, the fractional calcium excretion increases dramatically to approximately 6.5%, reflecting a combination of the increase in the filtered load of calcium from the calcium infusion and the suppression of endogenous PTH secretion. In the group receiving PTHrP, despite identical serum calcium concentration (and therefore an identical filtered load of calcium) to the calcium clamp group, fractional calcium excretion remains low, indicating that PTHrP is a potent stimulator of distal tubular calcium reabsorption. Studies comparing PTH with PTHrP indicate that the two peptides have equivalent effects in human renal calcium handling.[62-64] (Data from Syed MA, Horwitz MJ, Tedesco MB, et al: Parathyroid hormone-related protein [1-36] stimulates renal tubular calcium reabsorption in normal human volunteers: implications for the pathogenesis of humoral hypercalcemia of malignancy, J Clin Endocrinol Metab 86:1525–1531, 2001.)

Authentic Ectopic Hyperparathyroidism

As noted earlier, from the 1940s through the 1970s, ectopic hyperparathyroidism was believed to be a common cause of paraneoplastic hypercalcemia. By the 1980s, the term had fallen into disuse, and the existence of authentic ectopic hyperparathyroidism was in doubt; most authors believed that all cases of what had previously been considered to be ectopic hyperparathyroidism were in fact cases of HHM. With the advent of sensitive and specific immunoassays and molecular probes for PTH and PTHrP, the situation has changed. Now, approximately 15 case reports describe patients with diverse types of cancer (e.g., small cell carcinomas of the lung, squamous carcinoma of the lung, hepatoma, thymoma, neuroendocrine tumors, clear cell adenocarcinoma of the ovary, thyroid papillary carcinoma) who also displayed elevations in immunoreactive PTH in plasma with the use of modern two-site PTH immunoassays or expressed PTH mRNA in their tumor, or both.[75-82]

In one thoroughly studied case, reported by Nussbaum and associates,[75] immunoreactive PTH values were found to be elevated in plasma by a sensitive and specific two-site PTH immunoradiometric assay. At surgery, a fivefold gradient of PTH was demonstrated across the ovarian tumor. PTH values decreased precipitately after tumor resection, and the serum calcium concentration normalized (Fig. 8-9). Neck exploration before the ovarian surgery had revealed four normal parathyroid glands, and resection of three-and-a-half parathyroid glands had no effect on the serum calcium concentration. PTH mRNA was abundantly present in the tumor, whereas PTHrP mRNA was undetectable, as was PTHrP in plasma.

The basis of PTH gene overexpression in this tumor was found to be twofold. First, a clonal rearrangement in the upstream region of one copy of the PTH gene in the ovarian carcinoma apparently served to abolish a silencer in this region of the gene or included a promoter region of a normal ovarian gene. Second, the *PTH* gene was amplified in the tumor. In contrast, in the report by Yoshimoto and colleagues[76] describing ectopic hyperparathyroidism caused by a pulmonary small cell carcinoma, no such gene rearrangement or amplification events were identified, and the cause of the PTH expression was unexplained. In a recent report by VanHouten et al., ectopic production of PTH was documented from a pancreatic neuroendocrine tumor both in vivo and in vitro, and this was shown to be due not to a gene rearrangement or amplification, but to transcriptional activation of the *PTH* gene within the malignant neuroendocrine cells.[82]

These case reports demonstrate that authentic ectopic hyperparathyroidism, although rare, can occur. From a clinical standpoint, because of elevations in immunoreactive PTH, these patients may be misdiagnosed as having primary hyperparathyroidism. Unless the offending malignant neoplasm is obvious at the initial evaluation, such confusion may lead to unsuccessful parathyroidectomy.

Unusual Causes of Malignancy-Associated Hypercalcemia

The vast majority of patients with HHM are striking in their homogeneity. As was indicated earlier, the histologic findings

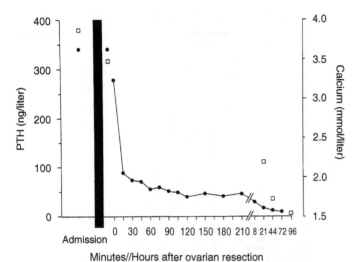

FIGURE 8-9. Serum calcium *(open squares)* and immunoreactive parathyroid hormone (PTH) *(solid circles)* in a patient with an ovarian carcinoma before and after oophorectomy, indicated by the *black bar.* The PTH immunoassay is that shown in Figure 8-2. Prior parathyroidectomy of 3.5 glands failed to influence her hypercalcemia or her elevated PTH concentration. (Data from Nussbaum SR, Gaz RD, Arnold A: Hypercalcemia and ectopic secretion of PTH by an ovarian carcinoma with rearrangement of the gene for PTH, N Engl J Med 323:1324–1328, 1990.)

(squamous, renal, bladder, and ovarian carcinomas) and biochemical findings (elevated NcAMP, reduced renal phosphorus thresholds, reduced 1,25[OH]$_2$D levels, suppressed immunoreactive PTH levels, elevated immunoreactive PTHrP concentrations) are so uniform that it seems inescapable that most cases of HHM are due to secretion of PTHrP.

It should be clear, however, that other humoral mediators undoubtedly exist in unusual patients. For example, a small number of patients with elevated PGE$_2$ levels or clear responsiveness to prostaglandin synthesis inhibitors or both have been described,[56,83] which suggests that in rare instances, PGE$_2$ may act as a humoral, systemic agent.

In addition, more than 40 patients with a variety of types of lymphoma have been described in whom hypercalcemia occurred in the absence of bone metastases and with reduced urinary cAMP or NcAMP excretion but elevated circulating levels of 1,25(OH)$_2$D[84-86] (Fig. 8-10). These observations suggest that tumor-derived 1,25(OH)$_2$D may have induced intestinal hyperabsorption of calcium or may have led to osteoclastic stimulation, or both. More recently, in patients harboring ovarian dysgerminomas, several groups have reported production and systemic elevations of 1,25(OH)$_2$D leading to hypercalcemia.[87,88]

Further, a patient with an ovarian dysgerminoma, no skeletal involvement, hypercalcemia in the presence of an elevated renal phosphorus threshold, and reduced levels of NcAMP and 1,25(OH)$_2$D has been described.[89] All these abnormalities

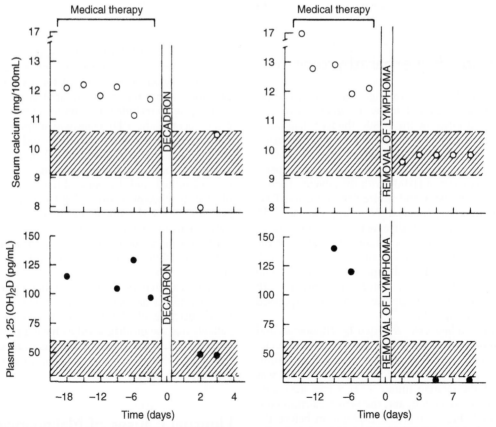

FIGURE 8-10. Serum calcium and plasma 1,25-dihydroxyvitamin (1,25[OH]$_2$D) concentrations in patients with the 1,25(OH)$_2$D-induced lymphoma syndrome before and after therapy. The patient shown in the two *left panels* was treated with dexamethasone (decadron) for systemic lymphoma. The patient in the two *right panels* had a splenectomy for a solitary splenic lymphoma. Note the decrease in plasma 1,25(OH)$_2$D concentration after therapy in both patients and the normalization of serum calcium. Also compare the plasma 1,25(OH)$_2$D concentrations in these patients versus those in patients with humoral hypercalcemia of malignancy and local osteolytic hypercalcemia shown in Figure 8-4. (Data from Rosenthal ND, Insogna KL, Godsall JW, et al: Elevations in circulating 1,25-dihydroxyvitamin D in three patients with lymphoma-associated hypercalcemia, J Clin Endocrinol Metab 60:29–33, 1985.)

promptly normalized after eradication of the patient's tumor, which suggests that the tumor produced a humoral agent distinct from PTH, PTHrP, or $1,25(OH)_2D$.

Finally, Bringhurst and others[90,91] described patients with hypercalcemia in the setting of metastatic malignant melanoma and bladder carcinoma. Excision of the tumor reversed the patients' hypercalcemia, thus indicating a humoral mechanism. In culture, the tumors were shown to produce a bone-resorbing protein devoid of adenylate cyclase–stimulating activity or PTH-like bioactivity. In the aggregate, these examples collectively indicate that humoral forms of MAHC can occur through the production of factors other than $1,25(OH)_2D$, PTHrP, or PTH; however, these examples appear to be rare.

Treatment of Hypercalcemia

OVERVIEW

This section summarizes treatment of hypercalcemia of any cause but with particular reference to that due to cancer. The treatment of hypercalcemia caused by cancer has received complete attention in several recent reviews.[92-94] As was noted earlier, the mean life expectancy in patients following a diagnosis of MAHC is 30 days.[14] The most effective long-term therapy for MAHC is successful antitumor therapy. This point should be borne in mind and acted on early in the management of any given patient. Therapies aimed at treatment of hypercalcemia in patients with MAHC per se are rarely effective over the long term. Hence, long-term control of hypercalcemia depends on tumor eradication or debulking through surgery, chemotherapy, or radiotherapy. It is therefore essential and urgent that a plan for chemotherapy, surgery, or radiotherapy be developed and acted upon very early on in the course of treatment for MAHC. Said another way, therapy aimed at correcting hypercalcemia is largely short term and palliative: it should be used only to temporize while a more concrete and effective long-term treatment plan is formulated.

Another important concept is that therapy should be aimed not at the serum calcium concentration, but at a given patient's overall status. For example, a patient with a calcium level of 11.5 mg/dL who has been stable and asymptomatic may need no treatment at all, whereas aggressive therapy for a calcium level of 11.0 may be appropriate in an elderly patient with symptoms of hypercalcemia, or when a rapid subsequent increase seems likely. Conversely, no antihypercalcemic therapy may be most appropriate in a patient with advanced cancer who has failed all attempts to control the malignancy.

It is useful to conceptualize short-term antihypercalcemic therapy in terms of the three organ systems that regulate calcium homeostasis and whose aggregate homeostatic failure leads to hypercalcemia: the intestine, the kidney, and the skeleton. Therapy should be tailored to a given patient's needs and with the factors in mind that may have precipitated development of the hypercalcemia. The development of hypercalcemia in a patient with MAHC may be primarily skeletal: it may be traced to tumor progression with progressive skeletal metastases, to increasing PTHrP levels in the circulation, or to recent immobilization. Therapy aimed at reducing tumor burden and/or reversing immobilization may be all that is necessary to correct such a patient's hypercalcemia. A previously normocalcemic patient with cancer may develop hypercalcemia as a result of dehydration due to anorexia or diarrhea. Simple rehydration may be all

that is required. As described previously, a patient with lymphoma or dysgerminoma may develop hypercalcemia owing to excessive intestinal absorption of calcium as a result of increased $1,25(OH)_2D$ concentrations (or with vitamin D intoxication). Reducing dietary calcium intake and vitamin D may be the best therapeutic option.

Finally, most often, combinations of the agents and measures described below are used. For example, a regimen designed to increase hydration and increase physical mobility, combined with a loop diuretic and a potent intravenous bisphosphonate, would be appropriate in most patients.

REHYDRATION

Patients with hypercalcemia of any cause but especially of malignancy are almost always markedly dehydrated and azotemic for several reasons. First, hypercalcemia leads to a state of nephrogenic diabetes insipidus that in turn augments renal free water losses, leading to the polyuria characteristic of hypercalcemia. Second, hypercalcemia induces afferent glomerular arteriolar vasoconstriction that limits glomerular blood flow. Third, patients with MAHC are routinely dehydrated as a result of poor oral intake of fluids consequent to altered mental status, cancer-induced cachexia, and inability to ambulate and access liquids. Dehydration may be worsened by diarrhea or diuretic use. The pathophysiologic consequences of dehydration are that glomerular perfusion declines, and along with it the ability of the kidney to filter serum calcium. This leads to a vicious cycle of hypercalcemia, leading to reduced GFR, leading to worsening hypercalcemia, leading to a further decline in renal calcium clearance, and thus the rapid upward spiral of serum calcium characteristic of patients with MAHC. This is quite different, for example, for patients with primary hyperparathyroidism, in whom serum calcium characteristically remains stable for years.

Thus, step one in treating hypercalcemia is to initiate a rehydration program.[92-96] This is done after careful review of the patient's clinical hydration status (lack of edema, neck vein distention, reduced skin turgor, and clinical and laboratory measures that might point to the presence of congestive heart failure or renal failure that might prevent aggressive rehydration). If no contraindications exist, intravenous hydration can be initiated with normal saline at a rate of between 200 and 1000 mL/hr, depending on the degree of dehydration and hypercalcemia and the ability to monitor the patient for congestive heart failure or other clinical syndromes of volume overload (with central venous pressure or pulmonary capillary wedge pressures as needed).

DIURESIS

Administration of intravenous saline will initiate or enhance calciuresis.[92-96] This is a result, in part, of an increase in glomerular blood flow and thus an increase in the filtered load of calcium. In addition, saline infusion inhibits calcium reabsorption in the proximal convoluted tubule. Renal calcium excretion can be further enhanced by the addition of a loop diuretic such as furosemide or ethacrynic acid, both of which inhibit calcium reabsorption in the thick ascending loop of Henle. However, because loop diuretics are also natriuretics and diuretics, they will exacerbate dehydration if they are initiated prematurely. Thus, loop diuretics should be initiated only after clinical evidence of adequate rehydration has accrued. Typically, therapy is initiated with furosemide at a dose of 20 mg IV every 2 to 12 hours, depending on the clinical circumstances, with careful monitoring of clinical volume status fluid balance, as well as potassium, magnesium, and electrolyte balance.

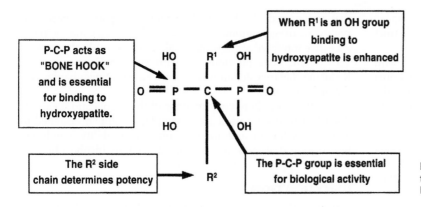

FIGURE 8-11. Structure of a bone-active bisphosphonate to show functional domains. (From Russell RG, Rogers MJ: Bisphosphonates: From the laboratory to the clinic and back again, Bone 25:97–106, 1999.)

It is important to remember that thiazide diuretics stimulate renal calcium retention in the distal renal tubule and thus worsen hypercalcemia: thiazides should not be employed as in the treatment of hypercalcemia. If they are being used for other reasons, they should be discontinued.

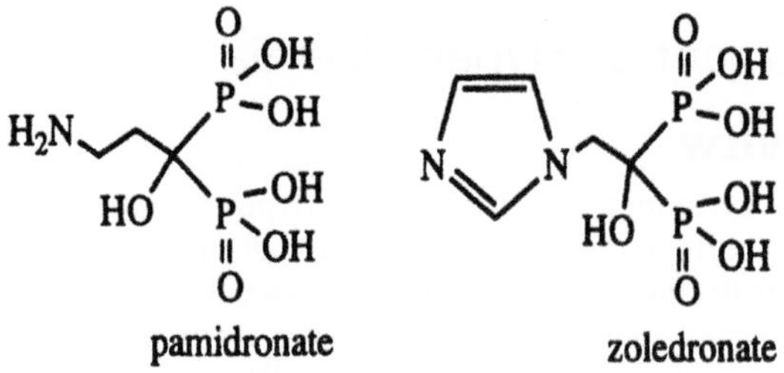

ANTIRESORPTIVE DRUGS

Historically, excess bone resorption in MAHC has been inhibited by the use of mithramycin (plicamycin), calcitonin, glucocorticoids, or gallium nitrate. More recently, the bisphosphonates have eclipsed these other agents because they are potent, safe, and easy to administer.

The Bisphosphonates

Bisphosphonates are structural analogues of pyrophosphate in which the two phosphate groups are joined by a carbon atom rather than an oxygen atom[97-101] (Fig. 8-11). The P-C-P bond is thus analogous to the P-O-P in pyrophosphate, a natural metabolite that can inhibit calcification but is rapidly metabolized. Because the bisphosphonates are resistant to cleavage by pyrophosphatases, they are stable in the body. The bisphosphonates were developed in the search for more stable bone-seeking compounds that could imitate pyrophosphate action.[97-101] The P-C-P bond is key for bone uptake; a hydroxyl group in the R_1 position (see Fig. 8-11) increases affinity for hydroxyapatite in bone. It is now established that the R_2 position is key to potency among the various bisphosphonates that have been developed. Once absorbed onto bone surface by the basic bisphosphonate pharmacophore, the nature of the substituent at the R_2 position determines antiosteoclast potency and inhibition of bone resorption (Fig. 8-12). Substituents that contain nitrogen generally are more potent, with the most potent being those with a nitrogen within a heterocyclic ring (see Fig. 8-12).

Bisphosphonates are concentrated in areas of high bone turnover, are taken up by osteoclasts, and are potent inhibitors of bone destruction.[97-101] Since their introduction almost 40 years ago, the precise cellular and biochemical mechanisms whereby the drugs act have been clarified, and successive generations of more potent compounds have been introduced.[97-101] The bisphosphonate cellular target is principally the osteoclast, which seems selectively to take up the compounds during the process of bone resorption. The cellular actions are probably multiple, with evidence of impaired differentiation of osteoclast precursors, reduced osteoclast function, and accelerated osteoclast apoptosis, the net result being reduction in bone resorption. Studies in vitro have established two distinct cellular pathways by which bisphosphonates act on osteoclasts. Nitrogen-containing bisphosphonates interfere with enzymes in the mevalonate pathway that

FIGURE 8-12. Structures of pamidronate and zoledronate.

catalyze the formation of geranyl diphosphate and farnesyl diphosphate, which are key to prenylation of signaling proteins, especially those that accelerate GTP hydrolysis (GTPases). Without normal prenylation, these small proteins cannot attach to the osteoclast cell membrane, thus interfering with osteoclast function. Impairment of protein prenylation may also promote osteoclast apoptosis. Farnesyl or geranylgeranyl pyrophosphate added in vitro can reverse the blockade caused by the nitrogen-containing bisphosphonates.

Although there has been speculation about a cellular receptor for bisphosphonate, more recent evidence favors a still unidentified specific cellular uptake channel.[102] In a series of experiments using osteoclasts and a related macrophage cell line, competition between several bisphosphonates for cellular uptake and biological effects was analyzed with varying doses of the two compounds administered to test for synergy at suboptimal doses of either, because the two bisphosphonates act by distinctive mechanisms. The overall results were interpreted as demonstrating competition for uptake through a common transport channel.[102]

At present, the two bisphosphonates most widely used for treatment of MAHC hypercalcemia are pamidronate (aminohydroxy-propylidene bisphosphonate) and zoledronate (zolendronic acid) (see Fig. 8-11).[97-101,103,104] Zoledronate is more potent on a milligram or molar basis and can be given more rapidly, thus facilitating inpatient and outpatient delivery. However, pamidronate is less expensive and displays similar efficacy.[103] In general, bisphosphonates of all types are absorbed from the gastrointestinal tract with extremely poor efficiency (less than 1% to 2%).[97-101] For this reason, zoledronate and pamidronate are administered intravenously.

Pamidronate, an aminobisphosphonate, is usually administered as a single intravenous infusion in a dosage of 60 to 90 mg over a 2-hour period intravenously, depending on the severity of the hypercalcemia.[97-101,103,105] Treatment must be repeated when hypercalcemia recurs, but efficacy may wane with repeated dosing.[32,35,36] The serum calcium normalizes in most patients with MAHC.[97-101,103,105] It is critical to remember that this response typically requires 3 to 7 days.[97-101,103,105] This means that once an initial dose is administered, a second dose generally should not be administered earlier than 3 to 4 days after the initial dose. The likelihood that the serum calcium level will normalize is related to both the dose of pamidronate administered and the severity of the initial hypercalcemia.

The most common side effect of intravenous pamidronate therapy is fever, which occurs in approximately 20% of patients and may be related to release of cytokines from osteoclasts, monocytes, and macrophages.[97-101,103,105,106] Fever is generally mild (<2°C) and typically occurs only once in a patient's lifetime, even if treatment is discontinued and restarted later. Other side effects of pamidronate include hypocalcemia (rare in patients with MAHC), hypophosphatemia, hypomagnesemia, and possibly reversible hepatotoxicity.[97-101,103,105] A recently reported complication of pamidronate therapy is glomerulosclerosis with renal insufficiency and nephrotic syndrome, which occurred in seven patients with cancer treated at higher than usual doses (180 or 360 mg/mo rather than the usual 90 mg/mo).[107] The interpretation was complicated by the use of other potent anticancer drugs, although high-dose pamidronate was the only common factor.[107]

Zoledronate generally is administered at a dose of 4 mg intravenously over a 15-minute period.[97-101,103,104] It may be slightly more effective than pamidronate for the treatment of hypercalcemia.[103] A randomized, double-blind study comparing zoledronic acid (at the recommended doses of 4 mg/5 minute infusion as well as 8 mg/5 minute infusion) with pamidronate (at the recommended 90 mg/2 hour infusion) in 250 patients with MAHC.[103] Both doses of zoledronic acid normalized serum calcium levels slightly faster with more sustained responses than pamidronate (32 or 43 days for 4 vs. 8 mg of zoledronic acid, respectively, as compared with 18 days for pamidronate). On the other hand, although these differences were statistically significant, they were quantitatively small, leaving one to wonder whether the added expense of zoledronate as compared with pamidronate is merited. Zoledronic acid has an adverse event profile similar to pamidronate with pyrexia and occasional reports of renal toxicity presumed to be secondary to precipitation of calcium bisphosphonate complexes.[108]

Mithramycin

Mithramycin (also called plicamycin) is a chemotherapeutic agent that has been used in the treatment of neuroendocrine tumors and testicular tumors.[109,110] It was found serendipitously to cause hypocalcemia as a result of its action to induce death in osteoclasts. Thus, for several decades it was used as a front-line treatment for MAHC, parathyroid carcinoma, and Paget's disease. However, its use, particularly in large and repeated doses, was associated with azotemia, hepatitis, and coagulation defects. It has been eclipsed in clinical practice by the intravenous bisphosphonates, because of their efficacy and safety. On the other hand, it is a particularly effective drug, and its use should be considered in special circumstances.

Calcitonin

Calcitonin is a naturally occurring peptide made by the parafollicular cells within the thyroid gland in humans; it inhibits bone resorption and decreases renal tubular calcium reabsorption.[111-115] Calcitonin has a rapid onset of action, but its calcium-lowering effect is limited because of rapid tachyphylaxis.[111-115] For example,

one early study reported that calcitonin lowered serum calcium levels by an average of 2 mg/dL with a peak effect in 6 hours.[114] In another report, calcitonin lowered serum calcium levels in 75% of subjects within 2 hours, half of whom became normocalcemic in several hours.[115] The calcium-lowering effect of calcitonin is clearly short-lived, however, with an increase in serum calcium levels often occurring within 48 to 96 hours despite continued calcitonin therapy.[111-115] Because of this rapid tachyphylaxis, calcitonin has limited utility beyond 1 to 2 days as a single agent for the treatment of hypercalcemia, and it should no longer be widely used. It may be useful in rare patients with severe hypercalcemia in whom the clinical situation cannot wait an extra 24 hours for the hypocalcemic effects of pamidronate or zoledronate. The usual dosage of salmon calcitonin is 4 U/kg every 12 hours, although doses as high as 8 U/kg have been given every 6 hours.[111-115] The most common side effects of calcitonin therapy are nausea and vomiting, which occur in approximately 10% to 15% of patients.[111-115] Other side effects include flushing and abdominal cramps.[111-115]

Gallium Nitrate

Gallium nitrate inhibits the release of ^{45}Ca from fetal rat bones in response to PTH and lymphokines and inhibits the ability of cultured osteoclasts to resorb cortical bone in vitro. It interacts with both hydroxyapatite and the cellular components of bone and accumulates preferentially in areas of active bone formation. Gallium nitrate has been shown to reduce the serum calcium in patients with MAHC,[116] but it must be given continuously intravenously to achieve these effects. Thus, its use is limited for practical reasons. Given their efficacy and superior convenience of use, bisphosphonates remain the standard therapy in most patients.

Glucocorticoids

Several decades ago, before the development of mithramycin, calcitonin, and the intravenous bisphosphonates, glucocorticoids were a therapeutic agent of choice for patients with MAHC and sometimes were used in vitamin D intoxication.[117,118] In large doses, glucocorticoids increase renal calcium clearance and urinary calcium excretion, directly decrease intestinal absorption of calcium, and inhibit tumor activity of 1-alpha hydroxylase, the enzyme that leads to production of 1,25(OH)$_2$D. They also may inhibit production of bone-resorbing cytokines by tumors. In some tumors, particularly hematologic tumors, glucocorticoids have antitumor effects as well. These effects of glucocorticoids on the tumor, the kidney, and the intestine lower serum calcium levels. Thus, they still have a place in the management of occasional patients with MAHC due to lymphomas, leukemias, and/or plasma cell dyscrasias, particularly if they are included as part of an antitumor chemotherapeutic regimen or protocol. Outside of this context, however, they are rarely used.

DIALYSIS

Dialysis may seem a heroic therapeutic measure in patients with advanced cancer, and in most cases, it is not appropriate clinically, economically, or perhaps ethically. On the other hand, there are exceptions to this rule, such as a recently diagnosed patient with estrogen receptor–positive, epidermal growth factor receptor–positive breast cancer who has not yet undergone chemotherapy, but who presents with hypercalcemia and in renal failure because of ureteral obstruction or nephrotoxic antibiotic use. Another example might be a patient with multiple myeloma who presents with light chain nephropathy and hypercalcemia. In these rare patients, the prognostic outlook is positive, but standard measures to lower calcium (hydration, loop diuretics, and IV bisphosphonates) may be ineffective or contraindicated because of the renal failure. Hemodialysis or peritoneal dialysis against a low calcium bath can lower serum calcium levels rapidly and dramatically in such patients,[119-121] and this can buy time for renal function to recover while an effective chemotherapeutic regimen is initiated. Dialysis membranes are quite permeable to calcium, and as much as 600 mg of calcium can be cleared per hour with hemodialysis. In a retrospective analysis of 33 patients with severe hypercalcemia of varying causes, calcium-free hemodialysis reduced serum calcium levels by an average of 6.9 mg/dL (1.71 mmol/L), but a partial rebound occurred in most patients within the first 24 hours.[119] Transient hypotension was noted in more than one third of patients but resolved with fluid replacement.[120] In another study of six patients with hypercalcemia of malignancy and renal failure, calcium-free hemodialysis reduced serum calcium levels without any adverse effects.[121] Peritoneal dialysis can remove 500 to 2000 mg of calcium and can lower the serum calcium level by 3 to 12 mg/dL in 24 to 48 hours if a calcium-free dialysis solution is used.[122-124]

PHOSPHORUS REPLACEMENT

Hypophosphatemia is common among patients with MAHC, as a result of many factors: the responsible tumor producing PTHrP; the therapeutic use of phosphaturic agents such as saline, diuretics, calcitonin, or phosphate-binding antacids; and anorexia and starvation. Hypophosphatemia may make it more difficult to treat hypercalcemia, because phosphate is required for the reentry of calcium, as calcium-phosphate, into the skeleton.

On the other hand, overzealous phosphate replacement can be hazardous in the extreme in patients with hypercalcemia, because it may be associated with abrupt and severe hypocalcemia and seizures, as well as with acute onset of renal failure due to nephrocalcinosis.[125] Thus, cautious phosphate replacement may be reasonable in subjects with serum phosphorus concentrations below 3.0 mg/dL. The authors' practice is to use oral phosphorus replacement, in an initial dose in the range of 250 mg four times per day.[93] Careful attention to both serum phosphorus and creatinine is required, as is withholding phosphorus replacement if the serum phosphorus rises above 3.0 mg/dL, or the serum creatinine rises above baseline values. In very rare patients who cannot receive oral medications but who have severe hypophosphatemia, it may be necessary to administer intravenous phosphorus as potassium phosphate. Small doses of phosphorus (e.g., 600 mg of phosphorus slowly over 24 hours) should be given, and extreme care should be taken to avoid hyperphosphatemia and increases in serum creatinine.

Future Therapies

The therapeutic armamentarium for treating hypercalcemia of malignancy is currently so effective and inexpensive that there may be little need for additional treatment modalities. On the other hand, at least a few potential agents may become available over the coming several years. These might include more potent or effective bisphosphonates, monoclonal antibodies directed against PTHrP,[126] and monoclonal antibodies directed against cellular pathways that lead to recruitment, differentiation, and activation of osteoclasts, such as the RANK-RANK-ligand system, or recombinant osteoprotegerin,[127] the natural decoy receptor for RANK-ligand. Among these, the most advanced in clinical trials is a monoclonal antibody, named denosumab, which binds to and inactivates RANK-ligand.[128-130] Denosumab has been shown to be effective in neutralizing RANK-ligand in vivo in humans and thereby markedly blocking osteoclastic bone resorption in patients with osteoporosis. Through this antiresorptive mechanism, denosumab markedly reduces fractures and increases bone mineral density in postmenopausal women with osteoporosis, and in animal studies, reverses HHM.[128-130] Because denosumab is at least as effective as bisphosphonates in osteoporosis, and because it is effective in animal models of MAHC,[130] it would seem to follow that denosumab may be similarly or more effective in treating hypercalcemia in patients with cancer. Time will tell whether this is true.

Acknowledgments

This work was supported by NIH grants DK51081 and DK073039. The authors wish to thank Arthur E. Broadus, MD, PhD, John T. Pottts, MD, and Joel S. Finkelstein, MD, for use of their contributions to these topics in earlier editions of *Endocrinology*.

REFERENCES

1. Zondek H, Petow H, Siebert W: Die bedeutung der calciumbestimmung im blute fur die diagnose der nie-reninsuffzientz, Z Klin Med 99:129–138, 1923.
2. Gutman AB, Tyson TL, Gutman EB: Serum calcium, inorganic phosphorus and phosphatase activity in hyperparathyroidism, Paget's disease, multiple myeloma and neoplastic disease of the bones, Arch Intern Med 57:379–413, 1936.
3. Case records of the Massachusetts General Hospital (case 27461), N Engl J Med 225:789–791, 1941.
4. Plimpton CH, Gelhorn A: Hypercalcemia in malignant disease without evidence of bone destruction, Am J Med 21:750–759, 1956.
5. Connors TB, Howard JF: The etiology of hypercalcemia associated with lung carcinoma, J Clin Invest 35:697–698, 1956.
6. Lafferty FW: Pseudohyperparathyroidism, Medicine (Baltimore) 45:247–260, 1966.
7. Rodman JS, Sherwood LM: Disorders of mineral metabolism in malignancy. In Avioli LV, Krane SM, editors: Metabolic Bone Disease, vol 2, New York, 1978, Academic Press, pp 555–631.

8. Myers WPL: Hypercalcemia in neoplastic disease, Arch Surg 80:308, 1960.
9. Besarab A, Caro JF: Mechanisms of hypercalcemia in malignancy, Cancer 41:2276–2285, 1978.
10. Powell D, Singer FR, Murray TM, et al: Nonparathyroid humoral hypercalcemia in patients with neoplastic diseases, N Engl J Med 289:176–181, 1973.
11. Stewart AF, Horst R, Deftos LJ, et al: Biochemical evaluation of patients with cancer-associated hypercalcemia: evidence for humoral and non-humoral groups, N Engl J Med 303:1377–1383, 1980.
12. Godsall JW, Burtis WJ, Insogna KL, et al: Nephrogenous cyclic AMP, adenylate cyclase–stimulating activity, and the humoral hypercalcemia of malignancy, Recent Prog Horm Res 40:705–750, 1986.
13. Stewart AF, Vignery A, Silvergate A, et al: Quantitative bone histomorphometry in humoral hypercalcemia of malignancy: uncoupling of bone cell activity, J Clin Metab 55:219–227, 1982.
14. Ralson SH, Gallagher SJ, Patel U, et al: Cancer-associated hypercalcemia: morbidity and mortality, Ann Intern Med 112:499–504, 1990.

15. Nierenberg DW, Ransil BJ: Q-aTc interval as a clinical indicator of hypercalcemia, Am J Cardiol 44:243–248, 1979.
16. Davis TME, Singh B, Choo KE, et al: Dynamic assessment of the electrocardiographic QT intervals during citrate infusion in healthy volunteers, Br Heart J 75:523–526, 1995.
17. Omenn GS, Roth SI, Baker WH: Hyperparathyroidism associated with malignant tumors of non-parathyroid origin, Cancer 24:1004–1012, 1969.
18. Skrabanek P, McPartlin J, Powell DM: Tumor hypercalcemia and ectopic hyperparathyroidism, Medicine (Baltimore) 59:262–282, 1980.
19. Burtis WJ, Brady TG, Orloff JJ, et al: Immunochemical characterization of circulating parathyroid hormone-related protein in patients with humoral hypercalcemia of malignancy, N Engl J Med 322:1106–1112, 1990.
20. Budayr AR, Nissenson RA, Klein RF, et al: Increased serum levels of PTH-like protein in malignancy-associated hypercalcemia, Ann Intern Med 111:807–810, 1989.

21. Blind E, Raue F, Gotzman J, et al: Circulating levels of mid-regional parathyroid hormone-related protein in hypercalcemia of malignancy, Clin Endocrinol 37:290–297, 1992.

22. Pandian MR, Morgan CH, Carlton E, et al: Modified immunoradiometric assay of parathyroid hormone-related protein: clinical application in the differential diagnosis of hypercalcemia, Clin Chem 38:282–288, 1992.

23. Bender RA, Hansen H: Hypercalcemia in bronchogenic carcinoma: a prospective study of 200 patients, Ann Intern Med 80:205–208, 1974.

24. Mahadevia PS, Pamaswamy A, Greenwald ES, et al: Hypercalcemia in prostatic carcinoma, Arch Intern Med 143:1339–1342, 1983.

25. Ralston S, Fogelman I, Gardner MD, et al: Hypercalcemia and metastatic bone disease: is there a link? Lancet 2:903–905, 1982.

26. Mundy GR, Raisz LG, Cooper RA, et al: Evidence for the secretion of an osteoclast stimulating factor in myeloma, N Engl J Med 290:1041–1046, 1974.

27. Mundy GR, Luben RA, Raisz LG, et al: Bone-resorbing activity in supernatants from lymphoid cell lines, N Engl J Med 290:867–871, 1974.

28. Callander NS, Roodman GD: Myeloma bone disease, Semin Hematol 38:276–285, 2001.

29. Horwitz MJ, Stewart AF: Malignancy-Associated Hypercalcemia. In Favus MJ, editor: The American Society for Bone and Mineral Research Primer on Metabolic Bone Diseases and Disorders of Mineral Metabolism, ed 6, Washington D.C., 2006, American Society for Bone and Mineral Research, pp 195–199.

30. Dewhirst FE, Stashenko PP, Mole JE, et al: Purification and partial sequence of human osteoclast activating factor: identity with human interleukin IB, J Immunol 135:2562, 1985.

31. Roodman GD: Mechanisms of bone metastasis, N Engl J Med 350:1655–1664, 2004.

32. Ross FP: Osteoclast Biology and Bone Resorption. In Favus M, editor: The American Society for Bone and Mineral Research Primer on Metabolic Bone Diseases and Disorders of Mineral Metabolism, ed 6, Washington D.C., 2006, American Society for Bone and Mineral Research, pp 30–35.

33. Tian E, Zhan F, Walker R, et al: The role of the Wnt/beta-catenin signaling antagonist DKK-1 in the development of osteolytic lesions in multiple myeloma, N Engl J Med 349:2483–2494, 2003.

34. Erlich LA, Chung HY, Ghobrial I, et al: IL-3 is a potent inhibitor of osteoblast differentiation in multiple myeloma, Blood 106:1407–1414, 2005.

35. Galasko CSB: Mechanisms of bone destruction in the development of skeletal metastases, Nature 263:507, 1976.

36. Guise TA, Yin JJ, Taylor SD, et al: Evidence for a causal role of parathyroid hormone–related protein in the pathogenesis of human breast cancer-mediated osteolysis, J Clin Invest 98:1544, 1996.

37. Southby J, Kissin MW, Danks JA, et al: Immunohistochemical localization of PTHrP in human breast cancer, Cancer Res 50:7710–7716, 1990.

38. Vargas SJ, Gillespie MT, Powell GJ, et al: Localization of PTHrP mRNA expression in breast cancer and metastatic lesions by in situ hybridization, J Bone Miner Res 7:971–979, 1992.

39. Sztern M, Barkan A, Rakowsky E, et al: Hypercalcemia in carcinoma of the breast without evidence of bone destruction, Cancer 48:2383–2385, 1981.

40. Legha SS, Powell K, Buzdar AU, et al: Tamoxifen-induced hypercalcemia in breast cancer, Cancer 47:2803–2806, 1981.

41. Valentin-Opran A, Eilon G, Saez S, et al: Estrogens stimulate release of bone-resorbing activity in cultured human breast cancer cells, J Clin Invest 72:726–731, 1985.

42. Nakayama K, Fukumoto S, Takeda S, et al: Differences in bone and vitamin D metabolism between primary hyperparathyroidism and malignancy-associated hypercalcemia, J Clin Endocrinol Metab 81:607–611, 1996.

43. Grill V, Ho P, Body JJ, et al: PTH-related protein: elevated levels in both humoral hypercalcemia of malignancy and hypercalcemia complicating metastatic breast cancer, J Clin Endocrinol 73:1309–1315, 1991.

44. Isales C, Carcangiu ML, Stewart AF: Hypercalcemia in breast cancer: a reassessment of the mechanism, Am J Med 82:1143–1147, 1987.

45. Fukumoto S, Matsumoto T, Ikeda T, et al: Clinical evaluation of adult T-cell lymphoma, Arch Intern Med 148:921–925, 1988.

46. Wantabe T, Yamaguchi K, Tatasuki K, et al: Constitutive expression of PTHrP gene in HTLV-1 carriers and adult T-cell leukemia patients that can be trans-activated by HTLV-1 tax gene, J Exp Med 172:759–765, 1990.

47. Mune T, Katakami H, Kato Y, et al: Production and secretion of parathyroid hormone-related protein in pheochromocytoma: participation of an α-adrenergic mechanism, J Clin Endocrinol Metab 76:757–762, 1993.

48. Stewart AF, Hoecker J, Segre GV, et al: Hypercalcemia in pheochromocytoma: evidence for a novel mechanism, Ann Intern Med 102:776–779, 1985.

49. Mao C, Carter P, Schaefer P, et al: Malignant islet cell tumor associated with hypercalcemia, Surgery 117:37–40, 1997.

50. Wu T-J, Lin C-L, Taylor RL, et al: Increased parathyroid hormone-related peptide in patients with hypercalcemia associated with islet cell carcinoma, Mayo Clin Proc 72:1111–1115, 1997.

51. Dagdelen S, Kalan I, Gurlek A: Humoral hypercalcemia of benignancy secondary to parathyroid hormone-related protein secreting uterine leiomyoma, Am J Med Sci 335:407–408, 2008.

52. Gordan GS, Fitzpatrick ME, Lubich WP: Identification of osteolytic sterols in human breast cancer, Trans Assoc Am Physicians 80:183–189, 1967.

53. Haddad JG, Couranz SJ, Avioli LV: Circulating phytosterols in normal females, lactating mothers, and breast cancer patients, J Clin Endocrinol Metab 30:174–180, 1970.

54. Klein DC, Raisz LG: Prostaglandins: stimulation of bone resorption in tissue culture, Endocrinology 86:1436–1440, 1970.

55. Tashjian AH: Role of prostaglandins in the production of hypercalcemia by tumors, Cancer Res 38:4138–4141, 1978.

56. Seyberth WJ, Segre GV, Morgan JL, et al: Prostaglandins as mediators of hypercalcemia associated with certain types of cancer, N Engl J Med 293:1278–1283, 1975.

57. Brenner D, Harvey HA, Lipton A, et al: A study of prostaglandin E$_2$ parathormone, and response to indomethacin in patients with hypercalcemia and malignancy, Cancer 49:556–561, 1982.

58. Benson RC, Riggs BL, Pickard BM, et al: Radioimmunoassay of parathyroid hormone in hypercalcemic patients with malignant disease, Am J Med 56:821–826, 1974.

59. Riggs BL, Arnaud CD, Reynolds JC, et al: Immunologic differentiation of primary hyperparathyroidism from hyperparathyroidism due to nonparathyroid cancer, J Clin Invest 50:2079–2083, 1971.

60. Everhart-Caye M, Inzucchi SE, Guinness-Henry J, et al: Parathyroid hormone-related protein(1–36) is equipotent with parathyroid hormone(1–34) in humans, J Clin Endocrinol Metab 81:199, 1996.

61. Henry JG, Mitnick MA, Dann PR, et al: Parathyroid hormone-related protein(1–36) is biologically active when administered subcutaneously to humans, J Clin Endocrinol Metab 82:900–906, 1997.

62. Syed MA, Horwitz MJ, Tedesco MB, et al: Parathyroid hormone-related protein (1–36) stimulates renal tubular calcium reabsorption in normal human volunteers: implications for the pathogenesis of humoral hypercalcemia of malignancy, J Clin Endocrinol Metab 86:1525–1531, 2001.

63. Horwitz MJ, Tedesco MB, Sereika S, et al: Direct comparison of sustained infusion of hPTHrP(1-36) versus hPTH(1-34) on serum calcium, plasma 1,25(OH)$_2$ vitamin D concentrations and fractional calcium excretion in healthy human volunteers, J Clin Endocrinol Metab 88:1603–1609, 2003.

64. Horwitz MJ, Tedesco MB, Sereika SM, et al: Continuous infusion of parathyroid hormone versus parathyroid hormone-related protein in humans: discordant effects on 1,25(OH)$_2$ vitamin D and prolonged suppression of bone formation, J Bone Miner Res 20:1792–1803, 2005.

65. Stewart A, Mangin M, Wu T, et al: A synthetic human parathyroid hormone-like protein stimulates bone resorption and causes hypercalcemia in rats, J Clin Invest 81:596–600, 1988.

66. Henderson J, Bernier S, D'Amour P, et al: Effects of passive immunization against PTH-like peptide in hypercalcemic tumor-bearing rats and normocalcemic controls, Endocrinology 127:1310–1316, 1990.

67. Kukreja SC, Shevrin DH, Wimbiscus SA, et al: Antibodies to PTH-related protein lower serum calcium in athymic mouse models of malignancy associated hypercalcemia due to human tumors, J Clin Invest 82:1798–1802, 1988.

68. Philbrick WM, Wysolmerski JJ, Galbraith S, et al: Defining the physiologic roles of parathyroid hormone-related protein in normal physiology, Physiol Rev 76:127–173, 1996.

69. Strewler GJ: The physiology of parathyroid hormone-related protein, N Engl J Med 342:177–185, 2000.

70. Nussbaum SR, Zahradnik RJ, Lavigne JR, et al: Highly sensitive two-site immunoradiometric assay of parathyrin and its clinical utility in evaluating patients with hypercalcemia, Clin Chem 33:1364–1367, 1987.

71. Dean T, Vilardaga J-P, Potts JT, et al: Altered selectivity of parathyroid hormone (PTH) and PTH-related protein (PTHrP) for distinct conformations of the PTH/PTHrP receptor, Mol Endocrinol 22:156–166, 2008.

72. Coombes RC, Ward MK, Greenberg PB, et al: Calcium metabolism in cancer. Studies using calcium isotopes and immunoassay for parathyroid hormone and calcitonin, Cancer 38:2111–2120, 1976.

73. Ralston SH, Fogelman I, Gardner MD, et al: Hypercalcemia of malignancy: evidence for a non-parathyroid humoral agent with an effect on renal tubular handling of calcium, Clin Sci 66:187–194, 1984.

74. Bonjour J-P, Phillipe J, Guelpa G, et al: Bone and renal components in hypercalcemia of malignancy and response to a single infusion of clodronate, Bone 9:123–130, 1988.

75. Nussbaum SR, Gaz RD, Arnold A: Hypercalcemia and ectopic secretion of PTH by an ovarian carcinoma with rearrangement of the gene for PTH, N Engl J Med 323:1324–1328, 1990.

76. Yoshimoto K, Yamasaki R, Sakai H, et al: Ectopic production of PTH by small cell lung cancer in a patient with hypercalcemia, J Clin Endocrinol Metab 68:976–981, 1989.

77. Strewler GJ, Budayr AA, Clark OH, et al: Production of parathyroid hormone by a malignant nonparathyroid tumor in a hypercalcemic patient, J Clin Endocrinol Metab 76:1373–1375, 1993.

78. Iguchi H, Miyagi C, Tomita K, et al: Hypercalcemia caused by ectopic production of parathyroid hormone in a patient with papillary adenocarcinoma of the thyroid gland, J Clin Endocrinol Metab 83:2653–2657, 1998.

79. Nielsen PK, Rasmussen AK, Feldt-Rasmussen U, et al: Ectopic production of intact parathyroid hormone by a squamous cell lung carcinoma in vivo and in vitro, J Clin Endocrinol Metab 81:3793–3796, 1996.

80. Rizzoli R, Pache J-C, Didierjean L, et al: A thymoma as a cause of true ectopic hyperparathyroidism, J Clin Endocrinol Metab 79:912–915, 1994.

81. Schmeltzer HJ, Hesch RD, Mayer H: Parathyroid hormone and PTH mRNA in a human small cell lung cancer, Recent Results Cancer Res 99:88–93, 1985.

82. VanHouten JN, Yu NY, Rimm D, et al: Hypercalcemia of malignancy due to ectopic transactivation of the parathyroid hormone gene, J Clin Endocrinol Metab 91:580–583, 2006.

83. Metz SA, McRae JR, Robertson RP: Prostaglandins as mediators of paraneoplastic syndromes: review and update, Metabolism 30:299–316, 1981.

84. Rosenthal N, Insogna KL, Godsall JW, et al: Elevations in circulating 1,25 dihydroxyvitamin D in three patients with lymphoma-associated hypercalcemia, J Clin Endocrinol Metab 60:29–33, 1985.

85. Breslau NA, McGuire JL, Zerwekh JE, et al: Hypercalcemia associated with increased serum 1,25 dihydroxyvitamin D in three patients with lymphoma, Ann Intern Med 100:1, 1984.

86. Seymour JF, Gagel RF, Hagemeister FB, et al: Calcitriol production in hypercalcemic and normocalcemic patients with non-Hodgkin lymphoma, Ann Intern Med 121:633–640, 1994.

87. Evans KN, Taylor H, Zehnder D, et al: Increased expression of 25-hydroxyvitamin D-1-alpha-hydroxy-

lase in dysgerminomas: a novel form of humoral hypercalcemia of malignancy, Am J Pathol 165:807–813, 2004.

88. Masahito H, Hara F, Tomishige H, et al: 1,25-Dihydroxyvitamin D–mediated hypercalcemia in ovarian dysgerminoma, Pediatr Hematol Oncol 25:73–78, 2008.

89. Stewart AF, Broadus AE, Schwartz PE, et al: Hypercalcemia in gynecologic neoplasms, Cancer 49:2389–2394, 1982.

90. Bringhurst FR, Bierer BE, Godeau F, et al: Humoral hypercalcemia of malignancy, J Clin Invest 77:456–464, 1986.

91. Bringhurst FR, Varner V, Segre GV: Cancer-associated hypercalcemia: characterization of a new bone-resorbing factor [Abstract], Clin Res 30:386, 1982.

92. Bilezikian JP: Management of acute hypercalcemia, N Engl J Med 326:1196–1203, 1992.

93. Stewart AF: Hypercalcemia associated with cancer, N Engl J Med 352:373–379, 2005.

94. Horwitz MJ, Hodak S, Stewart AF: Non-Parathyroid Hypercalcemia. In Rosen CJ, editor: The American Society for Bone and Mineral Research Primer on Metabolic Bone Diseases and Disorders of Mineral Metabolism, ed 7, Washington D.C., 2008, American Society for Bone and Mineral Research (in press).

95. Suki WN, Yium JJ, Von Minden M, et al: Acute treatment of hypercalcemia with furosemide, N Engl J Med 283:836–840, 1970.

96. Hosking DJ, Cowley A, Bucknall CA: Rehydration in the treatment of severe hypercalcaemia, Q J Med 50:473–481, 1981.

97. Fleisch H: Bisphosphonates: mechanism of action, Endocr Rev 19:80–100, 1998.

98. Russell RG, Rogers MJ: Bisphosphonates: from the laboratory to the clinic and back again, Bone 25:97–106, 1999.

99. Black D, Rosen CJ: Bisphosphonates for the Prevention and Treatment of Osteoporosis. In Favus M, editor: The American Society for Bone and Mineral Research Primer on Metabolic Bone Diseases and Disorders of Mineral Metabolism, ed 6, Washington D.C., 2006, American Society for Bone and Mineral Research, pp 30–35.

100. Rodan GA, Fleisch HA: Bisphosphonates: mechanisms of action, J Clin Invest 97:2692–2696, 1996.

101. Cheer SM, Noble S: Zolendronic acid, Drugs 61:799–805, 2001.

102. Frith JC, Rogers MJ: Antagonistic effects of different classes of bisphosphonates in osteoclasts and macrophages in vitro, J Bone Miner Res 18:204–212, 2003.

103. Major P, Lortholary A, Hon J, et al: Zoledronic acid is superior to pamidronate in the treatment of hypercalcemia of malignancy: A pooled analysis of two randomized controlled clinical trials, J Clin Oncol 19:558–567, 2001.

104. Body JJ, Lortholary A, Romieu G, et al: A dose-finding study of zoledronate in hypercalcemic cancer patients, J Bone Miner Res 14:1557–1561, 1999.

105. Nussbaum S, Younger J, VandePol C, et al: Single dose intravenous therapy with pamidronate for the treatment of hypercalcemia of malignancy: comparison of 30-, 60-, and 90-mg dosages, Am J Med 95:297–304, 1993.

106. Adami S, Bhalla AK, Dorizzi R, et al: The acute-phase response after bisphosphonate administration, Calcif Tissue Int 41:326–331, 1987.

107. Markowitz GS, Appel GB, Fine PL, et al: Collapsing focal segmental glomerulosclerosis following treatment with high-dose pamidronate, J Am Soc Nephrol 12:1164–1172, 2001.

108. Rosen LS, Gordon D, Kaminski M, et al: Long-term efficacy and safety of zoledonic acid compared with pamidronate disodium in the treatment of skeletal complications in patients with advanced multiple myeloma or breast carcinoma: a randomized, double-blind, multicenter, comparative trial, Cancer 98(8):1735–1744, 2003.

109. Perlia CP, Gubisch NJ, Wolter J, et al: Mithramycin treatment of hypercalcemia, Cancer 25:389–394, 1970.

110. Kennedy BJ: Metabolic and toxic effects of mithramycin during tumor therapy, Am J Med 49:494–503, 1970.

111. Hosking DJ, Gilson D: Comparison of the renal and skeletal actions of calcitonin in the treatment of severe hypercalcaemia of malignancy, Q J Med 53:359–368, 1984.

112. Cochran M, Peacock M, Sachs G, et al: Renal effects of calcitonin, BMJ 1:135–137, 1970.

113. Silva OL, Becker KL: Salmon calcitonin in the treatment of hypercalcemia, Arch Intern Med 132:337–339, 1973.

114. Kammerman S, Canfield RE: Effect of porcine calcitonin on hypercalcemia in man, J Clin Endocrinol Metab 31:70–75, 1970.

115. Wisneski LA, Croom WP, Silva OL, et al: Salmon calcitonin in hypercalcemia, Clin Pharmacol Ther 24:219–222, 1978.

116. Warrell RP Jr, Israel R, Frisone M, et al: Gallium nitrate for acute treatment of cancer-related hypercalcemia. A randomized, double-blind comparison to calcitonin, Ann Intern Med 108:669–674, 1988.

117. Fulmer DH, Dimich AB, Rothschild EO, et al: Treatment of hypercalcemia, comparison of intravenously administered phosphate, sulfate, and hydrocortisone, Arch Intern Med 129:923–930, 1972.

118. Percival RC, Yates AJ, Gray RE, et al: Role of glucocorticoids in management of malignant hypercalcaemia, BMJ 289:287, 1984.

119. Camus C, Charasse C, Jouannic-Montier I, et al: Calcium free hemodialysis: Experience in the treatment of 33 patients with severe hypercalcemia, Intensive Care Med 22:116–121, 1996.

120. Koo WS, Jeon DS, Ahn SJ, et al: Calcium-free hemodialysis for the management of hypercalcemia, Nephron 72:424–428, 1996.

121. Cardella CJ, Birkin BL, Rapoport A: Role of dialysis in the treatment of severe hypercalcemia: report of two cases successfully treated with hemodialysis and review of the literature, Clin Nephrol 12:285–290, 1979.

122. Nolph KD, Stoltz M, Maher JF: Calcium free peritoneal dialysis, treatment of vitamin D intoxication, Arch Intern Med 128:809–814, 1971.

123. Hamilton JW, Lasrich M, Hirszel P: Peritoneal dialysis in the treatment of severe hypercalcemia, J Dial 4:129–138, 1980.

124. Miach PJ, Dawborn JK, Martin TJ, et al: Management of the hypercalcaemia of malignancy by peritoneal dialysis, Med J Aust 1:782–784, 1975.

125. Goldsmith RS, Ingbar SH: Inorganic phosphate treatment of hypercalcemia of diverse etiologies, N Engl J Med 274:1–7, 1966.

126. Sato K, Onuma E, Yocum RC, et al: Treatment of malignancy-associated hypercalcemia and cachexia with humanized anti-parathyroid hormone-related protein antibody, Semin Oncol 30:167–173, 2003.

127. Body J-J, Greipp P, Coleman RE, et al: A phase I study of AMGN-00007, a recombinant osteoprotegerin construct, in patients with multiple myeloma or breast cancer related bone metastases, Cancer 97:887–892, 2003.

128. McClung MR, Leweicki EM, Cohen SB, et al: Denosumab in postmenopausal women with low bone mineral density, N Engl J Med 354:821–831, 2006.

129. Bone HG, Bolognese MA, Yuen CK, et al: Effects of denosumab on bone mineral density and bone turnover in postmenopausal women, J Clin Endocrinol Metab 93:2149–2157, 2008.

130. Moroney S, Warmington K, Adamu S, et al: The inhibition of RANKL causes greater suppression of bone resorption and hypercalcemia compared with bisphosphonates in two models of humoral hypercalcemia of malignancy, Endocrinology 146:3235, 2005.

Chapter 9

SURGICAL MANAGEMENT OF HYPERPARATHYROIDISM

JAMES H. ROSING and JEFFREY A. NORTON

Clinical Features and Indications for Surgery

Primary hyperparathyroidism (pHPT) is excessive secretion of parathyroid hormone (PTH) from one or more glands, resulting in hypercalcemia. The diagnosis of pHPT is based on concomitant measurement of elevated serum levels of calcium and intact PTH.

INDICATIONS FOR SURGERY

Patients with pHPT exist on a spectrum from being completely asymptomatic to morbidly symptomatic, based on duration and severity of hypercalcemia. For those who are symptomatic, there are several sited sequelae that remain clear indications for surgery: nephrolithiasis, osteoporosis which can result in pathologic bone fractures, progressive renal injury, neuromuscular and neurocognitive impairments such as fatigue, inability to concentrate, and depression, as well as the rare phenomenon of hypercalcemic crisis.[1-3]

The best treatment for totally asymptomatic patients is still a subject of controversy.[1-3] The 2008 Workshop on Primary Hyperparathyroidism recommended criteria for surgical treatment in these asymptomatic patients[4]:

- Age < 50 years
- Ca ≥ 1 mg/dL above normal
- 24-hour urinary calcium > 400 mg
- Creatinine clearance < 60 mL/min/1.73m^2
- Bone mineral density T score ≤ 2.5, any site
- Failure of medical management

This group certainly has no urgent need for surgery. Regular follow-up is indicated to avoid disease progression. Surgery is usually recommended for younger patients (<50 years), as symptoms will develop in approximately 20% of these patients with long-term follow-up.[3,5] Neuromuscular symptoms such as weakness (20% to 60%) occur in patients with pHPT, and successful surgery reverses these symptoms in most patients.[6]

In general, surgery is indicated for all patients with clear biochemical evidence of pHPT and documented signs or symptoms of the disease. In apparently asymptomatic patients with pHPT, surgery is indicated for younger patients who have a low operative risk and long temporal exposure to the disease. In apparently asymptomatic older patients, surgery is reserved for patients in whom evidence of progression and/or symptoms develop. Progression is measured by a decrease in bone density (T score ≤ 2.5 at any site), elevated serum calcium (≥1 mg/dL above normal), or urinary levels of calcium greater than 400 mg/24 hours.[4]

PROGNOSTIC INDICATORS OF PARATHYROID PATHOLOGY

Certain symptoms and signs are useful predictors of different types of parathyroid pathology. Parathyroid adenoma is seldom if ever palpable, but parathyroid carcinoma is usually palpable.[7] Exceptionally high concentrations of PTH or calcium in serum also may suggest parathyroid cancer.[7] The diagnosis of familial multiple endocrine neoplasia type 1 (MEN1) or MEN2a predicts parathyroid hyperplasia[7-9]; however, there is wide variation in the size of the abnormal parathyroid glands in patients with MEN1, so there might be a failure of the surgeon to recognize hyperplasia.[10] The presence of multiple lipomas can occur in MEN1. Studies have identified the genetic defect in patients with MEN1 to be a *MENIN* mutation on chromosome 11q13[11] and in patients with MEN2, a *RET* proto-oncogene mutation on chromosome 10.[12] MEN2 must be distinguished from familial

MEN2b, because hyperparathyroidism is not part of the latter. Familial hypocalciuric hypercalcemia (FHH) is an autosomal dominant trait usually manifested as asymptomatic hypercalcemia and relative hypocalciuria.[9,13] Mutations in the calcium-sensing receptor gene on chromosome 3 have been identified in a heterozygous form in benign FHH[9] but not in sporadic adenomas. In patients with FHH, the hypercalcemia is PTH dependent and associated with mild parathyroid hyperplasia; however, subtotal parathyroidectomy is not effective and contraindicated. In such cases, measurement of urinary calcium excretion and detection of relative hypocalciuria (<100 mg/24 hours) should lead to cancellation of surgery and testing for hypercalcemia and hypocalciuria in relatives.[13]

PARATHYROID CRISIS

Parathyroid crisis is an unusual state of progressive, marked hyperparathyroidism producing anorexia, vomiting, dehydration, decrease in renal function, progressive hypercalcemia, deterioration of mental status, confusion, coma, and if untreated, death.[14,15] Fatigue, muscle weakness, polyuria, and polydipsia are also frequent. Hypercalcemia may have been noted in the past but left untreated or inadequately treated. Often, no apparent reason can be found for the sudden worsening of hyperparathyroidism. Some cases are apparently precipitated by bacterial or viral infection, trauma, or recent surgery. Serum calcium should not be the only defining criterion for a hypercalcemic crisis, because asymptomatic patients with serum calcium of 20 mg/dL and patients in hypercalcemic crisis with serum calcium less than 14 mg/dL have been reported.[16] Severe hyperparathyroidism may also be a manifestation of parathyroid carcinoma, which should be considered in the differential diagnosis.[7]

Parathyroid crisis is a potentially life-threatening disorder that requires vigorous medical management in preparation for definitive surgery. Attention must first be directed toward hydration, reduction of the hypercalcemia, and stabilization of the clinical state. Large amounts of intravenous saline are administered to ensure rehydration. This is followed by furosemide, which further reduces the hypercalcemia. At the same time, the diagnosis of hyperparathyroidism is established by measuring serum levels of calcium and intact PTH. If hydration and treatment with furosemide intravenously are not effective in reducing the hypercalcemia, treatment with bisphosphonates, calcitonin, or cinacalcet might be necessary, but surgery is indicated as quickly as the patient can be stabilized, because the crisis can worsen rapidly.[14]

Minimally Invasive Parathyroidectomy: Procedures for Preoperative and Intraoperative Localization of Abnormal Parathyroid Glands

PARATHYROID LOCALIZATION BEFORE INITIAL SURGERY

The overall trend in surgery over the past 10 years is towards minimally invasive techniques. The objective is to minimize length of incisions and the associated increased pain, higher rate of infection, and longer duration of hospital stay. With the ability to now reliably localize abnormal parathyroid glands and confirm their removal intraoperatively, minimally invasive para-

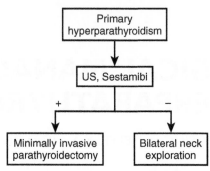

LOCALIZATION STRATEGY IN PREVIOUSLY UNOPERATED PATIENTS

FIGURE 9-1. Flow diagram for localization strategy in previously unoperated patients. *US*, Ultrasound.

thyroidectomy (MIP) has become the procedure of choice for pHPT.[17-23]

There is general consensus that the best localization procedures for initial parathyroid operations are the combination of ultrasound (US) and sestamibi scanning (Fig. 9-1). The single best preoperative localization study is sestamibi, which has a specificity of 98%, but there has been reported variation in localization sensitivity for pHPT from 43% to 91%.[24,25] It has been recently reported that sestamibi optimization of acquisition and processing parameters may improve scan sensitivity in pHPT.[26] Sestamibi is a monovalent lipophilic cation that diffuses passively across the cell membrane and concentrates in mitochondria. It is preferentially concentrated in abnormal parathyroid tissue because of increased blood supply, higher metabolic activity, and an absence of p-glycoprotein on the cell membrane. Sestamibi scans can be done preoperatively to plan a MIP (Fig. 9-2).[20,27-34] High-resolution ultrasound is also a useful study for preoperative parathyroid localization.[35-37] It images the abnormal parathyroid gland as a hypoechoic (sonolucent) mass compared to the more echo-dense thyroid tissue (Fig. 9-3). It is specific, but it is not as sensitive as sestamibi. Its specificity is 98% and sensitivity is 66%.[38] Further, if both sestamibi and ultrasound are positive in the same location, the patient is virtually assured that an abnormal parathyroid gland will be found and removed.

PARATHYROID LOCALIZATION BEFORE REPEAT SURGERY

In patients with persistent or recurrent (normocalcemia for 6 months or longer, then recurrent hypercalcemia) hyperparathyroidism, the chance of successful surgery is reduced,[39,40] and the incidence of complications is greater.[41-43] Therefore, maximum effort at parathyroid gland localization is made, commencing with the noninvasive procedures (US, computed tomography [CT], magnetic resonance imaging [MRI], and sestamibi scanning) and proceeding, if necessary, to the more invasive studies (Fig. 9-4). Currently, noninvasive techniques localize an abnormal gland in about 75% to 80% of patients requiring repeat surgery,[44] whereas invasive studies, such as venous sampling, selective angiography, or percutaneous ultrasound/CT-guided fine-needle aspiration, help with the remainder.[45,46]

Ultrasound

US, using a 10-MHz probe, is readily available, noninvasive, and the least expensive technique to preoperatively image abnormal parathyroid glands. It is particularly effective for localizing

Ant. TC99M MIBI

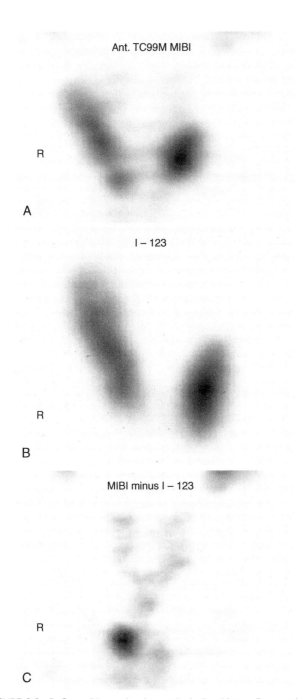

A

I – 123

B

MIBI minus I – 123

C

FIGURE 9-2. A, Sestamibi scan showing uptake in thyroid as well as parathyroid tissue. **B,** Thyroid uptake of I-123. **C,** Subtracted image of sestamibi without I-123.

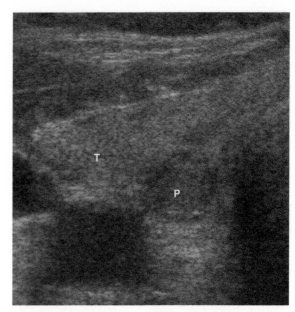

FIGURE 9-3. Hypoechoic mass *(P)* is an intrathyroidal parathyroid adenoma, with the more echogenic right superior thyroid lobe *(T)*.

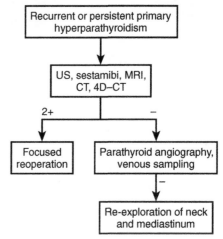

FIGURE 9-4. Flow diagram for localization strategy in previously operated patients.

enlarged parathyroid glands in the neck and can be used to identify 60% of the abnormal glands in patients requiring reoperation.[44] US identifies juxtathyroidal parathyroid glands (see Fig. 9-3).

US has some disadvantages. It is operator-dependent, making the accuracy variable.[35,37,38,47] It may fail to image posterior glands in the tracheoesophageal groove and glands in the anterior mediastinum. In multiple-gland hyperplasia, it generally demonstrates only the dominant gland.

Sestamibi Scintigraphy

Technetium 99m–labeled sestamibi scanning has superior resolution and sensitivity (80% to 90%) in detecting hypercellular parathyroid glands prior to reoperations.[48] Both the thyroid and

parathyroid will take up sestamibi, but the uptake will be stronger and the signal will persist longer in parathyroid adenomas or hyperplasia (see Fig. 9-2). The combination of single-photon emission CT (SPECT) with sestamibi has improved the sensitivity to about 85%, especially for deep cervical and mediastinal parathyroid tumors.[25] Sestamibi has been combined with the gamma probe for hand-held intraoperative localization of abnormal parathyroid glands.[27,29-34] Advocates suggest that this approach is less invasive and can be done under local anesthesia as an outpatient procedure through a smaller incision. Sestamibi scans facilitate the dissection and make the surgery easier, but they have not been shown to affect the outcome in previously unoperated patients. One study demonstrated that there was no significant difference in cure rate between patients who had preoperative sestamibi scan and those who did not. The cure rate was 97.5% and 99%, respectively. However, there was a significant difference in cure rate between the negative sestamibi scan group (92.7%) and both the no-scan group (99.3%) and the positive-scan group (100%). Thus sestamibi scan can be used to

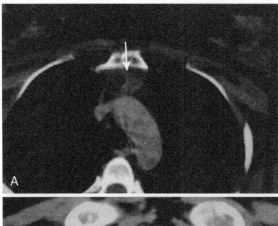
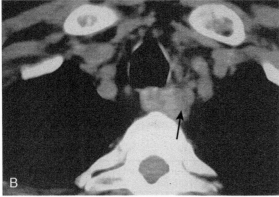

FIGURE 9-5. CT is the most useful imaging modality for identifying parathyroid adenomas located in the mediastinum **(A)** or in the tracheoesophageal groove **(B).**

identify those patients who are less likely to have successful surgery.[49]

Computed Tomography

CT is particularly effective for identifying ectopic glands in the anterior mediastinum and enlarged glands in the tracheoesophageal groove. Ectopic glands in the anterior mediastinum often lie within the fat-replaced thymus, and even small adenomas are readily visualized (Fig. 9-5A). Ectopic glands in the tracheoesophageal groove are detected as a solid mass adjacent to the esophagus (Fig. 9-5B). Undescended glands near the carotid bifurcation are also identified by CT, provided that the examination is carried up to the level of the hyoid bone. On the other hand, CT is poor at detecting intrathyroid or juxtathyroid tumors and exposes the patient to risks associated with contrast media and radiation.

Magnetic Resonance Imaging

Initial experience with MRI of abnormal parathyroid glands has been successful for large parathyroid adenomas, which on T2-weighted or stir-pulse sequences produce a bright signal.[50] In the mediastinum, this signal may be confused with fat, and a T1-weighted image is required to specifically identify the pathology. With gadolinium-enhanced MRI and T1- and T2-weighted images, MRI can now provide higher sensitivity than CT for identifying ectopic parathyroid tumors. It can be a useful study, and it may have more sensitivity than CT.

Angiography

The potential for morbidity associated with angiographic procedures to localize parathyroid glands limits its use to patients with symptomatic persistent or recurrent hyperparathyroidism requir-

ing reoperation. Intraarterial digital techniques have greatly simplified angiographic localization of parathyroid pathology. Because digital examination does not require highly selective catheter positioning, it can be accomplished expeditiously. The improved sensitivity of digital subtraction arteriography makes it possible to significantly reduce the total dose of water-soluble contrast material, thereby decreasing adverse effects on the kidney in a group of patients who may already have compromised renal function.

Selective Venous Sampling for Parathyroid Hormone

Selective venous sampling requires the greatest experience and is the most variably performed of all the localizing procedures in nonreferral centers. Contrast load, radiation exposure, and cost (15 to 20 PTH determinations), in addition to radiography costs, are all significant. Moreover, gradients determined by selective catheterization identify only the region of pathology (e.g., right side of the neck, mediastinum) but do not image the elusive gland. A new technique is to add the rapid PTH assay to selective venous sampling to provide a short turnaround time and allow the radiologist to obtain more selective samples in regions in which high concentrations of PTH are found. This combination of venous sampling and rapid PTH assay localized the abnormal parathyroid gland correctly in 6 of 7 patients who had negative noninvasive imaging and required reoperation for prior unsuccessful parathyroid surgery.[51] It is indicated in only a small proportion of reoperative patients who have significant primary hyperparathyroidism and no apparent localizing information after completing all noninvasive studies and angiography.

Positron Emission Tomography

Regional body fluorodeoxyglucose positron emission tomography (FDG-PET) has been evaluated as a means of localizing pathology in recurrent hyperparathyroidism. Regional PET imaging of the neck and upper chest was able to identify 79% of parathyroid adenomas in 20 patients.[52] PET appears to have potential; however, is relatively expensive compared to other more commonly utilized localization techniques. It is not used frequently for abnormal parathyroid gland localization.

Four-Dimensional Computed Tomography

4D-CT is the latest described technology for the preoperative evaluation of patients with parathyroid disease. 4D-CT adds to existing CT by detecting the perfusion characteristics of parathyroid and is able to differentiate between normal and hyperfunctioning glands (which have rapid uptake and quick washout). In a way, this is similar to CT angiography. This modality combines anatomic and functional localization in a single study, with preliminary data suggesting greater accuracy than sestamibi scan. Perhaps the greatest yield with 4D-CT imaging will be in localization of hyperfunctioning glands in the setting of persistent or recurrent parathyroid disease.[53]

Summary of Radiographic Localization

We suggest that sestamibi and US be used in patients undergoing initial exploration for pHPT. Accurate preoperative localization studies allow a minimally invasive parathyroidectomy that shortens hospital stay, minimizes scar, and provides a successful outcome. Furthermore, in patients undergoing reoperations, preoperative radiologic localization studies are necessary and helpful to plan the operative approach (see Fig. 9-4). We recommend liberal use of each of the noninvasive imaging studies (US, CT,

INTRAOPERATIVE PTH: ADENOMA

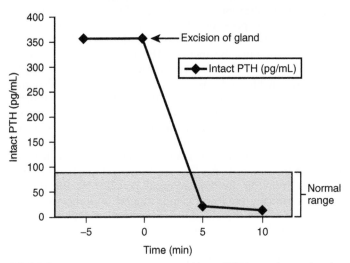

FIGURE 9-6. Intraoperative measurement of intact PTH in a patient undergoing surgery for an adenoma. After the parathyroid adenoma is removed, the serum PTH levels decrease more than 50% from the median baseline level, indicating a successful outcome, and the surgery is terminated.

INTRAOPERATIVE PTH: HYPERPLASIA

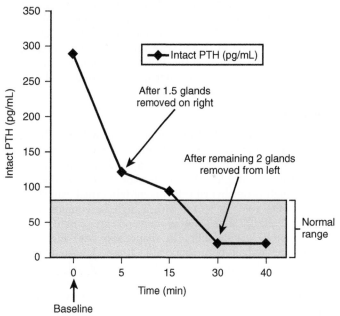

FIGURE 9-7. Intraoperative measurement of intact PTH in a patient who underwent neck exploration for pHPT. The right upper gland and half of the right lower gland were excised. Both appeared abnormally large, and frozen section analysis showed hypercellular tissue. The PTH decreased to less than 50% baseline, but it did not return to the normal range (<80 pg/mL). The left neck was explored, and both parathyroid glands were excised. The PTH level subsequently dropped within normal range.

^{99m}Tc-sestamibi, and MRI) as an initial imaging cluster. If two studies identify the abnormal parathyroid gland in the same location, we proceed with surgery. Our institution is currently establishing 4D-CT technology, but it is not yet available. As such, if the noninvasive studies are equivocal, we then perform arteriography. If that study is positive, we perform surgery; if negative, we recommend selective venous sampling for rapid PTH measurements (as discussed above).[51]

Intraoperative Determination of Parathyroid Hormone

Intraoperative determination of PTH allows rapid monitoring of parathyroid status during parathyroid surgery.[54] Generally, after successful removal of a single parathyroid adenoma or adequate resection of hyperplastic glands, serum PTH levels begin to fall immediately and reach a 50% drop from the baseline level or normal range within 10 to 15 minutes.[55] Studies demonstrate that serum levels of intact PTH decline rapidly, only 5 minutes after resection of a parathyroid adenoma (Fig. 9-6).[56,57] Furthermore, the rate of decline is less in patients with hyperplasia and may provide an additional intraoperative means of diagnosing hyperplasia (Fig. 9-7).[58] A serum sample for PTH should be obtained just after the induction of anesthesia. Repeated serum samples are obtained intraoperatively immediately following resection of an enlarged gland, and then 10 minutes following removal. This protocol has been designed to take into account the half-life of PTH, which is 1 to 4 minutes, and avoid misleading results from a spike in concentration that may occur during handling and removal of the adenoma.[57] A 50% reduction in the PTH level from the median baseline level indicates a successful outcome (see Fig. 9-6).[56] Some also recommend a second criterion of a normal serum level of PTH. The operation can be terminated on this result without identification of other parathyroid glands. Furthermore, the assay can be used to diagnose an abnormal parathyroid gland by performing fine needle aspiration (FNA) of a mass lesion and then diluting the sample with heparinized saline and measuring PTH levels—which will be very high if the mass is parathyroid tissue.[58]

Intraoperative determination of PTH levels appears to complement surgical skill and histopathologic information and has the potential to provide additional guidance regarding the extent and degree of neck exploration. However, false-negative results[57] or technical difficulties may be encountered, and this information may be difficult to interpret in the case of double adenoma or hyperplasia. Nevertheless, its use has greatly facilitated minimally invasive parathyroidectomy, and operative failure rates with the use of intraoperative PTH assay have decreased from 6% to 1.5% for initial operations[59] and from 24% to 6% for reoperations.[60]

Surgical Management of Primary Hyperparathyroidism

Surgery is the mainstay for treatment of pHPT. The methods of surgery are becoming less invasive. The possible causes of pHPT are adenoma (83%), hyperplasia (15%), double adenoma (1% to 2%), and carcinoma (1%).[61] Some argue that double adenomas might represent undetected hyperplasia. However, studies have shown that recurrent disease does not develop in patients with removed double adenomas after long follow-up.[62,63] This suggests that the diagnosis of double adenoma is real. A family history of parathyroid disease or associated endocrinopathies is associated with hyperplasia. A history of neck irradiation is associated with adenoma.[64]

Before performing surgery for pHPT, the surgeon must obtain informed consent, which requires careful discussion of the outcome and complications. A successful initial parathyroid surgery, using either minimally invasive techniques or bilateral cervical exploration, is expected in greater than 95% of patients undergoing initial operations[21,22,64] and in 78% to 90% of reoperations.[65,66] Udelsman et al.[42] recently reported a success rate for reoperative surgery for pHPT as high as 96%. Recurrent laryngeal nerve injury occurs in less than 1% of initial operations[64] and more than 5% of repeat operations.[41] Fortunately, the symptoms in many of these nerve injuries are temporary, and full recovery may be seen at the 3- to 6-month follow-up. Hypoparathyroidism rarely occurs after initial explorations but may occur in 2.7% to 16% of reoperations.[65,66]

ANATOMY

Facility in the surgical identification of normal and abnormal parathyroid glands is essential. Parathyroid glands vary in color from light yellow to reddish brown, and the consistency is usually soft and pliable.[67] A reddish color and dense consistency reflect a high parenchymal cell content (abnormal gland); a yellowish white color is found with a high fat content (normal gland).[67] Typically, four parathyroid glands are present.

Parathyroid glands differ in shape and size. Eighty-three percent are oval or bean-shaped, 11% are elongated, 5% are bilobate, and 1% are multilobated.[67] Normal glands tend to be flat and ovoid; with enlargement, they become globular. Normal measurements are 3 × 5 × 7 mm. The combined weight of all parathyroid glands is 90 to 130 mg, and the superior glands are usually smaller than the inferior glands.[64] Most parathyroid glands are suspended by a small vascular pedicle and enveloped by a pad of fatty tissue.[68]

Autopsy series demonstrate that four glands are found in 91% of subjects, five glands in 4%, and three glands in 5%.[69] In studies done by serial sectioning of embryos, at least four parathyroid glands are found in every specimen.[69] Approximately 5% of humans have supernumerary (more than four) parathyroid glands.[70] Supernumerary glands and fragments of parathyroid glands are most commonly found within the thymus.

Although gland distribution may deviate widely, the location of parathyroid glands is predictable from knowledge of embryology.[68] Originating from the fourth pharyngeal pouch,[71] the superior parathyroid glands are commonly found along the posterior surface of the upper two-thirds of the thyroid gland (92%)[67] (Fig. 9-8). Frequently (40%), superior parathyroid gland adenomas migrate posteriorly, behind the inferior thyroid artery to a posi-

tion along the esophagus.[61] Division of the superior thyroid artery and mobilization of the superior thyroid pole are usually unnecessary to expose the superior parathyroid glands, but the fascia connecting the lateral portion of the thyroid lobe to the carotid sheath must be incised. The location of the superior glands is relatively constant, and these glands can generally be identified quickly and easily. Superior parathyroid adenomas may have a unique relationship to the recurrent laryngeal nerve such that the nerve is embedded in the anterior medial capsule of the adenoma, or the gland can be rounded and tucked into the exact spot where the recurrent nerve enters the larynx.

The inferior parathyroid glands have a more variable distribution than the superior ones (see Fig. 9-8). With the thymus, they originate from the third pharyngeal pouch.[71] As the thymus migrates caudally, the lower glands migrate until they reach the lower pole of the thyroid gland. Seventeen percent of inferior parathyroid glands touch the inferior border of the thyroid, 44% are within 1 cm of the inferior border of the thyroid (also known as the *thyrothymic ligament*), 26% are within the superior horn of the thymus, and 2% are in the mediastinal thymus.[67,68] The remainder are either within the thyroid or are undescended in the upper portion of the neck near the carotid bifurcation[72] (see Fig. 9-8). This variable anatomic distribution makes the inferior glands more difficult to locate than the superior ones. An inferior parathyroid adenoma is generally bordered posteriorly and laterally by the recurrent laryngeal nerve and is inferior to the inferior thyroid artery.

GENERAL TECHNIQUE OF EXPLORATION

It appears that some form of minimally invasive parathyroid surgery has replaced standard bilateral neck exploration for pHPT. This is still controversial, and some recent studies suggest that standard bilateral neck exploration is just as good and less expensive.[73] However, most surgeons, endocrinologists, and patients now think that MIP is preferable because it is associated with similar excellent results, less pain, better cosmesis, and more rapid recovery.[74] We recommend the use of intraoperative rapid PTH assay to assess outcome intraoperatively without extensive exploration, but this has been controversial; one group has demonstrated that this is unnecessary if sestamibi demonstrates a single abnormal gland.[75] General endotracheal anesthesia is used, although regional block anesthesia has been advocated by some and is equally effective (Fig. 9-9).[76,77] Local anesthesia or regional block has been advocated for the elderly undergoing targeted parathyroidectomy.[76]

Intraoperative PTH assay is performed as described previously. The patient is positioned in a manner as for thyroid surgery. A 3-cm transverse cervical incision is made approximately 2 cm above the sternal notch in a skin crease. It is centered on the side of the localization studies and the anterior border of the sternocleidomastoid muscle. A focused approach directly to the abnormal parathyroid gland is made based on the preoperative imaging results. Alternatively, some recommend an approach based on a hand-held gamma probe to detect labeled sestamibi within the adenoma.[78] Because a high proportion (90%) of parathyroid adenomas are imaged by sestamibi scanning, the technique is used to guide intraoperative localization of the abnormal gland with a hand-held gamma detector.[27,30-33] Then under local anesthesia, an incision is made in the area of highest radioactivity, and dissection is focused on the abnormal "hot" adenoma. This technique can be combined with immediate PTH assay to quickly determine whether all the abnormal parathyroid tissue has been removed. The method relies on radioac-

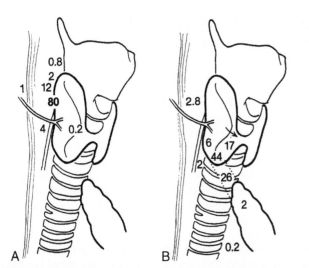

FIGURE 9-8. Diagram of potential locations of superior **(A)** and inferior **(B)** parathyroid glands. Numbers refer to the percentage of glands found at each location. (From Akerstrom G, Malmaeus J, Bergstrom R: Surgical anatomy of human parathyroid glands. Surgery 95:14, 1984.)

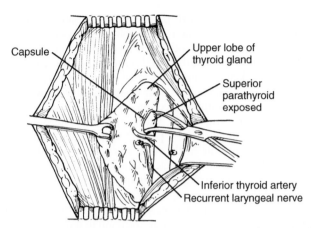

FIGURE 9-9. Identification of a left superior parathyroid adenoma. The thyroid gland is elevated with a Babcock clamp. The investing thyroid fascia is opened posterior to the upper pole of the left lobe. A left upper parathyroid adenoma is identified superior to the inferior thyroid artery and posterolateral to the recurrent laryngeal nerve. The left recurrent laryngeal nerve is shown in its usual location within the tracheoesophageal groove and posterior to the inferior thyroid artery.

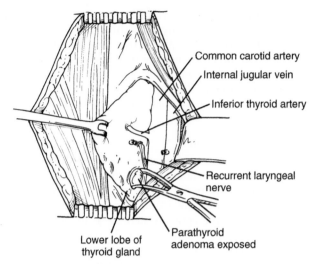

FIGURE 9-10. Identification of a left inferior parathyroid adenoma. The thyroid gland is elevated with a Babcock clamp. A left lower parathyroid adenoma is identified inferior to the inferior thyroid artery and anteromedial to the recurrent laryngeal nerve, which is the most common position for a left inferior parathyroid adenoma, although the inferior parathyroid gland can be located in other positions.

tive detection and PTH measurement to guide surgery rather than precise operative identification. It may be limited in identification of multiple abnormal glands and glands adjacent to the thyroid, which may also be hot. Limited sub-platysmal flaps are raised, since the goal of surgery is to remove a solitary adenoma and not to perform a standard neck exploration. Because of this, limited mobilization of the thyroid gland is performed, and retraction of the strap muscles on the side of the dissection is done. Dissection is focused on the preoperative localization studies, and the abnormal parathyroid gland is removed.

The surgeon should be aware of the relationship of the parathyroid glands to the recurrent laryngeal nerves and avoid injury to the nerve. The upper glands are posterior and lateral to the recurrent laryngeal nerve (see Fig. 9-9), while the lower glands are anterior and medial to it (Fig. 9-10). The vascular pedicle is either ligated, clipped, or controlled with the harmonic scalpel, and the specimen is sent to pathology. The intraoperative PTH blood levels are measured while the wound is closed. The procedure is not terminated until the levels drop 50% from the median baseline level and/or into the normal range (see Fig. 9-6). The success of MIP has been confirmed to be the same as bilateral standard neck exploration. For example, in 255 consecutive MIPs, the cure rate was 99%, and the complication rate was 1.2%. MIP has been associated with a 50% reduction in operating room time and shorter hospitalization (Table 9-1).[21] However, MIP may artificially increase the probability of adenoma and decrease the chance of detection of hyperplasia or multiple gland disease. Two recent independent studies documented that the rate of hyperplasia with MIP was lower than the expected rate of 15% for standard bilateral explorations.[79,80] If the serum levels of PTH do not drop or there is evidence for hyperplasia on the preoperative imaging studies or by family history, the conventional bilateral neck exploration is performed.

SPECIAL ISSUES IN SURGERY
Unsuccessful MIP

If focused MIP is unsuccessful, bilateral neck exploration is recommended. Essentially, this is the standard parathyroid exploration that was done for years with consistent high probability of success and low complication rate. Any enlarged or abnormal

Table 9-1. Success of Minimally Invasive Parathyroidectomy Compared to Bilateral Neck Exploration

656 Consecutive Parathyroidectomies 1990–2001	401 BNE	255 MIP
Complications	3%	1.2%
Cure rate	97%	99%
Operating time	2.4 hr	1.3 hr
Length of stay (days)	1.64	0.24
Mean cost savings	—	$2,693 per procedure

Abstracted from Udelsman R: Six hundred fifty-six consecutive explorations for primary hyperparathyroidism. Ann Surg 235:665–670; discussion 670–662, 2002.
BNE, Bilateral Neck Exploration; *MIP*, minimally invasive parathyroidectomy.

glands are removed.[64] The most important indicator of normal or abnormal parathyroid tissue is the appearance of the gland. Pathologists may find it difficult to differentiate normal from hypercellular parathyroid tissue or hyperplasia from adenoma, but they can reliably confirm that whatever tissue was biopsied is parathyroid.[77] If two glands are enlarged (double adenoma), both are removed. Long-term results with this method of management have been highly satisfactory.[63,64]

Hyperplasia

In generalized four-gland enlargement or hyperplasia, surgical management is more difficult and the results less satisfactory. Intraoperative PTH levels may help distinguish between adenoma and hyperplasia and help guide the amount of parathyroid resection. Abnormal parathyroid glands should be removed until the levels drop 50% from the median baseline preoperative level and into the normal range (see Figs. 9-6 and 9-7). Studies suggest that subtotal (3.5-gland) parathyroidectomy is the procedure of choice for hyperplasia. This is primarily because of an unacceptably high incidence of hypoparathyroidism with 4-gland parathyroidectomy and transplant. The cervical thymus should also be removed because supernumerary glands or fragments of parathyroid glands are commonly found within it. The results of subtotal parathyroidectomy have been variable, with a 13% incidence of persistent disease, a 15% incidence of recurrent disease, and a similar incidence of hypoparathyroidism. The surgical approach is removal of 3.5 parathyroid glands, with approximately 30 to 50 mg of the most normal-appearing parathyroid tissue left and marked with a surgical clip in the neck. If recurrent hypercalcemia develops, a portion of the remaining marked hyperplastic parathyroid gland can be removed at a reoperation.[81-84]

Mediastinal Exploration

If a patient undergoes an unsuccessful operation for hyperparathyroidism, the patient should be reevaluated, and localization procedures should be performed (see Fig. 9-4). Median sternotomy is indicated in only 1% to 2% of patients undergoing initial exploration and approximately 20% to 30% of those requiring reoperation. In our series of 33 patients who underwent median sternotomy as part of a reoperation for pHPT,[85] 30% did not have abnormal parathyroid tissue in the mediastinum.[86] Of the abnormal mediastinal glands found, most were discovered in the thymus (64%), and some were not visible during surgery. This mandates that a total thymectomy should be performed during any mediastinal exploration for pHPT. Wells and Cooper[86] have reported the ability to remove the entire thymus (including the mediastinal component) without dividing the sternum by using a special retractor to elevate the sternum. This procedure may be used to remove mediastinal parathyroid adenomas less invasively. Mediastinal parathyroid adenomas have also been reported in the aortopulmonary window.

Secondary and Tertiary Hyperparathyroidism

Almost all patients with advanced renal failure who are maintained by chronic dialysis have evidence of bone disease secondary to hyperparathyroidism and elevated serum levels of PTH.[87-89] Medical therapy has improved the course of these patients (see Chapter 14), but genetic evidence has shown that monoclonal transformations with specific genetic mutations sometimes arise in these patients, so that parathyroid gland growth independence has occurred that may explain resistant hypercalcemia. Clinically, additional potential indications for parathyroidectomy include (1) hypercalcemia in prospective renal transplant patients; (2) pathologic fractures secondary to renal osteodystrophy; (3) symptoms such as pruritus, bone pain, and extensive soft-tissue calcification and calciphylaxis; (4) hypercalcemia in patients with well-functioning renal transplants; and (5) a calcium-times-phosphate product greater than 70.[89] Improvements in medical management have reduced the need for surgery. Successful parathyroid surgery plus appropriate supplementation with vitamin D and calcium provide a marked increase in lumbar bone marrow density and a modest increase in radial bone marrow density in renal failure patients with secondary HPT.[90]

Reoperations for Primary Hyperparathyroidism

Reoperations for pHPT should be classified as operations for either persistent disease or recurrent disease. *Persistent disease* means that hypercalcemia never resolved after the initial neck exploration. *Recurrent disease* means that hypercalcemia recurs after 6 months of normalization of serum calcium. The complexity of repeat neck surgery for primary hyperparathyroidism makes it imperative to confirm the diagnosis and presence of symptoms and to order preoperative localization studies (see Fig. 9-4).[42,43,65] The prior operative record and pathology reports are reviewed.

The first operative report, pathology results, and localization studies are used to plan the re-exploration. For example, if two abnormal parathyroid glands were removed and the family history is positive for parathyroid disease, the working diagnosis is hyperplasia. A biopsy-proven normal gland found at the initial procedure and radiologic localization studies suggesting a mediastinal adenoma prompt a direct mediastinal approach. Designing the operation—right side, left side, median sternotomy, all or any—can be done only by putting all the data together. We use an alternative route in the neck along the medial border of the sternocleidomastoid muscle instead of between the strap muscles.[42,43,53,65] This technique requires a separate approach on each side of the neck. It is especially important to look for intrathyroid, intrathymic, and paraesophageal parathyroid adenomas because ectopic locations are more common in reoperations (Fig. 9-11).

It should be remembered that even during reoperations for primary hyperparathyroidism, most abnormal glands can be removed through a cervical incision[65] (see Fig. 9-11). Abnormal parathyroid glands may be retroesophageal or posterior along the tracheoesophageal groove, which is the most common missed position.[50,53] They may be intrathyroidal,[91] or they may be located in an undescended parathymic remnant high in the carotid sheath.[92] A missed adenoma may be located in pharyngeal or adjacent structures like the vagus nerve.[93] If these abnormal glands are not in the neck, they may be in the thymus. Slow, meticulous exploration in a bloodless field is generally necessary to find these "ectopic" glands (see Fig. 9-11).

Reoperative parathyroid disease remains a major challenge. It is clear that operative risk increases with each succeeding re-exploration. However, with careful attention to confirmation of the diagnosis, prior operative records, and judicious use of preoperative localization, a successful outcome may be achieved in approximately 90% of reoperations.[50,92]

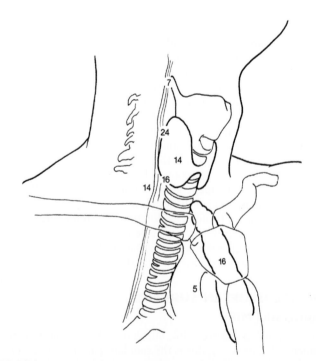

FIGURE 9-11. Location of abnormal parathyroid glands found during reoperations for pHPT. Numbers refer to the percentage of glands found at each location.

Parathyroid Carcinoma

Parathyroid carcinoma should be considered in the working diagnosis of patients with pHPT when the serum level of calcium is very high (>14 mg/dL), in patients with vocal cord paralysis, in patients with evidence of local recurrence of the abnormal gland, or when a palpable neck mass is present.[7,94] Parathyroid carcinoma may be familial.[95]

It is difficult to accurately assess the spectrum of clinical manifestations, degree of malignancy, and prognosis of parathyroid carcinoma. The incidence is very low, and the malignancy appears to be diagnosed at an earlier stage as a result of earlier detection of hypercalcemia. A major problem is failure to properly identify the correct pathologic diagnosis during the operation and, therefore, failure to perform adequate resection of the carcinomatous parathyroid tissue along with the ipsilateral lobe of the thyroid.[7,96] Unequivocal pathologic features of parathyroid carcinoma include the identification of mitoses in several high-power microscopic fields, fibrous bands or desmoplasia, and evidence of distant metastases or direct local invasion of the capsule, adjacent structures, and blood vessels.[97] However, not all patients with parathyroid carcinoma have all these features, so the diagnosis must be ascertained from clinical as well as pathologic evidence.[7] Furthermore, the natural history of patients with parathyroid cancer appears to be variable. Some tumors disseminate rapidly and have a poor prognosis,[98] whereas others tend to recur locally and have a long disease-free interval.[7]

Literature reports involving single cases tend to emphasize more serious tumors, either intrinsically malignant or longstanding, with clear evidence of extraglandular spread at the initial operation. The cancer is usually invading along the tracheoesophageal groove, and the patient may have hoarseness secondary to a recurrent laryngeal nerve injury. At neck exploration, the carcinomatous tissue appears gray with a thick, hard capsule. We recommend, based on suspicion (e.g., mass, local recurrence, high serum level of calcium), wide excision, including thyroid lobectomy in continuity with the tumor.[7,96,97] If one has doubt about the diagnosis, biopsy of tumor extrinsic from the main tumor mass, either within lymph nodes or invading local strap muscle, provides clear evidence of cancer. Recurrent laryngeal nerve injury, either from the tumor itself or from the surgeon attempting to completely resect the tumor mass with the ipsilateral thyroid lobe, is probable and occurs in 75% of patients.[7] Locally recurrent benign parathyroid adenomas may occur and be confused with parathyroid carcinomas. Recurrent adenomas generally have a longer disease-free interval, a lower serum level of calcium, and a history of either incomplete resection or spillage of tumor at the time of initial surgery.[7] Nevertheless, both locally recurrent parathyroid adenoma and cancer appear to respond favorably to aggressive local re-resection, and most patients can be rendered either hypocalcemic or normocalcemic for a reasonable period.[7] Once disease has spread to distant sites, surgery appears to have less of a role in treatment. Resection of pulmonary metastatic disease has been done without clear benefit.[98] In patients with distant metastases, dacarbazine (DTIC) chemotherapy has been effective in some instances.[97] Therapy for these patients has been primarily directed at controlling the severe hypercalcemia.

Postoperative Hypocalcemia

Most patients who have undergone successful surgery for pHPT have some (albeit mild) symptoms of hypocalcemia, and a posi-

tive Trousseau or Chvostek sign may develop. These symptoms should initiate measurement of the serum level of calcium and phosphorus. Treatment is guided primarily by the serum level of calcium, which should be maintained above 8.0 mg/dL. Initially, dietary calcium is used. However, dietary calcium, primarily milk products, is associated with a large phosphate load and may result in hyperphosphatemia. If this complication occurs, elemental calcium may be given in the usual oral doses of 1 to 2 g/day. Recently, patients have not been hospitalized after parathyroidectomy. Instead, they have been given prescriptions for oral calcium and calcitriol to minimize hypocalcemia and the symptoms from it. This practice has resulted in shorter hospitalizations and fewer symptoms of tetany.

If the symptoms of hypocalcemia are severe and the patient appears to be on the verge of tetany (occurring most frequently in patients with "hungry bone syndrome"), the clinician may need to treat with intravenous calcium. These symptoms can usually be rapidly corrected by the infusion of 2 mg/kg of elemental calcium over a 15-minute period. Symptoms return unless a longer infusion is used. Approximately 15 mg/kg of elemental calcium is then infused over a 24-hour period, with half the total amount administered in the initial 6 hours. Serum levels of calcium should be monitored closely during the infusion, and infusion rates and amounts may be adjusted accordingly. Only approximately 13% of patients have severe symptoms of hypoparathyroidism after surgery. These patients appear to be older; have higher preoperative serum levels of calcium, PTH, alkaline phosphatase, and urea nitrogen; and have large adenomas removed at surgery[16] and typically require intravenous calcium. Most patients do not need this type of calcium replacement.

When hypocalcemia persists despite maximal oral replacement doses, and hyperphosphatemia develops, $1,25(OH)_2D_3$ (calcitriol) is initiated.[99] This drug is recommended because of rapid onset of action and short duration of use. The usual initial dose of calcitriol is 0.25 to 1.0 μg/day given on a twice-daily schedule. The dose can be increased to a maximum of 2.0 μg/day, depending on the response in terms of serum levels of calcium and phosphorus. In general, the lowest possible dose that produces low normal serum levels and no hypocalcemic symptoms should be used. Serum levels of calcium should be monitored weekly after discharge to further adjust oral calcium and calcitriol doses.

Results of Surgery for Primary Hyperparathyroidism

Despite the complexity and decision making required, the results of surgery for pHPT are excellent. The success rate is between 95% and 100%, with a greater probability of success during initial procedures. Recurrent laryngeal nerve injuries have been reported in approximately 1% of patients undergoing initial operations and 5% undergoing reoperations. Chronic hypoparathyroidism occurs in less than 1% of patients undergoing initial operations and 10% undergoing reoperations. Successful surgery with reasonable morbidity appears to require experience, inasmuch as the results of larger series are better than those of smaller ones. Evidence indicates that the vast majority of patients with pHPT are cured by surgery, and few suffer complications.

REFERENCES

1. NIH conference: Diagnosis and management of asymptomatic primary hyperparathyroidism: consensus development conference statement, Ann Intern Med 114: 593–597, 1991.
2. Norton JA: Controversies and advances in primary hyperparathyroidism, Ann Surg 215:297–299, 1992.
3. Scholz DA, Purnell DC: Asymptomatic primary hyperparathyroidism. 10-year prospective study, Mayo Clin Proc 56:473–478, 1981.
4. Bilezikian JP, Khan AA, Potts JT Jr: Guidelines for the management of asymptomatic primary hyperparathyroidism: summary statement from the third international workshop, J Clin Endocrinol Metab 94(2):335–339, 2009.
5. Silverberg SJ, Brown I, Bilezikian JP: Age as a criterion for surgery in primary hyperparathyroidism, Am J Med 113:681–684, 2002.
6. Delbridge LW, Marshman D, Reeve TS, et al: Neuromuscular symptoms in elderly patients with hyperparathyroidism: improvement with parathyroid surgery, Med J Aust 149:74–76, 1988.
7. Fraker DL, et al: Locally recurrent parathyroid neoplasms as a cause for recurrent and persistent primary hyperparathyroidism, Ann Surg 213:58–65, 1991.
8. Keiser HR, Beaven MA, Doppman J, et al: Sipple's syndrome: medullary thyroid carcinoma, pheochromocytoma, and parathyroid disease. Studies in a large family. NIH conference, Ann Intern Med 78:561–579, 1973.
9. Rizzoli R, Green J 3rd, Marx SJ: Primary hyperparathyroidism in familial multiple endocrine neoplasia type I. Long-term follow-up of serum calcium levels after parathyroidectomy, Am J Med 78:467–474, 1985.
10. Marx SJ, et al: Heterogeneous size of the parathyroid glands in familial multiple endocrine neoplasia type 1, Clin Endocrinol (Oxf) 35:521–526, 1991.
11. The search for the MEN1 gene. The European Consortium on MEN-1, J Intern Med 243:441–446, 1998.
12. Lairmore TC, et al: Familial medullary thyroid carcinoma and multiple endocrine neoplasia type 2B map to the same region of chromosome 10 as multiple endocrine neoplasia type 2A, Genomics 9:181–192, 1991.
13. Hosokawa Y, Pollak MR, Brown EM, et al: Mutational analysis of the extracellular Ca(2+)-sensing receptor gene in human parathyroid tumors, J Clin Endocrinol Metab 80:3107–3110, 1995.
14. Bilezikian JP: Management of acute hypercalcemia, N Engl J Med 326:1196–1203, 1992.
15. Fitzpatrick LA, Bilezikian JP: Acute primary hyperparathyroidism, Am J Med 82:275–282, 1987.
16. Brasier AR, Nussbaum SR: Hungry bone syndrome: clinical and biochemical predictors of its occurrence after parathyroid surgery, Am J Med 84:654–660, 1988.
17. Chen H: Surgery for primary hyperparathyroidism: what is the best approach? Ann Surg 236:552–553, 2002.
18. Irvin GL 3rd, Carneiro DM, Solorzano CC: Progress in the operative management of sporadic primary hyperparathyroidism over 34 years, Ann Surg 239:704–708; discussion 708–711, 2004.
19. Palazzo FF, Delbridge LW: Minimal-access/minimally invasive parathyroidectomy for primary hyperparathyroidism, Surg Clin North Am 84:717–734, 2004.
20. Sosa JA, Udelsman R: Minimally invasive parathyroidectomy, Surg Oncol 12:125–134, 2003.
21. Udelsman R: Six hundred fifty-six consecutive explorations for primary hyperparathyroidism, Ann Surg 235:665–670; discussion 670–662, 2002.
22. Udelsman R, Donovan PI, Sokoll LJ: One hundred consecutive minimally invasive parathyroid explorations, Ann Surg 232:331–339, 2000.
23. Slepavicius A, Beisa V, Janusonis V, et al: Focused versus conventional parathyroidectomy for primary hyperparathyroidism: a prospective, randomized, blinded trial, Langenbecks Arch Surg 2008.
24. Denham DW, Norman J: Cost-effectiveness of preoperative sestamibi scan for primary hyperparathyroidism is dependent solely upon the surgeon's choice of operative procedure, J Am Coll Surg 186:293–305, 1998.
25. McBiles M, Lambert AT, Cote MG, et al: Sestamibi parathyroid imaging, Semin Nucl Med 25:221–234, 1995.
26. Pappu S, Donovan P, Cheng D, et al: Sestamibi scans are not all created equally, Arch Surg 140:383–386, 2005.
27. Rubello D, Mariani G: Hand-held gamma probe or hand-held miniature gamma camera for minimally invasive

28. Fuchs SP, et al: Minimally-invasive parathyroidectomy: a good operative procedure for primary hyperparathyroidism even without the use of intraoperative parathyroid-hormone assessment or a gamma probe, Ned Tijdschr Geneeskd 149:1463–1467, 2005.
29. Bekis R, et al: The role of gamma probe activity counts in minimally invasive parathyroidectomy. Preliminary results, Nuklearmedizin 43:190–194, 2004.
30. Ugur O, et al: Clinicopathologic and radiopharmacokinetic factors affecting gamma probe-guided parathyroidectomy, Arch Surg 139:1175–1179, 2004.
31. Bozkurt MF, Ugur O, Hamaloglu E, et al: Optimization of the gamma probe-guided parathyroidectomy, Am Surg 69:720–725, 2003.
32. Rubello D, et al: Importance of radio-guided minimally invasive parathyroidectomy using hand-held gamma probe and low (99m)Tc-MIBI dose. Technical considerations and long-term clinical results, Q J Nucl Med 47:129–138, 2003.
33. Burkey SH, et al: Will directed parathyroidectomy utilizing the gamma probe or intraoperative parathyroid hormone assay replace bilateral cervical exploration as the preferred operation for primary hyperparathyroidism? World J Surg 26:914–920, 2002.
34. Singer JA, Sardi A, Conaway G, et al: Minimally invasive parathyroidectomy utilizing a gamma detecting probe intraoperatively, MD Med J 48:55–58, 1999.
35. Davis ML, et al: Ultrasound facilitates minimally invasive parathyroidectomy in patients lacking definitive localization from preoperative sestamibi scan, Am J Surg 194:785–790; discussion 790–781, 2007.
36. Abraham D, et al: Utility of ultrasound-guided fine-needle aspiration of parathyroid adenomas for localization before minimally invasive parathyroidectomy, Endocr Pract 13:333–337, 2007.
37. Kell MR, et al: Minimally invasive parathyroidectomy with operative ultrasound localization of the adenoma, Surg Endosc 18:1097–1098, 2004.
38. Purcell GP, et al: Parathyroid localization with high-resolution ultrasound and technetium Tc 99m sestamibi, Arch Surg 134:824–828; discussion 828–830, 1999.
39. Carty SE, Norton JA: Management of patients with persistent or recurrent primary hyperparathyroidism, World J Surg 15:716–723, 1991.
40. Shen W, et al: Reoperation for persistent or recurrent primary hyperparathyroidism, Arch Surg 131:861–867; discussion 867–869, 1996.
41. Patow CA, Norton JA, Brennan MF: Vocal cord paralysis and reoperative parathyroidectomy. A prospective study, Ann Surg 203:282–285, 1986.
42. Udelsman R, Donovan PI: Remedial parathyroid surgery: changing trends in 130 consecutive cases, Ann Surg 244:471–479, 2006.
43. Wang TS, Udelsman R: Remedial surgery for primary hyperparathyroidism, Adv Surg 41:1–15, 2007.
44. Miller DL, et al: Localization of parathyroid adenomas in patients who have undergone surgery. Part I. Noninvasive imaging methods, Radiology 162:133–137, 1987.
45. Miller DL: Pre-operative localization and interventional treatment of parathyroid tumors: when and how? World J Surg 15:706–715, 1991.
46. MacFarlane MP, et al: Use of preoperative fine-needle aspiration in patients undergoing reoperation for primary hyperparathyroidism, Surgery 116:959–964; discussion 964–965, 1994.
47. Jaskowiak N, et al: A prospective trial evaluating a standard approach to reoperation for missed parathyroid adenoma, Ann Surg 224:308–320; discussion 320–321, 1996.
48. Wei JP, Burke GJ, Mansberger AR Jr: Preoperative imaging of abnormal parathyroid glands in patients with hyperparathyroid disease using combination Tc-99m-pertechnetate and Tc-99m-sestamibi radionuclide scans, Ann Surg 219:568–572; discussion 572–563, 1994.
49. Allendorf J, et al: The impact of sestamibi scanning on the outcome of parathyroid surgery, J Clin Endocrinol Metab 88:3015–3018, 2003.
50. Lange JR, Norton JA: Surgery for persistent or recurrent primary hyperparathyroidism, Curr Pract Surg 4:26, 1992.

51. Udelsman R, et al: Rapid parathyroid hormone analysis during venous localization, Ann Surg 237:714–719; discussion 719–721, 2003.
52. Neumann DR, et al: Regional body FDG-PET in postoperative recurrent hyperparathyroidism, J Comput Assist Tomogr 21:25–28, 1997.
53. Mittendorf EA, Perrier NP: Persistent or recurrent hyperparathyroidism. In Cameron JL, editor: Current Surgical Therapy, ed 9, St Louis, 2008, Mosby, p 630.
54. Patel PC, Pellitteri PK, Patel NM, et al: Use of a rapid intraoperative parathyroid hormone assay in the surgical management of parathyroid disease, Arch Otolaryngol Head Neck Surg 124:559–562, 1998.
55. Bergenfelz A, Isaksson A, Lindblom P, et al: Measurement of parathyroid hormone in patients with primary hyperparathyroidism undergoing first and reoperative surgery, Br J Surg 85:1129–1132, 1998.
56. Garner SC, Leight GS Jr: Initial experience with intraoperative PTH determinations in the surgical management of 130 consecutive cases of primary hyperparathyroidism, Surgery 126:1132–1137; discussion 1137–1138, 1999.
57. Yang GP, Levine S, Weigel RJ: A spike in parathyroid hormone during neck exploration may cause a false-negative intraoperative assay result, Arch Surg 136:945–949, 2001.
58. Westra WH, Pritchett DD, Udelsman R: Intraoperative confirmation of parathyroid tissue during parathyroid exploration: a retrospective evaluation of the frozen section, Am J Surg Pathol 22:538–544, 1998.
59. Boggs JE, Irvin GL 3rd, Carneiro DM, et al: The evolution of parathyroidectomy failures, Surgery 126:998–1002; discussion 1002–1003, 1999.
60. Irvin GL 3rd, Molinari AS, Figueroa C, et al: Improved success rate in reoperative parathyroidectomy with intraoperative PTH assay, Ann Surg 229:874–878; discussion 878–879, 1999.
61. Thompson NW, Eckhauser FE, Harness JK: The anatomy of primary hyperparathyroidism, Surgery 92:814–821, 1982.
62. Attie JN, Bock G, Auguste LJ: Multiple parathyroid adenomas: report of thirty-three cases, Surgery 108:1014–1019; discussion 1019–1020, 1990.
63. Roses DF, et al: Primary hyperparathyroidism associated with two enlarged parathyroid glands, Arch Surg 124:1261–1265, 1989.
64. Wells SA Jr, Leight GS, Ross AJ 3rd: Primary hyperparathyroidism, Curr Probl Surg 17:398–463, 1980.
65. Brennan MF, Norton JA: Reoperation for persistent and recurrent hyperparathyroidism, Ann Surg 201:40–44, 1985.
66. Grant CS, van Heerden JA, Charboneau JW, et al: Clinical management of persistent and/or recurrent primary hyperparathyroidism, World J Surg 10:555–565, 1986.
67. Akerstrom G, Malmaeus J, Bergstrom R: Surgical anatomy of human parathyroid glands, Surgery 95: 14–21, 1984.
68. Wang C: The anatomic basis of parathyroid surgery, Ann Surg 183:271–275, 1976.
69. Alveryd A: Parathyroid glands in thyroid surgery. I. Anatomy of parathyroid glands. II. Postoperative hypoparathyroidism—identification and autotransplantation of parathyroid glands, Acta Chir Scand 389:1–120, 1968.
70. Wang C, Mahaffey JE, Axelrod L, et al: Hyperfunctioning supernumerary parathyroid glands, Surg Gynecol Obstet 148:711–714, 1979.
71. Gilmour J: The gross anatomy of the parathyroid glands, J Pathology 46:133, 1938.
72. Edis AJ, Purnell DC, van Heerden JA: The undescended "parathymus." An occasional cause of failed neck exploration for hyperparathyroidism, Ann Surg 190:64–68, 1979.
73. Schell SR, Dudley NE: Clinical outcomes and fiscal consequences of bilateral neck exploration for primary idiopathic hyperparathyroidism without preoperative radionuclide imaging or minimally invasive techniques, Surgery 133:32–39, 2003.
74. Burkey SH, Snyder WH 3rd, Nwariaku F, et al: Directed parathyroidectomy: feasibility and performance in 100 consecutive patients with primary hyperparathyroidism, Arch Surg 138:604–608; discussion 608–609, 2003.
75. Goldstein RE, Billheimer D, Martin WH, et al: Sestamibi scanning and minimally invasive radioguided parathy-

roidectomy without intraoperative parathyroid hormone measurement, Ann Surg 237:722–730; discussion 730–731, 2003.

76. Biertho L, Chu C, Inabnet WB: Image-directed parathyroidectomy under local anaesthesia in the elderly, Br J Surg 90:738–742, 2003.

77. Saxe AW, Brown E, Hamburger SW: Thyroid and parathyroid surgery performed with patient under regional anesthesia, Surgery 103:415–420, 1988.

78. Norman J, Denham D: Minimally invasive radioguided parathyroidectomy in the reoperative neck, Surgery 124:1088–1092; discussion 1092–1083, 1998.

79. Genc H, et al: Differing histologic findings after bilateral and focused parathyroidectomy, J Am Coll Surg 196:535–540, 2003.

80. Lee NC, Norton JA: Multiple-gland disease in primary hyperparathyroidism: a function of operative approach? Arch Surg 137:896–899; discussion 899–900, 2002.

81. Wells SA Jr, Ellis GJ, Gunnells JC, et al: Parathyroid autotransplantation in primary parathyroid hyperplasia, N Engl J Med 295:57–62, 1976.

82. Wells SA Jr, Farndon JR, Dale JK, et al: Long-term evaluation of patients with primary parathyroid hyperplasia managed by total parathyroidectomy and heterotopic autotransplantation, Ann Surg 192:451–458, 1980.

83. Saxe AW, Brennan MF: Reoperative parathyroid surgery for primary hyperparathyroidism caused by multiple-gland disease: total parathyroidectomy and autotransplantation with cryopreserved tissue, Surgery 91:616–621, 1982.

84. Senapati A, Young AE: Parathyroid autotransplantation, Br J Surg 77:1171–1174, 1990.

85. Norton JA, Venzon DJ, Berna MJ, et al: Prospective study of surgery for primary hyperparathyroidism (HPT) in multiple endocrine neoplasia-type 1 and Zollinger-Ellison syndrome: long-term outcome of a more virulent form of HPT, Ann Surg 247(3):501–510, 2008.

86. Wells SA Jr, Cooper JD: Closed mediastinal exploration in patients with persistent hyperparathyroidism, Ann Surg 214:555–561, 1991.

87. Johnson WJ, et al: Results of subtotal parathyroidectomy in hemodialysis patients, Am J Med 84:23–32, 1988.

88. Arnold A, et al: Monoclonality of parathyroid tumors in chronic renal failure and in primary parathyroid hyperplasia, J Clin Invest 95:2047–2053, 1995.

89. Andress DL, Ott SM, Maloney NA, et al: Effect of parathyroidectomy on bone aluminum accumulation in chronic renal failure, N Engl J Med 312:468–473, 1985.

90. Yano S, et al: Effect of parathyroidectomy on bone mineral density in hemodialysis patients with secondary hyperparathyroidism: possible usefulness of preoperative determination of parathyroid hormone level for prediction of bone regain, Horm Metab Res 35:259–264, 2003.

91. Wang C, Gaz RD, Moncure AC: Mediastinal parathyroid exploration: a clinical and pathologic study of 47 cases, World J Surg 10:687–695, 1986.

92. Fraker DL, et al: Undescended parathyroid adenoma: an important etiology for failed operations for primary hyperparathyroidism, World J Surg 14:342–348, 1990.

93. Chan TJ, et al: Persistent primary hyperparathyroidism caused by adenomas identified in pharyngeal or adjacent structures, World J Surg 27:675–679, 2003.

94. Wang CA, Gaz RD: Natural history of parathyroid carcinoma. Diagnosis, treatment, and results, Am J Surg 149:522–527, 1985.

95. Streeten EA, Weinstein LS, Norton JA, et al: Studies in a kindred with parathyroid carcinoma, J Clin Endocrinol Metab 75:362–366, 1992.

96. Cohn K, Silverman M, Corrado J, et al: Parathyroid carcinoma: the Lahey Clinic experience, Surgery 98:1095–1100, 1985.

97. Calandra DB, Chejfec G, Foy BK, et al: Parathyroid carcinoma: biochemical and pathologic response to DTIC, Surgery 96:1132–1137, 1984.

98. Flye MW, Brennan MF: Surgical resection of metastatic parathyroid carcinoma, Ann Surg 193:425–435, 1981.

99. Reichel H, Koeffler HP, Norman AW: The role of the vitamin D endocrine system in health and disease, N Engl J Med 320:980–991, 1989.

Chapter 10

PSEUDOHYPOPARATHYROIDISM, ALBRIGHT'S HEREDITARY OSTEODYSTROPHY, AND PROGRESSIVE OSSEOUS HETEROPLASIA: Disorders Caused by Inactivating *GNAS* Mutations

MURAT BASTEPE and HARALD JÜPPNER

In 1942, Albright et al.[1] described a group of patients who displayed certain physical features—including obesity, short stature, brachydactyly, and cognitive impairment—combined with hypocalcemia and hyperphosphatemia. In these patients, exogenous, biologically active parathyroid hormone (PTH), extracted from parathyroid glands, failed to result in a full phosphaturic response; hence, the term pseudohypoparathyroidism (PHP) was introduced, indicating that hypocalcemia and hyperphosphatemia in these patients resulted from target organ resistance to, rather than deficiency of, PTH. Consistent with resistance to the actions of this hormone, it was later shown that patients affected by PHP have elevated concentrations of immunoreactive PTH.[2] Subsequently, it was shown that some patients affected by PHP have resistance toward additional hormones; however, PTH resistance is the most prominent feature of the disease.

The primary site of PTH resistance in PHP is the renal proximal tubule, as the actions of PTH in bone and in the distal tubule appear normal.[3-5] Patients with PHP have reduced serum concentrations of 1,25-dihydroxyvitamin D_3 [1,25(OH)$_2$D$_3$], which is the main cause of hypocalcemia.[6-9] Low serum 1,25(OH)$_2$D$_3$ and hyperphosphatemia are the direct results of PTH resistance at the proximal tubule. Hyperphosphatemia typically is worsened by the elevation of PTH in the circulation and the absence of resistance to bone resorptive actions of this hormone; on the other hand, serum PTH increase can prevent symptomatic hypocalcemia in some PHP patients largely by its unimpaired actions on the bone and the renal distal tubule.[10-14] However, at some point in their lives, most of these patients manifest hypocalcemia and therefore present with associated clinical findings.

Diagnosis, Progression, and Treatment of PTH Resistance

PTH exerts its actions by binding to a seven-transmembrane, G protein–coupled receptor (the PTH/PTH-related protein receptor, PTHR1).[15] Although PTHR1 can couple to several different G proteins,[16] most PTH actions are mediated primarily through the stimulatory G protein, which acts on adenylyl cyclases and thereby increases the formation of intracellular second messenger cyclic adenosine monophosphate (cAMP).[15,17] PTH-induced cAMP formation is used as an important indicator of renal tubular PTH function, because most PHP patients display an inadequate or absent increase in urinary cAMP in response to exogenous, biologically active PTH (Fig. 10-1).[18] In fact, the nephrogenous response to exogenously administered PTH is utilized as a test for establishing the diagnosis of PHP (Ellsworth-Howard test), although currently used high-sensitivity PTH assays often suffice to make the diagnosis when serum PTH is elevated in the presence of hypocalcemia and hyperphosphatemia. Nonetheless, depending on the nature of the nephrogenous response to exogenous PTH, PHP is subdivided into two main types. PHP type I is defined by blunted urinary excretion of both cAMP and phosphate, and PHP type II by blunted urinary excretion of phosphate only.[1,18,19]

Signs and symptoms of decreased serum calcium often reflect increased neuromuscular excitability. Although the most common manifestations of hypocalcemia include muscle tetany and spasms, findings vary markedly among patients. In more severe cases, patients present with seizures. Other neurologic symptoms can arise from hypocalcemia, and some patients with PHP initially have been diagnosed with movement disorders.[20-24] In one report,[25] two sisters with PHP Ib (see below) presented with paroxysmal kinesigenic choreoathetosis, and the diagnosis of PTH resistance in one sister was made through genetic testing and biochemical evaluation only after approximately 4 years of antiepileptic oral treatment.[25] Some patients presenting with seizures demonstrate epileptiform activity on electroencephalogram (EEG), and, because this activity typically responds to antiepileptic treatment, the diagnosis of PHP can be delayed.[26,27] As another complication of changes in serum calcium and phosphorus, brain imaging studies in PHP patients frequently show intracranial calcifications.[20,28-34]

PHP is a congenital disorder, and few reports describe findings consistent with PTH resistance during the neonatal period.[35,36] However, clinical manifestations of hypocalcemia typically occur only later in childhood. PTH resistance and resultant changes in serum calcium and phosphorus develop gradually.[37-40] In a longitudinal study of a child with PHP Ia (see below), cAMP response to PTH was found to be normal at age 3 months, although it was blunted at age 2.6 years.[38] In another PHP Ia case, a gradual decline in serum calcium, preceded by increasing serum phosphorus and PTH levels, was demonstrated.[37] In addition, a PHP Ib patient diagnosed by genetic analysis (see below) at birth was shown to have normal serum PTH levels until age 18 months, when an elevation in PTH was first detected despite normal serum calcium and phosphorus.[39] It thus appears that PTH responses are intact during the early postnatal period despite the existence of the molecular defect underlying PHP. The mechanisms that allow normal PTH signaling during this developmental stage remain unknown.

The primary goal of treatment entails correction of abnormal serum biochemistries that result from PTH and, in some cases, other hormone resistance. Regarding hypocalcemia, treatment involves oral calcium supplements and $1,25(OH)_2D$ (calcitriol) preparations. Note that the active form of vitamin D is required because of the lowered capacity of the proximal tubule to convert $25(OH)D$ into the biologically active $1,25(OH)_2D$. In addition, treatment for patients with PTH resistance should be aimed at keeping the serum PTH level within or close to the normal range, rather than simply avoiding symptomatic hypocalcemia, because persistent elevation of serum PTH will increase bone resorption and eventually may lead to hyperparathyroid bone disease, including osteitis fibrosa cystica.[41] PTH actions in the distal tubule, which are not impaired, provide sufficient calcium reabsorption from the glomerular filtrate; therefore, urinary calcium levels are usually low, and affected individuals do not have an increased risk of developing kidney stones and nephrocalcinosis. In fact, during the course of treatment, urinary calcium elevation typically does not occur. Nevertheless, blood chemistries and urinary calcium excretion in patients undergoing treatment should be monitored annually, but more frequently during pubertal development and once skeletal growth is completed, as the requirements for treatment with calcium and $1,25(OH)_2D$ may need adjustment.

Pseudohypoparathyroidism Type Ia

Among the two main PHP types, PHP type I is much more common. Clinical variants of PHP type I have been described, based on the presence or absence of clinical manifestations that coexist with PTH resistance, diminished stimulatory G protein activity in easily accessible cells, and imprinting abnormalities of the *GNAS* gene encoding the α subunit of the stimulatory G protein (Gsα) (Table 10-1).

As was described originally by Albright et al.,[1] some PHP patients exhibit characteristic physical features that may include obesity, round facies, short stature, brachydactyly, ectopic ossification, and mental impairment (Fig. 10-2). These features are

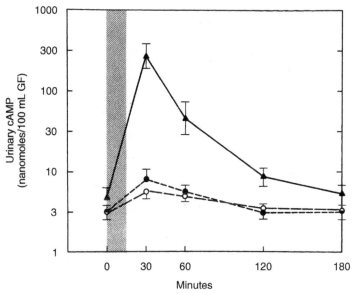

FIGURE 10-1. Urinary cyclic adenosine monophosphate (cAMP) excretion in response to an infusion of bovine parathyroid extract (300 USP units). The peak response in normal subjects (▲) and those with pseudopseudohypoparathyroidism (PPHP) *(not shown)* is 50- to 100-fold times basal. Subjects with PHP type Ia (o) or PHP type Ib (●) show only a two- to fivefold increase. Urinary cAMP is expressed as nanomoles per 100 mL of glomerular filtrate (GF), U_{cAMP} (nanomoles per 100 mL GF) = U_{cAMP} (nanomoles/dL) × S_{Cre} (mg/dL)/U_{Cre} (mg/dL). (Data from Levine et al., 1986.[65])

Table 10-1. Clinical and Molecular Features of PHP Forms and Variants

	PTH-Resistance	Additional Hormone Resistance	Typical AHO Features	GNAS Defects
PHP-Ia/Ic	Yes	Yes	Yes	Coding GNAS mutations
PPHP	No	No	Yes	Coding GNAS mutations
POH	No	No*	No	Coding GNAS mutations
PHP-Ib	Yes	Some cases	No†	Microdeletions affecting GNAS imprinting

* POH-like severe heterotopic-ossifications have been reported in some patients with homone resistance.
† Some recent studies have demonstrated co-existence of AHO features and GNAS imprinting defects.

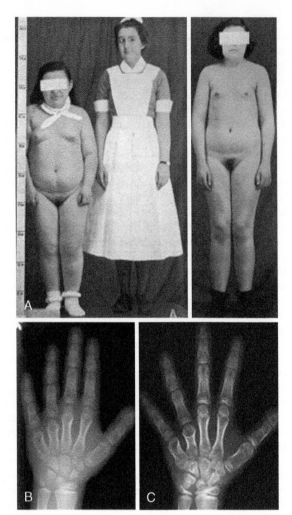

FIGURE 10-2. Albright's hereditary osteodystrophy (AHO). **A,** Short stature and obesity are among the typical features of AHO. **B,** Hand radiograph of a child with AHO demonstrating short fourth and fifth metacarpals at age $5\frac{1}{2}$ years. **C,** The same patient's hand radiograph at age $8\frac{1}{2}$ years. (**A** Adapted from Albright et al: Pseudohypoparathyroidism—an example of "Seabright-Bantam syndrome," Endocrinology 30:922–932, 1942).

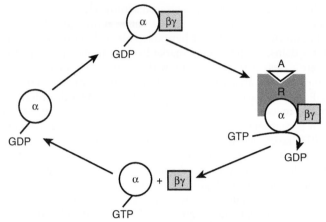

FIGURE 10-3. Heterotrimeric G protein activation cycle. The heterotrimeric complex is assembled at the basal state, with the α subunit associated with a guanosine diphosphate (GDP) molecule. Upon binding of an agonist (A) to its Gs-coupled receptor (R), the GDP molecule bound to the α subunit is replaced with a guanosine triphosphate (GTP) molecule, that is, the activated receptor acts as a guanine nucleotide exchange factor for the α subunit. The GTP-bound form of the α subunit dissociates from the βγ subunits and thereby stimulates its downstream effectors, which, in the case of Gsα, include adenylyl cyclase. Note that the free Gβγ dimer can also stimulate different downstream effectors. The intrinsic GTP hydrolase activity of the α subunit converts GTP into GDP, resulting in reassociation of the heterotrimer and, thus, termination of effector stimulation.

now termed Albright's hereditary osteodystrophy (AHO), and PHP patients who present with these features are classified as having pseudohypoparathyroidism type Ia (PHP Ia). The brachydactyly observed in patients with AHO typically involves the metacarpal and/or metatarsal bones; thus, the pattern of shortening of hand bones differs from that seen in other disorders with brachydactyly, such as familial brachydactyly and Turner's syndrome.[42] Because of shortened metacarpals, dimpling over the knuckles of a clenched fist (Archibald sign) is often observed.[43] Shortening of the distal phalanx of the thumb, however, is the most common skeletal abnormality (called "murderer's" or "potter's" thumb), and some patients have shortening of all digits.[44] Mental impairment is mild, often presenting as cognitive defects. It is possible that the cause of mental impairment is the deficiency of Gsα signaling in the brain. Although hypocalcemia and/or hypothyroidism may play a role in this phenotype, correction of these biochemical defects does not prevent mental impairment in all cases. Remarkable patient-to-patient variability is seen in AHO, even among patients who carry the same genetic mutation and belong to the same family (see below for discussion of the underlying genetic defect). Some patients may exhibit a single AHO feature only, such as obesity; others may present

with multiple different AHO features. Furthermore, the severity of each feature differs vastly among patients. In addition, individual AHO features are not unique to PHP, as they can be observed in other unrelated disorders. The variable expressivity and the lack of specificity of individual features can make the AHO diagnosis challenging. Although the coexistence of hormone resistance in PHP Ia patients is often helpful, it also can be misleading. This is particularly important in differential diagnosis of different PHP forms characterized by the presence of AHO features alone or hormone resistance alone (see below).

In addition to having PTH resistance and AHO, patients with PHP Ia show clinical evidence that is consistent with target organ resistance to other hormones. The most common additional hormone resistance involves the actions of thyroid-stimulating hormone (TSH) that lead to hypothyroidism.[45,46] In fact, unlike PTH resistance, which typically develops later in life, TSH resistance can be present at birth.[47-50] Resistance toward gonadotropins and growth hormone–releasing factor has been reported,[51-53] whereas resistance toward other peptide hormones that also mediate their actions through Gsα-coupled receptors, such as vasopressin or adrenocorticotropic hormone (ACTH), does not appear to become clinically overt.[52,54-58]

The genetic mutation that causes PHP Ia is located within Gsα-coding *GNAS* exons.[59,60] A protein that is essential for the actions of many hormones, Gsα primarily mediates agonist-induced generation of intracellular cAMP. Activation of a stimulatory G protein–coupled receptor by its agonist, such as PTH, leads to a guanosine diphosphate (GDP)-guanosine triphosphate (GTP) exchange on Gsα, causing dissociation of the latter from Gβγ subunits (Fig. 10-3). This allows both Gsα and Gβγ to stimulate their respective effectors. In its GTP-bound state, Gsα can directly activate several different effectors, such as Src tyrosine kinase,[61] and certain Ca channels.[62,63] Apart from these effectors, however, adenylyl cyclase is by far the most ubiquitous and the most extensively investigated effector molecule stimulated by Gsα. An integral membrane protein, adenylyl cyclase catalyzes the synthesis of the ubiquitous second messenger

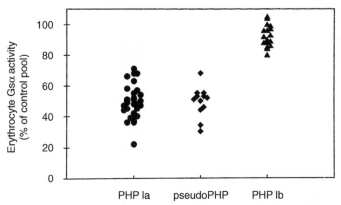

FIGURE 10-4. Gsα activity of erythrocyte membranes. Gsα is quantified in complementation assays with S49 cyc⁻ membranes, which genetically lack Gsα but retain all other components necessary for hormone responsive adenylyl cyclase activity. Activity is reduced by approximately 50% in patients with Albright's hereditary osteodystrophy (AHO) with pseudohypothyroidism (PHP) type Ia or pseudoPHP but is normal in patients with PHP type Ib.

cAMP, which then triggers various cell-specific responses. Activation of adenylyl cyclase and other effectors by Gsα is regulated by the intrinsic GTP hydrolase (GTPase) activity of Gsα. Conversion of GTP into GDP results in reassembly of the G protein heterotrimer and thereby prevents further effector stimulation (see Fig. 10-3).

Mutations identified in PHP-Ia patients are heterozygous and scattered throughout all 13 *GNAS* exons that encode Gsα, including missense and nonsense amino acid changes, insertions/deletions that cause frameshift, and nucleotide alterations that disrupt pre-mRNA splicing (an extensive list of these mutations can be found at OMIM entry #139320 at http://www.ncbi.nlm.nih.gov). Constitutional deletions of the chromosomal arm containing *GNAS* have also been identified.[64] Consistent with heterozygous mutations, Gsα level/activity is reduced by approximately 50% in easily accessible tissues from PHP Ia patients, such as erythrocytes, skin fibroblasts, and platelets.[45,65-78] Deficiency of Gsα has been demonstrated in renal membranes from a patient with PHP.[79] A complementation assay is typically used to examine Gsα activity, involving patient-derived erythrocyte membranes and membranes from turkey erythrocyte that lack endogenous Gsα (Fig. 10-4). The detection of reduced Gsα activity by this means is important for the establishment of PHP Ia diagnosis, particularly in cases where genetic analysis fails to reveal a *GNAS* mutation. Reduction of Gsα activity in PHP Ia is consistent with the fact that PTH and the other hormones with impaired actions in this disorder act via cAMP-mediated signaling pathways.

Among the many different inactivating *GNAS* mutations, a 4 bp deletion in exon 7 has been identified in numerous families, representing a genetic "hot spot." In addition, two different mutations are associated with additional phenotypes. A missense mutation in exon 13 (A366S) was identified in two unrelated boys who presented with PHP Ia and precocious puberty.[80] This mutant Gsα protein is temperature sensitive and thus rapidly degrades at normal body temperature. The amino acid substitution, however, renders the protein constitutively active, resulting in elevated cAMP signaling in the cooler temperature of the testis. Recently, another mutant Gsα protein was described in a unique case of familial PHP Ia and transient neonatal diarrhea.[81] The mutation, which entails a repeated AVDT sequence at residues 366 to 369, generates an unstable but constitutively active Gsα

mutant as the result of enhanced GDP-GTP exchange and reduced GTPase activity. Although hormone resistance results from the instability of the Gsα-AVDT mutant, diarrhea is attributed to increased plasma membrane localization of the mutant protein in the small intestinal epithelium.

PHP Ic has been described as a distinct variant of PHP Ia,[68] but the clinical features of patients with PHP Ic are indistinguishable from those with PHP Ia, in that they have both AHO and multihormone resistance. In contrast to PHP Ia, however, biochemical assays demonstrate no reduction in Gsα activity in erythrocytes obtained from PHP Ic patients, suggesting the absence of mutations within the *Gsα* gene. Nevertheless, recent molecular characterizations have revealed *Gsα* mutations in at least some PHP Ic patients. However, the *Gsα* mutants show impaired coupling to different G protein–coupled receptors, yet show normal Gsα activity in complementation assays that use nonhydrolyzable GTP analogues rather than a receptor agonist for stimulation of Gsα activity.[44,82] Thus, the mutant Gsα protein that causes PHP Ic allows basal cAMP formation but is unable to trigger an increase in response to hormones. Hence, at least some PHP Ic cases are allelic variants of PHP Ia. Although it remains possible that some patients who match the description of PHP Ic develop hormone resistance and AHO as the result of a novel gene mutation that affects cAMP production without functionally impairing Gsα itself (e.g., inactivating mutations that affect one of the adenylyl cyclases, or activating mutations in the phosphodiesterase), it appears unlikely that such putative mutations affect only a few G protein–coupled receptors and thus result in limited hormonal resistance as observed in PHP Ia and PHP Ic.

The Complex *GNAS* Locus

GNAS is a complex locus giving rise to multiple different coding and noncoding transcripts that show monoallelic, parent-of-origin specific expression profiles (Fig. 10-5). *GNAS* maps to the telomeric end of the long arm of chromosome 20 (20q13.2-20q13.3).[83-85] Gsα is encoded by 13 exons,[86] but because of alternative pre-mRNA splicing, the Gsα transcript has several variants. The long and short Gsα variants (Gsα-L and Gsα-S, respectively) differ from each other by the inclusion or exclusion of exon 3[86-88]; these Gsα variants are typically detected as 52 and 45 kDa protein bands on Western blots. Showing further complexity, each Gsα form either includes or excludes a CAG trinucleotide (encoding serine) at the start of exon 4. Small but potentially important differences have been reported between the activities of Gsα-L and Gsα-S. For example, Gsα-L has been shown to display a greater ability to mediate receptor signaling than Gsα-S when partially purified proteins from rabbit liver were examined,[89] although the opposite finding was reported upon the use of cultured pancreatic islet cells.[90] Furthermore, the GDP release rate from Gsα-L appears to be approximately twofold higher than that of Gsα-S,[91] and, accordingly, fusion proteins involving the β₂-adrenergic receptor and Gsα-L have shown higher constitutive activity than those involving the receptor and Gsα-S.[92] Moreover, differences have been reported in the subcellular targeting of these two Gsα variants.[93-95] Currently, it remains unclear whether these differences translate into biologically significant effects, such as divergence in the variety of effectors and/or the efficiency of effector activation. Nonetheless, a mutation in exon 3 has been identified recently in two siblings affected by a mild form of PHP Ia.[96] The mildness of the phenotype is consistent with the disruption of only one of the

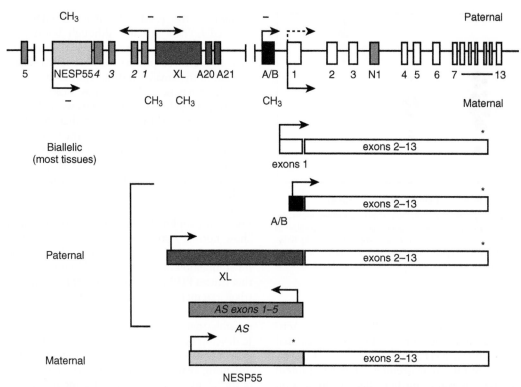

FIGURE 10-5. The *GNAS* locus. The complex *GNAS* locus gives rise to multiple transcripts. *Boxes* and *connecting lines* indicate exons and introns, respectively. *Arrows* show the direction of transcription for each transcript. The main transcriptions derived from *GNAS* and the utilized exons are depicted as *rectangles* below the gene schematic. Gsα is biallelically expressed, except in a small number of tissues, including renal proximal tubules, thyroid, gonads, and pituitary, in which expression from the paternal allele is silenced (*dashed arrow*). XLαs, A/B and antisense (AS) transcripts are derived from the paternal allele, and the NESP55 transcript from the maternal allele. Promoters of XLαs, A/B, antisense, and NESP55 transcripts are methylated on the silenced allele, as indicated by CH3 (methylated CpGs) and − (unmethylated CpGs).

two main Gsα variants—that is, Gsα-L. It remains unknown whether this exon 3 mutation impairs agonist responses in an effector- and tissue-specific manner; this possibility depends on the putative effector selectivity and relative expression levels of Gsα-L and Gsα-S in different tissues.

Recent studies have revealed that *GNAS* gives rise to multiple additional gene products that show parent-of-origin specific, monoallelic expression. Besides Gsα, at least two translated *GNAS* transcripts exist, using distinct upstream promoters and alternative first exons that splice onto exons 2 to 13 encoding Gsα. The most upstream promoter relative to the Gsα promoter drives expression of a neuroendocrine secretory protein with an apparent molecular mass of 55,000 (NESP55).[97] The paternal NESP55 promoter is methylated, and transcription occurs from the maternal allele.[98,99] In humans, the NESP55 protein is encoded by a single exon, so that Gsα exons 2 to 13 make up the 3′ untranslated region.[98,99] Expressed in neuroendocrine tissues, the peripheral and central nervous system, and some endocrine tissues,[97,100-103] NESP55 is a chromogranin-like protein that is associated with the constitutive secretory pathway.[104] Loss of NESP55 expression does not seem to have an overt clinical outcome in humans, as evidenced from patients with PHP type Ib (see below). However, its disruption in mice results in a subtle behavioral phenotype characterized by increased reactivity to novel environments.[105]

Another *GNAS* product is XLαs, which is expressed from the paternal allele.[99,106,107] XLαs also uses a distinct upstream promoter and a unique first exon that splices onto Gsα exons 2 to 13.[99,107] Unlike in NESP55 transcript, however, the latter portion of the XLαs transcript is included in the translated product, resulting in a protein that is partially identical to Gsα.[106] Con-

sistent with its structural similarity to Gsα, XLαs can mediate receptor-activated adenylyl cyclase stimulation in transfected cells.[44,108,109] However, the phenotype of mice with targeted disruption of the XL exon suggests that XLαs has unique, albeit as yet undefined, cellular functions. These mice show high early postnatal mortality as the result of poor adaptation to feeding and impairment in glucose and energy metabolism,[110] in contrast to Gsα knockout mice, which to a large extent recapitulate the findings in patients with PHP Ia.[111,112]

The paternal *GNAS* gives rise to two additional transcripts. From the sense strand originates the A/B transcript (also termed 1A or 1′), which, similar to NESP55 and XLαs, utilizes an upstream promoter and an alternative first exon (exon A/B) that splices onto Gsα exons 2 to 13.[113,114] Exon A/B does not comprise a translation initiation codon, but, as demonstrated in vitro, translation can be started through the use of an AUG located within exon 2, thereby giving rise to an N-terminally truncated protein that localizes to the plasma membrane.[114] However, no evidence currently supports the existence of endogenous A/B protein. It is thought instead that the A/B transcript is a noncoding RNA. Another paternal *GNAS* transcript is derived from the antisense strand.[115,116] The *GNAS* antisense transcript, which is formed in humans by several primary exons that show multiple alternative splicing patterns,[115,117] is also considered to be noncoding. The promoter of *GNAS* antisense transcript is immediately upstream of the promoter of XLαs. Although the promoters of XLαs and antisense transcript are located together within a large maternally methylated region, the female germline-specific imprint is established at the antisense promoter only.[118] The A/B promoter likewise is methylated in the female, but not in the male, germline.[119] Thus, the two germline imprint marks at the

GNAS locus include promoters of the antisense and A/B transcripts. Accordingly, data from different genetically manipulated mouse models show that these noncoding transcripts are essential for the regulation of imprinted gene expression from *GNAS*.[120-122] Imprinting of the A/B transcript is particularly important for the development of hormone resistance seen in patients with PHP Ib (see below).

Unlike the promoters of NESP55, antisense, XLαs, and A/B transcripts, the promoter of Gsα is not differentially methylated and, accordingly, Gsα expression is biallelic in most tissues.[98,107,123,124] Biallelic Gsα expression has been shown specifically in human bone and adipose tissue.[125] However, paternal Gsα expression is silenced in a small subset of tissues through as yet undefined mechanisms, so that the maternal allele is the predominant source of Gsα expression. These tissues include the renal proximal tubule, thyroid, pituitary, and gonads.[112,126-128] Although devoid of differential methylation, the Gsα promoter exhibits parent-of-origin specific histone modifications in those tissues in which it is monoallelic. The active maternal Gsα promoter shows a greater ratio of trimethylated to dimethylated histone-3 Lys[4] compared with the silenced paternal promoter in the proximal tubule, whereas the quantity of methylated histones is similar in maternal and paternal Gsα promoters in liver—a tissue in which Gsα is biallelic.[129] As is discussed below, tissue-specific, paternal Gsα silencing has a key role in the development of PTH resistance in patients with PHP Ia and PHP Ib.

Clinically Distinct, Genetically Related PHP Ia Variants

PSEUDOPSEUDOHYPOPARATHYROIDISM

Physical abnormalities similar to those observed in patients with PHP Ia but without evidence of an abnormal regulation of calcium and phosphate homeostasis were first reported in 1952.[130] Because of the lack of abnormal regulation of mineral ion homeostasis, the name pseudopseudohypoparathyroidism (PPHP) was coined to describe this disorder.[130] It is interesting to note that patients with PPHP also carry *GNAS* mutations that lead to diminished Gsα function, and these mutations can be found in the same kindred as those with PHP Ia. However, both disorders are never seen in the same sibling kinship, and careful analysis of multiple families has revealed that the mode of inheritance of each disorder depends on the gender of the parent who transmits the Gsα mutations.[131] Thus, an inactivating Gsα mutation causes PHP Ia (i.e., hormone resistance and AHO) after maternal inheritance, whereas the same mutation results in PPHP (AHO only). Because AHO appears to develop regardless of the parent of origin, it is primarily hormone resistance that displays an imprinted mode of inheritance. Recent findings regarding tissue-specific imprinting of Gsα expression (see above) now can explain the parent-of-origin specific inheritance of hormone resistance. In those tissues where Gsα expression is paternally silenced (i.e., Gsα is expressed exclusively or predominantly from the maternal allele), an inactivating mutation located on the paternal allele is not predicted to alter Gsα function, whereas the same mutation located on the maternal allele is predicted to abolish Gsα function completely (Fig. 10-6). Tissue-specific imprinting of Gsα expression also explains why the target organ resistance involves only a small subset of tissues despite the involvement of Gsα signaling in a multitude of physiologic responses. Hormone resistance is observed in those tissues where

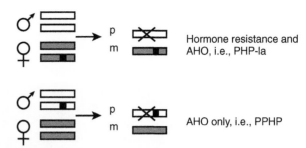

FIGURE 10-6. The effect of paternal Gsα silencing in the development of hormone resistance. Gsα is biallelic in most tissues; a heterozygous inactivating Gsα mutation therefore causes an approximately 50% reduction in Gsα activity/expression regardless of the parent of origin of the mutation. However, in some tissues, such as the proximal tubule and thyroid, the paternally inherited Gsα transcript is silenced (X). Thus, if a Gsα mutation (*black square*) is inherited from a female individual, this mutation nearly abolishes the expression or activity of Gsα in those tissues, thus leading to hormone resistance (PHP Ia). In contrast, upon paternal inheritance, the same mutation Gsα does not lead to a significant change in expression/activity, and thus, hormone responses are unimpaired. Paternal and maternal Gsα alleles are depicted by *white* or *gray rectangles*.

Gsα is imprinted, such as the proximal renal tubule and the thyroid; hormone responses are unimpaired in those tissues where Gsα is biallelic, such as the distal renal tubules. The role of tissue-specific Gsα imprinting in the development of PTH resistance has been demonstrated through the generation of mice heterozygous for maternal or paternal disruption of *Gnas*.[126]

Most AHO features develop regardless of the parent transmitting a Gsα mutation; this observation has led to the hypothesis that inheritance of AHO is due to Gsα haploinsufficiency in various tissues, which appears to be true in certain settings. PTH-related protein–induced cAMP generation is critical for proper control of hypertrophic differentiation of growth plate chondrocytes,[132] and Gsα haploinsufficiency has been demonstrated in this tissue through the study of mice chimeric for wild-type cells and mutant cells heterozygous for disruption of *Gnas* exon 2.[133] Regardless of the parental origin of the *Gnas* exon 2 disruption, mutant cells displayed premature hypertrophy compared with their wild-type neighbors, although paternal disruption (i.e., loss of one Gsα allele combined with a complete loss of XLαs) resulted in significantly more premature hypertrophy than did maternal disruption (loss of one Gsα allele only). Thus, the brachydactyly and/or short stature observed in the context of AHO likely results from diminished Gsα signaling in growth plate chondrocytes. Although these data correlate well with the notion that AHO develops after both maternal and paternal inheritance of a Gsα mutation, recent evidence suggests that individual AHO features can be subject to imprinting. Careful analysis of multiple patients with PHP Ia and PPHP revealed that obesity is primarily a feature of PHP Ia patients, which develops after maternal inheritance.[134] Given that Gsα is biallelic in white adipose tissue,[125] it was proposed that Gsα may also be imprinted—predominantly by maternal expression—in areas of the central nervous system that control satiety and body weight.[134] Recent reports have demonstrated that cognitive impairment is more prevalent in PHP Ia than PPHP, thus indicating that tissue-specific Gsα imprinting may involve additional brain regions.[135] On the other hand, imprinted inheritance has not been reported for short stature, despite the finding that Gsα is imprinted in the pituitary,[127,128] and that PHP Ia patients display growth hormone–releasing hormone (GHRH) resistance and growth hormone (GH) deficiency.[52,53] Future analyses of patients with PHP Ia and PPHP will be helpful in determining the relative roles of genomic

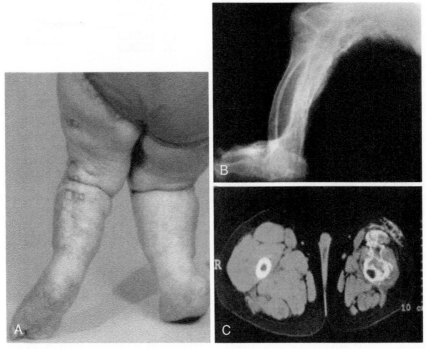

FIGURE 10-7. Clinical and radiographic appearance of progressive osseous heteroplasia (POH). **A,** Posterior view of the legs and feet of a 5-year-old girl with POH, showing severe maculopapular lesions caused by extensive dermal and subcutaneous ossification. **B,** A lateral radiogram of the right leg of an 11-year-old girl with POH demonstrating severe heterotopic ossification of the soft tissues. **C,** Computed tomographic image of the thighs of a 10-year-old boy with POH, showing atrophied soft tissues in the left leg and extensive ossification of the skin, subcutaneous fat, and quadriceps muscles. (Adapted from Shore EM, et al.[142])

imprinting and haploinsufficiency in the development of individual AHO features.

PROGRESSIVE OSSEOUS HETEROPLASIA

A disorder termed progressive osseous heteroplasia (POH) has been described in patients with severe extraskeletal ossifications that involve deep connective tissue and skeletal muscle (Fig. 10-7).[136,137] In POH, ectopic bone is primarily intramembranous, as opposed to a similar disease, termed fibrodysplasia ossificans progressiva (FOP), in which extraskeletal bone formation occurs via endochondral mechanisms and is accompanied by skeletal malformations.[138,139] Few patients with POH demonstrate AHO features and, consistent with the occasional coexistence of these two sets of clinical defects, heterozygous inactivating Gsα mutations have been identified as a cause of POH.[140-142] Several of the identified mutations are identical to those identified in PHP Ia/ PPHP kindreds.[141,142] Gsα activity and downstream signaling have been implicated in the control of osteogenic differentiation. Patients who are mosaic for heterozygous GNAS mutations that result in constitutive Gsα activity develop fibrous dyplasia of bone characterized by irregular woven bone disrupted by fibrous tissue.[143] Moreover, in human mesenchymal stem cells, reduction of Gsα protein levels has been shown to cause osteogenic differentiation, while inhibiting the formation of adipocytes.[144,145] In addition, Runx2, a key regulator of osteoblast-specific gene expression, appears to suppress Gsα expression.[146] Thus, osteoprogenitor formation and early stages of osteoblastic differentiation require reduced levels of cAMP signaling, consistent with the association of inactivating Gsα mutations with the severe ectopic bone formation observed in POH.

Because of the presence of GNAS mutations in both AHO and POH, it appears that POH is an extreme manifestation of AHO, and that additional factors, such as genetic background, epigenetic events, or environmental factors, may determine the pene-

trance and severity of ectopic ossifications in these patients that show approximately 50% loss of Gsα activity. Nevertheless, clinical and genetic data demonstrate several important differences between patients with AHO and those with POH. First, the ectopic bone in AHO is limited to subcutaneous tissue. In addition, in nearly all patients with POH, severe ectopic bone formation is isolated (i.e., other typical AHO features are not manifest).[142,147] Moreover, mutations leading to isolated POH are inherited from male obligate gene carriers only (i.e., the inheritance pattern is exclusively paternal).[142] In fact, in one large kindred, paternal inheritance of a GNAS mutation caused POH, and maternal inheritance of the same mutation caused typical AHO findings (without severe heterotopic ossification).[142] These findings suggest that the disease mechanism underlying POH is significantly different from that underlying AHO, and that a GNAS product with exclusive paternal expression, such as XLαs, contributes to the molecular pathogenesis of POH.

Pseudohypoparathyroidism Type Ib

Another form of PHP was described by Peterman and Garvey[148] and by Reynolds et al.[149] Now known as pseudohypoparathyroidism type Ib (PHP Ib), this PHP form is characterized by the presence of PTH-resistant hypocalcemia and hyperphosphatemia, but without evidence of AHO. In addition to increased serum PTH, patients with PHP Ib can demonstrate elevated serum alkaline phosphatase activity, which suggests normal PTH-dependent bone turnover.[150] In fact, hyperparathyroid bone disease sometimes is observed in association with PHP Ib, leading to the introduction of the term "pseudohypo-hyperparathyroidism" (PHP-HPT).[151-153] The intact PTH response in the bone is consistent with the lack of Gsα imprinting in bone.[125] Moreover, because the genetic defect underlying PHP Ib does not involve a coding Gsα mutation (see below), this intact response appears more likely to result in increased bone resorption as the result of elevated serum PTH in this PHP subtype compared with that in PHP Ia.

The hormone resistance observed in PHP Ib patients develops only after maternal inheritance of the genetic defect[154] (i.e., the mode of inheritance is identical to hormone resistance in PHP Ia). PTH resistance and related changes in calcium and phosphorous homeostasis are the major laboratory findings in PHP Ib, but recent reports have demonstrated that some PHP Ib patients also display mild hypothyroidism with slightly elevated TSH levels,[26,155-157] as well as some elevation in calcitonin level.[155] Hypothyroidism, as in patients with PHP Ia, likely results from mild TSH resistance and is consistent with the predominantly maternal expression of Gsα in the thyroid.[128,156] Nevertheless, evidence for resistance to other hormones, such as gonadotropins, whose actions also involve tissues in which Gsα is imprinted, has not been reported for PHP Ib patients. A recent study assessed growth hormone responsiveness to GHRH plus arginine stimulation in PHP Ib, revealing a normal response in 9 of 10 patients.[157] On the other hand, in addition to PTH and mild thyroid-stimulating hormone (TSH) resistance, hypouricemia due to increased fractional excretion of uric acid has been reported in the affected individuals of two unrelated PHP Ib kindreds.[27,159] Although this finding implicates impaired PTH actions in the development of hypouricemia in these patients, and this interpretation is consistent with two previous reports describing hyperuricemia in association with hyperparathyroidism,[160,161] the hypouricemia reported in one of the PHP Ib kindreds seemed to have resolved following treatment with calcium and calcitriol.[27]

Patients with PHP Ib display normal Gsα bioactivity/levels in easily accessible tissues. Accordingly, coding Gsα mutations are ruled out in these patients. In one family, however, a mutation located in exon 13 (in-frame deletion of Ile^{382}) was reported, leading to the uncoupling of Gsα from PTHR1 but not other receptors, including TSHR, LHR, and β-adrenergic receptor.[162] Analyses were performed in LLCPK cells, which are of renal origin and express endogenous Gsα. These findings are consistent with isolated PTH resistance seen in PHP Ib, and this mutation may represent a rare cause of PHP Ib. However, this conclusion has been questioned, as the use of transfected mouse embryonic fibroblasts null for endogenous Gsα showed that del382Ile leads to uncoupling from not only PTHR1 but also the β-adrenergic receptor.[44] Because of a lack of Gsα mutations, and because Gsα activity/levels in easily accessible tissues are normal in PHP Ib patients, inactivating mutations that affect the gene encoding PTHR1 were considered in the past.[163] However, several different studies have excluded such mutations as the cause of this disease.[164-167] Instead, inactivating mutations of PTHR1 have been revealed as the cause of Bloomstrand's chondrodysplasia, an embryonic lethal disorder with severe skeletal abnormalities.[168]

Based on genome-wide linkage analysis, the genetic defect underlying PHP Ib maps to a region of chromosome 20q13 that comprises the GNAS locus,[154] but the critical interval excludes all the coding GNAS exons, including those that encode Gsα.[26] On the other hand, patients with PHP Ib display epigenetic abnormalities within the GNAS locus.[26,169] The most consistent epigenetic defect is a loss of imprinting at exon A/B (also termed exon 1A), which is found primarily as an isolated defect in familial PHP Ib cases.[26,169] In addition, many sporadic and some familial PHP Ib cases show additional loss of imprinting at the DMR comprising the XLαs and antisense promoters and gain of imprinting at the differentially methylated region (DMR) comprising exon NESP55.[13,169] These abnormalities are associated with biallelic expression of A/B, XLαs, and antisense transcripts and the silencing of NESP55 transcript. Together with the genetic linkage data, these imprinting defects suggest that the mutation causing PHP Ib disrupts a regulatory element that controls GNAS imprinting. However, evidence for incomplete penetrance regarding GNAS imprinting defects has been reported in one kindred, in whom some individuals lacked loss of imprinting and were healthy despite maternally inheriting the disease-associated haplotype.[170] Thus, imprinting abnormalities of GNAS appear to be required for the development of PHP Ib. Consistent with the importance of imprinting in the disease mechanism, a patient with this disorder has been reported to have paternal uniparental isodisomy of chromosome 20q.[155] In addition to having a paternal-exclusive imprinting profile at the GNAS locus and PTH resistance, the patient presented with mild developmental delay and craniosynostosis, which may reflect unmasking of recessive mutations inherited from the father or disruption of gene expression at other imprinted loci in this genomic region, such as the gene encoding neuronatin (NNAT).

In multiple familial PHP Ib cases with isolated exon A/B loss of imprinting, a unique 3 kb microdeletion at the neighboring STX16 locus has been identified (Fig. 10-8).[171] The deleted region comprises STX16 exons 4 to 6 and is flanked by two direct repeats, which may underlie the mechanism whereby this deletion occurs. This is consistent with the presence of the same microdeletion in many unrelated families with different ethnic and racial origin.* In a single kindred, a different microdeletion within STX16 has been reported, removing exons 2 through 4 and overlapping with the 3 kb microdeletion by approximately 1.3 kb.[39] Thus, disruption of STX16 appears to be the common genetic defect in cases with isolated loss of exon A/B imprinting. The parental origin of these STX16 deletions correlates well with the mode of inheritance of PHP Ib. It is inherited maternally in affected individuals and is inherited paternally in unaffected carriers. This gene encodes syntaxin-16, a member of the SNARE family proteins. However, STX16 does not appear to be imprinted,[39,171] and it is therefore unlikely that the loss of one STX16 copy leads to PHP Ib. Instead, because maternal inheritance is associated with loss of exon A/B imprinting on the same allele, these deletions are presumed to disrupt a cis-acting element that controls the establishment or maintenance of exon A/B imprinting. Other than genetic evidence, however, no currently available data corroborate this prediction. A mouse model carrying a deletion equivalent to the 3-kb STX16 deletion in humans has been generated, but neither maternal nor paternal inheritance of this genetic alteration causes PTH resistance or any alterations in GNAS imprinting[174]; animals with the homozygous Stx16 deletion are also healthy. It thus appears plausible that the imprinting control element of GNAS located within STX16 in the human is not precisely at the same location in the mouse. Nonetheless, the absence of a phenotype in the Stx16 deletion mice argues against a model in which syntaxin 16, the product of this gene, is required in the oocyte for proper exon A/B imprinting.

In two unrelated familial cases of PHP Ib in which the affected individuals carried broad GNAS imprinting defects, maternally inherited deletions of the entire NESP55 DMR, including exons 3 and 4 of the antisense transcript, have been identified (see Fig. 10-8).[117] The deletions are 4 kb and 4.7 kb large and have break-

---

*References 13, 25, 27, 157, 159, 172, and 173.

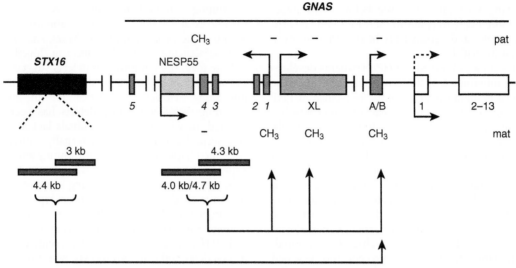

FIGURE 10-8. Mutations identified in patients with autosomal dominant PHP Ib (AD-PHP-Ib) and their effects on *GNAS* imprinting. The most frequent mutation is a 3 kb deletion within *STX16*, a gene located more than 200 kb upstream of *GNAS*. This deletion and another overlapping deletion in the same gene are predicted to disrupt a *cis*-acting control element of *GNAS* that is required for the imprint mark located at exon A/B. Deletions of the NESP55 DMR, including exons 3 and 4 of the antisense transcript and a recently identified deletion that includes only antisense transcript exons 3 and 4, have been identified in some AD-PHP-Ib kindreds. These reveal a *cis*-acting element that controls imprinting of the entire maternal *GNAS* allele. *Boxes* and *connecting lines* indicate exons and introns, respectively. *STX16* exons and *GNAS* exons 2 through 13 are shown as *single rectangles* for simplicity. Paternal (pat) and maternal (mat) methylation (CH3) and parental origin of transcription (*arrows*) are indicated. Tissue-specific silencing of the paternal Gsα transcription is depicted by a *dotted arrow*. Identified deletions are shown by *gray horizontal bars*.

points located in similar locations. Unaffected carriers in these families display an apparent loss of NESP55 methylation as the result of the loss of this region from the normally methylated paternal allele, but they do not show other imprinting *GNAS* defects. Affected individuals show loss of imprinting in the entire maternal allele. The presence of similarly large deletions at the NESP55 DMR has been excluded in a number of sporadic PHP Ib cases.[13,117] However, a different 4.2 kb deletion has been identified recently in the affected individuals of a different PHP Ib kindred who displayed broad *GNAS* imprinting defects[175] (see Fig. 10-8). This new deletion also includes antisense exons 3 and 4 but spares exon NESP55, overlapping with the previously identified two deletions by about 1.5 kb. Thus, these identified deletions reveal the putative location of another control element required for the imprinting of the entire maternal *GNAS* allele. The study of a mouse model in which Nesp55 transcription was prematurely truncated revealed loss of imprinting at exon 1A and, less consistently, the antisense promoter and exon XL.[176] Taken together with the genetic findings in patients with PHP Ib, it appears that the establishment of imprinting on the maternal *GNAS* allele, which allows expression of Gsα in the proximal renal tubule and other tissues in which this *GNAS* product is monoallelic, such as thyroid, requires transcription from the NESP55 promoter. It is thus possible that even small mutations that prevent the generation of NESP55 pre-mRNA can lead to PHP Ib.

In some sporadic PHP Ib cases that show *GNAS* methylation defects, the maternal allele is shared between affected and unaffected siblings, suggesting that these cases may carry small de novo mutations in this region. Alternatively, it is possible that some of the sporadic PHP Ib cases carry mutations in an entirely different genomic location with a putative autosomal recessive mode of inheritance. It has also been suggested that the broad *GNAS* imprinting defects observed in sporadic PHP Ib patients result from stochastic defects in the regulation of imprinting.[172]

Despite having distinct epigenetic abnormalities at the *GNAS* locus (i.e., isolated A/B loss of imprinting vs. broad imprinting

defects that involve exon A/B and at least one other *GNAS* DMR), PHP Ib patients seem to have similar clinical findings with respect to serum calcium, phosphate, and PTH levels.[13] Analysis of 20 families in which the affected individuals show an isolated loss of A/B imprinting reveals that a significant portion of such familial cases are asymptomatic at the time of diagnosis. In these cases, the diagnosis frequently is made only on the basis of elevated serum PTH. Comparison of male and female patients among sporadic PHP Ib cases that exhibit *GNAS* imprinting defects at two or more *GNAS* DMRs reveals that female patients have significantly higher serum PTH levels than male patients, suggesting that hormone resistance is more severe in females.[13]

By definition, PHP Ib patients do not show AHO features. However, some recent reports identified patients who carry genetic and epigenetic defects associated with PHP Ib, yet present with mild AHO features, particularly shortness of metacarpal bones.[27,173,177] This may suggest that Gsα imprinting occurs in more tissues than is currently recognized, although alternative explanations have been put forth. Given that individual AHO features can be observed in other disorders, the presence of AHO features may be unrelated to the molecular genetic defects underlying PHP Ib in these cases. In one case, the mother of two affected siblings with short metacarpals and loss of A/B imprinting also exhibited short metacarpals despite lacking any *GNAS* epigenetic abnormalities,[173] suggesting that the finding of short metacarpals is unrelated to the epigenetic defect in that family. In addition, the observed coexistence of *GNAS* imprinting defects and AHO can result from a large genomic deletion comprising at least the promoter of Gsα and one or more differentially methylated regions. Such deletions have been ruled out in some but not all cases.[27,173,177]

Pseudohypoparathyroidism Type II

Dissociation regarding the impairment of PTH-induced nephrogenous cAMP formation and phosphaturia (i.e., PHP II) appears to be the least common form of PHP. Although typically sporadic, a case with a familial form of PHP II type has been reported,[178] and several reports describe evidence of a self-limited form of this disease in newborns, which could indicate that it is transient in nature.[35,179-181] The molecular defect and pathophysiologic mechanisms underlying this PHP variant remains to be discovered. Because the defect underlying PHP II is associated with normal cAMP generation in response to exogenous PTH, it is possible that it is caused by molecular defects that involve downstream cAMP generation, such as protein kinase A.[19] Alternatively, the PTH signaling pathways that utilize G proteins other than Gs, such as Gq, may be defective in patients with PHP II. Signaling mediated by Gq involves activation of phopholipase C, which, in turn, leads to the formation of second messengers inositol 1,4,5-triphophate (IP3) and diacylglycerol (DAG). This signaling pathway results in stimulation of protein kinase C (PKC) and an increase in intracellular calcium ions. Serum calcium levels, which may affect the efficient utilization of intracellular calcium signaling pathways, appear to be important for restoring PTH responsiveness in PHP II, as shown in some patients who normalized their phosphaturic response to PTH following normalization of serum calcium.[182] It is also possible that sodium-phosphate transporters in the proximal renal tubule are nonresponsive to PTH, thus leading to a defective phosphaturic, but not cAMP, response to exogenous PTH. Such a defect, however, should preserve the action of PTH on 25(OH) D-1α-hydroxylase, leading to normal serum $1,25(OH)_2D$, unless it is combined with vitamin D deficiency. Hypocalcemia as a result of vitamin D deficiency has been associated with PTH resistance that entailed the phosphaturic effect of this hormone without altering its potential to raise urinary cAMP,[183] suggesting that some PHP II cases may in fact reflect vitamin D deficiency.[184,185]

Summary

PHP refers to a group of disorders characterized by PTH resistance associated with hypocalcemia, hyperphosphatemia, and elevated serum PTH. Proximal tubular resistance to PTH is the most prominent hormonal defect, but resistance to other hormones can also be observed. PTH and these other hormones all exert their actions via receptors that couple to Gsα. The primary genetic causes of PHP I and related disorders are mutations that affect the complex *GNAS* locus, the gene encoding Gsα. These mutations result in decreased expression/activity of Gsα but also affect some of the other gene products derived from *GNAS*. The nature and the parental origin of the *GNAS* mutation are important determinants of the clinical manifestations. Mutations that affect coding Gsα exons lead to broader clinical abnormalities than do mutations that disrupt *GNAS* imprinting. Because of the tissue-specific imprinting of Gsα, hormone resistance develops only after maternal inheritance. AHO typically occurs after both maternal and paternal inheritance of coding Gsα mutations, although some AHO features also follow an imprinted mode of inheritance. PPHP is used to describe those patients with AHO who lack hormone resistance. AHO features vary markedly. An extreme manifestation of AHO is progressive osseous heteroplasia, which appears to develop predominantly following paternal transmission of coding Gsα mutations. PHP II is rare, and the molecular determinants of this PHP form remain elusive.

REFERENCES

1. Albright F, Burnett CH, Smith PH, et al: Pseudohypoparathyroidism—an example of "Seabright-Bantam syndrome," Endocrinology 30:922–932, 1942.
2. Tashjian AH Jr, Frantz AG, Lee JB: Pseudohypoparathyroidism: assays of parathyroid hormone and thyrocalcitonin, Proc Natl Acad Sci U S A 56:1138–1142, 1966.
3. Ish-Shalom S, Rao LG, Levine MA, et al: Normal parathyroid hormone responsiveness of bone-derived cells from a patient with pseudohypoparathyroidism, J Bone Miner Res 11:8–14, 1996.
4. Murray T, Gomez Rao E, Wong MM, et al: Pseudohypoparathyroidism with osteitis fibrosa cystica: direct demonstration of skeletal responsiveness to parathyroid hormone in cells cultured from bone, J Bone Miner Res 8:83–91, 1993.
5. Stone M, Hosking D, Garcia-Himmelstine C, et al: The renal response to exogenous parathyroid hormone in treated pseudohypoparathyroidism, Bone 14:727–735, 1993.
6. Breslau NA, Weinstock RS: Regulation of $1,25(OH)_2D$ synthesis in hypoparathyroidism and pseudohypoparathyroidism, Am J Physiol 255:E730–E736, 1988.
7. Drezner MK, Neelon FA, Haussler M, et al: 1,25-Dihydroxycholecalciferol deficiency: the probable cause of hypocalcemia and metabolic bone disease in pseudohypoparathyroidism, J Clin Endocrinol Metab 42:621–628, 1976.
8. Braun JJ, Birkenhager JC, Visser TJ, et al: Lack of response of 1,25-dihydroxycholecalciferol to exogenous parathyroid hormone in a patient with treated pseudohypoparathyroidism, Clin Endocrinol (Oxf) 14:403–407, 1981.
9. Yamaoka K, Seino Y, Ishida M, et al: Effect of dibutyryl adenosine 3′,5′-monophosphate administration on plasma concentrations of 1,25-dihydroxyvitamin D in pseudohypoparathyroidism type I, J Clin Endocrinol Metab 53:1096–1100, 1981.
10. Drezner MK, Haussler MR: Normocalcemic pseudohypoparathyroidism, Association with normal vitamin D3 metabolism, Am J Med 66:503–508, 1979.
11. Balachandar V, Pahuja J, Maddaiah VT, et al: Pseudohypoparathyroidism with normal serum calcium level, Am J Dis Child 129:1092–1095, 1975.
12. Breslau NA, Notman DD, Canterbury JM, et al: Studies on the attainment of normocalcemia in patients with pseudohypoparathyroidism, Am J Med 68:856–860, 1980.
13. Linglart A, Bastepe M, Jüppner H: Similar clinical and laboratory findings in patients with symptomatic autosomal dominant and sporadic pseudohypoparathyroidism type Ib despite different epigenetic changes at the GNAS locus, Clin Endocrinol (Oxf) 67:822–831, 2007.
14. Tamada Y, Kanda S, Suzuki H, et al: A pseudohypoparathyroidism type Ia patient with normocalcemia, Endocr J 55:169–173, 2008.
15. Jüppner H, Abou-Samra AB, Freeman MW, et al: A G protein-linked receptor for parathyroid hormone and parathyroid hormone-related peptide, Science 254:1024–1026, 1991.
16. Gardella TJ, Jüppner H: Molecular properties of the PTH/PTHrP receptor, Trends Endocrinol Metab 12:210–217, 2001.
17. Abou-Samra AB, Jüppner H, Force T, et al: Expression cloning of a common receptor for parathyroid hormone and parathyroid hormone-related peptide from rat osteoblast-like cells: a single receptor stimulates intracellular accumulation of both cAMP and inositol triphosphates and increases intracellular free calcium, Proc Natl Acad Sci U S A 89:2732–2736, 1992.
18. Chase LR, Melson GL, Aurbach GD: Pseudohypoparathyroidism: defective excretion of 3′,5′-AMP in response to parathyroid hormone, J Clin Invest 48:1832–1844, 1969.
19. Drezner M, Neelon FA, Lebovitz HE: Pseudohypoparathyroidism type II: a possible defect in the reception of the cyclic AMP signal, N Engl J Med 289:1056–1060, 1973.
20. Siejka SJ, Knezevic WV, Pullan PT: Dystonia and intracerebral calcification: pseudohypoparathyroidism presenting in an eleven-year-old girl, Aust N Z J Med 18:607–609, 1988.
21. Dure L St, Mussell HG: Paroxysmal dyskinesia in a patient with pseudohypoparathyroidism, Mov Disord 13:746–748, 1998.
22. Huang CW, Chen YC, Tsai JJ: Paroxysmal dyskinesia with secondary generalization of tonic-clonic seizures in pseudohypoparathyroidism, Epilepsia 46:164–165, 2005.
23. Prashantha DK, Pal PK: Pseudohypoparathyroidism manifesting with paroxysmal dyskinesias and seizures, Mov Disord 24:623–624, 2009.
24. Kinoshita M, Komori T, Ohtake T, et al: Abnormal calcium metabolism in myotonic dystrophy as shown by the Ellsworth-Howard test and its relation to CTG triplet repeat length, J Neurol 244:613–622, 1997.
25. Mahmud FH, Linglart A, Bastepe M, et al: Molecular diagnosis of pseudohypoparathyroidism type Ib in a family with presumed paroxysmal dyskinesia, Pediatrics 115:e242–e244, 2005.
26. Bastepe M, Pincus JE, Sugimoto T, et al: Positional dissociation between the genetic mutation responsible for pseudohypoparathyroidism type Ib and the associated methylation defect at exon A/B: evidence for a long-range regulatory element within the imprinted GNAS1 locus, Hum Mol Genet 10:1231–1241, 2001.
27. Unluturk U, Harmanci A, Babaoglu M, et al: Molecular diagnosis and clinical characterization of pseudohypoparathyroidism type-Ib in a patient with mild Albright's hereditary osteodystrophy-like features, epileptic seizures, and defective renal handling of uric acid, Am J Med Sci 336:84–90, 2008.

28. Windeck R, Menken U, Benker G, et al: Basal ganglia calcification in pseudohypoparathyroidism type II, Clin Endocrinol (Oxf) 15:57–63, 1981.

29. Chen H, Tseng F, Su D, et al: Multiple intracranial calcifications and spinal compressions: rare complications of type Ia pseudohypoparathyroidism, J Endocrinol Invest 28:646–650, 2005.

30. Illum F, Dupont E: Prevalences of CT-detected calcification in the basal ganglia in idiopathic hypoparathyroidism and pseudohypoparathyroidism, Neuroradiology 27:32–37, 1985.

31. Manabe Y, Araki M, Takeda K, et al: Pseudohypoparathyroidism with striopallidodentate calcification—a case report and review of the literature, Jpn J Med 28:391–395, 1989.

32. Pearson DW, Durward WF, Fogelman I, et al: Pseudohypoparathyroidism presenting as severe Parkinsonism, Postgrad Med J 57:445–447, 1981.

33. Saito H, Saito M, Saito K, et al: Subclinical pseudohypoparathyroidism type II: evidence for failure of physiologic adjustment in calcium metabolism during pregnancy, Am J Med Sci 297:247–250, 1989.

34. Zachariah SB, Zachariah B, Antonios N, et al: Pseudohypoparathyroidism and cerebrovascular disease with dural calcification, J Fla Med Assoc 78:26–28, 1991.

35. Narang M, Salota R, Sachdev SS: Neonatal pseudohypoparathyroidism, Indian J Pediatr 73:97–98, 2006.

36. Sajitha S, Krishnamoorthy PN, Shenoy UV: Pseudohypoparathyroidism in newborn—a rare presentation, Indian J Pediatr 40:47–49, 2003.

37. Tsang R, Venkataraman P, Ho M, et al: The development of pseudohypoparathyroidism. Involvement of progressively increasing serum parathyroid hormone concentrations, increased 1,25-dihydroxyvitamin D concentrations, and "migratory" subcutaneous calcifications, Am J Dis Child 138:654–658, 1984.

38. Barr DG, Stirling HF, Darling JA: Evolution of pseudohypoparathyroidism: an informative family study, Arch Dis Child 70:337–338, 1994.

39. Linglart A, Gensure RC, Olney RC, et al: A novel STX16 deletion in autosomal dominant pseudohypoparathyroidism type Ib redefines the boundaries of a cis-acting imprinting control element of GNAS, Am J Hum Genet 76:804–814, 2005.

40. Gelfand IM, Eugster EA, Dimeglio LA: Presentation and clinical progression of pseudohypoparathyroidism with multi-hormone resistance and Albright hereditary osteodystrophy: a case series, J Pediatr 149:877–880, 2006.

41. Farfel Z: Pseudohypohyperparathyroidism-pseudohypoparathyroidism type Ib, J Bone Miner Res 14:1016, 1999.

42. Poznanski AK, Werder EA, Giedion A, et al: The pattern of shortening of the bones of the hand in PHP and PPHP—a comparison with brachydactyly E, Turner syndrome, and acrodysostosis, Radiology 123:707–718, 1977.

43. Archibald RM, Finby N, De Vito F: Endocrine significance of short metacarpals, J Clin Endocrinol Metab 19:1312–1322, 1959.

44. Linglart A, Mahon MJ, Kerachian MA, et al: Coding GNAS mutations leading to hormone resistance impair in vitro agonist- and cholera toxin-induced adenosine cyclic 3',5'-monophosphate formation mediated by human XLαs, Endocrinology 147:2253–2262, 2006.

45. Levine MA, Downs RW Jr, Moses AM, et al: Resistance to multiple hormones in patients with pseudohypoparathyroidism, Association with deficient activity of guanine nucleotide regulatory protein, Am J Med 74:545–556, 1983.

46. Mallet E, Carayon P, Amr S, et al: Coupling defect of thyrotropin receptor and adenylate cyclase in a pseudohypoparathyroid patient, J Clin Endocrinol Metab 54:1028–1032, 1982.

47. Yu D, Yu S, Schuster V, et al: Identification of two novel deletion mutations within the Gs alpha gene (GNAS1) in Albright hereditary osteodystrophy, J Clin Endocrinol Metab 84:3254–3259, 1999.

48. Levine MA, Jap TS, Hung W: Infantile hypothyroidism in two sibs: an unusual presentation of pseudohypoparathyroidism type Ia, J Pediatr 107:919–922, 1985.

49. Weisman Y, Golander A, Spirer Z, et al: Pseudohypoparathyroidism type 1a presenting as congenital hypothyroidism, J Pediatr 107:413–415, 1985.

50. Yokoro S, Matsuo M, Ohtsuka T, et al: Hyperthyrotropinemia in a neonate with normal thyroid hormone levels: the earliest diagnostic clue for pseudohypoparathyroidism, Biol Neonate 58:69–72, 1990.

51. Wolfsdorf JI, Rosenfield RL, Fang VS, et al: Partial gonadotrophin-resistance in pseudohypoparathyroidism, Acta Endocrinol (Copenh) 88:321–328, 1978.

52. Mantovani G, Maghnie M, Weber G, et al: Growth hormone-releasing hormone resistance in pseudohypoparathyroidism type Ia: new evidence for imprinting of the Gs alpha gene, J Clin Endocrinol Metab 88:4070–4074, 2003.

53. Germain-Lee EL, Groman J, Crane JL, et al: Growth hormone deficiency in pseudohypoparathyroidism type 1a: another manifestation of multihormone resistance, J Clin Endocrinol Metab 88:4059–4069, 2003.

54. Moses AM, Weinstock RS, Levine MA, et al: Evidence for normal antidiuretic responses to endogenous and exogenous arginine vasopressin in patients with guanine nucleotide-binding stimulatory protein-deficient pseudohypoparathyroidism, J Clin Endocrinol Metab 62:221–224, 1986.

55. Stirling HF, Barr DGD, Kelnar CJH: Familial growth hormone releasing factor deficiency in pseudohypoparathyroidism, Arch Dis Child 66:533–535, 1991.

56. Namnoum AB, Merriam GR, Moses AM, et al: Reproductive dysfunction in women with Albright's hereditary osteodystrophy, J Clin Endocrinol Metab 83:824–829, 1998.

57. Weinstein LS: Albright hereditary osteodystrophy, pseudohypoparathyroidism, and Gs deficiency, In Spiegel AM, editor: G Proteins, Receptors, and Disease. Totowa, NJ: Humana Press; 1998, pp 23–56.

58. Levine MA: Pseudohypoparathyroidism: from bedside to bench and back, J Bone Miner Res 14:1255–1260, 1999.

59. Weinstein LS, Gejman PV, Friedman E, et al: Mutations of the Gs alpha-subunit gene in Albright hereditary osteodystrophy detected by denaturing gradient gel electrophoresis, Proc Natl Acad Sci U S A 87:8287–8290, 1990.

60. Patten JL, Johns DR, Valle D, et al: Mutation in the gene encoding the stimulatory G protein of adenylate cyclase in Albright's hereditary osteodystrophy, N Engl J Med 322:1412–1419, 1990.

61. Ma YC, Huang J, Ali S, et al: Src tyrosine kinase is a novel direct effector of G proteins, Cell 102:635–646, 2000.

62. Yatani A, Imoto Y, Codina J, et al: The stimulatory G protein of adenylyl cyclase, Gs, also stimulates dihydropyridine-sensitive Ca2+ channels. Evidence for direct regulation independent of phosphorylation by cAMP-dependent protein kinase or stimulation by a dihydropyridine agonist, J Biol Chem 263:9887–9895, 1988.

63. Mattera R, Graziano MP, Yatani A, et al: Splice variants of the alpha subunit of the G protein Gs activate both adenylyl cyclase and calcium channels, Science 243:804–807, 1989.

64. Aldred MA, Aftimos S, Hall C, et al: Constitutional deletion of chromosome 20q in two patients affected with Albright hereditary osteodystrophy, Am J Med Genet 113:167–172, 2002.

65. Levine MA, Jap TS, Mauseth RS, et al: Activity of the stimulatory guanine nucleotide-binding protein is reduced in erythrocytes from patients with pseudohypoparathyroidism and pseudopseudohypoparathyroidism: biochemical, endocrine, and genetic analysis of Albright's hereditary osteodystrophy in six kindreds, J Clin Endocrinol Metab 62:497–502, 1986.

66. Miric A, Vechio JD, Levine MA: Heterogeneous mutations in the gene encoding the alpha-subunit of the stimulatory G protein of adenylyl cyclase in Albright hereditary osteodystrophy, J Clin Endocrinol Metab 76:1560–1568, 1993.

67. Farfel Z, Bourne HR: Deficient activity of receptor-cyclase coupling protein in platelets of patients with pseudohypoparathyroidism, J Clin Endocrinol Metab 51:1202–1204, 1980.

68. Farfel Z, Brothers VM, Brickman AS, et al: Pseudohypoparathyroidism: inheritance of deficient receptor-cyclase coupling activity, Proc Natl Acad Sci U S A 78:3098–3102, 1981.

69. Bourne HR, Kaslow HR, Brickman AS, et al: Fibroblast defect in pseudohypoparathyroidism, type I: reduced activity of receptor-cyclase coupling protein, J Clin Endocrinol Metab 53:636–640, 1981.

70. Spiegel AM, Levine MA, Aurbach GD, et al: Deficiency of hormone receptor-adenylate cyclase coupling protein: basis for hormone resistance in pseudohypoparathyroidism, Am J Physiol 243:E37–E42, 1982.

71. Motulsky HJ, Hughes RJ, Brickman AS, et al: Platelets of pseudohypoparathyroid patients: evidence that distinct receptor-cyclase coupling proteins mediate stimulation and inhibition of adenylate cyclase, Proc Natl Acad Sci U S A 79:4193–4197, 1982.

72. Farfel Z, Abood ME, Brickman AS, et al: Deficient activity of receptor-cyclase coupling protein is transformed lymphoblasts of patients with pseudohypoparathyroidism, type I, J Clin Endocrinol Metab 55:113–117, 1982.

73. Levine MA, Eil C, Downs RW Jr, et al: Deficient guanine nucleotide regulatory unit activity in cultured fibroblast membranes from patients with pseudohypoparathyroidism type I. A cause of impaired synthesis of 3',5'-cyclic AMP by intact and broken cells, J Clin Invest 72:316–324, 1983.

74. Levine MA, Ahn TG, Klupt SF, et al: Genetic deficiency of the alpha subunit of the guanine nucleotide-binding protein Gs as the molecular basis for Albright hereditary osteodystrophy, Proc Natl Acad Sci U S A 85:617–621, 1988.

75. Patten JL, Levine MA: Immunochemical analysis of the α-subunit of the stimulatory G-protein of adenylyl cyclase in patients with Albright's hereditary osteodystrophy, J Clin Endocrinol Metab 71:1208–1214, 1990.

76. Carter A, Bardin C, Collins R, et al: Reduced expression of multiple forms of the α subunit of the stimulatory GTP-binding protein in pseudohypoparathyroidism type Ia, Proc Natl Acad Sci U S A 84:7266–7269, 1987.

77. Farfel Z, Brickman AS, Kaslow HR, et al: Defect of receptor-cyclase coupling protein in pseudohypoparathyroidism, N Engl J Med 303:237–242, 1980.

78. Levine MA, Downs RW Jr, Singer M, et al: Deficient activity of guanine nucleotide regulatory protein in erythrocytes from patients with pseudohypoparathyroidism, Biochem Biophys Res Commun 94:1319–1324, 1980.

79. Downs RW Jr, Levine MA, Drezner MK, et al: Deficient adenylate cyclase regulatory protein in renal membranes from a patient with pseudohypoparathyroidism, J Clin Invest 71:231–235, 1983.

80. Iiri T, Herzmark P, Nakamoto JM, et al: Rapid GDP release from Gs in patients with gain and loss of function, Nature 371:164–168, 1994.

81. Makita N, Sato J, Rondard P, et al: Human G(salpha) mutant causes pseudohypoparathyroidism type Ia/neonatal diarrhea, a potential cell-specific role of the palmitoylation cycle, Proc Natl Acad Sci U S A 104:17424–17429, 2007.

82. Linglart A, Carel JC, Garabedian M, et al: GNAS1 lesions in pseudohypoparathyroidism Ia and Ic: genotype phenotype relationship and evidence of the maternal transmission of the hormonal resistance, J Clin Endocrinol Metab 87:189–197, 2002.

83. Gejman PV, Weinstein LS, Martinez M, et al: Genetic mapping of the Gs-α subunit gene (GNAS1) to the distal long arm of chromosome 20 using a polymorphism detected by denaturing gradient gel electrophoresis, Genomics 9:782–783, 1991.

84. Rao VV, Schnittger S, Hansmann I: G protein Gs alpha (GNAS 1), the probable candidate gene for Albright hereditary osteodystrophy, is assigned to human chromosome 20q12-q13.2, Genomics 10:257–261, 1991.

85. Levine MA, Modi WS, O'Brien SJ: Mapping of the gene encoding the alpha subunit of the stimulatory G protein of adenylyl cyclase (GNAS1) to 20q13.2-q13.3 in human by in situ hybridization, Genomics 11:478–479, 1991.

86. Kozasa T, Itoh H, Tsukamoto T, et al: Isolation and characterization of the human Gsα gene, Proc Natl Acad Sci U S A 85:2081–2085, 1988.

87. Bray P, Carter A, Simons C, et al: Human cDNA clones for four species of G alpha s signal transduction protein, Proc Natl Acad Sci U S A 83:8893–8897, 1986.

88. Robishaw JD, Smigel MD, Gilman AG: Molecular basis for two forms of the G protein that stimulates adenylate cyclase, J Biol Chem 261:9587–9590, 1986.

89. Sternweis PC, Northup JK, Smigel MD, et al: The regulatory component of adenylate cyclase: purification and properties, J Biol Chem 256:11517–11526, 1981.

90. Walseth TF, Zhang HJ, Olson LK, et al: Increase in Gs and cyclic AMP generation in HIT cells: evidence that the 45-kDa alpha-subunit of Gs has greater functional activity than the 52-kDa alpha-subunit, J Biol Chem 264:21106–21111, 1989.
91. Graziano MP, Freissmuth M, Gilman AG: Expression of Gs alpha in *Escherichia coli:* purification and properties of two forms of the protein, J Biol Chem 264:409–418, 1989.
92. Seifert R, Wenzel-Seifert K, Lee TW, et al: Different effects of Gsalpha splice variants on beta2-adrenoreceptor-mediated signaling: the beta2-adrenoreceptor coupled to the long splice variant of Gsalpha has properties of a constitutively active receptor, J Biol Chem 273:5109–5116, 1998.
93. Kvapil P, Novotny J, Svoboda P, et al: The short and long forms of the alpha subunit of the stimulatory guanine-nucleotide-binding protein are unequally redistributed during (−)-isoproterenol-mediated desensitization of intact S49 lymphoma cells, Eur J Biochem 226:193–199, 1994.
94. el Jamali A, Rachdaoui N, Jacquemin C, et al: Long-term effect of forskolin on the activation of adenylyl cyclase in astrocytes, J Neurochem 67:2532–2539, 1996.
95. Bourgeois C, Duc-Goiran P, Robert B, et al: G protein expression in human fetoplacental vascularization: functional evidence for Gs alpha and Gi alpha subunits, J Mol Cell Cardiol 28:1009–1021, 1996.
96. Thiele S, Werner R, Ahrens W, et al: A disruptive mutation in exon 3 of the GNAS gene with Albright hereditary osteodystrophy, normocalcemic pseudohypoparathyroidism, and selective long transcript variant Gsalpha-L deficiency, J Clin Endocrinol Metab 92:1764–1768, 2007.
97. Ischia R, Lovisetti-Scamihorn P, Hogue-Angeletti R, et al: Molecular cloning and characterization of NESP55, a novel chromogranin-like precursor of a peptide with 5-HT1B receptor antagonist activity, J Biol Chem 272:11657–11662, 1997.
98. Hayward BE, Moran V, Strain L, et al: Bidirectional imprinting of a single gene: GNAS1 encodes maternally, paternally, and biallelically derived proteins, Proc Natl Acad Sci U S A 95:15475–15480, 1998.
99. Peters J, Wroe SF, Wells CA, et al: A cluster of oppositely imprinted transcripts at the GNAS locus in the distal imprinting region of mouse chromosome 2, Proc Natl Acad Sci U S A 96:3830–3835, 1999.
100. Lovisetti-Scamihorn P, Fischer-Colbrie R, Leitner B, et al: Relative amounts and molecular forms of NESP55 in various bovine tissues, Brain Res 829:99–106, 1999.
101. Weiss U, Ischia R, Eder S, et al: Neuroendocrine secretory protein 55 (NESP55): alternative splicing onto transcripts of the GNAS gene and posttranslational processing of a maternally expressed protein, Neuroendocrinology 71:177–186, 2000.
102. Bauer R, Weiss C, Marksteiner J, et al: The new chromogranin-like protein NESP55 is preferentially localized in adrenaline-synthesizing cells of the bovine and rat adrenal medulla, Neurosci Lett 263:13–16, 1999.
103. Li JY, Lovisetti-Scamihorn P, Fischer-Colbrie R, et al: Distribution and intraneuronal trafficking of a novel member of the chromogranin family, NESP55, in the rat peripheral nervous system, Neuroscience 110:731–745, 2002.
104. Fischer-Colbrie R, Eder S, Lovisetti-Scamihorn P, et al: Neuroendocrine secretory protein 55: a novel marker for the constitutive secretory pathway, Ann N Y Acad Sci 971:317–322, 2002.
105. Plagge A, Isles AR, Gordon E, et al: Imprinted Nesp55 influences behavioral reactivity to novel environments, Mol Cell Biol 25:3019–3026, 2005.
106. Kehlenbach RH, Matthey J, Huttner WB: XLαs is a new type of G protein (Erratum in Nature 375:253, 1995), Nature 372:804–809, 1994.
107. Hayward B, Kamiya M, Strain L, et al: The human GNAS1 gene is imprinted and encodes distinct paternally and biallelically expressed G proteins, Proc Natl Acad Sci U S A 95:10038–10043, 1998.
108. Klemke M, Pasolli H, Kehlenbach R, et al: Characterization of the extra-large G protein alpha-subunit XLalphas, II, Signal transduction properties, J Biol Chem 275:33633–33640, 2000.
109. Bastepe M, Gunes Y, Perez-Villamil B, et al: Receptor-mediated adenylyl cyclase activation through XLalphas, the extra-large variant of the stimulatory G protein alpha-subunit, Mol Endocrinol 16:1912–1919, 2002.
110. Plagge A, Gordon E, Dean W, et al: The imprinted signaling protein XLalphas is required for postnatal adaptation to feeding, Nat Genet 36:818–826, 2004.
111. Chen M, Gavrilova O, Liu J, et al: Alternative Gnas gene products have opposite effects on glucose and lipid metabolism, Proc Natl Acad Sci U S A 102:7386–7391, 2005.
112. Germain-Lee EL, Schwindinger W, Crane JL, et al: A mouse model of Albright hereditary osteodystrophy generated by targeted disruption of exon 1 of the Gnas gene, Endocrinology 146:4697–4709, 2005.
113. Swaroop A, Agarwal N, Gruen JR, et al: Differential expression of novel Gs alpha signal transduction protein cDNA species, Nucleic Acids Res 19:4725–4729, 1991.
114. Ishikawa Y, Bianchi C, Nadal-Ginard B, et al: Alternative promoter and 5′ exon generate a novel $G_s\alpha$ mRNA, J Biol Chem 265:8458–8462, 1990.
115. Hayward B, Bonthron D: An imprinted antisense transcript at the human GNAS1 locus, Hum Mol Genet 9:835–841, 2000.
116. Wroe SF, Kelsey G, Skinner JA, et al: An imprinted transcript, antisense to Nesp, adds complexity to the cluster of imprinted genes at the mouse GNAS locus, Proc Natl Acad Sci U S A 97:3342–3346, 2000.
117. Bastepe M, Fröhlich LF, Linglart A, et al: Deletion of the NESP55 differentially methylated region causes loss of maternal GNAS imprints and pseudohypoparathyroidism type-Ib, Nat Genet 37:25–37, 2005.
118. Coombes C, Arnaud P, Gordon E, et al: Epigenetic properties and identification of an imprint mark in the Nesp-Gnasxl domain of the mouse GNAS imprinted locus, Mol Cell Biol 23:5475–5488, 2003.
119. Liu J, Yu S, Litman D, et al: Identification of a methylation imprint mark within the mouse GNAS locus, Mol Cell Biol 20:5808–5817, 2000.
120. Williamson CM, Ball ST, Nottingham WT, et al: A cis-acting control region is required exclusively for the tissue-specific imprinting of GNAS, Nat Genet 36:894–899, 2004.
121. Williamson CM, Turner MD, Ball ST, et al: Identification of an imprinting control region affecting the expression of all transcripts in the GNAS cluster, Nat Genet 38:350–355, 2006.
122. Liu J, Chen M, Deng C, et al: Identification of the control region for tissue-specific imprinting of the stimulatory G protein alpha-subunit, Proc Natl Acad Sci U S A 102:5513–5518, 2005.
123. Zheng H, Radeva G, McCann JA, et al: Gαs transcripts are biallelically expressed in the human kidney cortex: implications for pseudohypoparathyroidism type Ib, J Clin Endocrinol Metab 86:4627–4629, 2001.
124. Campbell R, Gosden CM, Bonthron DT: Parental origin of transcription from the human GNAS1 gene, J Med Genet 31:607–614, 1994.
125. Mantovani G, Bondioni S, Locatelli M, et al: Biallelic expression of the Gsalpha gene in human bone and adipose tissue, J Clin Endocrinol Metab 89:6316–6319, 2004.
126. Yu S, Yu D, Lee E, et al: Variable and tissue-specific hormone resistance in heterotrimeric G_s protein α-subunit ($G_s\alpha$) knockout mice is due to tissue-specific imprinting of the $G_s\alpha$ gene, Proc Natl Acad Sci U S A 95:8715–8720, 1998.
127. Hayward B, Barlier A, Korbonits M, et al: Imprinting of the G(s)alpha gene GNAS1 in the pathogenesis of acromegaly, J Clin Invest 107:R31–R36, 2001.
128. Mantovani G, Ballare E, Giammona E, et al: The Gsalpha gene: predominant maternal origin of transcription in human thyroid gland and gonads, J Clin Endocrinol Metab 87:4736–4740, 2002.
129. Sakamoto A, Liu J, Greene A, et al: Tissue-specific imprinting of the G protein Gsalpha is associated with tissue-specific differences in histone methylation, Hum Mol Genet 13:819–828, 2004.
130. Albright F, Forbes AP, Henneman PH: Pseudo-pseudohypoparathyroidism, Trans Assoc Am Physicians 65:337–350, 1952.
131. Davies AJ, Hughes HE: Imprinting in Albright's hereditary osteodystrophy, J Med Genet 30:101–103, 1993.
132. Kronenberg HM: Developmental regulation of the growth plate, Nature 423:332–336, 2003.
133. Bastepe M, Weinstein LS, Ogata N, et al: Stimulatory G protein directly regulates hypertrophic differentiation of growth plate cartilage in vivo, Proc Natl Acad Sci U S A 101:14794–14799, 2004.
134. Long DN, McGuire S, Levine MA, et al: Body mass index differences in pseudohypoparathyroidism type 1a versus pseudopseudohypoparathyroidism may implicate paternal imprinting of Galpha(s) in the development of human obesity, J Clin Endocrinol Metab 92:1073–1079, 2007.
135. Mouallem M, Shaharabany M, Weintrob N, et al: Cognitive impairment is prevalent in pseudohypoparathyroidism type Ia, but not in pseudopseudohypoparathyroidism: possible cerebral imprinting of Gsalpha, Clin Endocrinol (Oxf) 68:233–239, 2008.
136. Kaplan FS, Craver R, MacEwen GD, et al: Progressive osseous heteroplasia: a distinct developmental disorder of heterotopic ossification, Two new case reports and follow-up of three previously reported cases, J Bone Joint Surg Am 76:425–436, 1994.
137. Kaplan FS, Shore EM: Progressive osseous heteroplasia, J Bone Miner Res 15:2084–2094, 2000.
138. Buyse G, Silberstein J, Goemans N, et al: Fibrodysplasia ossificans progressiva: still turning into wood after 300 years? Eur J Pediatr 154:694–699, 1995.
139. Shore EM, Kaplan FS: Insights from a rare genetic disorder of extra-skeletal bone formation, fibrodysplasia ossificans progressiva (FOP), Bone 43:427–433, 2008.
140. Eddy MC, De Beur SM, Yandow SM, et al: Deficiency of the alpha-subunit of the stimulatory G protein and severe extraskeletal ossification, J Bone Miner Res 15:2074–2083, 2000.
141. Yeh GL, Mathur S, Wivel A, et al: GNAS1 mutation and Cbfa1 misexpression in a child with severe congenital platelike osteoma cutis, J Bone Miner Res 15:2063–2073, 2000.
142. Shore EM, Ahn J, Jan de Beur S, et al: Paternally inherited inactivating mutations of the GNAS1 gene in progressive osseous heteroplasia, N Engl J Med 346:99–106, 2002.
143. Weinstein LS, Yu S, Warner DR, et al: Endocrine manifestations of stimulatory G protein alpha-subunit mutations and the role of genomic imprinting, Endocr Rev 22:675–705, 2001.
144. Lietman SA, Ding C, Cooke DW, et al: Reduction in Gsalpha induces osteogenic differentiation in human mesenchymal stem cells, Clin Orthop Relat Res (434):231–238, 2005.
145. Zhao Y, Ding S: A high-throughput siRNA library screen identifies osteogenic suppressors in human mesenchymal stem cells, Proc Natl Acad Sci U S A 104:9673–9678, 2007.
146. Bertaux K, Broux O, Chauveau C, et al: Runx2 regulates the expression of GNAS on SaOs-2 cells, Bone 38:943–950, 2006.
147. Adegbite NS, Xu M, Kaplan FS, et al: Diagnostic and mutational spectrum of progressive osseous heteroplasia (POH) and other forms of GNAS-based heterotopic ossification, Am J Med Genet 146A:1788–1796, 2008.
148. Peterman MG, Garvey JL: Pseudohypoparathyroidism; case report, Pediatrics 4:790, 1949.
149. Reynolds TB, Jacobson G, Edmondson HA, et al: Pseudohypoparathyroidism: report of a case showing bony demineralization, J Clin Endocrinol Metab 12:560, 1952.
150. Elrick H, Albright F, Bartter FC, et al: Further studies on pseudo-hypoparathyroidism: report of four new cases, Acta Endocrinol 5:199–225, 1950.
151. Costello JM, Dent CE: Hypo-hyperparathyroidism, Arch Dis Child 38:397–407, 1963.
152. Allen EH, Millard FJC, Nassim JR: Hypo-hyperparathyroidism, Arch Dis Child 43:295–301, 1968.
153. Frame B, Hanson CA, Frost HM, et al: Renal resistance to parathyroid hormone with osteitis fibrosa: "pseudohypohyperparathyroidism." Am J Med 52:311–321, 1972.
154. Jüppner H, Schipani E, Bastepe M, et al: The gene responsible for pseudohypoparathyroidism type Ib is paternally imprinted and maps in four unrelated kindreds to chromosome 20q13.3, Proc Natl Acad Sci U S A 95:11798–11803, 1998.
155. Bastepe M, Lane AH, Jüppner H: Paternal uniparental isodisomy of chromosome 20q (patUPD20q)—and the resulting changes in *GNAS1* methylation—as a plausible cause of pseudohypoparathyroidism, Am J Hum Genet 68:1283–1289, 2001.

156. Liu J, Erlichman B, Weinstein LS: The stimulatory G protein α-subunit Gsα is imprinted in human thyroid glands: implications for thyroid function in pseudohypoparathyroidism types 1A and 1B, J Clin Endocrinol Metab 88:4336–4341, 2003.

157. Mantovani G, Bondioni S, Linglart A, et al: Genetic analysis and evaluation of resistance to thyrotropin and growth hormone-releasing hormone in pseudohypoparathyroidism type Ib, J Clin Endocrinol Metab 92:3738–3742, 2007.

158. Deleted in proofs.

159. Laspa E, Bastepe M, Jüppner H, et al: Phenotypic and molecular genetic aspects of pseudohypoparathyroidism type Ib in a Greek kindred: evidence for enhanced uric acid excretion due to parathyroid hormone resistance, J Clin Endocrinol Metab 89:5942–5947, 2004.

160. Pepersack T, Jabbour N, Fuss M, et al: Hyperuricemia and renal handling of urate in primary hyperparathyroidism, Nephron 53:349–352, 1989.

161. Westerdahl J, Valdemarsson S, Lindblom P, et al: Urate and arteriosclerosis in primary hyperparathyroidism, Clin Endocrinol (Oxf) 54:805–811, 2001.

162. Wu WI, Schwindinger WF, Aparicio LF, et al: Selective resistance to parathyroid hormone caused by a novel uncoupling mutation in the carboxyl terminus of Gαs: a cause of pseudohypoparathyroidism type Ib, J Biol Chem 276:165–171, 2001.

163. Silve C, Santora A, Breslau N, et al: Selective resistance to parathyroid hormone in cultured skin fibroblasts from patients with pseudohypoparathyroidism type Ib, J Clin Endocrinol Metab 62:640–644, 1986.

164. Schipani E, Weinstein LS, Bergwitz C, et al: Pseudohypoparathyroidism type Ib is not caused by mutations in the coding exons of the human parathyroid hormone (PTH)/PTH-related peptide receptor gene, J Clin Endocrinol Metab 80:1611–1621, 1995.

165. Suarez F, Lebrun JJ, Lecossier D, et al: Expression and modulation of the parathyroid hormone (PTH)/PTH-related peptide receptor messenger ribonucleic acid in skin fibroblasts from patients with type Ib pseudohypoparathyroidism, J Clin Endocrinol Metab 80:965–970, 1995.

166. Fukumoto S, Suzawa M, Takeuchi Y, et al: Absence of mutations in parathyroid hormone (PTH)/PTH-related protein receptor complementary deoxyribonucleic acid in patients with pseudohypoparathyroidism type Ib, J Clin Endocrinol Metab 81:2554–2558, 1996.

167. Jan de Beur S, Ding C, LaBuda M, et al: Pseudohypoparathyroidism 1b: exclusion of parathyroid hormone and its receptors as candidate disease genes, J Clin Endocrinol Metab 85:2239–2246, 2000.

168. Blomstrand S, Claësson I, Säve-Söderbergh J: A case of lethal congenital dwarfism with accelerated skeletal maturation, Pediatr Radiol 15:141–143, 1985.

169. Liu J, Litman D, Rosenberg M, et al: A GNAS1 imprinting defect in pseudohypoparathyroidism type IB, J Clin Invest 106:1167–1174, 2000.

170. Jan de Beur S, Ding C, Germain-Lee E, et al: Discordance between genetic and epigenetic defects in pseudohypoparathyroidism type 1b revealed by inconsistent loss of maternal imprinting at GNAS1, Am J Hum Genet 73:314–322, 2003.

171. Bastepe M, Fröhlich LF, Hendy GN, et al: Autosomal dominant pseudohypoparathyroidism type Ib is associated with a heterozygous microdeletion that likely disrupts a putative imprinting control element of GNAS, J Clin Invest 112:1255–1263, 2003.

172. Liu J, Nealon JG, Weinstein LS: Distinct patterns of abnormal GNAS imprinting in familial and sporadic pseudohypoparathyroidism type IB, Hum Mol Genet 14:95–102, 2005.

173. de Nanclares GP, Fernandez-Rebollo E, Santin I, et al: Epigenetic defects of GNAS in patients with pseudohypoparathyroidism and mild features of Albright's hereditary osteodystrophy, J Clin Endocrinol Metab 92:2370–2373, 2007.

174. Fröhlich LF, Bastepe M, Ozturk D, et al: Lack of GNAS epigenetic changes and pseudohypoparathyroidism type Ib in mice with targeted disruption of syntaxin-16, Endocrinology 148:2925–2935, 2007.

175. Chillambhi S, Turan S, Hwang D-Y, et al: Deletion of the GNAS antisense transcript results in parent-of-origin specific GNAS imprinting defects and phenotypes including PTH-resistance, Presented at: 30th

Annual Meeting of the American Society of Bone and Mineral Research, Montreal, September 12–26, 2008. Abstract No, 1052.

176. Chotalia M, Smallwood SA, Ruf N, et al: Transcription is required for establishment of germline methylation marks at imprinted genes, Genes Dev 23:105–117, 2009.

177. Mariot V, Maupetit-Mehouas S, Sinding C, et al: A maternal epimutation of GNAS leads to Albright osteodystrophy and parathyroid hormone resistance, J Clin Endocrinol Metab 93:661–665, 2008.

178. van Dop C: Pseudohypoparathyroidism: clinical and molecular aspects, Semin Nephrol 9:168–178, 1989.

179. Kruse K, Kustermann W: Evidence for transient peripheral resistance to parathyroid hormone in premature infants, Acta Paediatr Scand 76:115–118, 1987.

180. Lee CT, Tsai WY, Tung YC, et al: Transient pseudohypoparathyroidism as a cause of late-onset hypocalcemia in neonates and infants, J Formos Med Assoc 107:806–810, 2008.

181. Manzar S: Transient pseudohypoparathyroidism and neonatal seizure, J Trop Pediatr 47:113–114, 2001.

182. Kruse K, Kracht U, Wohlfart K, et al: Biochemical markers of bone turnover, intact serum parathyroid hormone and renal calcium excretion in patients with pseudohypoparathyroidism and hypoparathyroidism before and during vitamin D treatment, Eur J Pediatr 148:535–539, 1989.

183. Rao DS, Parfitt AM, Kleerekoper M, et al: Dissociation between the effects of endogenous parathyroid hormone on adenosine 3′,5′-monophosphate generation and phosphate reabsorption in hypocalcemia due to vitamin D depletion: an acquired disorder resembling pseudohypoparathyroidism type II, J Clin Endocrinol Metab 61:285–290, 1985.

184. Srivastava T, Alon US: Stage I vitamin D-deficiency rickets mimicking pseudohypoparathyroidism type II, Clin Pediatr (Phila) 41:263–268, 2002.

185. Shriraam M, Bhansali A, Velayutham P: Vitamin D deficiency masquerading as pseudohypoparathyroidism type 2, J Assoc Physicians India 51:619–620, 2003.

Chapter 11

GENETIC DEFECTS IN VITAMIN D METABOLISM AND ACTION

RENÉ ST-ARNAUD and FRANCIS H. GLORIEUX

Vitamin D is a key regulator of mineral homeostasis[1,2] and bone development,[3] and perturbation of the vitamin D endocrine system leads to rickets and/or osteomalacia (see Chapter 15). In order to gain a complete perspective of the clinical manifestations of genetic anomalies involving vitamin D endocrine function, this chapter will first present a short overview of the salient aspects of the vitamin D metabolic pathway. (An in-depth discussion of vitamin D metabolism and bone development and remodeling can be found in Chapters 3 and 4). The concepts presented here will lay the groundwork for the discussion of the clinical, pathophysiologic, and molecular aspects of hereditary rickets involving the vitamin D endocrine system.

Overview of Vitamin D Metabolism

Following exposure to sunlight, both plants and animals are able to synthesize vitamin D. Vitamin D_2 is generated in yeast and plants; vitamin D_3 is produced in fish and mammals. The slight differences in the chemical structure of the two compounds do not affect function or metabolism. The generic term of *vitamin D* (without subscript) will be used hereafter.

In humans, a sizeable proportion of vitamin D requirements can be produced endogenously in the skin upon exposure to ultraviolet (UV) light (sunlight). It has been shown, however, that at latitudes where vitamin D synthesis is reduced or absent during winter months, there is a seasonal variation in the photosynthesis of vitamin D.[4] People who receive an ample supply of sunlight during the rest of the year are not at risk of developing vitamin D deficiency, because excess cutaneously produced vitamin D is stored in fat and muscle and released at times of need.[5] Dietary sources such as fish, plants, and grains can help meet vitamin D requirements. In the absence of any exposure to sunlight, however (such as in elderly people), a daily multivitamin that contains 400 IU of vitamin D is indicated.[6,7]

Ultraviolet B (UVB) photons penetrate the epidermis and photolize 7-dehydrocholesterol into previtamin D, which rapidly becomes a more thermodynamically stable molecule, vitamin D. Vitamin D then exits the keratinocyte cells and enters the dermal capillary bed, where it becomes bound to the vitamin D binding protein, DBP. Once associated with DBP in the circulation, vitamin D is transported to the liver, where cytochrome P450 25-hydroxylase enzymes (CYP27A1 and/or CYP2R1) add a hydroxyl group on carbon 25 to produce 25-hydroxyvitamin D [25(OH)D]. Early studies using perfused rat liver revealed kinetics of vitamin D metabolism that supported two 25-hydroxylase activities: a microsomal high-affinity, low-capacity enzyme and a mitochondrial low-affinity, high-capacity form.[8] The mitochondrial enzyme is the bifunctional CYP27A1 sterol, 27-hydroxylase, that derives its name from its ability to both 27-hydroxylate the side chains of cholesterol-derived intermediates involved in bile acid biosynthesis and 25-hydroxylate vitamin D.[9] The microsomal, high-affinity vitamin D 25-hydroxylase was recently identified as CYP2R1, using an elegant expression-based screening strategy.[10] Based on specific activity determination, it is estimated that the microsomal enzyme is responsible for about 30% of the total 25-hydroxylation activity, while the mitochondrial enzyme is responsible for the remaining 70%.[11]

The 25(OH)D metabolite also circulates in the bloodstream bound to DBP. It is an abundant but relatively inactive vitamin D metabolite. Its circulating concentration provides the most readily available evaluation of the vitamin D status in a given individual. 25(OH)D must be further hydroxylated at a different site in the convoluted and straight portions of the proximal kidney tubule to gain hormonal bioactivity. Hydroxylation at position 1α by the mitochondrial cytochrome P450 enzyme 25-hydroxyvitamin D 1α-hydroxylase (CYP27B1) converts 25(OH)D to 1α,25-dihydroxyvitamin D [1,25(OH)$_2$D], the active, hormonal form of vitamin D that plays an essential role in mineral homeostasis, bone growth, and cellular differentiation.[12-14]

Upon reaching a target tissue, 1,25(OH)$_2$D binds a specific receptor (vitamin D receptor [VDR]) that is a member of the nuclear hormone receptor superfamily.[15] The VDR is considered a class II nuclear hormone receptor because it needs to form a heterodimer with the retinoid X receptor (RXR) to bind specific DNA sequence elements with high affinity. These target sequences are termed *vitamin D response elements* (VDRE), and the best characterized of these binding sites consist of two tandemly repeated hexanucleotide sequences separated by 3 base pairs (bp).[15] Transcriptional coactivators and components of the basal transcriptional machinery interact with the liganded, DNA-bound VDR-RXR heterodimer to activate the transcription of vitamin D target genes responsible for carrying out the physiologic actions of 1,25(OH)$_2$D.[13,15] Among several target genes, the 1,25(OH)$_2$D hormone induces in target cells the expression of the gene encoding the key effector of its catabolic breakdown: 25-hydroxyvitamin D 24-hydroxylase (*CYP24A1*).[16,17] This insures attenuation of the 1,25(OH)$_2$D biological signal inside target cells and helps regulate vitamin D homeostasis.

Rickets and Osteomalacia

The term *rickets* is often used to describe all of the skeletal abnormalities associated with defective mineralization in the growing skeleton, but it is more precise to restrict the term to changes in the growth plate and adjacent metaphysis. When mineralization is impaired, the accumulation of unmineralized osteoid at sites other than the growing metaphysis should be referred to as *osteomalacia*, not as rickets. Thus, defective mineralization can lead to both rickets and osteomalacia in the growing skeleton but only to osteomalacia in the mature skeleton.

Rickets is characterized by the inadequate calcification of the growth plate and adjacent metaphysis. The impaired mineralization of the growth plate cartilage in the zone of provisional calcification prevents this zone from being resorbed. As the cartilage continues to be formed but not resorbed, the growth plate begins to widen. Simultaneously, the trabecular bone directly underneath the cartilage fails to mineralize properly, and vascularization of this tissue becomes aberrant. These defects are accompanied by similar abnormalities in cortical bone, leading to the full spectrum of skeletal symptoms associated with the pathology (see following).

Vitamin D–Deficiency Rickets

It is evident from the brief overview presented earlier that vitamin D metabolism can be affected at several levels: inadequate exposure to sunlight; inadequate dietary intake; malabsorption of dietary vitamin D; impaired hepatic 25-hydroxylation; defects in renal 1α-hydroxylation; or defects in receptor function (Fig. 11-1). Reviews on the nonhereditary disorders of the vitamin D endocrine system have been published previously.[18] Only defects

in renal 1α-hydroxylation or receptor activity have been associated with several specific mutations in genes involved in regulating vitamin D metabolism and action; these will be discussed in this chapter. There is a single report[19] of mutations in both alleles of CYP2R1, the microsomal hepatic 25-hydroxylase,[10] in a patient with low serum calcium concentrations, low circulating levels of 25(OH)D, and rickets.[20] While obviously rare, this finding confirms CYP2R1 as a physiologically relevant vitamin D 25-hydroxylase and demonstrates that selective 25-hydroxylase deficiency can also cause a hereditary defect in vitamin D metabolism.

The prime metabolic consequence of vitamin D deficiency is reduced net intestinal absorption of calcium.[1,2] Calcium malabsorption leads to a fall in plasma calcium, secondary hyperparathyroidism, reduced renal tubular reabsorption of phosphate, hypophosphatemia, and thus a reduction in the calcium X phosphate product. Eventually, deposition of mineral in osteoid is impaired because the supply of the relevant ions is reduced. The impaired mineralization triggers the development of the rachitic and/or osteomalacic phenotype.

CLINICAL FEATURES OF PSEUDO–VITAMIN D–DEFICIENCY RICKETS (VITAMIN D–DEPENDENT RICKETS TYPE I)

The clinical symptoms of pseudo–vitamin D–deficiency rickets (PDDR), also referred to as *vitamin D–dependent rickets type I*, are similar to those of common vitamin D–deficiency rickets, including failure to thrive, hypotonia, and growth retardation. Affected babies lie supine because of severe muscle weakness and bone pain. At this age, gross skeletal deformities are rare; however, if diagnosis and treatment are delayed, severe deformities of the spine and long bones occur, together with generalized muscle weakness simulating myopathy. Motor problems translate into regression in head control and ability to stand. In some patients, the initial event is generalized convulsions, tremulations and Bravais-Jacksonian fits, or tetany. Pathologic fractures may occur (Fig. 11-2). The onset in most cases occurs early during the third trimester of life; the patients look healthy at birth.

Physical examination reveals a small, hypotonic child with wide anterior fontanel, frontal bossing, and frequent craniotabes (easy depression of the softened parieto-occipital region). Tooth eruption is delayed, and erupted teeth show evidence of enamel hypoplasia. A rachitic rosary is either visible or palpable. In limbs, widening of the metaphyseal areas is evidenced by enlargement of wrists and ankles, and there is a variable degree of deformity (bowing) of long-bone diaphyses. Deformities of the thorax may interfere with ventilation and predispose to pulmonary infection; infant death by pulmonary infections was not infrequent in the past, when the diagnosis was either missed (confused with a neurologic or respiratory condition) or made too late. The Chvostek sign (twitching of the upper lip upon light finger tapping of the facial nerve) reflects nerve irritability, a consequence of a rapid fall in serum calcium.

X-ray features include diffuse osteopenia (mild to severe hypomineralization of the skeleton) and classic rachitic metaphyseal changes: fraying, cupping, widening, and fuzziness of the zone of provisional calcification immediately under the growth plate (see Fig. 11-2). These changes are seen better and detected earlier in the most active growth plates—namely, the distal ulna and femur and the proximal and distal tibia. Changes in the diaphyses may not be evident when metaphyseal changes are first detected. However, they will appear a few weeks later as rarefaction, coarse trabeculation, cortical thinning, and subperi-

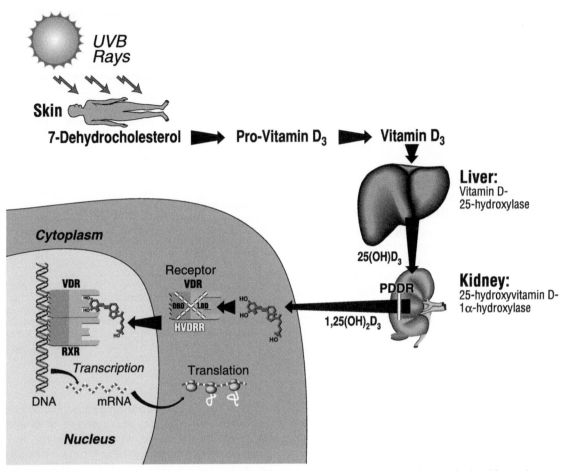

FIGURE 11-1. Schematic representation of the main steps of the vitamin D biosynthetic pathway, where genetic aberrations may lead to rickets and osteomalacia. The renal defect in pseudo–vitamin D–deficiency rickets (PDDR) is indicated by the break in the $1,25(OH)_2D_3$ arrow arising in the kidney. The mutation leads to insufficient synthesis of $1,25(OH)_2D$. The left part of the figure represents a target cell where schematic coupling of the ligand to its receptor (VDR) takes place in the cytosol or, more likely, in the nucleus. The VDR then heterodimerizes with the RXR receptor. For ease of representation, the RXR ligand (9-*cis* retinoic acid) is not depicted. The complex then binds to DNA to regulate gene transcription. Various mutations affecting either of the two VDR domains (*DBD*, DNA-binding domain; *LBD*, ligand-binding domain), depicted by the stippled X over the receptor complex, cause hereditary vitamin D–resistant rickets (HVDRR).

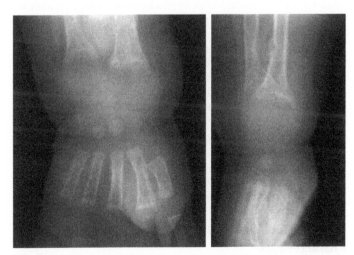

FIGURE 11-2. Radiograph of the wrist of a 19-month-old boy with pseudo–vitamin D–deficiency rickets (PDDR) at diagnosis. Severe rickets and demineralization are evident. Pronounced hypocalcemia and secondary hyperparathyroidism were documented, the latter causing a metaphyseal pseudofracture clearly seen on the lateral view.

osteal erosion. Looser-Milkman's pseudofractures and curvature of the shafts of long bones may be observed, especially in children older than 1 to 2 years.

Hypocalcemia is the main biochemical feature in PDDR. A rapid decrease in serum calcium concentration may give rise to tetany and convulsions, which may occur prior to any radiologic evidence of rickets. Prolonged hypocalcemia triggers secondary hyperparathyroidism and hyperaminoaciduria.[21] Urinary calcium excretion is very low, whereas fecal calcium is high as a consequence of impaired intestinal calcium absorption. Elevated urinary cyclic adenosine monophosphate (cAMP) is not a consistent finding, and normal values have been measured in PDDR patients, despite high circulating parathyroid hormone (PTH) levels.[22]

Serum phosphate concentrations may be normal or low. When reduced, the hypophosphatemia is usually of a lesser degree than that measured in X-linked hypophosphatemic rickets.[23] It results from the combination of impaired intestinal absorption and increased urinary loss induced by the secondary hyperparathyroidism. Serum alkaline phosphatase activity is consistently elevated, and its increase precedes the appearance of clinical symptoms.

Patients with PDDR have normal serum levels of 25(OH)D after exposure to sunlight or oral intake of small doses of vitamin

D; the concentrations increase if higher doses are given.[22] Circulating levels of 24,25-dihydroxyvitamin D [24,25(OH)$_2$D] are normal and correlate with those of 25(OH)D.[24] Serum levels of 1,25(OH)$_2$D are low in untreated patients.[22,25] This is evident immediately after birth, months before any clinical evidence of rickets appears. Even when patients are treated with high doses of vitamin D, causing major increases in circulating levels of 25(OH)D, the blood concentration of 1,25(OH)$_2$D does not reach the normal range. These characteristic features of serum vitamin D metabolites have provided key insight into the pathogenesis of PDDR.

CLINICAL FEATURES OF HEREDITARY VITAMIN D–RESISTANT RICKETS (VITAMIN D–DEPENDENT RICKETS TYPE II)

Many of the clinical findings in patients with hereditary vitamin D–resistant rickets (HVDRR), also termed *vitamin D–dependent rickets type II*, are identical to those described for PDDR, including bone pain, muscle weakness, hypotonia, and occasional convulsions.[26] Children are often growth retarded, and hypoplasia of the teeth is observed. The radiologic features of rickets are present. A major difference is that many children with HVDRR have sparse body hair, and some have total scalp and body alopecia, sometimes even including eyebrows and eyelashes. Hair loss may be evident at birth or occur during the first months of life. Patients with alopecia generally have more severe resistance to vitamin D. In families with a prior history of the disease, the absence of scalp hair in newborns can provide initial diagnostic clues for HVDRR. A defect in epithelial-mesenchymal communication that is required for normal hair cycling has been shown to be the cause of the alopecia in an animal model of HVDRR.[27]

Serum biochemistry includes low concentrations of calcium and phosphate and elevated alkaline phosphatase activity. Secondary hyperparathyroidism with elevated circulating PTH is measurable. The key difference concerns circulating levels of vitamin D metabolites. The 25(OH)D values are normal, and in the cases in which it has been measured, 24,25(OH)$_2$D levels have been low. Importantly, serum levels of 1,25(OH)$_2$D are elevated. This clinical feature clearly distinguishes HVDRR from PDDR, where circulating concentrations of 1,25(OH)$_2$D are depressed. Additionally, patients with HVDRR are resistant to supraphysiologic doses of all forms of vitamin D therapy. Table 11-1 outlines the similarities and differences between the two forms of hereditary rickets involving the vitamin D endocrine system.

Pseudo–Vitamin D–Deficiency Rickets

MOLECULAR ETIOLOGY

As previously mentioned, serum levels of 25(OH)D are normal in untreated patients with PDDR and elevated in patients receiving large daily amounts of vitamin D.[22] These results indicate that intestinal absorption of vitamin D and its hydroxylation in the liver are not impaired in PDDR. Circulating levels of 24,25(OH)$_2$D are also normal and highly correlated with those of 25(OH)D, indicating a fully functional 25(OH)D-24-hydroxylase enzyme.[24] However, serum concentrations of 1,25(OH)$_2$D are low in untreated patients and remain low even when they are treated with high doses of vitamin D.[22,25] This clearly identifies defective activity of the 25(OH)D-1α-hydroxylase enzyme (CYP27B1; hereafter referred to as *1α-hydroxylase*) as the basic abnormality in PDDR and differentiates it from HVDRR.

Table 11-1. Comparison of Pseudo–Vitamin D–Deficiency Rickets (Vitamin D–Dependent Rickets Type I) and Hereditary Vitamin D–Resistant Rickets (Vitamin D–Dependent Rickets Type II)

Feature	PDDR (or VDDR-I)	HVDRR (or VDDR-II)
Mutations	CYP27B1 (25[OH] D-1α-hydroxylase)	VDR (vitamin D receptor)
Genetic inheritance	Autosomal recessive	Autosomal recessive
Age of onset	Early	Early
Rickets	Yes	Yes
Hypocalcemia	Yes	Yes
Serum alkaline phosphatase	Elevated	Elevated
Secondary hyperparathyroidism	Yes	Yes
Alopecia	No	Yes
Serum 25(OH)D	Normal	Normal
Serum 1,25(OH)$_2$D	Low	Elevated
Response to 1,25(OH)$_2$D therapy	Yes	No

Reference range, serum biochemistry (child): calcemia (total calcium), 2.2–2.7 mmol/L; alkaline phosphatase, 20–150 U/L; 25(OH)D, 35–200 nmol/L; 1,25(OH)$_2$D, 12–46 μmol/L. *HVDRR,* Hereditary vitamin D–resistant rickets; *PDDR,* pseudo–vitamin D–deficiency rickets; *VDDR-I,* vitamin D–dependent rickets type I; *VDDR-II,* vitamin D–dependent rickets type II. From Favus MJ: Primer on the Metabolic Bone Diseases and Disorders of Mineral Metabolism, 3rd ed. Philadelphia: Lippincott-Raven, 1996, pp 451–452.

PDDR is inherited as a simple autosomal recessive trait.[28] No phenotypic abnormalities are observed in heterozygotes.[21] By taking advantage of the unusual frequency of PDDR in the French-Canadian population and the availability of sample material from relatively large kindreds, the PDDR locus was mapped to the region of band 14 on the long arm of chromosome 12 (12q13-14).[29,30]

Tremendous progress has been achieved in the study of the molecular etiology of PDDR through the cloning of the complementary DNA (cDNA) encoding for 1α-hydroxylase.[31-34] The human gene has also been cloned, sequenced, and mapped to 12q13.1-13.3 by fluorescence in situ hybridization,[33,35,36] consistent with the earlier mapping of the disease to this locus by linkage analysis.

The ultimate proof that mutations in the 1α-hydroxylase gene were responsible for the PDDR phenotype required the identification of such mutations in PDDR patients and carriers of the disease. The first identified mutation was reported by Fu et al.[31] in 1997; several additional mutations in various ethnic groups have since been published.[35-41] These findings unequivocally establish the molecular genetic basis of PDDR as inactivating mutation(s) in the 1α-hydroxylase gene (CYP27B1). Further proof was provided by developing valid animal models of the disease using targeted inactivation of the cyp27B1 gene in mice.[42,43]

25-HYDROXYVITAMIN D 1α-HYDROXYLASE
Characteristics

The 25(OH)D-1α-hydroxylase (CYP27B1; 1α-hydroxylase) enzyme catalyzes the addition of a hydroxyl group at position 1α of the secosteroid backbone of 25(OH)D. The 1α-hydroxylase is a mitochondrial cytochrome P450 enzyme that requires electrons from nicotinamide adenine dinucleotide phosphate (NADPH) to promote catalysis. These are delivered to the P450 moiety by the flavoprotein NADPH-ferredoxin reductase[44] and the nonheme iron protein, ferredoxin.[45] The expression of these cofactors is ubiquitous, and their genes were mapped to chromosomes 17 and 11,[44,45] respectively, excluding them rapidly in the search for the PDDR mutations, since the PDDR locus was mapped early on to chromosome 12.[30]

The main site for the 1α-hydroxylation of 25(OH)D is the proximal tubule of the renal cortex.[46] In the kidney, the expression of the 1α-hydroxylase gene is subject to complex regulation by PTH, calcitonin, calcium, phosphorus, and 1,25(OH)$_2$D itself.[47-49] The 1α-hydroxylase gene exists in a single copy in the human genome and contains nine exons spanning 5 kb of sequence. The ferredoxin-binding domain is encoded by sequences contained in exons 6 and 7, while the heme-binding domain is contained in exon 8.[50,51]

Mutations

To date, 35 different 1α-hydroxylase mutations have been described in PDDR patients and their parents (Table 11-2). All patients have mutations on both alleles, but a high frequency of compound heterozygosity (a different mutation on each allele) has been observed (23 compound heterozygotes out of 54 cases reported). Splice-site mutations, nucleotide deletions and duplications, and missense and nonsense mutations have been reported (see Table 11-2). The mutations are dispersed throughout the 1α-hydroxylase sequence, affecting all exons (Fig. 11-3).

The mutations detected at the highest frequency are 958ΔG, common among French-Canadian patients (owing to a founder effect),[29,36,38] and a mutation located at codons 438 to 442 in exon 8. These codons are composed of the duplicated 7-bp sequence 5′-CCCACCC CCCACCC-3′. In 11 families described to date,[36,38,39,41] three rather than two copies of the 7-bp sequence are present, which alters the downstream reading frame (Fig. 11-4). Careful analysis of the correlation between ethnic origin, microsatellite haplotyping, and the presence of the 7-bp duplication mutation suggested that the mutation has arisen by several independent de novo events.[36,38]

Structure/Function Relationships

An important aspect of the identification of mutations in the 1α-hydroxylase gene was to correlate the genotype of the patients with their phenotype—that is, the severity of the disease and the circulating levels of 1,25(OH)$_2$D. In several cases, although 1,25(OH)$_2$D serum levels are low, they are not undetectable,[22,25,37,40,52] suggesting some degree of residual 1α-hydroxylase activity. Presumably, some 1α-hydroxylase mutations affect the structural integrity of the enzyme, resulting in a modification of its kinetics. This reasoning cannot apply to the frameshift (deletions, insertions, and duplications) and nonsense mutations described to date. All such mutations eliminate the heme-binding site of the protein and thus completely abolish the 1α-hydroxylase enzymatic activity. The apparent residual 1α-hydroxylase activity observed in some patients could be attributable to missense mutations. Most of these missense mutations were entirely devoid of enzymatic activity in the assays used,[38,40] except for the L343F mutation (retained 2.3% of wild-type activity) and the E189G mutation (retained 22% of wild-type activity).[37] Thus some missense mutations contribute to the variable phenotype observed in patients with PDDR.

Early modeling efforts[16,38] compared the sequence of the 1α-hydroxylase protein (a mitochondrial class I cytochrome P450) with the sequence of bacterial class I cytochrome P450s for which x-ray crystallographic data were available. The tertiary structures of these enzymes show remarkable conservation

Table 11-2. *CYP27B1* (1α-Hydroxylase) Gene Mutations in Patients with Pseudo–Vitamin D–Deficiency Rickets (Vitamin D–Dependent Rickets Type I)

Mutation	Residue Function	Ethnic Group	Reference
212ΔG (codon 46)	N/A	Hispanic	38
Q65H	H-bond with substrate (inferred)	Chinese	38, 56
gggcg→cttcgg	N/A	African American	37
958ΔG (codon 88)	N/A	White American, French-Canadian	36, 38
R107H	Folding	Japanese	35, 54
P112L	Undetermined	Argentinian	41
G125E	Folding	Japanese	35, 54
IVS2+1g→a	N/A	Pakistani	37
P143L	Folding (inferred)	Japanese	40, 56
D164N	Folding	Japanese	40, 54
E189L	Folding (inferred)	Polish	38, 56
E189G	Folding (inferred)	Swiss	37, 56
IVS3+1g→a	N/A	Japanese	40
1921ΔG (codon 211)	N/A	White American	31, 38
1984ΔC (codon 231)	N/A	White American	31, 38
W241X	N/A	Polish	38
T321R	Oxygen activation	Japanese	40, 54
S323Y	Folding (inferred)	British	39, 56
W328X	N/A	Korean	41
R335P	Folding	Japanese	35, 56
L343F	Undetermined	Belgian	37
P382S	Folding (inferred)	Japanese	35, 56
R389H	Heme-propionate binding	White American, French-Canadian, African American, Belgian	37, 38, 54
R389C	Heme-propionate binding	Japanese	40, 54
R389G	Heme-propionate binding	Chilean	37, 54
IVS7+1g→a	N/A	African American	41
T409I	H-bond with substrate	Filipino, Chilean	37, 38, 57
R429P	Folding (inferred)	African American	38, 56
W433X	N/A	Japanese	40
7 bp duplication (codons 438-442)	N/A	Filipino, Polish, Chinese, British, White American, Hispanic, African American, Acadian, French-Canadian	36, 38, 39, herein
2 bp duplication (codon 442)	N/A	White American	38
R453C	Heme-propionate binding	Haitian	38, 54
V478G	Folding (inferred)	British	39, 56
P497R	Folding	Polish	38, 54
3922ΔA	N/A	Moroccan	41

The one-letter amino acid code is used. Δ, deletion; *bp*, base pairs; *IVS*, intervening sequence (intron); *X*, premature stop codon.

despite low amino acid sequence identity.[53] These sequence alignments yielded improper predictions of the functions of the residues mutated in PDDR patients.[54] Further modeling based on the first solved crystal structure of a eukaryotic cytochrome P450,[55] combined with extensive structure/function analysis of recombinant 1α-hydroxylase proteins, identified the functions of many residues mutated in PDDR patients (see Table 11-2).[54,56,57]

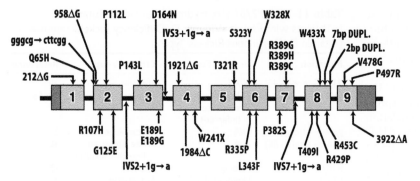

FIGURE 11-3. Mutations in pseudo–vitamin D–deficiency rickets (PDDR) patients. A schematic representation of the *CYP27B1* (25[OH] D-1α-hydroxylase) gene is shown. Exons are numbered from 1 to 9 with darker shaded regions representing 5'- and 3'-nontranslated regions. Mutations are presented above and below the gene map. *Numbers* refer to amino acid residue; the one-letter amino acid code is used. Δ, Deletion; *gggcg→cttcg*, deletion of gggcg and substitution of cttcgg beginning at nucleotide 897 in exon 2; *IVS2, IVS3, or IVS7+1 g→a*, splice-site mutation in intron (intervening sequence) 2, 3, or 7; *7bp dupl*, 7-base-pairs duplication; *2 bp dupl*, 2-base-pairs duplication.

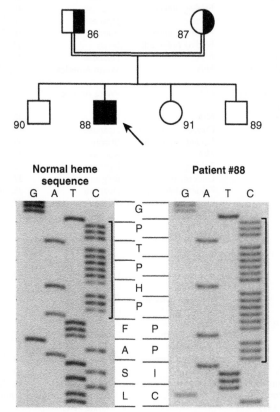

FIGURE 11-4. Identification of the molecular defect in a pseudo–vitamin D–deficiency rickets (PDDR) pedigree. *Upper panel*, The heterozygote parents are identified by *half-filled boxes* (male parent, *square symbol*, no. 86; female parent, *round symbol*, no. 87). The affected patient (male, no. 88) is identified by a *filled square symbol with an arrow*. *Lower panel*, DNA sequence analysis of the mutation within the heme-binding domain of the 25(OH)D-1α-hydroxylase (*CYP27B1*) gene. The 7-bp duplication is bracketed. The amino acid sequence (one-letter code) is highlighted in the center of the figure. Note the change of reading frame leading to an aberrant protein sequence and premature termination in the affected patient.

Most mutations affect folding and conformation.[54,56] Residue T321 is involved in oxygen activation, and amino acid R389 is essential for heme binding.[54,56] Spectroscopic analysis of wild-type and mutant 1α-hydroxylase proteins identified residue T409 as critical for binding of the 25(OH)D substrate.[57]

TREATMENT

Vitamin D_2, at high doses, was initially used to treat PDDR. Under such treatment, circulating levels of 25(OH)D increase sharply, and it is likely that massive concentrations of 25(OH)D can bind to the VDR and induce the response of the target organs to normalize calcium homeostasis. The risk of overdose is high because vitamin D progressively accumulates in fat and muscle, and the therapeutic doses are close to the toxic doses, ultimately placing the patient at risk for nephrocalcinosis and impaired renal function. The use of $25(OH)D_3$ as a therapeutic agent in PDDR has been reported.[58] The mechanism of action is likely to be similar to the one described earlier for vitamin D. The low availability and high cost of the metabolite have not encouraged its widespread use as long-term therapy for PDDR.

The treatment of choice is long-term (lifelong) replacement therapy with $1,25(OH)_2D_3$.[22,59] This results in rapid and complete correction of the abnormal phenotype, eliminating hypocalcemia, secondary hyperparathyroidism, and radiographic evidence of rickets. Strikingly, the myopathy disappears within days after initiation of therapy. The restoration of bone mineral content is equally rapid and histologic evidence of healing of the bone structure has been reported.[22] Correction of tooth enamel hypoplasia is only partial. An important aspect of treatment is to ensure adequate calcium intake during the bone-healing phase. Needs can be monitored by frequent assessment of urinary calcium excretion. It should be noted that hypercalciuria is common during treatment with $1,25(OH)_2D_3$, particularly during the first year of administration. Its close monitoring is used to adjust the needs in $1,25(OH)_2D_3$. The initial dose will be 1 to 2 μg/d, and the maintenance dose will vary between 0.5 and 1 μg/d. High levels of calcium excretion may amplify the pattern of calcium deposition in the kidney, so frequent renal imaging and assessment of renal function are essential during the course of treatment.

Before $1,25(OH)_2D_3$ became available from commercial sources, several investigators used the monohydroxylated analog, $1\alpha(OH)D_3$,[60] which only requires liver hydroxylation at position 25 to be activated to the hormonally active metabolite. The 25-hydroxylation step is not affected by the PDDR mutation. Response to treatment with $1\alpha(OH)D_3$ is rapid, with healing of rickets in 7 to 9 weeks, and this compound is still used in several countries. On a weight basis, $1\alpha(OH)D_3$ is about half as potent as $1,25(OH)_2D_3$, nullifying any possible economic advantage in favor of the monohydroxylated compound.

Hereditary Vitamin D–Resistant Rickets

MOLECULAR ETIOLOGY

Patients with HVDRR have normal 25(OH)D and low but measurable $24,25(OH)_2D$ serum values. The circulating levels of $1,25(OH)_2D$ are elevated from 3 to 5 times the normal values. These biochemical findings demonstrate that all the vitamin D metabolic enzymes (25-hydroxylase, 24-hydroxylase, and

1α-hydroxylase) are active in patients with HVDRR. Most patients with the disease are resistant to all forms of vitamin D therapy. This lack of response to vitamin D treatment led Albright et al.[61] to introduce the concept of hormonal resistance. The molecular basis of vitamin D end-organ resistance became clearer as the mechanism of action of the hormonal form of vitamin D was elucidated.

Ligand-binding studies first established that the $1,25(OH)_2D$ hormone, like other sex-steroid hormones studied at the time, binds to a high-affinity receptor located in the nucleus.[62] It was later discovered that this receptor could bind to DNA.[63] This property was utilized to purify sufficient quantities of the VDR to raise antibodies.[64,65]

The observation that binding sites for $1,25(OH)_2D$ could be detected in many tissues in addition to the classical vitamin D target tissues helped to define the etiology of HVDRR. Investigators began to study the VDR from cultured fibroblasts of patients and relatives, using ligand-binding assays, radioimmunoassays, and DNA-cellulose chromatography. Other fibroblast responses measured included induction of the 24-hydroxylase enzyme activity and vitamin D–mediated growth arrest. These methodologies led to several milestone observations. In the first studies reported, $[^3H]$-$1,25(OH)_2D_3$ binding was undetectable in fibroblasts from HVDRR patients, and high doses of $1,25(OH)_2D$ failed to induce the 24-hydroxylase bio-marker.[66] The diminished hormone binding provided a clear rationale for the end-organ resistance reported in patients. Subsequent reports continued to describe a lack of response of the patient's cells to $1,25(OH)_2D$, but some patients' fibroblasts exhibited normal $[^3H]$-$1,25(OH)_2D_3$ binding.[67] From these early reports, it was concluded that at least two classes of HVDRR patients could be recognized: "receptor-negative" patients and "receptor-positive" patients. The development of a sensitive radioimmunoassay for the VDR protein[68] demonstrated that these semantic differences were incorrect. Using this assay, it was shown that fibroblasts from so-called receptor-negative patients expressed normal levels of receptor protein. Pike et al.[69] hypothesized that the VDR defect in these patients' cells was due to a structural abnormality in the ligand-binding domain preventing $[^3H]$-$1,25(OH)_2D_3$ from binding to the receptor, not from defective synthesis of the VDR protein. The two classes of HVDRR were more adequately described by the terminology *ligand-binding positive* and *ligand-binding negative*.

A second type of VDR structural abnormality was identified in cultured cells from patients displaying the ligand-binding positive HVDRR phenotype. The VDR from these cells showed reduced affinity for heterologous DNA as measured by DNA-cellulose chromatography.[70] It was suspected that the defect in these patients would likely be a point mutation in the DNA-binding domain of the VDR. Interestingly, measurements of DNA binding affinities of the VDR from parents of ligand-binding positive patients clearly identified two forms of the VDR molecule, one with normal, wild-type affinity for DNA, and the second with reduced, defective DNA binding.[70] This was the first clear evidence establishing the heterozygous state of HVDRR parents. Binding and antibody-based assays had failed to reconcile genotype and phenotype of carriers in the past.

Eventually, the purified receptor was used to obtain monoclonal antibodies that led to the cloning of the VDR cDNA from various species.[71-73] In turn, the VDR genomic structure was analyzed. Eight exons comprise the entire coding region, spanning approximately 50 kb of genomic DNA.[74] The translation start site is contained within exon 2.

Analysis of the VDR cDNA sequence soon established that the VDR is a member of the nuclear hormone receptor superfamily, and its mechanism of action was subsequently unraveled.[15] The ligand-bound receptor forms a heterodimer with the retinoid X receptor (RXR), and the dimer contacts specific sites within the regulatory domains of responsive genes. This results in positive or negative modulation of the transcription of target genes. The VDR is essential to transduce the biological effects of $1,25(OH)_2D$, such as promoting calcium and phosphate transport across the small intestine and maintaining calcium homeostasis. The underlying molecular basis of the hormone resistance described in patients with HVDRR is mutation in the VDR which renders the receptor nonfunctional or less functional than the wild-type VDR. Several laboratories have independently engineered valid animal models of HVDRR by inactivating the *VDR* gene through gene targeting.[75]

HVDRR follows an autosomal recessive pattern of inheritance. Parents of patients, who are heterozygous for the mutation, show no symptoms and have normal bone development. In many cases, parental consanguinity is associated with the disease. Families often have several affected children, and males and females are affected equally.

VITAMIN D RECEPTOR

Characteristics

Structure/function analysis, sequence comparison alignments, and recent crystallographic studies have contributed to our understanding of the domain structure of the members of the nuclear hormone receptor superfamily to which the VDR belongs. The different domains of nuclear receptors have been labeled *A* to *F* (Fig. 11-5). Some of these domains exhibit high sequence similarity between individual family members, while others vary considerably or are altogether absent. This diversity is manifested most strongly in domains A/B, D, and F. Domain A/B includes all residues that are N-terminal to the receptor's DNA-binding domain (DBD). The size of this domain is highly variable, ranging from hundreds of residues in the progesterone receptor, for example, to only 24 amino acids in the VDR. The function of the A/B domain remains somewhat uncertain, but results suggest that polymorphisms in the VDR A/B segment could modulate its transcriptional activity.[76] Domain C comprises the highly conserved zinc-finger DBD, the hallmark feature of nuclear receptor family members, and will be discussed in detail later. Region D serves as a flexible hinge domain between the DBD and domain E and is the least conserved among nuclear receptors. Interestingly, because of the splicing in of an additional exon, the D segment of the VDR is longer by 50 amino acids when compared to classical steroid receptors.[77] Residues within the D domain of the VDR are subject to posttranslational modification in the form of reversible serine phosphorylation.[78,79] This regulation provides an additional degree of control of the VDR activity.[15] The E region encodes the ligand-binding domain (LBD) of ligand-activated receptors and also contributes to transactivation and dimerization. The small F domain is not highly conserved between nuclear receptor family members.

Structure/Function

The Vitamin D Receptor DNA-Binding Domain

The DNA-binding domain of the VDR consists of two zinc-finger motifs located between residues 24 and 90. The zinc fingers are of the C2C2 type, with two zinc atoms tetrahedrally coordinated

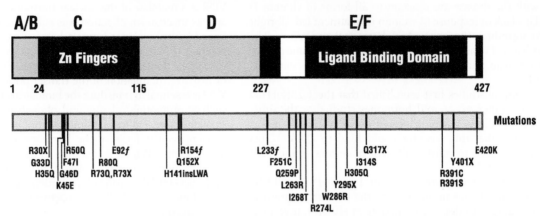

FIGURE 11-5. Natural mutations in hereditary vitamin D–resistant rickets (HVDRR). A schematic view of the vitamin D receptor is presented. The 427-amino-acid protein can be separated into domains, designated *A/B, C, D,* and *E/F.* The *white regions* represent helices within the E/F domain that are important for transcriptional activation. Point mutations in human patients with the HVDRR syndrome are indicated below (one-letter amino acid code). *f,* Frameshift mutation; *ins,* insertion; *X,* premature stop codon.

through four cysteine residues, each of which serves to stabilize the finger structure itself. The α-helical motifs residing on the C-terminal side of each zinc finger constitute the DNA-recognition and phosphate backbone–binding helices, respectively.[15] The region immediately C-terminal to the second zinc finger, covering residues 91 to 115, also forms an α-helical structure that could contribute to DNA contacts. The functional importance of those helical domains is confirmed by the analysis of the HVDRR mutations described in the Mutations section.

The VDR exhibits a unique characteristic when compared to other nuclear receptors: a cluster of five basic amino acids is located at residues 49 to 55 in the intervening sequence between the two zinc fingers. This domain is predicted to make DNA contact[80] and regulate the nuclear localization of the receptor.[81] Interestingly, this cluster contains residue serine-51, a site of posttranslational modification through phosphorylation by protein kinase C.[82,83]

Aside from their well-characterized role in the binding of the DNA response element, residues within the zinc-finger motifs of the VDR also contribute to association with the partner receptor, RXR, to form the functional heterodimer (see Fig. 11-1).[84,85] The α-helical domain immediately C-terminal to the second zinc finger also provides interactions with partner proteins.[85] These specific contact sites in the DBD of the VDR facilitate weak heterodimerization between VDR and RXR, while the stronger, ligand-dependent heterodimerization interactions are provided by residues located within the LBD.

The Vitamin D Receptor Ligand-Binding Domain

The E/F region of the VDR (see Fig. 11-5) represents a complex multifunctional domain involved in binding of the 1,25(OH)$_2$D ligand, heterodimerization with RXR, and transactivation. The structure of the LBD of the VDR has been modeled following x-ray crystallographic analysis.[86] It consists of 13 α-helices and several short β-strands organized as a "sandwich" around a lipophilic hormone-binding pocket. The LBD of the VDR is bordered by helices H3, H5, H7, H11, and residues Ser275 (loop H5-β), Trp286 (β-1), and Leu233 (helix H3). Once the ligand enters the pocket, a "lid" formed by H12 closes over the pocket. Several of the mutations characterized in HVDRR coincide with hormone contact sites.

It is hypothesized that ligand binding leads to conformational changes that expose, enhance, or produce novel dimerization and/or transactivation interfaces. Proteolytic digestion assays have provided indirect evidence that binding of 1,25(OH)$_2$D induces changes in the conformation of the VDR.[87,88] Interestingly, different vitamin D analogs induce different conformational changes.[86,87,89]

Two regions within the LBD of the VDR are involved in strong, ligand-dependent heterodimerization with RXR. These have been identified following mutagenesis experiments and by analogy to the RXR homodimer crystal.[90] These two subdomains consist of residues 244 to 263[91-93] and amino acids 317 to 395,[93,94] corresponding to portions of helices 3 to 4 and 7 to 10, respectively. Thus the ligand-binding and heterodimerization functions of the VDR are interrelated within the context of the tertiary structure of the molecule, presumably through allosteric effects that ultimately generate an active receptor conformation.

Transactivation

The regulation of gene transcription requires three classes of proteins. The first comprises the basal transcriptional machinery utilized to transcribe genes in every cell: RNA polymerase II and a series of basal factors that serve to insure transcription of protein-coding genes. The precise control of the transcription of particular genes then requires sequence-specific DNA-binding transcription factors. The VDR is such a factor, and its activity is further regulated through ligand binding. Finally, recent progress in our understanding of the molecular control of gene expression has unveiled a third class of proteins, generally known as *transcriptional coactivators,* that provide protein-protein contacts between the basal factors and the sequence-specific DNA-binding factors. Several performers involved in this tightly orchestrated choreography have been identified for VDR-mediated transcription.

As previously mentioned, ligand binding probably serves to induce conformational changes that allow the VDR to contact pertinent partners. Mutagenesis experiments have identified some of the key residues involved in these contacts. Two regions of the receptor are required exclusively for transcriptional activation. One of these regions is located between residues 244 and

263, a domain also involved in heterodimerization with RXR,[91-93] but residue lysine-246 is not involved in contacts with the RXR partner, and its alteration severely compromises transactivation.[92] This residue, highly conserved among nuclear receptors, must form part of the binding interface with transcriptional coactivators.[92,95]

The second region is known as *activation function 2*, or AF-2, and corresponds to helix 12 (residues 416 to 422).[96-98] Alteration of residues leucine-417 and glutamic acid-420 does not affect hormone binding or heterodimeric DNA binding but completely abrogates transactivation.[97,98] These residues also function to stimulate transcription by a mechanism involving coactivators. Some of the proteins interacting with the VDR to allow ligand-activated transcription have been identified. Within the basal transcriptional machinery, the VDR interacts with transcription factor TFIIB.[99,100] This contact involves the AF-2 domain of the VDR but also requires the wild-type residue arginine-391, located N-terminal to the AF-2 region within helix 10/11.[98]

Three categories of multicomponent transcriptional coactivator complexes that are involved in nuclear receptor–mediated transcription have been identified: those involved in ATP-dependent chromatin remodeling, those that physically interact with general transcription factors and RNA polymerase II, and complexes that modify histone tails covalently.[101] For VDR-mediated activation, the WINAC chromatin remodeling complex has been biochemically characterized.[102] The DRIP/TRAP complex that physically interacts with components of the general transcriptional machinery has been shown to be involved in ligand-dependent transcription by the VDR.[103,104] Finally, complexes that include histone acetyltransferase enzymes of the p160 family have been shown to coactivate the VDR.[105,106] Structure/function analysis of the AF-2 domain of the VDR identified residues that abolished interaction with p160 family members and DRIP components but retained ligand-dependant transcriptional activation. This suggests that yet uncharacterized coactivator complexes may participate in VDR-mediated transcription.[107] All of those categories of complexes transiently associate with the VDR, and their recruitment is thought to be cyclic and highly regulated.[105]

Mutations

Our understanding of the structural and functional consequences of HVDRR-causing mutations in the VDR has followed the introduction of molecular biological techniques as routine detection methods. For example, the amplification of mRNA by RT-PCR (reverse transcription-coupled polymerase chain reaction) has been of tremendous help for analysis of mutations (Fig. 11-6). Similarly, the functional consequences of particular mutations, first analyzed using ligand-binding assays and nonspecific binding to calf thymus DNA, can now be analyzed routinely using transient transfection assays on bona fide vitamin D–responsive promoter elements. Some laboratories have begun to test VDR protein-protein interactions. Finally, the availability of crystal structures for related nuclear receptors allows us to understand the consequences of particular mutations at the tertiary structure level.

Close to 30 mutations in the VDR have been described in HVDRR patients (see Fig. 11-5 and Table 11-3). Nine of these genetic alterations are nonsense (X) or frameshift (fs) mutations that introduce premature stop codons in the receptor: R30X (see Fig. 11-6), R73X, E92fs, Q152X, R154fs, L233fs, Y295X, Q317X, and Y401X. The premature translation termination codons lead to truncated VDRs that lack the DBD (R30X and R73X), the LBD

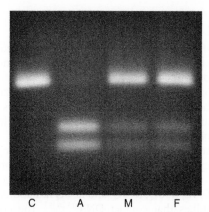

FIGURE 11-6. Prenatal diagnosis in a family where a first child had hereditary vitamin D–resistant rickets (HVDRR) caused by an *R30X* mutation. This mutation in the vitamin D receptor gene (C-to-T substitution in exon 2) has introduced a recognition site for the restriction endonuclease DdeI. Using primers internal to the affected exon, an 89-bp DNA fragment was amplified using PCR with 100 ng of genomic DNA prepared from amniotic cells (A), or from whole blood of an unrelated control (C), the mother (M), or the father (F). An aliquot of each amplimer was incubated with the restriction endonuclease DdeI. The digested fragments were visualized on a 2.5% agarose gel. The data show unambiguous homozygosity for the *R30X* mutation in the fetus, with both parents carriers for the mutation.

Table 11-3. Vitamin D–Receptor Mutations in Patients With Hereditary Vitamin D–Resistant Rickets (Vitamin D–Dependent Rickets Type II)

Mutation	VDR Domain	Ligand Binding	Reference
R30X	DBD	−	139, 140, herein
G33D	DBD	+	74
H35Q	DBD	+	141
K45E	DBD	+	111
G46D	DBD	+	142
F47I	DBD	+	111
R50Q	DBD	+	143
R73Q	DBD	+	74
R73X	DBD	−	112, 115
R80Q	DBD	+	144, 145
E92fs	Hinge	−	146
H141insLWA	Hinge	−	116
Q152X	Hinge	−	147
R154fs	Hinge	−	148
L233fs	LBD	−	112
F251C	LBD	−	117
Q259P	LBD	+	112
L263R	LBD	−	149
I268T	LBD	+/−	150
R274L	LBD	+	147
W286R	LBD	−	151
Y295X	LBD	−	108, 113-115
H305Q	LBD	+	124
I314S	LBD, dimer	+	123
Q317X	LBD	−	152
R391C	LBD, dimer	+	123
R391S	LBD, dimer	−	149
Y401X	LBD, AF-2	+/−	153
E420K	LBD, AF-2	+	118

The one-letter amino acid code is used. *AF-2,* Activating function 2; *DBD,* DNA-binding domain; *dimer,* domains involved in heterodimerization; *fs,* frameshift; *ins,* insertion; *LBD,* ligand-binding domain; *X,* premature stop codon.

(E92fs, Q152X, R154fs, L233fs, Y295X, and Q317X), or the AF-2 activation domain (Y401X); in most cases, the mRNAs for these truncated receptors are unstable.[108] The mutations involving amino acid substitutions (missense mutations) have been more revealing in terms of structure/function relationships.

DNA-Binding Domain Mutations

The first VDR mutation ever reported was described by Hughes et al.[74] and affected the DBD of the receptor. The mutation substitutes a polar uncharged glutamine for a positively charged arginine at position 73 (R73Q) within the second zinc finger of the DBD. The VDR mutation identified by Hughes et al.[74] was the first natural disease-causing mutation reported for the entire steroid-thyroid-retinoid receptor gene superfamily.

Several additional missense mutations affecting the DBD have been reported since (see Table 11-3). Based on the crystal structure of the related GR, RXR, and TR molecules,[90,109,110] the H35Q, K45E, R50Q, R73Q, and R80Q mutations are thought to affect residues that contact DNA.[15,26,111] The conversion of residue glycine-46 to aspartic acid (G46D) introduces a bulky, charged amino acid that would create unfavorable electrostatic interactions with the negatively charged phosphate backbone of the DNA helix.[112] The G33D mutation would be expected to have the same effect.[111] The F47I mutation is a relatively conserved substitution, but the loss of the phenylalanine ring structure may disrupt the hydrophobic core of the DBD and affect the proposed α-helical structure at the base of the first zinc finger.[111]

Ligand-Binding Domain Mutations

The first identified mutation affecting the LBD was the Y295X mutation reported by Ritchie et al.[113] This mutation truncates 132 amino acids from the carboxy-terminus of the VDR, which results in the deletion of a major portion of the LBD. This mutation has been described in seven families forming a large kindred in which consanguineous marriages occurred.[108] The mutation was also identified in three additional families unrelated to the extended kindred.[114,115] As previously mentioned, the mutant mRNA is unstable, and the truncated VDR is undetectable using immunology-based assays.[108]

The VDR crystallographic data[86] can be used to understand the structural consequences of the missense mutations in the VDR LBD described in HVDRR patients. The Q259P mutation (helix H4), the L263R and I268T (H4/5), the R274L mutation (H5), the W286R mutation (loop H5-H6), the H305Q mutation (loop H6-H7), the I314S mutation (H7), and the R391C or R391S mutations (positioned within H10) should perturb ligand binding and/or dimerization. Mutation H141ins-LWA consists of a unique 5-bp deletion combined with an 8-bp insertion in exon 4, leading to deletion of residues H141 and T142 and their substitution by mutant residues L141, W142, and A143 in helix H1.[116] The resulting mutant VDR does not bind ligand.[116]

Mutation F251C is located in the E1 region (amino acids 244 to 263) that overlaps helices 3 and 4 and loop 3 to 4 between them.[117] The mutation of residue F251 thus likely disrupts the ligand-binding pocket and perturbs optimal function of the VDR. Mutation E420K modifies a residue in helix H12 that provides coactivator dimerization interfaces, and thus it results in loss of transactivation.[118]

TREATMENT

Therapies with pharmacologic doses of vitamin D metabolites, including vitamin D itself, 25(OH)D, 1α(OH)D, and 1,25(OH)₂D, have been used to attempt to overcome the target-organ resistance to vitamin D associated with HVDRR. Patients with HVDRR without alopecia are generally more responsive to treatment with high doses of vitamin D preparations than patients with alope-

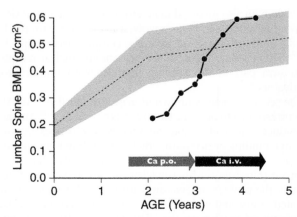

FIGURE 11-7. Bone mineral density (BMD) response in a patient with hereditary vitamin D–resistant rickets (HVDRR) treated with oral and intravenous (IV) calcium. BMD of the lumbar spine was measured by dual-energy x-ray absorptiometry (DXA). Patient received oral calcium, 2 g/d (Ca p.o.), for 17 months before treatment with IV calcium (Ca i.v.). The *shaded area* represents the reference values for the corresponding ages. Note the rapid correction of the BMD upon initiation of IV calcium therapy.

cia.[119] Reported effective doses range from 5000 to 40,000 IU/day for vitamin D, 20 to 200 μg/day for 25(OH)D, and 17 to 20 μg/day for 1,25(OH)₂D.[120-122] The efficacy of treatment with high doses of vitamin D metabolites can be reconciled with the molecular cause of HVDRR. When the resistance to vitamin D is caused by mutations in the VDR that moderately decrease the affinity of the receptor for its ligand, such as the H305Q or I314S mutations,[123,124] high doses of the hormone can apparently overcome the low-affinity binding defect and achieve adequate VDR occupancy to mediate normal 1,25(OH)₂D responses. A few patients with HVDRR with alopecia have also been treated successfully using vitamin D metabolites.[67,74,125-129]

When vitamin D therapy is proven ineffective, intensive calcium therapy is the alternative treatment of choice. Some success has been achieved with high-dose oral calcium (Fig. 11-7).[130] To bypass the calcium absorption defect in the intestine caused by the mutant VDR, long-term intravenous (IV) calcium infusions should be considered (see Fig. 11-7). High doses of IV calcium are infused during the night over a several-month period. Rapid disappearance of bone pains has been documented, and gradual improvement of calcemia and parathyroid function, followed by improvement of rickets (Fig. 11-8), and weight and height gains ensue.[131-134] The syndrome can recur when the IV infusions are discontinued.[131] After the serum calcium normalizes, and radiologic control of the rickets has been achieved with IV calcium infusions, high-dose oral calcium therapy is effective in maintaining normocalcemia.[133] For HVDRR patients who do not respond to high doses of vitamin D therapy, the two-step calcium protocol (IV infusions followed by high oral doses) appears to be the preferred therapeutic approach.

It is interesting to note several reports of spontaneous improvement in the disease of HVDRR patients.[67,135,136] This spontaneous healing of rickets usually happens between 7 and 15 years of age and has not been consistently associated with the onset of puberty. Spontaneous recovery does not appear to be related to treatment, since therapy was often ineffective, and improvement occurred after the treatment was discontinued. The patients appear to remain normocalcemic without therapy and show no evidence of rickets or osteomalacia. Spontaneous improvement has been reported for both ligand-binding-positive and ligand-

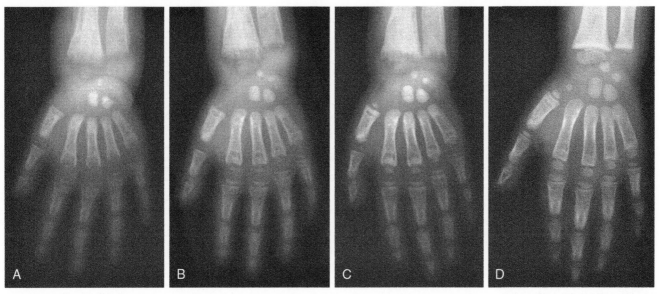

FIGURE 11-8. Radiographic analysis of response to calcium therapy in a patient with hereditary vitamin D–resistant rickets (HVDRR). **A,** At referral, the patient had been treated for 3 months with $1,25(OH)_2D_3$ (15 µg/d). Rickets is still active, and the bone is demineralized. **B,** After 6 months on $1,25(OH)_2D_3$ (30 µg/d) and oral calcium (2 g/d), no significant improvement. **C,** After 2 months of continuous intravenous calcium (without $1,25[OH]_2D_3$), mineralization is improved. **D,** Following 11 months of continuous infusion, mineralization is adequate, but the growth plate remains irregular. Clinical status is satisfactory and maintained with oral calcium (2 g/d).

binding-negative HVDRR patients.[67,135,136] The alopecia persists despite healing of the rickets.[67,135,136] It is not uncommon for children to "outgrow" genetic diseases, and the organism appears able to compensate for the loss of VDR function after skeletal growth has been completed. This apparent functional redundancy does not apply to the hair follicle, however, a situation analogous to what has been described in the VDR-ablated animal model of the disease.[137]

Perspectives

Conceptually, because the signal transduction pathway of $1,25(OH)_2D$ involves accessory molecules such as RXR, the coactivators, and components of the basic transcriptional machinery, it is possible that target-organ resistance to $1,25(OH)_2D$ may be due to mutations in other proteins involved in the transactivation process. When the proteins interact with numerous partners, like RXR, the phenotype associated with mutations would be expected to be broader than the clinical symptoms of HVDRR. The recent identification of transcriptional coactivators with specificity towards the VDR widens the range of putative targets for mutations that could cause HVDRR. It is interesting to note that Hewison et al.[138] described a case of HVDRR in an English patient in which a mutation could not be found in the VDR. The patient exhibited all of the clinical features of HVDRR, including alopecia. The patient's fibroblasts expressed wild-type VDR mRNA, and the receptor bound ligand with normal affinity. Ligand-dependent transcriptional activation by the VDR was deficient in the patient's cells but normal when the patient's VDR was expressed in heterologous cells. These results clearly demonstrate that the patient's VDR was normal and suggest that the vitamin D resistance is the result of a mutation affecting an accessory protein specific for $1,25(OH)_2D$-dependent transcriptional activation. The characterization of the molecular cause of these types of clinical manifestations will further enhance our understanding of vitamin D biology.

REFERENCES

1. Canadillas S, Rodriguez-Benot A, Rodriguez M: More on the bone-kidney axis—lessons from hypophosphataemia, Nephrol Dial Transplant 22:1521–1523, 2007.
2. DeLuca HF: Overview of general physiologic features and functions of vitamin D, Am J Clin Nutr 80:1689S–1696S, 2004.
3. St-Arnaud R: The direct role of vitamin D on bone homeostasis, Arch Biochem Biophys 473:225–230, 2008.
4. Webb AR, Kline L, Holick MF: Influence of season and latitude on the cutaneous synthesis of vitamin D₃: exposure to winter sunlight in Boston and Edmonton will not promote vitamin D₃ synthesis in human skin, J Clin Endocrinol Metab 67:373–378, 1988.
5. Mawer EB, Backhouse J, Holman CA, et al: The distribution and storage of vitamin D and its metabolites in human tissues, Clin Sci 43:413–431, 1972.
6. Chapuy M-C, Meunier PJ: Vitamin D insufficiency in adults and the elderly. In Feldman D, Glorieux FH,

Pike JW, editors: Vitamin D, San Diego, 1997, Academic Press, pp 679–693.
7. Holick MF: Photobiology of vitamin D. In Feldman D, Glorieux FH, Pike JW, editors: Vitamin D, San Diego, 1997, Academic Press, pp 33–39.
8. Guo YD, Strugnell S, Back DW, et al: Transfected human liver cytochrome P-450 hydroxylates vitamin D analogs at different side-chain positions, Proc Natl Acad Sci U S A 90:8668–8672, 1993.
9. Okuda KI, Usui E, Ohyama Y: Recent progress in enzymology and molecular biology of enzymes involved in vitamin D metabolism, J Lipid Res 36:1641–1652, 1995.
10. Cheng JB, Motola DL, Mangelsdorf DJ, et al: De-orphanization of cytochrome P450 2R1: a microsomal vitamin D 25-hydroxylase, J Biol Chem 278:38084–38093, 2003.
11. Bjorkhem I, Holmberg I: Assay and properties of a mitochondrial 25-hydroxylase active on vitamine D₃, J Biol Chem 253:842–849, 1978.

12. Bikle DD: What is new in vitamin D: 2006–2007? Curr Opin Rheumatol 19:383–388, 2007.
13. Christakos S, Dhawan P, Liu Y, et al: New insights into the mechanisms of vitamin D action, J Cell Biochem 88:695–705, 2003.
14. Sutton AL, MacDonald PN: Vitamin D: More than a "bone-a-fide" hormone, Mol Endocrinol 17:777–791, 2003.
15. Haussler MR, Whitfield GK, Haussler CA, et al: The nuclear vitamin D receptor: biological and molecular regulatory properties revealed, J Bone Miner Res 13:325–349, 1998.
16. Omdahl JL, Bobrovnikova EA, Choe S, et al: Overview of regulatory cytochrome P450 enzymes of the vitamin D pathway, Steroids 66:381–389, 2001.
17. Makin G, Lohnes D, Byford V, et al: Target cell metabolism of 1,25-dihydroxyvitamin D₃ to calcitroic acid. Evidence for a pathway in kidney and bone involving 24-oxidation, Biochem J 262:173–180, 1989.

18. Glorieux FH, Pettifor JM, Juppner H: Pediatric Bone: Biology and Diseases, San Diego, 2003, Academic Press, p 756.

19. Cheng JB, Levine MA, Bell NH, et al: Genetic evidence that the human CYP2R1 enzyme is a key vitamin D 25-hydroxylase, Proc Natl Acad Sci U S A 101:7711–7715, 2004.

20. Casella SJ, Reiner BJ, Chen TC, et al: A possible genetic defect in 25-hydroxylation as a cause of rickets, J Pediatr 124:929–932, 1994.

21. Arnaud C, Maijer R, Reade T, et al: Vitamin D dependency: An inherited postnatal syndrome with secondary hyperparathyroidism, Pediatrics 46:871–880, 1970.

22. Delvin EE, Glorieux FH, Marie PJ, et al: Vitamin D dependency: replacement therapy with calcitriol, J Pediatr 99:26–34, 1981.

23. Feldman D, Glorieux FH, Pike JW: Vitamin D, San Diego, 1997, Academic Press, p 1285.

24. Mandla S, Jones G, Tenenhouse HS: Normal 24-hydroxylation of vitamin D metabolites in patients with vitamin D-dependency rickets type I, Structural implications for the vitamin D hydroxylases, J Clin Endocrinol Metab 74:814–820, 1992.

25. Scriver CR, Reade TM, DeLuca HF, et al: Serum 1,25-dihydroxyvitamin D levels in normal subjects and in patients with hereditary rickets or bone disease, N Engl J Med 299:976–979, 1978.

26. Malloy PJ, Pike JW, Feldman D: The vitamin D receptor and the syndrome of hereditary 1,25-dihydroxyvitamin D–resistant rickets, Endocr Rev 20:156–188, 1999.

27. Sakai Y, Kishimoto J, Demay MB: Metabolic and cellular analysis of alopecia in vitamin D receptor knockout mice, J Clin Invest 107:961–966, 2001.

28. Scriver CR: Vitamin D dependency, Pediatrics 45:361–363, 1970.

29. Labuda M, Labuda D, Korab-Laskowska M, et al: Linkage disequilibrium analysis in young populations: pseudo–vitamin D–deficiency rickets and the founder effect in French Canadians, Am J Hum Genet 59:633–643, 1996.

30. Labuda M, Morgan K, Glorieux FH: Mapping autosomal recessive vitamin D–dependency type I to chromosome 12q14 by linkage analysis, Am J Hum Genet 47:28–36, 1990.

31. Fu GK, Lin D, Zhang MY, et al: Cloning of human 25-hydroxyvitamin D 1-alpha-hydroxylase and mutations causing vitamin D-dependent rickets type 1, Mol Endocrinol 11:1961–1970, 1997.

32. Shinki T, Shimada H, Wakino S, et al: Cloning and expression of rat 25-hydroxyvitamin D₃-1alpha-hydroxylase cDNA, Proc Natl Acad Sci U S A 94:12920–12925, 1997.

33. St-Arnaud R, Messerlian S, Moir JM, et al: The 25-hydroxyvitamin D 1alpha-hydroxylase gene maps to the pseudovitamin D-deficiency rickets (PDDR) disease locus, J Bone Miner Res 12:1552–1559, 1997.

34. Takeyama K, Kitanaka S, Sato T, et al: 25-Hydroxyvitamin D₃ 1alpha-hydroxylase and vitamin D synthesis, Science 277:1827–1830, 1997.

35. Kitanaka S, Takeyama K, Murayama A, et al: Inactivating mutations in the 25-hydroxyvitamin D₃ 1alpha-hydroxylase gene in patients with pseudovitamin D-deficiency rickets, N Engl J Med 338:653–661, 1998.

36. Yoshida T, Monkawa T, Tenenhouse HS, et al: Two novel 1alpha-hydroxylase mutations in French-Canadians with vitamin D dependency rickets type I, Kidney Int 54:1437–1443, 1998.

37. Wang X, Zhang MY, Miller WL, et al: Novel gene mutations in patients with 1alpha-hydroxylase deficiency that confer partial enzyme activity in vitro, J Clin Endocrinol Metab 87:2424–2430, 2002.

38. Wang JT, Lin CJ, Burridge SM, et al: Genetics of vitamin D 1alpha-hydroxylase deficiency in 17 families, Am J Hum Genet 63:1694–1702, 1998.

39. Smith SJ, Rucka AK, Berry JL, et al: Novel mutations in the 1alpha-hydroxylase (P450c1) gene in three families with pseudovitamin D-deficiency rickets resulting in loss of functional enzyme activity in blood-derived macrophages, J Bone Miner Res 14:730–739, 1999.

40. Kitanaka S, Murayama A, Sakaki T, et al: No enzyme activity of 25-hydroxyvitamin D₃ 1alpha-hydroxylase gene product in pseudovitamin D deficiency rickets, including that with mild clinical manifestation, J Clin Endocrinol Metab 84:4111–4117, 1999.

41. Kim CJ, Kaplan LE, Perwad F, et al: Vitamin D 1alpha-hydroxylase gene mutations in patients with 1alpha-hydroxylase deficiency, J Clin Endocrinol Metab 92:3177–3182, 2007.

42. Dardenne O, Prud'homme J, Arabian A, et al: Targeted inactivation of the 25-hydroxyvitamin D(3)-1(alpha)-hydroxylase gene (CYP27B1) creates an animal model of pseudovitamin D- deficiency rickets, Endocrinology 142:3135–3141, 2001.

43. Panda DK, Miao D, Tremblay ML, et al: Targeted ablation of the 25-hydroxyvitamin D 1alpha-hydroxylase enzyme: evidence for skeletal, reproductive, and immune dysfunction, Proc Natl Acad Sci U S A 98:7498–7503, 2001.

44. Solish SB, Picado-Leonard J, Morel Y, et al: Human adrenodoxin reductase: two mRNAs encoded by a single gene on chromosome 17cen–q25 are expressed in steroidogenic tissues, Proc Natl Acad Sci U S A 85:7104–7108, 1988.

45. Chang CY, Wu DA, Mohandas TK, et al: Structure, sequence, chromosomal location, and evolution of the human ferredoxin gene family, DNA Cell Biol 9:205–212, 1990.

46. Brunette MG, Chan M, Ferriere C, et al: Site of 1,25-(OH)2 vitamin D₃ synthesis in the kidney, Nature 276:287–289, 1978.

47. Murayama A, Takeyama K, Kitanaka S, et al: The promoter of the human 25-hydroxyvitamin D₃ 1 alpha-hydroxylase gene confers positive and negative responsiveness to PTH, calcitonin, and 1 alpha,25(OH)2D₃, Biochem Biophys Res Commun 249:11–16, 1998.

48. Murayama A, Takeyama K, Kitanaka S, et al: Positive and negative regulations of the renal 25-hydroxyvitamin D₃ 1alpha-hydroxylase gene by parathyroid hormone, calcitonin, and 1alpha,25(OH)2D₃ in intact animals, Endocrinology 140:2224–2231, 1999.

49. Yoshida T, Yoshida N, Monkawa T, et al: Dietary phosphorus deprivation induces 25-hydroxyvitamin D(3) 1alpha-hydroxylase gene expression, Endocrinology 142:1720–1726, 2001.

50. Fu GK, Portale AA, Miller WL: Complete structure of the human gene for the vitamin D 1alpha-hydroxylase, P450c1alpha, DNA Cell Biol 16:1499–1507, 1997.

51. Monkawa T, Yoshida T, Wakino S, et al: Molecular cloning of cDNA and genomic DNA for human 25-hydroxyvitamin D₃ 1 alpha-hydroxylase, Biochem Biophys Res Commun 239:527–533, 1997.

52. Rosen JF, Finberg L: Vitamin D-dependent rickets: actions of parathyroid hormone and 25- hydroxycholecalciferol, Pediatr Res 6:552–562, 1972.

53. Hasemann CA, Kurumbail RG, Boddupalli SS, et al: Structure and function of cytochromes P450: a comparative analysis of three crystal structures, Structure 3:41–62, 1995.

54. Sawada N, Sakaki T, Kitanaka S, et al: Structure-function analysis of CYP27B1 and CYP27A1. Studies on mutants from patients with vitamin D-dependent rickets type I (VDDR-I) and cerebrotendinous xanthomatosis (CTX), Eur J Biochem 268:6607–6615, 2001.

55. Williams PA, Cosme J, Sridhar V, et al: Mammalian microsomal cytochrome P450 monooxygenase: structural adaptations for membrane binding and functional diversity, Mol Cell 5:121–131, 2000.

56. Yamamoto K, Masuno H, Sawada N, et al: Homology modeling of human 25-hydroxyvitamin D₃ 1alpha-hydroxylase (CYP27B1) based on the crystal structure of rabbit CYP2C5, J Steroid Biochem Mol Biol 89–90:167–171, 2004.

57. Yamamoto K, Uchida E, Urushino N, et al: Identification of the amino acid residue of CYP27B1 responsible for binding of 25-hydroxyvitamin D₃ whose mutation causes vitamin D-dependent rickets type 1, J Biol Chem 280:30511–30516, 2005.

58. Balsan S, Garabedian M, Lieberherr M, et al: Serum 1,25-dihydroxyvitamin D concentrations in two different types of pseudo-deficiency rickets. In Norman AW, Schaefer K, von Herrath D, et al: Vitamin D: Basic Research and Its Clinical Application, Berlin, 1979, Walter de Gruyter, pp 1143–1149.

59. Glorieux FH: Calcitriol treatment in vitamin D-dependent and vitamin D-resistant rickets, Metabolism 39(suppl):10–12, 1990.

60. Reade TM, Scriver CR, Glorieux FH, et al: Response to crystalline 1alpha-hydroxyvitamin D₃ in vitamin D dependency, Pediatr Res 9:593–599, 1975.

61. Albright F, Buttler A, Bloomberg E: Rickets resistant to vitamin D therapy, Am J Dis Child 54:529–547, 1937.

62. Haussler MR, Norman AW: Chromosomal receptor for a vitamin D metabolite, Proc Natl Acad Sci U S A 62:155–162, 1969.

63. Pike JW, Haussler MR: Purification of chicken intestinal receptor for 1,25-dihydroxyvitamin D, Proc Natl Acad Sci U S A 76:5485–5489, 1979.

64. Pike JW, Marion SL, Donaldson CA, et al: Serum and monoclonal antibodies against the chick intestinal receptor for 1,25-dihydroxyvitamin D₃, Generation by a preparation enriched in a 64,000-dalton protein, J Biol Chem 258:1289–1296, 1983.

65. Dame MC, Pierce EA, Prahl JM, et al: Monoclonal antibodies to the porcine intestinal receptor for 1,25-dihydroxyvitamin D₃: interaction with distinct receptor domains, Biochemistry 25:4523–4534, 1986.

66. Feldman D, Chen T, Cone C, et al: Vitamin D resistant rickets with alopecia: cultured skin fibroblasts exhibit defective cytoplasmic receptors and unresponsiveness to 1,25(OH)2D₃, J Clin Endocrinol Metab 55:1020–1022, 1982.

67. Hirst MA, Hochman HI, Feldman D: Vitamin D resistance and alopecia: a kindred with normal 1,25-dihydroxyvitamin D binding, but decreased receptor affinity for deoxyribonucleic acid, J Clin Endocrinol Metab 60:490–495, 1985.

68. Dokoh S, Haussler MR, Pike JW: Development of a radioligand immunoassay for 1,25-dihydroxycholeclciferol receptors utilizing monoclonal antibody, Biochem J 221:129–136, 1984.

69. Pike JW, Dokoh S, Haussler MR, et al: Vitamin D₃-resistant fibroblasts have immunoassayable 1,25-dihydroxyvitamin D₃ receptors, Science 224:879–881, 1984.

70. Malloy PJ, Hochberg Z, Pike JW, et al: Abnormal binding of vitamin D receptors to deoxyribonucleic acid in a kindred with vitamin D-dependent rickets, type II, J Clin Endocrinol Metab 68:263–269, 1989.

71. Baker AR, McDonnell DP, Hughes M, et al: Cloning and expression of full-length cDNA encoding human vitamin D receptor, Proc Natl Acad Sci U S A 85:3294–3298, 1988.

72. Burmester JK, Maeda N, DeLuca HF: Isolation and expression of rat 1,25-dihydroxyvitamin D₃ receptor cDNA, Proc Natl Acad Sci U S A 85:1005–1009, 1988.

73. McDonnell DP, Mangelsdorf DJ, Pike JW, et al: Molecular cloning of complementary DNA encoding the avian receptor for vitamin D, Science 235:1214–1217, 1987.

74. Hughes MR, Malloy PJ, Kieback DG, et al: Point mutations in the human vitamin D receptor gene associated with hypocalcemic rickets, Science 242:1702–1705, 1988.

75. Bouillon R, Van Cromphaut S, Carmeliet G: Intestinal calcium absorption: molecular vitamin D mediated mechanisms, J Cell Biochem 88:332–339, 2003.

76. Arai H, Miyamoto K, Taketani Y, et al: A vitamin D receptor gene polymorphism in the translation initiation codon: effect on protein activity and relation to bone mineral density in Japanese women, J Bone Miner Res 12:915–921, 1997.

77. Miyamoto K, Kesterson RA, Yamamoto H, et al: Structural organization of the human vitamin D receptor chromosomal gene and its promoter, Mol Endocrinol 11:1165–1179, 1997.

78. Jurutka PW, Hsieh JC, MacDonald PN, et al: Phosphorylation of serine 208 in the human vitamin D receptor. The predominant amino acid phosphorylated by casein kinase II, in vitro, and identification as a significant phosphorylation site in intact cells, J Biol Chem 268:6791–6799, 1993.

79. Hilliard GMt, Cook RG, Weigel NL, et al: 1,25-dihydroxyvitamin D₃ modulates phosphorylation of serine 205 in the human vitamin D receptor: site-directed mutagenesis of this residue promotes alternative phosphorylation, Biochemistry 33:4300–4311, 1994.

80. Rastinejad F, Perlmann T, Evans RM, et al: Structural determinants of nuclear receptor assembly on DNA direct repeats, Nature 375:203–211, 1995.

81. Hsieh JC, Shimizu Y, Minoshima S, et al: Novel nuclear localization signal between the two DNA-binding zinc fingers in the human vitamin D receptor, J Cell Biochem 70:94–109, 1998.

82. Hsieh JC, Jurutka PW, Galligan MA, et al: Human vitamin D receptor is selectively phosphorylated by protein kinase C on serine 51, a residue crucial to its trans-activation function, Proc Natl Acad Sci U S A 88:9315–9319, 1991.

83. Hsieh JC, Jurutka PW, Nakajima S, et al: Phosphorylation of the human vitamin D receptor by protein kinase C. Biochemical and functional evaluation of the serine 51 recognition site, J Biol Chem 268:15118–15126, 1993.

84. Nishikawa J, Kitaura M, Imagawa M, et al: Vitamin D receptor contains multiple dimerization interfaces that are functionally different, Nucleic Acids Res 23:606–611, 1995.

85. Hsieh JC, Jurutka PW, Selznick SH, et al: The T-box near the zinc fingers of the human vitamin D receptor is required for heterodimeric DNA binding and trans-activation, Biochem Biophys Res Commun 215:1–7, 1995.

86. Rochel N, Wurtz JM, Mitschler A, et al: The crystal structure of the nuclear receptor for vitamin D bound to its natural ligand, Mol Cell 5:173–179, 2000.

87. Peleg S, Sastry M, Collins ED, et al: Distinct conformational changes induced by 20-epi analogues of 1 alpha,25-dihydroxyvitamin D_3 are associated with enhanced activation of the vitamin D receptor, J Biol Chem 270:10551–10558, 1995.

88. Allegretto EA, Pike JW, Haussler MR: Immunochemical detection of unique proteolytic fragments of the chick 1,25-dihydroxyvitamin D_3 receptor. Distinct 20-kDa DNA-binding and 45-kDa hormone-binding species, J Biol Chem 262:1312–1319, 1987.

89. Gardezi SA, Nguyen C, Malloy PJ, et al: A rationale for treatment of hereditary vitamin D-resistant rickets with analogs of 1 alpha,25-dihydroxyvitamin D(3), J Biol Chem 276:29148–29156, 2001.

90. Bourguet W, Ruff M, Chambon P, et al: Crystal structure of the ligand-binding domain of the human nuclear receptor RXR-alpha, Nature 375:377–382, 1995.

91. Rosen ED, Beninghof EG, Koenig RJ: Dimerization interfaces of thyroid hormone, retinoic acid, vitamin D, and retinoid X receptors, J Biol Chem 268:11534–11541, 1993.

92. Whitfield GK, Hsieh JC, Nakajima S, et al: A highly conserved region in the hormone-binding domain of the human vitamin D receptor contains residues vital for heterodimerization with retinoid X receptor and for transcriptional activation, Mol Endocrinol 9:1166–1179, 1995.

93. Jin CH, Kerner SA, Hong MH, et al: Transcriptional activation and dimerization functions in the human vitamin D receptor, Mol Endocrinol 10:945–957, 1996.

94. Nakajima S, Hsieh JC, MacDonald PN, et al: The C-terminal region of the vitamin D receptor is essential to form a complex with a receptor auxiliary factor required for high-affinity binding to the vitamin D-responsive element, Mol Endocrinol 8:159–172, 1994.

95. Henttu PM, Kalkhoven E, Parker MG: AF-2 activity and recruitment of steroid receptor coactivator 1 to the estrogen receptor depend on a lysine residue conserved in nuclear receptors, Mol Cell Biol 17:1832–1839, 1997.

96. Danielian PS, White R, Lees JA, et al: Identification of a conserved region required for hormone dependent transcriptional activation by steroid hormone receptors, EMBO J 11:1025–1033, 1992.

97. Jurutka PW, Hsieh JC, Remus LS, et al: Mutations in the 1,25-dihydroxyvitamin D_3 receptor identifying C-terminal amino acids required for transcriptional activation that are functionally dissociated from hormone binding, heterodimeric DNA binding, and interaction with basal transcription factor IIB, in vitro, J Biol Chem 272:14592–14599, 1997.

98. Masuyama H, Brownfield CM, St-Arnaud R, et al: Evidence for ligand-dependent intramolecular folding of the AF-2 domain in vitamin D receptor-activated transcription and coactivator interaction, Mol Endocrinol 11:1507–1517, 1997.

99. Blanco JC, Wang IM, Tsai SY, et al: Transcription factor TFIIB and the vitamin D receptor cooperatively activate ligand-dependent transcription, Proc Natl Acad Sci U S A 92:1535–1539, 1995.

100. MacDonald PN, Sherman DR, Dowd DR, et al: The vitamin D receptor interacts with general transcription factor IIB, J Biol Chem 270:4748–4752, 1995.

101. Glass CK, Rosenfeld MG: The coregulator exchange in transcriptional functions of nuclear receptors, Genes Dev 14:121–141, 2000.

102. Kitagawa H, Fujiki R, Yoshimura K, et al: The chromatin-remodeling complex WINAC targets a nuclear receptor to promoters and is impaired in Williams syndrome, Cell 113:905–917, 2003.

103. Gu W, Malik S, Ito M, et al: A novel human SRB/MED-containing cofactor complex, SMCC, involved in transcription regulation, Mol Cell 3:97–108, 1999.

104. Rachez C, Suldan Z, Ward J, et al: A novel protein complex that interacts with the vitamin D_3 receptor in a ligand-dependent manner and enhances VDR transactivation in a cell-free system, Genes Dev 12:1787–1800, 1998.

105. Kim S, Shevde NK, Pike JW: 1,25-Dihydroxyvitamin D_3 stimulates cyclic vitamin D receptor/retinoid X receptor DNA-binding, co-activator recruitment, and histone acetylation in intact osteoblasts, J Bone Miner Res 20:305–317, 2005.

106. Takeyama K, Masuhiro Y, Fuse H, et al: Selective interaction of vitamin D receptor with transcriptional coactivators by a vitamin D analog, Mol Cell Biol 19:1049–1055, 1999.

107. Yamaoka K, Shindo M, Iwasaki K, et al: Multiple coactivator complexes support ligand-induced transactivation function of VDR, Arch Biochem Biophys 460:166–171, 2007.

108. Malloy PJ, Hochberg Z, Tiosano D, et al: The molecular basis of hereditary 1,25-dihydroxyvitamin D_3 resistant rickets in seven related families, J Clin Invest 86:2071–2079, 1990.

109. Renaud JP, Rochel N, Ruff M, et al: Crystal structure of the RAR-gamma ligand-binding domain bound to all-trans retinoic acid, Nature 378:681–689, 1995.

110. Wagner RL, Apriletti JW, McGrath ME, et al: A structural role for hormone in the thyroid hormone receptor, Nature 378:690–697, 1995.

111. Rut AR, Hewison M, Kristjansson K, et al: Two mutations causing vitamin D resistant rickets: modelling on the basis of steroid hormone receptor DNA-binding domain crystal structures, Clin Endocrinol (Oxf) 41:581–590, 1994.

112. Cockerill FJ, Hawa NS, Yousaf N, et al: Mutations in the vitamin D receptor gene in three kindreds associated with hereditary vitamin D resistant rickets, J Clin Endocrinol Metab 82:3156–3160, 1997.

113. Ritchie HH, Hughes MR, Thompson ET, et al: An ochre mutation in the vitamin D receptor gene causes hereditary 1,25-dihydroxyvitamin D_3-resistant rickets in three families, Proc Natl Acad Sci U S A 86:9783–9787, 1989.

114. Malloy PJ, Hughes MR, Pike JW, et al: Vitamin D receptor mutations and hereditary 1,25-dihydroxyvitamin D resistant rickets. In Norman AW, Bouillon R, Thomasset M, editors: Vitamin D: Gene Regulation, Structure-Function Analysis, and Clinical Application. Eighth Workshop on Vitamin D, New York, 1991, Walter de Gruyter, pp 116–124.

115. Wiese RJ, Goto H, Prahl JM, et al: Vitamin D-dependency rickets type II: Truncated vitamin D receptor in three kindreds, Mol Cell Endocrinol 90:197–201, 1993.

116. Malloy PJ, Xu R, Cattani A, et al: A unique insertion/substitution in helix H1 of the vitamin D receptor ligand binding domain in a patient with hereditary 1,25-dihydroxyvitamin D-resistant rickets, J Bone Miner Res 19:1018–1024, 2004.

117. Malloy PJ, Zhu W, Zhao XY, et al: A novel inborn error in the ligand-binding domain of the vitamin D receptor causes hereditary vitamin D-resistant rickets, Mol Genet Metab 73:138–148, 2001.

118. Malloy PJ, Xu R, Peng L, et al: A novel mutation in helix 12 of the vitamin D receptor impairs coactivator interaction and causes hereditary 1,25-dihydroxyvitamin D-resistant rickets without alopecia, Mol Endocrinol 16:2538–2546, 2002.

119. Marx SJ, Bliziotes MM, Nanes M: Analysis of the relation between alopecia and resistance to 1,25-dihydroxyvitamin D, Clin Endocrinol (Oxf) 25:373–381, 1986.

120. Brooks MH, Bell NH, Love L, et al: Vitamin-D-dependent rickets type II. Resistance of target organs to 1,25-dihydroxyvitamin D, N Engl J Med 298:996–999, 1978.

121. Marx SJ, Spiegel AM, Brown EM, et al: A familial syndrome of decrease in sensitivity to 1,25-dihydroxyvitamin D, J Clin Endocrinol Metab 47:1303–1310, 1978.

122. Zerwekh JE, Glass K, Jowsey J, et al: An unique form of osteomalacia associated with end organ refractoriness to 1,25-dihydroxyvitamin D and apparent defective synthesis of 25-hydroxyvitamin D, J Clin Endocrinol Metab 49:171–175, 1979.

123. Whitfield GK, Selznick SH, Haussler CA, et al: Vitamin D receptors from patients with resistance to 1,25-dihydroxyvitamin D_3: point mutations confer reduced transactivation in response to ligand and impaired interaction with the retinoid X receptor heterodimeric partner, Mol Endocrinol 10:1617–1631, 1996.

124. Malloy PJ, Eccleshall TR, Gross C, et al: Hereditary vitamin D resistant rickets caused by a novel mutation in the vitamin D receptor that results in decreased affinity for hormone and cellular hyporesponsiveness, J Clin Invest 99:297–304, 1997.

125. Kudoh T, Kumagai T, Uetsuji N, et al: Vitamin D dependent rickets: decreased sensitivity to 1,25-dihydroxyvitamin D, Eur J Pediatr 137:307–311, 1981.

126. Balsan S, Garabedian M, Liberman UA, et al: Rickets and alopecia with resistance to 1,25-dihydroxyvitamin D: two different clinical courses with two different cellular defects, J Clin Endocrinol Metab 57:803–811, 1983.

127. Tsuchiya Y, Matsuo N, Cho H, et al: An unusual form of vitamin D-dependent rickets in a child: alopecia and marked end-organ hyposensitivity to biologically active vitamin D, J Clin Endocrinol Metab 51:685–690, 1980.

128. Castells S, Greig F, Fusi MA, et al: Severely deficient binding of 1,25-dihydroxyvitamin D to its receptors in a patient responsive to high doses of this hormone, J Clin Endocrinol Metab 63:252–256, 1986.

129. Takeda E, Kuroda Y, Saijo T, et al: 1 alpha-hydroxyvitamin D_3 treatment of three patients with 1,25-dihydroxyvitamin D-receptor-defect rickets and alopecia, Pediatrics 80:97–101, 1987.

130. Sakati N, Woodhouse NJ, Niles N, et al: Hereditary resistance to 1,25-dihydroxyvitamin D: clinical and radiological improvement during high-dose oral calcium therapy, Horm Res 24:280–287, 1986.

131. Balsan S, Garabedian M, Larchet M, et al: Long-term nocturnal calcium infusions can cure rickets and promote normal mineralization in hereditary resistance to 1,25-dihydroxyvitamin D, J Clin Invest 77:1661–1667, 1986.

132. Weisman Y, Bab I, Gazit D, et al: Long-term intracaval calcium infusion therapy in end-organ resistance to 1,25-dihydroxyvitamin D, Am J Med 83:984–990, 1987.

133. Hochberg Z, Tiosano D, Even L: Calcium therapy for calcitriol-resistant rickets, J Pediatr 121:803–808, 1992.

134. Bliziotes M, Yergey AL, Nanes MS, et al: Absent intestinal response to calciferols in hereditary resistance to 1,25-dihydroxyvitamin D: documentation and effective therapy with high dose intravenous calcium infusions, J Clin Endocrinol Metab 66:294–300, 1988.

135. Hochberg Z, Benderli A, Levy J, et al: 1,25-Dihydroxyvitamin D resistance, rickets, and alopecia, Am J Med 77:805–811, 1984.

136. Chen TL, Hirst MA, Cone CM, et al: 1,25-Dihydroxyvitamin D resistance, rickets, and alopecia: analysis of receptors and bioresponse in cultured fibroblasts from patients and parents, J Clin Endocrinol Metab 59:383–388, 1984.

137. Li YC, Amling M, Pirro AE, et al: Normalization of mineral ion homeostasis by dietary means prevents hyperparathyroidism, rickets, and osteomalacia, but not alopecia in vitamin D receptor-ablated mice, Endocrinology 139:4391–4396, 1998.

138. Hewison M, Rut AR, Kristjansson K, et al: Tissue resistance to 1,25-dihydroxyvitamin D without a mutation of the vitamin D receptor gene, Clin Endocrinol (Oxf) 39:663–670, 1993.

139. Zhu W, Malloy PJ, Delvin E, et al: Hereditary 1,25-dihydroxyvitamin D-resistant rickets due to an opal mutation causing premature termination of the vitamin D receptor, J Bone Miner Res 13:259–264, 1998.

140. Mechica JB, Leite MO, Mendonca BB, et al: A novel nonsense mutation in the first zinc finger of the vitamin D receptor causing hereditary 1,25-dihydroxyvitamin

D₃-resistant rickets, J Clin Endocrinol Metab 82:3892–3894, 1997.

141. Yagi H, Ozono K, Miyake H, et al: A new point mutation in the deoxyribonucleic acid-binding domain of the vitamin D receptor in a kindred with hereditary 1,25-dihydroxyvitamin D-resistant rickets, J Clin Endocrinol Metab 76:509–512, 1993.

142. Lin NU, Malloy PJ, Sakati N, et al: A novel mutation in the deoxyribonucleic acid-binding domain of the vitamin D receptor causes hereditary 1,25-dihydroxyvitamin D-resistant rickets, J Clin Endocrinol Metab 81:2564–2569, 1996.

143. Saijo T, Ito M, Takeda E, et al: A unique mutation in the vitamin D receptor gene in three Japanese patients with vitamin D-dependent rickets type II: utility of single-strand conformation polymorphism analysis for heterozygous carrier detection, Am J Hum Genet 49:668–673, 1991.

144. Malloy PJ, Weisman Y, Feldman D: Hereditary 1 alpha,25-dihydroxyvitamin D-resistant rickets resulting from a mutation in the vitamin D receptor deoxyribonucleic acid-binding domain, J Clin Endocrinol Metab 78:313–316, 1994.

145. Sone T, Marx SJ, Liberman UA, et al: A unique point mutation in the human vitamin D receptor chromosomal gene confers hereditary resistance to 1,25-dihydroxyvitamin D₃, Mol Endocrinol 4:623–631, 1990.

146. Hawa NS, Cockerill FJ, Vadher S, et al: Identification of a novel mutation in hereditary vitamin D resistant rickets causing exon skipping, Clin Endocrinol (Oxf) 45:85–92, 1996.

147. Kristjansson K, Rut AR, Hewison M, et al: Two mutations in the hormone binding domain of the vitamin D receptor cause tissue resistance to 1,25 dihydroxyvitamin D₃, J Clin Invest 92:12–16, 1993.

148. Katavetin P, Katavetin P, Wacharasindhu S, et al: A girl with a novel splice site mutation in VDR supports the role of a ligand-independent VDR function on hair cycling, Horm Res 66:273–276, 2006.

149. Nguyen M, d'Alesio A, Pascussi JM, et al: Vitamin D-resistant rickets and type 1 diabetes in a child with compound heterozygous mutations of the vitamin D receptor (L263R and R391S): dissociated responses of the CYP-24 and rel-B promoters to 1,25-dihydroxyvitamin D₃, J Bone Miner Res 21:886–894, 2006.

150. Malloy PJ, Xu R, Peng L, et al: Hereditary 1,25-dihydroxyvitamin D resistant rickets due to a mutation causing multiple defects in vitamin D receptor function, Endocrinology 145:5106–5114, 2004.

151. Nguyen TM, Adiceam P, Kottler ML, et al: Tryptophan missense mutation in the ligand-binding domain of the vitamin D receptor causes severe resistance to 1,25-dihydroxyvitamin D, J Bone Miner Res 17:1728–1737, 2002.

152. Malloy PJ, Zhu W, Bouillon R, et al: A novel nonsense mutation in the ligand binding domain of the vitamin D receptor causes hereditary 1,25-dihydroxyvitamin D-resistant rickets, Mol Genet Metab 77:314–318, 2002.

153. Malloy PJ, Wang J, Peng L, et al: A unique insertion/duplication in the VDR gene that truncates the VDR causing hereditary 1,25-dihydroxyvitamin D-resistant rickets without alopecia, Arch Biochem Biophys 460:285–292, 2007.

Chapter 12

HEREDITARY DISORDERS OF THE SKELETON

MICHAEL P. WHYTE

Sclerosing Bone Disorders
Osteopetrosis
Pycnodysostosis
Progressive Diaphyseal Dysplasia (Camurati-Engelmann Disease)
Endosteal Hyperostosis
Osteopoikilosis
Osteopathia Striata
Pachydermoperiostosis

Osteoporoses
Osteogenesis Imperfecta

Disorders of RANK/OPG/RANKL/NF-κB Signaling
Paget's Disease of Bone
Familial Expansile Osteolysis
Osteoprotegerin Deficiency (Juvenile Paget's Disease)

Endocrinologists can encounter a great diversity of heritable disorders of the skeleton.[1-4] Some are clinical curiosities; some are lethal. Some cause focal bony abnormalities; some feature generalized disturbances of skeletal growth, modeling (shaping), and remodeling (turnover).[3] A few are associated with overt derangements in mineral homeostasis. Cumulatively, the number of affected people is substantial.[1] Each of these entities is important because all harbor clues concerning specific genes and their products that influence skeletal biology. Furthermore, as individual conditions become understood molecularly, patients are being referred increasingly to endocrinologists.

This chapter describes a number of the more common or instructive of the hereditary disorders of the skeleton.

Sclerosing Bone Disorders

Increased skeletal mass is caused by many rare, often heritable osteochondrodysplasias,[1,4] and by a variety of endocrine, metabolic, dietary, hematologic, infectious, and neoplastic diseases (Table 12-1). *Osteosclerosis* and *hyperostosis* refer to trabecular versus cortical bone thickening, respectively. A radiographic skeletal survey of the genetic disorders shows where and sometimes how bone mass is increased, and often provides sufficient clues for diagnosis.[3,4]

OSTEOPETROSIS

Osteopetrosis (OPT; "marble bone disease") was reported first in 1904 by Albers-Schönberg.[5] Traditionally, two principal forms are discussed[6]: the autosomal recessive, infantile (malignant) type that is typically fatal during the first decade of life if untreated,[7] and the autosomal dominant, adult (benign) type with distinctly less severe complications.[8] Especially rare "intermediate" forms of OPT present during childhood, when the prognosis is poorly understood.[9]

Now, the gene defects that cause nearly all cases of OPT are known, greatly improving upon imprecise clinical nosologies.[10] Although there are different types of OPT, all true forms result from failure of osteoclasts to resorb skeletal tissue.[6] Consequently, the manifestations are largely predictable. Accumulation of primary spongiosa (calcified cartilage deposited during endochondral bone formation) represents the histopathologic hallmark.[11] It is understandable, however, that the term *osteopetrosis* persists generically for radiodense skeletons, but should henceforth be applied with precision based on pathogenesis because therapies for genuine OPTs may be inappropriate or harmful for other sclerosing bone disorders.[8]

Clinical Features

Infantile OPT manifests in babies.[7] There is failure to thrive. Cranial foramina do not widen, often compressing auditory, oculomotor, facial, and optic nerves. Blindness can result from retinal degeneration or raised intracranial pressure.[12] Some patients develop hydrocephalus or sleep apnea. Nasal stuffiness due to underdeveloped sinuses occurs early. Dentition is delayed. Recurrent infections and spontaneous bruising and bleeding are common and are due to myelophthisis from excessive bone tissue, osteoclasts, and fibrosis crowding marrow spaces. Extramedullary hematopoiesis with hypersplenism and hemolysis may exacerbate already severe anemia. A large head, frontal bossing, "adenoid" appearance, nystagmus, hepatosplenomegaly, short stature, and genu valgum are noted. Bones are fragile. Untreated patients succumb, usually during the first decade of life, to pneumonia, severe anemia, hemorrhage, or sepsis.[6,7]

Table 12-1. Disorders That Cause High Bone Mass

Dysplasias	Metabolic
Central osteosclerosis with ectodermal dysplasia	Carbonic anhydrase II deficiency
Craniodiaphyseal dysplasia	Fluorosis
Craniometaphyseal dysplasia	Heavy metal poisoning
Dysosteosclerosis	Hepatitis C-associated osteosclerosis
Endosteal hyperostosis	Hypervitaminosis A, D
Van Buchem disease	Hyper-, hypo-, and
Sclerosteosis	pseudohypoparathyroidism
Frontometaphyseal dysplasia	Hypophosphatemic osteomalacia
Hyperphosphatasia (juvenile Paget's disease)	Milk-alkali syndrome
	Renal osteodystrophy
Infantile cortical hyperostosis (Caffey disease)	**Other**
Lenz-Majewski syndrome	Axial osteomalacia
Melorheostosis	Fibrogenesis imperfecta ossium
Metaphyseal dysplasia (Pyle disease)	Ionizing radiation
Mixed-sclerosing bone dystrophy	Lymphoma
Oculodento-osseous dysplasia	Mastocytosis
Osteodysplasia of Melnick and Needles	Multiple myeloma
Osteopathia striata	Myelofibrosis
Osteopetrosis	Osteomyelitis
Osteopoikilosis	Osteonecrosis
Progressive diaphyseal dysplasia (Camurati-Engelmann disease)	Paget bone disease
	Sarcoidosis
Pycnodysostosis	Skeletal metastases
	Tuberous sclerosis

Modified from reference 6.

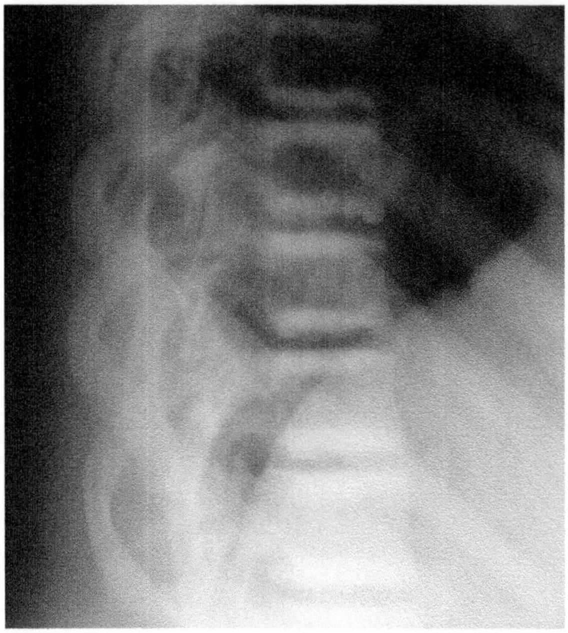

FIGURE 12-1. Osteopetrosis. This teenage girl with Albers-Schönberg disease has a "rugger-jersey" spine typical of adult ("benign") osteopetrosis. The vertebral end plates are markedly thickened.

Intermediate OPT causes macrocephaly and short stature, sometimes with cranial nerve palsies, ankylosed teeth leading to osteomyelitis of the jaw, recurrent fractures, and mild or occasionally moderately severe anemia.[9]

Autosomal dominant "benign" OPT (Albers-Schönberg disease) features brittle long bones and fractures within the axial and the appendicular skeleton, and sometimes compromised vision and hearing, facial nerve palsy, mandibular osteomyelitis,[13] psychomotor delay, carpal tunnel syndrome, slipped capital femoral epiphysis, or osteoarthritis.[14] Some affected individuals are asymptomatic,[8] and rare carriers show no radiographic findings.[15]

Carbonic anhydrase II (CA II) deficiency features OPT with renal tubular acidosis (RTA) and cerebral calcification.[16] Severity varies among affected families.[17] In infancy or early childhood, fractures, failure to thrive, developmental delay, or short stature manifest. Mental subnormality is common. Compression of the optic nerves and dental malocclusion are further complications. Metabolic acidosis presents as early as birth. Both proximal and distal RTA have been described,[18] although distal (type I) RTA seems better documented and may explain any hypotonia, apathy, and muscle weakness. Periodic hypokalemic paralysis can occur. Life expectancy is uncertain, with the oldest published cases reported in young adults.[19]

Neuronal storage disease with OPT features severe skeletal manifestations accompanying epilepsy and neurodegenerative disease.[20] Transient infantile OPT of unknown cause inexplicably resolves after the first months of life. OPT, lymphedema, anhidrotic ectodermal dysplasia, and immunodeficiency (OL-EDA-ID) is an X-linked recessive condition of boys.[21]

Radiographic Findings

A generalized, symmetrical increase in bone mass is the principal radiographic finding in OPT.[22] Cortical and trabecular bone is thickened. In severe disease, all components of skeletal development are disrupted: bone growth, modeling, and remodeling.

Furthermore, rachitic changes in growth plates may occur.[23] The skull, especially the base, is thickened and dense, and the paranasal and mastoid sinuses are underpneumatized. Vertebrae may show a "bone-in-bone" (endobone) configuration.[22]

In CA II deficiency, skeletal radiographs typically are abnormal at diagnosis, although findings can be subtle at birth. Remarkably, the osteosclerosis and defective skeletal modeling then diminish over years.[16] Cerebral calcification appears on computed tomography (CT) between ages 2 and 5 years and increases during childhood, affecting gray matter of the cortex and basal ganglia.[17]

In Albers-Schönberg disease, abnormalities appear during childhood. An especially dense skull base, a "rugger-jersey" spine, and enigmatic alternating sclerotic and lucent bands in the metaphyses of major long bones are characteristic (Fig. 12-1). Metaphyses are wide and may have a club shape or "Erlenmeyer flask" appearance.[8] Rarely, distal phalanges in the hands are eroded (more common in pycnodysostosis). Pathologic ("chalk-stick") fractures occur in major long bones.[22]

Skeletal scintigraphy reveals fractures and osteomyelitis.[24] Magnetic resonance imaging (MRI) helps assess patients undergoing bone marrow transplantation, because engraftment restores medullary spaces.[25]

Laboratory Findings

In infantile OPT, serum calcium concentrations depend largely upon gastrointestinal calcium absorption, because of the impaired bone resorption.[26] Secondary hyperparathyroidism with elevated serum levels of calcitriol is common.[26] Hypocalcemia can occur, especially with achlorhydria, and causes rickets.[23]

In adult OPT, biochemical indices of mineral homeostasis usually are unremarkable, although serum PTH levels can be increased.[27]

Serum acid phosphatase and the brain isoenzyme of creatine kinase often are elevated and seem to originate from the dysfunctional osteoclasts.[28]

Histopathologic Findings

Failure of osteoclast action provides a pathognomonic finding in OPT[6]—primary spongiosa synthesized during endochondral bone formation persists as "islands" of calcified cartilage encased within trabecular bone. Osteoclast numbers are increased, normal, or, rarely, decreased. In infantile OPT, these cells are usually abundant.[29] Their nuclei are especially numerous, but the "ruffled borders" and "clear zones" that characterize functioning osteoclasts are absent.[30] Fibrosis often crowds marrow spaces. Adult OPT shows increased amounts of osteoid, and osteoclasts can be few and may lack ruffled borders, or they can be especially numerous and large.[31]

Cause and Pathogenesis

Most patients with OPT have diminished osteoclast-mediated acidification at sites of bone resorption due to defects in CA II, the α3 subunit of the vacuolar proton pump, or chloride channel 7 (*CLCN7*).[32] Heterozygous loss-of-function mutation within CLCN7 causes Albers-Schönberg disease.[33] Homozygous or compound heterozygous *CLCN7* mutations lead to severe or intermediate OPT.[33] Malignant OPT usually is due to deactivating mutations in the gene *TCIRG1* (*ATP6i*), which encodes the α3 subunit of the vacuolar proton pump.[34] Defects in the "gray-lethal" and *OSTM1* genes cause especially severe OPT.[35] OL-EDA-ID represents disruption of an essential modulator of NF-κB.[21] Recently, loss-of-function mutations within the genes that encode the receptor activator of nuclear factor-κB (RANK) or its ligand (RANKL) were discovered in especially rare forms of autosomal recessive OPT.[36,37]

Ultimately, impaired skeletal resorption in OPT causes both myelophthisis and bone fragility resulting from the presence of fewer collagen fibrils interconnecting osteons.[11]

Treatment

Because the cause and pathogenesis, pattern of inheritance, and prognosis for the various forms of OPT can differ, a precise diagnosis is crucial before therapy is attempted. For example, infants or young children with CA II deficiency can have radiographic features of malignant OPT, yet sequential studies may show gradual resolution of bony sclerosis.[6] Until recently, the patient's family and investigation into the severity and progression of the disorder were the principal considerations. Now, diagnosis has been advanced greatly by mutation analysis.[38]

Bone Marrow Transplantation

Bone marrow transplantation from HLA-identical donors has improved remarkably some patients with infantile OPT.[32] However, this procedure is not always appropriate[6] (e.g., RANKL deficiency)[36] because the pathogenetic defect must be corrected by entry of donor cells into the osteoclast lineage.[32]

Because severely crowded medullary spaces appear less likely to engraft, early intervention is best.[39] Use of marrow from HLA-nonidentical donors warrants continued study. Purified progenitor cells in blood from HLA-haploidentical parents have been useful.[39a] Marked hypercalcemia can occur as osteoclast function begins.[40]

Dietary and Medical Therapy

Some success has been reported when a calcium-deficient diet is given. Conversely, calcium supplementation may be necessary for symptomatic hypocalcemia or rickets.[23] Large oral doses of calcitriol together with dietary calcium restriction (to prevent absorptive hypercalciuria/hypercalcemia) sometimes improves infantile OPT.[41] Calcitriol may stimulate defective osteoclasts, but resistance can occur.[41] Long-term infusion of PTH helped one infant,[42] perhaps by enhancing calcitriol synthesis. Diminished leukocyte production of superoxide serves as the basis for recombinant human interferon-γ-1b treatment for severely affected children.[41]

High-dose glucocorticoid treatment stabilizes pancytopenia and hepatomegaly. One case report describes inexplicable reversal of malignant OPT after prednisone therapy alone.[43] Prednisone and a low-calcium/high-phosphate diet may be effective.[44]

In CA II deficiency, the RTA has been treated with bicarbonate supplementation, but the long-term impact is unknown. Bone marrow transplantation corrects the OPT and slows cerebral calcification of CA II deficiency, but does not alter the RTA.[45]

Supportive Therapy

Hyperbaric oxygenation can be important for osteomyelitis of the jaw.[6] Surgical decompression of the optic and facial nerves may benefit some patients. Joint replacement can be helpful.[46] Internal fixation may be necessary for femoral fractures.[47]

Early prenatal diagnosis of OPT by ultrasound generally has been unsuccessful. Conventional radiographs occasionally reveal malignant OPT late in pregnancy. However, mutation analysis is now available in commercial laboratories and can be used to detect OPT in utero.[38]

PYCNODYSOSTOSIS

Pycnodysostosis was discovered in 1962.[48] Most reports have come from the United States or Europe, but its prevalence seems greatest in Japan.[49] Parental consanguinity with autosomal recessive inheritance explains ≈30% of cases. In 1996, loss-of-function mutation of the gene that encodes cathepsin K was identified.[50]

Clinical Features

Pycnodysostosis is diagnosed during infancy or early childhood because of disproportionate short stature and a relatively large cranium with fronto-occipital prominence, small facies and chin, beaked nose, high-arched palate, obtuse mandibular angle, dental malocclusion with retained deciduous teeth, proptosis, and bluish sclera.[51] The anterior fontanel and cranial sutures remain open. Mental retardation affects ≈10% of cases.[51] Hands are small and square and fingers are short and clubbed from acro-osteolysis or aplasia of terminal phalanges. Pectus excavatum may occur. Recurrent fractures typically involve the lower limbs and cause genu valgum deformity, although patients usually walk independently. Adult height ranges from 4 ft 3 in to 4 ft 11 in. Recurrent respiratory infections and right heart failure from upper airway obstruction caused by micrognathia trouble some patients.

Radiographic Findings

Pycnodysostosis shares many features with OPT.[22] Both cause generalized osteosclerosis and recurrent fractures. The osteosclerosis first appears in childhood, is uniform, and increases with age. The calvarium and the skull base are sclerotic, and orbital ridges are dense. Although long bones have narrow medullary canals, the striking modeling defects of OPT do not occur. Endobones and radiodense striations are absent.[22] Other distinguishing findings in pycnodysostosis include delayed closure of cranial sutures and fontanels (prominently the anterior), obtuse mandibular angle, wormian bones, gracile clavicles that are hypoplastic laterally, and hypoplasia or aplasia of the distal phalanges and ribs.[52] Hypoplasia of facial bones, sinuses, and terminal phalanges is characteristic. Vertebral bodies are dense with anterior and posterior concavities, but transverse processes are uninvolved. Lumbosacral spondylolisthesis is not uncommon, and lack of segmentation of the atlas and axis may be noted.[22]

Laboratory Findings

Anemia is not a concern. Serum calcium and inorganic phosphate levels and alkaline phosphatase activity usually are normal. Cortical bone appears unremarkable except for diminished osteoblastic and osteoclastic activity.[53] Abnormal inclusions have been described in chondrocytes. Electron microscopy suggests that degradation of collagen is defective.[53]

Cause and Pathogenesis

Deactivating mutations in the gene that encodes cathepsin K cause pycnodysostosis.[50] Cathepsin K is a lysosomal cysteine protease that is highly expressed in osteoclasts.[54] Hence, impaired collagen degradation is a fundamental defect. The rate of bone accretion and the size of the exchangeable calcium pool seem reduced. Bone remodeling and therefore quality are compromised.[55] Accordingly, pycnodysostosis can be thought of as a form of OPT.

Additionally, killing activity and interleukin-1 secretion by circulating monocytes is compromised.[56] Virus-like inclusions have been reported in osteoclasts.[57] Defective growth hormone secretion and low serum insulin-like growth factor 1 levels have been described.[58]

Treatment

No medical therapy is recognized. Bone marrow transplantation has not been reported.

The orthopedic challenges have been reviewed briefly.[59] Long bone fractures typically are transverse and heal at a satisfactory rate, but delayed union and massive formation of callus can occur. Intramedullary fixation of long bones is formidable because of their hardness.

Extraction of teeth is difficult, and mandibular fracture has occurred.[51] Osteomyelitis of the mandible may require antibiotic and surgical treatment.

PROGRESSIVE DIAPHYSEAL DYSPLASIA (CAMURATI-ENGELMANN DISEASE)

Progressive diaphyseal dysplasia (PDD) is an autosomal dominant disorder that affects all races. The condition was described by Cockayne in 1920.[60] Camurati discovered its heritable nature.[61] Engelmann characterized the severe, typical form in 1929.[61] In 2001, mutations that are activating defects were identified in the gene that encodes transforming growth factor (TGF)-β1.[62]

Characteristically in PDD, painful hyperostosis occurs gradually on both periosteal and endosteal surfaces of long bones.[22] However, the clinical and radiographic expression is quite variable.[63] In severe cases, osteosclerosis is widespread, including the skull and axial skeleton. Some carriers have no radiographic changes, but bone scintigraphy is abnormal.

Clinical Presentation

PDD typically presents during childhood with limping or a broad-based and waddling gait, leg pain, muscle wasting, and diminished subcutaneous fat in the extremities mimicking mus-

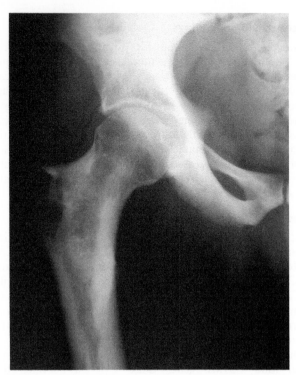

FIGURE 12-2. Progressive diaphyseal dysplasia. This man with Camurati-Engelmann disease has irregular hyperostosis (cortical thickening) of the proximal femur that characteristically does not extend to the end of the long bone.

cular dystrophy.[64] However, severely affected patients also have a characteristic body habitus that includes an enlarged head with prominent forehead, proptosis, and thin limbs with thickened bones. Cranial nerve palsies can develop when the skull is affected. Puberty sometimes is delayed. Raised intracranial pressure may occur. Palpable bony thickening, skeletal tenderness, and sometimes hepatosplenomegaly are present, as well as Raynaud's phenomenon and other findings suggestive of vasculitis.[65] Radiologic studies typically show progressive disease, but the course is variable and symptom remission sometimes occurs during adult life.

Radiologic Features

Hyperostosis of major long bone diaphyses, the principal finding, represents proliferation of new bone on both periosteal and endosteal surfaces.[22] Shafts of long bones gradually widen and develop irregular surfaces. Sclerosis is fairly symmetrical and spreads to involve metaphyses, but the epiphyses are characteristically spared (Fig. 12-2). Tibias and femurs most often are involved, less frequently the radii, ulnae, humeri, and, occasionally, the short tubular bones. Clavicles, scapulae, and the pelvis also may become thickened. Age of onset, rate of progression, and degree of bony involvement are highly variable. With mild disease, scintigraphic abnormalities may be confined to the lower limbs. Maturation of the new bone increases the hyperostosis. However, in severely affected children, some skeletal areas may appear osteopenic.

Clinical, radiographic, and scintigraphic findings are generally concordant.[66] Occasionally, however, bone scans are unremarkable despite marked radiographic changes. This seems to reflect advanced but quiescent disease. Increased radioisotope accumulation with few radiographic alterations can represent early skeletal involvement.

Laboratory Findings

Routine biochemical parameters of bone and mineral homeostasis typically are normal, although serum alkaline phosphatase levels can be elevated. Mild hypocalcemia and significant hypocalciuria may occur in severe disease, likely reflecting positive calcium balance.[67] Mild anemia and leukopenia and an elevated erythrocyte sedimentation rate seem to reflect the poorly characterized systemic disturbances.[65]

Histopathology shows new bone formation along diaphyses. Disorganized woven bone undergoes maturation and then incorporation into the cortex. Electron microscopy of muscle has revealed myopathic changes and vascular abnormalities.[64]

Cause and Pathogenesis

The clinical and laboratory features of severe PDD and its responsiveness to glucocorticoid treatment indicate an inflammatory connective tissue disease.[65] Now, the disorder is known to involve mutations in a specific region of the gene that encodes TGF-β1. Consequently, a "latency-associated peptide" encoded by this gene remains bound to TGF-β1, keeping this enhancer of bone formation active.[62] Aberrant differentiation of precursor cells to osteoblasts has been discussed as a pathogenetic mechanism.[68]

Treatment

PDD is a chronic and somewhat unpredictable disorder. Symptoms may remit during adolescence or adult life. Glucocorticoid therapy (typically small doses of prednisone on alternate days) can relieve bone pain and improve histologic abnormalities in bone.[69] Bisphosphonate therapy may increase skeletal pain.[70]

ENDOSTEAL HYPEROSTOSIS

In 1955, van Buchem et al.[71] described hyperostosis corticalis generalisata. Subsequently, additional forms of endosteal hyperostosis were characterized.[72] The hallmark of these disorders is thickening of cortical bone primarily on endosteal surfaces.[22]

Van Buchem disease is an autosomal recessive condition[71] that is considerably rarer than the number of case reports might suggest.[73] The principal clinical feature is progressive asymmetrical enlargement of the jaw during puberty. The mandible becomes markedly thickened with a wide angle, but no prognathism is noted. Dental malocclusion is uncommon. Affected individuals may be symptom free, but cranial sclerosis also occurs and recurrent facial nerve palsy, deafness, and optic atrophy from narrowing of cranial foramina are common and can develop during infancy. Long bones may hurt with applied pressure but are not fragile.[71] Endosteal cortical thickening leads to homogenously dense diaphyses with narrowed medullary canals. However, long bones are shaped properly. Osteosclerosis also affects the skull base, facial bones, vertebrae, pelvis, and ribs.[22] Serum alkaline phosphatase from bone may be increased, but calcium and inorganic phosphate levels are unremarkable.

Sclerosteosis, like van Buchem disease, is an autosomal recessive disorder that occurs primarily in people of Dutch ancestry.[72] However, sclerosteosis differs from van Buchem disease in that patients are excessively tall and have syndactyly.[72] At birth, only fused fingers may be noted.[73a] Syndactyly reflects cutaneous or bony fusion of the middle and index fingers. During early childhood, skeletal overgrowth involves especially the skull and causes facial disfigurement. Progressive bone thickening widens the jaw, resulting in prognathism.[74] Patients become tall and heavy. Deafness and facial palsy are prominent problems. A small

skull vault may increase intracranial pressure, causing headaches and compressing the brain stem.[75] Intelligence is normal. Life expectancy can be shortened.[76] Long bones become widened as cortices thicken. Vertebral pedicles, ribs, and the pelvis may become dense. Fusion of ossicles and narrowing of the internal auditory canals and cochlear aqueducts may occur.[72] Enhanced osteoblast activity with failure of osteoclasts to compensate explains the dense bone of sclerosteosis.[75] No abnormality of calcium homeostasis or of pituitary function has been documented.[77] No specific medical treatment is available. Surgical correction of syndactyly is difficult if there is bony fusion. Management of the neurologic dysfunction has been reviewed.[75]

Deactivating mutations in the gene that encodes sclerostin (SOST) cause sclerosteosis,[78,79] whereas van Buchem disease results from a 52-kb deletion that diminishes a downstream enhancer of SOST.[80] Sclerostin binds to LRP5/6, antagonizes canonical Wnt signaling,[81] and promotes the apoptosis of osteoblasts.[82] Accordingly, sclerostin deficiency in sclerosteosis and van Buchem disease enhances bone formation.

An autosomal dominant (Worth) type[83] of endosteal hyperostosis is relatively benign and was rediscovered recently as the "high bone mass phenotype."[84] Some affected individuals have torus palatineus.[85] Certain domain-specific, gain-of-function mutations of LRP5 encoding low-density lipoprotein receptor–related protein 5 cause this form of increased skeletal mass.[86] LRP5 activation may decrease the biosynthesis of systemic serotonin, leading to enhanced bone formation.[87] Despite excesses of good quality bone, the condition is not always benign, as cranial nerve palsies, skeletal pain, and oropharyngeal exostoses may occur.[88]

OSTEOPOIKILOSIS

Osteopoikilosis (spotted bones) is usually a radiographic curiosity transmitted as an autosomal dominant trait with a high degree of penetrance.[89] However, joint contractions and limb length inequality can occur, especially with accompanying radiographic changes of melorheostosis. When connective tissue nevi called dermatofibrosis lenticularis disseminata are present, this is the Buschke-Ollendorff syndrome.[90] The osteopoikilosis is asymptomatic, but if misunderstood can lead to studies for metastatic disease, etc.[91] Hence, family members at risk should be counseled. Radiographs show numerous small foci of usually round or oval osteosclerosis[22] involving the ends of the short tubular bones, the metaepiphyseal regions of the long bones, and the tarsal, carpal, and pelvic bones (Fig. 12-3). These are thickened trabeculae or islands of cortical bone and do not change appearance over decades. Radionuclide accumulation is not increased on bone scanning.[91]

The nevi usually appear before puberty, involve the lower trunk or extremities, and are small asymptomatic papules or yellow or white disks or plaques, deep nodules, or streaks.[90] They represent excessive, unusually broad, and markedly branched elastin fibers in the dermis.[90]

Heterozygous deactivating mutations in the LEMD3 gene cause osteopoikilosis and the Buschke-Ollendorff syndrome.[92] LEMD3 is an inner nuclear membrane protein that antagonizes TGF-β1 and bone morphogenetic protein signaling.

OSTEOPATHIA STRIATA

Osteopathia striata features linear striations at the ends of long bones and in the ileum[22] and is a curiosity if the skeletal findings occur alone as an autosomal dominant trait. However, osteopathia striata also occurs in clinically important syndromes.

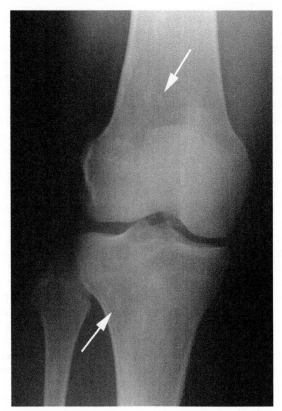

FIGURE 12-3. Osteopoikilosis. Faint, round or oval areas of osteosclerosis *(arrows)* are present in the metaphases of the distal femur and proximal tibia.

These include osteopathia striata with cranial sclerosis[93] due to *WTX* mutations,[94] where cranial nerve palsies are common.[93] Osteopathia striata with focal dermal hypoplasia (Goltz syndrome) is a serious X-linked dominant disorder featuring widespread linear areas of dermal hypoplasia through which adipose tissue herniates, together with bony defects in the limbs.[95]

Gracile striations affect trabecular bone, especially the meta-epiphyses of major long bones and the periphery of the iliac bones.[22] Lesions are unchanged for years. Radionuclide accumulation is not increased during bone scanning.[91]

PACHYDERMOPERIOSTOSIS

Pachydermoperiostosis (hypertrophic osteoarthropathy: primary or idiopathic) causes clubbing of the digits, hyperhidrosis, and thickening of the skin, especially involving the face and forehead (cutis verticis gyrata). Clubbing, periostitis, and pachydermia constitute the classic triad of features. However, some patients have just one or two of these findings. Radiographs reveal periosteal new bone formation, especially in the distal limbs. Autosomal dominant inheritance with variable expression is established,[96] but autosomal recessive transmission also seems to occur.[97]

Blacks seem to be affected more often than whites, and men more severely than women. Presentation is typically during adolescence, but variable.[96,97] Symptoms emerge over a decade, but then can abate.[98] Progressive enlargement of the hands and feet may cause a "paw-like" appearance. Palms may be wet. Arthralgias of the elbows, wrists, knees, and ankles are common. Acro-osteolysis has been reported. Stiffness of the appendicular and axial skeleton can develop. Compression of cranial or spinal nerves has been described. Cutaneous changes include coarsen-ing, thickening, furrowing, pitting, and oiliness of especially the scalp and face, with some affected individuals described as "acro-megalic." Fatigue is common. Myelophthisic anemia with extramedullary hematopoiesis may occur.

Radiologic Features

Severe periostitis thickens the distal portions of tubular bones—especially the radius, ulna, tibia, and fibula. Clubbing is obvious, and acro-osteolysis can occur. Ankylosis of joints, especially in the hands and in the feet, may trouble older patients.[22] The principal diagnostic challenge is secondary hypertrophic osteo-arthropathy (pulmonary or otherwise), but this presents a smooth, undulating appearance.[99] In pachydermoperiostosis, periosteal proliferation is more exuberant and irregular and often involves epiphyses. Bone scanning in either condition reveals symmetrical, diffuse, regular uptake along the cortical margins of long bones, especially in the legs, causing a "double-stripe" sign.

Laboratory Findings

Periosteal new bone roughens the surface of cortical bone.[100] The new osseous tissue undergoes cancellous compaction, rendering it difficult to distinguish from the original cortex on histopathologic examination.[100] Osteopenia of trabeculae reflects quiescent bone formation.[22] Mild cellular hyperplasia and thickening of subsynovial blood vessels occur near synovial membranes.[101,102]

Cause and Pathogenesis

In 2008, the cause of pachydermoperiostosis was discovered to be mutations in the gene that encodes 15-hydroxyprostaglandin dehydrogenase, the principal enzyme of prostaglandin degradation.[103]

Treatment

No specific medical treatment for pachydermoperiostosis is known, but recent identification of the gene defect will now allow targeting of prostaglandin excess. Painful synovial effusions may respond to nonsteroidal anti-inflammatory drugs.[103] Contractures or neurovascular compression may require surgical intervention.

Osteoporoses

OSTEOGENESIS IMPERFECTA

Osteogenesis imperfecta (OI), sometimes called brittle bone disease, is the most common heritable disorder of connective tissue.[2] The nosology for OI devised by Sillence[104] in 1981, according to clinical features and apparent modes of inheritance, has been the framework for prognostication and a foundation for biochemical/molecular studies. However, DNA-based findings subsequently have provided critical insights concerning genetic transmission patterns, especially for the severe forms, by revealing that autosomal dominant inheritance explains nearly all patients with OI.[105] Also, the clinical heterogeneity of OI is now better understood because a great number of mutations are recognized within the two large genes that encode the protein strands (the pro-α_1 and pro-α_2 chains) that combine to form the type 1 collagen heterotrimer.[105] All major clinical forms of OI represent quantitative and often qualitative abnormalities of this most abundant protein in bone.[2] The clinical hallmark is osteoporosis that leads to recurrent fractures and skeletal deformity.[106]

However, type I collagen also occurs in teeth, skin, ligaments, sclerae, and elsewhere, and many patients with OI have dental disease caused by defective formation of dentin (dentinogenesis imperfecta) and abnormalities of other tissues that contain this fibrillar protein.[4] It is understandable that the severity of OI is extremely variable and ranges from stillbirth to perhaps lifelong absence of symptoms.

Clinical Presentation

The differential diagnosis for OI in infants and children includes idiopathic juvenile osteoporosis, Cushing's syndrome, homocystinuria, congenital indifference to pain, and child abuse. However, OI usually features distinctive signs and symptoms that allow for a correct diagnosis based on the patient's medical history, physical features, and radiographic findings.[105,106] A positive family history is especially helpful, but many patients represent heterozygous, sporadic mutation.[105] Affected individuals can manifest ligamentous laxity with joint hypermobility, diaphoresis, susceptibility to bruises, fragile and discolored teeth, and hearing loss (≈50% of those <30 years, and nearly all who are older).[107] Deafness typically has a conductive or mixed pathogenesis but sometimes results from sensorineural defects.[107] Scleral discoloration ranges from a blue or gray tint that may be subtle or striking. Severe OI is characterized by a high-pitched voice, short stature, scoliosis, herniae, a disproportionately large head compared with body size, a triangular face, and chest deformity. Mitral valve "clicks" are not uncommon, but cardiac disease is unusual. Patients generally have normal intelligence. However, variable severity of OI can occur even within families.[106]

Type I OI features sclerae with bluish discoloration (especially apparent during childhood), relatively mild osteopenia with infrequent fractures (deformity is uncommon or slight), and deafness that manifests during early adult life. Approximately one third of cases represent new mutations. Elderly women with this type of OI can be mistaken as having postmenopausal osteoporosis alone. Type I OI has been subclassified into I-A and I-B disease depending on the absence or (more rarely) the presence, respectively, of dentinogenesis imperfecta.[105]

Type II OI is often fatal within the first weeks of life from respiratory complications. Affected newborns are frequently premature and small for gestational age and have short, bowed limbs, numerous fractures, markedly soft skulls, and small thoraces.

Type III OI features progressive skeletal deformity during childhood from recurrent fractures. Short stature results, in part, from fragmentation of growth plates. Dentinogenesis imperfecta is common. Thoracic distortion predisposes to pneumonia.

Type IV OI frequently explains multigenerational disease.[105] The sclerae are unremarkable, but skeletal deformity, dental disease, and hearing loss are typical.

Additional, rarer forms of OI have been reported, including severe autosomal recessive types now understood at the gene level to involve enzymatic defects in collagen cross-linking.[108]

Radiographic Features

Characteristic x-ray findings manifest in patients with severe OI,[22] including generalized osteopenia, modeling defects featuring gracile long bones, and deformities from recurrent fractures. Modeling abnormalities reflect impaired periosteal bone formation that retards circumferential widening of bones and their cortices. Multiple, recurrent fractures distort vertebrae as well as long bones.[22] In some severely affected infants, however, micromelia occurs where major long bones appear wide. Wormian

bones of significant number and size in the skull represent a common, but not pathognomonic, feature of OI.[109] Excessive pneumatization of the frontal and mastoid sinuses and platybasia that can progress to basilar impression are common in severely affected patients.[109] Osteoarthritis is a frequent problem for ambulatory adults with deformity.[22]

Radiographic abnormalities may worsen markedly during growth—a feature that helps to define progressively deforming, type III OI. Here, a characteristic is "popcorn" calcification. This finding appears in childhood as an acquired defect in the metaphyses of major long bones[110] and is believed to reflect traumatic fragmentation of growth plate cartilage. The complication impairs long-bone growth and contributes importantly to short stature, but then appears to resolve when endochondral cartilage becomes fully mineralized at skeletal maturity and is replaced by bone. When fractures occur in OI, they often heal at normal rates. Occasionally, exuberant callus has been mistaken for skeletal malignancy.

Laboratory Findings

Routine biochemical parameters of bone and mineral metabolism usually are unremarkable in OI, although hypercalciuria is common in severely affected children.[111] Fortunately, their renal function is intact.[111] Elevations in serum and urinary markers of bone turnover occur in severely affected patients.

Bone histology reflects the abnormal skeletal matrix, especially in severely affected patients. Polarized light microscopy often shows an abundance of disorganized (woven) bone, or abnormally thin collagen bundles in lamellar osseous tissue. Numerous osteocytes are found in the cortical bone of some patients.[112] This feature seems to reflect decreased amounts of bone produced by individual osteoblasts, yet many cells that are active simultaneously. Hence, the overall rate of skeletal turnover can be rapid, as assessed by in vivo tetracycline labeling before biopsy.[113]

Cause and Pathogenesis

The biochemical hallmark of OI is low levels of type I collagen synthesis that can be detected through the use of skin fibroblasts in culture.[105] Often, the collagen itself is also defective. Various types of heterozygous mutation occur within the pro-α_1 and pro-α_2 type I collagen genes.[105] The large size and complex nature of type I collagen are such that most OI families have unique ("private") mutations in either of these two genes.[105]

Treatment

Promising results are reported increasingly for bisphosphonate treatment, especially in growing children, but few trials have been blinded or placebo controlled.[114] The role of bisphosphonates or teriparatide is less certain or unknown, respectively, in adults with OI. Improving mouse models for OI provide new ways to test potential therapies. Patient management requires expert orthopedic, rehabilitative, and dental care. Rodding of long bones and bracing of the lower limbs have enabled some severely affected OI children to walk. Stapes surgery has been used for hearing loss.[115] The current management of OI has been reviewed.[116]

National support groups (e.g., Osteogenesis Imperfecta Foundation, Inc.) are important sources of comfort and lay language information for patients with OI and their families. Genetic counseling for OI is now based on gene mutation analysis. Although especially rare patients with severe OI represent autosomal recessive disease,[108] most sporadic cases result from new dominant mutations or reflect germline mosaicism for defects in the genes that encode type I collagen. The recurrence risk for type II OI is now estimated to be 5% to 10%[117] based on germline mosaicism. Some mildly affected individuals are mosaic and have had a severely affected child.

Prenatal diagnosis of severe OI is possible through ultrasound examination at 14 to 18 weeks' gestation.[117] Biochemical and especially mutation analysis is proving increasingly important.[117]

Disorders of RANK/OPG/RANKL/ NF-κB Signaling

Several extremely rare hereditary disorders of the skeleton feature osteoporosis from accelerated bone remodeling (and sometimes foci of osteolytic disease) due to disturbances of the receptor activator of nuclear factor-κB (RANK), osteoprotegerin (OPG), RANK ligand (RANKL), NF-κB signaling pathway.[118] Discovery of this principal regulatory system for osteoclast formation and action began with identification of new ligands and receptors in the tumor necrosis factor (TNF) superfamily, and then characterization of knockout and transgenic mouse models.[119] However, a full appreciation of this pathway in humans came from revelation of the genetic bases for several exceptional mendelian skeletal disorders. As is discussed below, the first represented constitutive activation of RANK, the second, deficiency of OPG.[120]

In the year 2000, heterozygous, gain-of-function, 18-bp and 27-bp tandem duplications in the gene that encodes RANK (*TNFRSF11A*) were discovered to cause familial expansile osteolysis (FEO) and early-onset Paget's disease of bone in Japan,[121] respectively. Soon after, a similar 15-bp duplication in RANK explained expansile skeletal hyperphosphatasia.[122] In 2002, homozygous selective deletion of the gene that encodes OPG (*TNFRSF11B*) was discovered in Navajo patients with juvenile Paget's disease (JPD).[123]

Before these particular disorders are discussed, a brief review of Paget's disease of bone (PDB) is in order to appreciate how such rare conditions have taught us about this second most common metabolic bone disease that is increasingly appreciated to involve a heritable predisposition.[118]

PAGET'S DISEASE OF BONE

PDB is common in the United States (i.e., prevalence at least 1%, and perhaps as much as 2%)[124] and features focally increased skeletal remodeling within axial or appendicular bones in adults.[125] Initially, a "wave" of osteoclast-mediated osteolysis moves slowly but relentlessly through a bone, and then is followed by disorganized skeletal repair leading to bony expansion, as well as to osteosclerosis and hyperostosis. Pagetic bone is unsound and can cause pain, fracture, and deformity. Deafness of multifactorial pathogenesis is common,[126] and dental problems include loosening and migration of teeth.[127] Rarely, malignant transformation of pagetic lesions to osteosarcoma or chondrosarcoma occurs.[125]

Although the precise cause of PDB remains unknown, evidence is accumulating for paramyxovirus acting in osteoclasts and their precursor cells within PDB lesions. Here, the marrow microenvironment is especially osteoclastogenic, together with measles virus proteins, transcripts, and inclusion bodies.[128] However, increasing evidence also indicates that PDB can be heritable. Its prevalence in first-degree relatives is now appreciated to be 12% to 40%, representing a sevenfold enhanced risk.[129] In fact, despite its classic focal appearance, PDB can manifest generalized acceleration in skeletal remodeling, which has been attributed previously to elevated circulating PTH levels.[130]

Clinical characterization of FEO with its similarity to PDB (see later) and obvious autosomal dominant inheritance resurrected interest in a possible genetic basis (or predisposition) for PDB.[131] Now, such predisposition is understood for patients with PDB to be genetically heterogeneous.[132] In 2001, PDB was mapped to chromosome 5 in French-Canadian families, leading to discovery in 2002 of a heterozygous loss-of-function mutation in the gene that encodes sequestosome (*SQSTM1*).[133] Additional *SQSTM1* defects then were identified worldwide in a large number of familial and some sporadic PDB cases.[134] Soon after, the rare autosomal dominant syndrome called inclusion body myopathy with early-onset PDB and frontotemporal dementia was shown to involve mutations in the gene that encodes valosin containing protein.[135] SQSTM1 and valosin containing protein both seem to participate in the intracellular process of ubiquination.[136]

FAMILIAL EXPANSILE OSTEOLYSIS

FEO is a remarkably instructive, autosomal dominant disorder.[132] Patients can manifest deafness early in life followed by focal, lytic expansion of one or more major appendicular bones, causing pain, fracture, deformity, and sometimes osteosarcoma. Osteolytic defects in FEO are especially common in the lower extremities, and a tibia most often is involved.[137] As in PDB, these lesions usually start at or near the end of a long bone and then slowly advance.[136,138] Deafness presents at as young as age 4 years, but more commonly in the second decade, and ultimately conductive deafness becomes of mixed type.[139] The long process of the incus disappears or becomes fibrous tissue. Loosening and pain and/or fracture of adult teeth can occur.[139] In FEO dentition, root resorption is extensive and the size of pulp chambers and root canals is reduced.[139] However, the most remarkable finding is "idiopathic external resorption" that destroys teeth.[140]

Skeletal lesions in FEO initially have the clinical, radiographic, and histopathologic appearance of PDB in its early osteolytic phase,[125] but affected bones eventually instead become expanded, shell-like, and fat-filled rather than exhibiting the osteosclerosis and hyperostosis of advanced PDB.[141] Furthermore, generalized osteopenia and a coarse trabecular pattern are present in adult life, suggesting that FEO is a systemic bone disease.[138] Elevation in serum alkaline phosphatase activity and other biochemical markers of bone remodeling in FEO is explained in part by this diffuse acceleration in skeletal turnover.[120] Light microscopy of FEO lesions early on shows filigree-like trabeculae of woven bone, abundant osteoclasts and osteoblasts lining trabeculae, giant osteoclasts with bizarre shapes and numerous nuclei, and fibrous marrow.[139] On electron microscopy, microcylindrical nuclear inclusion bodies with ultrastructure similar to paramyxoviridae can resemble PDB.[139,141] However, "mosaic bone," the hallmark of advanced PDB, is rare—perhaps reflecting the extreme rates of bone remodeling. Instead, woven bone seems to be deposited rapidly and does not mature or remodel into cortical bone.[138] Generally, little radiographic osteosclerosis occurs unless antiresorptive pharmaceuticals are administered.[138] Intermediate-stage disease, however, features scanty skeletal matrix with abundant fibrous tissue and vascularity. Advanced disease shows almost total loss of cortical and trabecular bone, as well as fat-occupied medullary spaces.[131,139]

The molecular defect causing FEO was discovered in 2000 through a candidate gene approach.[121] In three kindreds, an in-frame, 18-bp tandem duplication was identified in exon 1 of the *TNFRSF11A* gene encoding RANK. Transfection studies suggested increased NF-κB activity due to extension of the RANK signal peptide trapping this receptor intracellularly and causing constitutive activation.[121]

Treatment

In FEO, perhaps skeletal injury explains in part the focal nature of the bone lesions.[138] Microscopic or macroscopic fracture in FEO might initiate skeletal repair that becomes deranged because excessive RANK effect enhances osteoclast numbers and activity. Similar changes may be noted in other disorders of RANK excess and enhanced RANK/OPG/RANKL/NF-κB signaling (see later). Once osteolysis runs its course, expanded bone becomes fat-filled, perhaps because the mesenchymal stem cell pool has differentiated excessively to adipocytes.[141] It is understandable that advanced expansile lesions then are unresponsive to otherwise effective antiresorptive therapy.[138]

OSTEOPROTEGERIN DEFICIENCY

Juvenile Paget's disease (JPD), also called idiopathic or hereditary hyperphosphatasia, usually is diagnosed in infants or young children.[142] Occasionally, the disease presents later in childhood. A relatively mild form of JPD is associated with mental retardation.[142] In contrast to the autosomal dominant RANK activation disorders, all forms of JPD are considered to be autosomal recessive traits.[132]

JPD affects the entire skeleton.[143] This has prompted objection to the disorder being called a type of PDB; however, JPD and the RANK disorders seem increasingly to share features with PDB.

JPD causes bone pain, fracture, and deformity.[144] Premature loss of teeth and deafness are also typical. Radiographs show marked undertubulation of long bones with thin cortices (Fig. 12-4).[145] Rapid skeletal remodeling, confirmed by histopathologic findings, leads to substantially elevated biochemical markers of bone turnover.[123,142] In fact, the mosaic pattern of bone characteristic of advanced PDB is not found in JPD or the disorders of RANK excess.

Mild JPD features fewer fractures and less bony deformity, but radiographs show diffuse, acquired hyperostosis and osteosclerosis associated with biochemical and histologic evidence of accelerated skeletal turnover.[123,142]

Discovery in JPD of OPG deficiency from loss-of-function mutations in *TNFRSF11B* provided both a cause and a mechanism for this osteopathy.[123] OPG normally is released into the marrow space from preosteoblasts and osteoblasts, and it acts as a decoy receptor for RANKL.[119] Thus, OPG deficiency engenders

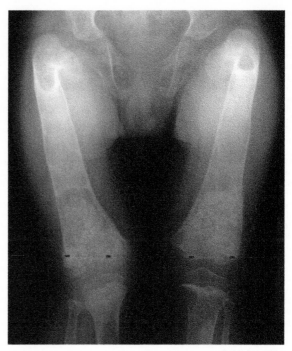

FIGURE 12-4. Osteoprotegerin deficiency. The femurs of this boy with juvenile Paget's disease are widened, and thin cortices and irregular ossifications are evident. Marked angular deformity is present proximally.

high levels of RANKL activity, which markedly accelerate osteoclastogenesis and bone turnover.[119]

Observations in JPD also complement findings in the *TNFRSF11B* knockout mouse model, which suggest a further role for OPG in preventing vascular calcification. In these mice, aorta and renal artery mineralization is found through histopathologic methods.[146] Although no calcifications are observed on radiographs or CT scans in patients with JPD, the literature describing JPD includes "calcifying arteriopathy" on histopathologic analysis.[147] Furthermore, striking changes consistent with pseudoxanthoma elasticum, including granular and coarse deposits of calcium in the membranes and intima of the muscular arteries and arterioles, were reported in all autopsy tissues from a young man with JPD.[148] Additionally, patients with OPG deficiency develop blindness from a retinopathy that seems to derive from microvascular calcification.[149]

Antiresorptive treatment using calcitonin or bisphosphonates has been beneficial for JPD.[144,149] Recombinant OPG has been effective for two affected adult siblings.[150] Anti-RANKL antibody could offer another therapeutic approach for the skeletal disease, but it might not slow vascular calcification.

REFERENCES

1. Online Mendelian Inheritance in Man, OMIM (TM): McKusick-Nathans Institute of Genetic Medicine, Johns Hopkins University (Baltimore, MD), and National Center for Biotechnology Information, National Library of Medicine (Bethesda, MD), June 3, 2009: http://www.ncbi.nlm.nih.gov/omim/.
2. Royce PM, Steinmann B, editors: Connective tissue and its heritable disorders, ed 2, New York, 2002, Wiley-Liss.
3. Castriota-Scanderbeg A, Dallapiccola B: Abnormal skeletal phenotypes: from simple signs to complex diagnoses, New York, 2005, Springer.
4. Rimoin DL, Connor JM, Pyeritz RE, et al: Emery and Rimoin's principles and practice of medical

genetics, ed 5, Philadelphia, 2007, Churchill Livingstone.
5. Albers-Schönberg H: Rontgenbilder einer seltenen, Knochenerkrankung, Meunch Med Wochenschr 51:365, 1904.
6. Whyte MP: Osteopetrosis. In Royce PM, Steinmann B, editors: Connective tissue and its heritable disorders, ed 2, New York, 2002, Wiley-Liss, pp 789–807.
7. Loria-Cortes R, Quesada-Calvo E, Cordero-Chaverri E: Osteopetrosis in children: a report of 26 cases, J Pediatr 91:43–47, 1977.
8. Johnston CC Jr, Lavy N, Lord T, et al: Osteopetrosis: a clinical, genetic, metabolic, and morphologic study of

the dominantly inherited, benign form, Medicine (Baltimore) 47:149–167, 1968.
9. Kahler SG, Burns JA, Aylsworth AS: A mild autosomal recessive form of osteopetrosis, Am J Med Genet 17:451–464, 1984.
10. Del Fattore A, Cappariello A, Teti A: Genetics, pathogenesis and complications of osteopetrosis, Bone 42:19–29, 2008.
11. Marks SC Jr: Osteopetrosis: multiple pathways for the interception of osteoclast function, Appl Pathol 5:172–183, 1987.
12. Vanier V, Miller R, Carson BS: Bilateral visual improvement after unilateral optic canal decompression and cranial vault expansion in a patient with osteopetrosis,

narrowed optic canals, and increased intracranial pressure, J Neurol Neurosurg Psychiatry 69:405–406, 2000.

13. Waguespack SG, Koller DL, White KE, et al: *Chloride channel 7 (ClCN7)* gene mutations and autosomal dominant osteopetrosis, type II, J Bone Miner Res 18:1513–1518, 2003.

14. Benichou OD, Lareo JD, De Verenjoul MC: Type II autosomal dominant osteopetrosis (Albers-Schönberg disease): clinical and radiological manifestations in 42 patients, Bone 26:87–93, 2000.

15. Campos-Xavier AB, Casanova JL, Doumaz Y, et al: Intrafamilial phenotypic variability of osteopetrosis due to *chloride channel 7 (CLCN7)* mutations, Am J Med Genet A 133:216–218, 2005.

16. Whyte MP, Murphy WA, Fallon MD, et al: Osteopetrosis, renal tubular acidosis and basal ganglia calcification in three sisters, Am J Med 69:64–74, 1980.

17. Sly WS, Whyte MP, Sundaram V, et al: Carbonic anhydrase II deficiency in 12 families with the autosomal recessive syndrome of osteopetrosis with renal tubular acidosis and cerebral calcification, N Engl J Med 313:139–145, 1985.

18. Sly WS, Whyte MP, Krupin T, et al: Positive renal response to acetazolamide in carbonic anhydrase II-deficient patients, Pediatr Res 19:1033–1036, 1985.

19. Awad M, Al-Ashwal AA, Sakati N, et al: Long-term follow up of carbonic anhydrase II deficiency syndrome, Saudi Med J 23:25–29, 2002.

20. Jagadha V, Halliday WC, Becker LE, et al: The association of infantile osteopetrosis and neuronal storage disease in two brothers, Acta Neuropathol (Berl) 75:233–240, 1988.

21. Dupuis-Girod S, Corradini N, Hadj-Rabia S, et al: Osteopetrosis, lymphedema, anhidrotic ectodermal dysplasia, and immunodeficiency in a boy and incontinentia pigmenti in his mother, Pediatrics 109:1–6, 2002.

22. Resnick D, Niwayama G: Diagnosis of bone and joint disorders, ed 4, Philadelphia, 2002, WB Saunders.

23. Di Rocco M, Buoncompagni A, Loy A, et al: Osteopetrorickets: case report, Eur J Paediatr Neurol 159:579–581, 2000.

24. Park H-M, Lambertus J: Skeletal and reticuloendothelial imaging in osteopetrosis: case report, J Nucl Med 18:1091–1095, 1977.

25. Rao VM, Dalinka MK, Mitchell DG, et al: Osteopetrosis: MR characteristics at 1.5 T, Radiology 161:217–220, 1986.

26. Cournot G, Trubert-Thil CL, Petrovic M, et al: Mineral metabolism in infants with malignant osteopetrosis: heterogeneity in plasma 1,25- dihydroxyvitamin D levels and bone histology, J Bone Miner Res 7:1–10, 1992.

27. Bollerslev J: Autosomal dominant osteopetrosis: bone metabolism and epidemiological, clinical and hormonal aspects, Endocr Rev 10:45–67, 1989.

28. Whyte MP, Chines A, Silva DP Jr, et al: Creatine kinase brain isoenzyme (BB-CK) presence in serum distinguishes osteopetrosis among the sclerosing bone disorders, J Bone Miner Res 11:1438–1443, 1996.

29. Flanagan AM, Massey HM, Wilson C, et al: Macrophage colony-stimulating factor and receptor activator NF-κB ligand fail to rescue osteoclast-poor human malignant infantile osteopetrosis in vitro, Bone 30:85–90, 2002.

30. Helfrich MH, Aronson DC, Everts V, et al: Morphologic features of bone in human osteopetrosis, Bone 12:411–419, 1991.

31. Bollerslev J, Steiniche T, Melsen F, et al: Structural and histomorphometric studies of iliac crest trabecular and cortical bone in autosomal dominant osteopetrosis: a study of two radiological types, Bone 10:19–24, 1986.

32. Tolar J, Teitelbaum SL, Orchard PJ: Osteopetrosis, N Engl J Med 351:2839–2849, 2004.

33. Campos-Xavier AB, Saraiva JM, Ribeiro LM, et al: *Chloride channel 7 (CLCN7)* gene mutations in intermediate autosomal recessive osteopetrosis, Hum Genet 112:186–189, 2003.

34. Taranta A, Migliaccio S, Recchia I, et al: Genotype-phenotype relationship in human ATP6i-dependent autosomal recessive osteopetrosis, Am J Pathol 162:57–68, 2003.

35. Ramirez A, Faupel J, Goebel I, et al: Identification of a novel mutation in the coding region of the grey-lethal gene *OSTM1* in human malignant infantile osteopetrosis, Hum Mutat 23:471–476, 2004.

36. Sobacchi C, Frattini A, Guerrini MM, et al: Osteoclast-poor human osteopetrosis due to mutations in the gene encoding RANKL, Nat Genet 39:960–962, 2007.

37. Guerrini MM, Sobacchi C, Cassani B, et al: Human osteoclast-poor osteopetrosis with hypogamma-globulinemia due to *TNFRSF11A* (RANK) mutations, Am J Hum Genet 83:64–76, 2008.

38. Segovia-Silvestre T, Neutzsky-Wulff AV, Sorensen MG, et al: Advances in osteoclast biology resulting from the study of osteopetrotic mutations, Hum Genet 124:561–577, 2009.

39a. Driessen GJ, Gerritsen EJ, Fischer A, et al: Long-term outcome of haematopoietic stem cell transplantation in autosomal recessive osteopetrosis: an EBMT report, Bone Marrow Transplant 32:657–663, 2003.

39. Tsuji Y, Ito S, Isoda T, et al: Successful nonmyeloablative cord blood transplantation for an infant with malignant infantile osteopetrosis, J Pediatr Hematol Oncol 27:495–498, 2005.

40. Rawlinson PS, Green RH, Coggins AM, et al: Malignant osteopetrosis: hypercalcaemia after bone marrow transplantation, Arch Dis Child 66:638–639, 1991.

41. Key LL, Rodriguiz RN, Willi SM, et al: Recombinant human interferon gamma therapy for osteopetrosis, N Engl J Med 332:1594–1599, 1995.

42. Glorieux FH, Pettifor JM, Marie PJ, et al: Induction of bone resorption by parathyroid hormone in congenital malignant osteopetrosis, Metab Bone Dis Relat Res 3:143–150, 1981.

43. Iacobini M, Migliaccio S, Roggini M, et al: Case report: apparent cure of a newborn with malignant osteopetrosis using prednisone therapy, J Bone Miner Res 16:2356–2360, 2001.

44. Dorantes LM, Mejia AM, Dorantes S: Juvenile osteopetrosis: effects of blood and bone of prednisone and low calcium, high phosphate diet, Arch Dis Child 61:666–670, 1986.

45. McMahon C, Will A, Hu P, et al: Bone marrow transplantation corrects osteopetrosis in the carbonic anhydrase II deficiency syndrome, Blood 97:1947–1950, 2001.

46. Gwynne Jones DP, Hodgson BF, Hung NA: Bilateral, uncemented total hip arthroplasty in osteopetrosis, J Bone Joint Surg Br 86:276–278, 2004.

47. Chhabra A, Westerlund LE, Kline AJ, et al: Management of proximal femoral shaft fractures in osteopetrosis: a case series using internal fixation, Orthopedics 28:587–592, 2005.

48. Maroteaux P, Lamy M: La pycnodysostose, Presse Med 70:999–1002, 1962.

49. Sugiura Y, Yamada Y, Koh J: Pycnodysostosis in Japan: report of six cases and a review of Japanese literature, Birth Defects 10:78–98, 1974.

50. Gelb BD, Brömme D, Desnick RJ: 2001 Pycnodysostosis: cathepsin K deficiency. In Scriver CR, Beaudet AL, Sly WS, editors: The metabolic and molecular bases of inherited disease, ed 8, New York, 2001, McGraw-Hill Book Company, pp 3453–3468.

51. Wolpowitz A, Matisson A: A comparative study of pycnodysostosis, cleidocranial dysostosis, osteopetrosis and acro-osteolysis, S Afr Med J 48:1011–1118, 1974.

52. Soto TJ, Mautalen CA, Hojman D, et al: Pycnodysostosis, metabolic and histologic studies, Birth Defects 5:109–115, 1969.

53. Everts V, Aronson DC, Beertsen W: Phagocytosis of bone collagen by osteoclasts in two cases of pycnodysostosis, Calcif Tissue Int 37:25–31, 1985.

54. Motyckova G, Fisher DE: Pycnodysostosis: role and regulation of cathepsin K in osteoclast function and human disease, Curr Mol Med 2:407–421, 2002.

55. Fratzl-Zelman N, Valenta A, Roschger P, et al: Decreased bone turnover and deterioration of bone structure in two cases of pycnodysostosis, J Clin Endocrinol Metab 89:1538–1547, 2004.

56. Karkabi S, Reis ND, Linn S, et al: Pyknodysostosis: imaging and laboratory observations, Calcif Tissue Int 53:170–173, 1993.

57. Beneton MNC, Harris S, Kanis JA: Paramyxovirus-like inclusions in two cases of pycnodysostosis, Bone 8:211–217, 1987.

58. Soliman AT, Rajab A, Al Salmi I, et al: Defective growth hormone secretion in children with pycnodysostosis and improved linear growth after growth hormone treatment, Arch Dis Child 75:242–244, 1996.

59. Edelson JG, Obad S, Geiger R, et al: Pycnodysostosis: orthopedic aspects, with a description of 14 new cases, Clin Orthop 280:263–276, 1992.

60. Cockayne EA: A case for diagnosis, Proc R Soc Med 13:132–136, 1920.

61. Engelmann G: Ein fall von osteopathia hyperostotica (sclerotisans) multiplex infantilis, Fortschr Geb Roentgen 39:1101–1106, 1929.

62. Saito T, Kinoshita A, Yoshiura KI, et al: Domain-specific mutations of a transforming growth factor (TGF)-β1 latency-associated peptide cause Camurati-Engelmann disease because of the formation of a constitutively active form of TGF-β1, J Biol Chem 276:11469–11472, 2001.

63. Wallace SE, Lachman RS, Mekikian PB, et al: Marked phenotypic variability in progressive diaphyseal dysplasia (Camurati-Engelmann disease): report of a four-generation pedigree, identification of a mutation in TGFβ1, and review, Am J Med Genet A 129:235–247, 2004.

64. Naveh Y, Ludatshcer R, Alon U, et al: Muscle involvement in progressive diaphyseal dysplasia, Pediatrics 76:944–949, 1985.

65. Crisp AJ, Brenton DP: Engelmann's disease of bone: a systemic disorder? Ann Rheum Dis 41:183–188, 1982.

66. Kumar B, Murphy WA, Whyte MP: Progressive diaphyseal dysplasia (Englemann's disease): scintigraphic-radiologic-clinical correlations, Radiology 140:87–92, 1981.

67. Smith R, Walton RJ, Corner BD, et al: Clinical and biochemical studies in Engelmann's disease (progressive diaphyseal dysplasia), Q J Med 46:273–294, 1977.

68. Labat ML, Bringuier AF, Seebold C, et al: Monocytic origin of fibroblasts: spontaneous transformation of blood monocytes into neo-fibroblastic structures in osteomyelosclerosis and Engelmann's disease, Biomed Pharmacother 45:289–299, 1991.

69. Naveh Y, Alon U, Kaftori JK, et al: Progressive diaphyseal dysplasia: evaluation of corticosteroid therapy, Pediatrics 75:321–323, 1985.

70. Inaoka T, Shuke N, Sato J, et al: Scintigraphic evaluation of pamidronate and corticosteroid therapy in a patient with progressive diaphyseal dysplasia (Camurati-Engelmann disease), Clin Nucl Med 26:680–682, 2001.

71. Van Buchem FSP, Prick JJG, Jaspar HHJ: Hyperostosis corticalis generalisata familiaris (van Buchem's disease), Amsterdam, 1976, Excerpta.

72. Beighton P, Barnard A, Hamersma H, et al: The syndromic status of sclerostenosis and van Buchem disease, Clin Genet 25:175–181, 1984.

73. Eastman JR, Bixler D: Generalized cortical hyperostosis (van Buchem disease): nosologic considerations, Radiology 125:297–304, 1977.

73a. Beighton P, Durr L, Hamersma H: The clinical features of sclerostenosis: a review of the manifestations in twenty-five affected individuals, Ann Intern Med 84:393–397, 1976.

74. Beighton P, Cremin BJ, Hamersma H: The radiology of sclerostenosis, Br J Radiol 49:934–939, 1976.

75. Stein SA, Witkop C, Hill S, et al: Sclerostenosis, neurogenetic and pathophysiologic analysis of an American kinship, Neurology 33:267–277, 1983.

76. Hamersma H, Gardner J, Beighton P: The natural history of sclerostenosis, Clin Genet 63:192–197, 2003.

77. Epstein S, Hamersma H, Beighton P: Endocrine function in sclerostenosis, S Afr Med J 55:1105–1110, 1979.

78. Brunkow ME, Gardner JC, Van Ness J, et al: Bone dysplasia sclerostenosis results from loss of the *SOST* gene product, a novel cystine knot-containing protein, Am J Hum Genet 68:577–589, 2001.

79. Kim CA, Honjo R, Bertola D, et al: A known SOST gene mutation causes sclerosteosis in a familial and an isolated case from Brazilian origin, Genet Test 12:475–479, 2008.

80. Balemans W, Patel N, Ebeling M, et al: Identification of a 52 kb deletion downstream of the *SOST* gene in patients with van Buchem disease, J Med Genet 39:91–97, 2002.

81. Li X, Zhang Y, Kang H, et al: Sclerostin binds to LRP5/6 and antagonizes canonical Wnt signaling, J Biol Chem 280:19883–19887, 2005.

82. Sutherland MK, Geoghegan JC, Yu C, et al: Sclerostin promotes the apoptosis of human osteoblastic cells: a

novel regulation of bone formation, Bone 35:828–835, 2004.

83. Perez-Vicente JA, Rodriguez de Castro E, Lafuente J, et al: Autosomal dominant endosteal hyperostosis: report of a Spanish family with neurological involvement, Clin Genet 31:161–169, 1987.

84. Whyte MP: Searching for gene defects that cause high bone mass (editorial), Am J Hum Genet 60:1309–1311, 1997.

85. Boyden LM, Mao J, Belsky J, et al: High bone density due to a mutation in LDL-receptor-related protein 5, N Engl J Med 345:1513–1521, 2002.

86. Van Wesenbeeck L, Cleiren E, Gram J, et al: Six novel missense mutations in the LDL receptor-related protein 5 (LRP5) gene in different conditions with an increased bone density, Am J Hum Genet 72:763–771, 2003.

87. Yadav VK, Ryu JH, Suda N, et al: Lrp5 controls bone formation by inhibiting serotonin synthesis in the duodenum, Cell 135:825–837, 2008.

88. Rickels MR, Zhang X, Mumm S: Oropharyngeal skeletal disease accompanying high bone mass and novel LRP5 mutation, J Bone Miner Res 20:878–885, 2005.

89. Berlin R, Hedensio B, Lilja B, et al: Osteopoikilosis: a clinical and genetic study, Acta Med Scand 18:305–314, 1967.

90. Uitto J, Santa Cruz DJ, Starcher BC, et al: Biochemical and ultrastructural demonstration of elastin accumulation in the skin of the Buschke-Ollendorff syndrome, J Invest Dermatol 76:284–287, 1981.

91. Whyte MP, Murphy WA, Seigel BA: 99m Tc-pyrophosphate bone imaging in osteopoikilosis, osteopathia striata, and melorheostosis, Radiology 127:439–443, 1978.

92. Hellemans J, Preobrazhenska O, Willaert A, et al: Loss-of-function mutations in LEMD3 result in osteopoikilosis, Buschke-Ollendorff syndrome and melorheostosis, Nat Genet 36:1213–1218, 2004.

93. Rabinow M, Unger F: Syndrome of osteopathia striata, macrocephaly, and cranial sclerosis, Am J Dis Child 138:821–823, 1984.

94. Jenkins ZA, van Kogelenberg M, Morgan T, et al: Germline mutations in WTX cause a sclerosing skeletal dysplasia but do not predispose to tumorigenesis, Nat Genet 41:95–100, 2008.

95. Clements SE, Wessagowit V, Lai-Cheong JE, et al: Focal dermal hypoplasia resulting from a new nonsense mutation, p.E300X, in the PORCN gene, J Dermatol Sci 49:39–42, 2008.

96. Rimoin DL: Pachydermoperiostosis (idiopathic clubbing and periostosis): genetic and physiologic considerations, N Engl J Med 272:923–931, 1965.

97. Matucci-Cerinic M, Lott T, Jajic IVO, et al: The clinical spectrum of pachydermoperiostosis (primary hypertrophic osteoarthropathy), Medicine 79:208–214, 1991.

98. Herman MA, Massaro D, Katz S: Pachydermoperiostosis: clinical spectrum, Arch Intern Med 116:919–923, 1965.

99. Ali A, Tetalman M, Fordham EW: Distribution of hypertrophic pulmonary osteoarthropathy, Am J Roentgenol 134:771–780, 1980.

100. Vogl A, Goldfischer S: Pachydermoperiostosis: primary or idiopathic hypertrophic osteoarthropathy, Am J Med 33:166–187, 1962.

101. Lauter SA, Vasey FB, Huttner I, et al: Pachydermoperiostosis: studies on the synovium, J Rheumatol 5:85–95, 1978.

102. Cooper RG, Freemont AJ, Riley M, et al: Bone abnormalities and severe arthritis in pachydermoperiostosis, Ann Rheum Dis 51:416–419, 1992.

103. Uppal S, Diggle CP, Carr IM, et al: Mutations in 15-hydroxyprostaglandin dehydrogenase cause primary hypertrophic osteoarthropathy, Nat Genet 40:789–793, 2008.

104. Sillence D: Osteogenesis imperfecta: an expanding panorama of variants, Clin Orthop 159:11–25, 1981.

105. Byers PH: Disorders of collagen biosynthesis and structure. In Striver CR, Beaudet AL, Sly WS, et al, editors: The metabolic and molecular bases of inherited disease, ed 8, New York, 2001, McGraw-Hill.

106. Albright JA, Millar EA: Osteogenesis imperfecta [symposium], Clin Orthop Relat Res 159:1–156, 1981.

107. Pedersen U: Hearing loss in patients with osteogenesis imperfecta, Scand Audiol 13:67–74, 1984.

108. Baldridge D, Schwarze U, Morello R, et al: CRTAP and LEPRE1 mutations in recessive osteogenesis imperfecta, Hum Mutat 29:1435–1442, 2008.

109. Cremin B, Goodman H, Prax M, et al: Wormian bones in osteogenesis imperfecta and other disorders, Skeletal Radiol 8:35–38, 1982.

110. Goldman AB, Davidson D, Pavlor H, et al: Popcorn calcifications: a prognostic sign in osteogenesis imperfecta, Radiology 136:351–358, 1980.

111. Chines A, Boniface A, McAlister W, et al: Hypercalciuria in osteogenesis imperfecta: a follow-up study to assess renal effects, Bone 16:333–339, 1995.

112. Falvo KA, Bullough PG: Osteogenesis imperfecta: a histometric analysis, J Bone Joint Surg Am 55:275–286, 1973.

113. Baron R, Gertner JM, Lang R, et al: Increased bone turnover with decreased bone formation by osteoblasts in children with osteogenesis imperfecta tarda, Pediatr Res 17:204–207, 1983.

114. Glorieux HI, Bishop NJ, Plotkin H, et al: Cyclic administration of pamidronate in children with severe osteogenesis imperfecta, N Engl J Med 339:947–952, 1998.

115. Kuurila K, Pynnönen S, Grénman R: Stapes surgery in osteogenesis imperfecta in Finland, Ann Otol Rhinol Laryngol 113:187–193, 2004.

116. Zeitlin L, Fassier F, Glorieux FH: Modern approach to children with osteogenesis imperfecta, J Pediatr Orthop B 12:77–87, 2003.

117. Pepin M, Atkinson M, Starman BJ, et al: Strategies and outcomes of prenatal diagnosis for osteogenesis imperfecta: a review of biochemical and molecular studies completed in 129 pregnancies, Prenat Diagn 17:559–570, 1997.

118. Whyte MP: Paget's disease of bone and genetic disorders of RANKL/OPG/RANK/NF-κB signaling, Ann NY Acad Sci 1068:143–164, 2006.

119. Martin TJ: Paracrine regulation of osteoclast formation and activity: milestones in discovery, J Musculoskel Neuron Interact 4:243–253, 2004.

120. Whyte MP, Mumm S: Heritable disorders of the RANKL/OPG/RANK signaling pathway, J Musculoskel Neuron Interact 4:254–267, 2004.

121. Hughes AE, Ralston SH, Marken J, et al: Mutations in TNFRSF11A, affecting the signal peptide of RANK, cause familial expansile osteolysis, Nat Genet 24:45–48, 2000.

122. Whyte MP, Hughes AE: Expansile skeletal hyperphosphatasia is caused by a 15-base pair tandem duplication in TNFRSF11A encoding RANK and is allelic to familial expansile osteolysis, J Bone Miner Res 17:26–29, 2002.

123. Whyte MP, Obrecht SE, Finnegan PM, et al: Osteoprotegerin deficiency and juvenile Paget's disease, N Engl J Med 347:174–184, 2002.

124. Altman RD, Bloch DA, Hochberg MC, et al: Prevalence of pelvic Paget's disease of bone in the United States, J Bone Miner Res 15:461–465, 2000.

125. Kanis JA: Pathophysiology and treatment of Paget's disease of bone, ed 2, Malden, MA, 1998, Blackwell Science.

126. Nager GT: Paget's disease of the temporal bone, Ann Otol Rhinol Laryngol 84:1–32, 1975.

127. Smith BJ, Eveson JW: Paget's disease of bone with particular reference to dentistry, J Oral Pathol 10:233–247, 1981.

128. Roodman GD, Windle JJ: Paget disease of bone, J Clin Invest 115:200–208, 2005.

129. Morales-Piga AA, Rey-Rey JS, Corres-Gonzalez J, et al: Frequency and characteristics of familial aggregation of Paget's disease of bone, J Bone Miner Res 10:663–670, 1995.

130. Meunier PJ, Coindre J, Edouard CM, et al: Bone histomorphometry in Paget's disease: quantitative and dynamic analysis of Paget's disease and non-pagetic bone tissue, Arthritis Rheum 23:1095–1103, 1980.

131. Singer FR, Leach RJ: Genetics of Paget's disease of bone. In Econs MJ, editor: The genetics of osteoporosis and metabolic bone disease, Totowa, NJ, 2000, Humana Press, pp 309–318.

132. McKusick VA: Mendelian inheritance in man: catalogs of human genes and genetic disorders, ed 12 (1998). Johns Hopkins University Press, Baltimore and Online Mendelian inheritance in man (2000). OMIM (TM) McKusick-Nathans institute for genetic Medicine, Johns Hopkins University, Baltimore and National Center for Biotechnology Information, National Library of Medicine, Bethesda, MD.

133. Laurin N, Brown JP, Morissette J, et al: Recurrent mutation of the gene encoding sequestosome 1 (SQSTM1/p62) in Paget disease of bone, Am J Hum Genet 70:1582–1588, 2002.

134. Good DA, Busfield F, Fletcher BH, et al: Identification of SQSTM1 mutations in familial Paget's disease in Australian pedigrees, Bone 35:277–282, 2004.

135. Watts GDJ, Wymer J, Kovach MJ, et al: Inclusion body myopathy associated with Paget disease of bone and frontotemporal dementia is caused by mutant valosin-containing protein, Nat Genet 10:1–5, 2004.

136. Asai T, Tomita Y, Nakatsuka S, et al: VCP (p97) regulates NFκB signaling pathway, which is important for metastasis of osteosarcoma cell line, Jpn J Cancer Res 93:296–304, 2002.

137. Hughes AE, Barr J: Familial expansile osteolysis: a genetic model of Paget's disease. In Sharpe PT, editor: The molecular biology of Paget's disease, Heidelberg, 1996, RG Landes, pp 179–199.

138. Whyte MP, Reinus WR, Podgornik MN, et al: Familial expansile osteolysis (excessive RANK effect) in a 5-generation American kindred, Medicine (Baltimore) 81:101–121, 2002.

139. Wallace RG, Barr RJ, Osterberg PH, et al: Familial expansile osteolysis, Clin Orthop 248:265–277, 1989.

140. Mitchell CA, Kennedy JG, Wallace RG: Dental abnormalities associated with familial expansile osteolysis: a clinical and radiographic study, Oral Surg Oral Med Oral Pathol Oral Radiol Endod 70:301–307, 1990.

141. Dickson GR, Shirodria PV, Kanis JA, et al: Familial expansile osteolysis: a morphological, histomorphometric and serological study, Bone 12:331–338, 1991.

142. Golob DS, McAlister WH, Mills BG, et al: Juvenile Paget disease: life-long features of a mildly affected young woman, J Bone Miner Res 11:132–142, 1996.

143. Caffey J: Familial hyperphosphatasemia with ateliosis and hypermetabolism of growing membranous bone: review of the clinical, radiographic and chemical features, Bull Hosp Joint Dis 33:81–110, 1972.

144. Cassinelli HR, Mautalen CA, Heinrich JJ, et al: Familial idiopathic hyperphosphatasia (FIH): response to long-term treatment with pamidronate (APD). Bone Miner 19:175–184, 1992.

145. Resnick D: Diagnosis of bone and joint disorders, ed 3, Philadelphia, 1995, WB Saunders.

146. Bucay N, Narosi I, Dunstan CR, et al: Osteoprotegerin-deficient mice develop early onset osteoporosis and arterial calcification, Genes Dev 12:260–268, 1998.

147. Silve C, Grosse B, Tau C, et al: Response to parathyroid hormone and 1,25-dihydroxyvitamin D3 of bone-derived cells isolated from normal children and children with abnormalities in skeletal development, J Clin Endocrinol Metab 62:583–590, 1986.

148. Mitsudo SM: Chronic idiopathic hyperphosphatasia associated with pseudoxanthoma elasticum, J Bone Joint Surg Am 53:303–314, 1971.

149. Whyte MP, Singhellakis P, Petersen MB, et al: Juvenile Paget's disease: the second reported, oldest patient is homozygous for the TNFRSF11B "Balkan" mutation (966_969delTGACinsCTT) which elevates circulating immunoreactive osteoprotegerin levels, J Bone Miner Res 22:938–946, 2007.

150. Cundy T, Davidson J, Rutland MD, et al: Recombinant osteoprotegerin for juvenile Paget's disease, N Engl J Med 353:918–923, 2005.

Chapter 13

BONE DENSITY AND IMAGING OF OSTEOPOROSIS

ROLAND D. CHAPURLAT, PIERRE D. DELMAS[†], and HARRY K. GENANT

Osteoporosis is defined as a systemic skeletal disease characterized by low bone mass and microarchitectural deterioration of bone tissue leading to enhanced bone fragility and consequent increase in fracture risk. The etymology is descriptive of the alteration in bone tissue: osteoporosis is derived from the Greek *osteon*, or "bone," and *poros*, "small hole." The term was first used in France and Germany in the 19th century to describe bone in the elderly, thus emphasizing its visible porosity.

An NIH conference[1] described osteoporosis as a "skeletal disorder characterized by compromised bone strength predisposing a person to an increased risk of fracture. Bone strength primarily reflects the integration of bone density and bone quality." *Bone density* corresponds to the amount of mineral within an area or a volume, and *bone quality* depends on architecture, bone turnover, damage accumulation, and mineralization. Compromised bone strength (bone fragility) increases the risk of fractures resulting from *moderate trauma*, defined as a fall from standing height or less, which has led to the concept of "fragility fracture." Therefore, osteoporosis is a risk factor for fracture.

The concept of osteoporosis has progressively evolved from criteria based on histology, to fracture occurrence, to assessment of bone mass, and currently to the individual assessment of fracture risk, including history of fracture, clinical risk factors for fracture, and bone mass evaluation. Indeed, a fracture-based diagnosis unacceptably delays intervention in a condition for which prevention of fracture is essential. Changes encountered in osteoporosis can be assessed by noninvasive techniques measuring bone mineral density (BMD), such as dual x-ray absorp-

[†]Deceased.

tiometry (DXA). BMD accounts for 75% to 85% of the variance in ultimate strength of bone tissue[2] and is well correlated with the load-bearing capacity of the skeleton in vitro.[3] Prospective studies demonstrate that the risk of fragility fractures increases as BMD declines, with a 1.5- to 3-fold increased risk of fracture for each standard deviation (SD) fall in BMD.[4] The main advantage of a density-based diagnosis is the possibility of an early intervention, before fractures. This approach was carried out by the World Health Organization (WHO) in its definition of osteoporosis in 1994.[5] In women, osteoporosis can be diagnosed if the BMD or the bone mineral content (BMC) at the spine, femoral neck, or forearm is 2.5 SD or more below the mean value of a reference population of young, healthy premenopausal women, with the following categories:

1. Normal: BMD higher than 1 SD below the young adult mean
2. Osteopenia, or low bone mass: BMD between 1 and 2.5 SD below the young adult mean
3. Osteoporosis: BMD lower than 2.5 SD below the young adult mean
4. Established (or severe) osteoporosis: BMD lower than 2.5 SD below the young adult mean and the presence of one or more fragility fractures

Thus, osteoporosis is defined in practice by a surrogate marker (i.e., BMD), not a health outcome (fracture), even if other factors can influence the likelihood of fractures. The relationship between BMD and fractures is very similar to that between hypertension and stroke and stronger than that between serum cholesterol and coronary heart disease (Fig. 13-1). The gradient of the risk of fracture with decreasing BMD is as steep as that between diastolic blood pressure and stroke.

It is estimated that with this 2.5 SD threshold, 30% of white women older than 50 years have osteoporosis,[6] a fraction that is similar to the lifetime risk of fracture at the hip, spine, and forearm for a 50-year-old woman.[7] By this definition, about 0.6% of young adult women have osteoporosis, and 16% have low bone mass. The prevalence of osteoporosis increases with age because of the decline in bone mass. Not all women who have osteoporosis by the WHO criteria will sustain fractures, and conversely, many women who do not have osteoporosis by this

definition may deserve treatment because of other risk factors that will increase their risk of fracture. Thus, this operational WHO definition of osteoporosis provided the concept of osteoporosis as a risk factor for fracture, which is important for assessing the number of affected individuals, but patient diagnosis must include other risk factors for fracture. This is the role of the individual fracture risk assessment of fracture.

Recently, a WHO Scientific Group issued a technical report including hierarchical levels of evidence for the ability of risk factors to identify individuals at risk for fracture.[8] Those risk factors were validated by meta-analyses of population-based cohorts from Asia, Australia, Europe, and North America. Those risk factors were BMD at the femoral neck, low body mass index, a prior fragility fracture, glucocorticoid exposure, a parental history of hip fracture, smoking, excessive intake of alcohol, and rheumatoid arthritis. The combination of those risk factors allowed for building fracture probability models, providing individual probabilities of fracture that will be the basis for therapeutic decision making, thus shifting the former therapeutic threshold paradigm, which was often based only on the BMD T score.

Epidemiology

MAGNITUDE OF THE PROBLEM

In women, osteoporosis is rare before menopause. With aging, more and more women are affected by osteoporosis; by the age of 80 years, 27% have low bone mass and 70% have osteoporosis at the hip, spine, or forearm.[7] Sixty percent of osteoporotic women will experience one or more fragility fractures. In the United States, it is estimated that 16.8 million (54%) of postmenopausal white women have low bone mass, and 9.4 million (30%) have osteoporosis.[7] These rates of prevalence are lower in nonwhite women and in men. NHANES III (Third National Health and Nutritional Examination Survey) data indicate that 10,103,000 Americans (8,021,000 women and 2,082,000 men) have osteoporosis and that 18,557,000 (15,434,000 women and 3,123,000 men) have low bone mass and thus an increased risk of osteoporosis in comparison to those who do not have low bone mass.[8] The prevalence of vertebral fractures can vary according to the definition of fracture used. Thus 10% to 25% of women older than 50 years are estimated to have vertebral fractures.[9,10] In 1990, 1.66 million hip fractures were estimated worldwide in those older than 35 years.[11]

Osteoporosis results in high rates of morbidity. In 1986 in the United States, osteoporosis was responsible for an estimated 321,909 hospitalizations in white women 45 years and older—167,421 for hip fractures, 35,106 for fragility vertebral fractures, 120,636 for wrist fractures, and 20,369 for humerus fractures.[12] Osteoporosis-related fractures also significantly contribute to the economic burden of health care. In 1995, direct costs for osteoporosis fractures were estimated to be $13.8 billion,[13] whereas it was 5 to 6 billion annually 10 years earlier.[12] Being elderly, patients with hip fractures often have other medical conditions, thus increasing their risk of complications such as pressure sores or infections. Hip fractures often result in admission to nursing homes.[14] The number of hip fractures and their associated costs are expected to sharply increase and could triple by the year 2040. Indeed, the number of elderly people is quickly growing, and fracture incidence rates increase with age.[15] This phenomenon is observed in developed countries, but the projected rapid

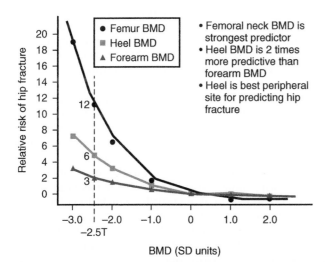

FIGURE 13-1. Hip fracture incidence as a function of BMD measured at the hip, spine, and forearm in postmenopausal women. (Data from Cummings SR, Black DM, Nevitt MC, et al: Bone density at various sites for prediction of hip fractures, Lancet 341:72–75, 1993.)

expansion of the elderly populations of Latin America and Asia could lead to an increase in hip fractures from 1.66 million worldwide in 1990 to 6.26 million in 2050, with only 25% occurring in North America and Europe.[11] Osteoporosis is also associated with mortality. For each standard deviation decrease in bone mineral density, the mortality risk is increased 1.5-fold.

The lifetime risk of fractures can be estimated, given the probability of fracture and the odds of reaching a given age. Most data have been generated in white populations of Western countries. The lifetime risk of sustaining an osteoporotic fracture has been estimated in the United States to be close to 40% for women and 13% for men. For vertebral fractures, the estimated risk is 15.6% for women and 5% for men. The risk of hip fracture is 17.5% for women and 6% for men and for wrist fracture, 16% for women and 2.5% for men.[7]

SITE-SPECIFIC FRACTURES

Hip Fracture

Hip fracture is the most serious complication of osteoporosis. It results in high morbidity and sometimes mortality. The most striking characteristic of hip fractures is that they are associated with a 12% to 20% reduction in expected survival.[16] Many of the deaths after hip fractures are related to other diseases.[17] Few deaths are actually due to or hastened by the fracture, but the risk of dying of another disease is sometimes increased by the hip fracture. About 5% of women sustaining a hip fracture die during the following year as a consequence of fracture. In women living in nursing homes, 36% of those having a hip fracture will die within a year. Thirty percent to 50% of these patients are unable to regain the level of function they had before the hip fracture. The patient's physical condition before the fracture may be the best predictor of postfracture functional outcome.

The incidence of hip fracture increases exponentially with age in both genders. In women younger than 35 years, the incidence is 2 per 100,000 person years, whereas it is 3032 per 100,000 person years in women older than 85 years.[18] In men the rates are 4 and 1909 per 100,000 person years, respectively. Most hip fractures occur in elderly people: 52% after age 80 years and 90% after age 50 years.[18] The decline in BMD and the increase in frequency of falls in elderly people are responsible for this high incidence of hip fracture. Only 1% of falls lead to a hip fracture, but 90% of hip fractures are related to a fall from standing height or less.[19] Hip fractures tend to be the consequence of falls on hard surfaces, the fall not being stopped by protective reflexes of upper limbs.[20] Fifty percent of the falls leading to hip fractures result from slipping or tripping, 20% from loss of consciousness, and 20% to 30% of loss of balance and other factors.

Vertebral Fracture

The epidemiology of vertebral fractures is less well characterized than that for hip fractures because symptoms after vertebral fracture are unidentified in up to 70% of cases, and standardized radiographic diagnostic criteria for vertebral fractures are lacking. Less than a third of patients with vertebral deformities seek medical assistance, and 2% to 8% need hospital admission.[23] In women, 90% of vertebral deformities are a consequence of mild to moderate trauma, whereas this proportion is only 50% in men.[24]

The incidence of clinical vertebral fractures increases gradually with age in both genders. The age-adjusted prevalence is thought to be between 8% and 25% in women older than 50

years. The difference in prevalence figures is due to the definition used.[24] Early definitions of vertebral fracture were based on the type of deformity and thus had poor precision. New techniques using vertebral morphometry give more reliable results.[25] Vertebral deformities are mostly noted in women, with a ratio of 2:1, but this ratio becomes narrower in elderly people older than 80 years. It has been suggested in a large epidemiologic study involving 15,570 European men and women that the incidence of vertebral deformities might be equal in both genders. In the same cohort, vertebral fracture incidence in women over 50 was estimated at 10.7/1000 person years in women and 5.7/1000 per person years in men.[26] Changes in the gross appearance of the vertebral body encompass a wide range of morphologic characteristics, from increased endplate concavity to complete destruction of the vertebral anatomy in vertebral crush fractures.[27] It must be kept in mind that vertebral deformity is not synonymous with vertebral fracture; for example, Scheuermann's disease is frequently discussed as a differential diagnosis.[28]

New vertebral fractures, even those not recognized clinically, are associated with substantial increases in back pain and functional limitation due to back pain, at least in elderly women.[29] Ten percent to 20% of elderly women with worsening of their functional status because of back pain have had a vertebral fracture. Common complications of vertebral deformities are chronic back pain, back disability, height loss, limitations in activity, emotional difficulties stemming from physical appearance, and more medical consumption. Kyphosis from vertebral fractures adds to the overall back pain. For instance, after adjustment for age, a 15% increase in kyphosis increases the odds ratio of severe upper back pain 2.1-fold. However, no association has been found between the number of fractures and impairment in quality of life. The occurrence of vertebral fracture is predictive of new fracture, with RR = 5 to 11. Vertebral fractures are associated with increased mortality at 5 years, as for hip fracture. The increase in mortality is progressive over this period, as opposed to hip fracture. The risk of death appears to be much higher for clinically apparent vertebral fracture, and the presence of multiple vertebral fractures further increases this risk.[30,31]

Wrist Fracture

Wrist fractures, also called *distal forearm fractures* or *Colles' fractures*, are very common. The incidence of wrist fracture is hard to calculate because only a minority of patients is hospitalized. A Norwegian study showed that it was the most common fracture responsible for admission to a local university hospital.[32] Incidence varies among different ethnic groups. Wrist fracture risk is lower in black people than white people.[33] Increasing incidence was observed between 1950 and 1982,[34] but this trend seemed to have leveled off during the second part of the 1980s.

The pattern of incidence of wrist fracture is different from that of hip or vertebral fractures. The age-adjusted female-to-male ratio is 4:1, with a linear increase in incidence in women from ages 40 to 60 years, followed by a plateau.[35] In men, the incidence is almost constant between the ages of 20 and 80 years, for unknown reasons. Wrist fractures are not associated with an increase in mortality and are usually thought to be free of long-term poor outcome.[36] Other data, however, suggest that half of the patients do not report good functional status at 6 months because of complications such as algodystrophy, neuropathies, and posttraumatic osteoarthritis.[37]

Wrist fractures must be considered as an important predictor of subsequent vertebral and hip fractures. Indeed, it has been shown that men and women with distal forearm fractures have on average a twofold increase in the risk of sustaining a hip fracture.[38] Previous wrist fractures are also significant predictors of overall osteoporotic fractures, with a doubled risk. In younger women, the predictive value of a previous wrist fracture for subsequent osteoporotic fractures seems even more important, with a relative risk of 2.67 (1.02 to 6.94) for women aged 40 to 49 years. This predictive value is of the same magnitude as that provided by a 1-SD decrease in BMD measured by bone densitometry.[39] Thus, the occurrence of a wrist fracture in an early postmenopausal woman is suggestive of osteoporosis and should trigger appropriate investigation such as BMD measurement.

Other Fractures

Other fractures include proximal humerus, pelvis, proximal tibia, and rib fractures. An excess of these fractures is noted in postmenopausal women, their rates increase with aging, and they are often a consequence of minimal trauma. These fractures are related to low bone mass, similar to hip and vertebral fracture, and they should also motivate BMD measurement because any of them could be the first symptom of osteoporosis.

VARIABILITY IN FRACTURE INCIDENCE

The incidence of hip fracture is markedly lower in black and Asian people and varies among different countries and populations. Rates are higher in Scandinavia than in Western Europe and Oceania.[21] A north-south gradient in age-standardized risk is found in Europe and the United States,[22] with a higher rate in the north. The age-adjusted increase in incidence that has been observed in several countries over the past 50 years appears to have leveled off in some of these countries. The incidence increases with socioeconomic difficulties, decreased winter sunlight, and water fluoridation. Fractures are more frequent in winter months. This seasonal trend could be due to altered neuromuscular coordination and vitamin D deficiency in winter months, because most fractures occur indoors and thus cannot be explained only by slippery winter conditions.[22] About 80% of hip fractures occur in women, because the age-adjusted incidence in men is two times lower than in women, and more elderly women are alive than are elderly men.

COSTS

In the United States, direct medical expenditures for osteoporotic fractures were estimated at $20 billion in 2000,[40] two-thirds of which are accounted for by hip fracture alone. An important determinant of rising cost is increased age. The estimated cost for care in the United States during the first year after a hip fracture is $21,000 per person and is much higher in women older than 80 years. If the cost of the subsequent nursing home is attributed to the hip fracture, the cost of care for those who stay in nursing homes after 1 year is $93,378 per person. The average cost for vertebral fracture during the first year is $1200 per patient, and it is $800 for Colles' fracture. Costs are expected to double in 2050, due to the increasing number of fractures resulting from the aging population.

OSTEOPOROSIS: A NEGLECTED DISEASE

It has been shown in recent years that even after marketing of several effective therapies for osteoporosis, most patients who have sustained an osteoporotic fracture (forearm fracture, vertebral fracture, and even hip fracture) do not receive adequate secondary prevention for future fractures, whereas the risk of repeated fractures is markedly increased, including that of second hip fracture.[41]

Table 13-1. Risk Factors for Hip Fracture With and Without Adjustment for Calcaneal Bone Density and History of Prior Fracture

Factor	Relative Risk (95% Confidence Interval)	
	Base Model	Adjustment for Fracture and BMD
Age (per 5 yr)	1.5 (1.3-1.7)	1.4 (1.2-1.6)
History of maternal hip fracture	2.0 (1.4-2.9)	1.8 (1.2-2.7)
Increase in weight since age 25 yr	0.6 (0.5-0.7)	0.8 (0.6-0.9)
Height at age 25 yr	1.2 (1.1-1.4)	1.3 (1.1-1.5)
Self-rated health	1.7 (1.3-2.2)	1.6 (1.2-2.1)
Previous hyperthyroidism	1.8 (1.2-2.6)	1.7 (1.2-2.5)
Current use of long-acting benzodiazepines	1.6 (1.1-2.4)	1.6 (1.1-2.4)
Current use of anticonvulsant drugs	2.8 (1.2-6.3)	2.0 (0.8-4.9)
Current caffeine intake	1.3 (1.0-1.5)	2.0 (0.8-4.9)
Walking for exercise	0.7 (0.5-0.9)	1.2 (1.0-1.5)
On feet <4 hr/day	1.7 (1.2-2.4)	0.7 (0.5-1.0)
Inability to rise from chair	2.1 (1.3-3.2)	1.7 (1.2-2.4)
Lowest quartile for distant depth perception	1.5 (1.1-2.0)	1.4 (2.0-1.9)
Low-frequency contrast sensibility	1.2 (1.0-1.5)	1.2 (1.0-1.5)
Resting pulse rate >80 beats/min	1.8 (1.3-2.5)	1.7 (1.2-2.4)
Any fracture since age 50 yr	1.5 (1.1-2.0)	
Calcaneal bone density (per 1-SD decrease)	1.6 (1.3-1.9)	

Data from Study of Osteoporotic Fractures.
BMD, Bone mineral density.

Pathogenesis

Osteoporosis is a multifactorial disease. Most but not all risk factors influence the level of bone mass. Some may have an impact on bone structure (the so-called quality of bone), and some increase the risk of fragility fracture through extraskeletal mechanisms. One should distinguish risk factors for falls from risk factors for bone fragility.

CLINICAL RISK FACTORS

Clinical risk factors can shed light on the pathophysiology of fragility fractures. Bone mineral density is a key risk factor for fracture,[42] but numerous studies have evaluated other risk factors for fractures.[16,43-50] The use of such factors (Table 13-1) to identify high-risk subjects is frequently advocated. Different types of fractures have different risk-factor profiles.[44]

Estrogen Deficiency

Estrogen deficiency has been associated with osteoporosis since first suggested by Fuller Albright in the 1940s. It is the main cause of bone loss in women after menopause. Premature menopause—natural or surgically induced—extends the period during which a woman is exposed to a hypogonadal state, thus increasing the total duration of bone loss occurring after menopause.[51] Similarly, late menarche and primary or secondary amenorrhea also increase the risk for osteoporosis.[52] Luteal deficiency in premenopausal women has been suggested to be associated with bone loss,[53] but the evidence is still controversial. Estrogen deficiency is also associated with bone loss during the 3 to 4 years preceding the actual menopause—the perimenopause—with a rate similar to that observed in the early postmenopausal years.[54] It is likely that women with the lowest concentrations of residual estrogen have faster bone loss and fracture more often, although this might be confounded by the effect of body weight or other sex steroids.[55-57] Also, women receiving aromatase inhibitors as adjuvant therapy for breast cancer lose bone more rapidly and sustain an increased rate of fragility fracture.[58]

Other Factors

Many factors increase the risk of fracture. For instance, the Study of Osteoporotic Fractures[49] identified 16 independent risk factors for hip fracture in addition to low BMD (see Table 13-1). Numerous studies have described risk factors such as female gender, white or Asian race, age, previous fractures, thinness, cigarette smoking, family history of hip fracture, use of sedative hypnotics, and impairment in visual and neuromuscular function. Lack of physical activity may also be an important cause of bone loss,[59,60] and it has been hypothesized that some of the age-related bone loss and the burden of skeletal fragility result from a decline in physical activity, in particular, in Western societies. Black people have less osteoporosis and fewer fractures than white and Asian people do. Excessive alcohol consumption increases the risk of fractures, whereas moderate intake might exert a protective effect. Undernutrition in the elderly may contribute to bone loss, the risk of falling, or the response to injury.[61] It is widely believed that inadequate calcium intake throughout life is a significant risk factor.[62]

In a cohort of 7575 French women aged 75 years or older, the risk of subsequent hip fracture was significantly increased (even after adjustment for femoral hip BMD) in women with a slow gait speed, in women who had difficulty performing a tandem (heel-to-toe) walk (i.e., neuromuscular impairment), and in women with visual acuity less than 2/10.[63] The incidence of hip fracture among women classified as being at high risk because of both a high fall risk status and a low BMD was found to be 29 per 1000 women years. It was 11 per 1000 in women at risk because of either a high fall risk status or low BMD, and the risk was 5.4 per 1000 women years in those at low risk according to both criteria. Even with this combined approach, about a third of women with a hip fracture had not been identified as being at high risk, thus indicating that other factors are important in the pathogenesis of hip fracture. Although these clinical risk factors can be easily assessed with a rapid questionnaire and physical examination, they are probably of limited value in younger women. A personal history of hip fracture is still predictive, but its prevalence is much lower in women younger than 65 years. Fall-related factors have not been tested but are likely to be poor discriminants in younger and healthier women.

Candidate risk factors have been examined by a WHO working group in individual data meta-analyses of 12 prospective population-based cohorts. Data were collected from 60,000 men and women participating in the Rotterdam study in the Netherlands; the European Vertebral Osteoporosis Study and the European Prospective Osteoporosis Study; the Canadian Multicenter Osteoporosis Study; the Dubbo Osteoporosis Epidemiology Study in Australia; the EPIDOS and OFELY cohorts in France; and cohorts from Rochester, Minnesota; Sheffield, England; Kuopio, Finland; Hiroshima, Japan; and Gothenburg, Sweden. Several risk factors have been selected on the basis of the possibility to modify them and ease of use in clinical practice: BMD at the femoral neck, low body mass index, a prior fragility fracture, glucocorticoid exposure, a parental history of hip fracture, smoking, excessive intake of alcohol, and rheumatoid arthritis.[64-68] Those factors are modeled to provide individual probabilities of fracture that can be easily calculated using the computer-driven WHO fracture risk assessment tool called *FRAX* (available at Internet websites such as http://www.shef.ac.uk/FRAX/).[69]

PEAK BONE MASS

Peak bone mass is the amount of bone acquired at the end of skeletal growth, and it is followed by bone loss throughout the rest of life. Bone mass at a given age is a function of the peak bone mass achieved and the amount of bone lost as a consequence of menopause and aging. Peak bone mass, which is reached in early adult life, primarily depends on genetic factors. It is also influenced by dietary calcium intake during adolescence and by physical activity.

Blacks achieve higher peak bone mass than whites do, who have greater peak bone mass than Asians, particularly Japanese. Twin studies have shown a strong correspondence of peak bone mass in monozygotic twins, who have closer concordance in BMD than dizygotic twins.[70] Which genes are the most important is still unknown. It has been reported by Morrison et al. that polymorphism of a noncoding sequence of the vitamin D receptor gene was associated with peak bone mass variance in monozygotic twins, and that these polymorphisms accounted for most of the genetic effect.[71] This association has not been confirmed by most subsequent studies[72-74] but has initiated searches for other candidate genes, including the estrogen receptor, interleukin 6 (IL-6), transforming growth factor β (TGF-β), and type I collagen. For example, the collagen Iα1 Sp1 polymorphism is moderately associated with BMD and fracture, as shown in a meta-analysis of 13 studies involving 3642 patients.[75] More recently, some variants of *LRP5* have been found associated with BMD and fracture.[76-78] Even if many advances have been made in understanding the role of genetic factors in the last 10 years, a great deal of additional research is required to identify the genes relevant to the pathogenesis of osteoporotic fracture. Indeed, most studies so far have been underpowered. In the future, it is likely that a combination of large-scale studies and technologic improvements such as genomewide associations will help identify candidate genes in the regulation of bone strength.[77-79]

Dietary calcium intake may be important for attaining optimal peak bone mass. Three placebo-controlled trials in children or adolescents, including one performed in twins, have shown a modest but significant increase in BMD in those receiving calcium supplementation.[80-82] Children with very low calcium intake are more likely to benefit from an increase in calcium, preferably from a dietary source.

Other factors may be important, such as those influencing the progression of puberty. Exercise during growth may contribute to the level of peak bone mass. It has been shown that intensive exercise before puberty may enhance bone acquisition that might persist in adulthood,[83] but the role of exercise in the normal physiologic range is unknown. In girls, areal BMD gains stop around ages 16 to 20 and in boys around ages 20 to 22. Bone width, however, will continue to increase throughout life, even after linear growth cessation, to maintain bending strength despite areal BMD decline.[84] Diet, physical activity, and toxic substances exposure, including maternal cigarette smoking during pregnancy (programming), may also influence the level of peak bone mass.[85,86]

BONE LOSS WITH AGING

Changes in bone mass as a function of age are presented in Fig. 13-2. Throughout life, women lose 35% to 50% of their bone mass, depending on the skeletal site. Although osteoporosis is a

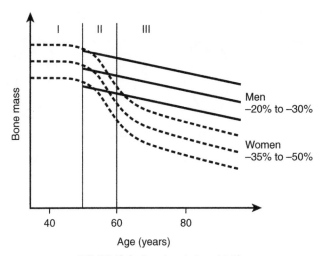

FIGURE 13-2. Bone loss during adult life.

systemic disease affecting the whole skeleton (with the exception of the bones of the skull and face), the pattern of bone loss differs slightly and depends on the type of bone. It has been generally believed that bone loss starts around menopause. In fact, a recent study showed that trabecular bone loss—assessed at the distal forearm with high-resolution peripheral quantitative computed tomography (HR-pQCT)—starts in young adults of both sexes, accounting for a third of the total trabecular bone loss over the entire life.[87] Menopause induces accelerated bone loss within 5 to 8 years, followed by a linear rate of bone loss that may accelerate after the age of 75 years.[88] Because of a much slower rate of bone remodeling, cortical bone loss may start later, but the total amount of cortical bone mass that is lost in women in their 80s is probably similar to the amount of cancellous bone lost. The proportion of overall bone loss related to menopause and to the estrogen-independent aging process is debated, but clearly bone loss in the elderly is still under the influence of estrogen deficiency and can be prevented by hormone replacement therapy (HRT).[89]

Two major mechanisms underlie bone loss in women. First, an age-related decrease in osteoblast activity occurs and leads to an imbalance between the amount of bone resorbed and the amount of bone formed within a remodeling unit (BMU). Second, menopause induces a marked increase in the number of remodeling units activated within the cancellous and cortical bone envelopes per unit of time, which will amplify the small deficits observed at each BMU. This overall increase in bone turnover peaks within the first 2 to 3 years after menopause but persists throughout life, even in women in their 80s, as shown by the sustained increase in bone markers of resorption and formation in elderly postmenopausal women. The mechanism by which estrogen deficiency results in increased bone resorption and bone loss is not yet completely understood, but evidence indicates that estrogens act indirectly through cytokines and growth factors such as IL-1α, IL-1 receptor antagonist, tumor necrosis factor α (TNF-α), IL-7, and TGF-β. Estrogen also stimulates production of osteoprotegerin—a decoy receptor that is a potent inhibitor of osteoclast activity—in osteoblastic cells and is also an inhibitor of receptor activator of nuclear factor κB (RANKL) and RANKL-stimulated osteoclastogenesis, thus explaining a large part of the antiresorptive action of estrogen in bone.[90-92] Estrogen results in an increase in IL-7 in target organs such as bone, thymus, and spleen, at least in part through decreases in TGF-β and increased IGF-1 production, leading to a first wave

of T-cell activation.[93] Those activated T cells release IFN-γ, increasing antigen presentation by dendritic cells and macrophages as a result of up-regulation of MHCII expression through the transcription factor CIIA.[94] Estrogen deficiency also amplifies osteoclastogenesis and T cell activation by down-regulating antioxidant pathways, resulting in an upswing in ROS, which in turn stimulates antigen presentation and TNF production by mature osteoclasts. As a result, T-cell activation is again amplified and promotes release of the osteoclastogenic factors RANKL and TNF. In addition, TNF stimulates osteoblastic RANKL and M-CSF production, in part by up-regulating IL-1, thus leading to osteoclastic formation.[95,96] TNF and IL-7 also directly blunt bone formation through their effects on osteoblasts.

Bone turnover in osteoporosis, however, varies widely with patients with high, normal, and low bone turnover.[97] In osteoporosis, trabecular plates are perforated and transform into rods, leading to thinning of trabeculae and loss of connectivity, with increased risk of fracture as a result. Cortices also thin because of reduced periosteal apposition failing to compensate for bone loss at the endosteal surfaces. Modifications in collagen matrix (e.g., variations in the proportions of various crosslinks and isomerization of C-telopeptide) and the degree of mineralization may also influence bone strength.

Serum intact parathyroid hormone (PTH) levels increase with advanced age in both genders. This hyperparathyroidism is secondary to the calcium and/or vitamin D deficiency commonly found in the elderly, especially in those institutionalized, and may contribute to bone loss in both women and men. A classification of osteoporotic fractures based on clinical features and underlying mechanisms has been used. Type I osteoporosis includes mainly wrist and vertebral fractures, occurring mostly in women younger than 70 years, and is predominantly due to loss of cancellous bone because of estrogen deficiency. Type II osteoporosis includes mainly hip fractures that occur in both elderly men and women as a result of cancellous and cortical bone loss driven primarily by secondary hyperparathyroidism. It has been proposed that this model should be unitary, with bone loss caused by estrogen deficiency in both phases and in both genders.[43] In this model, the accelerated phase of bone loss after menopause involves a disproportionate loss of cancellous bone, mainly due to estrogen deficiency. Compared to normal postmenopausal women, osteoporotic women seem to have impaired responsiveness to postmenopausal low levels of estrogen. The subsequent phase of slow bone loss involves proportionate losses of cancellous and cortical bone and is associated with secondary hyperparathyroidism. In aging men, low testosterone and estrogen levels contribute to bone loss. In the elderly, decreased bone formation also contributes to bone loss, probably due to stem cells which tend to differentiate toward the adipocyte lineage rather than the osteoblastic lineage.

BONE QUALITY

Bone strength is determined by its material composition and structure.[98] Bone must be stiff to resist deformation, thereby making loading possible, and it must also be flexible to absorb energy by deforming. Bones shorten and widen when compressed, and lengthen and narrow in tension. When bone is brittle (i.e., too stiff and unable to deform a little), the energy imposed during loading leads to structural failure, initially by the development of microcracks and then by complete fracture. When bone is too flexible and deforms beyond its peak strain, it breaks. Long bones are mainly made of cortical bone, favoring rigidity over flexibility, whereas mainly trabecular vertebrae can absorb more energy by deforming more before breaking. Differences in bone dimensions explain the better tolerance to load in men compared with women and in some races compared with others.[99] Men and women generally have similar vertebral trabecular volumetric density and similar vertebral heights. The larger vertebral cross-sectional area in men contributes to sex-based differences in bone strength. Black people tend to have wider but shorter vertebral bodies and higher trabecular volumetric density than do white people, owing to thicker trabeculae. The geometry of the hip (hip axis length) influences the risk of hip fractures. Femoral neck length is a predictor of future fracture, and individuals with particularly long femoral necks are more likely to have hip fractures. This feature has been noted in white women from the United States[100] and France.[101] The increase in height over the second part of the 20th century could partly explain the increase in the incidence of hip fracture during this period.[102] Bone modeling (construction) produces a change in size and shape of bone when new bone is deposited without previous bone resorption. During bone remodeling (reconstruction), resorption by osteoclasts precedes bone formation by osteoblasts. Bone modeling and remodeling modify the external size and contours of bone and its internal architecture by the deposition or removal of bone from the surface of bone. They result in cortical and trabecular thickening during growth and thinning during aging. Bone loss occurring with menopause and aging is associated with disturbances in bone microarchitecture.[103] Osteoclastic resorption leads to focal perforations in cancellous bone plates, which results in loss of connection of the horizontal plates, along with detachment of vertical bars throughout the bone marrow cavity. Thus the probability of crush fracture is increased in bones rich in cancellous bone, such as vertebrae. The thickness of cancellous bone plates is about 100 to 150 μm, and osteoclasts dig resorption defects of 50 to 100 μm during normal remodeling. Perforations in cancellous plates can be a consequence of increased osteoclast activity and lead to impairment in bone mechanical properties and therefore to an increased risk of fracture. With continued remodeling, trabeculae perforate and some disappear completely. Active endocortical and intracortical remodeling "trabecularizes" cortical bone (i.e., creates cortical bone with more surface area).[104] Older, more densely mineralized interstitial bone distant from surface remodeling has a reduced number of osteocytes and accumulates microdamage.[105] Both cortical thinning and cortical porosity reduce the resistance of bone to the propagation of cracks, leading to complete fracture in case of a fall. The loss of bone strength due to cortical thinning and porosity is partially offset by deposition of new bone on the external surface (periosteal apposition), so cortical thickness is better maintained than would occur without periosteal apposition (Fig. 13-3).[106,107] However, details of changes in periosteal apposition with aging—along with the effects of site, sex, and race—are difficult to evaluate prospectively, given the small magnitude of periosteal apposition throughout adult life. The notion that periosteal apposition is greater in men than in women remains controversial.[108] More recent studies suggest that sex-based differences may occur at some but not all sites.[99,109] Sex-based differences may also vary across races.

ROLE OF FALLS

Skeletal determinants of bone strength do not reflect all the factors related to fracture risk. For any given bone density, the risk of fracture is greater in the elderly. The increased frequency of falling, the type of fall that occurs among the elderly, and the

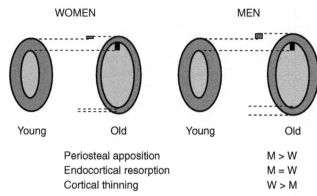

FIGURE 13-3. Bone morphology as a function of age and gender.

loss of protective soft tissue may all explain the larger contribution of age and the less important role of bone mass in the elderly. Among postmenopausal women in the United States, the frequency of at least one annual fall rises from about one in five at 60 to 64 years of age to one in three at 80 to 84 years of age.[110] Propensity for falling has been assessed in several studies[48] with parameters such as gait speed, inability to rise from a chair without using one's arms, and of course, visual impairment. These parameters are associated with a risk of falling. The increase in falling is nevertheless not sufficient to account for the increasing incidence of fractures, because only 5% to 6% of falls result in a fracture (1% of hip fractures and 4% to 5% for other fractures). Fracture risk is also related to the seriousness of the trauma on the femur and the direction of the fall. Indeed, the risk of hip fracture is 13 times higher when the impact is delivered directly over the hip.[110] A great amount of force can be dissipated by the thickness of soft tissue over the femur, and patients with low fat mass may be at higher risk of hip fracture.

Clinical Features

POSTMENOPAUSAL OSTEOPOROSIS

The most common clinical form of osteoporosis is postmenopausal. Typically, women sustain a wrist fracture about 10 years after menopause, a vertebral fracture 15 to 20 years after menopause, and eventually, after 75 years of age, a hip fracture.

Wrist fractures or distal forearm fractures are mainly of two types: a Colles' fracture is a consequence of dorsal angulation, and the less frequent type, a Smith fracture, results from volar angulation. These fractures usually have a favorable outcome, but some patients suffer from algodystrophy, osteoarthritis, or neuropathies.[36]

Two types of hip fracture are cervical and trochanteric. The femoral trochanter is composed of more cancellous bone than the femoral neck is. It seems that the predictive value of BMD and ultrasonic parameters may be higher for trochanteric fracture than for cervical fracture.[111] Hip fractures are associated with more morbidity and mortality, and the prefracture functional state is restored in less than half of patients (see earlier in Epidemiology).

Vertebral fracture requires separate consideration. Vertebral fracture results in back pain, which often appears after some strain on the back, such as lifting a suitcase or working in the garden. The pain is commonly severe and often confines the patient to bed. This pain localizes to the back and rarely radiates to the legs; cord compression is exceptional, and in this latter case, one must consider other diagnoses such as metastases or myeloma. Pain from the fracture usually eases over a period of 6 to 8 weeks and disappears. Nevertheless, it has been estimated that about two-thirds of vertebral fractures are not diagnosed at the time they occur because they are considered by patients or physicians as nonspecific back pain. Loss of height is another main feature of vertebral fracture, but often patients do not report it spontaneously, so it needs to be sought by asking about the individual's height in early adulthood and measuring the current height. Therefore, it is worthwhile to record the patient's height at each clinical visit. Height loss of 3 cm or more should alert the physician to the possibility of a new vertebral fracture. Detection of asymptomatic vertebral fractures is clinically relevant because they are associated with a threefold to fivefold increased risk of new vertebral fractures, independent of the level of BMD. In addition, the incidence of new vertebral fracture in the year following a vertebral fracture has been estimated to be 20%.[112] Kyphosis is generally a consequence of vertebral crush fractures in the thoracic spine and sometimes results in decreased lung capacity. Vertebral fractures in the lumbar spine result in decreased abdominal volume, which causes protrusion of the abdomen and impingement of the costal margin on the iliac crest. This iliocostal contact provokes pain and a grating sensation.

DISEASES AND TREATMENTS CONTRIBUTING TO OSTEOPOROSIS

A variety of disorders are associated with an increased risk of osteoporosis (Table 13-2). In most of these cases, osteoporosis appears to be multifactorial and cannot be attributed to only a specific disease ("secondary osteoporosis"). We will discuss only the most common disorders associated with osteoporosis.

Glucocorticoid-Induced Osteoporosis

Consistent evidence indicates that glucocorticoids impair bone formation[113] by directly inhibiting osteoblastic activity. Osteoblastic synthesis of type I collagen, osteocalcin, and alkaline phosphatase is decreased; the production of insulin-like growth factor 1 (IGF-1) and IGF-2 is also inhibited by glucocorticoids. Measurement of serum osteocalcin provides a good index of this osteoblast inhibition by glucocorticoids. The effect of corticosteroids on bone resorption is less clear. High doses have been associated (in some but not all studies) with an increased rate of bone resorption resulting from decreased intestinal calcium absorption, increased urine calcium excretion, decreased osteoprotegerin levels, and hypogonadism. Glucocorticoids contribute to adrenal and gonadal deficiency because of inhibition of pituitary hormone secretion, with a dose-dependent reduction in free testosterone in men. Consequently, exposure to supraphysiologic doses of glucocorticoids leads to substantial and rapid bone loss in most individuals, especially in the first year of therapy and with doses above 7.5 mg of prednisone. Thus fractures are very common, especially vertebral fractures, which occur in 30% to 50% of corticosteroid-treated patients; the risk of vertebral and hip fractures is generally more than doubled.[114] Patients undergoing organ transplantation may have a higher fracture risk than other steroid-treated patients, perhaps because of the preexisting condition and the osteopenic effect of other immunosuppressive drugs. One of the main problems with corticosteroid treatment is the minimal effective dose to avoid side effects. Some evidence suggests that corticosteroid-induced inhi-

Table 13-2. Diseases and Treatments Contributing to Osteoporosis

Endocrine disorders
  Hyperthyroidism
  Hyperparathyroidism
  Type 1 diabetes mellitus
Conditions associated with hypogonadism
  Hemochromatosis
  Turner's syndrome
  Klinefelter's syndrome
  Postchemotherapy
  Hypopituitarism
  Anorexia nervosa
Inflammatory disorders
  Rheumatoid arthritis
  Ankylosing spondyloarthritis
  Lupus erythematosus
Disorders associated with malabsorption
  Celiac disease
  Gastrectomy
  Chronic liver diseases
  Total parenteral nutrition
  Inflammatory bowel disease
Conditions associated with immobilization
  Parkinson's disease
  Poliomyelitis
  Cerebral palsy
  Paraplegia
Bone marrow disorders
  Multiple myeloma
  Mastocytosis
  Leukemia
Disorders of connective tissues
  Osteogenesis imperfecta
  Marfan's syndrome
  Homocystinuria
Drugs
  Corticosteroids
  Medroxyprogesterone acetate
  Anticonvulsants
  Methotrexate
  Heparin
Cyclosporine
Miscellaneous
  Pregnancy/lactation
  Hypercalciuria
  Alcohol
  Caffeine

bition of bone formation occurs even with low doses of inhaled corticosteroids, with a marked decrease in serum osteocalcin.[115] With oral corticosteroids, the increase in fracture risk starts as low as 2.5 mg/day.[116] Data from cross-sectional and prospective studies suggest that the bone mass of asthmatic patients treated with inhaled corticosteroids is lower than that of controls, in a dose-dependent fashion.[117] The increased fracture risk rapidly offsets on cessation of therapy.[118] BMD values are not good predictors of fracture risk in patients on corticosteroids, since the risks start to rise with T score around 0.0.[119]

Endocrine Diseases

Sex hormone deficiency in both genders results in bone loss. All diseases and drugs that reduce sex hormone levels are associated with bone loss, and the list includes athletic amenorrhea, anorexia nervosa, hemochromatosis, Turner's syndrome, Klinefelter's syndrome, numerous chemotherapeutic regimens, hypopituitarism, or treatment with luteinizing hormone–releasing hormone analogs for endometriosis. In type 1 diabetes mellitus, small and variable decreases in bone density have been reported. In type 2 diabetes, BMD seems to be increased, perhaps because of increased body weight and hyperinsulinemia, but fracture risk seems to rise, perhaps due to impairment in bone quality. Cushing's syndrome leads to bone loss that is reversible after treatment of the disease. Thyroid hormones are major activators of bone remodeling.

Patients with hyperthyroidism are subject to high-turnover osteoporosis with or without mild hypercalcemia, and they have an increased risk of fracture.[49] The decrease in BMD in thyrotoxic patients is reversible after treatment of the hyperthyroidism.[120] The deleterious effects of supraphysiologic doses of thyroid hormone on bone may also occur (but to a lesser extent) in patients who receive suppressive doses of thyroxin for the treatment of thyroid carcinomas and nontoxic goiter. Conversely, hypothyroidism does not seem to significantly affect BMD. The potential role of calcitonin deficiency in bone loss after thyroidectomy is unclear.

Studies by DXA in mild primary hyperparathyroidism have shown that bone density is reduced in regions of cortical bone but is normal in areas of cancellous bone. This decrease in BMD is likely to increase the risk of fracture. Skeletal recovery after surgical treatment of parathyroid adenoma is very significant, with an increased BMD of about 6% at the femoral neck and 8% at the spine 1 year after surgery.[121] This improvement is sustained 10 years after surgery. These patients were the more severely affected patients whose surgery was dictated by the guidelines of the National Institutes of Health.

Gastrointestinal Diseases

All diseases associated with impairment in calcium and/or vitamin D absorption may induce bone loss and include disorders such as celiac disease, inflammatory bowel syndromes, jejuno-ileal bypasses, pancreatic insufficiency, gastrectomy, chronic liver diseases, or prolonged total parenteral nutrition. The decrease in bone density is sometimes due to osteomalacia rather than osteoporosis per se. The origin of gastrointestinal-induced osteoporosis can be multifactorial and could include, for example, the role of corticosteroid therapy in the case of inflammatory bowel diseases.

Bone Marrow Diseases

Multiple myeloma is generally characterized by osteolytic lesions but often induces generalized bone loss. Vertebral crush fractures are also very common. Histomorphometric studies of bone have shown a marked uncoupling between increased resorption and decreased formation that may be due to the secretion of IL-1, IL-6, Dickkopf 1 (DKK1), and TNF-β by plasma cells and other cells of the marrow environment. Corticosteroid therapy and immobilization can also contribute to this bone loss. Acute leukemia in children and adolescents, rather than lymphomas, is sometimes associated with generalized osteoporosis with or without osteolytic lesions. Systemic mastocytosis is a rare disease caused by the proliferation of mast cells infiltrating the skin, bone marrow, spleen, liver, and lymph nodes. Skeletal involvement may be focal or generalized, and about 70% of patients have radiographic abnormalities, including osteosclerotic lesions but also generalized osteopenia and vertebral fractures. In the absence of typical skin lesions, bone biopsy is often the only way to diagnose mastocytosis.

Other Conditions

Rheumatologic conditions such as rheumatoid arthritis and ankylosing spondylitis are associated with osteoporosis and an increased rate of fracture. Pregnancy is very uncommonly associated with bone loss in the last trimester. At intakes higher than 40 g of ethanol per day, alcoholism increases the risk of osteoporotic fractures, particularly in men. In addition to the direct effect of alcohol on osteoblasts, the role of hypogonadism and liver disease may be of importance. Caffeine consumption has also been associated with reduced bone mass and hip fracture risk in some studies.[49,59] Medroxyprogesterone acetate is a progestational agent that suppresses gonadotropin, thus causing anovulation and hypoestrogenemia. Its prolonged use is associated with decreased spinal bone density in about 10%. Other drugs, such as some anticonvulsants, methotrexate, heparin, and cyclosporine, may increase the risk of osteoporosis. More recently, aromatase inhibitors[58] and the thiazolidinediones used in the treatment of type 2 diabetes have been found to increase fracture risk.[122]

OSTEOPOROSIS IN YOUNG ADULTS

A few young adults have osteoporotic fractures corresponding to either mild osteogenesis imperfecta or idiopathic osteoporosis. Osteogenesis imperfecta is an inherited syndrome characterized by fragile bones and recurrent fractures that can lead to skeletal deformities.[123] Inheritance and phenotypic expression are very heterogeneous. Clinical features of osteogenesis imperfecta also include short stature, blue sclerae, dentinogenesis imperfecta, hearing loss, scoliosis, and joint laxity. Osteogenesis imperfecta generally results from mutations of type I collagen.

Idiopathic juvenile osteoporosis is a very rare condition[123] of children and adolescents before puberty. This disease does not seem to be of familial origin. Vertebral fractures usually occur over a 2- to 4-year period. In severe cases, patients may have deformities of the extremities and kyphoscoliosis.

Idiopathic adult osteoporosis is more often recognized because bone densitometry is more widely available. Although the condition may resemble mild osteogenesis imperfecta, these patients do not have dentinogenesis imperfecta, blue sclerae, or hearing loss. They do, however, have joint laxity and mild scoliosis, and a familial history is sometimes found.[123]

OSTEOPOROSIS IN MEN

Fractures are more prevalent in men than in women from childhood to middle life, probably because of a higher incidence of trauma. After 40 years of age, fractures are less common in men than in women, but the incidence of fracture as a result of mild trauma increases with aging. The incidence of hip fracture in men rises exponentially with age, as in women. The sex ratio (female to male) is about 2 : 1 in northern Europe, but it may vary in other areas and reflects the lower life expectancy of men. Mortality related to hip fracture is significantly higher in men than in women. Although vertebral deformities are common in men, many of them are unrelated to osteoporosis. Vertebral fractures in men are associated with height loss, kyphosis, and increased disability, as in women. The incidence of osteoporotic vertebral fractures seems to be half that in women.[23] Vertebral fracture in men is associated with lower BMD than in controls.[124] The incidence of limb fracture begins to rise at a later age in men than in women.

As in women, osteoporosis in men can result from an inadequate peak bone mass and/or accelerated bone loss. As discussed later, gonadal status may be critical for the achievement of peak bone mass in the male. Age-related bone loss is less pronounced in men than in women, around 15% to 20% from 30 to 80 years of age. The mechanisms underlying bone loss with aging in men are unknown, but some evidence indicates decreased osteoblastic activity in males with idiopathic osteoporosis.[125] In elderly men, secondary hyperparathyroidism may contribute to bone loss.

The same risk factors for fragility fractures have been described in men and women and include smoking and excessive alcohol intake; these factors are often combined in a man with osteoporosis. About 50% of men with osteoporosis are considered to have secondary osteoporosis. The most common causes are chronic glucocorticoid therapy, hypogonadism, alcoholism, gastrectomy, and other gastrointestinal disorders. Male hypogonadism has a major influence on the occurrence of osteoporosis. Peak bone mass may be impaired by disorders of puberty, and men with abnormal or delayed puberty have reduced bone mass.[126] Estrogen status is believed to be critical for the acquisition of peak bone mass in men since the observation that aromatase deficiency in a man, resulting in estrogen deficiency, led to the absence of epiphyseal closure and to osteopenia, abnormalities that can be successfully treated with estrogen.[127] Androgens are also essential for the maintenance of bone mass in adult men insofar as hypogonadism in men is associated with low bone mass. Osteoporosis is encountered in many forms of hypogonadism, such as hyperprolactinemia, castration, anorexia, hemochromatosis, and Klinefelter's syndrome. Prolonged abuse of alcohol has detrimental effects on the skeleton, with reduced bone mass resulting mainly from impaired osteoblast activity, nutritional deficiencies, and hypogonadism. Gastrointestinal disorders, particularly gastrectomy, are also associated with osteoporosis in men. Some but not all studies have linked nephrolithiasis or hypercalciuria with reduced bone mass, but their impact on the mechanisms of bone loss remains unclear.

The absolute risk of various osteoporotic fractures is similar in men and women with the same BMD level, but fewer men than women have a low BMD, and men are generally older if they reach such low levels.[128] This difference in age and biomechanical factors such as bone size may also modulate the influence of BMD on fracture risk. There is currently no consensus on T scores that may be used as thresholds for therapeutic decision making in men. The −2.5 cutoff T score (if the reference values are obtained from a male population) is often used, given the similar relationship between BMD and fracture in men and women. The FRAX calculator[69] can also be used in men to assess the individual probability of fracture, but the T score to enter in the software must be calculated using a reference curve obtained with women data (NHANES III database).

Pathology

HISTOMORPHOMETRY

Bone histomorphometry of the iliac crest allows an assessment of bone structure and turnover and is usually performed on transiliac bone biopsy samples. The specimen is processed without prior decalcification and analyzed with standardized histomorphometric methods. Histomorphometry is the only method to differentiate the cell and tissue level of remodeling. Nowadays, noninvasive techniques such as DXA and bone markers are sufficient for most clinical situations involving osteoporosis, and very few indications for bone biopsy still remain. Histomorphometry should be restricted to patients whose history, examination, radiographs, or biochemical profile suggests the possibility of atypical osteomalacia, mast cell bone

disease, nonsecreting myeloma, sarcoidosis, or other rare conditions.

Diagnosis

Investigation of patients with osteoporosis is intended to fulfill the following purposes:

- To establish the diagnosis and eliminate the possibility of conditions mimicking osteoporosis
- To identify factors contributing to osteoporosis
- To determine the prognosis of the disease, with quantification of bone mass, identification of previous fractures, identification of factors that influence the risk of fractures independently of bone mass, and assessment of the rate of bone loss with biochemical markers
- To select the most appropriate treatment
- To obtain baseline measurements that can be useful for monitoring treatment efficacy

DIFFERENTIAL DIAGNOSIS AND CAUSES OF OSTEOPOROSIS

Evaluation of a patient suspected of having osteoporosis includes an adequate history and physical examination, and it must assess the potential causes of secondary osteoporosis and diseases mimicking osteoporosis. Biological abnormalities are commonly found in osteoporotic women, but few major medical problems are identified with screening,[129] and routine laboratory testing may not be cost effective.[130] However, a biochemical profile is necessary in patients with vertebral fractures, including assays of serum calcium, phosphate, creatinine, 25-hydroxycholecalciferol [25(OH)D], and alkaline phosphatase; serum protein electrophoresis; test for proteinuria; urine calcium; and in some cases, urine protein immunoelectrophoresis and blood cell count. Thyroid-stimulating hormone measurement and, in men, total and bioavailable testosterone and prolactin assays may be useful in some cases. In the elderly, 25(OH)D and PTH assays are appropriate when vitamin D deficiency is suspected. Assessment is guided by the clinical findings because some patients with apparent primary osteoporosis turn out to have mild hyperparathyroidism, osteomalacia, systemic mastocytosis, or late appearance of atypical osteogenesis imperfecta.

A complete examination of the spine is often necessary in patients with osteoporosis and includes height measurement and assessment of pain, paraspinal muscle contraction, thoracic kyphosis and lumbar lordosis, scoliosis, and the gap between the costal margin and the iliac crest, as well as the abdomen protrusion that can result from multiple vertebral fractures. Blue sclerae, joint hyperelasticity, and signs in favor of hyperthyroidism or hyperadrenocorticism should be looked for. A general examination is also important to rule out a neoplasm (e.g., lymph node and breast palpation) or other conditions.

RADIOLOGIC EVALUATION

The estimation of spine BMD on conventional radiographs is insensitive and inaccurate because the subjective assessment is dependent on radiographic exposure, patient size, and film-processing techniques. BMD has to decline by as much as a third before it can be detected on plain radiographs. The radiographic manifestation of osteopenia of the axial skeleton includes increased radiolucency of the vertebrae, sometimes vertical striation, framed appearance of the vertebrae ("empty box" or "picture framing") and increased concavity of the vertebral endplates

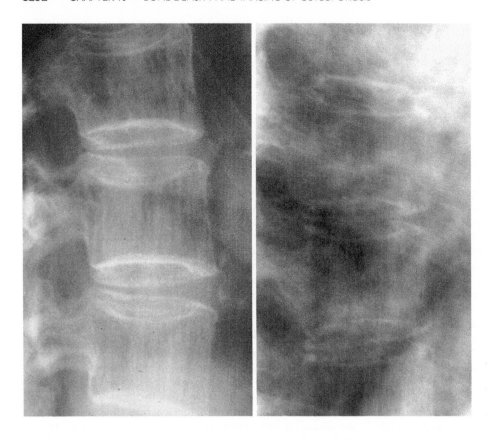

FIGURE 13-4. Reinforcement of the vertical primary trabeculae and loss of the horizontal trabeculae in postmenopausal osteoporosis led to vertical striations on a radiograph of the lumbar and thoracic spine, combined with an overall radiolucency and "empty box" appearance.

resulting from protrusion of the intervertebral disk into the weakened vertebral body (Fig. 13-4).[131] Those signs of osteopenia, however, do not reflect the bone mineral status accurately, so they have been replaced by bone densitometry.

Radiographs are important tools to confirm fractures and their potential etiology. Plain radiographs with anteroposterior and lateral views are required for both the thoracic and lumbar spine. Vertebral fractures include wedge deformities, endplate ("biconcave") deformities, and compression (or crush) fractures (Fig. 13-5). Some vertebral deformities unrelated to osteoporosis include Scheuermann's disease, malignancies, and osteomalacia. The diagnosis of mild vertebral fracture can be difficult because of the overlap with the normal range of vertebral body shape. Algorithms to define vertebral fractures that were developed for epidemiologic studies and clinical trials have led to a consensus proposal for the radiologic diagnosis of vertebral fractures.[132]

Vertebral fracture evaluation, however, may be challenging because of a considerable variability in fracture identification if clinicians or radiologists interpret radiographs without specific training. Several qualitative and quantitative methods have been developed to standardize visual vertebral fracture evaluation, but the most widely used currently is Genant's semiquantitative assessment.[133] Vertebral fractures are distinguished from other nonfracture deformities, and the severity of the vertebral fracture is assessed by visual determination of the magnitude of vertebral height reduction and morphologic change. The type of deformity (wedge, biconcave, compression) is not linked to the extent of vertebral height reduction—that is, the grading of the fracture. Vertebrae from T4 to L4 are graded on visual inspection as normal (grade 0), mildly deformed (grade 1, 20% to 25% in anterior, middle, and/or posterior height), moderately deformed (grade 2, 25% to 40% in anterior, middle, and/or posterior height), and severely deformed (grade 3, >40% in anterior, middle, and/or posterior height) (Fig. 13-6). Semiquantitative

interpretation has excellent intraobserver and interobserver precision, provided careful training and standardization have been applied.[133,134]

The axial skeleton is not the only site where changes due to osteoporosis can be observed. Widening of the medullary canal and thinning of the cortices is commonly described in older individuals as a result of longstanding endosteal bone resorption in the appendicular skeleton (Fig. 13-7). Conventional radiographs can also be used to assess the bone structure, with image procedures relying on texture or fractal analyses.[135]

A variety of diseases and medications are associated with bone loss, but some differences can be seen in the appearance of those secondary osteoporoses compared with postmenopausal or senile osteoporosis. The characteristic radiographic appearance of Cushing's or corticosteroid-induced osteoporosis, in the extreme, consists of a marginal condensation of the fractured vertebral bodies, resulting from exuberant callus formation (Fig. 13-8). Primary hyperparathyroidism may affect all bone surfaces and result in subperiosteal, intracortical, endosteal, subchondral, and trabecular bone resorption. Those signs, however, are seldom encountered because most patients with primary hyperparathyroidism have mild forms of the disease. In osteomalacia, radiographic abnormalities include osteopenia, non-sharp delineation of cortical bone, deformities, and stress and true fractures. Hyperparathyroidism secondary to renal insufficiency associates vertebral osteosclerosis, amyloid deposits, avascular necrosis, and vascular calcifications (Fig. 13-9A,B). The typical radiographic appearance of steroid-induced osteoporosis consists of a marginal condensation of the fractured vertebral bodies secondary to exuberant callus formation. In multiple myeloma, the radiographic appearance of spine radiographs can imitate osteoporosis, and other diagnostic procedures like skull radiographs (Fig. 13-10) or protein electrophoresis will make the diagnosis. Additional imaging techniques such as computed tomography

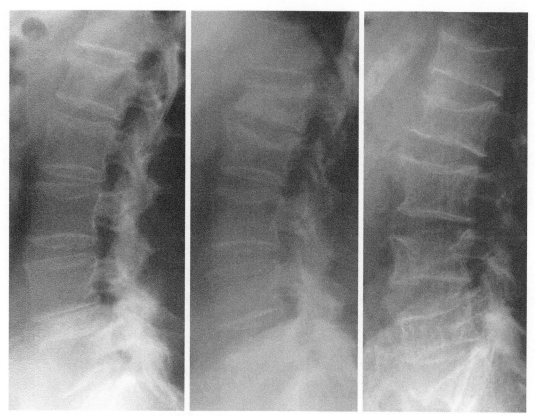

FIGURE 13-5. Progressive evolution of spinal osteoporosis in a postmenopausal woman with vertebral fracture cascade, at baseline, 10, and 20 years.

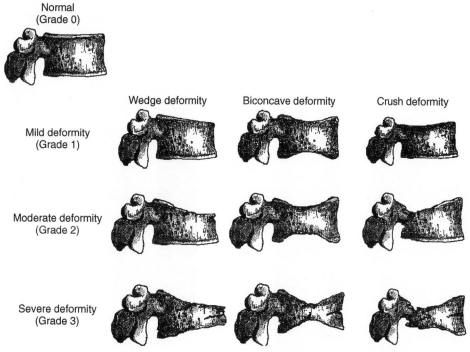

FIGURE 13-6. Schematic representations of wedge, biconcave, and crush vertebral deformities with grading normal to severe deformity. The figure illustrates the semiquantitative visual grading system of Genant. (Drawn by C.Y. Wu.)

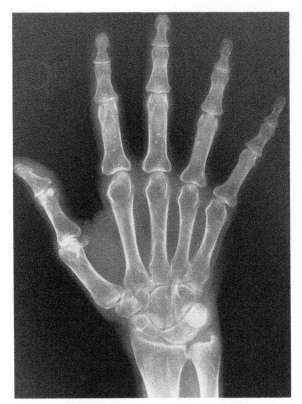

FIGURE 13-7. PA radiograph of the hand in an elderly osteoporotic woman showing severe diffuse cortical thinning, principally by endosteal resorption.

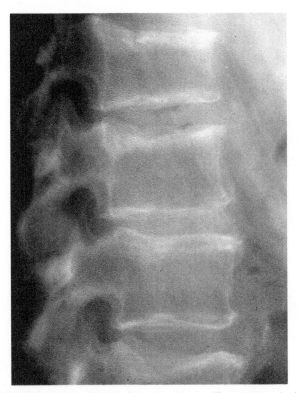

FIGURE 13-8. Lateral radiograph of the spine showing diffuse osteoporosis, dense thickened endplate, or marginal sclerosis, all characteristic of Cushing's- or steroid-induced secondary osteoporosis.

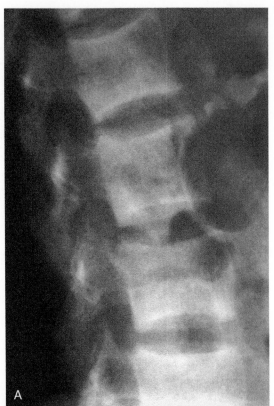

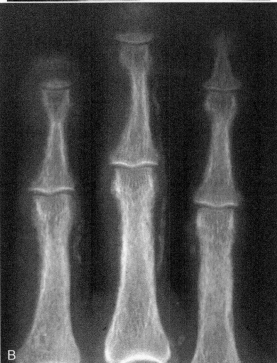

FIGURE 13-9. **A,** Lateral radiograph of the lumbar spine showing typical changes of renal osteodystrophy with rugger jersey spine. **B,** PA radiograph of the fingers shows tuft and subperiosteal resorption and vascular calcification.

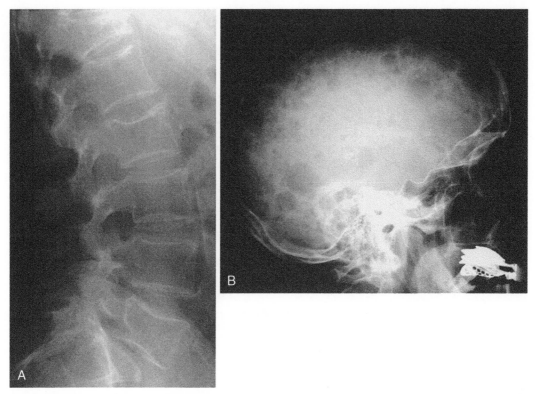

FIGURE 13-10. Changes in the spine in multiple myeloma **(A),** here seen with increased radiolucency and vertebral deformities, may easily be confused with osteoporotic changes. However, additional typical lesions at other sites (besides clinical features and relatively typical laboratory values) may reveal the nature of the underlying disease. In this example, multiple osteolytic lesions in the skull **(B)** support the diagnosis of multiple myeloma.

(CT), magnetic resonance imaging (MRI), and bone scintigraphy may be useful in the differential diagnosis of the various conditions associated with osteoporosis or vertebral fractures (e.g., trauma [Fig. 13-11], multiple myeloma [Fig. 13-12], storage diseases, leukemia, sickle cell anemia, and thalassemia). Bone scintigraphy or MRI are the ideal techniques to diagnose sacrum stress fracture (Fig. 13-13) that may be encountered in elderly patients with osteoporosis or osteomalacia.

BONE MASS MEASUREMENTS

Measurement of bone mass is a critical step in the investigation of an osteoporotic patient to (1) confirm the reduction in bone mass and (2) assess the magnitude of bone loss and therefore the risk of further fracture. Some of the terms may be confusing, so they need to be defined.[136] What is measured with the various densitometric techniques is an apparent density, including the bone itself and the bone marrow. The term *bone mineral density* is related to the mass of bone tissue. The true bone mineral density—the mass of bone per unit volume, excluding the marrow and non-bone tissue—is not determined. DXA provides an areal apparent bone density because of a two-dimensional image, so the density is expressed as the bone density per unit area, not per volume, in g/cm^2. Even if QCT provides a volumetric bone density, usually expressed in mg/cm^3, it is also an apparent density, because it includes the marrow spaces of vertebrae.

DUAL X-RAY ABSORPTIOMETRY

Technical Principles

The physical principle of DXA is to measure the attenuation of x-rays with two different energies through the body, thus accounting for variable soft-tissue thickness and composition, at sites like the axial skeleton, the hip, and the whole body. The dual x-ray can be generated by either K-edge filters or kVp switching. The preferred anatomic sites for BMD measurement are the lumbar spine (L1 to L4) and the proximal femur (Fig. 13-14), although the whole body and peripheral sites can also be scanned (calcaneus, distal forearm). Measurement of attenuation of the x-ray photons of two distinct energies also allows accurate assessment of body fat content.[137] The areal density that is measured by DXA is an integral of both cortical and trabecular BMC normalized to the size of the projected area. Scan times have been shortened from about 5 to 10 minutes for pencil-beam scanners to 10 to 30 seconds for the fan-beam systems, which perform a single sweep across the patient instead of a two-dimensional raster scan. Fan-beam systems also allow for easier identification of vertebral structures and artifacts because of better image resolution, but at the expense of greater x-ray exposure.

The x-ray tube, the detectors, and the hardware are never perfectly stable, so there is a need to compensate for day-to-day variations in measurements. A set of stable calibration standards are acquired each day before assessing patient data; some machines have internal calibration systems to monitor the densitometer performance continuously.

The radiation dose to patients is small (0.08 to 4.6 μSv) compared with other techniques using ionizing radiation. Fan-beam technology has increased the dose (6.7 to 31 μSv), which is still acceptable. Measuring vertebral morphometry by DXA also delivers less radiation (<60 μSv) than do lateral radiographs. The greater scatter dose from fan-beam DXA systems approaches limits set by regulatory bodies for occupational exposure.

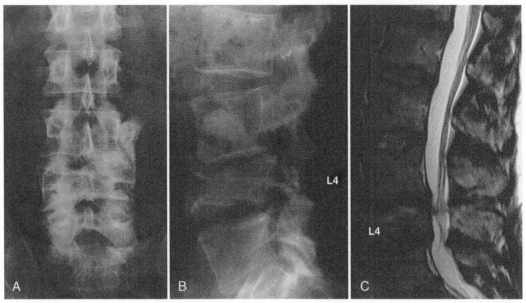

FIGURE 13-11. Conventional radiographs of the lumbar spine in the anteroposterior **(A)** and lateral **(B)** views reveal an old traumatic fracture of the fourth lumbar vertebra, resulting in instability of the lumbar spine and modest spinal stenosis, as shown on the corresponding MRI **(C)**.

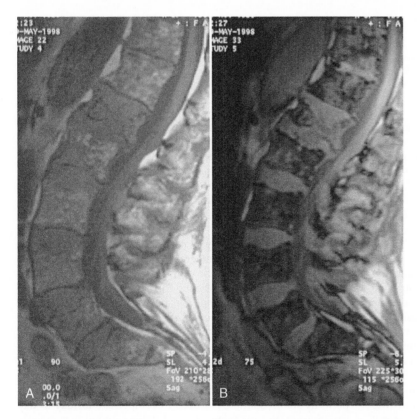

FIGURE 13-12. MRI of the spine in patients with multiple myeloma may give information on the infiltration of spinal bone marrow. In this patient, a diffuse infiltration pattern may be seen on T1-weighted spin echo **(A)** and gradient echo **(B)** images. In addition, the patient has a pathologic fracture of the first lumbar vertebra.

Diagnostic Use

Several sites can be measured with DXA. The spine measurement is limited to the lumbar spine, because the thoracic spine evaluation would be compounded by air in the lungs and ribs and sternum overlying the scan field. The scan usually includes L1 to L4 (sometimes L2 to L4). The spine should be centered in the scan field and properly aligned. One should remain alert to artifacts such as those induced by patient movement. The presence of vertebral fracture, deformities, osteoarthritis, aortic cal-

cification, or curvature such as scoliosis modifies BMD,[138] so in individuals older than 65 or 70 years, those commonly affected by osteoarthritis, the spine measurement is often of limited clinical utility. On the DXA report, large differences in vertebral height, area, BMC, and/or BMD suggest fracture or degenerative changes. Affected vertebral bodies should be excluded from the analysis; the entire spine scan is often discarded because of these kinds of artifacts. The hip DXA scan includes the proximal end of the femur and a portion of the pelvis. Only the proximal femur bone is assessed. Small changes in femur rotation can induce

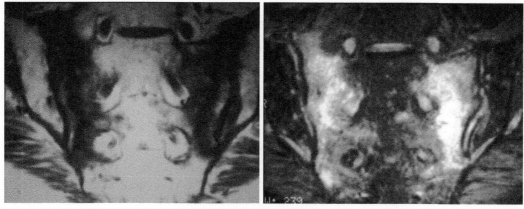

FIGURE 13-13. Coronal T1-weighted and T2-weighted images of the sacrum show bilateral sacral insufficiency fractures in an elderly osteoporotic woman.

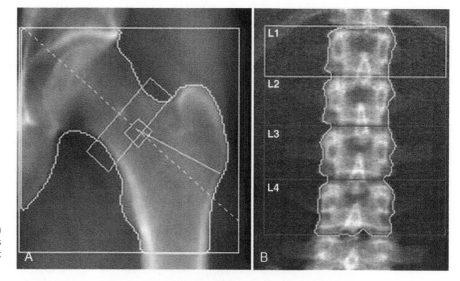

FIGURE 13-14. Fan-beam dual x-ray absorptiometry (DXA) scan of **(A)** the hip (*oblong box*, femoral neck; *box*, Ward's area; trochanter, shaft, and total), and **(B)** regions of interest analyzed in the spine (L1-4).

significant changes in hip BMD,[139] so special positioning devices are typically used to position the measured limb at 15 to 30 degrees inward rotation. This way, the femoral neck is visible because it is aligned to the table and perpendicular to the x-ray beam. The right and left hips being similar within an individual, one can choose either side and repeat measurements on the same side. If degenerative changes, previous fracture, localized bone disease (hip osteonecrosis, Paget's disease of bone, etc,) affect only one hip, the scan will be performed on the opposite side. On the report image, the lesser trochanter should be only slightly visible, indicating an appropriate rotation. Machines evaluate different regions of the hip, including the femoral neck, the trochanteric region, Ward's triangle, and the total region. The diagnosis relies on the femoral neck and total regions values. The forearm can also be measured, typically on the nondominant side. The radial shaft is a good indicator of cortical bone density. Total body scans mainly reflect the cortical bone and are very precise. They are generally performed to assess body composition parameters such as lean and fat mass.

Several prospective studies have shown that BMD measured by DXA at various skeletal sites (spine, hip, forearm, calcaneus, total body) predicts the risk of fragility fractures, with a relative risk of 1.5 to 3.0 for each 1-SD decrease in BMD.[4] The prediction of fracture is higher when BMD is measured at the site of fracture—for example, measuring hip BMD for hip fracture.

Although BMD is commonly measured at the spine and hip, measuring multiple sites has little advantage.

The most convenient way to describe BMD is by T scores and Z scores. The *T score* is the number of standard deviations above or below the mean for young adults. The WHO definition of osteoporosis is based on the T score (see earlier). The T score declines with aging. The *Z score* is the number of standard deviations above or below the mean for people of the same age. The Z score permits a comparison of patients with a reference population of the same age and therefore allows detection of bone loss that is excessive for age. The high prevalence of osteoporosis in the elderly, however, as well as the difficulty in selecting a population adequate to establish a reference range of values in the elderly, limits use of the Z score. From a practical perspective, the diagnostic thresholds proposed by the WHO can be applied effectively to spine and hip DXA measurement. Therapeutic thresholds should include not only the BMD T score but also age and risk factors that predict the risk of fracture independently of BMD.

Observed changes on follow-up should not be due to precision errors. The bone content and area should be checked for consistency. The precision error—expressed as a coefficient of variation (CV)—is usually around 1% at the spine and 1.5% to 2% at the hip. This precision error should be evaluated in a group of subjects representative of the clinic population setting.

The precision error can be estimated by measuring a group of 14 individuals, each at least three times, with interim repositioning.[140] The least significant change—the minimal BMD variation considered statistically significant within an individual—is calculated as $2 \times \sqrt{2} \times CV$. Thus, the least significant change in BMD is generally around 3% at the spine and 5% to 6% at the femoral neck. The precision error can also be expressed as an absolute BMD value difference, which is more accurate for extreme BMD values.

Limitations

First, measurement of the spine is often more difficult to interpret in persons older than 65 years because of the high prevalence of degenerative osteoarthritic changes, which will increase the apparent BMD reading without accurately measuring trabecular bone. Second, the accuracy of the technique is reduced in obese subjects. Third, repeated measurements may have limited value in assessing the rate of change in BMD because the expected percent change in BMD is the same magnitude as the precision error of the technique. Variations in technologist performance will adversely affect the precision of the exam. The same scan mode and parameters should be used at follow-up as those on the baseline examination. A 3- to 5-year interval between two measurements may be necessary in untreated postmenopausal women to detect fast BMD losers. In patients treated with antiresorptive therapy, a 2-year interval is usually necessary to detect a significant increase in BMD.

Contraindications

Pregnancy, recent administration of oral contrast media or radioisotopes, spinal deformity, and orthopedic hardware contraindicate DXA. BMD results can also be affected by metal objects such as belts and buttons. Severe obesity and small stature also undermine the interpretation of BMD results.

OTHER TECHNIQUES
Quantitative Computed Tomography

QCT measures the volumetric BMD of the lumbar spine and proximal femur, allows differentiation between cortical and trabecular BMD, and provides a sensitive measure of compartmental changes; however, it has several drawbacks, including relatively high radiation exposure and a higher precision error than that of DXA.[136,141] QCT was originally implemented to determine bone mineral density in single slices through the midsections of the lumbar vertebral bodies (Fig. 13-15) or the distal radius.[136,141,142] With the advent of whole body multislice/multidetector (spiral) CT, a technique in which the examination table is continually advanced during data acquisition and one that allows more rapid scanning of large sections of the body, three-dimensional volumetric QCT (vQCT) techniques were developed. These advances improved the precision for measuring spine or hip from approximately 2% to 3% for single-slice to approximately 1% to 2% for volumetric measurements and enhanced the sensitivity and accuracy of the original approach by covering larger volumes.[143-145] As a volumetric technique, vQCT can determine BMD or bone mineral content of the entire bone or of specified subregions and, similar to single-slice QCT, can provide a separate analysis of the trabecular or cortical components. Geometric measurements, such as cross-sectional area or hip axis length, and derivation of mechanical properties, such as cross-sectional moment of inertia, are possible (Fig. 13-16). For further central skeletal analyses, the vQCT data can be used for high-resolution imaging of bone structure[146,147] and for finite

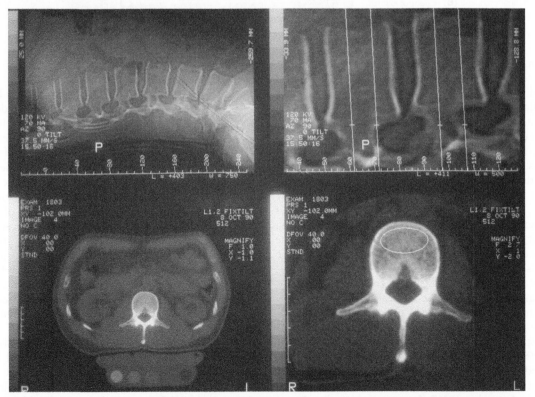

FIGURE 13-15. Traditional quantitative computed tomography (QCT) with single slice per vertebra is illustrated, along with the scout localization, the simultaneously scanned phantom, and the ellipse region of interest in the vertebral centrum.

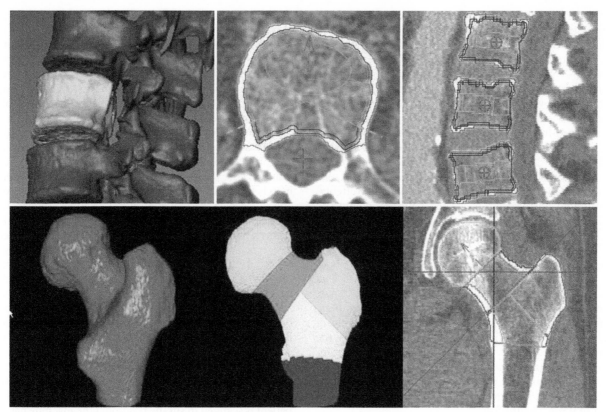

FIGURE 13-16. Volumetric quantitative computed tomography of the spine *(top)* and hip *(bottom)* may be used to analyze bone mineral density (BMD) in various bone compartments and to accurately measure BMD and geometry. *Top left,* Segmented vertebral body selected for analysis with removed processes. *Top center and right,* Integral and trabecular and peeled trabecular volumes of interest along with the traditional elliptical and Pacman volumes of interest (VOIs). *Bottom left,* Segmented proximal femur. *Bottom center and right,* Analysis VOIs in the hip.

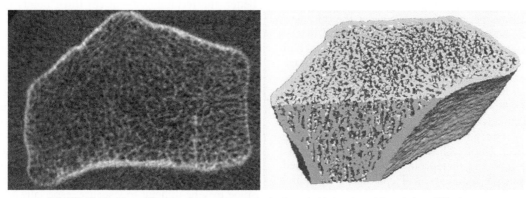

FIGURE 13-17. Micro-CT of the distal radial metaphysic at nominal isotropic spatial resolution of 90 microns.

element analysis (FEA).[148,149] This technique computes distributions of mechanical stress and strain throughout the bone under simulated loading conditions in an iterative process. Finite element modeling may improve the assessment of bone strength and the prediction of fracture healing, because it integrates the geometric and densitometric information that has been acquired from the QCT scan.

High-Resolution Peripheral Quantitative Computed Tomography

HR-pQCT allows for three-dimensional evaluation of BMD and quantification of architecture. These devices were introduced more than 10 years ago, but their performance has been improved

more recently, with machines evaluating trabecular architecture and volumetric BMD at the distal radius and tibia with a nominal isotropic voxel size of 82 μm (Fig. 13-17). Precision of HR-pQCT measurements was 0.7% to 1.5% for total, trabecular, and cortical densities and 2.5% to 4.4% for trabecular architecture.[150] In the OFELY cohort, postmenopausal women had lower density, trabecular number, and cortical thickness than premenopausal women at both radius and tibia. Osteoporotic women had lower density, cortical thickness, and increased trabecular separation than osteopenic women at both sites. Furthermore, although spine and hip BMD were similar, fractured osteopenic women had lower trabecular density and more heterogeneous trabecular distribution at the radius compared with unfractured osteopenic women.[150] At the distal radius, women with fractures had lower volumetric total (D tot), trabecular (D trab) BMDs, trabecular bone volume (BV/TV), cortical thickness (Cort Th), trabecular number (TbN), trabecular thickness (TbTh), and higher trabecular separation (TbSp) and distribution of trabecular separation (TbSpSd) than controls without fractures. In a logistic model, each SD decrease of volumetric total and trabecular densities was associated with a significantly increased risk of fracture at both sites (ORs ranged from 2.00 to 2.47). After adjusting for aBMD measured by DXA at the ultradistal radius, differences between cases and controls remained significant for D trab, and there was a similar trend for TbN, TbSp, and TbSpSd, with adjusted ORs ranging from 1.32 to 1.50. In postmenopausal women, vertebral and nonvertebral fractures are associated with low volumetric BMD and architectural alterations of trabecular and cortical bone that can be assessed noninvasively and that are partially independent of aBMD assessed by DXA.[151] Assessment of bone mechanical properties by FEA may improve identification of those at high risk for fracture. The three-dimensional data obtained with HR-pQCT may help to achieve this goal. Thus, the proportion of load carried by cortical versus trabecular bone seemed to be associated with wrist fracture independently of BMD and microarchitecture in the same set of women from the OFELY cohort. These results suggest that bone mechanical properties assessed by microFE may provide information about skeletal fragility and fracture risk not assessed by BMD or architecture measurements alone and are therefore likely to enhance the prediction of wrist fracture risk.[152]

Quantitative Ultrasonography

Quantitative ultrasonography may be a surrogate technique for DXA and may provide additional information on the material properties of bone. Ultrasound velocity (speed of sound) and ultrasound attenuation through bone (broadband attenuation) are recorded at various peripheral bones such as the calcaneus, patella, phalanges, and tibia.[153] In general, ultrasound devices have a low precision error, but their accuracy is unknown. Both speed of sound and broadband attenuation decrease with age, with a magnitude that varies considerably from device to device. Prospective studies have shown that ultrasound measurement of the os calcis is a valid predictor of hip fracture risk in elderly women.[153,154] Quantitative ultrasonography is a technique for the broad diagnosis of osteoporosis, with the availability of cheap and portable devices. Until each device is adequately validated and precise diagnostic and therapeutic thresholds are defined, quantitative ultrasound should be still considered a research tool.

WHO SHOULD BE SCREENED WITH DXA?

Even if BMD is an important predictor of fracture risk, it is too insensitive to be used solely as an indication for treatment, so targeted BMD testing of postmenopausal women who have clinical risk factors for fracture or low BMD is generally recommended, rather than universal testing.[155] The U.S. Preventive Services Task Force has concluded that the benefits of BMD testing are clear for all women 65 and older.[156] The use of other risk factors such as smoking, family history, race, decreased physical activity, alcohol or caffeine use, or low calcium intake could not be used to identify women at high risk. Most North American guidelines consider that BMD testing is appropriate in all women aged 65 and older. In younger women, BMD testing should be limited to those with BMD-independent risk factors. In other regions of the world, specifically in Europe, a case

finding strategy is often adopted, so that BMD testing is proposed in women who have risk factors for low bone mass; for example, low BMI, smoking, excessive alcohol consumption, history of steroid use, personal or familial history of fragility fracture, diseases associated with accelerated bone loss (hyperparathyroidism, uncontrolled hyperthyroidism, osteogenesis imperfecta, malabsorption), or premature menopause, regardless of age.

According to the latest recommendations of the U.S. National Osteoporosis Foundation (NOF), the decision to perform bone density assessment should be based on an individual's fracture risk profile and skeletal health assessment. The results of the test must be able to influence the treatment decision. NOF recommends testing of all women aged 65 and older and men aged 70 and older, regardless of clinical risk factors. Younger postmenopausal women and men aged 50 to 69 with clinical risk factors, adults who sustain fracture after age 50, adults with a condition (e.g., rheumatoid arthritis) or taking a medication (e.g., glucocorticoids in a daily dose ≥5 mg prednisone or equivalent for ≥3 months) associated with low bone mass or bone loss should be tested. BMD measurement is not recommended in children or adolescents and is not routinely indicated in healthy young men or premenopausal women. In patients treated for osteoporosis, BMD may be used to monitor treatment effect.

VERTEBRAL FRACTURE ASSESSMENT

With most recent DXA systems, it is possible to scan the entire thoracic and lumbar spine to evaluate vertebral height.[157] The patient is scanned in supine position if the machine has a rotating arm, or in the lateral position. Vertebral bodies can be assessed qualitatively to screen for vertebral deformities, typically using the semiquantitative scoring method also applied to radiographs.[133,134] Those deformities can be quantified with a software that measures the height of vertebral bodies. The computer—or better, the technologist—places three points on the posterior, mid-, and anterior margins of both endplates of each vertebra from T4 to L4 to calculate the vertebral heights. Significant changes in vertebral height are indicative of vertebral fracture. This technique is attractive because evaluation of vertebral fracture prevalence can be performed without a conventional radiograph at the same time as the BMD measurement, thus saving time, unnecessary irradiation, and cost. This is an important advantage because vertebral fractures are often overlooked. The interpretation must be cautious, however, because the image quality is variable across individuals, so the observation of deformities is not synonymous for vertebral fracture and should lead to radiographs for confirmation. In addition, the upper thoracic spine may be difficult to visualize, especially among older individuals, with false-negative readings as a result. The specificity and the negative predictive value remain high despite these limitations, because most vertebral fractures occur at lumbar and lower thoracic levels where the image quality is still acceptable.[158] VFA is now widely used as a screening tool for vertebral fracture.

Biochemical Markers

DIFFERENT TYPES OF MARKERS

Bone markers are usually classified as markers of bone formation and markers of bone resorption (Table 13-3), but in diseases in which both processes are coupled and disclose similar variation, markers reflect the overall rate of bone turnover. Markers cannot

Table 13-3. Biochemical Markers of Bone Turnover

Formation	Resorption
Serum	Plasma or serum
Osteocalcin	Tartrate-resistant acid phosphatase
Bone alkaline phosphatase (total and bone-specific)	Free deoxypyridinoline
Procollagen N-terminal extension peptides (PINPs)	Type I collagen N- and C-telopeptide breakdown products (NTX and CTX)
	Urine
	Free deoxypyridinoline
	Type I collagen N- and C-telopeptide breakdown products (NTX and CTX)

distinguish between bone turnover changes originating in the cortical or in the trabecular envelopes.

Bone Formation Markers

Markers of bone formation are serum total and bone measurements of alkaline phosphatase, osteocalcin, and procollagen I extension peptides. Serum alkaline phosphatase is the most commonly used marker of bone formation but lacks sensitivity and specificity. New assays have been developed to improve specificity in order to separate bone and liver isoenzymes—in particular, immunoassays using monoclonal antibodies with a cross-reactivity of only 15% to 20%.[159] Thus, bone alkaline phosphatase is a sensitive marker of increased turnover in postmenopausal women, and since it is an enzyme activity and not a protein that is cleared by the kidney, it is also a marker of choice in the evaluation of bone turnover in chronic kidney failure.

Serum osteocalcin, also called *bone Gla protein*, is a small (49 amino acids) noncollagenous protein that is specific for bone tissue and dentin and produced only by osteoblasts and odontoblasts. Serum osteocalcin levels correlate with skeletal growth during puberty, as well as with increase in bone formation rate in conditions characterized by increased bone turnover, such as primary and secondary hyperparathyroidism, hyperthyroidism, or acromegaly. Conversely, osteocalcin is decreased in hypothyroidism, hypoparathyroidism, and glucocorticoid-treated patients, conditions associated with a decreased rate of bone formation. When resorption and formation are coupled, serum osteocalcin is a good marker of bone turnover. The most robust and sensitive assays measure both the intact molecule and the N-midfragment (which is the largest product of degradation of osteocalcin).[160] Although osteocalcin was discovered 30 years ago, its function remains elusive.[161] It might be involved in the regulation of energy metabolism, its action depending on its degree of gamma-carboxylation.[162]

Propeptides of type I procollagen (N-terminal and C-terminal extension peptides of type I collagen [PINP and PICP, respectively]) are cleaved during the extracellular processing of collagen. They also reflect bone formation, because type I collagen is the most abundant organic component of bone matrix. PICP exhibits smaller variations in postmenopausal osteoporosis than other markers, so it is probably less useful. However, it seems valuable in the monitoring of growth hormone treatment.[163] After the menopause, PINP augments to a similar extent that osteocalcin and bone alkaline phosphatase does. It is the most sensitive marker to monitor PTH treatment.[164]

Bone Resorption Markers

Markers of bone resorption are fasting urinary calcium and hydroxyproline, plasma tartrate-resistant acid phosphatase (TRAP), and collagen pyridinium cross-links. Fasting urinary

calcium, corrected by creatinine excretion, is the cheapest marker of bone resorption but lacks sensitivity in osteoporosis. Hydroxyproline is derived from the degradation of collagen and has long been used as a routine marker of resorption, but it also lacks sensitivity and specificity.

The most specific of the osteoclasts fraction of TRAP is the b subform of the isoenzyme 5 (TRAP5b). It is the only available marker of the osteoclast metabolic activity. Several drawbacks (e.g., influence of clotting, temperature instability) limit its practical use.

Pyridinoline (Pyr) and deoxypyridinoline (D-Pyr) are nonreducible pyridinium cross-links in the mature form of collagen (Fig. 13-18). This posttranslational covalent cross-linking creates interchain bonds stabilizing the molecule of collagen. Concentration of Pyr and D-Pyr in biological fluids is derived predominantly from bone. Pyr and D-Pyr are released from bone matrix during osteoclastic bone resorption. They are excreted in urine in a free form (around 40%) and in a peptide-bound form (60%). Enzyme-linked immunosorbent assays have been developed against the N-telopeptide to helix (NTX) and against breakdown products of type I collagen C-telopeptide (CTX) in urine and serum. These cross-links are markedly increased at the time of menopause and return to premenopausal levels with estrogen and bisphosphonate therapy.[165]

CLINICAL USE OF BONE MARKERS
Bone Markers for Assessment of Bone Loss

A sharp increase in bone markers occurs after menopause. This increase is sustained long after the start of menopause, even in elderly women, and markers are negatively correlated with bone mass assessed by DXA,[166] which suggests that a high bone turnover rate is associated with increased bone loss. A long-term study suggested that the rate of bone loss measured over 12 years by densitometry is increased in women classified as rapid losers at baseline and significantly higher than that of slow losers.[167] Thus a combination of markers and BMD measurement could be useful in assessment of the risk of osteoporosis.[168]

Bone Markers for Assessment of Fracture Risk

It has been reported that women classified as fast losers have a vertebral and wrist fracture risk double that of those classified as normal or slow losers.[169] Large prospective studies have shown that increased bone resorption (i.e., above the premenopausal values) is associated with an increased risk in vertebral and peripheral fractures, independently of BMD.[170,171] Women with both a low BMD and increased bone resorption had a fourfold to fivefold increase in the risk of hip fracture. Measurements of bone resorption markers may be combined with other risk factors for fracture to calculate individual probability of fracture, but markers do not enter into the calculation of individual probabilities of fracture in the FRAX calculator, because data were not available in most cohorts used in model building.

Bone Markers for Monitoring Treatment of Osteoporosis

Antiresorptive therapies such as calcitonin, estrogen, and bisphosphonates induce a significant decrease in markers, which return to the premenopausal range within 3 to 6 months for resorption markers and within 6 to 9 months for formation markers. The significant decrease in bone turnover seen after treatment of osteoporotic women with a bisphosphonate signifi-

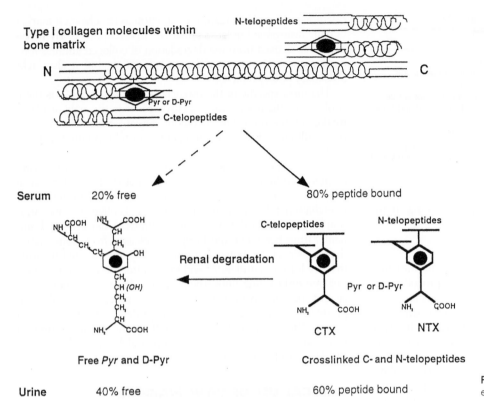

FIGURE 13-18. Degradation of type I collagen and excretion of type I collagen cross-links.

cantly correlates with an increase in BMD at the lumbar spine after 2 years, with a low rate of false-positive and false-negative results.[172] There is also an association between the decrease in bone turnover markers in response to antiresorptive agents such as bisphosphonates or raloxifene and the degree of reduction in fracture risk.[173,174] Given the precision of bone mass measurement with DXA and the expected change induced by antiresorptive treatment, it is usually necessary to wait for 2 years to determine whether the treatment is effective in an individual patient. Determination of markers after a few months of treatment is likely to provide useful information on efficacy and may improve compliance.[175] Therapies stimulating bone formation, such as teriparatide, may be monitored using bone formation markers (e.g., PINP).

Treatment

NONPHARMACOLOGIC INTERVENTION

Lifestyle

Patients who have sustained vertebral fractures need specific guidelines in their daily activities to prevent additional fractures. They should avoid weightlifting and learn how to bend to avoid excessive strain on their spine. All lifestyle factors that might be deleterious to bone metabolism should be corrected. Thus patients should not smoke, they should consume moderate amounts of alcohol, and conditions predisposing to osteoporosis should be treated. Although no controlled trial has shown that cessation of smoking increases BMD or reduces the risk of osteoporotic fractures, sufficient evidence indicates that smoking is a risk factor for vertebral and hip fractures.[48] Drugs predisposing to osteoporosis should be avoided as much as possible.

Nutrition

No universal consensus has been reached on the daily calcium requirement by age, but according the Dietary Reference Intake (DRI) published in 1997,[176] 1300 mg/day is the recommended dose for adolescents, 1000 to 1200 mg/day for adults up to 70 years, and 1200 mg/day after the age of 70 years. Although most studies have shown a beneficial effect of calcium supplementation, as discussed later, the long-term effect of high dietary calcium intake on bone health is unknown. Conversely, there seems to be a threshold of calcium intake—around 400 mg/day—under which increasing calcium intake appears to be beneficial and necessary, both in children and in women older than 60 years.

Several nutritional factors influence the calcium requirement, such as sodium, protein, caffeine, fiber, and vitamin D status. The effect of fiber and caffeine is relatively small, whereas sodium and protein intake may be more relevant because they increase urinary excretion of calcium. A sodium-rich diet has been associated with increased incidence of kidney stones. The effects of phosphorus and fat intake do not substantially influence bone metabolism. Vitamin D promotes calcium absorption and thereby influences calcium requirements. Vitamin D status commonly deteriorates in older people, with serum levels of 25(OH)D lower than those in young adults because of low vitamin D intake and decreased sunlight exposure (see Chapters 3 and 15). NOF recommends an intake of 800 to 1000 international units (IU) of vitamin D per day for adults aged 50 and older. This intake will bring the average adult's serum 25(OH)D concentration to the desired level of 30 ng/mL (75 nmol/L) or higher.[176-179] The low levels of 25(OH)D commonly seen in the elderly, especially those institutionalized, contribute to secondary hyperparathyroidism, which may play a role in bone loss in the elderly.

Exercise

Immobilization induces bone loss, as documented after prolonged bedrest, space flight, paralysis from spinal cord injury, and casting of limbs. The beneficial effect of exercise on bone mass and bone strength in normal and osteoporotic individuals, however, is still unclear. Several controlled trials have looked at the effect of various exercise programs on BMD, including walking, weight training, aerobics, and high-impact and low-impact exercise. Most of them show a small (1% to 2%) increase in BMD in comparison to either baseline or the control group at some but not all skeletal sites; the increase is not sustained once the exercise program is stopped. Both clinical trials and observational studies suggest that load-bearing exercise is more effective in preserving or increasing bone mass than other types of exercise are. The dominant arm of tennis players or the limbs of gymnasts usually have higher bone mass than other sites do.[180] Skeletal sites must be directly strained to be affected by exercise. In addition, it is likely that fitness might indirectly preserve individuals from fractures by improving mobility and reducing the risk of falls. No randomized controlled trial has been conducted to assess the effect of exercise on fracture risk. Because of the many nonskeletal benefits of exercise, it seems appropriate to recommend regular and moderate exercise in postmenopausal women, but it cannot replace pharmacologic prevention. After vertebral fracture, a supervised exercise program to maintain strength and flexibility of the thoracic and lumbar spine is recommended in the elderly.

It is critical to develop specific interventions aimed at preventing falls and their consequences in the elderly. So far, few studies have shown that specific strategies prevent falls. For example, one trial has shown that older men and women trained to practice tai chi regularly (better balance training) were less prone to fall than untrained counterparts.[181]

Given the multifactorial etiology of falls, interventions have to be multidimensional. An adequate exercise program may decrease the risk of falling in the elderly, who should be encouraged to walk at least half an hour per day. Indeed, a sedentary lifestyle leads to low muscle mass, postural alterations, and deconditioning of lower limbs and increases the incidence of falls. Visual impairment is a risk factor for falls and fractures because it results in tripping or slipping accidents and decreases postural stability. Therefore, glasses should be checked regularly and cataracts detected early. Whenever possible, the use of drugs that increase the risk of falling should be reduced; such drugs include benzodiazepines, hypnotics, antidepressant agents, and medications that can induce hypotension. Patients should be instructed to avoid slippery floors and to have adequate lights and handrails in bathrooms and on stairs at home.

Experimental studies have shown that the soft tissues covering the hip may have an impact on energy absorption of the fall. Some clinical trials have shown that hip protectors substantially decrease the risk of hip fracture in elderly people living in institution (up to 80%), but those results were not found in all trials, and poor compliance remains an issue in all studies.[182,183]

PHARMACOLOGIC INTERVENTION

Evaluation of Drug Efficacy

The goal of therapy is to prevent fragility fractures, and drugs for osteoporosis should demonstrate their ability to significantly decrease the incidence of fractures in adequately powered, prospective, randomized placebo-controlled studies. Conducting such placebo-controlled trials has been debated, but they remain the cornerstone of sound drug evaluation.[184] The diagnosis of nonvertebral fractures is easy, whereas the diagnosis of existing and new vertebral fractures requires adequate morphometric evaluation of spinal radiographs to exclude vertebral deformities unrelated to osteoporosis. Changes in BMD are commonly monitored and are usually seen as a surrogate marker of treatment efficacy. Actually, most drugs that inhibit bone turnover induce a small increase in BMD (i.e., 2% to 10% according to the skeletal site of measurement) that does not account for their marked reduction in fracture rate (i.e., 30% to 50% for vertebral fractures). In addition, some drugs—such as fluoride—may induce a marked increase in BMD without decreasing the fracture rate. Bone turnover markers are another surrogate for treatment efficacy of antiresorptive drugs. Their diminution in response to antiresorptive therapies is associated with the decreased fracture rate. High bone turnover is associated with an increased risk of fractures that is independent of the level of BMD,[170] and antiresorptive therapy such as raloxifene and bisphosphonates induces a dose-dependent decrease in bone markers that is sustained throughout treatment. Anabolic therapies such as PTH induce a substantial increase in markers of bone formation (e.g., PINP).

Anticatabolic Agents

Estrogen

Several controlled trials have shown that estrogen stops bone loss in early and late postmenopausal women by inhibiting bone resorption and that it results in a small increment in BMD (5% to 10% over a period of 1 to 3 years). Estrogen reduces bone turnover and increases bone density in postmenopausal women of all ages, as well as improving calcium homeostasis. Results from observational studies[185] and randomized placebo-controlled trials[186-188] show that estrogen decreased the risk of hip fracture by about 30% and the risk of spine fracture by 30% to 50%. So, HRT has been a standard treatment for prevention and treatment of postmenopausal osteoporosis for years. The reduction in fracture risk exceeds that expected by BMD alone. Calcium supplements enhance the effect of estrogen on BMD.[189] When HRT is stopped, bone loss resumes at the same rate as after menopause. In the Study of Osteoporotic Fractures,[190] the relative risk for nonspinal fracture was 0.66 in postmenopausal women currently taking HRT as compared with those not taking HRT, but it was not decreased in previous users regardless of the duration of treatment. This positive effect was not affected by age and was more significant for women who started HRT soon after menopause (within 5 years).

The long-term risks of HRT, however, outweigh the benefits, as has been shown in a large randomized placebo-controlled trial, the Women's Health Initiative (WHI) randomized trial.[191] Indeed, among more than 16,000 women aged 50 to 79 followed for an average 5.2 years, treated using conjugated equine estrogen and medroxyprogesterone acetate, although hip fracture and colon cancer risks were reduced,[191] increased risks of coronary heart disease (CHD) (nonfatal myocardial infarction or death due to CHD),[192] stroke,[193] breast cancer,[194] and dementia[195] were observed. In addition, in this trial, estrogen plus progestin did not have clinically meaningful effect on health-related quality of life, such as sleep disturbance or vasomotor symptoms.[196] Those results in primary prevention are consistent with those obtained in secondary CHD prevention in a well-conducted randomized placebo-controlled trial.[197] More recent subgroup analyses from

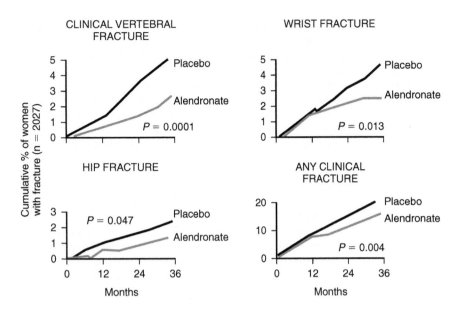

FIGURE 13-19. Effects of alendronate (aln) on the risk of fragility fracture. (Data from Black DM, Cummings SR, Karpf DB, et al: Randomized trial of effect of alendronate on risk of fracture in women with existing vertebral fractures, Lancet 348:1535–1541, 1996.)

the WHI trial have suggested that women who initiated hormone therapy closer to menopause (<10 years) tended to have reduced CHD risk compared with the increase in CHD risk among women more distant from menopause, but this trend did not meet strict criteria for statistical significance. A similar non-significant trend was observed for total mortality, but the risk of stroke was elevated regardless of years since menopause. These data should be considered in regard to the short-term treatment of menopausal symptoms.[198] The fall in HRT prescription observed after the release of the WHI results has been associated with a decline in new breast cancer incidence in several countries.[199] Thus, estrogen replacement therapy is no longer recommended as a first-line therapy for prevention and treatment of osteoporosis. It should be used only to relieve menopausal symptoms for as short a time and at the lowest dose possible.

Bisphosphonates

Bisphosphonates are stable analogs of pyrophosphate characterized by two P-C-P bonds. By substituting for hydrogens on the carbon atom, a variety of bisphosphonates have been synthesized, the potency of which depends on the length and structure of the side chain. Bisphosphonates have a strong affinity for bone apatite, both in vitro and in vivo, which is the basis for their clinical use. Bisphosphonates are potent inhibitors of bone resorption and produce their effect by reducing the recruitment and activity of osteoclasts and increasing their apoptosis. This activity varies greatly from compound to compound and ranges from 1 to 10,000. The mechanism of action on osteoclasts includes inhibition of the proton vacuolar ATPase of some phosphatases and alteration of the cytoskeleton and the ruffled border. Aminobisphosphonates also inhibit several steps of the mevalonate pathway, thereby modifying the isoprenylation of guanosine triphosphatate–binding proteins.[200]

Oral bioavailability is low, between 1% and 3% of the dose ingested, and is impaired by food, calcium, iron, coffee, tea, and orange juice. Bisphosphonates are quickly cleared from plasma, about 50% being deposited in bone and the remainder excreted in urine. Their half-life in bone is very prolonged. Aminobisphosphonates can induce a 24- to 48-hour period of fever when administered intravenously and, rarely, esophagitis when given orally.

Etidronate, given in an intermittent regimen, has led to an increase of about 3.5% in spine BMD after 2 years, with a reduction in the vertebral fracture rate,[201] but this reduction in vertebral fracture rate was no longer significant after 3 years of treatment. Etidronate does not appear to be effective in preventing bone loss at the hip and in reducing nonvertebral fractures.[202] Inhibition of mineralization can occur when etidronate is given in high dose.

Alendronate at 5 mg/day is effective in preventing bone loss in postmenopausal women to nearly the same extent as HRT.[203] In women with vertebral fractures, alendronate given for 3 years resulted in an 8.8% increase in BMD at the lumbar spine and hip[204] (Fig. 13-19). This treatment reduced the incidence of new vertebral, wrist, and hip fractures by half and prevented height loss. Alendronate also reduces fracture risk in postmenopausal women at the highest risk of fracture (i.e., those older than 75 years or those with very low BMD).[205] In women without preexisting vertebral fracture but with a hip T score lower than 2.5, alendronate is able to decrease clinical fractures of all types.[206] Alendronate is approved in most countries for the treatment of osteoporosis at the 10-mg/day dose and for the prevention of osteoporosis at the 5-mg/day dose in the United States. Alendronate is safe but can induce mild upper gastrointestinal tract disturbances and heartburn; on rare occasions, these side effects are related to the esophagitis sometimes caused by inappropriate administration of the drug. The antifracture efficacy of another oral nitrogen-containing bisphosphonate, risedronate, has been established in randomized placebo-controlled trials. This compound has been able to halve the rate of vertebral fracture in postmenopausal women in two studies.[207,208] A trial in elderly women has shown a reduction of about a third of the incidence of hip fracture in women with hip BMD in the osteoporosis range, whereas women selected using clinical risk factors for fracture—and who generally were not osteoporotic—did not benefit from the treatment.[209] Although these drugs were developed with daily dosages, they are now prescribed to be taken only on a weekly basis. Compliance has been slightly improved by weekly regimens, using 70 mg for alendronate and 35 mg for risedronate.

Ibandronate, given either daily (2.5 mg) or intermittently (20 mg every other day for the first 24 days, followed by 9 weeks without the treatment) has reduced the incidence in vertebral fracture of about 50% in a randomized trial involving postmenopausal osteoporotic women.[210] It has been marketed as a monthly 150-mg tablet and a 3-mg, every-3-months IV injection.

Intravenous zoledronate (e.g., 4 mg once a year or 1 mg every 3 months) has been shown to decrease bone turnover and increase BMD with the same magnitude as alendronate in a randomized phase II trial.[211] Two phase III trials have been published on the antifracture efficacy of annual IV zoledronic acid 5 mg. In the HORIZON Prevention Fracture Trial,[212] the rate of vertebral fracture was reduced by 65% at 3 years, hip fracture by 40%, and nonvertebral fracture by 25%. In the Recurrent Fracture Trial,[213] men and women with a recent hip fracture who received annual 5 mg zoledronic acid had a 35% reduction in clinical fractures and a 28% reduction in all-cause mortality. Other bisphosphonates have been studied in the treatment of osteoporosis. Pamidronate can increase BMD, but no valuable data on its antifracture efficacy have been presented. Clodronate may have an antifracture efficacy, but no adequate data have been published so far.[214]

Bisphosphonates can also be used in secondary osteoporosis, such as corticosteroid-induced osteoporosis. Etidronate prevents bone loss at the spine in men and women receiving corticosteroids, but not entirely at the femoral neck.[215] At a dose of 5 or 10 mg/day, alendronate is an effective therapy for the prevention and treatment of glucocorticoid-induced osteoporosis, preventing bone loss at all skeletal sites in men and women and reducing the rate of new vertebral fractures in postmenopausal women.[216] Risedronate (5 mg daily) also increases BMD in patients receiving long-term treatments with corticosteroids and may have favorable effects on fracture rate.[217] Annual IV zoledronic acid has also shown favorable effects in prevention of steroid-induced osteoporosis.

Selective Estrogen Receptor Modulators

Selective estrogen receptor modulators (SERMs), also called *estrogen analogs,* act as estrogen agonists or antagonists, depending on the target tissue. Tamoxifen, which has long been used for the adjuvant treatment of breast cancer, is an estrogen antagonist in breast tissue but a partial agonist on bone, cholesterol metabolism, and endometrium. Tamoxifen does not entirely prevent bone loss in postmenopausal women and increases the risk of endometrial cancer, which precludes its use in healthy postmenopausal women. Raloxifene is a benzothiophene that competitively inhibits the action of estrogen in the breast and the endometrium and also acts as an estrogen agonist of bone and lipid metabolism. In a large 2-year randomized placebo-controlled trial of raloxifene in postmenopausal women,[218] raloxifene increased lumbar spine (2.4%), total hip (2.4%), and total body (2.0%) BMD and significantly reduced markers of bone turnover. Serum cholesterol concentrations and its low-density lipoprotein (LDL) fraction were reduced without stimulation of the endometrium. Results of the MORE trial (Multiple Outcomes of Raloxifene Evaluation),[219] performed in 7705 osteoporotic women randomized to receive either raloxifene or placebo, showed that the incidence of estrogen receptor–positive breast cancer is reduced by two-thirds in postmenopausal women. In this study, raloxifene also lowered the incidence of vertebral fractures in osteoporotic women with (−30%) or without (−50%) existing fracture but had no significant effect on nonvertebral fractures.[220,221] In a post hoc analysis of women with prevalent vertebral fractures that were at highest risk of subsequent fractures, raloxifene has decreased the risk of both vertebral and nonvertebral fractures.[222] In another subgroup post hoc analysis of this trial,[223] women at higher cardiovascular risk were also protected by raloxifene compared to those on placebo; but in the RUTH trial,[224] in which the primary endpoint was cardiovascular events, raloxifene did not reduce cardiovascular events or mortality in a high-cardiovascular-risk population of postmenopausal women. In addition, two trials with incidence of breast cancer as the primary endpoint have confirmed the reduction in receptor-positive breast cancer incidence that was suggested in the MORE trial.[224,225]

In a 3-year randomized trial,[226] arzoxifene was compared to placebo and raloxifene among 6847 postmenopausal osteoporotic women. A vertebral fracture risk reduction of 42% was obtained with arzoxifene compared to placebo, which was similar to that observed with raloxifene. It is only in a subgroup analysis of patients at high risk that nonvertebral fracture risk was diminished. The incidence of breast cancer was low and did not differ between groups. The adverse events profile was comparable to that of raloxifene.

In a 5-year randomized placebo-controlled trial,[227] lasofoxifene 0.5 mg/day use was associated with a 42% reduction in vertebral fracture risk and a 22% reduction in nonvertebral fracture risk. The risk of estrogen receptor–positive breast cancer decreased by 67%.

Denosumab

Denosumab is a human monoclonal anti-RANKL antibody. It is a potent antiresorptive agent which is administered by a 60-mg subcutaneous injection every 6 months. In a large randomized placebo-controlled trial involving postmenopausal women with osteoporosis,[228] denosumab has been shown to reduce the risk of vertebral fracture by 68% at 3 years. The risk of hip fracture was diminished by 40% and nonvertebral fractures by 20%. The compound was well tolerated. In a trial among 1189 postmenopausal osteoporotic women randomized to receive either weekly alendronate or denosumab 60 mg every 6 months, the increase in BMD and the decrease in markers of bone resorption was larger in the denosumab group than in the alendronate group.[229] In a trial conducted in 252 women at high risk of rapid loss because of an antiaromatase inhibitor therapy prescribed for nonmetastatic breast cancer over 24 months, twice-yearly administration of denosumab led to significant increases in BMD over 24 months at trabecular and cortical bone, with overall adverse events rates similar to those of placebo.[230] In another trial, postmenopausal women with low BMD were randomized to denosumab every 3 months (Q3M; 6, 14, or 30 mg) or every 6 months (Q6M; 14, 60, 100, or 210 mg); placebo; or open-label oral alendronate weekly.[231] After 24 months, patients receiving denosumab either continued treatment at 60 mg Q6M for an additional 24 months, discontinued therapy, or discontinued treatment for 12 months then reinitiated denosumab (60 mg Q6M) for 12 months. The placebo cohort was maintained. Alendronate-treated patients discontinued alendronate and were followed. The main finding was that the effects on bone turnover were fully reversible with discontinuation of denosumab, and its effects were restored with subsequent retreatment.

Calcitonin

Calcitonin, a peptide produced by thyroid C cells, reduces bone resorption by inhibiting osteoclast activity. It is traditionally given by subcutaneous or intramuscular injection, with poor tolerance (nausea, facial flushes, diarrhea). The development of intranasal salmon calcitonin has made this therapy more acceptable, with fewer side effects. The minimum intranasal dose to have an effect on BMD is 200 IU/day. Calcitonin is less effective in preventing cortical bone loss than cancellous bone loss in postmenopausal women.[232] A small controlled study in osteoporotic women suggested a reduction in new vertebral fractures.[233] In the PROOF (Prevent Recurrence of Osteoporotic Fractures) study,[234] which is a 5-year double-blind, randomized, placebo-controlled study of 1255 postmenopausal women with osteoporosis, 200 IU/day of intranasal salmon calcitonin significantly reduced the rate of vertebral (but not peripheral) fractures by about 30% in comparison to placebo, but doses of 100 and 400 IU had no effect, and no consistent effect on BMD and bone turnover markers was seen in this trial with a high dropout rate. Thus the role of nasal calcitonin in the management of postmenopausal osteoporosis is not yet clearly documented.[235] Studies examining the effect of oral calcitonin are ongoing.

Anabolic Agents

Parathyroid Hormone

When administered intermittently, PTH stimulates bone formation. It can be administered as the intact hormone (1-84) or as the 1-34 fragment (teriparatide). Teriparatide increases osteoblast birth rate and prevents osteoblasts apoptosis, thereby increasing the number of osteoblasts and the rate of new bone formation. When given once daily subcutaneously, teriparatide increases BMD and improves trabecular architecture, cortical geometry, and strength. In a randomized placebo-controlled trial involving 1637 postmenopausal women with severe osteoporosis, the risk of vertebral fracture was reduced by 65% in those receiving 20 μg/day compared to those on placebo, and their reduction in peripheral fracture risk was of 53% after a median duration of treatment of 21 months (see Fig. 13-16).[236] Treatment was well tolerated, with a transient rise in serum calcium in fewer than 10% of patients.

PTH is prescribed mostly in patients with severe osteoporosis. Those women, however, have often received other therapies for osteoporosis (e.g., raloxifene or bisphosphonates) before PTH may be started because they continue to fracture. In an observational prospective study, Ettinger et al.[237] have treated osteoporotic women who had been either on raloxifene or alendronate for 18 to 36 months, with teriparatide 20 μg/day for 18 months. They found that teriparatide stimulated bone turnover in patients pretreated with raloxifene and alendronate, but the increase in markers of bone formation was blunted during the first months among those on prior alendronate. Moreover, among those on prior raloxifene, the teriparatide-induced increase in BMD was comparable to that reported in treatment-naïve patients, whereas prior treatment with alendronate delayed increase in BMD, particularly during the first 6 months. One may think that activated bone resorption is a prerequisite for an effect of PTH on bone formation. Thus, in old female sheep treated with the bisphosphonate tiludronate, PTH, or PTH and tiludronate, it has been shown that in the combined-therapy PTH and tiludronate group, the anabolic effect of PTH—as assessed using biochemical markers of bone formation and bone histomorphometry—was abolished.[238] Comparable findings have been made in clinical trials in humans. In postmenopausal women treated with both alendronate and PTH(1-84), the increase in volumetric density was comparable to that observed in those receiving alendronate alone and significantly lower than that of women taking PTH alone, suggesting that concurrent use of alendronate and PTH may reduce the anabolic effects of PTH.[239] Similar findings have

been made in men taking alendronate, PTH(1-34), or PTH plus alendronate.[240]

Such results suggest that PTH and bisphosphonates should not be prescribed simultaneously because the bisphosphonate reduces the anabolic effect of PTH. In contrast, in patients who have taken raloxifene before, the effect of PTH does not appear to be modified, and in those who have taken a bisphosphonate before, the anabolic effect of PTH is still obtained but delayed. This initial blunting of anabolic effect seems to depend on the potency of the antiresorptive agent preceding the PTH treatment, (1) since the increase in markers of bone formation is greater in patients who have taken risedronate previously compared to those who have taken alendronate[241] and (2) because there is no blunting after raloxifene.[237,242]

The antifracture efficacy of intact PTH(1-84) has also been tested. In a trial among 2532 postmenopausal women with mildly severe osteoporosis, PTH could reduce the risk of vertebral fracture by 40%, but not that of nonvertebral fracture. Study results interpretation was hampered by a high dropout rate. The incidence of hypercalcemia among patients on PTH was 23%.[243] This form of PTH is marketed in some European countries but not in the United States.

Other Medications

Calcium

Calcium partially decreases the rate of bone loss, especially in women in late postmenopause. It is generally prescribed as an adjunct to other drugs such as bisphosphonates, and in most clinical trials, both the active and placebo groups receive calcium supplements.

Calcium is likely to be partially effective in preventing bone loss, particularly in older women and those with low calcium intake. Two studies[244,245] have shown a slight reduction in the incidence of fractures in patients receiving calcium supplements. In one study,[246] women older than 60 years were supplemented with 1200 mg/d when their calcium intake was below 1000 mg/d, and this regimen resulted in prevention of bone loss from the forearm over a 4-year period and decreased the rate of vertebral fractures by 59% in women who had vertebral fractures at baseline but not in those without existing vertebral fractures. Calcium supplementation on the order of 500 to 1500 mg/day is safe. Mild gastrointestinal disturbances such as constipation are commonly reported. The risk of kidney stone disease related to hypercalciuria appears to be minimally increased. Bioavailability is greater during meals and varies with different calcium salts, but this factor is probably of little clinical significance.

Vitamin D

In a French study of 3270 institutionalized women with a mean age of 84 years who were treated with calcium (1200 mg/d) and vitamin D (800 IU/day) for 1.5 years, the risk of hip fracture and other nonvertebral fractures was decreased 43% and 32%, respectively, when compared with the placebo group.[178] Treatment increased serum 25(OH)D, decreased serum PTH, and increased femoral neck BMD. However, in a Dutch study of 2578 women of similar age treated with 400 IU of vitamin D or placebo for 3.5 years but without supplemental calcium because of higher dietary calcium intake, the rate of hip fracture was the same in the two groups.[247] These women were healthier and more ambulatory, and the hip fracture rate was much lower than in the French study. In a more recent smaller study, 389 men and women older than 63 years were treated with vitamin D (700 IU/

day) and calcium (500 mg/day); the study noted a trend toward a decrease in nonvertebral fractures.[248] Another study showed a decrease in nonvertebral fractures when vitamin D was given annually by intramuscular injection.[249] These studies show the utility of adequate calcium (500 to 1500 mg/day) and vitamin D (700 IU or equivalent) in calcium-deficient and vitamin D–deficient elderly women and probably men. A reduction of about 25% has also been found in men and women aged 65 and older living in the community, after receiving 100,000 IU of vitamin D every 4 months for 5 years.[250] In elderly women recovering from a first hip fracture, a supplement in vitamin D has been able to increase BMD and reduce the incidence of falls, these effects being more marked with the addition of calcium.[251]

Vitamin D should be used routinely in institutionalized patients because they have low vitamin D intake, low sunshine exposure, and impaired vitamin D synthesis in the skin. When compliance is reduced, oral or intramuscular dosing of 150,000 to 300,000 U can be administered twice a year. Vitamin D is safe and does not require monitoring. The utility of calcium and vitamin D supplementation in healthy elderly persons with adequate intake and normal BMD has not been established.

Strontium Ranelate

Strontium ranelate is a compound containing two atoms of non-radioactive strontium; it improves bone mass by inhibiting bone resorption while preserving bone formation. Strontium ranelate prevents bone loss induced by estrogen deficiency and immobilization in animal models and also improves bone strength in those models. In phase II trials, this compound has been able to prevent bone loss at the dose of 1 g/day.[252,253] In a randomized placebo-controlled trial conducted in 1649 postmenopausal women with osteoporosis (mean age 69) treated for 3 years, strontium ranelate use has been associated with a 41% reduction in vertebral fracture risk, this diminution being apparent as early as the first year.[254] In another randomized trial, the primary endpoint being incidence of nonvertebral fracture, all peripheral fractures were significantly but slightly reduced (−16%). The reduction in the incidence of hip fracture did not reach statistical significance in the intent-to-treat analysis but only in a per-protocol analysis (−41%, P = 0.025).[255] In those trials, strontium ranelate has been well tolerated. An analysis based on preplanned pooling of data from these two international phase III, randomized, placebo-controlled, double-blind studies included 1488 women between 80 and 100 years of age followed for 3 years. In this study, treatment with strontium ranelate reduced the risk of vertebral (−59%) and nonvertebral (−41%) fractures in women 80 years and older with osteoporosis.[256] Strontium ranelate is not approved by the U.S. Food and Drug Administration.

Others

Ipriflavone is a synthetic compound that belongs to the family of isoflavones. In a large randomized placebo-controlled trial, it failed to demonstrate prevention of bone loss.[257] In addition, a sizeable proportion of women on ipriflavone had lymphopenia.

Tibolone is a synthetic analog of anabolic steroids with estrogen-like, androgen-like, and progestin-like properties. It is marketed in some countries and generally used as HRT in postmenopausal women. It prevents postmenopausal bone loss and has positive effects on hot flashes. In the randomized LIFT study,[258] 4538 women who were between the ages of 60 and 85 years and had a BMD T score of −2.5 or less at the hip or spine or a T score of −2.0 or less and radiologic evidence of a vertebral fracture were assigned to receive once-daily tibolone (at a dose

of 1.25 mg) or placebo. Tibolone reduced the risk of vertebral fracture (−45%), nonvertebral fracture (−26%), and invasive breast cancer (−68%) and possibly colon cancer, but increased the risk of stroke.

Growth hormone has been used for its alleged bone and muscle anabolic properties. However, growth hormone has produced conflicting results in the prevention of bone loss in postmenopausal osteoporosis.[259]

Thiazide diuretics reduce tubular reabsorption of calcium and slow cortical bone loss in normal postmenopausal women, so they should not be used as a monotherapy in the treatment of postmenopausal osteoporosis.[260]

WHO SHOULD BE TREATED?

Indications

Therapeutic recommendations for women rely on results of clinical trials whose main endpoint was the reduction in fracture risk.[261] There was no clinical trial in which the main endpoint was reduction in fracture risk in men, although bisphosphonates clearly increase BMD, reduce levels of biochemical markers, and are likely to reduce fracture risk to the same extent as in women. Similarly, teriparatide has shown beneficial effects in men with surrogates, but without the fracture outcome. The decision-making process should be based on an analysis of the patient's individual risk of fracture and the efficacy and tolerance of the drugs to be prescribed. This decision should rely on age, the existence of clinical risk factors, the magnitude of bone loss as assessed by the level of BMD, and the presence or not of previous fragility fractures.

Most recent therapeutic recommendations rely at least partly on the use of the FRAX algorithm. Each country can adapt the available models to its public health priorities. For example, in the United Kingdom, a cost-effectiveness analysis using the probabilities of fracture calculated with the FRAX algorithm at various ages and the cost of medications in the United Kingdom found that treatment is cost effective at all ages when the 10-year probability of a major fracture exceeds 7%.[262] The intervention threshold at the age of 50 years corresponds to a 10-year probability of a major osteoporotic fracture of 7.5% and rises progressively with age up to 30% at the age of 80 years, so that intervention is cost effective at all ages. The use of these thresholds in a case-finding strategy would identify 23% to 46% as eligible for treatment, depending on age. The same threshold can be used in men.

In a United States–specific cost-effectiveness analysis,[263] osteoporosis treatment was considered cost effective when the 10-year hip fracture probability reached approximately 3%. Although the RR at which treatment became cost effective varied markedly between genders and by race/ethnicity, the absolute 10-year hip fracture probability at which intervention became cost effective was similar across race/ethnicity groups and tended to be slightly higher for men than for women. The new WHO fracture prediction algorithm has been combined with an updated economic analysis to evaluate existing NOF guidance for osteoporosis prevention and treatment.[264] The WHO fracture prediction algorithm was calibrated to the U.S. population using national age-, sex- and race-specific death rates and age- and sex-specific hip fracture incidence rates. Thus, it is cost effective to treat patients with a fragility fracture and those with osteoporosis by WHO criteria, as well as older individuals at average risk and osteopenic patients with additional risk factors. However, the estimated 10-year fracture probability was lower in men and nonwhite women compared to postmenopausal white women. This analysis generally endorsed existing clinical practice recommendations and concluded that specific treatment decisions must be individualized. So, in the latest NOF recommendations, postmenopausal women and men aged 50 and older presenting with the following should be considered for treatment:

- A hip or vertebral (clinical or morphometric) fracture
- T score ≤−2.5 at the femoral neck or spine after appropriate evaluation to exclude secondary causes
- Low bone mass (T score between −1.0 and −2.5 at the femoral neck or spine) and a 10-year probability of a hip fracture ≥3% or a 10-year probability of a major osteoporosis-related fracture ≥20% based on the U.S.-adapted WHO algorithm.

WHICH DRUG FOR WHICH PATIENT?

Patients With Previous Fragility Fractures

The existence of a previous fragility fracture requires, as an initial diagnostic step, investigation of the differential diagnosis and measurement of BMD. The first-line treatment, based on the current evidence for antifracture efficacy, may be a second-generation bisphosphonate (alendronate, risedronate, ibandronate, zoledronic acid), strontium ranelate, or raloxifene. Calcitonin might be another option, although evidence of efficacy is limited. In patients with severe osteoporosis (low bone mass and several prevalent fractures) teriparatide may be indicated. General measures including fall prevention and adequate nutrition should be implemented. The potential benefits of osteoporosis therapy may be limited if life expectancy is short, and the decision may be to not treat in very elderly women. Whatever the treatment option, adequate calcium and vitamin D supplementation is warranted.

Patients Without Fractures

Women with a T score lower than −2.5 at the spine and hip have osteoporosis and should be treated as indicated, unless their life expectancy is short, and therefore their lifetime risk of fracture is low. For example, women older than 80 years with no additional risk factor for fractures may be treated with calcium and vitamin D alone. Women with a T score above −1 have normal BMD and should not be treated.

Management of women with a low bone mass, that is, with a T score ranging between 1 and 2.5, is more complex. The decision to treat or not is based on the individual's probability of fracture, as assessed in FRAX, which depends on the magnitude of the deficit in BMD (the fracture risk at a T score of −2 is double the risk of fracture at a T score of −1) and on additive risk factors such as age, parental history of hip fracture, low body weight, history of steroid therapy, and rheumatoid arthritis. Increased bone resorption as assessed by a biochemical marker

may also be of interest in some patients. Although treating elderly women with low bone mass might be more cost effective than treating younger ones, treating women in their late 50s and 60s who have a high lifetime risk of fracture is recommended. Raloxifene, strontium ranelate, or bisphosphonates may be proposed.

Treatment Monitoring

MONITORING OF TREATMENT WITH DENSITOMETRY

Whether the long-term antifracture efficacy of antiosteoporotic drugs will depend on the extent to which treatment can increase or maintain BMD is controversial. In one meta-analysis, 16% of vertebral fracture risk reduction after treatment with alendronate was attributed to an increase in BMD at the lumbar spine.[265] For patients treated with risedronate or raloxifene, changes in BMD predict even more poorly the degree of reduction in vertebral (raloxifene) or nonvertebral (risedronate) fractures. In women taking alendronate and losing BMD (0 to −4%) at the spine during the first or second year of treatment, the effect of alendronate on vertebral fracture risk reduction is similar to that observed in those women who gained BMD.[266] For bone-forming agents, increases in BMD account for approximately one-third of the vertebral fracture risk reduction with teriparatide.[267] Further data are needed on the role of BMD in monitoring patients treated with bone-forming agents, but it appears to be of greater value than its use with inhibitors of bone resorption.

MONITORING OF TREATMENT WITH BIOCHEMICAL MARKERS OF BONE TURNOVER

Antiresorptive therapies such as calcitonin, estrogen, SERMs, and bisphosphonates induce a significant decrease in bone markers that return to the premenopausal range within 3 to 6 months for the resorption markers and within 6 to 9 months for markers of formation. A significant association has been reported between the short-term decrease and the absolute level of markers of bone turnover with the use of antiresorptive agents (raloxifene and bisphosphonates) on the one hand, and the magnitude of the reduction of the risk of vertebral and nonvertebral fractures on the other hand.[173,174,268] In addition, a large prospective study suggests that the use of markers of bone turnover in the monitoring of bisphosphonate therapy is associated with a greater persistence with therapy than in those not monitored.[175] Thus, measurement of markers of bone turnover after a few months of treatment may provide useful information on efficacy and improve persistence. Changes in markers of bone turnover with strontium ranelate are of small magnitude and are unlikely to be clinically useful for the monitoring of treatment.

REFERENCES

1. NIH Consensus development panel on osteoporosis prevention, diagnosis and therapy. Osteoporosis prevention diagnosis and therapy, JAMA 285:785–795, 2001.
2. Hayes WC: Biomechanics of fractures. In Riggs BL, Melton LJ III, editors: Osteoporosis diagnosis and management, ed 2, Philadelphia, 1995, Lippincott-Raven, pp 93–114.
3. Mosekilde L, Bentzen SM, Ortoft G, et al: The predictive value of quantitative computed tomography for vertebral body compressive strength and ash density, Bone 10:465–470, 1989.

4. Cummings SR, Black DM, Nevitt MC, et al: Bone density at various sites for prediction of hip fractures, Lancet 341:72–75, 1993.
5. World Health Organization: Assessment of fracture risk and its application to screening for postmenopausal osteoporosis, World Health Organ Tech Rep Ser 1994.
6. Kanis JA, Melton LJ III, Christiansen C, et al: The diagnosis of osteoporosis, J Bone Miner Res 9:1137–1141, 1994.
7. Melton LJ III: How many women have osteoporosis now? J Bone Miner Res 10:175–177, 1995.

8. Kanis JA on behalf of the World health Organization scientific Group: Assessment of osteoporosis at the primary health-care level. Technical report. World Health organization collaborating centre for metabolic bone diseases, University of Sheffield, UK, 2007.
9. National Osteoporosis Foundation: 1996 and 2015: Osteoporosis prevalence figures: state-by-state report, Washington, DC, 1997, National Osteoporosis Foundation.
10. O'Neill TW, Felsenberg D, Varlow J, et al: The prevalence of vertebral deformity in European men and

women: the European vertebral osteoporosis study, J Bone Miner Res 11:1010–1018, 1996.

11. Spector TD, McCloskey EV, Doyle DV, et al: Prevalence of vertebral fractures in women and the relationship with bone density and symptoms: the Chingford study, J Bone Miner Res 7:817–822, 1993.

12. Cooper C, Campion G, Melton LJ III: Hip fractures in the elderly: a worldwide projection, Osteoporos Int 2:285–289, 1992.

13. Phillips S, Fox N, Jacobs J, et al: The direct medical costs for osteoporosis for American women aged 45 and older, 1986, Bone 9:271–279, 1988.

14. Ray NF, Chan JK, Thaemer M, et al: Medical expenditures for the treatment of osteoporotic fractures in the United States in 1994, J Bone Miner Res 12:24–35, 1997.

15. Jensen JS, Bagger J: Long-term social prognosis after hip fractures, Acta Orthop Scand 53:97–101, 1982.

16. Schneider EL, Guralnik JM: The aging of America: impact on health care costs, JAMA 263:2335–2350, 1990.

17. Cummings SR, Kelsey JL, Nevitt MC, et al: Epidemiology of osteoporosis and osteoporotic fractures, Epidemiol Rev 7:178–208, 1985.

18. Browner WS, Pressman AR, Nevitt MC, et al: Mortality following fractures in older women: the Study of Osteoporotic Fractures, Arch Intern Med 156:1521–1525, 1996.

19. Cooper C, Melton LJ III: Epidemiology of osteoporosis, Trends Endocrinol Metab 314:224–229, 1992.

20. Gallagher JC, Melton LJ, Riggs BL, et al: Epidemiology of fractures of the proximal femur in Rochester, Minnesota, Clin Orthop 150:163–171, 1980.

21. Nevitt MC, Cummings SR, Study of Osteoporotic Fractures Research Group: type of fall and risk of hip and wrist fractures: the study of osteoporotic fractures, Am J Geriatr Soc 41:1226–1234, 1993.

22. Melton LJ III: Differing patterns of osteoporosis across the world. In Chesnut CH III, editor: New dimensions in osteoporosis in the 1990s. Asia Pacific Conference Series No 125. Hong Kong, 1991, Excerpta Medica, pp 13–18.

23. Melton LJ III: Epidemiology of age-related fractures. In Avioli LV, editor: The osteoporotic syndrome: detection, prevention and treatment, New York, 1993, Wiley-Liss, pp 17–18.

24. Cooper C, Atkinson EJ, O'Fallon WM, et al: The incidence of clinically diagnosed vertebral fractures: a population-based study in Rochester, Minnesota, 1985–1989, J Bone Miner Res 7:221–227, 1992.

25. Melton LJ III, Lane AW, Cooper C, et al: Prevalence and incidence of vertebral deformities, Osteoporos Int 3:113–119, 1993.

26. EPOS Group: Incidence of vertebral fracture in Europe: results from the European Prospective Osteoporosis Study, J Bone Miner Res 17:716–724, 2002.

27. McCloskey EV, Spector TD, Eyres KS, et al: The assessment of vertebral deformity. A method for use in population studies and clinical trials, Osteoporos Int 3:138–147, 1993.

28. Hedlund LR, Gallagher JC: Vertebral morphometry in diagnosis of spinal fractures, Bone Miner 5:59–67, 1988.

29. Kleerekoper M, Nelson DA: Vertebral fracture or vertebral deformity? Calcif Tissue 50:5–6, 1992.

30. Kado DM, Browner WS, Palermo L, et al: Vertebral fractures and mortality in older women: a prospective study. Study of Osteoporotic Fractures Research Group, Arch Intern Med 159:1215–1220, 1999.

31. Center JR, Nguyen TV, Pocock NA, et al: Mortality after all major types of osteoporotic fracture in men and women: an observational study, Lancet 353:878–882, 1999.

32. Nevitt MC, Ettinger B, Black DM, et al: The association of radiographically detected vertebral fractures with back pain and function: a prospective study, Ann Intern Med 128:793–800, 1998.

33. Sahlin Y: Occurrence of fractures in a defined population: a 1-year study, Injury 21:158–160, 1990.

34. Baron JA, Barrett J, Malenka D, et al: Racial differences in fracture risk, Epidemiology 5:42–47, 1994.

35. Bengnér U, Johnell O: Increasing incidence of forearm fractures, Acta Orthop Scand 56:158–160, 1985.

36. Owen RA, Melton LJ III, Johnson KA, et al: Incidence of Colles fracture in a North American community, Am J Public Health 72:605–607, 1982.

37. Cooper C, Atkinson EJ, Jacobsen SJ, et al: Population-based study of survival following osteoporotic fractures, Am J Epidemiol 137:1001–1005, 1993.

38. Kaukonen JP, Karaharju EO, Porras M, et al: Functional recovery after fractures of the distal forearm, Ann Chir Gynaecol 77:27–31, 1988.

39. Klotzbuecher CM, Ross PD, Landsmann PB, et al: Patients with prior fractures have an increased risk of future fractures: a summary of the literature and statistical synthesis, J Bone Miner Res 15:721–739, 2000.

40. Woolf AD, Akesson K: Preventing fractures in elderly people, BMJ 327:89–95, 2003.

41. Chapurlat RD, Bauer DC, Nevitt M, et al: Incidence and risk factors for a second hip fracture: the Study of Osteoporotic Fractures, Osteoporos Int 14:130–136, 2003.

42. Cummings SR, Black DM, Nevitt MC, et al: Bone densitometry at various sites for prediction of hip fractures, Lancet 341:72–75, 1993.

43. Riggs BL, Khosla S, Melton LJ III: A unitary model for involutional osteoporosis: estrogen deficiency causes both type I and type II osteoporosis in postmenopausal women and contributes to bone loss in aging men, J Bone Miner Res 13:763–773, 1998.

44. Kelsey JL, Browner WS, Seeley DG, et al: Risk factors for fractures of the distal forearm and proximal humerus, Am J Epidemiol 135:477–489, 1992.

45. Cooper C, Barker DJP, Wickham C: Physical activity, muscle strength, and calcium intake in fracture of the proximal femur in Britain, BMJ 297:1443–1446, 1988.

46. Farmer ME, Harris T, Madans JH, et al: Anthropometric indicators and hip fracture: The NHANES I epidemiologic follow-up study, J Am Geriatr Soc 37:9–16, 1989.

47. Paganini-Hill A, Chao A, Ross RK, et al: Exercise and other factors in the prevention of hip fracture: The Leisure World study, Epidemiology 2:16–25, 1991.

48. Grisso JA, Kelsey JL, Strom BL, et al: Risk factors for falls as a cause for hip fractures in women, N Engl J Med 324:1326–1331, 1991.

49. Cummings SR, Nevitt MC, Browner WS, et al: Risk factors for hip fracture in white women, N Engl J Med 332:767–773, 1995.

50. Johnell O, Gullberg B, Kanis JA, et al: Risk factors for hip fracture in European women—the MEDOS study, J Bone Miner Res 10:1802–1815, 1995.

51. Ohta H, et al: Which is more osteoporosis-inducing, menopause or oophorectomy? Bone Miner 19:273–285, 1992.

52. Davies MC, Hall ML, Jacobs HS: Bone mineral loss in young women with amenorrhea, BMJ 301:790–793, 1990.

53. Prior JC, Vigna YM, Schechter MT, et al: Spinal bone loss and ovulatory disturbances, N Engl J Med 323:1211–1227, 1990.

54. Chapurlat RD, Garnero P, Sornay-Rendu E, et al: Longitudinal study of bone loss in pre- and perimenopausal women: evidence for bone loss in perimenopausal women, Osteoporos Int 11:493–498, 2000.

55. Cummings SR, Browner WS, Bauer DC, et al: Endogenous hormones and the risk of hip and vertebral fractures among older women. Study of Osteoporotic Fractures Research Group, N Engl J Med 339:733–738, 1998.

56. Chapurlat RD, Garnero P, Bréart G, et al: Serum estradiol and sex hormone-binding globulin and the risk of hip fracture in elderly women: the EPIDOS study, J Bone Miner Res 15:1835–1841, 2000.

57. Lee JS, LaCroix AZ, Lu S, et al: Associations of serum sex hormone-binding globulin and sex hormone concentrations with hip fracture risk in postmenopausal women, J Clin Endocrinol Metab 93:1796–1803, 2008.

58. Eastell R, Adams JE, Coleman RE, et al: Effect of anastrozole on bone mineral density: 5-year results from the anastrozole, tamoxifen, alone or in combination trial 18233230, J Clin Oncol 26:1051–1057, 2008.

59. Bauer DC, Browner WS, Cauley JA, et al: Factors associated with appendicular bone mass in older women, Ann Intern Med 118:657–665, 1993.

60. Mosekilde L: Osteoporosis and exercise, Bone 17:193–195, 1995.

61. Tinetti ME, Speechley M, Ginter SF: Risk factors for falls among persons living in the community, N Engl J Med 319:1701–1707, 1988.

62. Nordin BEC, Heaney RP: Calcium supplementation of the diet: justified by the present evidence, BMJ 300:1056–1060, 1990.

63. Dargent-Molina P, Favier F, Grandjean H, et al: Fall-related factors and risk for hip fracture: the EPIDOS prospective study, Lancet 348:145–149, 1996.

64. Kanis JA, Johansson H, Oden O, et al: A family history of fracture and fracture risk, Bone 35:1029–1037, 2004.

65. Kanis JA, Johnell O, De Laet C, et al: A meta-analysis of previous fracture and subsequent fracture risk, Bone 35:375–382, 2004.

66. Kanis JA, Oden O, Johnell O, et al: The burden of osteoporotic fracture: a method for setting intervention thresholds, Osteoporos Int 12:417–424, 2001.

67. Higgins JP, Thompson SG, Deeks JJ, et al: Measuring inconsistency in meta-analyses, BMJ 327:557–560, 2003.

68. Kanis JA, Johnell O, Oden O, et al: Ten year probabilities of osteoporotic fractures according to BMD and diagnostic thresholds, Osteoporos Int 12:989–995, 2001.

69. http://www.shef.ac.uk/FRAX.

70. Smith DM, Nance WE, Kang KW, et al: Genetic factors in determining bone mass, J Clin Invest 52:2800–2808, 1973.

71. Morrison NA, Qi JC, Tokita A, et al: Prediction of bone density from vitamin D receptor alleles, Nature 367:284–287, 1994.

72. Morrison NA, Qi JC, Tokita A, et al: Prediction of bone density from vitamin D alleles, Nature 387:106, 1997.

73. Peacock M: Vitamin D receptor gene alleles and osteoporosis: a contrasting view, J Bone Miner Res 10:1294–1297, 1995.

74. Garnero P, Borel O, Sornay-Rendu E, et al: Vitamin D receptor gene polymorphisms are not related to bone turnover, rate of bone loss, and bone mass in postmenopausal women: The OFELY study, J Bone Miner Res 11:827–834, 1996.

75. Efstathiadou Z, Tsatsoulis A, Ioannidis JP: Association of collagen I alpha 1 Sp1 polymorphism with the risk of prevalent fractures: a meta-analysis, J Bone Miner Res 16:1586–1592, 2001.

76. Tran BN, Nguyen ND, Eisman JA, et al: Association between LRP5 polymorphism and bone mineral density: a Bayesian meta-analysis, BMC Med Genet 9:55, 2008.

77. van Meurs JB, Trikalinos TA, Ralston SH, et al: Large-scale analysis of association between LRP5 and LRP6 variants and osteoporosis, JAMA 299:1277–1290, 2008.

78. Richards JB, Rivadeneira F, Inouye M, et al: Bone mineral density, osteoporosis, and osteoporotic fractures: a genome-wide association study, Lancet 371:1505–1512, 2008.

79. Langdahl BL, Uitterlinden AG, Ralston SH, et al: Large-scale analysis of association between polymorphisms in the transforming growth factor beta 1 gene (TGFB1) and osteoporosis: the GENOMOS study, Bone 42:969–981, 2008.

80. Bonjour J-P, Carrie A-L, Ferrari S, et al: Calcium-enriched foods and bone mass growth in prepubertal girls: a randomized, double-blind, placebo-controlled trial, J Clin Invest 99:1287–1294, 1997.

81. Cadogan J, Eastell R, Jones N, et al: Milk intake and bone mineral acquisition in adolescent girls: randomised, controlled intervention trial, BMJ 315:1255–1260, 1997.

82. Johnston CC, Miller JZ, Slemenda CW, et al: Calcium supplementation and increases in bone mineral density in children, N Engl J Med 327:82–87, 1992.

83. Bass S, Pearce G, Bradney M, et al: Exercise before puberty may confer residual benefits in bone density in adulthood: studies in active prepubertal and retired female gymnasts, J Bone Miner Res 13:500–507, 1998.

84. Ahlborg HG, Johnell O, Turner CH, et al: Bone loss and bone size after menopause, N Engl J Med 349:327–334, 2003.

85. Lanham SA, Roberts C, Cooper C, et al: Intrauterine programming of bone. Part 1: alteration of the osteogenic environment, Osteoporos Int 19:147–156, 2008.

86. Lanham SA, Roberts C, Perry MJ, et al: Intrauterine programming of bone. Part 2: alteration of skeletal structure, Osteoporos Int 19:157–167, 2008.

87. Riggs BL, Melton LJ, Robb RA, et al: A population-based assessment of rates of bone loss at multiple skel-

etal sites: evidence for substantial trabecular bone loss in young adult women and men, J Bone Miner Res 23:205–214, 2008.
88. Riggs BL, Wahner HW, Dunn WL, et al: Differential changes in bone mineral density of the appendicular and axial skeleton with ageing: relationship to spinal osteoporosis, J Clin Invest 67:328–335, 1981.
89. Lindsay R, Hart DM, Forrest C, et al: Prevention of spinal osteoporosis in oophorectomised women, Lancet 2:1151–1153, 1980.
90. Hofbauer LC, Khosla S, Dunstan CR, et al: Estrogen stimulates gene expression and protein production of osteoprotegerin in human osteoblastic cells, Endocrinology 140:4367–4370, 1999
91. Shevde NK, Bendixen AC, Dienger KM, et al: Estrogens suppress RANK ligand-induced osteoclast differentiation via a stromal cell independent mechanism involving c-Jun repression, Proc Natl Acad Sci U S A 97:7829–7834, 2000.
92. Eghbali-Faterouchi G, Khosla S: Role of RANK ligand in mediating bone resorption in early postmenopausal women, J Clin Invest 111:1221–1230, 2003.
93. Weitzmann MN, Roggia G, Toraldo L, et al: Increased production of IL-7 uncouples bone formation from bone resorption during estrogen deficiency, J Clin Invest 110:1643–1650, 2002.
94. Cenci S, Toraldo G, Weitzmann MN, et al: Estrogen deficiency induces bone loss by increasing T cell proliferation and life-span through IFN-gamma-induced class II transactivator, Proc Nat Acad Sci U S A 100:10405–10410, 2003.
95. Lam J, Takeshita S, Barker JE, et al: TNF-alpha induces osteoclastogenesis by direct stimulation of macrophages exposed to permissive levels of RANL ligand, J Clin Invest 106:1229–1237, 2000.
96. Wei S, Kitaura H, Zhou P, et al: IL-1 mediates TNF-induced osteoclastogenesis, J Clin Invest 115:282–290, 2005.
97. Chavassieux P, Seeman E, Delmas PD: Insights into material and structural basis of bone fragility from diseases associated with fractures: how determinants of the biomechanical properties of bone are compromised by disease, Endocr Rev 28:151–164, 2007.
98. Seeman E, Delmas PD: Bone quality—the material and structural basis of bone strength and fragility, N Engl J Med 354:2250–2261, 2006.
99. Duan Y, Wang XF, Evans A, et al: Structural and biomechanical basis of racial and sex differences in vertebral fragility in Chinese and Caucasians, Bone 36:987–998, 2005.
100. Faulkner KG, Cummings SR, Black D, et al: Simple measurement of femoral geometry predicts hip fracture: The study of osteoporotic fractures, J Bone Miner Res 8:1211–1217, 1993.
101. Duboeuf F, Hans D, Schott AM, et al: Different morphometric and densitometric parameters predict cervical and trochanteric hip fracture: the EPIDOS Study, J Bone Miner Res 12:1895–1902, 1997.
102. Reid IR, Chin K, Evans MC, et al: Relation between increase in length of hip axis in older women between 1950s and 1990s and increase in age specific rates of hip fracture, BMJ 309:508–509, 1994.
103. Parfitt AM, Matthews CHE, Villanueva AR, et al: Relationship between surface, volume and thickness of iliac trabecular bone on aging and in osteoporosis: implications for the micro-anatomic and cellular mechanism of bone loss, J Clin Invest 72:1396–1409, 1983.
104. Foldes J, Parfitt AM, Shih M-S, et al: Structural and geometric changes in iliac bone: relationship to normal aging and osteoporosis, J Bone Miner Res 6:759–766, 1991.
105. Qiu S, Rao DS, Fyhrie DP, et al: The morphological association between microcracks and osteocyte lacunae in human cortical bone, Bone 37:10–15, 2005.
106. Seeman E: Periosteal bone formation—a neglected determinant of bone strength, N Engl J Med 349:320–323, 2003.
107. Ahlborg HG, Johnell O, Turner CH, et al: Bone loss and bone size after menopause, N Engl J Med 349:327–334, 2003.
108. Riggs BL, Melton LJ III, Robb RA, et al: A population-based study of age and sex differences in bone volumetric density, size, geometry and structure at different skeletal sites, J Bone Miner Res 19:1945–1954, 2004.
109. Wang XF, Duan Y, Beck T, et al: Varying contributions of growth and ageing to racial and sex differences in femoral neck structure and strength in old age, Bone 36:978–986, 2005. [Erratum, Bone 2005; 37:599.]
110. Berry SD, Kiel DP: Falls as risk factors for fracture. In Marcus R, Feldman D, Nelson DA, et al, editors: Osteoporosis, ed 3, San Diego, 2008, Academic press, pp 911–922.
111. Hans D, Dargent-Molina P, Schott AM, et al: Ultrasonographic heel measurements to predict hip fracture in elderly women: The EPIDOS prospective study, Lancet 348:511–514, 1996.
112. Lindsay R, Silverman SL, Cooper C, et al: Risk of new vertebral fracture in the year following a fracture, JAMA 17(285):320–323, 2001.
113. Dempster DW: Bone histomorphometry in glucocorticoid-induced osteoporosis, J Bone Miner Res 4:137–141, 1989.
114. Van Staa TP, Leufkens HGM, Cooper C: The epidemiology of corticosteroid-induced osteoporosis: a meta-analysis, Osteoporos Int 13:777–787, 2002.
115. Teelucksingh S, Padfield PL, Tibi L, et al: Inhaled corticosteroids, bone formation, and osteocalcin, Lancet 338:60–61, 1991.
116. van Staa TP, Gueusens P, Pols HA, et al: A simple score for estimating the long-term risk of fracture in patients using oral glucocorticoids, QJM 98:191–198, 2005.
117. Israel E, Banerjee TR, Fitzmaurice GM, et al: Effects of inhaled glucocorticoids on bone density in premenopausal women, N Engl J Med 345:941–947, 2001.
118. van Staa TP, Leufkens HG, Abenhaim M, et al: Use of oral corticosteroids and risk of fractures, J Bone Miner Res 15:993–1000, 2000.
119. van Staa TP, Laan RF, Barton IP, et al: Bone density threshold and other predictors of vertebral fracture in patients receiving oral glucocorticoid therapy, Arthritis Rheum 48:3224–3229, 2003.
120. Toh SH, Claunch BC, Brown PH: Effect of hyperthyroidism and its treatment on bone mineral content, Arch Intern Med 145:883–886, 1985.
121. Silverberg SJ, Shane E, Jacobs TP, et al: A 10-year prospective study of primary hyperparathyroidism with or without parathyroid surgery, N Engl J Med 341:1249–1255, 1999.
122. McDonough AK, Rosenthal RS, Cao X, et al: The effect of thiazolidinediones on BMD and osteoporosis, Nat Clin Pract Endocrinol Metab 4:507–513, 2008.
123. Shapiro JR: Osteogenesis imperfecta and other defects of bone development as occasional causes of adult osteoporosis. In Marcus R, Feldman D, Nelson DA et al, editors: Osteoporosis. San Diego, CA, 2008, Academic, pp 1247–1281.
124. Mann T, Oviatt SK, Wilson D, et al: Vertebral deformity in men, J Bone Miner Res 7:1259–1265, 1992.
125. Marie PJ, De Vernejoul MC, Connes C, et al: Decreased DNA synthesis by cultures of osteoblastic cells in eugonadal osteoporotic men with defective bone formation, J Clin Invest 88:1167–1172, 1991.
126. Finkelstein JS, Klibanski A, Neer RM, et al: Osteoporosis in men with idiopathic hypogonadotrophic hypogonadism, Ann Intern Med 106:354–361, 1987.
127. Bilezikian JP, Morishima A, Bell J, et al: Increased bone mass as a result of estrogen therapy in a man with aromatase deficiency, N Engl J Med 339:599–603, 1998.
128. Melton LJ III, Orwoll ES, Wasnich RD: Does bone density predict fractures comparably in men and women? Osteoporos Int 12:707–709, 2001.
129. Tannenbaum C, Clark J, Schwartzmann K, et al: Yield of laboratory testing to identify secondary contributors to osteoporosis in otherwise healthy women, J Clin Endocrinol Metab 87:4431–4437, 2002.
130. Jamal SA, Leiter RE, Bayoumi AM, et al: Clinical utility of laboratory testing in women with osteoporosis, Osteoporos Int 16:534–540, 2005.
131. Twomey LT, Taylor JR: Age changes in lumbar vertebrae and intervertebral discs, Clin Orthop Relat Res 224:97–104, 1987.
132. National Osteoporosis Foundation Working Group on Vertebral Fractures: assessing vertebral fractures, J Bone Miner Res 10:518–523, 1995.
133. Genant HK, Wu CY, van Kuijk C, et al: Vertebral fracture assessment using a semi-quantitative technique, J Bone Miner Res 8:1137–1148, 1993.
134. Wu CY, Li J, Jergas M, et al: Comparison of semi-quantitative and quantitative techniques for the assessment of prevalent and incident fractures, Osteoporos Int 5:354–370, 1995.
135. Benhamou CL, Lespessailles E, Jacquet G, et al: Fractal organization of trabecular bone images on calcaneus radiographs, J Bone Miner Res 9:1909–1918, 1994.
136. Genant HK, Engelke K, Fuerst T, et al: Noninvasive assessment of bone mineral and structure: state of the art, J Bone Miner Res 11:707–730, 1996.
137. Faulkner KG, Miller PD: Clinical use of bone densitometry. In Marcus R, Feldman D, Nelson DA, Rosen CJ, editors: Osteoporosis, ed 3, San Diego, CA, 2007, Academic Press, San Diego, pp 1493–1518.
138. Reid IR, Evans MC, Ames R, et al: The influence of osteophytes and aortic calcification on spinal mineral density. The influence of osteophytes and aortic calcification on spinal mineral density in postmenopausal women, J Clin Endocrinol Metab 72:1372–1374, 1991.
139. Goh JCH, Low SL, Bose K: Effect of femoral rotation on bone mineral density measurements with dual x-ray absorptiometry, Calcif Tissue Int 57:340–343, 1995.
140. Gluer CC, Blake G, Lu Y, et al: Accurate assessment of precision errors: how to measure the reproducibility errors of bone densitometry techniques, Osteoporos Int 5:262–270, 1995.
141. Genant H, Cann C, Ettinger B, et al: Quantitative computed tomography of vertebral spongiosa: a sensitive method for detecting early bone loss after oophorectomy, Ann Intern Med 97:699–705, 1982.
142. Rüegsegger P, Koller B, Müller R: A microtomographic system for the non-destructive evaluation of bone architecture, Calcif Tis Int 58:24–29, 1996.
143. Kang Y, Engelke K, Fuchs S, et al: Anatomic coordinate system of the femoral neck for highly reproducible BMD measurements using 3D QCT, Comput Med Imaging Graph 29:533–541, 2005.
144. Lang TF, Li J, Harris ST, et al: Assessment of vertebral bone mineral density using volumetric quantitative CT, J Comput Assist Tomogr 23:130–137, 1999.
145. Bousson V, LeBras A, Roqueplan F, et al: Volumetric quantitative computed tomography of the proximal femur: relationships linking geometric and densitometric variables to bone strength. Role for compact bone, Osteoporos Int 17:855–864, 2006.
146. Gordon C, Lang T, Augat P, et al: Image-based assessment of spinal trabecular bone structure from high-resolution CT images, Osteoporos Int 8:317–325, 1998.
147. Ito M, Ikeda K, Nishiguchi M, et al: Multi-detector row CT imaging of vertebral microstructure for evaluation of fracture risk, J Bone Miner Res 20:1828–1836, 2005.
148. Kevak JH, Rossi SA, Jones KA, et al: Prediction of femoral fracture load using automated finite element modelling, J Biomech 31:125–133, 1998.
149. Crawford RP, Cann CE, Keaveny TM: Finite element models predict in vitro vertebral body compressive strength better than quantitative computed tomography, Bone 33:44–50, 2003.
150. Boutroy S, Bouxsein ML, Munoz F, et al: In vivo assessment of trabecular bone microarchitecture by high-resolution peripheral quantitative computed tomography, J Clin Endocrinol Metab 90:6508–6515, 2005.
151. Sornay-Rendu E, Boutroy S, Munoz F, et al: Alterations of cortical and trabecular architecture are associated with fractures in postmenopausal women, partially independent of decreased BMD measured by DXA: the OFELY study, J Bone Miner Res 22:425–433, 2007.
152. Boutroy S, Van Rietbergen B, Sornay-Rendu E, et al: Finite element analysis based on in vivo HR-pQCT images of the distal radius is associated with wrist fracture in postmenopausal women, J Bone Miner Res 23:392–399, 2008.
153. Hans D, Gluer CC, Njeh CF: Ultrasonic evaluation of osteoporosis. In Meunier PJ editor: Osteoporosis, Diagnosis and management. London, 1998, Martin Dunitz, pp 59–78.
154. Bauer DC, Gluer CC, Cauley JA, et al: Bone ultrasound predicts fractures strongly and independently of densitometry in older women: a prospective study, Arch Intern Med 157:629–634, 1997.
155. Kanis JA: Diagnosis of osteoporosis and assessment of fracture risk, Lancet 359:1929–1936, 2002.
156. Nelson HD, Helfand M, Woolf SH, et al: Screening for postmenopausal osteoporosis: a review of the evidence for the US preventive Services Task Force, Ann Int Med 137:529–541, 2002.

157. Duboeuf F, Bauer DC, Chapurlat RD, et al: Assessment of vertebral fracture using densitometric morphometry, J Clin Densitom 8:362–368, 2005.
158. Chapurlat RD, Duboeuf F, Marion-Audibert HO, et al: Effectiveness of instant vertebral assessment to detect prevalent vertebral fracture, Osteoporos Int 17:1189–1195, 2006.
159. Garnero P, Delmas PD: Assessment of the serum levels of bone alkaline phosphatase with a new immunometric assay in patients with metabolic bone disease, J Clin Endocrinol Metab 77:1046–1053, 1993.
160. Garnero P, Grimaux M, Demiaux B, et al: Measurement of serum osteocalcin with a human-specific two-site immunoradiometric assay, J Bone Miner Res 7:1389–1398, 1992.
161. Ducy P, Desbois C, Boyce B, et al: Increased bone formation in osteocalcin-deficient mice, Nature 382:448–452, 1986.
162. Lee NK, Sowa H, Hinoi E, et al: Endocrine regulation of energy metabolism by the skeleton, Cell 130:456–469, 2007.
163. Szulc P, Seeman E, Delmas PD: Biochemical measurements of bone turnover in children and adolescents, Osteoporos Int 11:281–294, 2000.
164. Chen P, Satterwhite JH, Licata AA, et al: Early changes in biochemical markers of bone formation predict BMD response to teriparatide in postmenopausal women with osteoporosis, J Bone Miner Res 20:962–970, 2005.
165. Uebelhart D, Schlemmer A, Johansen J, et al: Effect of menopause and hormone replacement therapy on the urinary excretion of pyridinium crosslinks, J Clin Endocrinol Metab 72:367–373, 1991.
166. Garnero P, Sornay-Rendu E, Chapuy MC, et al: Increased bone turnover in late post-menopausal women is a major determinant of osteoporosis, J Bone Miner Res 11:337–349, 1996.
167. Hansen MA, Kirsten O, Riis BJ, et al: Role of peak bone mass and bone loss in postmenopausal osteoporosis: 12 years study, BMJ 303:961–964, 1991.
168. Garnero P, Dargent-Molina P, Hans D, et al: Do markers of bone resorption add to bone mineral density and ultrasonographic heel measurement for the prediction of hip fracture in elderly women? The EPIDOS prospective study, Osteoporos Int 8:563–569, 1998.
169. Riis SBL, Hansen AM, Jensen K, et al: Low bone mass and fast rate of bone loss at menopause—equal risk factors for future fracture. A 15 year follow-up study, Bone 19:9–12, 1996.
170. Garnero P, Hausher M, Chapuy C, et al: Markers of bone resorption predict hip fracture in elderly women: the EPIDOS prospective study, J Bone Miner Res 11:1531–1538, 1996.
171. Chapurlat RD, Garnero P, Bréart PJ, et al: serum type I collagen breakdown products (serum CTX) predicts hip fracture risk in elderly women: the EPIDOS study, Bone 27:283–286, 2000.
172. Garnero P, Shih WJ, Gineyts E, et al: Comparison of new biochemical markers of bone turnover in late postmenopausal osteoporotic women in response to alendronate treatment, J Clin Endocrinol Metab 79:1693–1700, 1994.
173. Bjarnason NH, Sarkar S, Duong T, et al: Six and twelve months changes in bone turnover are related to reduction in vertebral fracture risk during 3 years of raloxifene treatment in postmenopausal osteoporosis, Osteoporos Int 12:922–930, 2001.
174. Eastell R, Barton I, Hannon RA, et al: Relationship of early changes in bone resorption in fracture risk with risedronate, J Bone Miner Res 18:1051–1056, 2003.
175. Delmas PD, Vrijens B, Eastell R, et al: Effect of monitoring bone turnover markers on persistence with risedronate treatment of postmenopausal osteoporosis: the IMPACT study, J Clin Endocrinol Metab 92:1296–1304, 2007.
176. Institute of Medicine: Dietary references intakes for calcium, phosphorus, magnesium vitamin D and fluoride, Washington DC, 1997, National Academy Press.
177. Ooms ME, Roos JC, Bezemer PD, et al: Prevention of bone loss by vitamin D supplementation in elderly women: a randomized double-blind trial, J Clin Endocrinol Metab 80:1052–1058, 1995.
178. Chapuy MC, Arlot ME, Duboeuf, et al: Vitamin D_3 and calcium to prevent hip fractures in elderly women, N Engl J Med 237:1637–1642, 1992.
179. Dawson-Hughes B, Dallal GE, Krall EA, et al: Effects of vitamin D supplementation on overall bone loss in healthy postmenopausal women, Ann Intern Med 115:505–512, 1991.
180. Kannus P, Haapasalo H, Sankelo M, et al: Effect of starting age of physical activity on bone mass in the dominant arm of tennis and squash players, Ann Intern Med 123:27–31, 1995.
181. Wolf SL, Barnhart HX, Kutner NJ, et al: Reducing frailty and falls in older persons: an investigation of tai chi and computerized balance training, J Am Geriatr Soc 44:489–497, 1996.
182. Kannus P, Parkkari J, Niemi S, et al: Prevention of hip fracture in elderly people with use of hip protector, N Engl J Med 343:1506–1513, 2000.
183. van Schoor NM, Smit JH, Twisk JWR, et al: Prevention of hip fractures by external hip protectors. a randomized controlled trial, JAMA 289:1957–1962, 2003.
184. Kanis JA, Oden A, Johnell O, et al: Uncertain future of trials in osteoporosis, Osteoporos Int 13:443–449, 2002.
185. Grady D, Rubin SM, Pettiti DB, et al: Hormone therapy to prevent disease and prolong life in postmenopausal women, Ann Intern Med 117:1016–1037, 1992.
186. Cauley JA, Robbins J, Chen Z, et al: Effects of estrogen plus progestin on risk of fracture and bone mineral density. The Women's Health Initiative randomized trial, JAMA 290:1729–1738, 2003.
187. Torgerson DJ, Bell-Syer SEM: Hormone replacement therapy and prevention of vertebral fractures: a meta-analysis of randomized trials, BMC Musculoskelet Disord 2:2–7, 2001.
188. Torgerson DJ, Bell-Syer SEM: Hormone replacement therapy and prevention of nonvertebral fractures. A met-analysis of randomized trials, JAMA 285:2891–2897, 2001.
189. Nieves JW, Komar L, Cosman F, et al: Calcium potentiates the effect of estrogen and calcitonin on bone mass: review and analysis, Am J Clin Nutr 67:18–24, 1998.
190. Cauley JA, Seeley DJ, Ensrud K, et al: Estrogen replacement therapy and fractures in older women: study of Osteoporotic Fractures Research Group, Ann Intern Med 122:9–16, 1995.
191. Writing group for the Women's Health Initiative investigators: risks and benefits of estrogen plus progestin in healthy postmenopausal women. Principal results from the Women's Health Initiative randomized controlled trial, JAMA 288:321–333, 2002.
192. Manson JE, Hsia J, Johnson KC, et al: Estrogen plus progestin and the risk of coronary heart disease, N Engl J Med 349:523–534, 2003.
193. Wassertheil-Smoller S, Hendrix SL, Limacher M, et al: Effect of estrogen plus progestin on stroke in postmenopausal women. The Women's Health Initiative: a randomized trial, JAMA 289:2673–2684, 2003.
194. Chlebowski RT, Hendrix SL, Langer RD, et al: Influence of estrogen plus progestin on breast cancer and mammography in healthy postmenopausal women. The Women's Health Initiative randomized trial, JAMA 289:3243–3253, 2003.
195. Schumaker SA, Legault C, Rapp SR, et al: Estrogen plus progestin and the incidence of dementia and mild cognitive impairment in postmenopausal women. The Women's Health Initiative Memory study: a randomized controlled trial, JAMA 289:2651–2662, 2003.
196. Hays J, Ockene JK, Brunner RL, et al: Effects of estrogen plus progestin on health-related quality of life, N Engl J Med 348:1839–1854, 2003.
197. Hulley S, Grady D, Bush T, et al: Randomized trial of estrogen plus progestin for secondary prevention of coronary heart disease in postmenopausal women, JAMA 280:605–613, 1998.
198. Rossouw JE, Prentice RL, Manson JE, et al: Postmenopausal hormone therapy and risk of cardiovascular disease by age and years since menopause, JAMA 297:1465–1477, 2007.
199. Kumle M: Declining breast cancer incidence and decreased HRT use, Lancet 372:608–610, 2008.
200. Chapurlat RD, Delmas PD: Drug insight: Bisphosphonates for postmenopausal osteoporosis, Nat Clin Pract Endocrinol Metab 2:211–219, 2006.
201. Watts NB, Harris ST, Genant HK, et al: Intermittent cyclical etidronate treatment of postmenopausal osteoporosis, N Engl J Med 323:73–79, 1990.
202. Cranney A, Guyatt G, Krolicki N, et al: A meta-analysis of etidronate for the treatment of postmenopausal osteoporosis, Osteoporos Int 12:140–151, 2001.
203. Hosking D, Chilvers CED, Christiansen C, et al: Prevention of bone loss with alendronate in postmenopausal women under 60 years of age, N Engl J Med 338:485–492, 1998.
204. Black DM, Cummings SR, Karpf DB, et al: Randomised trial of effect of alendronate on risk of fracture in women with existing vertebral fractures, Lancet 348: 1535–1541, 1996.
205. Ensrud KE, Black DM, Palermo L, et al: Treatment with alendronate prevents fractures in women at highest risk, Arch Intern Med 157:2617–2624, 1997.
206. Cummings SR, Black DM, Thompson DE, et al: Effect of alendronate on risk of fracture in women with low bone density but without vertebral fractures, JAMA 280:2077–2082, 1998.
207. Harris ST, Watts N, Genant HK, et al: Effects of risedronate treatment on vertebral and nonvertebral fractures in women with postmenopausal osteoporosis, JAMA 282:1344–1352, 1999.
208. Reginster J-Y, Minne HW, Sorensen OH, et al: Randomized trial of the effects of risedronate on vertebral fractures in women with established postmenopausal osteoporosis, Osteoporos Int 11:83–91, 2000.
209. McClung MR, Geusens P, Miller PD, et al: Effect of risedronate on the risk of hip fracture in elderly women, N Engl J Med 344:333–340, 2001.
210. Chestnut CHIII, Skag A, Christiansen C, et al: Effects of oral ibandronate administered daily or intermittently on fracture risk in postmenopausal osteoporosis, J Bone Miner Res 19:1241–1249, 2004.
211. Reid IR, Brown JP, Burckardt P, et al: Intravenous zoledronic acid in postmenopausal women with low bone mineral density, N Engl J Med 346:653–661, 2002.
212. Black DM, Delmas PD, Eastell R, et al: Once-yearly zoledronic acid for treatment of postmenopausal osteoporosis, N Engl J Med 356:1809–1822, 2006.
213. Lyles KW, Colon-Emeric CS, Magaziner JS, et al: Zoledronic acid and clinical fractures and mortality after hip fracture, N Engl J Med 357:1799–1809, 2007.
214. McCloskey E, Selby P, de Takats D, et al: Effects of clodronate on vertebral fracture risk in osteoporosis: a 1-year interim analysis, Bone 28:310–315, 2001.
215. Adachi JD, Bensen WG, Brown J, et al: Intermittent etidronate therapy to prevent corticosteroid-induced osteoporosis, N Engl J Med 337:382–387, 1997.
216. Saag KG, Emkey R, Schnitzer TJ, et al: Alendronate for the prevention and treatment of glucocorticoid-induced osteoporosis, N Engl J Med 339:292–299, 1998.
217. Wallach S, Cohen S, Reid DM, et al: Effects of risedronate treatment on bone density and vertebral fracture in patients on corticosteroid therapy, Calcif Tissue Int 67:277–285, 2000.
218. Delmas PD, Bjarnason NH, Mitlak BH, et al: Effects of raloxifene on bone mineral density, serum cholesterol concentrations and uterine endometrium in postmenopausal women, N Engl J Med 337:1641–1647, 1997.
219. Cummings SR, Eckert S, Krueger KA, et al: The effect of raloxifene on risk of breast cancer in postmenopausal women: results from the MORE randomized trial. Multiple outcomes on raloxifene evaluation, JAMA 281:2189–2197, 1999.
220. Ettinger B, Black DM, Mitlack BH, et al: Reduction of vertebral fracture risk in postmenopausal women with osteoporosis treated with raloxifene, JAMA 282:637–645, 1999.
221. Delmas PD, Ensrud KE, Adachi JD, et al: Efficacy of raloxifene on vertebral fracture risk reduction in postmenopausal women with osteoporosis: four-year results from a randomized clinical trial, J Clin Endocrinol Metab 87:3609–3617, 2002.
222. Delmas PD, Genant HK, Crans GG, et al: Severity of prevalent vertebral fractures and the risk of subsequent vertebral and non vertebral: results from the MORE trial, Bone 33:522–532, 2003.
223. Barrett-Connor E, Grady D, Sashegyi A, et al: Raloxifene and cardiovascular events in osteoporotic postmenopausal women. Four-year results from the MORE randomized trial, JAMA 287:847–857, 2002.
224. Barrett-Connor E, Mosca L, Collins P, et al: Effects of raloxifene on cardiovascular events and breast cancer

in postmenopausal women, N Engl J Med 355:125–137, 2006.

225. Vogel VG, Costantino JP, Wickerham DL, et al: Effects of tamoxifen vs raloxifene on the risk of developing invasive breast cancer and other disease outcomes: the NSABP Study of Tamoxifen and Raloxifene (STAR) P-2 trial, JAMA 295:2727–2741, 2006.

226. Silverman SL, Christiansen C, Genant HK, et al: Efficacy of bazedoxifene in reducing new vertebral fracture risk in postmenopausal women with osteoporosis: results of a 3-year randomized placebo-, and active-controlled clinical trial, J Bone Miner Res 23:1923–1934, 2008.

227. Cummings SR, Eastell R, Ensrud K, et al: The effects of lasofoxifene on fractures and breast cancer: 3-year results from the PEARL Trial, J Bone Miner Res 23(Suppl 1):S81, 2008.

228. Cummings SR, McClung MR, Christiansen C, et al: A phase III study of the effects of denosumab on vertebral, non vertebral, and hip fracture in women with osteoporosis: results from the FREEDOM Trial, J Bone Miner Res 23(Suppl 1):S80, 2008.

229. Brown JP, Prince RL, Deal C, et al: Comparison of the effect of denosumab and alendronate on bone mineral density and biochemical markers of bone turnover in postmenopausal women with low bone mass: a randomized, blinded, phase 3 trial, J Bone Miner Res 24:153–161, 2009.

230. Ellis GK, Bone HG, Chlebowski R, et al: Randomized trial of denosumab in patients receiving adjuvant aromatase inhibitors for nonmetastatic breast cancer, J Clin Oncol 26:4875–4882, 2008.

231. Miller PD, Bolognese MA, Liewecki EM, et al: Effect of denosumab on bone density and turnover in postmenopausal women with low bone mass after long-term continued, discontinued, and restarting of therapy: a randomized blinded phase 2 clinical trial, Bone 43:222–229, 2008.

232. Overgaard K, Riis BJ, Christiansen C, et al: Effect of salcatonin given intranasally on early postmenopausal bone loss, BMJ 299:477–479, 1989.

233. Overgaard K, Hansen MA, Jensen SB, et al: Effect of salcatonin given intranasally on bone mass and fracture rates in established osteoporosis: a dose-response study, BMJ 305:556–561, 1992.

234. Chestnut CH 3rd, Silverman S, Andriano K, et al: A randomized trial of nasal spray salmon calcitonin in postmenopausal women with established osteoporosis: the Prevent Recurrence of Osteoporotic Fractures study. PROOF Study Group, Am J Med 109:267–276, 2000.

235. Cummings SR, Chapurlat RD: What PROOF proves about calcitonin and clinical trials, Am J Med 109:330–331, 2000.

236. Neer RM, Arnaud CD, Zanchetta JR, et al: Effect of parathyroid hormone (1–34) on fractures and bone mineral density in postmenopausal women with osteoporosis, N Engl J Med 344:434–441, 2001.

237. Ettinger B, San Martin J, Crans G, et al: Differential effects of teriparatide on BMD after treatment with raloxifene or alendronate, J Bone Miner Res 2004; 19:745–751.

238. Delmas PD, Vergnaud P, Arlot ME, et al: The anabolic effect of human PTH (1–34) on bone formation is blunted when bone resorption in inhibited by the bisphosphonate tiludronate—Is activated resorption a prerequisite for the in vivo effect of PTH on formation in a remodeling system? Bone 16:603–610, 1995.

239. Black DM, Greenspan SL, Ensrud KE, et al: The effects of parathyroid hormone and alendronate alone or in combination in postmenopausal osteoporosis, N Engl J Med 349:1207–1215, 2003.

240. Finkelstein JS, Hayes A, Hunzelman JL, et al: The effects of parathyroid hormone, alendronate, or both, in men with osteoporosis, N Engl J Med 349:1216–1226, 2003.

241. Miller PD, Delmas PD, Lindsay R, et al: Early responsiveness of women with osteoporosis to teriparatide after therapy with alendronate or risedronate, J Clin Endocrinol Metab 93:3785–3793, 2008.

242. Obermayer-Pietsch BM, Marin F, McCloskey EV, et al: Effects of two years of daily teriparatide treatment on BMD in postmenopausal women with severe osteoporosis with and without prior antiresorptive treatment, J Bone Miner Res 23:1591–1600, 2008.

243. Geenspan SL, Bone HG, Ettinger MP, et al: Effect of recombinant human parathyroid hormone (1–84) on vertebral fracture and bone mineral density in postmenopausal women with osteoporosis: a randomized trial, Ann Intern Med 146(5):326–339, 2007.

244. Dawson-Hughes B, Dallal GE, Krall EA, et al: A controlled trial of the effect of calcium supplementation on bone density in postmenopausal women, N Engl J Med 323:878–883, 1990.

245. Reid IR, Ames RW, Evans MC, et al: Long-term effects of calcium supplementation on bone loss and fractures in postmenopausal women: a randomized controlled trial, Am J Med 98:331–335, 1995.

246. Recker RR, Hinders S, Davies KM, et al: Correcting calcium nutritional deficiency prevents spine fractures in elderly women, J Bone Miner Res 11:1961–1966, 1996.

247. Lips P, Graafmans WC, Ooms ME, et al: Vitamin D supplementation and fracture incidence in elderly persons: a randomized, placebo-controlled clinical trial, Ann Intern Med 124:400–406, 1996.

248. Dawson-Hughes B, Harris SS, Krall EA, et al: Effect of calcium and vitamin D supplementation on bone density in men and women 65 years of age or older, N Engl J Med 337:670–676, 1997.

249. Heikinheimo RJ, Inkovaraa JA, Harju EJ, et al: Annual injection of vitamin D and fractures of aged bones, Calcif Tissue Int 51:105–110, 1992.

250. Trivedi DP, Doll R, Khaw KY: Effect of four monthly oral vitamin D3 (cholecalciferol) supplementation on fractures and mortality in men and women living in the community: randomized double blind controlled trial, BMJ 326:469–475, 2003.

251. Harwood RH, Sahota O, Gaynor K, et al: A randomized, controlled comparison of different calcium and vitamin D supplementation regimens in elderly women after hip fracture: the Nottingham neck of femur (NONOF) study, Age Ageing 33:45–51, 2004.

252. Meunier PJ, Slosman DO, Delmas PD, et al: Strontium ranelate: dose-dependent effects in established postmenopausal osteoporosis—a two-year randomized placebo controlled trial, J Clin Endocrinol Metab 87:2060–2066, 2002.

253. Reginster JY, Deroisy R, Dougados M, et al: Prevention of early postmenopausal bone loss by strontium ranelate: the randomized, two-year, double-masked, dose ranging, placebo-controlled PREVOS trial, Osteoporos Int 13:925–931, 2002.

254. Meunier PJ, Roux C, Seeman E, et al: The effects of strontium ranelate on the risk of vertebral fracture in women with postmenopausal osteoporosis, N Engl J Med 350:459–468, 2004.

255. Reginster JY, Seeman E, De Vernejoul MC, et al: Strontium ranelate reduces the risk of nonvertebral fractures in postmenopausal women with osteoporosis: Treatment of Peripheral Osteoporosis (TROPOS) study, J Clin Endocrinol Metab 90(5):2816–2822, 2005.

256. Seeman E, Vellas B, Benhamou C, et al: Strontium ranelate reduces the risk of vertebral and nonvertebral fractures in women eighty years of age and older, J Bone Miner Res 21:1113–1120, 2006.

257. Alexandersen P, Toussaint A, Christiansen C, et al: Ipriflavone in the treatment of postmenopausal osteoporosis: a randomized controlled trial, JAMA 285:1482–1488, 2001.

258. Cummings SR, Ettinger B, Delmas PD, et al: The effects of tibolone in older postmenopausal women, N Engl J Med 359:697–708, 2008.

259. Holloway L, Kohlmeier L, Kent K, et al: Skeletal effects of cyclic recombinant human growth hormone and salmon calcitonin on osteopenic postmenopausal women, J Clin Endocrinol Metab 82:1111–1117, 1997.

260. Reid IR, Ames RW, Orr-Walker BJ, et al: Hydrochlorothiazide reduces loss of cortical bone in normal postmenopausal women: a randomized controlled trial, Am J Med 109:362–370, 2000.

261. Delmas PD: Treatment of postmenopausal osteoporosis, Lancet 359:2018–2026, 2002.

262. Kanis JA, McCloskey EV, Johansson H, et al: Case finding for the management of osteoporosis with FRAX-assessment and intervention thresholds for the UK, Osteoporos Int 19:1395–1408, 2008.

263. Tosteson ANA, Melton LJ III, Dawson-Hugues B, et al: Cost-effective osteoporosis treatment thresholds: the United States perspective, Osteoporos Int 19:437–447, 2008.

264. Dawson-Hughes B, Tosteson ANA, Melton LJ III, et al: Implications of absolute fracture risk assessment for osteoporosis practice guidelines in the USA, Osteoporos Int 19:449–458, 2008.

265. Cummings SR, Karpf DB, Harris F, et al: Improvement in spine bone density and reduction in risk of vertebral fractures during treatment with antiresorptive drugs, Am J Med 112:281–289, 2002.

266. Chapurlat RD, Palermo L, Ramsay P, et al: Risk of fracture among women who lose bone density during treatment with alendronate, The Fracture Intervention Trial Osteoporos Int 16:842–848, 2005.

267. Chen P, Satterwhite JH, Licata AA, et al: Early changes in biochemical markers of bone formation predict BMD response to teriparatide in postmenopausal women with osteoporosis, J Bone Miner Res 20:962–970, 2005.

268. Bauer DC, Black DM, Garnero P, et al: Change in bone turnover and hip, non-spine, and vertebral fracture in alendronate-treated women: the Fracture Intervention Trial, J Bone Miner Res 19:1250–1258, 2004.

Chapter 14

CHRONIC KIDNEY DISEASE MINERAL AND BONE DISORDER

KATHERINE WESSELING-PERRY and ISIDORO B. SALUSKY

Pathogenesis of CKD-MBD
Abnormalities of Calcium, Phosphorous, FGF-23, Vitamin D, and PTH Metabolism

Pathogenesis of Renal Bone Disease
Abnormalities in Bone Turnover, Mineralization, and Volume

Clinical Manifestations
Bone Pain
Muscle Weakness
Skeletal Deformities
Growth Retardation
Extraskeletal Calcification
Calciphylaxis
Dialysis-Related Amyloidosis

Diagnostic Evaluations
Biochemical Determinations
Radiography
Bone Biopsy

Treatment of CKD-MBD
Dietary Manipulation of Calcium and Phosphorus
Phosphate-Binding Agents
Vitamin D Therapy
Calcimimetics
Parathyroidectomy
Growth Hormone Therapy

Bone Disease After Successful Kidney Transplantation

The kidney plays a major role in bone and mineral homeostasis by regulating calcium, phosphorous, parathyroid hormone (PTH), fibroblast growth factor-23 (FGF-23), and calcitriol [1,25-dihydroxyvitamin D_3, $1,25(OH)_2D_3$] metabolism. Disordered regulation of mineral metabolism occurs early in the course of chronic kidney disease (CKD) and results in alterations in bone modeling and remodeling. A growing body of evidence demonstrates that cardiovascular calcifications accompany CKD, that cardiovascular disease is the leading cause of mortality in patients with CKD, and that therapies designed to treat the skeletal consequences of CKD affect the progression of vascular pathology; this has led to reclassification of the mineral, skeletal, and vascular complications associated with progressive kidney disease. Together, these alterations are termed CKD mineral and bone disorder (CKD-MBD).[1]

CKD-MBD is defined as a systemic disorder of mineral and bone metabolism due to CKD that is manifested by one or a combination of the following: (1) abnormalities of calcium, phosphorous, PTH, or vitamin D metabolism; (2) abnormalities in bone histology, linear growth, or strength; or (3) vascular or other soft tissue calcification. Renal osteodystrophy is the specific term used to describe the bone pathology that occurs as a complication of CKD and therefore is one aspect of CKD-MBD. Traditionally, such lesions have been defined according to alterations in bone turnover, ranging from high bone turnover (secondary hyperparathyroidism, osteitis fibrosa) to low bone turnover (adynamic bone disease and osteomalacia). However, alterations in skeletal mineralization and volume are common in patients in CKD[1] and may contribute to such outcomes as fractures and skeletal deformities, which may persist despite normalization of bone turnover.[2] Bone histomorphometry continues to be the gold standard for the assessment of three essential aspects of bone histology: turnover, mineralization, and volume.[1] This chapter summarizes major aspects of the pathogenesis, clinical manifestations, histologic features, and therapeutic interventions currently used in the management of CKD-MBD. Clinical and histologic features of bone disease after successful kidney transplantation are also described.

Pathogenesis of CKD-MBD

ABNORMALITIES OF CALCIUM, PHOSPHOROUS, FGF-23, VITAMIN D, AND PTH METABOLISM

Calcium and Phosphorus

$1,25(OH)_2D_3$, the most active form of vitamin D, regulates serum calcium levels by increasing intestinal calcium absorption. The kidney generates most circulating $1,25(OH)_2D_3$, converting $25(OH)D$ to $1,25(OH)_2D_3$ by means of the enzyme 1α-hydroxylase. As renal failure progresses, calcitriol levels and

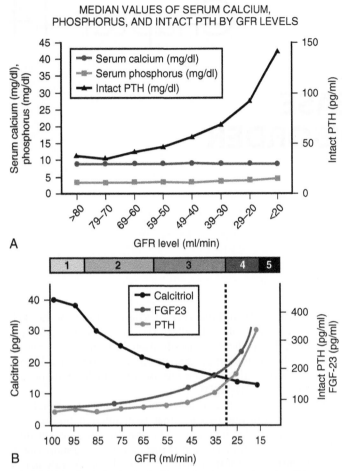

A, MEDIAN VALUES OF SERUM CALCIUM, PHOSPHORUS, AND INTACT PTH BY GFR LEVELS

FIGURE 14-1. **A,** Median levels of calcium, phosphorus, and parathyroid hormone (PTH) per stage of chronic kidney disease (CKD). Median serum levels of calcium and phosphorus stay constant until late in the course of CKD; PTH levels rise before any changes are seen in calcium and phosphorus. **B,** In patients with CKD, serum $1,25(OH)_2D_3$ levels decline early in the course of kidney dysfunction, before changes in serum calcium or phosphorous concentrations occur and prior to any rise in serum PTH levels. (**A,** Data from Levin A, et al: Kidney Int 71:31–38, 2007.[3])

intestinal calcium absorption decline. However, at the same time, rising PTH levels increase 1α-hydroxylase activity, release calcium and phosphorus from bone, and promote renal conservation of calcium, thus maintaining serum calcium levels within the normal range until late in the course of CKD.[3,4]

Likewise, serum phosphorous levels usually are maintained in the normal range throughout mild to moderate CKD. Elevated serum PTH and FGF-23 levels increase phosphate excretion, thus maintaining overall phosphate balance until the glomerular filtration rate (GFR) declines to 25% to 30% of normal.[5,6] In late (stage 4) CKD, hyperphosphatemia ensues and contributes to secondary hyperparathyroidism (Fig. 14-1A).[3]

Fibroblast Growth Factor-23

A recently described phosphaturic hormone, FGF-23, was first identified in patients with tumor-induced osteomalacia[7] and autosomal dominant hypophosphatemic rickets.[8] In these conditions and in patients with X-linked hypophosphatemia, elevated circulating levels of FGF-23 result in renal phosphate wasting and suppression of $1,25(OH)_2D_3$ production.[8,9] FGF-23 is made within bone,[10,11] and the presence of a cofactor, Klotho, is essential for its action.[12] Serum values increase as CKD progresses,

becoming markedly elevated in individuals with end-stage kidney disease (Fig. 14-1B).[13,14] In patients with CKD, $1,25(OH)_2D_3$ levels are inversely related to levels of circulating FGF-23, suggesting that increases in FGF-23 early in the course of CKD may play a role in declining active vitamin D levels.[14] FGF-23 levels increase in response to vitamin D sterol therapy,[15] and levels may be regulated by phosphorous intake.[16,17] FGF-23 levels have been implicated in parathyroid gland regulation (vide infra).[18,19]

Vitamin D

Serum $1,25(OH)_2D_3$ levels decline early in the course of kidney dysfunction, before any changes in serum calcium or phosphorous concentrations and prior to any rise in serum PTH levels.[3,20] In late stages of CKD, phosphate retention and increased serum phosphorous levels directly suppress 1α-hydroxylase activity.[16] However, although these factors contribute to declining 1α-hydroxylase activity, current evidence demonstrates that rising FGF-23 levels may be of even greater importance.[14]

Low circulating levels of $1,25(OH)_2D_3$ have consequences for many tissues. Aside from its effect on intestinal calcium absorption, $1,25(OH)_2D_3$ plays a direct role in the suppression of PTH gene transcription (vide infra). Animal studies also indicate that $1,25(OH)_2D_3$ is essential for normal skeletal physiology— particularly in growing animals—and that this effect may not be mediated by the vitamin D receptor (VDR). Mice who lack the VDR [i.e., mice unable to respond to the actions of $1,25(OH)_2D_3$ through its classical receptor] are phenotypically similar to those lacking the 1α-hydroxylase gene itself [i.e., mice unable to generate $1,25(OH)_2D_3$]; both sets of mice are hypocalcemic with markedly elevated serum PTH levels, parathyroid gland hyperplasia, and rickets.[21] However, a diet replete in calcium, phosphorus, and lactate is sufficient to normalize serum calcium, phosphorous, and PTH levels and to prevent the development of rickets in VDR-deficient animals.[22] By contrast, this "rescue diet" is unable to completely reverse growth plate abnormalities in 1α-hydroxylase–deficient mice, suggesting that $1,25(OH)_2D_3$, acting through a receptor other than the classical VDR, may be essential for proper growth plate development.[23] $1,25(OH)_2D_3$ has been shown to regulate the renin-angiotensin system; 1α-hydroxylase–deficient mice demonstrate cardiac hypertrophy and dysfunction, which are reversed with angiotensin-converting enzyme blockade.[24,25] Thus, $1,25(OH)_2D_3$ may be essential for cardiac health—a finding that could explain observational data suggesting that active vitamin D sterol therapy improves survival in patients treated with maintenance dialysis.[26,27]

Native 25-hydroxyvitamin D [25(OH)D] deficiency is prevalent in patients with CKD; low levels of this form of the hormone also contribute to altered mineral metabolism. Vitamin D may be made in the skin or ingested from the diet.[28,29] Ultraviolet B (UVB) (290 to 315 nm) photons penetrate the skin and are absorbed by 7-dehydrocholesterol to form previtamin D_3, which then spontaneously converts to vitamin D_3. Vitamin D_3 is extruded from the skin cell into the extracellular space, where it binds vitamin D–binding protein.[30] Although vitamin D created in the skin is exclusively of the D_3 form, dietary sources of vitamin D and food supplements may contain vitamin D_2 (created through UV irradiation of ergosterol in yeast) or D_3 (from animal sources, particularly fish). Vitamin D (both D_2 and D_3) undergoes hydroxylation by the liver, forming 25(OH)D.[31] Subsequently, 25(OH)D is taken up by renal tubular cells through a megalin-dependent process and undergoes a second hydroxylation, facilitated by renal 1α-hydroxylase, to $1,25(OH)_2D_3$, a more potent stimulator of gut calcium absorption.[32,33] Conversion of $25(OH)D$ to $1,25(OH)_2D_3$ is independent of $25(OH)D$ stores in the general population but becomes a substrate-dependent process in patients with CKD.[34] Although the actions of $25(OH)D$ have been underemphasized in CKD, extrarenal 1α-hydroxylase activity may significantly contribute to $1,25(OH)_2D_3$ production, even in anephric patients.[35-37] Thus low levels of the precursor, $25(OH)D$, exacerbate $1,25(OH)_2 D_3$ deficiency in the context of CKD.

Levels of $25(OH)D$ below 32 ng/mL are associated with increased PTH levels, reduced bone mineral density (BMD),[38] and increased rates of hip fracture[39] in the general population and therefore represent insufficient vitamin D storage. It is interesting to note that $25(OH)D$ levels in the vast majority of the general population meet the definition of D insufficiency, and a large percentage—as many as 57% in one series of medical inpatients[40]—have serum levels less than 15 ng/mL, thus qualifying as vitamin D deficient. Prevalence is higher in individuals with darker skin pigmentation, with 52% of Hispanic and black adolescents from the same cohort meeting the criteria for vitamin D deficiency.[41]

Several recent studies have documented a high prevalence of $25(OH)D$ deficiency in patients with CKD.[42,43] Patients with CKD are at increased risk for vitamin D deficiency for several reasons. Many are chronically ill with little outdoor (sunlight) exposure, and CKD dietary restrictions, particularly of dairy products, curtail the intake of vitamin D–rich food.[44] When compared with individuals with normal kidney function, patients with CKD display decreased skin synthesis of vitamin D_3 in response to sunlight.[45] This is exacerbated in individuals with darker skin.[46] Proteinuria also contributes to D deficiency in the CKD population; $25(OH)D$, in combination with vitamin D–binding protein, is lost in the urine.[47,48]

Parathyroid Hormone

The human *PTH* gene is located on chromosome 11 and contains two introns, which separate three exons encoding the 5′ untranslated region (UTR), the prepro region and PTH, and the 3′ untranslated region. The initial translational product of the mRNA is prepro-PTH, a 115 amino acid single-chain polypeptide, which undergoes conversion to pro-PTH (90 amino acids) in the rough endoplasmic reticulum. Six additional residues are removed from the N-terminal of pro-PTH in the Golgi apparatus to form the biologically active 1-84 PTH. PTH then is stored in secretory granules prior to release into the bloodstream.[49-51] Sustained increases in PTH secretion occur with progression of CKD. This prolonged stimulation leads to high turnover bone disease and to the development of parathyroid gland hyperplasia.

PTH levels increase in response to alterations in metabolism of calcium, $1,25(OH)_2 D_3$, phosphorus, $25(OH)D$, and FGF-23 (Fig. 14-2). With the progression of CKD, additional factors develop that sustain high production of PTH. Among these factors are alterations in the regulation of *prepro-PTH* gene transcription, post-transcriptional modifications of PTH mRNA, reductions in calcium-sensing receptor (CaSR) and vitamin D receptor expression in the parathyroids, autonomous activity of adenomatous parathyroid glands, and skeletal resistance to the calcemic actions of PTH.

Calcium is the primary stimulus for PTH release. Calcium directly regulates PTH release via activation of the CaSR (vide

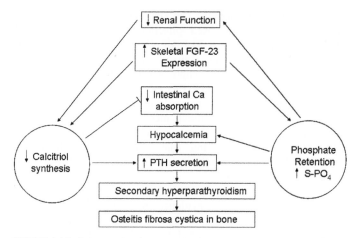

FIGURE 14-2. Pathogenesis of disordered mineral metabolism in chronic kidney disease (CKD). *Dark arrows* indicate effects of altered parathyroid hormone regulation; *open arrows* depict changes in fibroblast growth factor (FGF)-23 metabolism.

infra). Activation of the CaSR decreases PTH release; deactivation increases PTH secretion. Serum calcium levels also regulate pre-pro PTH transcription via two negative calcium-response elements (nCaRE) located far upstream (−2.4 kbp and −3.5 kbp) of the *PTH* gene,[52] and low serum calcium levels increase the stability of PTH mRNA by increasing levels of cytosolic parathyroid proteins, including AUF1,[53] which binds to the 3′ UTR of the PTH mRNA. Thus, low levels of serum calcium present in CKD increase the amount of PTH release and the longevity of the PTH transcript. However, serum calcium levels are maintained within the normal range until late in the course of CKD, but serum PTH levels begin to rise much earlier, before any changes in serum calcium are evident.[3] This suggests that factors other than calcium are important for the development of secondary hyperparathyroidism. Altered $1,25(OH)_2 D_3$ metabolism may, in fact, be the initiating event early in the course of CKD.[54-56]

Apart from its effects on serum calcium levels, $1,25(OH)_2D$ directly suppresses PTH levels. In conjunction with the VDR, $1,25(OH)_2D_3$ binds negative vitamin D response elements in the promoter region of the *PTH* gene, thus inhibiting *prepro-PTH* gene transcription.[57,58] In a positive-feedback loop, $1,25(OH)_2D_3$ itself increases *VDR* gene expression in the parathyroid gland, further suppressing *PTH* gene transcription. $1,25(OH)_2D_3$ also increases the expression of the CaSR, the expression of which is reduced in hyperplastic parathyroid tissues obtained from patients with secondary hyperparathyroidism.[59] Vitamin D deficiency in animals is associated with decreased expression of CaSR mRNA in parathyroid tissue; $1,25(OH)_2D_3$ therapy increases CaSR mRNA levels in a dose-dependent manner.[60] Because $1,25(OH)_2D_3$ is a potent inhibitor of cell proliferation, disturbances in renal calcitriol production and/or changes in VDR expression may be particularly important determinants of the degree of parathyroid hyperplasia and the extent of parathyroid gland enlargement in CKD.[61]

Phosphorous retention and hyperphosphatemia have been recognized for many years as important factors in the pathogenesis of secondary hyperparathyroidism. Phosphorous retention and hyperphosphatemia indirectly promote the secretion of PTH in several ways. Hyperphosphatemia lowers blood ionized calcium levels as free calcium ions complex with excess inorganic phosphate. The ensuing hypocalcemia stimulates PTH release. Increased phosphorus also impairs renal 1α-hydroxylase activity, which diminishes the conversion of 25(OH)D to 1,25(OH)$_2$D$_3$.[16] Finally, phosphorus can directly enhance PTH synthesis. High serum phosphorous levels decrease cytosolic phospholipase A2 (normally increased by CaSR activation), leading to a decrease in arachidonic acid production with a subsequent increase in PTH secretion.[62] Hypophosphatemia also decreases PTH mRNA transcript stability in vitro,[63] suggesting that phosphorus itself affects serum PTH levels, probably by increasing the stability of the PTH mRNA transcript.

Although the actions of 25(OH)D have been underemphasized in dialyzed patients, evidence suggests that levels of this so-called "storage" form of vitamin D have both indirect and direct effects on PTH secretion. Extrarenal 1α-hydroxylase activity may contribute significantly to calcitriol production, even in anephric patients.[35-37] Furthermore, recent evidence suggests the presence of 1α-hydroxylase in the parathyroid glands. 25(OH)D is converted inside the gland to 1,25(OH)$_2$D, thereby suppressing PTH.[64] 25(OH)D administration suppresses PTH synthesis even when parathyroid gland 1α-hydroxylase is inhibited, indicating that 25(OH)D contributes to PTH suppression independent of its conversion to calcitriol.[64] Indeed, recent studies have demonstrated that supplementation with ergocalciferol decreases serum PTH levels in patients with CKD.[65,66] Such findings suggest that assessment of vitamin D status should be routinely performed in this patient population.[67]

Altered FGF-23 synthesis and secretion may contribute to increasing PTH levels through both indirect and direct mechanisms. Levels of FGF-23 rise as CKD progresses[13,14] and contribute to declining 1,25(OH)$_2$D levels. Lower 1,25(OH)$_2$D levels, in turn, result in increasing PTH release. FGF-23 levels have been implicated in direct regulation of parathyroid gland function. In vitro and in vivo analysis of parathyroid glands from animals with normal renal function demonstrates that FGF-23 suppresses PTH secretion through a mechanism independent of its actions on vitamin D metabolism (vide infra).[18,19]

Alterations in parathyroid gland CaSR expression also occur in secondary hyperparathyroidism and may contribute to parathyroid gland hyperplasia. The CaSR is a seven-transmembrane G protein–coupled receptor with a large extracellular N-terminus, which binds acidic amino acids and divalent cations.[68] Low extracellular calcium levels result in decreased calcium binding to the receptor, conformational relaxation of the receptor, and a resultant increase in PTH secretion,[69] while activation of the receptor by high levels of serum calcium decreases PTH secretion.[70,71] Expression of the CaSR is reduced by 30% to 70%, as judged by immunohistochemical methods in hyperplastic parathyroid tissue obtained from human subjects with renal failure.[59,72] Decreased expression and activity of CaSR have been linked to decreased responsiveness in PTH secretion due to altered calcium levels.[73] This decreased expression of the CaSR results in insensitivity to serum calcium levels with subsequent uncontrolled secretion of PTH. Increased stimulation of the CaSR by calcimimetics has been shown to decrease PTH cell proliferation, implicating the CaSR as a regulator of cell proliferation and PTH secretion.[74]

The link between the CaSR and vitamin D in cell cycling in the parathyroid gland is incompletely understood. However, some evidence suggests that vitamin D may decrease parathyroid hyperplasia by activating the CaSR. CaSR gene transcription is regulated by vitamin D through two distinct vitamin D response elements in the gene's promoter region,[75] suggesting that alterations in vitamin D metabolism in renal failure could account for changes in calcium sensing by the parathyroid glands, and that vitamin D may act upstream of the CaSR in preventing parathyroid cell hyperplasia.[21]

Once established, parathyroid enlargement is difficult to reverse because the rate of apoptosis in parathyroid glands is low, and the half-life of parathyroid cells is approximately 30 years.[76] Chronic stimulation of parathyroid glands may lead to chromosomal changes that ultimately result in autonomous, unregulated growth and hormone release.[77] Hyperplastic parathyroid tissue has been shown to develop inactivation of tumor suppressor genes MEN1, the retinoblastoma protein,[78-80] and/or activating mutations of the RET proto-oncogene (MEN2a).[81] Chromosomal translocations resulting in the parathyroid promoter driving cell cycle proteins (particularly cyclin D$_1$) have been shown to be present in parathyroid adenomas.[82] Even in the absence of somatic mutations, PTH secretion from enlarged parathyroid glands may become uncontrollable owing to the nonsuppressible component of PTH release from a large number of parathyroid cells. This alone may be sufficient to produce hypercalcemia and progressive bone disease in patients with end-stage renal disease.

Pathogenesis of Renal Bone Disease

ABNORMALITIES IN BONE TURNOVER, MINERALIZATION, AND VOLUME

Evaluation of skeletal histology by bone histomorphometry provides a method for understanding the pathophysiology of renal bone disease and a guide to its proper management. As recently recommended by the Kidney Disease Improving Global Outcomes (KDIGO) workgroup, three areas of bone histology are examined: bone turnover, mineralization, and volume, all of which may be altered in patients with CKD.[1]

Turnover

Traditionally, renal osteodystrophy has been classified primarily by alterations in bone turnover. Because PTH activates the PTH-related protein (PTHrP) receptor on osteocytes and osteoblasts, increasing cellular activity of both osteoblasts and osteoclasts,[83,84] excessive levels of circulating PTH result in increased bone turnover (Figs. 14-3A and 14-3B).[85] Serum PTH levels are inversely correlated with GFR, and most patients with GFR less than 50 mL/min have increased serum PTH levels and high turnover bone disease.[86-88] The presence of CKD, however, markedly attenuates the effects of PTH on bone.[89-90] Indeed, serum levels of PTH that are three to five times the normal range are associated with normal bone turnover in patients treated with maintenance dialysis, while similar PTH values in patients with mild to moderate kidney disease are associated with high turnover osteodystrophy.[87,91,92] Although the precise mechanisms are poorly understood, uremia has been associated with this "skeletal resistance" to the actions of PTH. Uremic animals and humans display decreased PTH/PTHrP receptor mRNA expression in bone and growth plate.[93,94] Hyperphosphatemia and alterations in vitamin D metabolism, among other factors, have been implicated in these changes, and calcitriol administration has been shown to partially restore the calcemic response to PTH in both experimental animals and patients with moderate CKD.[95] Despite this "skeletal resistance" to PTH, many patients with end-stage kidney disease display bone biopsy evidence of PTH excess.

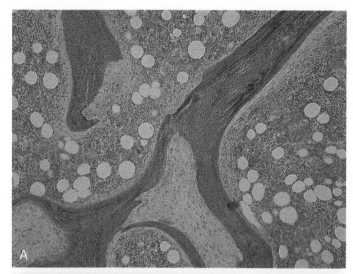

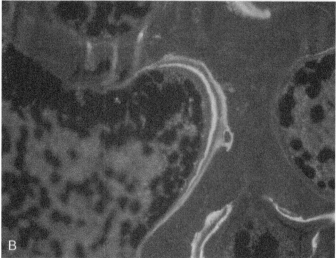

FIGURE 14-3. Bone histology, osteitis fibrosa. **A,** Under light microscopy, an increase in cellular activity, osteoid accumulation, erosion, and fibrosis are visible. **B,** An increase in double tetracycline labeling signifies an increase in bone turnover rate.

The bone in secondary hyperparathyroidism exhibits a marked increase in turnover with increased numbers of osteoblasts and osteoclasts and variable degrees of peritrabecular fibrosis. Activation of osteoclasts is mediated through PTH[96-99]; the result is increased resorption of both mineral and matrix along the trabecular surface and within the haversian canals of cortical bone.[100] Such increased cellular activity can occur secondary to a nonspecific reaction to local factors, such as insulin-like growth factor-1 (IGF-1), cytokines, or fracture, or as the result of systemic stimuli, such as increased thyroxine or PTH. One characteristic of high bone turnover is increased quantities of woven osteoid, exhibiting haphazard arrangements of collagen fibers in contrast to the usual lamellar pattern of osteoid in normal bone. Woven osteoid can become mineralized in patients with advanced kidney disease in the absence of vitamin D; however, the calcium may be deposited as amorphous calcium phosphate rather than hydroxyapatite.[101]

At the other end of the spectrum of bone turnover, adynamic bone disease is characterized by normal osteoid volume, an absence of fibrosis, and a reduced bone formation rate, as indicated by a reduced or absent double tetracycline label on bone histomorphometry (Fig. 14-4).[102,103] A paucity of osteoblasts and

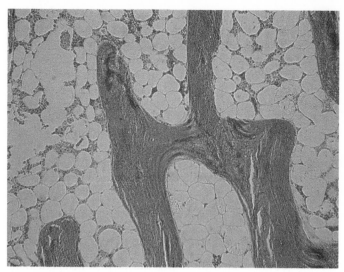

FIGURE 14-4. Bone histology, adynamic bone. Under light microscopy, decreased cellular activity occurs with minimal osteoid accumulation.

osteoclasts is observed.[85] The histologic features of adynamic renal osteodystrophy, in the absence of aluminum deposition in bone, cannot be distinguished from the histologic features of corticosteroid-induced osteoporosis or age-related or postmenopausal osteoporosis. Therefore, it is not possible to determine whether osteoporosis accounts for decreases in osteoblastic activity and bone formation in patients with adynamic renal osteodystrophy unless the amount of trabecular bone is reduced. Decreases in bone mass and histologic evidence of trabecular bone loss are not integral features of the adynamic lesion of renal osteodystrophy when other causes of osteoporosis can be excluded. Adynamic bone is associated with low PTH levels, low alkaline phosphatase levels, high serum calcium levels, and a propensity for increased vascular calcification.[104,105]

In the 1970s and 1980s, aluminum intoxication was largely responsible for the development of adynamic bone and osteomalacia in patients with CKD. Two distinct patterns of aluminum intoxication were identified: (1) absorbed from the aluminum content of water used to prepare dialysate solution,[106-108] and (2) intestinal aluminum absorption after ingestion of large doses of aluminum hydroxide.[109-115] The neurologic syndrome of "dialysis encephalopathy" and a bone disease manifested by fractures, pain, persistent hypercalcemia, and osteomalacia were the main clinical features. Although the prevalence of aluminum bone disease in developed countries is now very low, the prevalence of adynamic renal osteodystrophy not associated with aluminum intoxication has increased substantially over the past few years in adult patients receiving regular dialysis.[116] Currently, adynamic renal osteodystrophy is commonly associated with disorders such as age-related or postmenopausal osteoporosis, steroid-induced osteoporosis, hypoparathyroidism (idiopathic or surgically induced), and diabetes mellitus, and with overtreatment with calcium and vitamin D therapy.[117]

Because PTH is the major determinant of bone formation and skeletal remodeling in renal failure, oversuppression of PTH secretion can result in adynamic renal osteodystrophy. Approximately 40% of those treated with hemodialysis and more than half of adult patients undergoing peritoneal dialysis have serum PTH levels that are only minimally elevated or that fall within the normal range; such values are typically associated with normal or reduced rates of bone formation and turnover.[103] Prolonged treatment with calcium-containing phosphate-binding medications and the use of high-dialysate calcium concentrations also contribute to low bone turnover.[118] Calcitriol may directly suppress osteoblastic activity when given intermittently in large doses to patients receiving regular dialysis.[119]

The long-term consequences of adynamic renal osteodystrophy not attributable to aluminum toxicity remain to be determined, but concerns have been raised about increases in the risk for skeletal fracture and delayed fracture healing due to low rates of bone remodeling.[119] The development of soft tissue and vascular calcifications has been associated with adynamic bone disease in cross-sectional studies.[105] In prepubertal children, adynamic renal osteodystrophy has been associated with a reduction in linear growth.[117]

Mineralization

Although renal osteodystrophy has traditionally been defined by lesions in bone turnover, alterations in skeletal mineralization are also prevalent in CKD.[92] Increases in unmineralized bone (osteoid) in conjunction with delayed rates of mineral deposition are common.[92,100] Defective mineralization associated with low to normal bone turnover is termed osteomalacia.[1] Histomorphometric characteristics of osteomalacia include the presence of wide osteoid seams, an increased number of osteoid lamellae, an increase in the trabecular surface covered with osteoid, and a diminished rate of mineralization or bone formation, as assessed by double tetracycline labeling. Fibrosis is often absent.[85] In patients on long-term dialysis, osteomalacia that is refractory to vitamin D therapy is most commonly a result of aluminum intoxication.[120]

Although the mechanisms of skeletal mineralization are incompletely understood, factors such as 25(OH)D deficiency and altered FGF-23 metabolism have been implicated in their pathogenesis. In the general population, nutritional 25(OH)D deficiency results in osteomalacia, and a similar phenotype may occur in patients with CKD. FGF-23 may play a role; both overexpression[121-123] and ablation of FGF-23[124,125] in mice with normal renal function are associated with abnormal mineralization of osteoid, although by different mechanisms. The phosphaturic effects of increased FGF-23 may cause rickets and osteomalacia through an insufficiency of mineral substrate. The mechanisms leading to impaired mineralization in FGF-23–null animals, which have severe hyperphosphatemia and normal or elevated serum calcium levels, remain uncertain; however, osteomalacia in these animals suggests that FGF-23 may play a direct role in skeletal mineral deposition. Although the ramifications of defective mineralization remain to be established, increased fracture rates and bone deformities are prevalent in patients with CKD despite adequate control of bone turnover. These complications may be due, in part, to alterations in bone mineralization.

Treatment with anticonvulsant therapy may contribute to the development of osteomalacia in patients with kidney disease. Long-term ingestion of phenytoin and/or phenobarbital is associated with a high incidence of osteomalacia in nonuremic patients.[126] These findings may be due in part to alterations in vitamin D metabolism.[127]

Osteitis fibrosa cystica, a finding of secondary hyperparathyroidism, can coexist with defective mineralization in some patients; this pattern is called a "mixed" lesion.[128] Patients with mixed lesions often display high serum PTH and alkaline phosphatase levels, along with lower serum calcium levels. Mixed lesions are seen with high turnover bone disease in patients who are developing aluminum toxicity, or in patients with low turn-

over aluminum-related bone disease during desferoxamine (DFO) therapy (vide infra).[129] In these cases, mixed lesions represent a transitional stage between high turnover and low turnover bone disease.

Volume

Because PTH is anabolic at the level of trabecular bone, high levels of serum PTH are typically associated with increases in bone volume, trabecular volume, and trabecular width.[92,116,130,131] However, bone volume may also be low (termed osteoporosis), particularly in individuals with underlying age-related bone loss and in those treated with corticosteroids. Osteoporosis in the general population is associated with increased risk for hip fractures and mortality.[132] Thus, bone volume is considered a critically important parameter of bone histology. The impact of osteoporosis on morbidity and mortality in the CKD population, however, remains to be defined.

Clinical Manifestations

The symptoms and signs of renal osteodystrophy are usually nonspecific, and laboratory and radiographic abnormalities generally pre-date clinical manifestations. Some specific symptoms and syndromes do occur, however.

BONE PAIN

Bone pain is a common manifestation of severe bone disease in patients with advanced kidney disease. It usually is insidious in appearance and often is aggravated by weight bearing or a change in posture. Physical findings are often absent. Pain is most common in the lower part of the back, hips, and legs but may occur in the peripheral skeleton. Occasionally, sudden appearance of pain around the knee, ankle, or heel can suggest acute arthritis; such pain is not usually relieved by massage or local heat. Bone pain is more common and often is more marked in patients with aluminum-related bone disease than in those with osteitis fibrosa cystica, but marked variability may be seen from one patient to another.[133]

In patients on long-term dialysis, carpal tunnel syndrome and chronic arthralgias often occur in association with the deposition of β_2-microglobulin amyloid in articular and periarticular structures.[134] Arthralgias usually are bilateral and most commonly affect the shoulders, knees, wrists, and small joints of the hand; symptoms typically are worse with inactivity and at night.[135,136]

MUSCLE WEAKNESS

Proximal myopathy can be marked in patients with advanced kidney disease. Symptoms appear slowly. Patients may note difficulty climbing stairs or rising from a low chair, or they may have difficulty raising their arms to comb their hair. This proximal muscle weakness resembles that found in 25(OH)D deficiency and in primary hyperparathyroidism. Plasma levels of muscle enzymes usually are normal, and electromyographic changes are nonspecific.

The pathogenesis of this myopathy is not clear, and several different mechanisms, including secondary hyperparathyroidism, phosphate depletion,[137] abnormal vitamin D metabolism, and aluminum intoxication, have been implicated.[138] Improvement in gait posture has been reported in children with moderate renal failure after treatment with $1,25(OH)_2D_3$, and muscle weakness improves rapidly in affected adult patients with end-stage kidney disease.[139] Improvement in muscular strength has been observed after treatment with 25(OH)D₃, after subtotal parathyroidectomy, after successful renal transplantation, and after chelation therapy with deferoxamine for aluminum intoxication.

SKELETAL DEFORMITIES

Bone deformities are common in uremic children because their bones undergo growth, modeling, and remodeling. In adult patients, skeletal deformities also arise from abnormal remodeling or recurrent fractures.[140] In children, bone deformities of the femora and wrists arise from slipped epiphyses.[141] This problem is most common during the preadolescent period and is most frequent in patients with long-standing congenital kidney disease. In adults with kidney disease, particularly those with aluminum-related bone disease, skeletal deformities may be characterized by lumbar scoliosis, kyphosis, and deformities of the thoracic cage.[140]

GROWTH RETARDATION

Growth retardation is the hallmark of CKD in children. Protein and calorie malnutrition, metabolic acidosis, end-organ growth hormone resistance, and renal bone disease are most commonly implicated in growth failure.[142] Despite correction of acidosis and anemia, normalization of serum calcium and phosphorous levels, and vitamin D sterol therapy replacement, most children with CKD continue to grow poorly. Growth failure worsens as renal function declines; the average height of children with even mild CKD (GFR 50 to 70 mL/minute/1.73 m²) is 1 standard deviation (SD) below the average for healthy children. Moderate CKD (GFR 25 to 49 mL/minute/1.73 m²) is associated with a height SD of −1.5, and, at the time of initiation of dialysis, the mean height SD is −1.8. Boys, younger patients, and those with prior renal transplants are at greatest risk for growth failure.[143]

Acidosis has been linked to delayed linear growth in patients with renal tubular acidosis and normal renal function, and correction of metabolic acidosis often leads to acceleration in growth velocity.[144] Acidotic rats have been found to have decreased growth hormone (GH) secretion, serum insulin-like growth factor 1 (IGF-1), and hepatic IGF-1 mRNA expression. Moreover, metabolic acidosis has been shown to inhibit the effects of GH in rats with normal and decreased renal function.[145-147] Growth plate mRNA levels of GH receptor, IGF-1 receptor, and IGF-1 expression are downregulated, and IGF-binding proteins are upregulated.[148] In adults treated with maintenance dialysis, correction of acidosis has been shown to decrease the progression of secondary hyperparathyroidism and to improve skeletal mineralization.[149]

Calcitriol deficiency has been thought to contribute to growth retardation and bone disease in children with CKD. Secondary hyperparathyroidism remains prevalent in children with advanced renal disease, and osteitis fibrosa continues to be the most common skeletal lesion of renal osteodystrophy in those undergoing regular dialysis despite treatment with daily doses of oral calcitriol.[116,150] Secondary hyperparathyroidism contributes to growth retardation, although optimal target values for PTH in children at all stages of CKD remain controversial. In children with moderate CKD, some data indicate that normal growth velocity is achieved when PTH levels are maintained within the normal range[151]; others have demonstrated a linear correlation between growth and PTH levels in the same patient population, with those with the highest PTH values displaying the highest growth velocity.[152] Treatment for secondary hyperparathyroidism with large, intermittent doses of calcitriol and calcium-based

phosphate binders has been shown to significantly reduce bone formation and suppress osteoblastic activity in both adults and children.[95,153] However, adynamic bone disease may develop and linear bone growth decrease, despite serum PTH levels in the K/DOQI[117,154] recommended range during intermittent vitamin D sterol therapy. Maintaining serum PTH levels at between 300 and 500 pg/mL reduces the frequency of these complications.[131] The mechanisms by which calcitriol inhibits epiphyseal growth plate cartilage remain poorly understood. However, it is well known that calcitriol exerts dose-dependent inhibitory effects on cell proliferation of chondrocytes and osteoblasts in vitro. In addition, vitamin D sterols increase expression of a number of IGF-binding proteins (IGFBPs). IGFBP-2, -3, -4, and -5 sequester IGF-1 and may exert IGF-1–independent antiproliferative effects through their own receptors.[155-159]

GH resistance also contributes to impaired linear growth in renal failure. In CKD, poor growth develops despite normal or increased serum GH levels.[160,161] Uremia has been associated with diminished hepatic GH receptor and IGF-1 mRNA expression, defects in postreceptor GH-mediated signal transduction,[162,163] reductions in serum GH-binding protein levels,[164] and increased synthesis and reduced clearance of IGF binding proteins.[138,164,165] Improved growth velocity during recombinant human GH (rhGH) therapy has been ascribed to increased bioavailability of IGF-1 to target tissues. Children who are treated with maintenance dialysis respond less well to rhGH therapy than do children with less severe CKD, but the mechanisms for differences in response to GH therapy remain to be determined.

EXTRASKELETAL CALCIFICATION

Extraskeletal calcification has been associated with uremia for many years[166] and has been included recently in the definition of CKD-MBD.[1] Vascular calcifications are associated with increased mortality. These lesions have their origins in CKD prior to dialysis and begin in childhood (Fig. 14-5).[167,169] The mortality rate in adults and children with CKD is markedly higher than that in the general population, and cardiovascular disease is the leading cause of death in both children and adults treated with maintenance dialysis.[168,170] In contrast to the calcified atherosclerotic plaques that develop in the vascular intima of aging individuals with normal kidney function, uremia facilitates calcification of the tunica media. This form of calcification is associated with decreased distensibility of blood vessels, causing a rigid

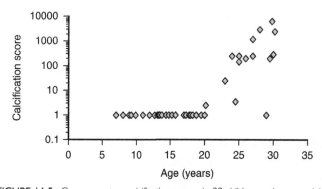

FIGURE 14-5. Coronary artery calcification scores in 39 children and young adults with end-stage renal disease who were treated by dialysis, according to age. Coronary artery calcification was assessed by electron beam computed tomography. The scale on the y-axis is logarithmic. (Data from Goodman WG, et al: Coronary artery calcification in young adults with end-stage renal disease who are undergoing dialysis, N Engl J Med 106:100–105, 2000.)

"lead pipe" pathology that is associated with increased risk for congestive heart failure.[1] Electron beam computed tomography (EBCT) is used in assessment of vascular calcifications in the adult population, and measurements in young adults who were treated with maintenance dialysis as children demonstrated that a significant proportion of this population has evidence of vascular calcification.[168] Carotid ultrasound measurement of intima medial thickness (IMT) has been validated for the assessment of cardiovascular pathology in children, with increased thickness associated with worsening disease.[169,171]

Hypercalcemia, hyperphosphatemia, elevated levels of the calcium x phosphorous product, and high doses of vitamin D sterols[167,168] all have been implicated in the pathogenesis of cardiovascular calcification. However, 40% of adult patients with stage 3 CKD, without these risk factors, show evidence of calcification,[172] suggesting a role for uremic factors other than high levels of calcium and phosphorus. Indeed, vascular tissues in the uremic milieu express osteoblast differentiation factors.[173] Osteoblasts and vascular smooth muscle cells have a common mesenchymal origin; core binding factor-1 (Cbfa1) is thought to trigger mesenchymal cell-to-osteoblast transformation. Mice that are deficient in Cbfa1 fail to mineralize bone,[174] and arteries obtained from patients undergoing renal transplantation show increased levels of this protein.[173] Upregulation of the sodium-dependent phosphate transporter PIT-1 likely also contributes to increased calcification,[175] and upregulation of pro-mineralization factors such as osteopontin, bone sialoprotein, osteonectin, alkaline phosphatase, type I collagen, and bone morphogenic protein-2 (BMP-2) is potentiated by the uremic milieu.[176-179] By contrast, expression of calcification inhibitors such as fetuin A, matrix gla protein, and klotho is suppressed.[180-183] Levels of circulating FGF-23 also may contribute, as high levels of the protein are associated with increased mortality in adult dialysis patients.[184] Klotho, the cofactor necessary for the actions of FGF-23, has been implicated in vascular calcification. Animals lacking the *Klotho* gene display elevated levels of calcium, phosphorus, and vitamin D, along with vascular calcification and premature aging. CKD is associated with low circulating levels of Klotho,[183] which has been implicated in the regulation of sodium/phosphate co-transport in the aorta.[185]

Because the pathophysiology of cardiovascular disease in CKD is multifactorial, treatment strategies are also multifaceted and vary according to stage of CKD. Therapies that are effective in early CKD may not be effective in later stages—lipid-lowering agents decrease mortality in adults with CKD[186] and in those with stable renal allografts[187] but have not been shown to benefit patients treated with dialysis.[188] By contrast, normalization of mineral metabolism (attained by avoiding hypercalcemia and hyperphosphatemia, limiting calcium intake, and avoiding adynamic bone) is effective at slowing the progression of cardiovascular calcification in patients treated with maintenance dialysis.[154,168,189,190] Thus, at different stages of CKD, the relative importance of individual risk factors and the value of different biomarkers may vary.

CALCIPHYLAXIS

This unique syndrome, which is characterized by ischemic necrosis of the skin, subcutaneous fat, and muscles, can develop in patients with advanced renal failure not yet treated by dialysis, in those treated with regular dialysis, and in patients with well-functioning kidney transplants.[191] The pathogenesis of this syndrome is uncertain. Extensive medial calcifications of medium-sized arteries are noted; such calcifications

commonly exist in patients with renal disease without causing gangrene or ulcerations, and it is not clear that vascular calcifications per se are the cause of the ischemic necrosis. Two distinct types of the syndrome are recognized: proximal calciphylaxis, which affects the thighs, abdomen, and chest wall, and acral calciphylaxis, which involves sites distal to the knees and elbows, such as the toes, fingers, and ankles.[192] The former has a terrible prognosis, with death occurring in more than 80% to 90% of affected patients. This syndrome is often accompanied by morbid obesity and hypoalbuminemia. Many patients have severe secondary hyperparathyroidism, and most have a history of severe and uncontrolled hyperphosphatemia.[192] Some patients may have defective regulation of coagulation.[193] The appearance of this syndrome in renal transplant recipients receiving glucocorticoids suggests that steroids may also play a role. Patients with calciphylaxis frequently die of secondary infection.

A significant number of patients improve after parathyroidectomy, and a few have healed after substantial reductions in levels of serum phosphorus. Parathyroidectomy and aggressive control of serum phosphate levels therefore are indicated in those with evidence of severe secondary hyperparathyroidism. However, although ischemic lesions and medial vascular calcifications are common in uremic patients with diabetes, such lesions rarely improve after parathyroidectomy. Thus, parathyroid surgery should be reserved for those diabetic patients with calciphylaxis who have clear evidence of severe secondary hyperparathyroidism. Calcimimetics,[194] as well as sodium-thiosulfate (a calcium chelating agent) and pamidronate,[195] have been used effectively in some individuals. Hyperbaric oxygen therapy also has been advocated.[195]

DIALYSIS-RELATED AMYLOIDOSIS

Several clinical syndromes that arise as a consequence of dialysis-related amyloidosis can mimic the clinical features of renal osteodystrophy, or amyloidosis can occur concurrently with uremic bone disease. Dialysis-related amyloidosis arises from the deposition in bone and periarticular structures of a specific type of amyloid composed of β_2-microglobulin.[196] In addition to β_2-microglobulin, the amyloid deposits contain advanced glycosylation end products, which may account for their uptake by certain collagen-rich structures.[197,198] The frequency of its clinical manifestation rises markedly in patients treated with regular dialysis for longer than 5 to 10 years, and it is much more common in patients who start dialysis when older than 50 years.[199] Blood levels of β_2-microglobulin are strikingly elevated in all patients with end-stage renal disease because of failure of normal renal clearance and catabolism. Clinical manifestations include (1) carpal tunnel syndrome; (2) destructive or erosive arthropathy involving the large and medium-sized joints, with shoulder, knee, hip, or back pain being common manifestations; (3) spondyloarthropathy, most commonly affecting the cervical spine; and (4) subchondral, thin-walled cysts of bone, most commonly affecting the carpal bones, the humoral and femoral heads, the distal end of the radius, the acetabulum, and the tibial plateau. These subchondral cysts at times are confused with brown tumors of secondary hyperparathyroidism, although their location and occurrence in multiple sites make them quite different from brown tumors. Nonetheless, in a patient who has undergone long-term dialysis, this syndrome may be a potential cause of neuromuscular and periarticular symptoms usually considered to be due to secondary hyperparathyroidism or aluminum accumulation. Parathyroid surgery should be avoided in dialysis patients whose severe musculoskeletal symptoms have not improved with calcitriol therapy; symptoms in these patients actually may be due to dialysis-related amyloidosis. Specific diagnosis of the latter is made from the biopsy demonstration of amyloid composed of β_2-microglobulin; however, the diagnosis can be strongly suspected from the clinical features, the presence of multiple thin-walled cysts, or the demonstration in periarticular sites of presumed amyloid tissue on ultrasonography.[200] Its management is difficult and largely unsatisfactory, but successful renal transplantation leads to rapid disappearance of symptoms and no further progression of the bone lesions on radiographs.[201] In patients who remain on maintenance dialysis, the use of high-flux dialyzer membranes may decrease amyloid accumulation[202]; the long-term effects of this form of therapy on symptoms remain to be determined.

Diagnostic Evaluations

BIOCHEMICAL DETERMINATIONS

Phosphorus

Hyperphosphatemia has been found to be an independent risk factor for mortality in patients treated with maintenance dialysis.[203] Hemodialysis and continuous ambulatory peritoneal dialysis (CAPD) remove phosphate, but dietary phosphate restriction and the use of phosphate-binding agents are required by 90% to 95% of patients undergoing treatment with dialysis. To prevent the development and progression of secondary hyperparathyroidism and vascular calcification, such measures as dietary phosphate restriction and the use of phosphate-binding medications should be initiated to maintain serum phosphorous levels within age-appropriate levels and calcium phosphorous products lower than 55 mg^2/dL.[67,204]

Calcium

Hypocalcemia often resolves during treatment with calcium-containing phosphate binders, with vitamin D, and with initiation of dialysis. The development of hypercalcemia in patients undergoing regular dialysis warrants prompt and thorough investigation. Conditions associated with hypercalcemia include marked hyperplasia of the parathyroid glands as a result of severe secondary hyperparathyroidism, aluminum-related bone disease, therapy with calcitriol or other vitamin D sterols, administration of large doses of calcium carbonate or other calcium-containing compounds, immobilization, malignancy, and granulomatous disorders, such as sarcoidosis or tuberculosis in which extrarenal production of 1,25(OH)D occurs.[102,205,206] Basal serum calcium levels are also higher in patients with adynamic bone than in subjects with other lesions of renal osteodystrophy, and episodes of hypercalcemia are common.[92] Because skeletal calcium uptake is limited in adynamic lesions, calcium entering the extracellular fluid from dialysate or after intestinal absorption cannot be buffered adequately in bone, and serum calcium levels rise.[207] Maintaining total calcium intake at between 1500 and 2000 mg per day, the use of new-generation vitamin D sterols, and treatment with calcimimetic agents help to limit episodes of hypercalcemia.

Magnesium

The net intestinal absorption of magnesium generally is normal or only very slightly reduced in patients with renal failure,[204] yet serum magnesium levels often increase with advanced kidney disease as the result of reduced renal excretion. During hemodialysis, serum magnesium levels generally are increased if the dialysate magnesium concentration is maintained at 1.75 mEq/L; however, magnesium levels remain within the upper range of normal with dialysate magnesium concentrations of 0.5 mEq/L. The use of magnesium-containing laxatives or antacids should be avoided as these may cause an abrupt increase in serum magnesium levels in patients with kidney disease.[208] Serum magnesium levels should be measured frequently and regularly if magnesium-containing medications are used. Rarely, hypomagnesemia can develop in uremic patients with severe malabsorption or diarrhea.[204]

Alkaline Phosphatase

Serum alkaline phosphatase values are fair markers of the severity of secondary hyperparathyroidism in patients with renal failure. Osteoblasts normally express large amounts of the bone isoenzyme of alkaline phosphatase, and serum levels usually are elevated when osteoblastic activity and bone formation rates are increased. High levels generally reflect the extent of histologic change in patients with high turnover lesions of renal osteodystrophy, and values frequently correlate with serum PTH levels.[209] Serum total alkaline phosphatase measurements are also useful for monitoring the skeletal response to treatment with vitamin D sterols in patients with osteitis fibrosa; values that decrease over several months usually indicate histologic improvement.[117] Bone-specific alkaline phosphatase activity may be useful in predicting the histologic lesions of renal osteodystrophy, but whether these values are superior to total alkaline phosphatase levels remains to be demonstrated. Serum alkaline phosphatase levels may increase early in the course of treatment for aluminum-related bone disease with the chelating agent deferoxamine. Levels also may increase during therapy with recombinant human growth hormone in pediatric patients with renal failure.[210]

Assays for bone-specific alkaline phosphatase and measurements of serum osteocalcin levels provide additional information about the level of osteoblastic activity in patients with CKD.[211] Osteocalcin levels generally are elevated in renal failure, but values may help distinguish between patients with high turnover and those with low turnover skeletal lesions.[211,212] If these assays are not available, measurement of the heat-stabile and heat-labile fractions of alkaline phosphatase helps to separate skeletal from hepatic causes of elevated total alkaline phosphatase levels.

Parathyroid Hormone

Over the past few years, a series of observations have highlighted important shortcomings of the first-generation immunometric assays (IMAs) for measuring PTH (1st PTH-IMAs). Studies by D'Amour et al.[213-215] demonstrated that 1st PTH-IMAs detect not only the intact hormone, but also PTH fragments truncated at the aminoterminus. Indeed, most of the detection antibodies, which usually are directed against epitopes within the aminoterminus of the hormone, detect not only PTH(1-84), but also one or several amino-truncated fragments of the PTH molecule, some of which co-elute from reverse-phase high-performance liquid chromatography (HPLC) columns with synthetic PTH(7-84).[214] By contrast, a more recently developed second-generation immunometric PTH assay (2nd PTH-IMA), using detection antibodies, which interact with epitopes comprising the first four aminoterminal amino acids of human PTH, recognizes only PTH(1-84) and possibly PTH fragments that are truncated at the carboxyterminus, but not PTH(7-84).[69,216,217] PTH levels determined by

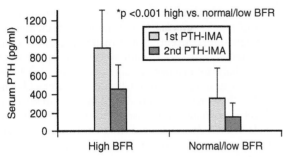

FIGURE 14-6. Parathyroid hormone (PTH) levels by different assays according to bone histology in patients treated with maintenance dialysis.

1st PTH-IMAs overestimate the concentration of PTH(1-84) by 40% to 50% in healthy individuals with normal renal function and in those with varying degrees of CKD (Fig. 14-6). Unlike 1st PTH-IMAs, more recently developed 2nd PTH-IMAs do not detect these large PTH fragments.[69,216-219] Consistent with this assessment, human PTH(1-34), but not human PTH(2-34) or other aminoterminally truncated fragments of human PTH(1-34), cross-react with the detection antibody.[69,216,217] Faugere et al.[218] suggested that 2nd PTH-IMAs and, mainly, the ratio between PTH(1-84) and amino-truncated PTH fragments (calculated from the differences in PTH levels determined between 1st and 2nd PTH-IMAs) could be better predictors of bone turnover than 1st PTH-IMA[218]; however, these findings were not confirmed by subsequent investigations.[130,219] When the crucial role of serum PTH concentrations in the diagnosis and treatment of renal osteodystrophy is considered, 2nd PTH-IMA may provide important new insights into the physiology of parathyroid gland function. At present, however, measurements of PTH using 1st or 2nd PTH-IMAs have shown similar accuracy for predicting bone turnover in patients undergoing maintenance dialysis. Current data do not yet support the claim that 2nd PTH-IMAs provide an advantage over 1st PTH-IMAs in the diagnosis of different subtypes of renal bone disease.[218]

Although these molecules detected by PTH-IMAs are still uncharacterized, in vitro and in vivo experimental data indicate that one or more aminoterminally truncated PTH(1-84) fragments antagonize the calcemic actions of PTH(1-84) and diminish bone cell activity, and therefore may modulate bone metabolism. Indeed, synthetic PTH(7-84), which appears to be similar to naturally occurring circulating aminoterminally truncated PTH fragments,[220] has hypocalcemic properties in vivo.[216] Furthermore, PTH(7-84) inhibits the formation of TRAP-positive bone resorbing cells in vitro,[221] and it inhibits bone formation in vivo.[222] In addition, Nguyen-Yamamoto et al.[223] demonstrated that PTH(7-84), with or without a mixture of other carboxyterminal PTH-fragments, inhibited the calcemic effects of PTH(1-34) in vivo, indicating that these actions are not mediated through the PTH/PTHrP receptor, but instead via a receptor that interacts only with carboxyterminal portions of PTH. Thus, a growing body of evidence suggests that at least some of the different carboxyterminal PTH fragments have biological activity.

Aluminum

Aluminum toxicity occurs in dialysis patients or patients with CKD with GFR less than 30 mL/min/1.73 m^2 because aluminum that is absorbed from the gut, from the dialysate, or from parenteral infusions is inadequately excreted by the diseased kidney. Accumulation occurs in various tissues, including bone, liver, brain, and parathyroid glands, and can produce toxicity such as

dialysis encephalopathy, osteomalacia, and microcytic anemia. The gold standard for the diagnosis of aluminum bone disease is a bone biopsy demonstrating increased aluminum staining of the bone surface (>15% to 25%) with histologic evidence of adynamic bone or osteomalacia. The presence of aluminum deposits in the bone and liver does not correlate with plasma levels[224]; however, plasma aluminum levels are useful for monitoring patients who are undergoing long-term dialysis therapy and receiving aluminum-containing phosphate-binding agents for prolonged periods. DFO should be administered to symptomatic patients with aluminum levels between 60 and 200 μg/L or a positive DFO test. The DFO infusion test is performed by infusing 5 mg/kg of DFO during the last hour of the dialysis session. Serum aluminum is measured before DFO infusion and 2 days later, before the next dialysis session. To prevent DFO-induced neurotoxicity, DFO should not be administered if serum aluminum concentrations are greater than 200 μg/L.[130,225]

RADIOGRAPHY

Radiographic Features of Osteitis Fibrosa Cystica

The most consistent radiographic feature of secondary hyperparathyroidism is the presence of subperiosteal erosions.[226,227] The degree of subperiosteal erosion can correlate with serum PTH and alkaline phosphatase levels, but radiographs can be normal in patients with moderate to severe histologic features of osteitis fibrosa cystica on bone biopsy.[228]

In pediatric patients, metaphyseal changes (i.e., growth zone lesions that are termed "rickets-like lesions") are common.[226] Radiographic changes arising from secondary hyperparathyroidism may be difficult to differentiate from true rachitic abnormalities. However, the radiographic features of slipped epiphyses resulting from osteitis fibrosa are present in uremic children but absent in rickets resulting from vitamin D deficiency.[141] These findings are best detected by hand radiographs, and several techniques, including the use of fine-grain films and magnification with a hand lens, are used to enhance sensitivity.[229] Subperiosteal erosions also occur in the distal ends of clavicles, on the surface of the ischium and pubis, at the sacroiliac joints, and at the junction of the metaphysis and diaphysis of long bones.[227,228] Subperiosteal erosions can be found in patients with aluminum-related bone disease.[230] This finding represents the residuals of earlier hyperparathyroidism with osteitis fibrosa cystica, which, owing to aluminum toxicity, are unable to remineralize during treatment with vitamin D sterols or with parathyroidectomy.[230]

Radiographic abnormalities of the skull in secondary hyperparathyroidism may include (1) a diffuse "ground-glass" appearance, (2) a generalized mottled or granular appearance, (3) focal radiolucencies, and (4) focal sclerosis.

Radiographic Features of Osteomalacia

Radiographic features of osteomalacia are less specific and less common than those of secondary hyperparathyroidism. Typical rachitic lesions, with widening of the epiphyseal growth plate and other deformities, can occur in children with open epiphyses.[226] Looser's zones or pseudofractures, the only pathognomonic radiographic features of osteomalacia in adult patients, are rare in renal patients with osteomalacia; they occur as straight, wide bands of radiolucency that are perpendicular to the long axis of the bone. Fractures, particularly of the ribs, vertebral bodies, and hips, are more common in patients with osteomalacia than in patients with osteitis fibrosa cystica or mixed osteodystrophy.[231] Decreased bone density is another common radiographic feature present in patients with advanced kidney disease and may arise from secondary hyperparathyroidism, osteomalacia, or osteoporosis.[232] Paradoxically, localized osteosclerosis is common in patients with kidney disease and is more frequent in patients with osteitis fibrosa cystica.

BONE BIOPSY

Although not routinely performed in the clinical setting, a bone biopsy should be considered in all patients with CKD who have fractures with minimal trauma (pathologic fractures), suspected aluminum bone disease, or persistent hypercalcemia despite serum PTH levels between 400 and 600 pg/mL.[154] For bone labeling, a 2 day course of tetracycline is administered at 15 mg/kg/day (divided into twice- or thrice-daily doses). Phosphate binders should be held during labeling because they may interfere with gut absorption of tetracycline. Fourteen days later, the 2 day course is repeated. For children younger than 8 years, tetracycline dosage usually is kept below 10 mg/kg/day to avoid toxicity. Histochemical staining procedures demonstrate the deposition of abnormal components such as iron, aluminum, and oxalate within bone.[116,233]

Treatment of CKD-MBD

To minimize complications in the skeleton and to prevent extraskeletal calcifications, particular attention must be made to alterations of bone and mineral metabolism in CKD. The specific aims of management of CKD-MBD are (1) to maintain blood levels of serum calcium and phosphorus near normal limits, (2) to prevent hyperplasia of the parathyroid glands and to maintain serum PTH at levels appropriate for stage of CKD, (3) to avoid the development of extraskeletal calcifications, and (4) to prevent or reverse the accumulation of toxic substances such as aluminum and β_2-microglobulin.

DIETARY MANIPULATION OF CALCIUM AND PHOSPHORUS

As active vitamin D levels fall during the progression of renal disease, calcium absorption in the gut and kidney diminishes and hypocalcemia often develops. Patients with untreated CKD commonly ingest as little as 400 to 700 mg of elemental calcium per day in their diet. Calcium-rich foods such as dairy products, unfortunately, also are high in phosphorus. Thus, increasing dietary consumption of calcium to meet daily needs is accompanied by excessive intake of phosphorus, which cannot be excreted in the face of renal failure. As a result, calcium supplementation in the form of calcium-containing salts is often required. The total amount of calcium supplementation provided, however, must be monitored carefully, because overly aggressive supplementation (as is common when calcium-containing salts are used as the sole means of binding phosphorus) may lead to hypercalcemia and vascular calcification.

The development of hyperphosphatemia occurs in the vast majority of patients with advanced renal insufficiency. Hyperphosphatemia and an elevated calcium-phosphorous ion product have been reported as independent risk factors for vascular calcification and mortality in adult dialysis patients.[189,190,203] Thus, treatment goals include maintaining serum phosphorous levels within normal limits for age and avoiding a calcium-phosphorous ion product above 55 mg^2/dL^2. The average phosphorous intake of both adults and children in the U.S. population is

approximately 1500 to 2000 mg/day, and 60% to 70% of the dietary intake is absorbed. In the early stages of renal failure, dietary phosphate restriction is sufficient in preventing hyperphosphatemia. However, strict adherence to dietary phosphate restriction is often difficult because low-phosphate diets are unpalatable, especially to older children and adults, and because phosphorous intake is directly linked to protein intake, with 10 to 12 mg of phosphorus accompanying each gram of protein. Adequate protein intake is necessary for growth in children and for maintenance of lean body mass in adults. Current dietary recommendations suggest that adults with CKD ingest between 0.8 to 1 g/kg/day of protein, and that children, depending on age, ingest anywhere from 1 to 2.5 g/kg/day.[67,154] This translates to a minimum phosphate ingestion of 800 mg/day in an 80 kg person.

Patients treated with dialysis require dietary phosphorous restriction, in addition to phosphate-binder therapy (vide infra), because standard prescription peritoneal dialysis and hemodialysis remove insufficient amounts of phosphate (300 to 400 mg/day for peritoneal dialysis and 800 mg/treatment for hemodialysis) to maintain normal serum phosphorous levels. The use of daily, slow, continuous hemodialysis in some centers has been associated with excellent control of serum phosphorous levels, often allowing phosphate-binding agents to be discontinued.[234,235] Indeed, some patients have developed hypophosphatemia and have required the addition of phosphorus to the dialysate solution to prevent the long-term consequences of hypophosphatemia.[234,235]

PHOSPHATE-BINDING AGENTS

Phosphate-binding agents reduce intestinal phosphate absorption by forming poorly soluble complexes with phosphorus in the intestinal tract. Aluminum-containing phosphate binders were used frequently in the past, but long-term treatment led to bone disease, encephalopathy, and anemia.[236] The use of aluminum-containing phosphate binders, therefore, should be restricted to the treatment of patients with severe hyperphosphatemia (>7 mg/dL) associated with hypercalcemia or an elevated calcium-phosphorous ion product, because both conditions will be aggravated by calcium-containing compounds. In such cases, the dose of aluminum hydroxide should not exceed 30 mg/kg/day, and the lowest possible dose should be given only for a limited period of approximately 4 to 6 weeks.[237] Plasma aluminum levels should be monitored regularly. Concomitant intake of citrate-containing compounds should be avoided, because citrate increases intestinal aluminum absorption[238] and increases the risk for acute aluminum intoxication.[239,240] Constipation is a common adverse effect and can be relieved by stool softeners.

To avoid aluminum-related bone disease and encephalopathy, the use of aluminum-free phosphate binders has been advocated. Among these, calcium-containing salts are used worldwide for control of hyperphosphatemia and serve as a source of supplemental calcium. Several calcium salts, including calcium carbonate, calcium acetate, and calcium citrate, are commercially available. Calcium carbonate is the most commonly used compound, and studies in adults and children have shown its efficacy in controlling serum phosphorous levels.[102,241,242] The recommended dose is proportional to the phosphorous content of the meal and is adjusted to achieve acceptable serum levels of calcium and phosphorus. Large doses of calcium carbonate may lead to hypercalcemia, particularly in patients treated with vitamin D or those with adynamic bone.[243,244] Hypercalcemia usually is reversible with reductions in the dose of oral calcium salts, dose of vitamin D sterol, and dialysate calcium concentrations. To avoid the development and progression of cardiovascular calcifications, it is currently recommended that elemental calcium intake should not exceed 2 g/day, with less than 1500 mg of calcium given as calcium-containing phosphorous binders.[67]

Comparison studies between calcium carbonate and calcium acetate have demonstrated that an equivalent dose of calcium acetate binds twice as much phosphorus, but the relative incidence of hypercalcemia varies among studies.[245-247] Calcium citrate is an effective phosphate-binding agent but should be used with caution in patients with renal failure because of enhanced intestinal aluminum absorption when given in combination with aluminum-containing phosphate binders.[248] Calcium ketoglutarate is less calcemic than calcium carbonate and has anabolic benefits, but gastrointestinal side effects and high cost of therapy often limit its use.[249]

To limit the vascular calcification risks associated with the use of calcium salts and the bone and neurologic toxicity associated with aluminum hydroxide, alternative phosphate binders have been developed. Sevelamer hydrochloride (RenaGel), a calcium- and aluminum-free hydrogel of cross-linked poly-allylamine, has been shown to lower serum phosphorus, the calcium-phosphorous ion product, and PTH without inducing hypercalcemia in adult patients treated with hemodialysis.[250-252] Sevelamer also halts the progression of vascular calcification, although such lesions increase during calcium-containing binder therapy in adult hemodialysis patients.[253] In addition to its effects on serum phosphorous levels, sevelamer has been shown to decrease concentrations of total serum cholesterol and low-density lipoprotein cholesterol, but to increase high-density lipoprotein levels.[252] These effects may offer additional benefits in reducing cardiovascular complications in patients with end-stage renal disease. Acidosis may occur in patients treated with sevelamer; thus, a new form of sevelamer, sevelamer carbonate, has been introduced recently. This new compound is as effective a phosphate binder as sevelamer hydrochloride, with less potential to induce acidosis.[254]

Other alternative phosphate-binding agents include magnesium, iron, and lanthanum compounds. Magnesium carbonate lowers serum phosphorous levels, but magnesium-free dialysate solutions should be used in those treated with dialysis.[139,255] Large doses, however, result in diarrhea, limiting the use of this compound as a single agent. Iron compounds, such as stabilized polynuclear iron hydroxide and ferric polymaltose complex, have proved to be effective phosphate binders in short-term studies in adults with CKD.[256,257] Clinical trials have demonstrated that lanthanum carbonate also effectively controls serum phosphorous and PTH levels without increasing serum calcium values. Lanthanum carbonate lowers serum phosphorous and PTH levels without causing hypercalcemia, adynamic bone disease, or osteomalacia.[258-260] However, lanthanum is a heavy metal that accumulates in animal livers.[261] Lanthanum also accumulates in the bone of dialysis patients, where its presence persists despite discontinuation for as long as 2 years.[262] Additional long-term studies therefore needed to confirm the absence of toxicity before this agent is recommended for widespread use.

VITAMIN D THERAPY

Despite dietary phosphate restriction, the intake of phosphate-binding agents, the use of an appropriate level of calcium in dialysate solution, and an adequate intake of calcium, progressive osteitis fibrosa cystica due to hyperparathyroidism develops in a significant number of uremic patients. Treatment with vitamin D is aimed at controlling serum PTH levels and the resultant high turnover bone disease. Current evidence indicates that two main issues exist in vitamin D therapy. First, treatment for 25(OH)D deficiency, a common finding in patients with renal disease, in itself may reverse hyperparathyroidism. Second, treatment with active vitamin D sterols, by inhibiting the formation of prepro-PTH and by activating the CaSR, is useful in pharmacologically reducing PTH levels.

Assessment and Treatment of 25(OH)D Deficiency

Measurement of 25(OH)D levels and treatment of vitamin D deficiency are an important part of the management of hyperparathyroidism in patients with CKD. The current classification system stratifies vitamin D deficiency into three categories[67]: (1) severe deficiency, defined as a serum level less than 5 ng/mL; (2) mild deficiency, equivalent to serum concentrations of 5 to 15 ng/mL; and (3) vitamin D insufficiency, with levels between 16 and 30 ng/mL. Thus, ergocalciferol treatment should be initiated in patients with CKD when 25(OH)D levels fall below 30 ng/mL. Severe deficiency (<5 ng/mL) should be treated with 50,000 IU orally, once a week for 12 weeks, then 50,000 IU orally once a month for a total of 6 months. Alternatively, 500,000 IU may be given as a single intramuscular dose. Serum 25(OH)D levels in the range of 5 to 15 ng/mL (so-called mild deficiency) should be treated with 50,000 IU of ergocalciferol orally once a week for 4 weeks, followed by 50,000 IU orally once a month for a total of 6 months. Vitamin D insufficiency (serum levels between 16 and 30 ng/mL) should be treated with 50,000 IU of ergocalciferol orally once a month for 6 months. In D-deficient patients, serum 25(OH)D levels should be rechecked after completion of the 6 month course of therapy.[67]

Treatment With Active Vitamin D Sterols

As mentioned previously, active vitamin D sterols act through a variety of pathways to decrease PTH production—by increasing calcium absorption in the gut and kidney, by binding to the CaSR, by increasing skeletal sensitivity to PTH, and by altering prepro-PTH transcription. Calcitriol (Rocaltrol) has been widely used for many years to control secondary hyperparathyroidism in both adults and children. The efficacy of daily oral doses of calcitriol for the treatment of patients with symptomatic renal osteodystrophy has been documented in several clinical trials.[263,264] Bone pain diminishes, muscle strength and gait-posture improve, and osteitis fibrosa frequently resolves partially or completely.[120] When measured by reliable assays, serum PTH levels decrease in patients who respond favorably to treatment. Doses of oral calcitriol in most clinical trials have ranged from 0.25 to 1.5 μg/day. In patients with CKD, initial doses are determined by target PTH levels and specific stage of kidney disease.[206] In dialysis patients, $1,25(OH)_2D_3$ given thrice weekly by IV injection or by oral pulse therapy is effective in reducing serum PTH levels.[153,265] Dosage regimens range from 0.5 to 1.0 μg to 3.5 to 4.0 μg three times weekly or 2.0 to 5.0 μg twice weekly. Low doses should be used initially, and dosage adjustments should be based on frequent measurements of serum calcium, phosphorous, and PTH levels.

Oral 1α-$(OH)D_3$ (alfacalcidol) undergoes 25-hydroxylation in the liver to form calcitriol,[266,267] and this agent is used widely in Europe, Japan, and Canada. Calcitriol and 1α-$(OH)D_3$ are similarly effective for the treatment of secondary hyperparathyroidism in patients with CKD.

Although calcitriol and alfacalcidol are effective in decreasing PTH levels and preventing osteitis fibrosis cystica, treatment with these sterols in combination with calcium-based binders often results in hypercalcemia and hyperphosphatemia, which limits their use and contributes to the development of soft tissue calcification. Thus, new vitamin D analogues have been developed to prevent or minimize intestinal calcium and phosphorous absorption, while suppressing PTH levels as effectively as calcitriol. Three of these new vitamin D analogues are already on the market for use in patients with CKD: 22-oxacalcitriol (maxacalcitol) in Japan and 19-nor-1,25-$(OH)_2D_2$ (paricalcitol) and 1α-$(OH)D_2$ (doxercalciferol) in the United States.

19-Nor-1α,25$(OH)_2D_2$ (paricalcitol) is effective in controlling serum PTH levels in adult patients with stages 3 and 4 CKD,[268] as well as in dialysis patients. The long-term consequences of therapy with paricalcitol in conjunction with the use of calcium-containing binders for vascular calcification and cardiovascular complications remain to be determined. However, in a large cohort of patients undergoing hemodialysis, higher survival rates were observed in dialyzed patients treated with paricalcitol when compared with those receiving calcitriol.[269]

Another new vitamin analogue, 1α-$(OH)D_2$ (1α-D_2, doxercalciferol), is equipotent to 1α-$(OH)D_3$ in intestinal calcium absorption and bone calcium mobilization in rats.[270] A comparative trial of calcitriol and doxercalciferol in the control of secondary hyperparathyroidism in pediatric patients revealed no differences between the two vitamin D sterols in the control of secondary hyperparathyroidism or the development of hypercalcemia.[131] Doxercalciferol also effectively controls secondary hyperparathyroidism in adult patients with stable CKD.[271] Similar to paricalcitol, a survival advantage has been observed in adult hemodialysis patients receiving paricalcitol over those treated with calcitriol.[272]

Active vitamin D therapy has been associated with protective effects on both the heart and the kidney. Active vitamin D sterols ameliorate cardiac hypertrophy in animals,[24] and calcitriol therapy improves cardiac systolic function in hemodialysis patients.[273] Administration of active vitamin D sterols reduces proteinuria, fibrosis, and podocyte hypertrophy in subtotally nephrectomized rats,[274] and paricalcitol treatment decreases proteinuria in CKD patients.[275] These effects may be mediated by suppression of the renin-angiotensin system (RAS); indeed in vitro studies have demonstrated that calcitriol, paricalcitol, and doxercalciferol all suppress the RAS to a similar degree.[276] However, all activated vitamin D analogues may also increase FGF-23 secretion. Although the consequences of these increased levels in dialyzed patients remain to be completely determined, current evidence suggests that excessive circulating FGF-23 is associated with increased mortality rates.[184]

A growing body of evidence suggests additional health benefits of 25(OH)D therapy, primarily due to its immune regulatory role. Current observations also suggest a role for 25(OH)D in improving survival in patients treated with maintenance dialysis.[277]

CALCIMIMETICS

Cinacalcet, an allosteric activator of the calcium-sensing receptor, is now available for the treatment of secondary hyperparathyroidism. This small organic molecule reduces serum PTH levels and has been shown to decrease the calcium-phosphorous ion product in adult patients treated with maintenance dialysis, regardless of the specific phosphate-binding agent.[74,278] Experiments in uremic rats have demonstrated that calcimimetics are able to halt the progression of parathyroid cell hyperplasia[74]; the antiproliferative effect of this agent shows promise for use of the

molecule as a "medical parathyroidectomy." Studies in animals suggest that the use of calcimimetic agents may play a role in reversing the process of vascular calcification[279]; however, such effects need to be further evaluated in humans. Owing to the presence of the calcium-sensing receptor on the growth plate, these agents are not approved and should be used with caution in growing children.

PARATHYROIDECTOMY

In many cases when parathyroid surgery is needed and undertaken, the tumor has become monoclonal and growth autonomous.[77,280] Patients with severe hyperparathyroidism often are unresponsive to vitamin D therapy, developing hypercalcemia and hyperphosphatemia without reduction in PTH values or parathyroid gland size.[280] Clinical features that indicate the need for parathyroidectomy are as follows: the presence of hyperplasia and/or hypertrophy of the parathyroid glands (as documented by the presence of biochemical and radiographic features and, if necessary, the findings of osteitis fibrosa cystica on bone biopsy), elevated serum PTH levels unresponsive to vitamin D sterol therapy, persistent hypercalcemia, pruritus unresponsive to dialysis or other medical treatment, progressive extraskeletal calcification, severe skeletal pain or fractures, and calciphylaxis. Aluminum-related bone disease must be ruled out first in patients receiving low-dose calcitriol with persistent hypercalcemia.[281] Other causes of hypercalcemia, such as sarcoidosis, malignancy-related hypercalcemia, intake of calcium supplements, and the presence of adynamic/aplastic bone lesions not related to aluminum, should also be considered.[100,282]

When the decision has been made to perform parathyroid surgery, it is essential to avoid a marked postoperative fall in serum calcium levels caused by the "hungry bone" syndrome. Because of the severity of the bone disease, this fall can be much more marked and prolonged than after parathyroidectomy for primary hyperparathyroidism. Renal patients should receive daily oral calcitriol (0.5 to 1.0 μg) or some sort of intravenous active vitamin D sterol for 2 to 6 days before parathyroid surgery and during the postoperative period to stimulate intestinal calcium absorption and to maximize the effectiveness of oral calcium salts. Within 24 to 36 hours after surgery, marked hypocalcemia with serum calcium levels below 7 to 8 mg/dL may develop. This condition may be associated with serious symptoms, including seizures resulting in fractures and tendon avulsion. For reasons that are still unclear, these seizures most often occur during the last 1 to 2 hours of a hemodialysis procedure or immediately thereafter. To reduce the risk for convulsions, an infusion containing calcium gluconate should be started in the operating room, upon removal of the parathyroid glands. Calcium gluconate should be initiated at a rate of 100 mg of calcium ion per hour. Serum calcium should be measured every 4 to 6 hours and the calcium gluconate infusion rate increased if the serum calcium level continues to fall. The infusion rate may exceed 200 mg/hr. Enteral calcium carbonate is initiated once the patient is able to tolerate oral intake, and doses as high as 1.0 g (elemental calcium) given four to six times daily, along with vitamin D sterol in excess of 1.0 to 2.0 μg/day (for calcitriol, doses of other agents vary according to their potency), are often needed for patients with marked hypocalcemia. The intravenous calcium drip is weaned as soon as the oral intake of calcium salts is able to maintain normal serum calcium levels. The duration of intravenous calcium requirements varies greatly between patients—most patients require IV therapy for 2 to 3 days, but severe hypocalcemia may persist for several weeks or months, necessitating permanent central catheter access for daily home infusions of 800 to 1000 mg of calcium ion. Serum phosphorous levels may fall to subnormal levels postoperatively; phosphate treatment will markedly aggravate the hypocalcemia, and patients should not be treated with phosphate unless serum phosphorus falls to below 2.0 mg/dL.[283-286]

Hyperplastic parathyroid glands may be infiltrated with ethanol or calcitriol to cause sclerosis of the parathyroid tissue. This technique has been used at some centers[287,288] with variable efficacy in reducing hyperplastic tissue. This technique is used currently by only a few centers worldwide.

GROWTH HORMONE THERAPY

Recombinant human growth hormone (rhGH) should be considered in children with growth failure that does not respond to optimization of nutrition, correction of acidosis, and control of renal osteodystrophy. Serum phosphorous and PTH levels should be well controlled prior to the initiation of rhGH in children with CKD. Serum phosphorous levels should be less than 1.5 times the upper limit for age and PTH-IMA-1 levels less than 1.5 times the upper target values for the CKD stage before rhGH therapy is begun.[154] GH therapy will increase serum PTH levels during the first months of therapy; therefore, serum PTH levels should be monitored monthly. GH therapy should be discontinued temporarily if PTH levels exceed three times the upper target value for the CKD stage.[154]

Bone Disease After Successful Kidney Transplantation

Successful kidney transplantation corrects many of the abnormalities associated with renal osteodystrophy, but disorders of bone and mineral metabolism remain a major problem in such patients. Several factors, including persistent secondary hyperparathyroidism, prolonged immobilization, graft function, and, most important, use of different immunosuppressive agents, have been implicated in the development of bone disease after organ transplantation.

Hypercalcemia is not uncommon after renal transplantation. During the first several months, it can be quite severe, and patients with severe secondary hyperparathyroidism before renal transplantation are at greatest risk. More often, hypercalcemia may be less severe, with serum calcium levels between 10.5 and 12.0 mg/dL, and usually resolves within the first 12 months.[289] Parathyroidectomy should be considered when serum calcium levels are persistently above 12.5 mg/dL for longer than 1 year after transplantation.[290] Calcimimetic agents may be useful in preventing the need for parathyroidectomy in these patients.[291]

Hypophosphatemia may occur early in the post-transplant period, mainly in patients with severe secondary hyperparathyroidism, although persistent post-transplant elevation of serum FGF-23 levels also may contribute.[292,293] The clinical manifestations are variable; some patients complain of malaise, fatigue, and muscle weakness.[294,295] Phosphorous supplementation is required when values are persistently below 2.0 mg/dL, primarily in pediatric patients.

Significant bone loss has been shown to occur as early as 3 to 6 months after kidney transplantation.[296,297] Several factors, including persistent alterations in mineral metabolism, prolonged immobilization, and the use of immunosuppressive

agents required to maintain graft function, have been implicated in the development of bone disease after transplantation. Osteonecrosis, or avascular necrosis, is by far the most debilitating skeletal complication associated with organ transplantation. In approximately 15% of patients, osteonecrosis will develop within 3 years of renal transplantation.[298,299] The occurrence of osteonecrosis in inpatients after cardiac, hepatic, and bone marrow transplantation suggests that glucocorticoids play a critical role in the pathogenesis of this disorder.[300,301]

In both adult and pediatric kidney recipients, bone histologic changes associated with secondary hyperparathyroidism have been shown to resolve within 6 months after kidney transplantation.[297] However, some patients have persistently elevated rates of bone turnover, and others develop adynamic lesions, despite moderately elevated serum PTH levels.[302] Bone biopsy data from pediatric kidney recipients indicate that 67% of patients with stable graft function have features of normal bone formation; 10% have adynamic bone lesion, and 23% have bone lesions characteristic of secondary hyperparathyroidism.[303] Bone resorption typically is increased,[304] leading to a net loss of bone mass over time. Serum PTH levels are unable to discriminate between adynamic, normal, and increased bone turnover in the pediatric transplant population.[303] The use of maintenance corticosteroids has been implicated in these alterations; steroids decrease intestinal calcium absorption, enhance urinary calcium excretion, inhibit osteoblastic activity, decrease bone formation, and increase osteoclastic activity and bone resorption.[305-308] Likewise, cyclosporine has been reported to increase both bone formation and bone resorption and to reduce cancellous bone volume in the rat.[309,310] By contrast, azathioprine has been shown to have minimal impact on skeletal remodeling.[311] The role of other immunosuppressive agents, such as mycophenolate mofetil, as potential modifiers of bone formation and bone resorption has not been evaluated.

Although bone turnover may return to normal, defective skeletal mineralization is present in most pediatric transplant recipients.[303] Osteoid volume is increased, and mineral apposition rate is markedly reduced.[303] Although the factors responsible for the persistent increase in osteoid formation remain to be fully explained, corticosteroid use may contribute, as may persistent imbalances in PTH, vitamin D, and FGF-23 metabolism.[293]

After successful kidney transplantation with standard immunosuppressive regimens (daily corticosteroids, calcineurin inhibitor, and anti-metabolite), growth may be accelerated by an improvement in kidney function, but catch-up growth may not be observed even in children who undergo transplantation very early in life.[143] Moreover, height deceleration occurs in approximately 75% of patients who undergo transplantation before the age of 15 years.[312] The cause of persistent growth retardation is not completely understood, but immunosuppressive agents, persistent secondary hyperparathyroidism, altered vitamin D and FGF-23 metabolism, and the persistence of defective skeletal mineralization all may contribute. Children receiving steroid-free immunosuppressive regimens, those treated with alternate-day steroids, and those with better height SD at the time of transplant attain the greatest final adult height.[143,312-314] Used in children with significant height deficit after kidney transplantation, rhGH has produced a substantial increase in linear growth within the first year of therapy, but the magnitude of growth response may decline thereafter.[315]

Cardiovascular disease continues to be the leading cause of death after renal transplantation. In the post-transplant period, the presence of hypertension is strongly linked to increased IMT and poor vessel distensibility in children.[316] Alterations in bone and mineral metabolism also may contribute, as impaired kidney function persists in most patients during the post-transplant period.[67,143] Indeed, EBCT data indicate that vascular calcifications do not regress posttransplantation and do contribute to the burden of cardiovascular disease in this population.[317]

REFERENCES

1. Moe S, Drueke T, Cunningham J, et al: Definition, evaluation, and classification of renal osteodystrophy: a position statement from Kidney Disease: Improving Global Outcomes (KDIGO), Kidney Int 69:1945–1953, 2006.
2. Groothoff JW, Offringa M, Van Eck-Smit BL, et al: Severe bone disease and low bone mineral density after juvenile renal failure, Kidney Int 63:266–275, 2003.
3. Levin A, Bakris GL, Molitch M, et al: Prevalence of abnormal serum vitamin D, PTH, calcium, and phosphorus in patients with chronic kidney disease: results of the study to evaluate early kidney disease, Kidney Int 71:31–38, 2007.
4. Avasthi G, Singh HP, Katyal JC, et al: Copper, zinc, calcium and magnesium in chronic renal failure, J Assoc Physicians India 39:531–534, 1991.
5. Goldman R, Bassett SH: Phosphorus excretion in renal failure, J Clin Invest 33:1623–1628, 1954.
6. Coburn JW, Popovtzer MM, Massry SG, et al: The physicochemical state and renal handling of divalent ions in chronic renal failure, Arch Intern Med 124:302–311, 1969.
7. Shimada T, Mizutani S, Muto T, et al: Cloning and characterization of FGF23 as a causative factor of tumor-induced osteomalacia, Proc Natl Acad Sci U S A 98:6500–6505, 2001.
8. Autosomal dominant hypophosphataemic rickets is associated with mutations in FGF23, Nat Genet 26:345–348, 2000.
9. Larsson T, Zahradnik R, Lavigne J, et al: Immunohistochemical detection of FGF-23 protein in tumors that cause oncogenic osteomalacia, Eur J Endocrinol 148:269–276, 2003.
10. Mirams M, Robinson BG, Mason RS, et al: Bone as a source of FGF23: regulation by phosphate? Bone 35:1192–1199, 2004.
11. Yoshiko Y, Wang H, Minamizaki T, et al: Mineralized tissue cells are a principal source of FGF23, Bone 40:1565–1573, 2007.
12. Urakawa I, Yamazaki Y, Shimada T, et al: Klotho converts canonical FGF receptor into a specific receptor for FGF23, Nature 444:770–774, 2006.
13. Larsson T, Nisbeth U, Ljunggren O, et al: Circulating concentration of FGF-23 increases as renal function declines in patients with chronic kidney disease, but does not change in response to variation in phosphate intake in healthy volunteers, Kidney Int 64:2272–2279, 2003.
14. Gutierrez O, Isakova T, Rhee E, et al: Fibroblast growth factor-23 mitigates hyperphosphatemia but accentuates calcitriol deficiency in chronic kidney disease, J Am Soc Nephrol 16:2205–2215, 2005.
15. Kolek OI, Hines ER, Jones MD, et al: 1alpha,25-Dihydroxyvitamin D₃ upregulates FGF23 gene expression in bone: the final link in a renal-gastrointestinal-skeletal axis that controls phosphate transport, Am J Physiol Gastrointest Liver Physiol 289:G1036–G1042, 2005.
16. Portale AA, Booth BE, Halloran BP, et al: Effect of dietary phosphorus on circulating concentrations of 1,25-dihydroxyvitamin D and immunoreactive parathyroid hormone in children with moderate renal insufficiency, J Clin Invest 73:1580–1589, 1984.
17. Antoniucci DM, Yamashita T, Portale AA: Dietary phosphorus regulates serum fibroblast growth factor-23 concentrations in healthy men, J Clin Endocrinol Metab 91:3144–3149, 2006.
18. Krajisnik T, Bjorklund P, Marsell R, et al: Fibroblast growth factor-23 regulates parathyroid hormone and 1alpha-hydroxylase expression in cultured bovine parathyroid cells, J Endocrinol 195:125–131, 2007.
19. Ben-Dov IZ, Galitzer H, Lavi-Moshayoff V, et al: The parathyroid is a target organ for FGF23 in rats, J Clin Invest 117:4003–4008, 2007.
20. Martinez I, Saracho R, Montenegro J, et al: A deficit of calcitriol synthesis may not be the initial factor in the pathogenesis of secondary hyperparathyroidism, Nephrol Dial Transplant 11(suppl 3):22–28, 1996.
21. Li YC, Pirro AE, Amling M, et al: Targeted ablation of the vitamin D receptor: an animal model of vitamin D-dependent rickets type II with alopecia, Proc Natl Acad Sci U S A 94:9831–9835, 1997.
22. Amling M, Priemel M, Holzmann T, et al: Rescue of the skeletal phenotype of vitamin D receptor-ablated mice in the setting of normal mineral ion homeostasis: formal histomorphometric and biomechanical analyses, Endocrinology 140:4982–4987, 1999.
23. Panda DK, Miao D, Bolivar I, et al: Inactivation of the 25-hydroxyvitamin D 1alpha-hydroxylase and vitamin D receptor demonstrates independent and interdependent effects of calcium and vitamin D on skeletal and mineral homeostasis, J Biol Chem 279:16754–16766, 2004.
24. Bodyak N, Ayus JC, Achinger S, et al: Activated vitamin D attenuates left ventricular abnormalities induced by dietary sodium in Dahl salt-sensitive animals, Proc Natl Acad Sci U S A 104:16810–16815, 2007.
25. Zhou C, Lu F, Cao K, et al: Calcium-independent and 1,25(OH)₂D₃-dependent regulation of the renin-angiotensin system in 1alpha-hydroxylase knockout mice, Kidney Int 74:170–179, 2008.
26. Teng M, Wolf M, Ofsthun MN, et al: Activated injectable vitamin D and hemodialysis survival: a historical cohort study, J Am Soc Nephrol 16:1115–1125, 2005.
27. Teng M, Wolf M, Lowrie E, et al: Survival of patients undergoing hemodialysis with paricalcitol or calcitriol therapy, N Engl J Med 349:446–456, 2003.
28. Holick MF, Garabedian M: Vitamin D: photobiology, metabolism, mechanism of action, and clinical applications. In Favus MJ, editor: Primer on the metabolic bone diseases and disorders of mineral metabolism, Washington, DC, 2006, American Society for Bone and Mineral Research, pp 129–137.
29. DeLuca HF: Overview of general physiologic features and functions of vitamin D, Am J Clin Nutr 80S:1689S–1696S, 2004.
30. Holick MF: Resurrection of vitamin D deficiency and rickets, J Clin Invest 116:2062–2072, 2006.
31. Holick MF: Vitamin D deficiency, N Engl J Med 357:266–281, 2007.
32. Nykjaer A, Dragun D, Walther D, et al: An endocytic pathway essential for renal uptake and activation of the steroid 25-(OH) vitamin D₃, Cell 96:507–515, 1999.
33. Leheste JR, Melsen F, Wellner M, et al: Hypocalcemia and osteopathy in mice with kidney-specific megalin gene defect, FASEB J 17:247–249, 2003.
34. Zehnder D, Landray MJ, Wheeler DC, et al: Cross-sectional analysis of abnormalities of mineral homeostasis, vitamin D and parathyroid hormone in a cohort of pre-dialysis patients. The Chronic Renal Impairment in Birmingham (CRIB) study, Nephron Clin Pract 107:c109–c116, 2007.
35. Lambert PW, Stern PH, Avioli RC, et al: Evidence for extrarenal production of 1 alpha,25-dihydroxyvitamin D in man, J Clin Invest 69:722–725, 1982.
36. Dusso A, Lopez-Hilker S, Rapp N, et al: Extra-renal production of calcitriol in chronic renal failure, Kidney Int 34:368–375, 1988.
37. Dusso AS, Finch J, Brown A, et al: Extrarenal production of calcitriol in normal and uremic humans, J Clin Endocrinol Metab 72:157–164, 1991.
38. Khaw KT, Sneyd MJ, Compston J: Bone density parathyroid hormone and 25-hydroxyvitamin D concentrations in middle aged women, BMJ 305:273–277, 1992.
39. LeBoff MS, Kohlmeier L, Hurwitz S, et al: Occult vitamin D deficiency in postmenopausal US women with acute hip fracture, JAMA 281:1505–1511, 1999.
40. Thomas MK, Lloyd-Jones DM, Thadhani RI, et al: Hypovitaminosis D in medical inpatients, N Engl J Med 338:777–783, 1998.
41. Gordon CM, DePeter KC, Feldman HA, et al: Prevalence of vitamin D deficiency among healthy adolescents, Arch Pediatr Adolesc Med 158:531–537, 2004.
42. Stavroulopoulos A, Porter CJ, Roe SD, et al: Relationship between vitamin D status, parathyroid hormone levels and bone mineral density in patients with chronic kidney disease stages 3 and 4, Nephrology (Carlton) 13:63–67, 2008.
43. Reichel H, Deibert B, Schmidt-Gayk H: Calcium metabolism in early chronic renal failure: implications for the pathogenesis of hyperparathyroidism, Nephrol Dial Transplant 6:162–169, 1991.
44. Coburn JW, Koppel MH, Brickman AS, et al: Study of intestinal absorption of calcium in patients with renal failure, Kidney Int 3:264–272, 1973.
45. Holick MF: Vitamin D and the kidney, Kidney Int 32:912–929, 1987.
46. Clemens TL, Adams JS, Henderson SL, et al: Increased skin pigment reduces the capacity of skin to synthesise vitamin D3, Lancet 1:74–76, 1982.
47. Koenig KG, Lindberg JS, Zerwekh JE, et al: Free and total 1,25-dihydroxyvitamin D levels in subjects with renal disease, Kidney Int 41:161–165, 1992.
48. Saha H: Calcium and vitamin D homeostasis in patients with heavy proteinuria, Clin Nephrol 41:290–296, 1994.
49. Vasicek TJ, McDevitt BE, Freeman MW, et al: Nucleotide sequence of the human parathyroid hormone gene, Proc Natl Acad Sci U S A 80:2127–2131, 1983.
50. Reis A, Hecht W, Groger R, et al: Cloning and sequence analysis of the human parathyroid hormone gene region, Hum Genet 84:119–124, 1990.
51. Fraser RA, Kronenberg HM, Pang PK, et al: Parathyroid hormone messenger ribonucleic acid in the rat hypothalamus, Endocrinology 127:2517–2522, 1990.
52. Okazaki T, Ando K, Igarashi T, et al: Conserved mechanism of negative gene regulation by extracellular calcium. Parathyroid hormone gene versus atrial natriuretic polypeptide gene, J Clin Invest 89:1268–1273, 1992.
53. Moallem E, Kilav R, Silver J, et al: RNA-Protein binding and post-transcriptional regulation of parathyroid hormone gene expression by calcium and phosphate, J Biol Chem 273:5253–5259, 1998.
54. Saggese G, Federico G, Cinquanta L: In vitro effects of growth hormone and other hormones on chondrocytes and osteoblast-like cells, Acta Paediatr Suppl 82(suppl 391):54–59, 1993.
55. Scharla SH, Strong DD, Mohan S, et al: 1,25-Dihydroxyvitamin D₃ differentially regulates the production of insulin-like growth factor I (IGF-I) and IGF-binding protein-4 in mouse osteoblasts, Endocrinology 129:3139–3146, 1991.
56. Akiyama H, Hiraki Y, Shigeno C, et al: 1 alpha,25-dihydroxyvitamin D₃ inhibits cell growth and chondrogenesis of a clonal mouse EC cell line, ATDC5, J Bone Miner Res 11:22–28, 1996.
57. Silver J, Russell J, Sherwood LM: Regulation by vitamin D metabolites of messenger ribonucleic acid for pre-proparathyroid hormone in isolated bovine parathyroid cells, Proc Natl Acad Sci U S A 82:4270–4273, 1985.
58. Silver J, Naveh-Many T, Mayer H, et al: Regulation by vitamin D metabolites of parathyroid hormone gene transcription in vivo in the rat, J Clin Invest 78:1296–1301, 1986.
59. Kifor O, Moore FD Jr, Wang P, et al: Reduced immunostaining for the extracellular Ca2+-sensing receptor in primary and uremic secondary hyperparathyroidism, J Clin Endocrinol Metab 81:1598–1606, 1996.
60. Brown AJ, Zhong M, Finch J, et al: Rat calcium-sensing receptor is regulated by vitamin D but not by calcium, Am J Physiol 270(3 Pt 2):F454–F460, 1996.
61. Szabo A, Merke J, Beier E, et al: 1,25(OH)2 vitamin D₃ inhibits parathyroid cell proliferation in experimental uremia, Kidney Int 35:1049–1056, 1989.
62. Almaden Y, Canalejo A, Ballesteros E, et al: Regulation of arachidonic acid production by intracellular calcium in parathyroid cells: effect of extracellular phosphate, J Am Soc Nephrol 13:693–698, 2002.

63. Silver J, Kilav R, Sela-Brown A, et al: Molecular mechanisms of secondary hyperparathyroidism, Pediatr Nephrol 14:626–628, 2000.

64. Ritter CS, Armbrecht HJ, Slatopolsky E, et al: 25-Hydroxyvitamin D(3) suppresses PTH synthesis and secretion by bovine parathyroid cells, Kidney Int 70:654–659, 2006.

65. Zisman AL, Hristova M, Ho LT, et al: Impact of ergocalciferol treatment of vitamin D deficiency on serum parathyroid hormone concentrations in chronic kidney disease, Am J Nephrol 27:36–43, 2007.

66. Chandra P, Binongo JN, Ziegler TR, et al: Cholecalciferol (vitamin D3) therapy and vitamin D insufficiency in patients with chronic kidney disease: a randomized controlled pilot study, Endocr Pract 14:10–17, 2008.

67. K/DOQI clinical practice guidelines for bone metabolism and disease in chronic kidney disease, Am J Kidney Dis 42(4 suppl 3):S1–S201, 2003.

68. Brown EM, Gamba G, Riccardi D, et al: Cloning and characterization of an extracellular Ca(2+)-sensing receptor from bovine parathyroid, Nature 366:575–580, 1993.

69. John MR, Goodman WG, Gao P, et al: A novel immunoradiometric assay detects full-length human PTH but not amino-terminally truncated fragments: implications for PTH measurements in renal failure, J Clin Endocrinol Metab 84:4287–4290, 1999.

70. Freichel M, Zink-Lorenz A, Holloschi A, et al: Expression of a calcium-sensing receptor in a human medullary thyroid carcinoma cell line and its contribution to calcitonin secretion, Endocrinology 137:3842–3848, 1996.

71. Kirkwood JR, Ozonoff MB, Steinbach HL: Epiphyseal displacement after metaphyseal fracture in renal osteodystrophy, Am J Roentgenol Radium Ther Nucl Med 115:547–554, 1972.

72. Martin-Salvago M, Villar-Rodriguez JL, Palma-Alvarez A, et al: Decreased expression of calcium receptor in parathyroid tissue in patients with hyperparathyroidism secondary to chronic renal failure, Endocr Pathol 14:61–70, 2003.

73. Brown AJ, Zhong M, Ritter C, et al: Loss of calcium responsiveness in cultured bovine parathyroid cells is associated with decreased calcium receptor expression, Biochem Biophys Res Commun 212:861–867, 1995.

74. Wada M, Furuya Y, Sakiyama J, et al: The calcimimetic compound NPS R-568 suppresses parathyroid cell proliferation in rats with renal insufficiency. Control of parathyroid cell growth via a calcium receptor, J Clin Invest 100:2977–2983, 1997.

75. Canaff L, Hendy GN: Human calcium-sensing receptor gene. Vitamin D response elements in promoters P1 and P2 confer transcriptional responsiveness to 1,25-dihydroxyvitamin D, J Biol Chem 277:30337–30350, 2002.

76. Lloyd HM, Parfitt AM, Jacobi JM, et al: The parathyroid glands in chronic renal failure: a study of their growth and other properties made on the basis of findings in patients with hypercalcemia, J Lab Clin Med 114:358–367, 1989.

77. Arnold A, Brown MF, Urena P, et al: Monoclonality of parathyroid tumors in chronic renal failure and in primary parathyroid hyperplasia, J Clin Invest 95:2047–2053, 1995.

78. Agarwal SK, Guru SC, Heppner C, et al: Menin interacts with the AP1 transcription factor JunD and represses JunD-activated transcription, Cell 96:143–152, 1999.

79. Chandrasekharappa SC, Guru SC, Manickam P, et al: Positional cloning of the gene for multiple endocrine neoplasia-type 1, Science 276:404–407, 1997.

80. Cryns VL, Thor A, Xu HJ, et al: Loss of the retinoblastoma tumor-suppressor gene in parathyroid carcinoma, N Engl J Med 330:757–761, 1994.

81. Mulligan LM, Marsh DJ, Robinson BG, et al: Genotype-phenotype correlation in multiple endocrine neoplasia type 2: report of the International RET Mutation Consortium, J Intern Med 238:343–346, 1995.

82. Motokura T, Bloom T, Kim HG, et al: A novel cyclin encoded by a bcl1-linked candidate oncogene, Nature 350:512–515, 1991.

83. Atkins D, Peacock M: A comparison of the effects of the calcitonins, steroid hormones and thyroid hormones on the response of bone to parathyroid hormone in tissue culture, J Endocrinol 64:573–583, 1975.

84. Lee K, Deeds JD, Bond AT, et al: In situ localization of PTH/PTHrP receptor mRNA in the bone of fetal and young rats, Bone 14:341–345, 1993.

85. Sherrard DJ: Renal osteodystrophy, Semin Nephrol 6:56–67, 1986.

86. Malluche HH, Ritz E, Lange HP, et al: Changes of bone histology during maintenance hemodialysis at various levels of dialysate Ca concentration, Clin Nephrol 6:440–447, 1976.

87. Hamdy NA, Kanis JA, Beneton MN, et al: Effect of alfacalcidol on natural course of renal bone disease in mild to moderate renal failure, BMJ 310:358–363, 1995.

88. Norman ME, Mazur AT, Borden S, et al: Early diagnosis of juvenile renal osteodystrophy, J Pediatr 97:226–232, 1980.

89. Massry SG, Friedler RM, Coburn JW: Excretion of phosphate and calcium. Physiology of their renal handling and relation to clinical medicine, Arch Intern Med 131:828–859, 1973.

90. Galceran T, Martin KJ, Morrissey JJ, et al: Role of 1,25-dihydroxyvitamin D on the skeletal resistance to parathyroid hormone, Kidney Int 32:801–807, 1987.

91. Mathias R, Salusky I, Harman W, et al: Renal bone disease in pediatric and young adult patients on hemodialysis in a children's hospital, J Am Soc Nephrol 3:1938–1946, 1993.

92. Salusky IB, Ramirez JA, Oppenheim W, et al: Biochemical markers of renal osteodystrophy in pediatric patients undergoing CAPD/CCPD, Kidney Int 45:253–258, 1994.

93. Urena P, Ferreira A, Morieux C, et al: PTH/PTHrP receptor mRNA is down-regulated in epiphyseal cartilage growth plate of uraemic rats, Nephrol Dial Transplant 11:2008–2016, 1996.

94. Sanchez CP, Salusky IB, Kuizon BD, et al: Growth of long bones in renal failure: roles of hyperparathyroidism, growth hormone and calcitriol, Kidney Int 54:1879–1887, 1998.

95. Massry SG, Stein R, Garty J, et al: Skeletal resistance to the calcemic action of parathyroid hormone in uremia: role of 1,25 (OH)2 D3, Kidney Int 9:467–474, 1976.

96. Parfitt AM: The actions of parathyroid hormone on bone: relation to bone remodeling and turnover, calcium homeostasis, and metabolic bone disease. Part IV of IV parts: The state of the bones in uremic hyperparathyroidism—the mechanisms of skeletal resistance to PTH in renal failure and pseudohypoparathyroidism and the role of PTH in osteoporosis, osteopetrosis, and osteofluorosis, Metabolism 25:1157–1188, 1976.

97. Parfitt AM: The actions of parathyroid hormone on bone: relation to bone remodeling and turnover, calcium homeostasis, and metabolic bone disease. Part I of IV parts: Mechanisms of calcium transfer between blood and bone and their cellular basis: morphological and kinetic approaches to bone turnover, Metabolism 25:809–844, 1976.

98. Parfitt AM: The actions of parathyroid hormone on bone: relation to bone remodeling and turnover, calcium homeostasis, and metabolic bone disease. Part III of IV parts: PTH and osteoblasts, the relationship between bone turnover and bone loss, and the state of the bones in primary hyperparathyroidism, Metabolism 25:1033–1069, 1976.

99. Parfitt AM: The actions of parathyroid hormone on bone: relation to bone remodeling and turnover, calcium homeostasis, and metabolic bone diseases. Part II of IV parts: PTH and bone cells: bone turnover and plasma calcium regulation, Metabolism 25:909–955, 1976.

100. Malluche H, Faugere MC: Renal bone disease 1990: an unmet challenge for the nephrologist, Kidney Int 38:193–211, 1990.

101. El-Husseini AA, El-Agroudy AE, El-Sayed M, et al: A prospective randomized study for the treatment of bone loss with vitamin D during kidney transplantation in children and adolescents, Am J Transplant 4:2052–2057, 2004.

102. Salusky IB, Coburn JW, Foley J, et al: Effects of oral calcium carbonate on control of serum phosphorus and changes in plasma aluminum levels after discontinuation of aluminum-containing gels in children receiving dialysis, J Pediatr 108(5 Pt 1):767–770, 1986.

103. Goodman WG, Ramirez JA, Belin TR, et al: Development of adynamic bone in patients with secondary hyperparathyroidism after intermittent calcitriol therapy, Kidney Int 46:1160–1166, 1994.

104. Ott SM, Maloney NA, Klein GL, et al: Aluminum is associated with low bone formation in patients receiving chronic parenteral nutrition, Ann Intern Med 98:910–914, 1983.

105. London GM, Marty C, Marchais SJ, et al: Arterial calcifications and bone histomorphometry in end-stage renal disease, J Am Soc Nephrol 15:1943–1951, 2004.

106. Ward MK, Feest TG, Ellis HA, et al: Osteomalacic dialysis osteodystrophy: evidence for a water-borne aetiological agent, probably aluminium, Lancet 1:841–845, 1978.

107. Parkinson IS, Ward MK, Feest TG, et al: Fracturing dialysis osteodystrophy and dialysis encephalopathy. An epidemiological survey, Lancet 1:406–409, 1979.

108. Pierides AM, Edwards WG Jr, Cullum UX Jr, et al: Hemodialysis encephalopathy with osteomalacic fractures and muscle weakness, Kidney Int 18:115–124, 1980.

109. Nathan E, Pedersen SE: Dialysis encephalopathy in a non-dialysed uraemic boy treated with aluminium hydroxide orally, Acta Paediatr Scand 69:793–796, 1980.

110. Felsenfeld AJ, Gutman RA, Llach F, et al: Osteomalacia in chronic renal failure: a syndrome previously reported only with maintenance dialysis, Am J Nephrol 2:147–154, 1982.

111. Griswold WR, Reznik V, Mendoza SA, et al: Accumulation of aluminum in a nondialyzed uremic child receiving aluminum hydroxide, Pediatrics 71:56–58, 1983.

112. Kaye M: Oral aluminum toxicity in a non-dialyzed patient with renal failure, Clin Nephrol 20:208–211, 1983.

113. Andreoli SP, Bergstein JM, Sherrard DJ: Aluminum intoxication from aluminum-containing phosphate binders in children with azotemia not undergoing dialysis, N Engl J Med 310:1079–1084, 1984.

114. Sedman AB, Miller NL, Warady BA, et al: Aluminum loading in children with chronic renal failure, Kidney Int 26:201–204, 1984.

115. Kaehny WD, Hegg AP, Alfrey AC: Gastrointestinal absorption of aluminum from aluminum-containing antacids, N Engl J Med 296:1389–1390, 1977.

116. Salusky IB, Coburn JW, Brill J, et al: Bone disease in pediatric patients undergoing dialysis with CAPD or CCPD, Kidney Int 33:975–982, 1988.

117. Kuizon BD, Goodman WG, Jüppner H, et al: Diminished linear growth during intermittent calcitriol therapy in children undergoing CCPD, Kidney Int 53:205–211, 1998.

118. Cohen-Solal ME, Sebert JL, Boudailliez B, et al: Non-aluminic adynamic bone disease in non-dialyzed uremic patients: a new type of osteopathy due to overtreatment? Bone 13:1–5, 1992.

119. Atsumi K, Kushida K, Yamazaki K, et al: Risk factors for vertebral fractures in renal osteodystrophy, Am J Kidney Dis 33:287–293, 1999.

120. Ott SM, Maloney NA, Coburn JW, et al: The prevalence of bone aluminum deposition in renal osteodystrophy and its relation to the response to calcitriol therapy, N Engl J Med 307:709–713, 1982.

121. De Beur SM, Finnegan RB, Vassiliadis J, et al: Tumors associated with oncogenic osteomalacia express genes important in bone and mineral metabolism, J Bone Miner Res 17:1102–1110, 2002.

122. Jonsson KB, Zahradnik R, Larsson T, et al: Fibroblast growth factor 23 in oncogenic osteomalacia and X-linked hypophosphatemia, N Engl J Med 348:1656–1663, 2003.

123. Nelson AE, Bligh RC, Mirams M, et al: Clinical case seminar: Fibroblast growth factor 23: a new clinical marker for oncogenic osteomalacia, J Clin Endocrinol Metab 88:4088–4094, 2003.

124. Shimada T, Kakitani M, Yamazaki Y, et al: Targeted ablation of FGF23 demonstrates an essential physiological role of FGF23 in phosphate and vitamin D metabolism, J Clin Invest 113:561–568, 2004.

125. Sitara D, Razzaque MS, Hesse M, et al: Homozygous ablation of fibroblast growth factor-23 results in hyperphosphatemia and impaired skeletogenesis, and reverses hypophosphatemia in Phex-deficient mice, Matrix Biol 23:421–432, 2004.

126. Genuth SM, Klein L, Rabinovich S, et al: Osteomalacia accompanying chronic anticonvulsant therapy, J Clin Endocrinol Metab 35:378–386, 1972.

127. Pierides AM, Ellis HA, Ward M, et al: Barbiturate and anticonvulsant treatment in relation to osteomalacia with haemodialysis and renal transplantation, Br Med J 1:190–193, 1976.

128. Wang M, Hercz G, Sherrard DJ, et al: Relationship between intact 1-84 parathyroid hormone and bone histomorphometric parameters in dialysis patients without aluminum toxicity, Am J Kidney Dis 26:836–844, 1995.

129. NIDDK. USRDS 1994 Annual Report. 2008.

130. Salusky IB, Goodman WG, Kuizon BD, et al: Similar predictive value of bone turnover using first- and second-generation immunometric PTH assays in pediatric patients treated with peritoneal dialysis, Kidney Int 63:1801–1808, 2003.

131. Salusky IB, Goodman WG, Sahney S, et al: Sevelamer controls parathyroid hormone-induced bone disease as efficiently as calcium carbonate without increasing serum calcium levels during therapy with active vitamin D sterols, J Am Soc Nephrol 16:2501–2508, 2005.

132. Ho AY, Kung AW: Determinants of peak bone mineral density and bone area in young women, J Bone Miner Metab 23:470–475, 2005.

133. Bouillon R, Van CS, Carmeliet G: Intestinal calcium absorption: Molecular vitamin D mediated mechanisms, J Cell Biochem 88:332–339, 2003.

134. Noel LH, Zingraff J, Bardin T, et al: Tissue distribution of dialysis amyloidosis, Clin Nephrol 27:175–178, 1987.

135. Kleinman KS, Coburn JW: Amyloid syndromes associated with hemodialysis, Kidney Int 35:567–575, 1989.

136. Hampl H, Lobeck H, Bartel-Schwarze S, et al: Clinical, morphologic, biochemical, and immunohistochemical aspects of dialysis-associated amyloidosis, ASAIO Trans 33:250–259, 1987.

137. Baker LR, Ackrill P, Cattell WR, et al: Iatrogenic osteomalacia and myopathy due to phosphate depletion, Br Med J 3:150–152, 1974.

138. Powell DR: Effects of renal failure on the growth hormone-insulin-like growth factor axis, J Pediatr 131(1 Pt 2):S13–S16, 1997.

139. Zanello SB, Collins ED, Marinissen MJ, et al: Vitamin D receptor expression in chicken muscle tissue and cultured myoblasts, Horm Metab Res 29:231–236, 1997.

140. Wright RS, Hunt SM: A radioimmunoassay for 17-alpha 20 beta-dihydroxy-4-pregnen-3-one: its use in measuring changes in serum levels at ovulation in Atlantic salmon (Salmo salar), coho salmon (Oncorhynchus kisutch), and rainbow trout (Salmo gairdneri), Gen Comp Endocrinol 47:475–482, 1982.

141. Mehls O, Ritz E, Krempien B, et al: Slipped epiphyses in renal osteodystrophy, Arch Dis Child 50:545–554, 1975.

142. Tonshoff B, Schaefer F, Mehls O: Disturbance of growth hormone–insulin-like growth factor axis in uraemia. Implications for recombinant human growth hormone treatment, Pediatr Nephrol 4:654–662, 1990.

143. North American Pediatric Renal Transplant Cooperative Study (NAPRTCS) 2006 Annual Report. 2006.

144. Nash MA, Torrado AD, Greifer I, et al: Renal tubular acidosis in infants and children. Clinical course, response to treatment, and prognosis, J Pediatr 80:738–748, 1972.

145. Challa A, Chan W, Krieg RJ Jr, et al: Effect of metabolic acidosis on the expression of insulin-like growth factor and growth hormone receptor, Kidney Int 44:1224–1227, 1993.

146. Maniar S, Kleinknecht C, Zhou X, et al: Growth hormone action is blunted by acidosis in experimental uremia or acid load, Clin Nephrol 46:72–76, 1996.

147. Challa A, Krieg RJ Jr, Thabet MA, et al: Metabolic acidosis inhibits growth hormone secretion in rats: mechanism of growth retardation, Am J Physiol 265(4 Pt 1):E547–E553, 1993.

148. Green J, Maor G: Effect of metabolic acidosis on the growth hormone/IGF-I endocrine axis in skeletal growth centers, Kidney Int 57:2258–2267, 2000.

149. Lefebvre A, de Vernejoul MC, Gueris J, et al: Optimal correction of acidosis changes progression of dialysis osteodystrophy, Kidney Int 36:1112–1118, 1989.

150. Goodman WG, Salusky IB: Evolution of secondary hyperparathyroidism during oral calcitriol therapy in pediatric renal osteodystrophy, Contrib Nephrol 90:189–195, 1991.

151. Waller SC, Ridout D, Cantor T, et al: Parathyroid hormone and growth in children with chronic renal failure, Kidney Int 67:2338–2345, 2005.

152. Schmitt CP, Ardissino G, Testa S, et al: Growth in children with chronic renal failure on intermittent versus daily calcitriol, Pediatr Nephrol 18:440–444, 2003.

153. Martin KJ, Ballal HS, Domoto DT, et al: Pulse oral calcitriol for the treatment of hyperparathyroidism in patients on continuous ambulatory peritoneal dialysis: preliminary observations, Am J Kidney Dis 19:540–545, 1992.

154. K/DOQI clinical practice guidelines for bone metabolism and disease in children with chronic kidney disease, Am J Kidney Dis 46(4 suppl 1):S1–S121, 2005.

155. Nickerson T, Huynh H: Vitamin D analogue EB1089-induced prostate regression is associated with increased gene expression of insulin-like growth factor binding proteins, J Endocrinol 160:223–229, 1999.

156. Miyakoshi N, Richman C, Kasukawa Y, et al: Evidence that IGF-binding protein-5 functions as a growth factor, J Clin Invest 107:73–81, 2001.

157. Richman C, Baylink DJ, Lang K, et al: Recombinant human insulin-like growth factor-binding protein-5 stimulates bone formation parameters in vitro and in vivo, Endocrinology 140:4699–4705, 1999.

158. Longobardi L, Torello M, Buckway C, et al: A novel insulin-like growth factor (IGF)-independent role for IGF binding protein-3 in mesenchymal chondroprogenitor cell apoptosis, Endocrinology 144:1695–1702, 2003.

159. Collard TJ, Guy M, Butt AJ, et al: Transcriptional upregulation of the insulin-like growth factor binding protein IGFBP-3 by sodium butyrate increases IGF-independent apoptosis in human colonic adenoma-derived epithelial cells, Carcinogenesis 24:393–401, 2003.

160. Samaan NA, Freeman RM: Growth hormone levels in severe renal failure, Metabolism 19:102–113, 1970.

161. Tonshoff B, Veldhuis JD, Heinrich U, et al: Deconvolution analysis of spontaneous nocturnal growth hormone secretion in prepubertal children with preterminal chronic renal failure and with end-stage renal disease, Pediatr Res 37:86–93, 1995.

162. Tonshoff B, Sammet A, Sanden I, et al: Outcome and prognostic determinants in the hemolytic uremic syndrome of children, Nephron 68:63–70, 1994.

163. Schaefer F, Chen Y, Tsao T, et al: Impaired JAK-STAT signal transduction contributes to growth hormone resistance in chronic uremia, J Clin Invest 108:467–475, 2001.

164. Tonshoff B, Cronin MJ, Reichert M, et al: Reduced concentration of serum growth hormone (GH)-binding protein in children with chronic renal failure: correlation with GH insensitivity. The European Study Group for Nutritional Treatment of Chronic Renal Failure in Childhood. The German Study Group for Growth Hormone Treatment in Chronic Renal Failure, J Clin Endocrinol Metab 82:1007–1013, 1997.

165. Powell DR, Liu F, Baker BK, et al: Modulation of growth factors by growth hormone in children with chronic renal failure. The Southwest Pediatric Nephrology Study Group, Kidney Int 51:1970–1979, 1997.

166. Conger JD, Hammond WS, Alfrey AC, et al: Pulmonary calcification in chronic dialysis patients. Clinical and pathologic studies, Ann Intern Med 83:330–336, 1975.

167. Milliner DS, Zinsmeister AR, Lieberman E, et al: Soft tissue calcification in pediatric patients with end-stage renal disease, Kidney Int 38:931–936, 1990.

168. Goodman WG, Goldin J, Kuizon BD, et al: Coronary-artery calcification in young adults with end-stage renal disease who are undergoing dialysis, N Engl J Med 342:1478–1483, 2000.

169. Oh J, Wunsch R, Turzer M, et al: Advanced coronary and carotid arteriopathy in young adults with childhood-onset chronic renal failure, Circulation 106:100–105, 2002.

170. Chavers BM, Li S, Collins AJ, et al: Cardiovascular disease in pediatric chronic dialysis patients, Kidney Int 62:648–653, 2002.

171. Mitsnefes MM, Kimball TR, Kartal J, et al: Cardiac and vascular adaptation in pediatric patients with chronic kidney disease: role of calcium-phosphorus metabolism, J Am Soc Nephrol 16:2796–2803, 2005.

172. Russo D, Palmiero G, De Blasio AP, et al: Coronary artery calcification in patients with CRF not undergoing dialysis, Am J Kidney Dis 44:1024–1030, 2004.

173. Moe SM, Duan D, Doehle BP, et al: Uremia induces the osteoblast differentiation factor Cbfa1 in human blood vessels, Kidney Int 63:1003–1011, 2003.

174. Ducy P, Zhang R, Geoffroy V, et al: Osf2/Cbfa1: a transcriptional activator of osteoblast differentiation, Cell 89:747–754, 1997.

175. Jono S, McKee MD, Murry CE, et al: Phosphate regulation of vascular smooth muscle cell calcification, Circ Res 87:E10-E17, 2000.

176. Ahmed S, O'Neill KD, Hood AF, et al: Calciphylaxis is associated with hyperphosphatemia and increased osteopontin expression by vascular smooth muscle cells, Am J Kidney Dis 37:1267–1276, 2001.

177. Bostrom K: Insights into the mechanism of vascular calcification, Am J Cardiol 88(2A):20E–22E, 2001.

178. Moe SM, O'Neill KD, Duan D, et al: Medial artery calcification in ESRD patients is associated with deposition of bone matrix proteins, Kidney Int 61:638–647, 2002.

179. Chen NX, O'Neill KD, Duan D, et al: Phosphorus and uremic serum up-regulate osteopontin expression in vascular smooth muscle cells, Kidney Int 62:1724–1731, 2002.

180. Schafer C, Heiss A, Schwarz A, et al: The serum protein alpha 2-Heremans-Schmid glycoprotein/fetuin-A is a systemically acting inhibitor of ectopic calcification, J Clin Invest 112:357–366, 2003.

181. Schinke T, Amendt C, Trindl A, et al: The serum protein alpha2-HS glycoprotein/fetuin inhibits apatite formation in vitro and in mineralizing calvaria cells. A possible role in mineralization and calcium homeostasis, J Biol Chem 271:20789–20796, 1996.

182. Sweatt A, Sane DC, Hutson SM, et al: Matrix Gla protein (MGP) and bone morphogenetic protein-2 in aortic calcified lesions of aging rats, J Thromb Haemost 1:178–185, 2003.

183. Koh N, Fujimori T, Nishiguchi S, et al: Severely reduced production of klotho in human chronic renal failure kidney, Biochem Biophys Res Commun 280:1015–1020, 2001.

184. Gutierrez O, Mannstadt M, Isakova T, et al: Fibroblast growth factor 23 and mortality among patients undergoing hemodialysis, N Engl J Med 359:584–592, 2008.

185. Miyamoto K, Ito M, Segawa H, Kuwahata M: Molecular targets of hyperphosphataemia in chronic renal failure, Nephrol Dial Transplant 18(suppl 3):iii79–iii80, 2003.

186. Tonelli M, Keech A, Shepherd J, et al: Effect of pravastatin in people with diabetes and chronic kidney disease, J Am Soc Nephrol 16:3748–3754, 2005.

187. Holdaas H, Fellstrom B, Cole E, et al: Long-term cardiac outcomes in renal transplant recipients receiving fluvastatin: the ALERT extension study, Am J Transplant 5:2929–2936, 2005.

188. Wanner C, Krane V, Marz W, et al: Atorvastatin in patients with type 2 diabetes mellitus undergoing hemodialysis, N Engl J Med 353:238–248, 2005.

189. Block GA, Spiegel DM, Ehrlich J, et al: Effects of sevelamer and calcium on coronary artery calcification in patients new to hemodialysis, Kidney Int 68:1815–1824, 2005.

190. Block GA, Raggi P, Bellasi A, et al: Mortality effect of coronary calcification and phosphate binder choice in incident hemodialysis patients, Kidney Int 71:438–441, 2007.

191. Gipstein RM, Coburn JW, Adams DA, et al: Calciphylaxis in man. A syndrome of tissue necrosis and vascular calcification in 11 patients with chronic renal failure, Arch Intern Med 136:1273–1280, 1976.

192. Bleyer AJ, Choi M, Igwemezie B, et al: A case control study of proximal calciphylaxis, Am J Kidney Dis 32:376–383, 1998.

193. Goldsmith DJ: Calciphylaxis, thrombotic diathesis and defects in coagulation regulation, Nephrol Dial Transplant 12:1082–1083, 1997.

194. Mohammed IA, Sekar V, Bubtana AJ, et al: Proximal calciphylaxis treated with calcimimetic "Cinacalcet." Nephrol Dial Transplant 23:387–389, 2008.

195. Rogers NM, Teubner DJ, Coates PT: Calcific uremic arteriolopathy: advances in pathogenesis and treatment, Semin Dial 20:150–157, 2007.
196. Bardin T, Kuntz D, Zingraff J, et al: Synovial amyloidosis in patients undergoing long-term hemodialysis, Arthritis Rheum 28:1052–1058, 1985.
197. Hou FF, Chertow GM, Kay J, et al: Interaction between beta 2-microglobulin and advanced glycation end products in the development of dialysis related-amyloidosis, Kidney Int 51:1514–1519, 1997.
198. Miyata T, Inagi R, Iida Y, et al: Involvement of beta 2-microglobulin modified with advanced glycation end products in the pathogenesis of hemodialysis-associated amyloidosis. Induction of human monocyte chemotaxis and macrophage secretion of tumor necrosis factor-alpha and interleukin-1, J Clin Invest 93:521–528, 1994.
199. Van Ypersele de Strihou C, Jadoul M, Malghem J, et al: Effect of dialysis membrane and patient's age on signs of dialysis-related amyloidosis. The Working Party on Dialysis Amyloidosis, Kidney Int 39:1012–1019, 1991.
200. McMahon LP, Radford J, Dawborn JK: Shoulder ultrasound in dialysis related amyloidosis, Clin Nephrol 35:227–232, 1991.
201. Bindi P, Chanard J: Destructive spondyloarthropathy in dialysis patients: an overview, Nephron 55:104–109, 1990.
202. Ayli M, Ayli D, Azak A, et al: The effect of high-flux hemodialysis on dialysis-associated amyloidosis, Ren Fail 27:31–34, 2005.
203. Block GA, Hulbert-Shearon TE, Levin NW, et al: Association of serum phosphorus and calcium x phosphate product with mortality risk in chronic hemodialysis patients: a national study, Am J Kidney Dis 31:607–617, 1998.
204. Alfrey AC, Miller NL, Butkus D: Evaluation of body magnesium stores, J Lab Clin Med 84:153–162, 1974.
205. Brown EM, Wilson RE, Eastman RC, et al: Abnormal regulation of parathyroid hormone release by calcium in secondary hyperparathyroidism due to chronic renal failure, J Clin Endocrinol Metab 54:172–179, 1982.
206. Salusky IB, Fine RN, Kangarloo H, et al: "High-dose" calcitriol for control of renal osteodystrophy in children on CAPD, Kidney Int 32:89–95, 1987.
207. Kurz P, Monier-Faugere MC, Bognar B, et al: Evidence for abnormal calcium homeostasis in patients with adynamic bone disease, Kidney Int 46:855–861, 1994.
208. Guillot AP, Hood VL, Runge CF, et al: The use of magnesium-containing phosphate binders in patients with end-stage renal disease on maintenance hemodialysis, Nephron 30:114–117, 1982.
209. Sherrard DJ, Hercz G, Pei Y, et al: The spectrum of bone disease in end-stage renal failure—an evolving disorder, Kidney Int 43:436–442, 1993.
210. Van Renen MJ, Hogg RJ, Sweeney AL, et al: Accelerated growth in short children with chronic renal failure treated with both strict dietary therapy and recombinant growth hormone, Pediatr Nephrol 6:451–458, 1992.
211. Charhon SA, Delmas PD, Malaval L, et al: Serum bone Gla-protein in renal osteodystrophy: comparison with bone histomorphometry, J Clin Endocrinol Metab 63:892–897, 1986.
212. Epstein S, Traberg H, Raja R, et al: Serum and dialysate osteocalcin levels in hemodialysis and peritoneal dialysis patients and after renal transplantation, J Clin Endocrinol Metab 60:1253–1256, 1985.
213. Brossard JH, Cloutier M, Roy L, et al: Accumulation of a non-(1–84) molecular form of parathyroid hormone (PTH) detected by intact PTH assay in renal failure: importance in the interpretation of PTH values, J Clin Endocrinol Metab 81:3923–3929, 1996.
214. Lepage R, Roy L, Brossard JH, et al: A non-(1–84) circulating parathyroid hormone (PTH) fragment interferes significantly with intact PTH commercial assay measurements in uremic samples, Clin Chem 44:805–809, 1998.
215. Brossard JH, Yamamoto LN, D'Amour P: Parathyroid hormone metabolites in renal failure: bioactivity and clinical implications, Semin Dial 15:196–201, 2002.
216. Slatopolsky E, Finch J, Clay P, et al: A novel mechanism for skeletal resistance in uremia, Kidney Int 58:753–761, 2000.
217. Gao P, Scheibel S, D'Amour P, et al: Development of a novel immunoradiometric assay exclusively for biologically active whole parathyroid hormone 1-84: implications for improvement of accurate assessment of parathyroid function, J Bone Miner Res 16:605–614, 2001.
218. Monier-Faugere MC, Geng Z, Mawad H, et al: Improved assessment of bone turnover by the PTH-(1–84)/large C-PTH fragments ratio in ESRD patients, Kidney Int 60:1460–1468, 2001.
219. Coen G, Bonucci E, Ballanti P, et al: PTH 1-84 and PTH "7-84" in the noninvasive diagnosis of renal bone disease, Am J Kidney Dis 40:348–354, 2002.
220. D'Amour P, Brossard JH, Rousseau L, et al: Structure of non-(1-84) PTH fragments secreted by parathyroid glands in primary and secondary hyperparathyroidism, Kidney Int 68:998–1007, 2005.
221. Divieti P, John MR, Jüppner H, et al: Human PTH-(7-84) inhibits bone resorption in vitro via actions independent of the type 1 PTH/PTHrP receptor, Endocrinology 143:171–176, 2002.
222. Langub MC, Monier-Faugere MC, Wang G, et al: Administration of PTH-(7-84) antagonizes the effects of PTH-(1-84) on bone in rats with moderate renal failure, Endocrinology 144:1135–1138, 2003.
223. Nguyen-Yamamoto L, Rousseau L, Brossard JH, et al: Synthetic carboxyl-terminal fragments of parathyroid hormone (PTH) decrease ionized calcium concentration in rats by acting on a receptor different from the PTH/PTH-related peptide receptor, Endocrinology 142:1386–1392, 2001.
224. Alfrey AC: Aluminum metabolism, Kidney Int Suppl 18:S8–S11, 1986.
225. Andress DL, Endres DB, Maloney NA, et al: Comparison of parathyroid hormone assays with bone histomorphometry in renal osteodystrophy, J Clin Endocrinol Metab 63:1163–1169, 1986.
226. Wright RS, Mehls O, Ritz E, et al: Musculoskeletal manifestation of chronic renal failure, dialysis and transplantation. In Bacon P, Hadler N, editors: Renal Manifestations in Rheumatic Disease, London, 1982, Butterworth Publishers, p. 352.
227. Dent CE, Hodson CJ: Radiological changes associated with certain metabolic bone diseases, Br J Radiol 27:605–618, 1954.
228. Parfitt AM, Kleerekoper M, Cruz C: Reduced phosphate reabsorption unrelated to parathyroid hormone after renal transplantation: implications for the pathogenesis of hyperparathyroidism in chronic renal failure, Miner Electrolyte Metab 12:356–362, 1986.
229. Meema HE, Rabinovich S, Meema S, et al: Improved radiological diagnosis of azotemic osteodystrophy, Radiology 102:1–10, 1972.
230. Shimada H, Nakamura M, Marumo F: Influence of aluminium on the effect of 1 alpha (OH)D3 on renal osteodystrophy, Nephron 35:163–170, 1983.
231. Simpson W, Ellis HA, Kerr DN, et al: Bone disease in long-term haemodialysis: the association of radiological with histological abnormalities, Br J Radiol 49:105–110, 1976.
232. Parfitt AM, Massry SG, Winfield AC: Osteopenia and fractures occurring during maintenance hemodialysis. A new form of renal osteodystrophy, Clin Orthop Relat Res 87:287–302, 1972.
233. Mallette LE, Patten BM, Engel WK: Neuromuscular disease in secondary hyperparathyroidism, Ann Intern Med 82:474–483, 1975.
234. Mucsi I, Hercz G, Uldall R, et al: Control of serum phosphate without any phosphate binders in patients treated with nocturnal hemodialysis, Kidney Int 53:1399–1404, 1998.
235. Fischbach M, Terzic J, Menouer S, et al: Intensified and daily hemodialysis in children might improve statural growth, Pediatr Nephrol 21:1746–1752, 2006.
236. Goodman WG: Aluminum and renal osteodystrophy. In Bushinsky DA, editor: Renal Osteodystrophy, Philadelphia, 1998, Lippincott-Raven, p. 317.
237. Salusky IB, Foley J, Nelson P, et al: Aluminum accumulation during treatment with aluminum hydroxide and dialysis in children and young adults with chronic renal disease, N Engl J Med 324:527–531, 1991.
238. Coburn JW, Mischel MG, Goodman WG, et al: Calcium citrate markedly enhances aluminum absorption from aluminum hydroxide, Am J Kidney Dis 17:708–711, 1991.
239. Bakir AA, Hryhorczuk DO, Berman E, et al: Acute fatal hyperaluminemic encephalopathy in undialyzed and recently dialyzed uremic patients, ASAIO Trans 32:171–176, 1986.
240. Portale AA, Booth BE, Tsai HC, et al: Reduced plasma concentration of 1,25-dihydroxyvitamin D in children with moderate renal insufficiency, Kidney Int 21:627–632, 1982.
241. Alon U, Davidai G, Bentur L, et al: Oral calcium carbonate as phosphate-binder in infants and children with chronic renal failure, Miner Electrolyte Metab 12:320–325, 1986.
242. Andreoli SP, Dunson JW, Bergstein JM: Calcium carbonate is an effective phosphorus binder in children with chronic renal failure, Am J Kidney Dis 9:206–210, 1987.
243. Salusky IB, Kuizon BD, Belin TR, et al: Intermittent calcitriol therapy in secondary hyperparathyroidism: a comparison between oral and intraperitoneal administration, Kidney Int 54:907–914, 1998.
244. Salusky IB, Goodman WG: Adynamic renal osteodystrophy: is there a problem? J Am Soc Nephrol 12:1978–1985, 2001.
245. Pflanz S, Henderson IS, McElduff N, et al: Calcium acetate versus calcium carbonate as phosphate-binding agents in chronic haemodialysis, Nephrol Dial Transplant 9:1121–1124, 1994.
246. Caravaca F, Santos I, Cubero JJ, et al: Calcium acetate versus calcium carbonate as phosphate binders in hemodialysis patients, Nephron 60:423–427, 1992.
247. Wallot M, Bonzel KE, Winter A, et al: Calcium acetate versus calcium carbonate as oral phosphate binder in pediatric and adolescent hemodialysis patients, Pediatr Nephrol 10:625–630, 1996.
248. Cushner HM, Copley JB, Lindberg JS, et al: Calcium citrate, a nonaluminum-containing phosphate-binding agent for treatment of CRF, Kidney Int 33:95–99, 1988.
249. Birck R, Zimmermann E, Wassmer S, et al: Calcium ketoglutarate versus calcium acetate for treatment of hyperphosphataemia in patients on maintenance haemodialysis: a cross-over study, Nephrol Dial Transplant 14:1475–1479, 1999.
250. Slatopolsky EA, Burke SK, Dillon MA: RenaGel, a nonabsorbed calcium- and aluminum-free phosphate binder, lowers serum phosphorus and parathyroid hormone. The RenaGel Study Group, Kidney Int 55:299–307, 1999.
251. Bleyer AJ, Burke SK, Dillon M, et al: A comparison of the calcium-free phosphate binder sevelamer hydrochloride with calcium acetate in the treatment of hyperphosphatemia in hemodialysis patients, Am J Kidney Dis 33:694–701, 1999.
252. Chertow GM, Burke SK, Dillon MA, et al: Long-term effects of sevelamer hydrochloride on the calcium x phosphate product and lipid profile of haemodialysis patients, Nephrol Dial Transplant 14:2907–2914, 1999.
253. Chertow GM, Burke SK, Raggi P: Sevelamer attenuates the progression of coronary and aortic calcification in hemodialysis patients, Kidney Int 62:245–252, 2002.
254. Delmez J, Block G, Robertson J, et al: A randomized, double-blind, crossover design study of sevelamer hydrochloride and sevelamer carbonate in patients on hemodialysis, Clin Nephrol 68:386–391, 2007.
255. O'Donovan R, Baldwin D, Hammer M, et al: Substitution of aluminium salts by magnesium salts in control of dialysis hyperphosphataemia, Lancet 1:880–882, 1986.
256. Hergesell O, Ritz E: Phosphate binders on iron basis: a new perspective? Kidney Int Suppl 73:S42–S45, 1999.
257. Hergesell O, Ritz E: Stabilized polynuclear iron hydroxide is an efficient oral phosphate binder in uraemic patients, Nephrol Dial Transplant 14:863–867, 1999.
258. Hutchison AJ, Speake M, Al-Baaj F: Reducing high phosphate levels in patients with chronic renal failure undergoing dialysis: a 4-week, dose-finding, open-label study with lanthanum carbonate, Nephrol Dial Transplant 19:1902–1906, 2004.
259. Finn WF, Joy MS, Hladik G: Efficacy and safety of lanthanum carbonate for reduction of serum phosphorus in patients with chronic renal failure receiving hemodialysis, Clin Nephrol 62:193–201, 2004.
260. D'Haese PC, Spasovski GB, Sikole A, et al: A multicenter study on the effects of lanthanum carbonate (Fosrenol) and calcium carbonate on renal bone disease in dialysis patients, Kidney Int Suppl (85):S73–S78, 2003.

261. Slatopolsky E, Liapis H, Finch J: Progressive accumulation of lanthanum in the liver of normal and uremic rats, Kidney Int 68:2809–2813, 2005.

262. Spasovski GB, Sikole A, Gelev S, et al: Evolution of bone and plasma concentration of lanthanum in dialysis patients before, during 1 year of treatment with lanthanum carbonate and after 2 years of follow-up, Nephrol Dial Transplant 21:2217–2224, 2006.

263. Baker LR, Muir JW, Sharman VL, et al: Controlled trial of calcitriol in hemodialysis patients, Clin Nephrol 26:185–191, 1986.

264. Berl T, Berns AS, Hufer WE, et al: 1,25 dihydroxycholecalciferol effects in chronic dialysis. A double-blind controlled study, Ann Intern Med 88:774–780, 1978.

265. Fukagawa M, Okazaki R, Takano K, et al: Regression of parathyroid hyperplasia by calcitriol-pulse therapy in patients on long-term dialysis, N Engl J Med 323:421–422, 1990.

266. Pierides AM, Ellis HA, Simpson W, et al: Variable response to long-term 1alpha-hydroxycholecalciferol in haemodialysis osteodystrophy, Lancet 1:1092–1095, 1976.

267. Kanis JA, Henderson RG, Heynen G, et al: Renal osteodystrophy in nondialysed adolescents. Long-term treatment with 1alpha-hydroxycholecalciferol, Arch Dis Child 52:473–481, 1977.

268. Coyne D, Acharya M, Qiu P, et al: Paricalcitol capsule for the treatment of secondary hyperparathyroidism in stages 3 and 4 CKD, Am J Kidney Dis 47:263–276, 2006.

269. Dobrez DG, Mathes A, Amdahl M, et al: Paricalcitol-treated patients experience improved hospitalization outcomes compared with calcitriol-treated patients in real-world clinical settings, Nephrol Dial Transplant 19:1174–1181, 2004.

270. Sjoden G, Smith C, Lindgren U, et al: 1 alpha-hydroxyvitamin D_2 is less toxic than 1 alpha-hydroxy-vitamin D_3 in the rat, Proc Soc Exp Biol Med 178:432–436, 1985.

271. Andress DL, Norris KC, Coburn JW, et al: Intravenous calcitriol in the treatment of refractory osteitis fibrosa of chronic renal failure, N Engl J Med 321:274–279, 1989.

272. Tentori F, Hunt WC, Stidley CA, et al: Mortality risk among hemodialysis patients receiving different vitamin D analogs, Kidney Int 70:1858–1865, 2006.

273. Singh NP, Sahni V, Garg D, et al: Effect of pharmacological suppression of secondary hyperparathyroidism on cardiovascular hemodynamics in predialysis CKD patients: A preliminary observation, Hemodial Int 11:417–423, 2007.

274. Schwarz U, Amann K, Orth SR, et al: Effect of 1,25(OH)₂ vitamin D_3 on glomerulosclerosis in subtotally nephrectomized rats, Kidney Int 53:1696–1705, 1998.

275. Agarwal R, Acharya M, Tian J, et al: Antiproteinuric effect of oral paricalcitol in chronic kidney disease, Kidney Int 68:2823–2828, 2005.

276. Nakane M, Ma J, Ruan X, et al: Mechanistic analysis of VDR-mediated renin suppression, Nephron Physiol 107:35–44, 2007.

277. Wolf M, Shah A, Gutierrez O, et al: Vitamin D levels and early mortality among incident hemodialysis patients, Kidney Int 72:1004–1013, 2007.

278. Wada M, Nagano N: Control of parathyroid cell growth by calcimimetics, Nephrol Dial Transplant 18(suppl 3):iii13–iii17, 2003.

279. Lopez I, Guilera-Tejero E, Mendoza FJ, et al: Calcimimetic R-568 decreases extraosseous calcifications in uremic rats treated with calcitriol, J Am Soc Nephrol 17:795–804, 2006.

280. Quarles LD, Yohay DA, Carroll BA, et al: Prospective trial of pulse oral versus intravenous calcitriol treatment of hyperparathyroidism in ESRD, Kidney Int 45:1710–1721, 1994.

281. Froment DP, Molitoris BA, Buddington B, et al: Site and mechanism of enhanced gastrointestinal absorption of aluminum by citrate, Kidney Int 36:978–984, 1989.

282. Jorna FH, Tobe TJ, Huisman RM, et al: Early identification of risk factors for refractory secondary hyperparathyroidism in patients with long-term renal replacement therapy, Nephrol Dial Transplant 19:1168–1173, 2004.

283. Andress DL, Ott SM, Maloney NA, et al: Effect of parathyroidectomy on bone aluminum accumulation in chronic renal failure, N Engl J Med 312:468–473, 1985.

284. De Vernejoul MC, Marchais S, London G, et al: Increased bone aluminum deposition after subtotal parathyroidectomy in dialyzed patients, Kidney Int 27:785–791, 1985.

285. Kurokawa K, Akizawa T, Suzuki M, et al: Effect of 22-oxacalcitriol on hyperparathyroidism of dialysis patients: results of a preliminary study, Nephrol Dial Transplant 11(suppl 3):121–124, 1996.

286. Charytan C, Coburn JW, Chonchol M, et al: Cinacalcet hydrochloride is an effective treatment for secondary hyperparathyroidism in patients with CKD not receiving dialysis, Am J Kidney Dis 46:58–67, 2005.

287. De Barros Gueiros JE, Chammas MC, Gerhard R, et al: Percutaneous ethanol (PEIT) and calcitrol (PCIT) injection therapy are ineffective in treating severe secondary hyperparathyroidism, Nephrol Dial Transplant 19:657–663, 2004.

288. Fukagawa M, Kitaoka M, Tominaga Y, et al: Guidelines for percutaneous ethanol injection therapy of the parathyroid glands in chronic dialysis patients, Nephrol Dial Transplant 18(suppl 3):iii31–iii33, 2003.

289. Diethelm AG, Edwards RP, Whelchel JD: The natural history and surgical treatment of hypercalcemia before and after renal transplantation, Surg Gynecol Obstet 154:481–490, 1982.

290. D'Alessandro AM, Melzer JS, Pirsch JD, et al: Tertiary hyperparathyroidism after renal transplantation: operative indications, Surgery 106:1049–1055, 1989.

291. Bergua C, Torregrosa JV, Fuster D, et al: Effect of cinacalcet on hypercalcemia and bone mineral density in renal transplanted patients with secondary hyperparathyroidism, Transplantation 86:413–417, 2008.

292. Bhan I, Shah A, Holmes J, et al: Post-transplant hypophosphatemia: Tertiary "Hyper-Phosphatoninism"? Kidney Int 70:1486–1494, 2006.

293. Evenepoel P, Naesens M, Claes K, et al: Tertiary "hyperphosphatoninism" accentuates hypophosphatemia and suppresses calcitriol levels in renal transplant recipients, Am J Transplant 7:1193–1200, 2007.

294. Bonomini V, Feletti C, Di Felica A, et al: Bone remodelling after renal transplantation (RT), Adv Exp Med Biol 178:207–216, 1984.

295. Nielsen HE, Melsen F, Christensen MS: Aseptic necrosis of bone following renal transplantation. Clinical and biochemical aspects and bone morphometry, Acta Med Scand 202:27–32, 1977.

296. Grotz WH, Mundinger FA, Gugel B, et al: Bone mineral density after kidney transplantation. A cross-sectional study in 190 graft recipients up to 20 years after transplantation, Transplantation 59:982–986, 1995.

297. Julian BA, Laskow DA, Dubovsky J, et al: Rapid loss of vertebral mineral density after renal transplantation, N Engl J Med 325:544–550, 1991.

298. Slatopolsky E, Martin K: Glucocorticoids and renal transplant osteonecrosis, Adv Exp Med Biol 171:353–359, 1984.

299. Parfrey PS, Farge D, Parfrey NA, et al: The decreased incidence of aseptic necrosis in renal transplant recipients—a case control study, Transplantation 41:182–187, 1986.

300. Isono SS, Woolson ST, Schurman DJ: Total joint arthroplasty for steroid-induced osteonecrosis in cardiac transplant patients, Clin Orthop Relat Res (217):201–208, 1987.

301. Enright H, Haake R, Weisdorf D: Avascular necrosis of bone: a common serious complication of allogeneic bone marrow transplantation, Am J Med 89:733–738, 1990.

302. Velasquez-Forero F, Mondragon A, Herrero B, et al: Adynamic bone lesion in renal transplant recipients with normal renal function, Nephrol Dial Transplant 11(suppl 3):58–64, 1996.

303. Sanchez CP, Salusky IB, Kuizon BD, et al: Bone disease in children and adolescents undergoing successful renal transplantation, Kidney Int 53:1358–1364, 1998.

304. Lindberg JS, Culleton B, Wong G, et al: Cinacalcet HCl, an oral calcimimetic agent for the treatment of secondary hyperparathyroidism in hemodialysis and peritoneal dialysis: a randomized, double-blind, multicenter study, J Am Soc Nephrol 16:800–807, 2005.

305. Allen DB, Goldberg BD: Stimulation of collagen synthesis and linear growth by growth hormone in glucocorticoid-treated children, Pediatrics 89:416–421, 1992.

306. Root AW, Bongiovanni AM, Eberlein WR: Studies of the secretion and metabolic effects of human growth hormone in children with glucocorticoid-induced growth retardation, J Pediatr 75:826–832, 1969.

307. Ortoft G, Oxlund H: Qualitative alterations of cortical bone in female rats after long-term administration of growth hormone and glucocorticoid, Bone 18:581–590, 1996.

308. Wehrenberg WB, Bergman PJ, Stagg L, et al: Glucocorticoid inhibition of growth in rats: partial reversal with somatostatin antibodies, Endocrinology 127:2705–2708, 1990.

309. Aubia J, Serrano S, Marinoso L, et al: Osteodystrophy of diabetics in chronic dialysis: a histomorphometric study, Calcif Tissue Int 42:297–301, 1988.

310. Movsowitz C, Epstein S, Fallon M, et al: Cyclosporin-A in vivo produces severe osteopenia in the rat: effect of dose and duration of administration, Endocrinology 123:2571–2577, 1988.

311. Bryer HP, Isserow JA, Armstrong EC, et al: Azathioprine alone is bone sparing and does not alter cyclosporin A-induced osteopenia in the rat, J Bone Miner Res 10:132–138, 1995.

312. Hokken-Koelega AC, van Zaal MA, van Bergen W, et al: Final height and its predictive factors after renal transplantation in childhood, Pediatr Res 36:323–328, 1994.

313. Sarwal MM, Yorgin PD, Alexander S, et al: Promising early outcomes with a novel, complete steroid avoidance immunosuppression protocol in pediatric renal transplantation, Transplantation 72:13–21, 2001.

314. Sarwal MM, Vidhun JR, Alexander SR, et al: Continued superior outcomes with modification and lengthened follow-up of a steroid-avoidance pilot with extended daclizumab induction in pediatric renal transplantation, Transplantation 76:1331–1339, 2003.

315. Fine RN, Yadin O, Nelson PA, et al: Recombinant human growth hormone treatment of children following renal transplantation, Pediatr Nephrol 5:147–151, 1991.

316. Mitsnefes MM, Kimball TR, Witt SA, et al: Abnormal carotid artery structure and function in children and adolescents with successful renal transplantation, Circulation 110:97–101, 2004.

317. Ishitani MB, Milliner DS, Kim DY, et al: Early subclinical coronary artery calcification in young adults who were pediatric kidney transplant recipients, Am J Transplant 5:1689–1693, 2005.

Chapter 15

DISORDERS OF CALCIFICATION:
Osteomalacia and Rickets

MARIE B. DEMAY and STEPHEN M. KRANE

Osteomalacia and rickets are disorders of mineralization. Osteomalacia is a failure to mineralize the newly formed organic matrix (osteoid) of bone. In rickets, a disease of children, the growth plate at the epiphysis is involved in a process that is characterized by delay in the maturation of chondrocytes in the growth plate and disorganization of these chondrocytes, resulting in expansion of the growth plate. While rickets is associated with impaired mineralization of cartilage matrix, hypophosphatemia is thought to play a predominant role in the etiology of rickets.[1] A number of different disorders are associated with osteomalacia in adults and rickets in children.[2-4] The pathogenesis of the mineralization defect, the biochemical alterations, the clinical manifestations, and the therapeutic approaches differ in these conditions, so a systematic approach to the diagnosis and treatment of these disorders is essential.

Mineralization Defect

Mineralization of bone is a complex process in which the calcium-phosphate inorganic mineral phase is deposited in relation to the organic matrix in a highly ordered fashion. Optimal mineralization can take place at bone-forming surfaces only if cellular activity of bone-forming cells is adequate, matrix is normal in composition and is synthesized at a normal rate, the supply of mineral ions (calcium and inorganic phosphate) from the extracellular fluid is sufficient, the pH at sites of mineralization is appropriate (approximately 7.6), and the concentration of inhibitors of calcification is controlled. Structural and regulatory aspects of biological mineralization have been considered in numerous reviews.[5-8] Clinical disorders of mineralization can be attributed to defects at several of these control steps, examples of which are shown in Table 15-1. Overall features of mineralization in normal and abnormal bone remodeling and the relevance to mineralization disorders have been comprehensively reviewed.[4]

The determinants for the deposition of the mineral phase in normally mineralized tissues—cartilage, bone, and teeth—and the precise mechanisms that govern the process of biological mineralization have yet to be elucidated. It is thought that deposition of the initial mineral phase takes place within the collagen fibrils in the gap formed by the packing of the trimeric type I collagen molecules, the most abundant organic component of bone.[7] The earliest calcium-phosphate (Ca-P) mineral phase is thought to be composed of very small apatite crystals, less than 9 nmol in length, that can fit into the channels formed by adjacent gaps.[9] These initial Ca-P crystals appear to form complexes with phosphoproteins of the organic matrix.[10] As the bone and minerals mature, additional Ca-P crystals are deposited between collagen macromolecules. Other proteins that are abundant in mineralized tissues and thought to play a role in mineralization include the sialic acid–rich proteins such as osteopontin and bone sialoprotein (BSP).[11] The ultimate size and shape of the Ca-P crystals are also influenced by anionic electrolytes in the environment.[12]

The major driving force for mineralization is the concentration of inorganic phosphate (Pi), which at normal sites of

Table 15-1. Examples of Disorders with Different Causes of Impaired Mineralization

Disorder	Mechanism
Postoperative hyperparathyroidism	Rate of matrix synthesis exceeds rate of mineralization
Fibrogenesis imperfecta ossium	Defective collagenous matrix
Adult phosphate diabetes	Phosphate concentration deficient at mineralization sites
Vitamin D deficiency	Insufficient calcium and phosphate
Systemic acidosis	pH inadequate for mineralization
Hypophosphatasia	Excess inhibitor (? inorganic pyrophosphate)

mineralization is derived predominantly from the plasma. Therefore, control of Pi reabsorption in the renal tubular lumen is the most important process regulating mineralization. It is also possible that tissue-nonspecific alkaline phosphatase (TNAP), which functions as an inorganic pyrophosphatase localized on the surface of osteoblasts, generates additional Pi to drive mineralization.[13] Osteomalacia is seen in loss-of-function mutations in the *TNAP* gene, but decreased TNAP also results in accumulation of inorganic pyrophosphate (PPi), which acts as a potent inhibitor of mineralization.[13,14] It is likely that this pyrophosphatase function of TNAP is the most critical. PPi is generated by osteoblasts and chondrocytes through the action of two enzymes: the ectonucleoside, pyrophosphatase phosphodiesterase 1 (NNP1/PC-1), which releases PPi from nucleoside triphosphates[13,14] and the transmembrane protein, ANK, which shuttles PPi between intracellular and extracellular compartments.[15,16] Ectopic mineralization due to decreased local concentrations of PPi accompanies spontaneous deficiency of these proteins in humans and mice. In cartilage, there is evidence that matrix vesicles (MVs) formed from chondrocyte plasma membranes play a role in the regulation of mineralization.[5,6] These extracellular MVs are approximately 100 nm in diameter and contain enzymes such as TNAP, NNP1, and Ca-binding proteins as well as Ca-P crystals at the inner surface of the membranes. They are thought to play a role in the initial mineralization of growth plate cartilage matrix by exposing preformed apatite crystals to the extracellular fluid, where further crystal growth can occur. MVs have also been found in bone near sites of mineralization, but it is difficult to assign them a function, since the initial crystallites are deposited in association with collagen fibers in bone. An explanation for the specificity of normal mineralization of bone is provided by the exclusive coexpression in bone of the genes encoding the predominant organic matrix protein, type I collagen, and the enzyme that hydrolyzes the inhibitor, PP$_i$. Furthermore, the protein mineralization inhibitor, matrix GLA protein (MGP), that is expressed in cells in several other tissues is not expressed in bone.[17,18]

The mechanism of defective mineralization is not the same in all disorders associated with osteomalacia and rickets, and biochemical indices such as serum levels of calcium and phosphorus also differ. Moreover, the relative imbalance in matrix synthesis and its mineralization varies depending on the underlying disease mechanism. Estimates from tetracycline labeling indicate that the appositional growth rate in normal bone is about 1 μm/day.[19] It has also been suggested[20] that complete mineralization of the osteoid in normal bone requires approximately 10 to 21 days. Thus the thickness of the osteoid seam normally does not exceed 15 to 20 μm, the surface of bone that is covered by osteoid is normally less than 20%, and the active surface that is covered

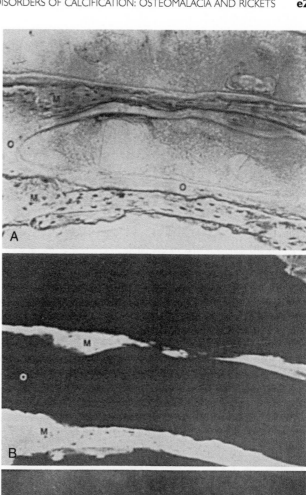

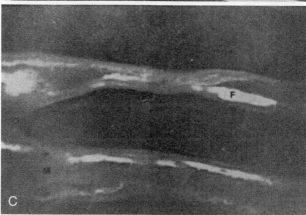

FIGURE 15-1. Undecalcified sections of a bone biopsy from a patient with an adult-onset renal phosphate leak. **A,** Unstained. **B,** Microradiograph. **C,** Ultraviolet photomicrograph demonstrating fluorescence (F) of tetracycline administered 14 days prior to biopsy. Mineralized bone (M) and osteoid (O) are noted. (From Case 1 in Baylink D, Stauffer M, Wergedal J et al: Formation, mineralization, and resorption of bone in vitamin D–deficient rats, J Clin Invest 49:1122–1134, 1970.)

by osteoid is considerably less. The major histologic criteria for the diagnosis of osteomalacia are the increased osteoid surface and the increased thickness of the osteoid seam (Fig. 15-1). The mineralization front at the junction of mineralized bone and osteoid is also abnormal in osteomalacia.[21] In applying kinetic criteria to the diagnosis of osteomalacia, it has been suggested that a mean osteoid seam width greater than 15 μm and a mineralization lag time greater than 100 days are appropriate diagnostic criteria.[22] However, other investigators[23,24] have suggested that more stringent criteria be applied to establish the diagnosis of osteomalacia, based on the observation that reduced mineral

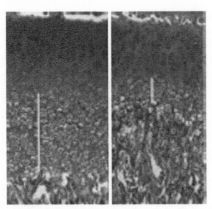

FIGURE 15-2. Histology of the growth plate in a mouse model of renal phosphate wasting *(left)* and control normal mouse *(right)*. The extent of the hypertrophic chondrocyte layer is indicated by the *white bar*.

apposition rate, reduced fractional extent of the mineralization front, and prolongation of the mineralization lag time are indices that reflect impaired matrix synthesis by osteoblasts rather than specific features of osteomalacia. The diagnosis of osteomalacia must include evidence of an absolute increase in the total osteoid volume and an increased number of osteoid lamellae. A detailed consideration of the kinetics of remodeling as specifically applicable to osteomalacia is found in a review by Parfitt.[4]

The architecture of the bone cells and matrix in osteomalacic bone is usually normal. The collagen of the osteoid is largely lamellar, although foci of woven bone are occasionally seen. Hypomineralized periosteocytic lesions have been observed in some affected individuals with hypophosphatemic rickets.[25] The persistence of this defect in patients in whom the abnormality in bone mineralization was corrected with therapy supports the hypothesis that osteocyte function may be abnormal. In contrast, there are clear abnormalities in the cells of the rachitic growth plate. The characteristic changes occur in the maturation zone of hypertrophic chondrocytes, whereas the resting and proliferative zones show normal histologic features (Fig. 15-2). In the maturation zone, the number of cells per column is increased, and the cells are irregularly aligned. This is also accompanied by an increase in the transverse diameter, which may extend beyond the ends of the bone, resulting in characteristic cupping or flaring. In experimental rickets, the water content of the growth plate is increased, and a number of metabolic abnormalities have been observed, including decreased glycogen content and an altered pattern of glycolysis.[26] When bone is examined histologically, it is essential that undemineralized sections be used. In usual practice, however, with classic clinical, radiologic, and biochemical findings, bone biopsy is not necessary to arrive at the diagnosis of osteomalacia. The most commonly biopsied site is the iliac crest; sample size ranges from 5 to 10 mm in diameter and should include both inner and outer cortices. Growth plates from long bones in children are usually not biopsied, although an open-wedge biopsy of growth cartilage of the iliac apophysis may occasionally be obtained without the hazard of altering growth of long bones. Mineralized specimens of bone are most satisfactorily embedded in plastic media—which provide preservation of tissue architecture not usually attained with paraffin-embedding techniques—because the distinction between mineralized and unmineralized bone is lost with decalcification of the specimen. A number of different staining techniques can then be used to demonstrate the osteoid and apply quantitative morphometric analysis.[23-25] In normal bone, the mineralization

front is seen at the junction of the osteoid seam and newly mineralized bone. This region can be identified by an intense fluorescence of tetracycline, deposited in this zone when administered prior to obtaining the biopsy (see Fig. 15-1). In normal persons, the osteoid seam/bone junctions fluoresce intensely; in osteomalacia, the fluorescence is less well defined (more diffuse) or even absent. In addition to impaired matrix mineralization, matrix biosynthesis may be abnormal in osteomalacia. In osteomalacia observed with vitamin D deficiency, a decreased rate of matrix formation is observed.[23,24,27] Osteoblast function may be impaired in many forms of human rickets and osteomalacia, which may result in abnormal matrix formation. Notably, the hydroxylation of certain collagen lysyl residues is increased in vitamin D–deficient bone, as well as in other experimental hypocalcemic states.[28-30]

Clinical Features of Rickets and Osteomalacia

The clinical manifestations of rickets are mainly related to skeletal pain and deformity, slippage of epiphyses, disturbances in growth, and fracture of the osteomalacic bones. Hypocalcemia, when it occurs, may be symptomatic. Depending on the degree of hypophosphatemia, muscular weakness and hypotonia may be prominent features. Dent and Stamp[31] have indicated nine factors that underlie the clinical manifestations of rickets and osteomalacia, modified here as follows:

1. Failure of mineralization affects predominantly those parts of the skeleton in which growth is most rapid.
2. Endochondral bone is more affected than intramembranous bone, possibly because of the more rapid growth of the former.
3. Proximal and distal ends of bones do not grow at the same rate, and rickets affects the most rapidly growing area.
4. Because different bones grow at different rates at different stages of development, the time when rickets is active determines the clinical expression. For example, the skull is growing rapidly at birth, so craniotabes is a manifestation of congenital rickets. During the first year, the upper limbs and rib cage grow rapidly, so abnormalities at these sites are prominent—for example, rachitic rosary. Signs of rickets at the wrist are usually seen at the ulnar side because the growth rate of the distal ulnar epiphysis is greater than that of the distal radial epiphysis.
5. Deformities in mild chronic rickets are most often due to disordered growth at the epiphysial plate rather than to bending at the shafts.
6. In some forms of rickets, the radiologic changes include those of secondary hyperparathyroidism (subperiosteal resorption, most commonly at the metaphyses).
7. Deformities that occur before the age of 4 years correct themselves if the rickets is cured; if rickets persists to a later age, the deformities are permanent (dwarfism, bowleg, and knock-knee).
8. "Late" rickets, which occurs at the time of the pubescent growth spurt, produces dramatic disturbances and results in knock-knee.
9. Adult manifestations of osteomalacia, such as Looser's zones and increased biconcavity of vertebral bodies, are seen in young children only when the rickets is very severe.

In infants and young children, especially in severe, classic rickets, listlessness and irritability are common. In infants, myopathy is characteristic and is manifested by hypotonia. In older children, the weakness may present as a proximal myopathy similar to that observed in the adult. Other findings in infants include parietal flattening or frontal bossing, softening of the calvarium (craniotabes), and widening of the sutures. The thickened growth plates may be evident clinically as the rachitic rosary at the rib ends and may even simulate juvenile rheumatoid arthritis when areas such as the wrists are involved. Indentation of the lower ribs at the site of attachment of the diaphragm is known as *Harrison's groove* or *sulcus*. Pelvic deformities also occur, and the skeleton is more prone to fractures. Pain, when present, is greater at the knees and other weight-bearing joints. Dental eruption may be delayed, and enamel defects are common.

In contrast, osteomalacia in adults may be difficult to detect on clinical grounds alone. Diffuse skeletal pain and muscular weakness may be present. Pain, often prominent about the hips and in association with hypophosphatemic myopathy, may produce a waddling or antalgic gait. Fractures may occur in the ribs and vertebral bodies, as well as in long bones, leading to progressive deformities. Affected individuals may also have localized pain and swelling in one or more joints. Synovial fluid is noninflammatory and free of crystals. Symmetric polyarthralgias resembling those of rheumatoid arthritis or polymyalgia rheumatica may also be observed.[32] Muscular weakness is quite common,[33,34] is primarily proximal in distribution (which contributes to the waddling gait), and is often associated with wasting and hypotonia with preservation of brisk reflexes.[35] This is thought to be a consequence of hypophosphatemia and responds to phosphate repletion.[36] The molecular basis remains elusive, with no difference observed in the relative concentrations of skeletal muscle phosphocreatine, adenosine triphosphate, or inorganic phosphate estimated by phosphorus nuclear magnetic resonance spectroscopy.[37] Although the etiology of the neuromuscular features of osteomalacia is not clearly defined, therapy of the underlying disorder, such as vitamin D in nutritional osteomalacia, alkalinization in acidosis, and phosphate

repletion in hypophosphatemic osteomalacia, results in resolution of these features. The role of hypophosphatemia per se in muscular weakness is discussed in Chapter 6.

Radiologic Features

Radiologic features of rickets and osteomalacia reflect the histopathologic changes. In rickets, the alterations are most evident at the epiphyseal growth plate, which is increased in thickness, cupped, and reveals haziness at the diaphyseal border due to decreased mineralization of the hypertrophic zone and inadequate mineralization of the primary spongiosa (Fig. 15-3). Variation in the pattern of rachitic changes is influenced by differences in the rates of growth of individual bones. The trabecular pattern of the metaphyses is abnormal, the cortices of the diaphyses may be thinned, and bowing of the shafts may be present.

Osteomalacia is due to decreased mineralization and is therefore associated with a decrease in bone density, loss of trabecular patterning, and variable degrees of thinning of the cortices.[38,39] In some patients, radiologic changes are indistinguishable from those seen in osteoporosis. The characteristic finding that specifically suggests osteomalacia is the presence of radiolucent bands known as *pseudofractures*, *Looser's zones*, or *umbauzonen*, ranging from a few millimeters to several centimeters in length and usually oriented perpendicularly to the surface of the bone. (Fig. 15-4). They tend to occur symmetrically and are particularly common at the inner aspects of the femur near the femoral neck, in the pelvis, in the outer edge of the scapula, in the upper fibula, and in the metatarsals.

Pseudofractures are most often seen at sites where major arteries cross the bones. Arteriography in some[36,40,41] but not all cases[42] suggests that the origins of the pseudofractures correspond to the locations of major arteries (Fig. 15-5). Trauma of some sort, whether related to arterial pulsation or other factors (e.g., weight-bearing stress), is likely responsible for the symmetry of the lesions and their predilection for the described sites. Pseudofractures are often multiple, occasionally occurring at 10

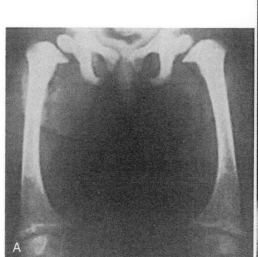
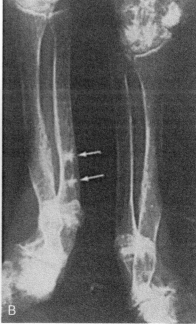

FIGURE 15-3. A, Rickets in a child with Fanconi's syndrome, showing typical cupping of distal femoral epiphyses. **B,** Osteomalacia in an 80-year-old woman who had a history compatible with hypophosphatemic rickets dating to early childhood. Note multiple pseudofractures *(arrows).*

to 15 sites in a single individual; such multiple symmetric pseudofractures in osteomalacic individuals have been referred to as *Milkman's syndrome*.[43-46] The abnormalities in Milkman's original case were also considered by Albright and Reifenstein[43] to be manifestations of osteomalacia. The histopathology of Looser's zones is that of premalacic lamellar bone, some of which is surrounded by lamellar osteoid at the edge of the defect.[47] In addition, there are foci of woven bone, some of which is mineralized and some not. This accounts for the lower radiologic mineral density of the pseudofracture compared with the surrounding bone. Subperiosteal erosions along the diaphyseal cortices extending to the metaphyses may be seen when secondary hyperparathyroidism is present. Widening (or pseudowidening) of the sacroiliac joints and the appearance of hazy margins has also been observed, sometimes suggesting ankylosing spondylitis, which osteomalacia may mimic clinically.[36]

In some patients with osteomalacia, increased rather than decreased radiologic density of bones may be observed.[48] This is seen particularly in patients with renal tubular phosphate leaks, as opposed to vitamin D deficiency (Fig. 15-6). In such patients, there may be a striking degree of thickening of the cortices and trabeculae of the spongy bone, at times associated with exostotic spurs. This hyperostosis has been noted in untreated patients. It is not usually observed in patients with generalized defects in proximal renal tubular reabsorption. Despite the increase in mass of bone per unit volume, microscopically the trabeculae are covered with abnormally thickened osteoid seams typical of osteomalacia. Similar findings may be noted in patients with chronic renal failure. The reason for the hyperostosis is unknown; the bone is still architecturally abnormal and subject to fracture with relatively minimal trauma.

In patients with X-linked hypophosphatemic osteomalacia and rickets, an additional finding has been the presence of a

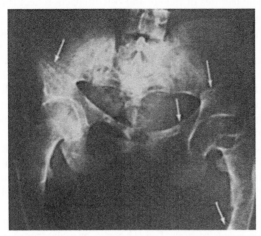

FIGURE 15-4. Radiograph of the pelvis and proximal femora in an adult with renal phosphate wasting. Note pseudofractures, also known as *Looser's zones (arrows)*. (From Case 2 in Jaworski ZFG, Kloswvych S, Cameron E: Proceedings of the First Workshop on Bone Morphometry. Ottawa: University of Ottawa Press, 1973.)

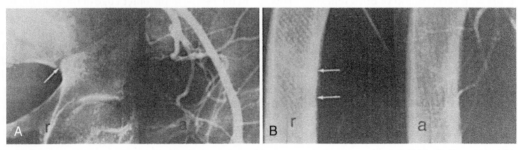

FIGURE 15-5. Radiograph (r) and corresponding arteriograms (a) of a patient with adult-onset renal phosphate wasting. **A,** Pelvis. **B,** Femur. Note that the origin of Looser's zones *(arrows)* corresponds with crossing of major vessels. (From Case 2 in Jaworski ZFG, Kloswvych S, Cameron E: Proceedings of the First Workshop on Bone Morphometry. Ottawa: University of Ottawa Press, 1973.)

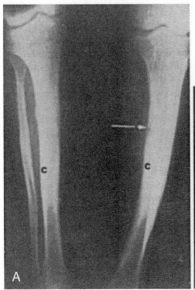

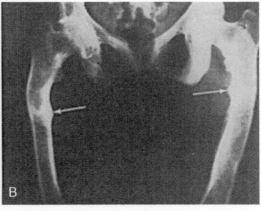

FIGURE 15-6. Increased bone mass in patients with osteomalacia. **A,** Radiographs of femora of a 15-year-old boy with X-linked hypophosphatemia. Note the thick tibial cortex (c) and Looser's zone *(arrow)*. **B,** Radiograph of pelvis and femora of a 38-year-old woman with hypophosphatemia present since childhood. Note Looser's zones *(arrows)*.

Table 15-2. Classification of Rickets and Osteomalacia

I. Nutritional
  A. Vitamin D lack
    1. Dietary deficiency
    2. Deficient endogenous synthesis
      a. Inadequate solar irradiation
      b. Sunscreen
      c. Other factors, e.g., genetic, aging
  B. Calcium lack
    1. Dietary deficiency
II. Gastrointestinal
  A. Intestinal
    1. Small intestine diseases with malabsorption, e.g., celiac disease (gluten-sensitive enteropathy)
    2. Partial or total gastrectomy
    3. Intestinal bypass
  B. Hepatobiliary
    1. Cirrhosis
    2. Biliary fistula
    3. Biliary atresia
  C. Pancreatic
    1. Chronic pancreatic insufficiency
III. Disorders of vitamin D metabolism
  A. Hereditary
    1. Isolated 25-hydroxyvitamin D deficiency
    2. Pseudo–vitamin D–deficiency rickets
    3. Hereditary vitamin D–resistant rickets
  B. Acquired
    1. Hypoparathyroidism
    2. Anticonvulsants
    3. Renal insufficiency (see below)
IV. Acidosis
  A. Distal renal tubular acidosis (classic or type I)
    1. Primary (specific cause not determined)
      a. Sporadic
      b. Familial
    2. Secondary
      a. Galactosemia (after galactose ingestion)
      b. Hereditary fructose intolerance with nephrocalcinosis (after chronic fructose ingestion)
      c. Fabry's disease
    3. Hypergammaglobulinemic states
    4. Medullary sponge kidney
    5. Following renal transplantation
  B. Acquired
    1. Ureterosigmoidostomy
    2. Drug-induced
      a. Chronic acetazolamide administration
      b. Chronic ammonium chloride administration
V. Chronic renal failure

VI. Phosphate depletion
  A. Dietary
    1. Low phosphate intake
    2. Aluminum hydroxide ingestion (or other nonabsorbable hydroxides)
  B. Impaired renal tubular phosphate reabsorption (intestinal)
    1. Hereditary
      a. X-linked hypophosphatemic rickets (vitamin D–resistant rickets)—dominant inheritance
      b. Adult-onset vitamin D–resistant hypophosphatemic osteomalacia—dominant inheritance
    2. Acquired
      a. Sporadic hypophosphatemic osteomalacia (phosphate diabetes)
      b. Tumor-associated rickets and osteomalacia (includes neurofibromatosis and fibrous dysplasia)
VII. General renal tubular disorders (Fanconi's syndrome)
  A. Primary renal
    1. Idiopathic
      a. Sporadic
      b. Familial
    2. Associated with systemic metabolic process
      a. Cystinosis
      b. Glycogenesis
      c. Lowe's syndrome
  B. Systemic disorder with associated renal disease (prerenal)
    1. Hereditary
      a. Inborn errors
        i. Wilson's disease
        ii. Tyrosinemia
      b. Neurofibromatosis
    2. Acquired
      a. Multiple myeloma
      b. Nephrotic syndrome
      c. Transplanted kidney
    3. Intoxications
      a. Heavy metals
        i. Cadmium
        ii. Lead
      b. Drugs
        i. Outdated tetracycline
VIII. Primary mineralization defects
  A. Hereditary
    1. Hypophosphatasia
IX. States of rapid bone formation with or without a relative defect in bone resorption
  A. Postoperative hyperparathyroidism with osteitis fibrosa cystica
  B. Osteopetrosis
X. Defective matrix synthesis
  A. Fibrogenesis imperfecta ossium
XI. Miscellaneous
  A. Aluminum intoxication
    1. Chronic renal failure
    2. Total parenteral nutrition

generalized involvement of the entheses, with exuberant calcification (more likely ossification) of tendon and ligament insertions.[49,50] The absence of inflammatory cells, as well as other clinical features, differentiates this disorder from degenerative joint disease and the seronegative spondyloarthropathies. A comprehensive classification of rickets and osteomalacia is shown in Table 15-2. A detailed discussion of all these conditions is not included here.

Nutritional Osteomalacia and Rickets

In 17th century Scotland and England, the association of poverty and malnutrition with the occurrence of infantile rickets was vividly documented. The widespread prevalence of infantile rickets in the industrialized regions of Britain was further docu-mented in reports from Glasgow in the late 1800s and early 1900s. The link between rickets, dietary deficiency of vitamin D, and correction of vitamin D deficiency by solar radiation was finally established in 1923 by the work of the Vienna Council. Following this discovery, fortification of certain foods with vitamin D reduced the incidence of nutritional rickets in Europe and the United States to negligible levels, and by the 1940s, vitamin D deficiency was no longer regarded as an important cause of osteomalacia and rickets.[43] Vitamin D metabolism and the role of specific metabolites in bone development, mineralization, and remodeling are discussed elsewhere (see Chapter 3). Nevertheless, the role of vitamin D in the prevention of osteomalacia and rickets is relevant to the discussion in this chapter.

Studies in Glasgow[51-53] and London[54] documented the reappearance of nutritional osteomalacia and rickets as a public health problem in the United Kingdom. Since the 1950s, the population at risk primarily involves East Asian immigrants whose unique dietary and social customs have led to the development of osteomalacia and rickets.[52,54-58] Other groups at risk include housebound and elderly subjects and food faddists, especially those on vegetarian or fat-free diets.[52,54-58] An unexpectedly high prevalence of osteomalacia was also observed in elderly women with rheumatoid arthritis who were housebound and had poor nutritional status.[59]

Gastrointestinal and Hepatic Diseases

Another population at risk for development of nutritional osteomalacia are morbidly obese individuals[60] and those who have undergone intestinal bypass surgery for treatment of severe obesity.[61-63] In one bypass surgery series, iliac bone biopsies revealed the presence of osteomalacia in nearly a third of 21 patients studied.[63] Treatment with vitamin D_2 (36,000 IU/day), as well as supplemental calcium (27 mmol/day), was required to promote a more positive calcium balance in some individuals.[61] An increased frequency of osteomalacia also was observed in patients after gastrectomy,[64-66] the severity of the mineralization defect being positively correlated with serum 25-hydroxyvitamin D [25(OH)D] but not with serum 1,25-dihydroxyvitamin D [1,25(OH)$_2$D].

Malabsorption associated with diseases of the small intestine, hepatobiliary tree, and pancreas is the most common cause of severe vitamin D deficiency in the United States. Disorders of the small intestine causing malabsorption of vitamin D and resultant osteomalacia include celiac disease or sprue, regional enteritis, scleroderma, multiple jejunal diverticula, and blind-loop syndrome. Impaired absorption of calcium in association with, or as a consequence of, vitamin D malabsorption contributes to the development of osteomalacia.

Rickets occurs in infants and children with cholestatic liver disease.[67] Children with biliary atresia develop biliary cirrhosis, jaundice, and ascites. Intestinal absorption of vitamin D is markedly impaired, and serum values are low. Bone disease has been attributed to vitamin D deficiency, and pharmacologic doses of 1,25(OH)$_2$D$_3$ are required for treatment of the bone disease.[68]

Low-birthweight infants are at risk for rickets, with the reported incidence ranging from 13% to 32%. Insufficient intake of calcium, phosphorus, and vitamin D have been implicated. The condition should be detected early, since prompt nutritional supplementation is required.[69] Infants of vitamin D–deficient mothers are at greatest risk for neonatal rickets,[70] which can be averted by maternal vitamin D supplementation during pregnancy. Special consideration should be given to screening for vitamin D deficiency during pregnancy in women whose social and dietary history reveal inadequate sun exposure and food sources of vitamin D. Infants who are entirely breastfed and have inadequate exposure to sunlight are also at risk for rickets, because the amount of vitamin D and 25(OH)D in human milk is inadequate.[71]

Vitamin D sources include dietary supplementation with ergocalciferol (vitamin D_2), an irradiation product obtained from plants, and cholecalciferol (vitamin D_3), produced in human skin by the action of ultraviolet light on the physiologic precursor, 7-dehydrocholesterol. Because most foods (with the exception of fatty fish) contain only small amounts of vitamin D_3, individuals must rely on either adequate sunlight exposure or dietary supplements to avoid vitamin D deficiency. There is marked seasonal

variation in plasma 25(OH)D, independent of age and sex.[72-74] These variations parallel changes in duration and intensity of sun exposure, with higher values in late summer months in the northern hemisphere. Plasma 25(OH)D is almost twice as high in American women of Caucasian descent than in those of African descent during winter months, and the increment during summer months is also greater.[75] Plasma 25(OH)D and parathyroid hormone (PTH) are inversely correlated, implying that the changes in circulating 25(OH)D are metabolically significant.[76] In a study of patients who were hospitalized in a general medical ward, plasma 25(OH)D was low in over half of the subjects, consistent with a high prevalence of vitamin D deficiency.[77] Thus, adequate vitamin D supplementation is essential when exposure to sunlight is marginal.

Vitamin D requirements are greater in the elderly than in young adults. This difference is attributed to an age-related decline in dermal production of 7-dehydrocholesterol, the precursor for vitamin D_3,[78] diminished renal production of 1,25(OH)$_2$D,[79] and diminished intestinal absorption of calcium caused by lower levels of the vitamin D receptor in the intestine.[80] Other contributing factors include previous gastric surgery and occult malabsorption in addition to altered vitamin D metabolism. To determine optimal plasma 25(OH)D and how much vitamin D is required to achieve optimal values, Vieth,[81] in an exhaustive review, and Heaney in another[82] concluded that total daily intake and production of vitamin D of 2.5 to 5.0 mg (100 to 200 IU) and plasma 25(OH)D values greater than 20 to 25 nmol/L are sufficient to prevent clinical rickets or osteomalacia. Higher intakes or production of vitamin D would be necessary, however, to prevent secondary hyperparathyroidism, bone loss, and subclinical osteomalacia. Therefore, it may be necessary to maintain serum 25(OH)D levels of 100 nmol/L or greater to avoid bone loss, subclinical osteomalacia, and osteoporosis. The amount of vitamin D supplementation necessary to attain these levels varies widely, based on dietary factors and solar exposure.

In the East Asian immigrant populations of Britain, rickets and osteomalacia secondary to vitamin D deficiency are seen most commonly in neonates, infants, and adolescents during pubertal growth and less frequently among adults.[51,83-85] Multiple factors have been implicated in the development of bone disease, including insufficient intake of calcium and vitamin D, skin pigmentation,[86] which attenuates ultraviolet transmission through the epidermis, genetic factors,[87-89] and social customs, such as avoidance of sun exposure and consumption of chapati, a dietary staple flatbread high in phytate, which binds calcium in the gut and interferes with its absorption.[90] Furthermore, studies in rats demonstrated that the rate of inactivation of vitamin D in the liver was increased by a calcium-restricted diet.

Studies by Dent and colleagues[91] strongly suggest that insufficient sunlight exposure plays a pivotal role in the development of nutritional rickets and osteomalacia, in addition to the rickets and osteomalacia observed in patients on long-term anticonvulsant therapy.[92] In two carefully studied individuals, they demonstrated healing of rickets and positive calcium balance following therapy with ultraviolet light, despite a vitamin D–deficient, high-phytate diet. Substitution of a low-phytate diet did not affect the plasma biochemical abnormalities or the calcium balance.[91]

Scriver[93] divides the evolution of vitamin D deficiency in infancy into three stages. In stage 1, serum calcium tends to be low, serum phosphorus normal, and aminoaciduria absent. Without treatment, stage 2 develops, and aminoaciduria and hypophosphatemia appear as a consequence of diminished tubular reabsorption. In this stage, serum calcium tends to return to normal, and serum alkaline phosphatase increases, presumably related to the increased PTH and resultant increase in bone turnover. Renal tubular dysfunction (aminoaciduria, phosphaturia) has, at least in part, been attributed to the increased PTH.[94,95] Stage 3 is characterized by the return of hypocalcemia. The effect of lowered concentrations of serum phosphorus in stage 2 and lowered concentrations of serum calcium and serum phosphorus in stage 3 presumably account for development of the mineralization defect.

Rao et al.[96] reviewed the histomorphometric findings in a series of 65 patients with vitamin D depletion diagnosed on the basis of plasma levels of 25(OH)D less than 10 ng/mL. They found that in early vitamin D depletion, the effects on bone are manifested principally by the occurrence of secondary hyperparathyroidism. With increasing severity or duration of the vitamin D deficiency, the mineralization process becomes progressively impaired, bone formation rates decline, and osteoid surface and thickness increase.

In summary, rickets and osteomalacia are being recognized with increasing frequency in selected populations. Serum 1,25(OH)$_2$D is not a reliable indicator of vitamin D nutrition, since values may be normal in individuals with vitamin D deficiency.[97,98] The availability of serum 25(OH)D assays has also permitted detection of those at risk, prior to the development of overt clinical disease.

Acidosis and Osteomalacia

Acidosis resulting from a number of different causes has been associated with osteomalacia. The mechanism of bone loss and the mineralization defects are complex and not completely understood. Albright and Reifenstein[43] originally suggested that acidosis produces slow dissolution of the mineral phase of bone in an attempt to buffer retained hydrogen ion. This process is associated with hypercalciuria. Support for this suggestion has been obtained in studies of patients with renal tubular acidosis in whom retention of hydrogen ion is greater than that theoretically required to produce the observed decrease in plasma bicarbonate concentrations.[99] On the basis of measurements in normal subjects in whom metabolic acidosis is induced, it has been proposed that excess retained hydrogen ion is balanced by bone buffering and loss of bone calcium in the urine.[100-102] Since the hypercalciuria and increased bone resorption that accompany most acidotic states do not directly result in osteomalacia, other mechanisms must be invoked to explain the occurrence of clinically significant skeletal mineralization defects. Osteoclasts function optimally at a pH of approximately 6.9 and are inactive at a pH greater than 7.3; therefore, it is probable that the calcium release from bone induced by acidosis can be ascribed to increased osteoclast activity rather than to simple physicochemical buffering.[103] Chronic acidosis activates vacuolar hydrogen ion pumps in isolated osteoclasts and stimulates osteoclastic bone resorption.[104] In addition, activation of the voltage-gated H$^+$ channel through protein kinase C in osteoclasts can sense changes in pH.[105]

In parallel, metabolic acidosis inhibits the function of osteoblasts: in osteoblast culture systems, lowering pH to 6.9 decreases formation of mineralized nodules.[106] Acidosis increases expression of osteoblastic RANK-L via a cyclooxygenase-dependent mechanism, leading to enhanced osteoclastogenesis.[107] Another potential proton-sensing mechanism in the osteoblast is G protein–coupled receptors OGR1 and OGR2.[108] OGR1 is inactive at pH 7.8 and fully activated at pH 6.8, signals through the phosphoinositol pathway, and is expressed in osteosarcoma lines and primary osteoblasts. OGR2 signals through the cyclic adenosine monophosphate (cAMP) pathway but has not yet been shown to be expressed in bone cells. Maintenance of pH within a critical range is thus essential for bone-cell function and for mineralization to proceed normally.

Acidosis can also affect phosphate metabolism by altering renal tubular handling of the anion. In patients with chronic acidosis, treatment with alkali to correct the acidosis can normalize serum phosphate by increasing renal tubular phosphate reabsorption and phosphate maximal tubular excretory capacity.[109,110] Secondary hyperparathyroidism may be another factor involved in the altered phosphate handling in systemic acidosis,[109] and acidosis can impair intestinal calcium absorption in response to exogenous vitamin D,[106] as well as activation of 25(OH)D.[111] Rickets and osteomalacia secondary to acidosis are most frequently a complication of inherited distal renal tubular acidosis (RTA).[112] Clinical manifestations vary widely in type as well as severity. Autosomal-dominant as well as autosomal-recessive forms have been described. As a rule, the dominant form is usually recognized in adults who present with relatively mild disease characterized by nephrolithiasis and acidosis. Osteomalacia occurs infrequently. In contrast, the autosomal-recessive form is recognized in infancy or early childhood, is usually severe, and rickets is common. In dominant RTA, the causal mutation is in the *SLC4A1:AE1* gene that encodes the heterotopic Cl$^-$/HCO$_3^-$ exchanger located in the α-intercalated cells of the distal tubules. In recessive RTA, the causal mutations are in the B1 or A4 subunits of the H$^+$/ATPase encoded by *ATP6V1B1* and *ATP6V0A4* genes, respectively. Rarely, mutations in the *SLC4A1:AE1* gene occur in recessive RTA as well. In most of the cases described in early reports,[113-115] healing of the bone disease resulted from correction of the acidosis with sodium bicarbonate alone (5 to 10 g/day). Nevertheless, healing is slow, and the response may be hastened by the addition of vitamin D or 1,25(OH)$_2$D$_3$. Occasionally, vitamin D toxicity can develop unexpectedly, so patients must be monitored carefully. Although chronic treatment with vitamin D is not necessary once the osteomalacia is cured, continued use of vitamin D may be required to complete healing in those individuals in whom the glomerular filtration rate is low.[115,116]

Another form of inherited mixed distal/proximal RTA is associated with osteopetrosis and cerebral calcifications. The osteopetrosis, due to inadequate osteoclast function secondary to defects in acidification in the extracellular space adjacent to the ruffled border, is caused by mutations in the gene that encodes carbonic anhydrase II (CAII).[117-119] This RTA is characterized by defective urinary acidification and bicarbonate wasting, and the syndrome is explained by the fact that CAII is expressed not only in osteoclasts but in both proximal and distal segments of the nephron. It is of interest that bone marrow transplantation does not affect the acidosis but reverses the osteopetrosis (by radiologic and histologic criteria), since osteoclasts are of hematopoietic origin.[120]

In several of the syndromes associated with more widespread renal tubular reabsorptive defects, systemic acidosis may contribute to the pathogenesis of osteomalacia. Some of these are inherited, such as various forms of Fanconi's syndrome and Lowe's syndrome (oculocerebrorenal syndrome). Some patients with renal tubular phosphate leaks may also have mild acidosis.[121-125]

Other aspects of these syndromes are considered elsewhere in this chapter.

Osteomalacia may also be a complication of the acidosis produced by ureterosigmoidostomy, a procedure formerly used in the treatment of patients with carcinoma of the bladder. Reabsorption of chloride and hydrogen ions from urine in the colon is responsible for the acidosis. Keeping the rectosigmoid empty by frequent drainage corrects the acidosis and thus prevents the development of osteomalacia. Typical osteomalacia has also been observed in a patient with acidosis presumably resulting from chronic acetazolamide therapy. This patient was receiving phenobarbital, as well as phenytoin, for a severe seizure disorder, but when the acetazolamide alone was discontinued and the plasma bicarbonate increased, radiologic and clinical healing of osteomalacia was observed. Acetazolamide has direct inhibitory effects on bone resorption in animals independent of pH, and carbonic anhydrase inhibitors do prevent bone loss in humans.[126,127]

Dietary Phosphate Depletion

In humans, phosphate depletion and resultant hypophosphatemia may lead to the development of rickets or osteomalacia by mechanisms that were discussed earlier. It is difficult to produce selective deficiency of phosphorus by dietary means alone, because most foods contain this element in concentrations that are sufficient to prevent hypophosphatemia and bone disease (see Chapter 6). However, hypophosphatemia has been reported in patients who ingest large quantities of nonabsorbable antacids, usually as a form of self-medication for dyspepsia.[128-132] This is accompanied by a marked increase in fecal phosphorus content, presumably related to binding of dietary phosphate by the antacid, resulting in a complex that is poorly absorbed from the gastrointestinal tract. In addition to the changes in phosphorus handling, these individuals also develop hypercalciuria. Most of the affected individuals show no evidence of increased bone resorption, although a small increase in osteoclastic surface and number of osteoclasts has been reported in one patient studied.[133] It is more likely that the rise in urinary calcium excretion is related primarily to impaired bone mineralization, a concept that is supported by the association of this syndrome with osteomalacia. Elevated levels of serum $1,25(OH)_2D$ are observed in patients with antacid-induced osteomalacia, a normal response to hypophosphatemia. Clinically significant bone disease is rare, suggesting that an ample supply of dietary phosphorus compensates for the absorptive defect. A similar syndrome of phosphate depletion has been described in patients with renal failure receiving large quantities of aluminum hydroxide gel, but osteomalacia in these patients may be related to aluminum intoxication and/or renal insufficiency.

Hypophosphatemia has also been observed in both chronic and acute alcoholism (see Chapter 6).[134,135] Bone densitometric studies and tetracycline-labeled bone biopsies obtained from chronic alcoholic patients have revealed an increased frequency of bone disease compared to sex- and race-matched controls.[136] Bone abnormalities include changes consistent with mixtures of osteoporosis, osteomalacia, and osteitis fibrosa. Multiple factors, including hypomagnesemia, metabolic alkalosis or acidosis, and renal tubular phosphate wasting contribute to the hypophosphatemia and bone disease.[137] Bone disease in alcoholism may be part of the generalized skeletal disorder associated with chronic liver disease of diverse origin, which has been termed *hepatic*

osteodystrophy.[137] The syndrome comprises osteomalacia, osteitis fibrosa, osteoporosis, and periosteal new bone formation in the presence of chronic liver disease. Osteomalacia is most common in patients with cholestasis (particularly primary biliary cirrhosis) but is also observed in patients with alcoholic liver disease and other forms of cirrhosis. In most patients, the serum levels of 25(OH)D are low, ascribable to impaired intestinal absorption of vitamin D, but reduced exposure to ultraviolet light and reduced dietary intake also contribute.[138] Treatment with vitamin D metabolites can heal hepatic osteomalacia.

Dietary Calcium Deficiency

Nutritional rickets caused by calcium deficiency was first reported in 1978 by Pettifor and co-workers,[139] who described findings in nine rural South African children. Although they had spent extensive time outdoors, the children showed obvious clinical features of rickets, including progressive bone deformities, decreased growth, and typical radiographic changes. Four of the children had hypocalcemia, and all of them had normal serum 25(OH)D values but increased serum alkaline phosphatase and serum $1,25(OH)_2D$ values. Calcium-balance studies showed that calcium absorption was not impaired. The biochemical and radiographic changes of rickets were entirely corrected by treatment with calcium alone.

In a prospective, randomized, double-blind study of 123 Nigerian children with nutritional rickets, Thacher et al.[140] compared treatment with calcium alone, vitamin D alone, and the combination of calcium and vitamin D together. Treatment with calcium alone or calcium and vitamin D together was more effective than treatment with vitamin D alone. Baseline calcium intake was similar in patients and in a control group. It was concluded that although calcium deficiency was an important contributor to nutritional rickets, other unidentified factors might have been involved. Calcium deficiency is also prevalent in North American children and can contribute to nutritional rickets. Review of the records of 43 infants and toddlers who presented with rickets in New Haven, Connecticut (86% of whom were of African, Hispanic, or Middle Eastern descent and more than 93% of whom had been breastfed), revealed serum 25(OH)D levels less than 15 ng/mL in only 22%. However, 86% of those with a food history had been weaned to diets with minimal calcium content.[141]

Impaired Renal Tubular Phosphate Reabsorption

In 1937, Albright and co-workers[142] reported their studies of a 16-year-old boy with longstanding rickets in whom standard doses of vitamin D failed to produce clinical improvement. Healing of the bone disease eventually occurred, but only after administration of extremely high doses of vitamin D. The results of their studies led to the introduction of the concept of "vitamin D resistance" in certain types of rickets. Since this initial report, so-called vitamin D–resistant rickets has been classified into several clinical and biochemical subtypes, the most common of which is the X-linked, dominantly inherited form discussed in detail in Chapter 11. Affected individuals usually present with clinical and radiographic evidence of rickets within the second or third year of life. The cardinal biochemical disturbance is hypophosphatemia due to renal phosphate wasting, associated with elevated levels of fibroblast growth factor (FGF-23).[143] Other causes of osteomalacia (see Table 15-2) must be excluded, particularly primary vitamin D deficiency, malabsorption, renal insufficiency, generalized renal tubular disorders, and the presence of certain mesenchymal tumors.

The mode of presentation of patients with adult hypophosphatemic osteomalacia or *phosphate diabetes*, as it has occasionally been termed, is characteristic. In contrast to individuals with the X-linked form, patients with the sporadic disease often develop prominent myopathy similar to that seen in other forms of rickets or osteomalacia. Deformities of the limbs are usually absent (possibly indicating normophosphatemia during the growth period), but these patients experience severe bone pain related to vertebral body collapse or femoral neck fractures. As in other forms of osteomalacia, radiographs commonly reveal extensive pseudofractures. Some subjects may also have isolated renal hyperglycinuria and occasionally renal glycosuria in addition to the hypophosphatemia. Generalized aminoaciduria or acidification defects are not seen in these individuals. Evaluation of patients with possible adult-onset hypophosphatemic osteomalacia should include general tests of renal function (creatinine clearance, acidification, concentrating ability, and analysis of urinary amino acid excretion), evaluation for malabsorption, and a search for the presence of occult tumors.

A positional cloning approach was utilized by a consortium of investigators to identify the gene for X-linked hypophosphatemia.[144] The gene was structurally similar to a group of membrane-bound metalloendopeptidases and was termed *PEX*, but renamed *PHEX* to avoid confusion with other genes. Several inactivating mutations have been shown in the *PHEX* genes of patients with X-linked hypophosphatemia as well as in the murine *Phex* gene in the Hyp mouse.[145-148] It is still not clear how the mutations in the *PHEX* gene account for the excessive renal tubular phosphate losses, but it has been suggested that *PHEX* might function to directly or indirectly degrade FGF-23 or regulate its expression.

Another disorder with isolated renal tubular phosphate wasting and inappropriately normal plasma 1,25(OH)$_2$D levels has been termed *autosomal-dominant hypophosphatemic rickets* (ADHR). In contrast to X-linked hypophosphatemia, ADHR displays variable and incomplete penetrance, as well as other clinical manifestations.[149-151] Positional cloning was used to identify FGF-23 as the abnormal gene associated with ADHR.[152] In individuals with ADHR, mutations in FGF-23 that are localized to a subtilisin-like proprotein convertase cleavage site lead to elevated levels of FGF-23, which results in increased renal phosphate clearance.

A mutation in the phosphate transporter SLC34A3 (NptIIc) is the genetic basis for hereditary hypophosphatemic rickets with hypercalciuria (HHRH). This disorder is due to hypophosphatemia secondary to renal phosphate wasting and presents with rickets, muscle weakness and bone pain. Hypercalciuria, secondary to increased 1,25(OH)$_2$D (which leads to increased intestinal calcium absorption), distinguishes it from other forms of hypophosphatemic rickets.[153]

In patients with X-linked hypophosphatemia, serum levels of 25(OH)D are normal, whereas the levels of 1,25(OH)$_2$D are in the low-normal range, inappropriately low for the level of serum phosphorus. Treatment of affected patients with 1,25(OH)$_2$D$_3$ and oral phosphate (1 to 2 g/day phosphorus equivalent) results in healing of rickets and osteomalacia; however, hypercalcemia and hypercalciuria may complicate therapy.[154,155] Of note is that heterozygous girls appear to respond better to therapy than

hemizygous boys.[156] A variety of neutral phosphate salts are available for oral supplementation, including sodium and potassium salts or mixtures of the two. Greater elevations in serum phosphorus levels are observed with the potassium salt, likely related to the effects of the sodium ion on increasing renal phosphate clearance.[157] The precise amount of phosphate must be individualized for each patient. In individuals with severe renal phosphate leaks, as much as 1000 mg of elemental phosphorus is required every 4 to 6 hours to effect sustained elevations of serum phosphorus levels. The rise in serum phosphorus level after a single oral dose of phosphate is transient, so phosphate supplements must be administered at frequent intervals. The efficacy of therapy cannot be assessed with a single fasting determination of serum phosphate; multiple measurements of serum levels at various times after each dose are required. Emptying the capsules and dissolving the salt in water or other liquid may improve intestinal absorption and enhance serum phosphorus levels. Most patients experience some degree of gastrointestinal distress, such as cramps and diarrhea, when therapy is initiated; therefore, initial doses should be low and increments gradually introduced as tolerated. Simultaneous use of phosphate and vitamin D has resulted in accelerated healing in children with the X-linked form of hypophosphatemic osteomalacia.[158] Vitamin D itself or various analogues have a "phosphate-sparing" effect, allowing the use of lower doses of oral phosphate supplements. Whether the improved serum phosphorus levels seen with vitamin D or 1,25(OH)$_2$D$_3$ are accounted for by increased intestinal absorption of phosphate or decreased renal loss (due to decreased secondary hyperparathyroidism) has not been established. After fusion of the growth plates, patients are no longer at risk for rickets or growth retardation, raising the question as to whether treatment should be continued in affected adults. Healing of osteomalacia with therapy has been documented in adults, but close monitoring is required to avert the potential development of parathyroid hyperplasia and hypercalcemia resulting in nephrocalcinosis and renal insufficiency.[159,160]

Tumor-Associated Rickets and Osteomalacia

In 1959, Prader et al. described the case of an 11-year-old girl who, over the course of a year, developed severe symptomatic rickets accompanied by hypophosphatemia, increased renal phosphate clearance, and mild hypocalcemia.[161] The child was found to have a large tumor in the left chest that on biopsy was interpreted as a reparative giant cell granuloma of a rib. Following excision of the tumor, the rickets healed without any specific therapy. It was postulated that the giant cell reparative granuloma may have produced a "rachitogenic substance."

Since that time, numerous patients have been described in whom osteomalacia has been associated with the presence of various types of tumor. One review[162] reported that of 72 tumors, 40 were localized to bone and 31 to soft tissues; two-thirds of the tumors occurred in the extremities. More than a third of the tumors were classified as vascular tumors, and half of these were hemangiopericytomas. Other common pathologic diagnoses were nonossifying fibromas and mesenchymal and giant cell tumors. All of the tumors exhibited prominent vascularity, multinucleated giant cells, and primitive stromal cells. Ten of the tumors were classified as malignant. Whereas most neoplasms associated with this syndrome have been exclusively of mesenchymal origin, two cases of hypophosphatemic osteomalacia associated with prostate carcinoma have been reported.[163] As in other forms of tumor-associated osteomalacia, serum 1,25(OH)$_2$D levels were low. In most of the reported cases, the removal of the tumor results in clinical cure of the osteomalacia or rickets, but the size of the tumors is usually small, and in several instances, the tumor is not detected until years after development of clinical osteomalacia.[164] Recurrence of the tumor or inadequate removal of the malignancy may prevent a complete clinical response. In a patient with hypophosphatemia due to a malignant giant cell sarcoma, resection of the tumor resulted in a clinical remission that lasted 4 years, at which time hypophosphatemia recurred, associated with the reappearance of pulmonary metastases.

Patients with tumor-induced osteomalacia exhibit hypophosphatemia, high renal phosphate clearance, and normal serum calcium levels. Serum immunoreactive PTH levels have been variable, but low or undetectable levels of serum 1,25(OH)$_2$D are observed because these tumors release products that impair renal 1α-hydroxylation of 25(OH)D and phosphate transport, including FGF-23, the serum level of which normalizes after tumor resection.[143] Oncogenic osteomalacia tumors have also been shown to express FGF-23 mRNA and/or protein,[152,165,166] as well as other phosphaturic factors, including complementary DNAs (cDNAs) encoding dentin matrix protein 1, secreted frizzled-related protein 4 (sFRP-4) and matrix extracellular phosphoglycoprotein (MEPE). Studies have shown that sFRP-4 decreases sodium-dependent phosphate transport in kidney cells, and infusion of sFRP-4 into mice produces renal phosphate excretion.[167] These results suggest that other factors in addition to FGF-23 may participate in the pathogenesis of oncogenic osteomalacia.

Dent and Gertner[168] also described three patients with fibrous dysplasia who had concomitant hypophosphatemic osteomalacia or rickets. Two of the patients were adults with polyostotic fibrous dysplasia; the third was an 8-year-old with fibrous dysplasia of the facial bones and rickets. In the child, resection of most of the dysplastic bone was accompanied by improvement in the metabolic bone disease. The immunoreactive PTH levels were not elevated, leading the authors to postulate that the hypophosphatemia and resultant osteomalacia in patients with fibrous dysplasia was analogous to other forms of oncogenic osteomalacia. Subsequent investigations revealed that dysplastic tissue produced FGF-23, implicating this hormone in the pathogenesis of the renal phosphate leak.[169]

General Renal Tubular Disorders

Another subset of patients with rickets or osteomalacia of renal origin are classified under the general heading of de Toni-Debré-Fanconi syndrome, renal Fanconi's syndrome, or type II RTA. Characteristic findings are a generalized dysfunction of the proximal renal tubules, with excessive loss of amino acids, glucose, phosphate, uric acid, and bicarbonate in the absence of abnormal glomerular function. This results in systemic acidosis, hypophosphatemia, and dehydration, which leads to growth disturbance, rickets, or osteomalacia. The abnormal gene(s) causing autosomal-dominant renal Fanconi's syndrome has not been identified. However, genetic and physical mapping studies have identified a locus at chromosome 15q15.3.[170]

The disorders with features of Fanconi's syndrome may be further classified into primary renal abnormalities, in which the

underlying defect is located within the renal tubular cells, and prerenal disorders, in which toxic metabolic substances from outside the kidney lead to derangements in tubular function (see Table 15-2). These disorders occur in adults as well as children.

Distal or type I RTA is caused by impaired secretion of hydrogen ions from the distal nephron, with resultant metabolic acidosis, nephrocalcinosis, hypokalemia, rickets, and osteomalacia. Autosomal-dominant distal RTA is caused by mutations in the SLC4A1 gene that encodes the polytopic chloride-bicarbonate exchanger AE1, which is normally expressed in red cells and at the basolateral surface of α-intercalated cells in the distal nephron.[171-173] Ovalocytosis may occur. Autosomal-recessive distal RTA is caused by mutations in the ATP6VB1 and ATP6V0A4 genes that encode the B1 and A4 subunits of the collecting duct apical proton pump, vacuolar H$^+$/ATPase, and may be associated with progressive bilateral sensorineural hearing loss.[174] An additional locus at chromosome 7q33-34 was found in patients with distal RTA and no hearing loss.[112]

Dent's disease is an X-linked renal tubular disorder characterized by low-molecular-weight proteinuria, hypercalciuria, nephrocalcinosis, nephrolithiasis, rickets, and renal failure and may include other features of Fanconi's syndrome.[31] The disease results from mutations of the X-linked CLCN5 gene that encodes a 746-amino-acid protein chloride channel with 12 to 13 transmembrane domains.[175,176] Patients usually present at age 40 with signs and symptoms of hypokalemia and osteomalacia. Healing of the bone disease has occurred by treatment with vitamin D, alkali, and potassium. Sporadic idiopathic Fanconi's syndrome may also present with muscle weakness and bone pain attributable to osteomalacia.[177]

In cystinosis (Lignac-de Toni-Fanconi syndrome),[178] Fanconi-Bickel syndrome,[177,179] and Lowe's syndrome,[180] the renal disease is associated with a more generalized systemic metabolic disorder. In Wilson's disease, tyrosinemia,[181] and the other inborn errors of metabolism outlined in Table 15-2, Fanconi's syndrome may accompany the generalized systemic disease and lead to the development of bone disease.

Nephropathic cystinosis is an autosomal-recessive lysosomal storage disease characterized by renal failure by 10 years of age and other complications, including Fanconi's syndrome. The disease is caused by mutation of the CTNS gene that encodes a 367-amino-acid protein with seven transmembrane domains that is thought to transport cystine out of lysosomes.[182-184] In cystinosis, accumulation of cystine occurs in many tissues, including the kidneys, resulting in tubular dysfunction and later in glomerular failure. Recent experience with renal transplantation in patients with cystinosis has shown reaccumulation of cystine in the transplanted kidney without the reappearance of Fanconi's syndrome, suggesting that a primary renal tubular cell defect might exist in these patients, or alternatively, that cystine deposition has different effects on the developing and mature kidney.[185]

Fanconi-Bickel syndrome is an autosomal-recessive disorder of carbohydrate metabolism characterized by hepatorenal glycogen accumulation, Fanconi nephropathy, impaired utilization of glucose and galactose, and rickets. The disorder results from mutations of the GLUT2 gene that encodes a glucose transporter that is present in plasma membrane of pancreatic islet β cells, hepatocytes, and absorptive epithelial cells in intestine and kidney.[179]

Lowe's syndrome is a rare X-linked disorder that involves the eyes, kidney, and nervous system and is manifested by congenital cataracts, mental retardation, and renal tubular dysfunction.[180]

The disorder results from mutations of the *OCRL* gene that encodes the OCRL-1 protein, a phosphatidylinositol 4,5-bisphosphonate 5-phosphatase localized in the Golgi apparatus.[186,187] Studies with kidney proximal tubules indicate that *OCRL* might function in membrane trafficking by regulating a specific pool of phosphatidylinositol-4,5-bisphosphonate that is associated with lysosomes, since it accumulates in the mutant kidney cells.[188]

Wilson's disease is an autosomal-recessive disease caused by mutations in the *ATP7B* gene encoding a copper-transporting P-type ATPase that localizes to the trans-Golgi network of hepatocytes and is required to move copper into the secretory pathway, where the metal is incorporated into ceruloplasmin and excreted into bile.[189,190] Clinical and pathologic manifestations in Wilson's disease are attributed to the toxic effects of excessive accumulation of copper in liver, kidney, brain, and cornea. Most patients present with signs and symptoms secondary to liver disease, hemolytic anemia, or neurologic disease. Fanconi's syndrome, renal dysfunction, and associated rickets and osteomalacia may predominate or be the presenting feature. Although the bone disease responds to vitamin D supplementation, renal tubular dysfunction persists, including aminoaciduria, glucosuria, uricosuria, hypercalciuria, and RTA.[191] The presence of hypercalciuria and the frequent occurrence of nephrolithiasis are consistent with studies demonstrating that the defect in acidification is related to a distal rather than a proximal tubular defect.[192] Treatment of Wilson's disease with D-penicillamine significantly improves the renal tubular acidification defect,[193] whereas healing of the bone disease requires oral vitamin D supplements.

Hereditary tyrosinemia type I is an autosomal recessive disease caused by mutations in the fumarylacetoacetate hydrolase (*FAH*) gene that encodes an enzyme involved in the last step of tyrosine degradation.[194] Tyrosine accumulates in the kidney, peripheral nerves, and liver, leading to the development of cirrhosis and hepatoma.

The development of Fanconi's syndrome in plasma cell myeloma has been attributed to the toxic effects of Bence Jones protein on the proximal renal tubule.[195] Although extremely rare, osteomalacia may develop as a consequence of the renal phosphate wasting and hypophosphatemia. Osteomalacia associated with RTA has also been reported in a patient with Sjögren's syndrome with increased urinary β2-microglobulin and retinol-binding protein.[196] The patient showed clinical improvement after treatment with oral potassium citrate, calcium supplements, and glucocorticoids.

Fanconi's syndrome and osteomalacia occur in patients with heavy-metal poisoning, particularly cadmium[197] and lead,[198] as well as in patients who have been exposed to outdated tetracycline.[199] The bone disease is attributed to hypophosphatemia and systemic acidosis produced by impaired tubular function.

Hypophosphatasia

Hypophosphatasia is a heritable disorder characterized by deficiency in the tissue-nonspecific (bone/liver/kidney) isoenzyme of alkaline phosphatase (TNSALP), increased urinary excretion of phosphorylethanolamine, and skeletal disease that includes osteomalacia and rickets.[200-203] The disease may present in infancy with hypercalcemia, renal failure, and increased intracranial pressure. Skeletal features include enlarged sutures in the skull, craniostenosis, delayed dentition, enlarged epiphyses, and prominent costochondral junctions. Genu valgum or varum may develop. The histologic picture is indistinguishable from that of other forms of rickets. Disease that presents in infancy may be fatal. Bone marrow transplants have been performed for life-threatening disease.[204,205]

When hypophosphatasia presents in older children, it is less severe and may present as rickets alone. In this group, serum calcium and phosphorus levels are usually normal. In the infantile forms, the disorder is inherited as an autosomal-recessive trait. The disorder in the adult, however, is probably distinct from the infantile and childhood forms and is inherited as an autosomal-dominant trait with variable penetrance. In adults, even though osteopenia may be seen, the disorder tends to be mild, and osteomalacia is not always the most prominent finding. By definition, in hypophosphatasia, enzymatic activity of TNSALP in blood and tissues is reduced. TNSALP has broad substrate activity, thus in patients with hypophosphatasia, phosphorylated molecules such as phosphorylethanolamine and phosphorylcholine are excreted in excessive amounts in the urine, and circulating levels of pyridoxal-5′-phosphate, another TNSALP substrate, are markedly elevated.[206-209] Serum phosphorus levels are usually normal, and it is not clear how the biochemical findings are related to the inadequate skeletal mineralization. TNSALP, tethered through a glycophosphoinositol moiety to the osteoblast cell surface, generates inorganic phosphate (Pi) locally by cleaving various substrates even at neutral pH. One such substrate is inorganic pyrophosphate (PPi), and TNSALP is a pyrophosphatase that can generate additional Pi from PPi to drive mineralization.[13] PPi, however, is also a potent inhibitor of mineralization, and it is likely that this pyrophosphatase function of TNALP is the most critical.[13,14] It is probable that the concentrations of PPi are too high to allow normal mineralization at sites of bone formation.[210,211]

Since the alkaline phosphatase cDNA was cloned, it has been possible to study the defects in the *TNSALP* gene in patients with hypophosphatasia. Characterization of the patterns of clinical expression with the specific mutation in humans has provided insight into the molecular basis for the high degree of phenotypic heterogeneity in this disorder. The results indicate that the extreme heterogeneity in phenotype among patients with hypophosphatasia is due to residual enzyme activity in some individuals.[127,212]

Hyperparathyroidism, Hypoparathyroidism, and Pseudohypoparathyroidism

In individuals with primary hyperparathyroidism who have excessive bone resorption and high rates of bone formation, thick osteoid seams may be seen. This may present clinically as hungry bone syndrome following surgical cure of the hyperparathyroidism. It is associated with histologic changes in bone.[43] However, frank vitamin D deficiency and osteomalacia may coexist with primary hyperparathyroidism, as well as with hypophosphatemic rickets and osteomalacia.

Hypoparathyroidism is a rare cause of osteomalacia.[213,214] The bone disease is attributed to a decrease in formation of 1,25(OH)2D and hypocalcemia, both a consequence of lack of PTH; thus, appropriate therapy of hypoparathyroidism should prevent the mineralization defect. Osteomalacia occurs infrequently in pseudohypoparathyroidism, owing to decreased 1,25(OH)2D, a consequence of impaired renal response to PTH-induced formation of cAMP as well as hypocalcemia.[215,216]

Osteopetrosis

Rickets also may occur in the severe (recessive) form of osteopetrosis.[217] Affected children may have low levels of serum phosphorus and calcium and increased alkaline phosphatase activity.[218] In addition to rickets, decreased osteoclastic resorption and abnormal-appearing osteoclasts are observed.[219] This disorder is heterogeneous, and several different cellular or biochemical defects may lead to similar clinical manifestations. It is not clear why abnormal matrix mineralization should occur in these patients. One possible explanation is a decreased local supply of mineral ions, secondary to decreased resorption in the face of relatively high rates of bone formation. Absence of the isoenzyme II of carbonic anhydrase leads to autosomal-recessive osteopetrosis with RTA and cerebral calcification.[117] Reduced levels of isoenzyme II were also detected in obligate heterozygotes. A consanguineous kindred with a similar presentation was found to have a mutation in two genes, thus manifesting two separate disorders: osteopetrosis due to mutation of the osteoclast vacuolar H$^+$/ATPase (*TCIRG1*) and mutation of the B1 subunit of the renal H$^+$/ATPase (*ATP6V1B1*).[220]

Fibrogenesis Imperfecta Ossium

Described in men over age 50, fibrogenesis imperfecta ossium is a rare disorder characterized by progressively disabling skeletal pain and tenderness, forced immobilization, muscular weakness, atrophy, and contractures.[221] Levels of calcium and phosphorus in the serum are normal, but alkaline phosphatase activity is increased. The radiographic abnormalities include thickened and amorphous-appearing trabeculae with spotty increases in density, reduced cortical thicknesses, and occasional pseudofractures. The abnormal "fishnet" trabecular pattern seen on conventional radiographs, combined with MR imaging of low signal intensity bone marrow on T1- and T2-weighted images, is helpful in diagnosis.[222] Histologically, there is an increase in thickness of "osteoid," which occurs diffusely on bone surfaces. Its appearance is distinctive in that this osteoid lacks the lamellar structure and typical birefringence that is characteristic of the other osteomalacic states. Electron microscopic studies reveal immature, small-diameter collagen fibers that are arranged in loops, as well as dense areas that have been termed *whorls*.[223] A study of bone from a single patient with fibrogenesis imperfecta ossium has revealed that the collagen was more soluble in neutral salt and dilute acetic acid, suggesting defective cross-linking.[224] However, direct evidence for defective cross-linking or the chemical nature of the putative defect has not been obtained. Of interest are observations that among the 17 cases of fibrogenesis imperfecta ossium reported by 1996, 5 had associated monoclonal gammopathy.[225] Melphalan and calcitriol were ineffective therapy.

Renal Osteodystrophy and Aluminum Intoxication

Renal osteodystrophy comprises a heterogeneous group of skeletal disorders associated with chronic kidney disease. Prior to the introduction of hemodialysis for the therapy of chronic renal failure, the major accompanying skeletal disorder was a high turnover state, ascribable to secondary hyperparathyroidism.[226]

Bone formation rates were very high, and the bone surfaces covered by osteoid were also increased.

Following the introduction of hemodialysis for treatment of chronic renal failure and the widespread use of aluminum-containing gels as phosphate binders, two patterns of osteomalacia were described (see also Chapter 14). The first (type I) was associated with high-turnover bone disease, and the second (type II) was associated with "adynamic" bone disease. In osteomalacia type I, there were increased osteoid seams, accompanied by low circulating calcium and phosphorus levels. In osteomalacia type II, the osteoid seams were thinner, and there was often a dramatic reduction in tetracycline-labeled double surfaces, reflecting a low mineralization rate.[227-230] In contrast to patients with osteomalacia type I, patients with osteomalacia type II tended to have normal or slightly elevated circulating concentrations of calcium and phosphorus and clinically manifested a high frequency of skeletal pain and fractures.

The presence of true osteomalacia (type I) with high turnover was ascribed to factors such as accompanying acidosis and functional vitamin D deficiency with low circulating levels of 1,25(OH)$_2$D.[226] It has now been conclusively demonstrated that although 1,25(OH)$_2$D can modulate bone cell function, the skeletal consequences of vitamin D deficiency and even the absence of vitamin D receptors in receptor-null mice can be reversed by maintaining sufficient extracellular concentrations of calcium and phosphate.[231,232] Therefore, in chronic kidney disease where serum levels of phosphate are usually high and calcium levels only slightly reduced or normal, it is difficult to ascribe mineralization defects to vitamin D deficiency alone. Circulating mineralization inhibitors—for example, inorganic pyrophosphate and others not identified—may have a role. In the past, most cases of osteomalacia type II described in patients with chronic renal failure were associated with aluminum deposition in bone at osteoid-bone interfaces. Aluminum was also implicated as a factor in pathogenesis of a significant proportion of cases of mixed uremic osteodystrophy (type I) and even some cases of predominantly hyperparathyroid bone disease.[229,233] Early observations suggested that deposition of aluminum at the calcification front interfered with the mineralization process per se and impaired osteoblast proliferation and function.[234] Alternatively, these observations could reflect deposition of aluminum in pre-existing osteomalacic bone without direct effects on the mineralization process. Notable in this respect, in vitamin D–deficient dogs fed aluminum chloride, aluminum is deposited at the osteoid-bone interface of the osteomalacic bone[235]; however, the continued administration of aluminum did not impair healing of osteomalacia with vitamin D repletion.

In the past, more than two-thirds of patients on maintenance dialysis had stainable aluminum in bone. Currently, with better control of aluminum content of dialysates and replacing aluminum-based phosphate binders with calcium salts or sevelamer hydrochloride (a nonabsorbed metal-free, calcium-free phosphate binder),[236-238] fewer than 10% of patients have stainable aluminum in bone.

Heritable Disorders of Vitamin D Metabolism

Rickets or osteomalacia can be caused by gene mutations of enzymes responsible for 25-hydroxylation of vitamin D, for 1α-hydroxylation of 25(OH)D, or mutations of the vitamin D receptor (see Chapter 11). Isolated deficiency of 25(OH)D is a rare autosomal-recessive disorder with rickets caused by impaired hepatic production of 25(OH)D. It is attributed to deficiency of the 25(OH)D-hydroxylase, the enzyme that modulates conversion of vitamin D to 25(OH)D.[239-241] The disease is characterized by a low serum 25(OH)D, a normal serum $1,25(OH)_2D$, hypocalcemia, increases in serum alkaline phosphatase, secondary hyperparathyroidism, and early onset of rickets that responds to physiologic doses of $1\alpha(OH)D_3$ or pharmacologic doses of vitamin D; the condition relapses when treatment is discontinued. Recently, the CYP2R1 gene that encodes a hepatic microsomal vitamin D-25-hydroxylase that hydroxylates both vitamin D_2 and vitamin D_3 was cloned and sequenced. A homozygous L99P inactivating mutation of the CYP2R1 gene was the cause of the deficiency of 25(OH)D and rickets in a Nigerian boy with the disorder.[242] These findings provide evidence that CYP2R1 is a key vitamin D 25-hydroxylase.

Pseudo–vitamin D–deficiency rickets is an autosomal recessive disorder caused by impaired renal production of $1,25(OH)_2D$. The disease is caused by mutations of the CYP27B1 gene that encodes the 25(OH)D 1α-hydroxylase, the mitochondrial enzyme responsible for conversion of 25(OH)D to $1,25(OH)_2D$.[243-245] Affected individuals are apparently normal at birth and develop the clinical and biochemical changes of rickets during the first year of life. Hypocalcemia, hypophosphatemia, and elevated serum immunoreactive PTH and alkaline phosphatase are consistent findings. The diagnosis is made by demonstration of a normal serum 25(OH)D and low or undetectable serum $1,25(OH)_2D$ in a patient with rickets who responds to physiologic doses of $1,25(OH)_2D_3$.

Hereditary vitamin D–resistant rickets is a rare autosomal disorder characterized by resistance of target organs to $1,25(OH)_2D$.[246] The disease is caused by mutations of the vitamin D receptor (VDR) gene.[247] Onset of symptoms can occur at any age from infancy to adolescence, and occurrence is usually familial. Patients have hypocalcemia, hypophosphatemia, elevation of serum alkaline phosphatase and immunoreactive PTH, normal or increased serum 25(OH)D, and marked elevation of serum $1,25(OH)_2D$. The disorder is transmitted as an autosomal-recessive trait and often results from consanguineous parentage. Patients may also develop alopecia. Because the pathophysiologic abnormality underlying this disorder is a receptor defect, no treatment has been uniformly successful. Therapeutic responses to pharmacologic doses of vitamin D metabolites and oral calcium supplements vary. Although 1α-hydroxylated metabolites have been the favored treatment, the high levels of circulating $1,25(OH)_2D$ demonstrate that formation of this metabolite is not impaired and suggest that treatment with vitamin D or 25(OH)D would be effective. In some severely affected individuals, hypocalcemia persists, as do the rachitic and osteomalacic lesions. Because the main physiologic effect of $1,25(OH)_2D$ is thought to be the promotion of intestinal calcium absorption, treatment with parenteral calcium infusions, circumventing the intestinal resistance to $1,25(OH)_2D$, can normalize the biochemical abnormalities and lead to clinical and radiologic remission of the osteomalacic lesions.[248]

Treatment

There is growing evidence that the recommended daily intake (RDI) by the Institute of Medicine's Food and Nutrition Board for 200 IU of vitamin D in young adults is inadequate. The American Academy of Pediatrics has suggested an RDI of 400 IU/day for children 0 to 18 years of age. Similarly, the definition of vitamin D deficiency is unclear: the value for the lower limit of the normal range for serum 25(OH)D has never been established on a scientific basis. Assigned reference values were determined in subjects, based on the fact that they did not have overt rickets or osteomalacia.[82] Three degrees of hypovitaminosis D bone disease have been defined.[4] Stage 1 is characterized by decreased intestinal absorption of calcium resulting in osteoporosis without histologic skeletal changes; stage 2 by decreased calcium absorption, osteoporosis, and early histologic features of osteomalacia and no clinical or laboratory features of osteomalacia; and stage 3 by clinical and histologic osteomalacia. Currently, recommended doses of vitamin D prevent changes found in stages 2 and 3 but not those found in stage 1.

Vitamin D deficiency leads to impaired intestinal calcium absorption, secondary hyperparathyroidism, and bone loss. A number of studies indicate that the change in PTH secretion occurs at a value of approximately 80 nmol/L for serum 25(OH)D. Further, increasing the serum 25(OH)D from approximately 50 nmol/L to 80 nmol/L, values that are well within the normal range, increases calcium absorption by nearly two-thirds[249] and reduces the risk of osteoporotic fracture by one-third.[250] Importantly, in a large cohort of subjects in the Second National Health and Nutrition Examination Survey (NHANES II),[251] bone mineral density of the hip varied directly with serum 25(OH)D values throughout the normal range. This was notable in both pre- and postmenopausal women of Caucasian, Hispanic, and African descent. For these reasons, it is apparent that the current RDI for vitamin D is not adequate for accrual of peak bone mass. These results have profound implications for defining the optimal RDI for vitamin D. A study in normal men by Heaney et al.,[252] the first to attempt to define optimal requirements, indicated that daily requirement of vitamin D from all sources during winter months (supplement, food, tissue stores) is on the order of approximately 3800 IU (95 µg). In other studies,[81] administration of a dose of vitamin D of 4000 IU (100 µg) per day was not associated with abnormal increases in serum 25(OH)D, serum calcium, or urinary calcium in any of the normal subjects; however, calcium intake was not factored in. A comprehensive review of the literature showed that hypercalcemia did not occur when extended doses of vitamin D as high as 10,000 IU (250 µg) per day were administered. The need for higher intake of vitamin D is also supported by the inverse relationship that exists between sun exposure and a number of cancers, including colon, prostate, and breast.[253,254] These findings should be kept in mind while considering the recommended doses of vitamin D and its analogues for treatment of patients with osteomalacia and rickets outlined later. The goals for treatment of patients with osteomalacia or rickets are to correct hypocalcemia if it exists, to reverse skeletal deformities and secondary hyperparathyroidism, and to prevent vitamin D intoxication which may lead to hypercalcemia, hypercalciuria, nephrocalcinosis, and nephrolithiasis.

Vitamin D, $1,25(OH)_2D_3$ and 1α-hydroxyvitamin D_2 [$1\alpha(OH)D_2$] are available in the United States, and $1\alpha(OH)D_3$ is available in a number of other countries. The requirements vary from patient to patient, so the dose must be tailored for a given individual. Vitamin D is marketed in 50,000 IU (1.25 mg) capsules of vitamin D_2 for oral administration and in propylene glycol (250 IU or 6.25 µg per drop) for oral administration. The advantages of vitamin D are its low cost and the endogenous regulation of activation to $1,25(OH)_2D$. The disadvantages of its use are that an optimal therapeutic response may take several weeks, and in cases of toxicity, its biological activity persists for several weeks after it is discontinued, because it is stored in fat and has a long half-life.

$1,25(OH)_2D_3$ is available in 0.25 μg and 0.50 μg capsules and in oral and intravenous preparations containing 1 μg/mL. The advantages of calcitriol are its rapid onset and offset of action. The half-life of the drug is less than 6 hours.[255] One disadvantage is that hypercalcemia may occur even long after an apparently optimal dose has been used.[256] Since the occurrence of hypercalcemia during treatment with $1,25(OH)_2D_3$ cannot be predicted, patients must be monitored closely. $1\alpha(OH)D_2$ is approved for use in the treatment of secondary hyperparathyroidism in patients with kidney failure.[257] It is marketed in 2.5 μg capsules and 1-mL solutions containing 2 μg/mL. After administration, it undergoes conversion to $1,25(OH)_2D_2$.[258]

In children with nutritional rickets caused by calcium deficiency, increasing the calcium intake to between 800 and 1500 mg/day was shown to heal the bone disease.[139,259] Several protocols are recommended for treatment of vitamin D–deficient bone disease; however, most of these have reversal of rickets and osteomalacia as an end point. They do not have as a goal the achievement of 25(OH)D levels that are "optimal" for bone mass accrual and fracture prevention. A trial with small daily oral doses of vitamin D, 50 μg (2000 IU), for 3 to 4 weeks is suggested because a clear biochemical response occurs in classic rickets and osteomalacia resulting from simple vitamin D deficiency. However, based on the study of Heaney et al.,[252] this intake is insufficient to maintain normal levels of vitamin D in healthy men. Furthermore, this dose is insufficient to treat the metabolic forms of rickets that are associated with renal insufficiency, malabsorption, and various hereditary and acquired forms of vitamin D resistance or dependency. Current recommendations include treatment with 50,000 to 500,000 IU over 1 to 3 months, followed by maintenance doses of 400 IU to 1200 IU/day, to achieve a normal circulating 25(OH)D level. Patients on chronic anticonvulsant therapy may require higher maintenance doses.[260] Unlike adults in whom the effects of anticonvulsant drugs in producing osteomalacia may be self-limited, children may require persistent therapy because long-term anticonvulsant therapy has a greater effect on the skeleton of growing children than that of adults. Osteomalacia can also be corrected with relatively low doses of 1α-hydroxylated metabolites.[261] However, these more potent analogues should be reserved for patients with more pronounced forms of calcium malabsorption or with impaired 1α-hydroxylation. Administration of vitamin D to patients with vitamin D–deficiency rickets or osteomalacia invariably results in healing of the bone disease, although the patterns of response, particularly with regard to changes in serum calcium, phosphorus, alkaline phosphatase, and immunoreactive PTH, show marked variation. There may be an initial increase in serum alkaline phosphatase, indicative of healing of the osteomalacic lesions, followed by a gradual fall in both alkaline phosphatase and immunoreactive PTH.

$1,25(OH)_2D_3$ is often most useful in treatment of diseases in which renal synthesis of the metabolite is diminished or impaired (hypoparathyroidism, pseudohypoparathyroidism, renal insufficiency, vitamin D–dependent rickets type I, tumor-induced osteomalacia, hypophosphatemic rickets) or there is resistance to its effects at the cellular level. Sometimes osteomalacia or rickets associated with hereditary vitamin D–resistant rickets responds to treatment with vitamin D.[246] However, in instances of a more profound resistance, $1,25(OH)_2D_3$ may be beneficial. Doses as high as 15 to 20 μg per day are sometimes required

and even so may not be effective. Under these circumstances, long-term parenteral administration of calcium can be used to heal the bone disease.[248]

Hypercalcemia and hypercalciuria are potential complications of treatment with vitamin D.[262,263] Hypercalcemia resulting from vitamin D intoxication is caused by a combination of increased intestinal absorption of calcium and increased osteoclastic bone resorption. Impairment in kidney function may develop and lead to nephrocalcinosis, nephrolithiasis, and even death.[263] Patients may be asymptomatic or have anorexia, nausea, vomiting, weight loss, headache, constipation, polyuria, polydipsia, and altered mental status. Treatment with intravenous fluids is sometimes effective, but elevated serum 25(OH)D and serum calcium values may persist. In addition to hydration, glucocorticoids may be effective in lowering serum calcium levels, and additional benefit may be obtained by impairing osteoclastic bone resorption with intravenous bisphosphonates. Patients on long-term treatment with vitamin D should be carefully followed with measurement of serum and urinary calcium and serum creatinine. This is critical, since there is no way of predicting when or in whom vitamin D intoxication will develop and/or recur.

Treatment of hypophosphatemia, not associated with vitamin D deficiency, involves oral supplementation with neutral phosphate salts, including sodium or potassium salts. Greater elevations in serum phosphorus values have been reported in individuals receiving the potassium salt.[36] The less favorable results with the sodium salt are most likely related to the effects of the sodium ion on increasing renal phosphate clearance. The rise in serum phosphorus after a single oral dose of phosphate is transient,[157] so phosphate supplements must be administered at frequent intervals. The precise amount of phosphate must be individualized for each patient and is a reflection of the degree of renal loss. In individuals with severe leaks, as much as 1000 mg of elemental phosphorus is required every 4 to 6 hours to effect sustained elevations of serum phosphorus values. Optimal treatment of tumor-induced osteomalacia requires removal of the tumor.

The efficacy of therapy cannot be assessed with a single fasting determination of serum phosphorus; multiple measurements of serum values at various times after each dose are required. Emptying the capsules and dissolving the salt in water or other liquid may improve intestinal absorption. When therapy is initiated, most patients experience some degree of gastrointestinal distress, including cramps and diarrhea. Therefore, initial doses should be low, and increments should be gradually introduced as tolerated. Simultaneous use of phosphate and vitamin D metabolites accelerated healing in children with the X-linked form of hypophosphatemic osteomalacia.[159] Whether the improved serum phosphorus values that are seen with vitamin D or $1,25(OH)_2D_3$ are accounted for by increased intestinal absorption of phosphate or decreased renal loss due to reductions in PTH has not been established. However, the use of a calcimimetics to decrease PTH secretion has been used as adjuvant treatment for hereditary and acquired hypophosphatemia associated with impaired tubular reabsorption.[264,265]

In the various types of pre-renal Fanconi's syndrome, the specific treatment of the underlying disorder often results in disappearance or improvement in the renal tubular dysfunction, thus allowing healing of the associated bone disease. In several of the above disorders, improvement in the bone disease can also be achieved by correcting the acidosis and hypophosphatemia (i.e., supplementation with alkali, oral phosphate, and vitamin D).

Hypophosphatasia presents a treatment challenge. Unless there is deficiency of vitamin D, treatment with vitamin D metabolites and calcium is contraindicated, since serum calcium, phosphorus, 25(OH)D, and 1,25(OH)$_2$D are usually normal,[205] and such treatment may exaggerate any tendency to develop hypercalcemia and hypercalciuria. Bone marrow transplantation has been reported to improve the bone disease in the infantile form.[205] Similarly, in osteomalacia associated with osteopetrosis, the most effective treatment is bone marrow or stem cell transplant to provide normally functioning osteoclasts.[266]

REFERENCES

1. Sabbagh Y, Carpenter TO, Demay MB: Hypophosphatemia leads to rickets by impairing caspase-mediated apoptosis of hypertrophic chondrocytes, Proc Natl Acad Sci U S A 102:9637–9642, 2005.
2. Hutchison FN, Bell NH: Osteomalacia and rickets, Semin Nephrol 12:127–145, 1992.
3. Mankin HJ: Rickets, osteomalacia, and renal osteodystrophy. Part II, J Bone Joint Surg Am 56:352–386, 1974.
4. Parfitt AM: Osteomalacia and related disorders. In Avioli LV, Krane SM, editors: Metabolic Bone Disease, San Diego, 1998, Academic Press, pp 328–386.
5. Anderson HC: Matrix vesicles and calcification, Curr Rheumatol Rep 5:222–226, 2003.
6. Boskey AL: Mineral analysis provides insights into the mechanism of biomineralization, Calcif Tissue Int 72:533–536, 2003.
7. Glimcher M: The nature of the mineral phase in bone: biological and clinical implications. In Metabolic Bone Disease, San Diego, 1998, Academic Press, pp 23–50.
8. Slavkin H, Price P: Chemistry and Biology of Mineralized Tissues, Amsterdam, 1992, Excerpta Medica.
9. Tong W, Glimcher MJ, Katz JL, et al: Size and shape of mineralites in young bovine bone measured by atomic force microscopy, Calcif Tissue Int 72:592–598, 2003.
10. Wu Y, Ackerman JL, Strawich ES, et al: Phosphate ions in bone: identification of a calcium-organic phosphate complex by 31P solid-state NMR spectroscopy at early stages of mineralization, Calcif Tissue Int 72:610–626, 2003.
11. Qin C, Brunn JC, Jones J, et al: A comparative study of sialic acid-rich proteins in rat bone and dentin, Eur J Oral Sci 109:133–141, 2001.
12. Eanes ED, Hailer AW: Anionic effects on the size and shape of apatite crystals grown from physiological solutions, Calcif Tissue Int 66:449–455, 2000.
13. Hessle L, Johnson KA, Anderson HC, et al: Tissue-nonspecific alkaline phosphatase and plasma cell membrane glycoprotein-1 are central antagonistic regulators of bone mineralization, Proc Natl Acad Sci U S A 99:9445–9449, 2002.
14. Timms AE, Zhang Y, Russell RG, et al: Genetic studies of disorders of calcium crystal deposition, Rheumatology (Oxford) 41:725–729, 2002.
15. Ho AM, Johnson MD, Kingsley DM: Role of the mouse ank gene in control of tissue calcification and arthritis, Science 289:265–270, 2000.
16. Pendleton A, Johnson MD, Hughes A, et al: Mutations in ANKH cause chondrocalcinosis, Am J Hum Genet 71:933–940, 2002.
17. Murshed M, Harmey D, Millan JL, et al: Unique coexpression in osteoblasts of broadly expressed genes accounts for the spatial restriction of ECM mineralization to bone, Genes Dev 19:1093–1104, 2005.
18. Murshed M, Schinke T, McKee MD, et al: Extracellular matrix mineralization is regulated locally; different roles of two GLA-containing proteins, J Cell Biol 165:625–630, 2004.
19. Lee WR: Bone formation in Paget's disease. A quantitative microscopic study using tetracycline markers, J Bone Joint Surg Br 49:146–153, 1967.
20. Frost HM: Tetracycline-based histological analysis of bone remodeling, Calcif Tissue Res 3:211–237, 1969.
21. Bordier P, Tun Chot S: Quantitative histology of metabolic bone disease, Clin Endocrinol Metab 1:197–215, 1972.
22. Rao DS, Villanueva A, Mathews M: Histological evolution of vitamin D-depletion in patients with intestinal malabsorption or dietary deficiency. In Frame B, Potts JJ, editors: Clinical Disorders of Bone and Mineral Metabolism, Amsterdam, 1983, Excerpta Medica, pp 224–226.

23. Boyce BF, Smith L, Fogelman I, et al: Focal osteomalacia due to low-dose diphosphonate therapy in Paget's disease, Lancet 1:821–824, 1984.
24. Frame B, Parfitt AM: Osteomalacia: current concepts, Ann Intern Med 89:966–982, 1978.
25. Marie PJ, Glorieux FH: Relation between hypomineralized periosteocytic lesions and bone mineralization in vitamin D-resistant rickets, Calcif Tissue Int 35:443–448, 1983.
26. Howell DS: Histologic observations and biochemical composition of rachitic cartilage with special reference to mucopolysaccharides, Arthritis Rheum 8:337–354, 1965.
27. Baylink D, Stauffer M, Wergedal J, et al: Formation, mineralization, and resorption of bone in vitamin D-deficient rats, J Clin Invest 49:1122–1134, 1970.
28. Barnes MJ, Constable BJ, Morton LF, et al: Bone collagen metabolism in vitamin D deficiency, Biochem J 132:113–115, 1973.
29. Barnes MJ, Constable BJ, Morton LF, et al: The influence of dietary calcium deficiency and parathyroidectomy on bone collagen structure, Biochim Biophys Acta 328:373–382, 1973.
30. Toole BP, Kang AH, Trelstad RL, et al: Collagen heterogeneity within different growth regions of long bones of rachitic and non-rachitic chicks, Biochem J 127:715–720, 1972.
31. Dent CE: Rickets (and osteomalacia), nutritional and metabolic (1919–69), Proc R Soc Med 63:401–408, 1970.
32. Reginato AJ, Falasca GF, Pappu R, et al: Musculoskeletal manifestations of osteomalacia: report of 26 cases and literature review, Semin Arthritis Rheum 28:287–304, 1999.
33. Prineas JW, Mason AS, Henson RA: Myopathy in metabolic bone disease, Br Med J 1:1034–1036, 1965.
34. Smith R, Stern G: Myopathy, osteomalacia and hyperparathyroidism, Brain 90:593–602, 1967.
35. Schott GD, Wills MR: Muscle weakness in osteomalacia, Lancet 1:626–629, 1976.
36. Nagant de Deuxchaisnes C, Krane SM: The treatment of adult phosphate diabetes and Fanconi syndrome with neutral sodium phosphate, Am J Med 43:508–543, 1967.
37. Smith R, Newman RJ, Radda GK, et al: Hypophosphataemic osteomalacia and myopathy: studies with nuclear magnetic resonance spectroscopy, Clin Sci (Lond) 67:505–509, 1984.
38. Dent CE, Stamp TC: Vitamin D, rickets and osteomalacia. In Avioli LV, Krane SM, editors: Metabolic Bone Disease, New York, 1977, Academic Press.
39. Krane SM, Parsons V, Kunin AS: Studies of the metabolism of epiphyseal cartilage. In Basset C, editor: Cartilage Degradation and Repair, Washington DC, 1967, National Research Council, p 43.
40. Le May M, Blunt JW Jr: A factor determining the location of pseudofractures in osteomalacia, J Clin Invest 28:521–525, 1949.
41. Steinbach HL, Kolb FO, Gilfillan R: A mechanism of the production of pseudofractures in osteomalacia (Milkman's syndrome), Radiology 62:388–395, 1954.
42. Jackson WP, Dowdle E, Linder GC: Vitamin-D-resistant osteomalacia, Br Med J 1:1269–1274, 1958.
43. Albright F, Reifenstein EJ: Parathyroid Glands and Metabolic Bone Disease. Baltimore, 1948, The Williams and Wilkins Company.
44. de Seze S, Lichtwitz A, Ryckewaert A, et al: The Looser-Milkman syndrome. Study of 60 cases, Sem Hop 38:2005–2025, 1962.
45. Milkman L: Pseudofractures (hungry osteopathy, late rickets, osteomalacia): Report of a case, Am J Roentgenol 24:29–37, 1930.

46. Milkman L: Multiple spontaneous idiopathic symmetrical fractures, Am J Roentgenol 32:622–634, 1934.
47. Ball J, Garner A: Mineralisation of woven bone in osteomalacia, J Pathol Bacteriol 91:563–567, 1966.
48. Steinbach HL, Noetzli M: Roentgen appearance of the skeleton in osteomalacia and rickets, Am J Roentgenol Radium Ther Nucl Med 91:955–972, 1964.
49. Burnstein MI, Lawson JP, Kottamasu SR, et al: The enthesopathic changes of hypophosphatemic osteomalacia in adults: radiologic findings, Am J Roentgenol 153:785–790, 1989.
50. Polisson RP, Martinez S, Khoury M, et al: Calcification of entheses associated with X-linked hypophosphatemic osteomalacia, N Engl J Med 313:1–6, 1985.
51. Arneil GC: Nutritional rickets in children in Glasgow, Proc Nutr Soc 34:101–109, 1975.
52. Arneil GC, Crosbie JC: Infantile rickets returns to Glasgow, Lancet 2:423–425, 1963.
53. Dunnigan MG, Paton JP, Haase S, et al: Late rickets and osteomalacia in the Pakistani community in Glasgow, Scott Med J 7:159–167, 1962.
54. Benson PF, Stroud CE, Mitchell NJ, et al: Rickets in immigrant children in London, Br Med J 1:1054–1056, 1963.
55. Chanarin I, Malkowska V, O'Hea AM, et al: Megaloblastic anaemia in a vegetarian Hindu community, Lancet 2:1168–1172, 1985.
56. Finch PJ, Ang L, Colston KW, et al: Blunted seasonal variation in serum 25-hydroxy vitamin D and increased risk of osteomalacia in vegetarian London Asians, Eur J Clin Nutr 46:509–515, 1992.
57. Henderson JB, Dunnigan MG, McIntosh WB, et al: Asian osteomalacia is determined by dietary factors when exposure to ultraviolet radiation is restricted: a risk factor model, Q J Med 76:923–933, 1990.
58. Shaunak S, Colston K, Ang L, et al: Vitamin D deficiency in adult British Hindu Asians: a family disorder, Br Med J (Clin Res Ed) 291:1166–1168, 1985.
59. Ralston SH, Willocks L, Pitkeathly DA, et al: High prevalence of unrecognized osteomalacia in hospital patients with rheumatoid arthritis, Br J Rheumatol 27:202–205, 1988.
60. Botella-Carretero JI, Alvarez-Blasco F, Villafruela JJ, et al: Vitamin D deficiency is associated with the metabolic syndrome in morbid obesity, Clin Nutr 26:573–580, 2007.
61. Charles P, Mosekilde L, Sondergard K, et al: Treatment with high-dose oral vitamin D2 in patients with jejunoileal bypass for morbid obesity. Effects on calcium and magnesium metabolism, vitamin D metabolites, and faecal lag time, Scand J Gastroenterol 19:1031–1038, 1984.
62. Crowley LV, Seay J, Mullin G: Late effects of gastric bypass for obesity, Am J Gastroenterol 79:850–860, 1984.
63. Parfitt AM, Podenphant J, Villanueva AR, et al: Metabolic bone disease with and without osteomalacia after intestinal bypass surgery: a bone histomorphometric study, Bone 6:211–220, 1985.
64. Basha B, Rao DS, Han ZH, et al: Osteomalacia due to vitamin D depletion: a neglected consequence of intestinal malabsorption, Am J Med 108:296–300, 2000.
65. Bisballe S, Eriksen EF, Melsen F, et al: Osteopenia and osteomalacia after gastrectomy: interrelations between biochemical markers of bone remodelling, vitamin D metabolites, and bone histomorphometry, Gut 32:1303–1307, 1991.
66. Tovey FI, Godfrey JE, Lewin MR: A gastrectomy population: 25–30 years on, Postgrad Med J 66:450–456, 1990.
67. Daum F, Rosen JF, Roginsky M, et al: 25-Hydroxycholecalciferol in the management of rickets associated with extrahepatic biliary atresia, J Pediatr 88:1041–1043, 1976.

68. Heubi JE, Tsang RC, Steichen JJ, et al: 1,25-Dihydroxyvitamin D₃ in childhood hepatic osteodystrophy, J Pediatr 94:977–982, 1979.

69. Roberts WA, Badger VM: Osteomalacia of very-low-birth-weight infants, J Pediatr Orthop 4:593–598, 1984.

70. Heckmatt JZ, Peacock M, Davies AE, et al: Plasma 25-hydroxyvitamin D in pregnant Asian women and their babies, Lancet 2:546–548, 1979.

71. Specker BL, Tsang RC, Hollis BW: Effect of race and diet on human-milk vitamin D and 25-hydroxyvitamin D, Am J Dis Child 139:1134–1137, 1985.

72. Haddad JG, Stamp TC: Circulating 25-hydroxyvitamin D in man, Am J Med 57:57–62, 1974.

73. Lester E, Skinner RK, Wills MR: Seasonal variation in serum-25-hydroxyvitamin-D in the elderly in Britain, Lancet 1:979–980, 1977.

74. Stamp TC, Round JM: Seasonal changes in human plasma levels of 25-hydroxyvitamin D, Nature 247:563–565, 1974.

75. Dawson-Hughes B, Dallal GE, Krall EA, et al: Effect of vitamin D supplementation on wintertime and overall bone loss in healthy postmenopausal women, Ann Intern Med 115:505–512, 1991.

76. Harris SS, Dawson-Hughes B: Seasonal changes in plasma 25-hydroxyvitamin D concentrations of young American black and white women, Am J Clin Nutr 67:1232–1236, 1998.

77. Thomas MK, Lloyd-Jones DM, Thadhani RI, et al: Hypovitaminosis D in medical inpatients, N Engl J Med 338:777–783, 1998.

78. MacLaughlin J, Holick MF: Aging decreases the capacity of human skin to produce vitamin D₃, J Clin Invest 76:1536–1538, 1985.

79. Tsai KS, Heath H 3rd, Kumar R, et al: Impaired vitamin D metabolism with aging in women. Possible role in pathogenesis of senile osteoporosis, J Clin Invest 73:1668–1672, 1984.

80. Ebeling PR, Sandgren ME, DiMagno EP, et al: Evidence of an age-related decrease in intestinal responsiveness to vitamin D: relationship between serum 1,25-dihydroxyvitamin D₃ and intestinal vitamin D receptor concentrations in normal women, J Clin Endocrinol Metab 75:176–182, 1992.

81. Vieth R: Vitamin D supplementation, 25-hydroxyvitamin D concentrations, and safety, Am J Clin Nutr 69:842–856, 1999.

82. Heaney RP: Lessons for nutritional science from vitamin D, Am J Clin Nutr 69:825–826, 1999.

83. Goel KM, Sweet EM, Logan RW, et al: Florid and subclinical rickets among immigrant children in Glasgow, Lancet 1:1141–1145, 1976.

84. Lawson M, Thomas M: Vitamin D concentrations in Asian children aged 2 years living in England: population survey, BMJ 318:28, 1999.

85. Stanbury SW, Torkington P, Lumb GA, et al: Asian rickets and osteomalacia: patterns of parathyroid response in vitamin D deficiency, Proc Nutr Soc 34:111–117, 1975.

86. Loomis WF: Skin-pigment regulation of vitamin-D biosynthesis in man, Science 157:501–506, 1967.

87. Doxiadis S, Angelis C, Karatzas P, et al: Genetic aspects of nutritional rickets, Arch Dis Child 51:83–90, 1976.

88. Ford JA, Colhoun EM, McIntosh WB, et al: Rickets and osteomalacia in the Glasgow Pakistani community, 1961–71, Br Med J 2:677–680, 1972.

89. Heaney RP: Long-latency deficiency disease: insights from calcium and vitamin D, Am J Clin Nutr 78:912–919, 2003.

90. Wills MR, Phillips JB, Day RC, et al: Phytic acid and nutritional rickets in immigrants, Lancet 1:771–773, 1972.

91. Dent CE, Round JM, Rowe DJ, et al: Effect of chapattis and ultraviolet irradiation on nutritional rickets in an Indian immigrant, Lancet 1:1282–1284, 1973.

92. Dent CE, Richens A, Rowe DJ, et al: Osteomalacia with long-term anticonvulsant therapy in epilepsy, Br Med J 4:69–72, 1970.

93. Scriver CR: Rickets and the pathogenesis of impaired tubular transport of phosphate and other solutes, Am J Med 57:43–49, 1974.

94. Arnaud C, Glorieux F, Scriver CR: Serum parathyroid hormone levels in acquired vitamin D deficiency of infancy, Pediatrics 49:837–840, 1972.

95. Muldowney FP, Freaney R, McGeeney D: Renal tubular acidosis and amino-aciduria in osteomalacia of dietary or intestinal origin, Q J Med 37:517–539, 1968.

96. Rao DS, Parfitt AM, Kleerekoper M, et al: Dissociation between the effects of endogenous parathyroid hormone on adenosine 3′,5′-monophosphate generation and phosphate reabsorption in hypocalcemia due to vitamin D depletion: an acquired disorder resembling pseudohypoparathyroidism type II, J Clin Endocrinol Metab 61:285–290, 1985.

97. Adams JS, Clemens TL, Parrish JA, et al: Vitamin-D synthesis and metabolism after ultraviolet irradiation of normal and vitamin-D-deficient subjects, N Engl J Med 306:722–725, 1982.

98. Eastwood JB, de Wardener HE, Gray RW, et al: Normal plasma-1,25-(OH)2-vitamin-D concentrations in nutritional osteomalacia, Lancet 1:1377–1378, 1979.

99. Goodman AD, Lemann J Jr, Lennon EJ, et al: Production, excretion, and net balance of fixed acid in patients with renal acidosis, J Clin Invest 44:495–506, 1965.

100. Lemann J Jr, Bushinsky DA, Hamm LL: Bone buffering of acid and base in humans, Am J Physiol Renal Physiol 285:F811–F832, 2003.

101. Lemann J Jr, Lennon EJ, Goodman AD, et al: The net balance of acid in subjects given large loads of acid or alkali, J Clin Invest 44:507–517, 1965.

102. Lemann J Jr, Litzow JR, Lennon EJ: The effects of chronic acid loads in normal man: further evidence for the participation of bone mineral in the defense against chronic metabolic acidosis, J Clin Invest 45:1608–1614, 1966.

103. Arnett T: Regulation of bone cell function by acid-base balance, Proc Nutr Soc 62:511–520, 2003.

104. Nordstrom T, Shrode LD, Rotstein OD, et al: Chronic extracellular acidosis induces plasmalemmal vacuolar type H⁺ ATPase activity in osteoclasts, J Biol Chem 272:6354–6360, 1997.

105. Mori H, Sakai H, Morihata H, et al: Regulatory mechanisms and physiological relevance of a voltage-gated H⁺ channel in murine osteoclasts: phorbol myristate acetate induces cell acidosis and the channel activation, J Bone Miner Res 18:2069–2076, 2003.

106. Harrison HE, Harrison HC: Physiology of vitamin D. In Rodahl K, Nicholson JT, Brown EMJ, editors: Bone as a Tissue, New York, 1960, McGaw-Hill, p 300.

107. Frick KK, Bushinsky DA: Metabolic acidosis stimulates RANKL RNA expression in bone through a cyclo-oxygenase-dependent mechanism, J Bone Miner Res 18:1317–1325, 2003.

108. Ludwig MG, Vanek M, Guerini D, et al: Proton-sensing G-protein-coupled receptors, Nature 425:93–98, 2003.

109. Donohoe JF, Freaney R, Muldowney FP: Osteomalacia in ureterosigmoidostomy, Ir J Med Sci 8:523–530, 1969.

110. Tschopp AB, Lippuner K, Jaeger P, et al: No evidence of osteopenia 5 to 8 years after ileal orthotopic bladder substitution, J Urol 155:71–75, 1996.

111. Lee SW, Russell J, Avioli LV: 25-hydroxycholecalciferol to 1,25-dihydroxycholecalciferol: conversion impaired by systemic metabolic acidosis, Science 195:994–996, 1977.

112. Karet FE: Inherited distal renal tubular acidosis, J Am Soc Nephrol 13:2178–2184, 2002.

113. Morris RC Jr: Renal tubular acidosis. Mechanisms, classification and implications, N Engl J Med 281:1405–1413, 1969.

114. Morris RC Jr, McSherry E: Symposium on acid-base homeostasis. Renal acidosis, Kidney Int 1:322–340, 1972.

115. Richards P, Chamberlain MJ, Wrong OM: Treatment of osteomalacia of renal tubular acidosis by sodium bicarbonate alone, Lancet 2:994–997, 1972.

116. York SE, Yendt ER: Osteomalacia associated with renal bicarbonate loss, Can Med Assoc J 94:1329–1342, 1966.

117. Sly WS, Hewett-Emmett D, Whyte MP, et al: Carbonic anhydrase II deficiency identified as the primary defect in the autosomal recessive syndrome of osteopetrosis with renal tubular acidosis and cerebral calcification, Proc Natl Acad Sci U S A 80:2752–2756, 1983.

118. Sly WS, Whyte MP, Sundaram V, et al: Carbonic anhydrase II deficiency in 12 families with the autosomal recessive syndrome of osteopetrosis with renal tubular acidosis and cerebral calcification, N Engl J Med 313:139–145, 1985.

119. Whyte MP, Murphy WA, Fallon MD, et al: Osteopetrosis, renal tubular acidosis and basal ganglia calcification in three sisters, Am J Med 69:64–74, 1980.

120. McMahon C, Will A, Hu P, et al: Bone marrow transplantation corrects osteopetrosis in the carbonic anhydrase II deficiency syndrome, Blood 97:1947–1950, 2001.

121. Dent CE, Harris H: Hereditary forms of rickets and osteomalacia, J Bone Joint Surg Br 38-B:204–226, 1956.

122. Henneman PH, Dempsey EF, Carroll EL, et al: Acquired vitamin D-resistant osteomalacia: a new variety characterized by hypercalcemia, low serum bicarbonate and hyperglycinuria, Metabolism 11:103–116, 1962.

123. Kallmeyer J, Dunea G, Schwartz FD: Hypophosphatemic osteomalacia with hyperglycinuria, Ann Intern Med 66:136–141, 1967.

124. Rico H, Gomez-Castresana F, Hernandez ER, et al: Adult hypophosphatemic osteomalacia: report of two cases, Clin Rheumatol 4:325–334, 1985.

125. Scriver CR, Goldbloom RB, Roy CC: Hypophosphatemic rickets with renal hyperglycinuria, renal glucosuria, and glycyl-prolinuria: a syndrome with evidence for renal tubular secretion of phosphorus, Pediatrics 34:357–371, 1964.

126. Pierce WM Jr, Nardin GF, Fuqua MF, et al: Effect of chronic carbonic anhydrase inhibitor therapy on bone mineral density in white women, J Bone Miner Res 6:347–354, 1991.

127. Waite LC, Volkert WA, Kenny AD: Inhibition of bone resorption by acetazolamide in the rat, Endocrinology 87:1129–1139, 1970.

128. Baker LR, Ackrill P, Cattell WR, et al: Iatrogenic osteomalacia and myopathy due to phosphate depletion, Br Med J 3:150–152, 1974.

129. Bloom W, Flinchum D: Osteomalacia with pseudofractures caused by ingestion of aluminum hydroxide, JAMA 174:1327–1330, 1960.

130. Dent CE, Winter CS: Osteomalacia due to phosphate depletion from excessive aluminium hydroxide ingestion, Br Med J 1:551–552, 1974.

131. Levy Y, Bansal M, Zackson DA, et al: Phosphate depletion syndrome: case report with bone and muscle histology findings and review of the literature, JPEN J Parenter Enteral Nutr 12:313–317, 1988.

132. Lotz M, Zisman E, Bartter FC: Evidence for a phosphorus-depletion syndrome in man, N Engl J Med 278:409–415, 1968.

133. Godsall JW, Baron R, Insogna KL: Vitamin D metabolism and bone histomorphometry in a patient with antacid-induced osteomalacia, Am J Med 77:747–750, 1984.

134. Stein JH, Smith WO, Ginn HE: Hypophosphatemia in acute alcoholism, Am J Med Sci 252:78–83, 1966.

135. Territo MC, Tanaka KR: Hypophosphatemia in chronic alcoholism, Arch Intern Med 134:445–447, 1974.

136. de Vernejoul MC, Bielakoff J, Herve M, et al: Evidence for defective osteoblastic function. A role for alcohol and tobacco consumption in osteoporosis in middle-aged men, Clin Orthop Relat Res 107–115, 1983.

137. Elisaf MS, Siamopoulos KC: Mechanisms of hypophosphataemia in alcoholic patients, Int J Clin Pract 51:501–503, 1997.

138. Klein GL, Soriano H, Shulman RJ, et al: Hepatic osteodystrophy in chronic cholestasis: evidence for a multifactorial etiology, Pediatr Transplant 6:136–140, 2002.

139. Pettifor JM, Ross P, Wang J, et al: Rickets in children of rural origin in South Africa: is low dietary calcium a factor? J Pediatr 92:320–324, 1978.

140. Thacher TD, Fischer PR, Pettifor JM, et al: A comparison of calcium, vitamin D, or both for nutritional rickets in Nigerian children, N Engl J Med 341:563–568, 1999.

141. DeLucia MC, Mitnick ME, Carpenter TO: Nutritional rickets with normal circulating 25-hydroxyvitamin D: a call for reexamining the role of dietary calcium intake in North American infants, J Clin Endocrinol Metab 88:3539–3545, 2003.

142. Albright F, Butler AM, Bloomberg E: Rickets resistant to vitamin D therapy, J Clin Dis Child 54:529–547, 1937.

143. Jonsson KB, Zahradnik R, Larsson T, et al: Fibroblast growth factor 23 in oncogenic osteomalacia and X-linked hypophosphatemia, N Engl J Med 348:1656–1663, 2003.

144. A gene (PEX) with homologies to endopeptidases is mutated in patients with X-linked hypophosphatemic rickets. The HYP Consortium, Nat Genet 11:130–136, 1995.

145. Sabbagh Y, Boileau G, Campos M, et al: Structure and function of disease-causing missense mutations in the PHEX gene, J Clin Endocrinol Metab 88:2213–2222, 2003.

146. Sabbagh Y, Boileau G, DesGroseillers L, et al: Disease-causing missense mutations in the PHEX gene interfere with membrane targeting of the recombinant protein, Hum Mol Genet 10:1539–1546, 2001.

147. Sabbagh Y, Gauthier C, Tenenhouse HS: The X chromosome deletion in HYP mice extends into the intergenic region but does not include the SAT gene downstream from Phex, Cytogenet Genome Res 99:344–349, 2002.

148. Sabbagh Y, Jones AO, Tenenhouse HS: PHEXdb, a locus-specific database for mutations causing X-linked hypophosphatemia, Hum Mutat 16:1–6, 2000.

149. Brame LA, White KE, Econs MJ: Renal phosphate wasting disorders: clinical features and pathogenesis, Semin Nephrol 24:39–47, 2004.

150. Econs MJ: New insights into the pathogenesis of inherited phosphate wasting disorders, Bone 25:131–135, 1999.

151. Econs MJ, McEnery PT: Autosomal dominant hypophosphatemic rickets/osteomalacia: clinical characterization of a novel renal phosphate-wasting disorder, J Clin Endocrinol Metab 82:674–681, 1997.

152. White KE, Jonsson KB, Carn G, et al: The autosomal dominant hypophosphatemic rickets (ADHR) gene is a secreted polypeptide overexpressed by tumors that cause phosphate wasting, J Clin Endocrinol Metab 86:497–500, 2001.

153. Bergwitz C, Roslin NM, Tieder M, et al: SLC34A3 mutations in patients with hereditary hypophosphatemic rickets with hypercalciuria predict a key role for the sodium-phosphate cotransporter NaPi-IIc in maintaining phosphate homeostasis, Am J Hum Genet 78:179–192, 2006.

154. Harrell RM, Lyles KW, Harrelson JM, et al: Healing of bone disease in X-linked hypophosphatemic rickets/osteomalacia. Induction and maintenance with phosphorus and calcitriol, J Clin Invest 75:1858–1868, 1985.

155. Verge CF, Lam A, Simpson JM, et al: Effects of therapy in X-linked hypophosphatemic rickets, N Engl J Med 325:1843–1848, 1991.

156. Petersen DJ, Boniface AM, Schranck FW, et al: X-linked hypophosphatemic rickets: a study (with literature review) of linear growth response to calcitriol and phosphate therapy, J Bone Miner Res 7:583–597, 1992.

157. Frame B, Manson G: Refractory rickets and osteomalacia, Henry Ford Hosp Med Bull 8:293–298, 1960.

158. Glorieux FH, Scriver CR, Reade TM, et al: Use of phosphate and vitamin D to prevent dwarfism and rickets in X-linked hypophosphatemia, N Engl J Med 287:481–487, 1972.

159. Glorieux FH: Calcitriol treatment in vitamin D-dependent and vitamin D-resistant rickets, Metabolism 39:10–12, 1990.

160. Sullivan W, Carpenter T, Glorieux F, et al: A prospective trial of phosphate and 1,25-dihydroxyvitamin D$_3$ therapy in symptomatic adults with X-linked hypophosphatemic rickets, J Clin Endocrinol Metab 75:879–885, 1992.

161. Prader A, Illig R, Uehlinger E, et al: Rickets following bone tumor, Helv Paediatr Acta 14:554–565, 1959.

162. Nuovo MA, Dorfman HD, Sun CC, et al: Tumor-induced osteomalacia and rickets, Am J Surg Pathol 13:588–599, 1989.

163. Lyles KW, Berry WR, Haussler M, et al: Hypophosphatemic osteomalacia: association with prostatic carcinoma, Ann Intern Med 93:275–278, 1980.

164. Linovitz RJ, Resnick D, Keissling P, et al: Tumor-induced osteomalacia and rickets: a surgically curable syndrome. Report of two cases, J Bone Joint Surg Am 58:419–423, 1976.

165. Jan De Beur SM, Finnegan RB, Vassiliadis J, et al: Tumors associated with oncogenic osteomalacia express genes important in bone and mineral metabolism, J Bone Miner Res 17:1102–1110, 2002.

166. Shimada T, Mizutani S, Muto T, et al: Cloning and characterization of FGF23 as a causative factor of tumor-induced osteomalacia, Proc Natl Acad Sci U S A 98:6500–6505, 2001.

167. Berndt T, Craig TA, Bowe AE, et al: Secreted frizzled-related protein 4 is a potent tumor-derived phosphaturic agent, J Clin Invest 112:785–794, 2003.

168. Dent CE, Gertner JM: Hypophosphataemic osteomalacia in fibrous dysplasia, Q J Med 45:411–420, 1976.

169. Imel EA, Econs MJ: Fibrous dysplasia, phosphate wasting and fibroblast growth factor 23, Pediatr Endocrinol Rev 4(Suppl 4):434–439, 2007.

170. Lichter-Konecki U, Broman KW, Blau EB, et al: Genetic and physical mapping of the locus for autosomal dominant renal Fanconi syndrome, on chromosome 15q15.3, Am J Hum Genet 68:264–268, 2001.

171. Bruce L, Wrong O, Toye A, et al: Band 3 mutations, renal tubular acidosis and South East Asian ovalocytosis in Malaysia and Papua New Guinea: loss of up to 95% band 3 transport in red cells, Biochem J 350:41–51, 2003.

172. Cheidde L, Vieira TC, Lima PR, et al: A novel mutation in the anion exchanger 1 gene is associated with familial distal renal tubular acidosis and nephrocalcinosis, Pediatrics 112:1361–1367, 2003.

173. Devonald MA, Smith AN, Poon JP, et al: Non-polarized targeting of AE1 causes autosomal dominant distal renal tubular acidosis, Nat Genet 33:125–127, 2003.

174. Smith AN, Borthwick KJ, Karet FE: Molecular cloning and characterization of novel tissue-specific isoforms of the human vacuolar H$^+$-ATPase C, G and D subunits, and their evaluation in autosomal recessive distal renal tubular acidosis, Gene 297:169–177, 2002.

175. Carballo-Trujillo I, Garcia-Nieto V, Moya-Angeler FJ, et al: Novel truncating mutations in the ClC-5 chloride channel gene in patients with Dent's disease, Nephrol Dial Transplant 18:717–723, 2003.

176. Cox JP, Yamamoto K, Christie PT, et al: Renal chloride channel, CLCN5, mutations in Dent's disease, J Bone Miner Res 14:1536–1542, 1999.

177. Brodehl J: Tubular Fanconi syndromes with bone involvement. In Bickel H, Stern J, editors: Inborn Errors of Calcium and Bone Metabolism, Baltimore, 1976, University Park Press, pp 191–213.

178. Schneider JA, Seegmiller JE: Cystinosis and the Fanconi syndrome. In Stanbury JB, Wyngaarden JB, Frederickson D, editors: The Metabolic Basis of Inherited Disease, New York, 1972, McGraw-Hill, p 1581.

179. Sakamoto O, Ogawa E, Ohura T, et al: Mutation analysis of the GLUT2 gene in patients with Fanconi-Bickel syndrome, Pediatr Res 48:586–589, 2000.

180. Lowe CU, Terrey M, Mac LE: Organic-aciduria, decreased renal ammonia production, hydrophthalmos, and mental retardation; a clinical entity, AMA Am J Dis Child 83:164–184, 1952.

181. Rosenberg LE, Scriver CR: Disorders of amino acid metabolism. In Bondy PK, editor: Duncan's Disease of Metabolism, Philadelphia, 1969, WB Saunders, pp 366–515.

182. Anikster Y, Shotelersuk V, Gahl WA: CTNS mutations in patients with cystinosis, Hum Mutat 14:454–458, 1999.

183. McGowan-Jordan J, Stoddard K, Podolsky L, et al: Molecular analysis of cystinosis: probable Irish origin of the most common French Canadian mutation, Eur J Hum Genet 7:671–678, 1999.

184. Shotelersuk V, Larson D, Anikster Y, et al: CTNS mutations in an American-based population of cystinosis patients, Am J Hum Genet 63:1352–1362, 1998.

185. Briggs WA, Kominami N, Wilson RE, et al: Kidney transplantation in Fanconi syndrome, N Engl J Med 286:25, 1972.

186. Monnier N, Satre V, Lerouge E, et al: OCRL1 mutation analysis in French Lowe syndrome patients: implications for molecular diagnosis strategy and genetic counseling, Hum Mutat 16:157–165, 2000.

187. Roschinger W, Muntau AC, Rudolph G, et al: Carrier assessment in families with lowe oculocerebrorenal syndrome: novel mutations in the OCRL1 gene and correlation of direct DNA diagnosis with ocular examination, Mol Genet Metab 69:213–222, 2000.

188. Zhang X, Hartz PA, Philip E, et al: Cell lines from kidney proximal tubules of a patient with Lowe syndrome lack OCRL inositol polyphosphate 5-phosphatase and accumulate phosphatidylinositol 4,5-bisphosphate, J Biol Chem 273:1574–1582, 1998.

189. Huster D, Hoppert M, Lutsenko S, et al: Defective cellular localization of mutant ATP7B in Wilson's disease

190. Majumdar R, Al Jumah M, Fraser M: 4193delC, a common mutation causing Wilson's disease in Saudi Arabia: rapid molecular screening of patients and carriers, Mol Pathol 56:302–304, 2003.

191. Morgan HG, Stewart WK, Lowe KG, et al: Wilson's disease and the Fanconi syndrome, Q J Med 31:361–384, 1962.

192. Wilson DM, Goldstein NP: Bicarbonate excretion in Wilson's disease (hepatolenticular degeneration), Mayo Clin Proc 49:394–400, 1974.

193. Walshe JM: Effect of penicillamine on failure of renal acidification in Wilson's disease, Lancet 1:775–778, 1968.

194. Bergeron A, D'Astous M, Timm DE, et al: Structural and functional analysis of missense mutations in fumarylacetoacetate hydrolase, the gene deficient in hereditary tyrosinemia type 1, J Biol Chem 276:15225–15231, 2001.

195. Snaper I, Kahn A: Determination of Bence Jones protein in urine and serum. In Myelomatosis, Fundamentals and Clinical Features, Baltimore, 1971, University Park Press, pp 203–204.

196. Monte Neto JT, Sesso R, Kirsztajn GM, et al: Osteomalacia secondary to renal tubular acidosis in a patient with primary Sjogren's syndrome, Clin Exp Rheumatol 9:625–627, 1991.

197. Adams RG, Harrison JF, Scott P: The development of cadmium-induced proteinuria, impaired renal function, and osteomalacia in alkaline battery workers, Q J Med 38:425–443, 1969.

198. Chisolm JJ Jr: Aminoaciduria as a manifestation of renal tubular injury in lead intoxication and a comparison with patterns of aminoaciduria seen in other diseases, J Pediatr 60:1–17, 1962.

199. Gross JM: Fanconi syndrome (adult type) developing secondary to the ingestion of outdated tetracycline, Ann Intern Med 58:523–528, 1963.

200. Bethune JE, Dent CE: Hypophosphatasia in the adult, Am J Med 28:615–622, 1960.

201. Fraser D: Hypophosphatasia, Am J Med 22:730–746, 1957.

202. Rathbun JC: Hypophosphatasia; a new developmental anomaly, Am J Dis Child 75:822–831, 1948.

203. Sobel EH, Clark LC Jr, Fox RP, et al: Rickets, deficiency of alkaline phosphatase activity and premature loss of teeth in childhood, Pediatrics 11:309–322, 1953.

204. Cahill RA, Wenkert D, Perlman SA, et al: Infantile hypophosphatasia: transplantation therapy trial using bone fragments and cultured osteoblasts, J Clin Endocrinol Metab 92:2923–2930, 2007.

205. Whyte MP, Kurtzberg J, McAlister WH, et al: Marrow cell transplantation for infantile hypophosphatasia, J Bone Miner Res 18:624–636, 2003.

206. Birtwell WM Jr, Riggs L, Peterson LF, et al: Hypophosphatasia in an adult, Arch Intern Med 120:90–93, 1967.

207. McCance R, Morrison AB, Dent CE: The excretion of phosphoethanolamine and hypophosphatasia, Lancet 268:131, 1955.

208. Whyte MP: Hypophosphatasia. In Scriver CR, Beaudet AL, Sly WS, et al, editors: The Metabolic and Molecular Bases of Inherited Disease, ed 8, New York, 2001, McGraw-Hill, pp 5313–5329.

209. Whyte MP, Mahuren JD, Vrabel LA, et al: Markedly increased circulating pyridoxal-5'-phosphate levels in hypophosphatasia. Alkaline phosphatase acts in vitamin B$_6$ metabolism, J Clin Invest 76:752–756, 1985.

210. Fleish H, Neuman WF: Mechanisms of calcification: role of collagen, polyphosphates, and phosphatase, Am J Physiol 200:1296–1300, 1961.

211. Russell RG: Metabolism of inorganic pyrophosphate (PPi), Arthritis Rheum 19(Suppl 3):465–478, 1976.

212. Henthorn PS, Raducha M, Fedde KN, et al: Different missense mutations at the tissue-nonspecific alkaline phosphatase gene locus in autosomal recessively inherited forms of mild and severe hypophosphatasia, Proc Natl Acad Sci U S A 89:9924–9928, 1992.

213. Albright F: Hypoparathyroidism as a cause of osteomalacia, J Clin Endocrinol Metab 16:419–425, 1956.

214. Drezner MK, Neelon FA, Jowsey J, et al: Hypoparathyroidism: a possible cause of osteomalacia, J Clin Endocrinol Metab 45:114–122, 1977.

215. Epstein S, Meunier PJ, Lambert PW, et al: 1 alpha,25-dihydroxyvitamin D₃ corrects osteomalacia in hypoparathyroidism and pseudohypoparathyroidism, Acta Endocrinol (Copenh) 103:241–247, 1983.

216. Wilson JD, Hadden DR: Pseudohypoparathyroidism presenting with rickets, J Clin Endocrinol Metab 51:1184–1189, 1980.

217. Whyte MP, Murphy WA: Osteopetrosis and other sclerosing bone disorders. In Avioli LV, Krane SM, editors: Metabolic Bone Disease, Philadelphia, 1990, WB Saunders, pp 616–658.

218. Pincus JB, Gittleman IF, Karamer B: Metabolic studies in two cases and further observations on the composition of bones in this disease, Am J Dis Child 73:458–472, 1947.

219. Bonucci E, Sartori E, Spina M: Osteopetrosis fetalis. Report on a case, with special reference to ultrastructure, Virchows Arch A Pathol Anat Histol 368:109–121, 1975.

220. Borthwick KJ, Kandemir N, Topaloglu R, et al: A phenocopy of CAII deficiency: a novel genetic explanation for inherited infantile osteopetrosis with distal renal tubular acidosis, J Med Genet 40:115–121, 2003.

221. Frame B, Frost HM, Pak CY, et al: Fibrogenesis imperfecta ossium. A collagen defect causing osteomalacia, N Engl J Med 285:769–772, 1971.

222. Coursey C, Weber T, Dodd L, et al: Fibrogenesis imperfecta ossium: MR imaging of the axial and appendicular skeleton and correlation with a unique radiographic appearance, Skeletal Radiol 36:1077–1084, 2007.

223. Swan CHJ, Cooke WT: Fibrogenesis imperfect ossium. In Frame B, Parfitt AM, Duncan H, editors: Clinical Aspects of Metabolic Bone Disease, Amsterdam, 1973, Excerpta Medica, p 465.

224. Henneman DH, Pak CY, Bartter FC: Collagen composition, solubility and biosynthesis in fibrogenesis imperfecta ossium. In Frame B, Parfitt AM, Duncan H, editors: Clinical Aspects of Metabolic Bone Disease, Amsterdam, 1973, Excerpta Medica, p 469.

225. Lafage-Proust M, Schaeverbeke T, Dehais J: Fibrogenesis imperfecta ossium: ineffectiveness of melphalan, Calcif Tissue Int 59:240–244, 1996.

226. Martin KJ, Gonzalez E, Slatopolsky E: Renal Osteodystrophy. In Brenner BM, editor: Brenner and Rector's the Kidney, Philadelphia, 2004, WB Saunders, pp 2255–2304.

227. Charhon SA, Berland YF, Olmer MJ, et al: Effects of parathyroidectomy on bone formation and mineralization in hemodialyzed patients, Kidney Int 27:426–435, 1985.

228. Dunstan CR, Hills E, Norman AW, et al: The pathogenesis of renal osteodystrophy: role of vitamin D, aluminium, parathyroid hormone, calcium and phosphorus, Q J Med 55:127–144, 1985.

229. Goodman WG: Bone disease and aluminum: pathogenic considerations, Am J Kidney Dis 6:330–335, 1985.

230. Hodsman AB, Sherrard DJ, Alfrey AC, et al: Bone aluminum and histomorphometric features of renal osteodystrophy, J Clin Endocrinol Metab 54:539–546, 1982.

231. Li YC, Amling M, Pirro AE, et al: Normalization of mineral ion homeostasis by dietary means prevents hyperparathyroidism, rickets, and osteomalacia, but not alopecia in vitamin D receptor-ablated mice, Endocrinology 139:4391–4396, 1998.

232. Li YC, Pirro AE, Amling M, et al: Targeted ablation of the vitamin D receptor: an animal model of vitamin D-dependent rickets type II with alopecia, Proc Natl Acad Sci U S A 94:9831–9835, 1997.

233. Malluche HH: Aluminium and bone disease in chronic renal failure, Nephrol Dial Transplant 17(Suppl 2):21–24, 2002.

234. Parisien M, Charhon SA, Arlot M, et al: Evidence for a toxic effect of aluminum on osteoblasts: a histomorphometric study in hemodialysis patients with aplastic bone disease, J Bone Miner Res 3:259–267, 1988.

235. Quarles LD, Dennis VW, Gitelman HJ, et al: Aluminum deposition at the osteoid-bone interface. An epiphenomenon of the osteomalacic state in vitamin D-deficient dogs, J Clin Invest 75:1441–1447, 1985.

236. Bleyer AJ, Burke SK, Dillon M, et al: A comparison of the calcium-free phosphate binder sevelamer hydrochloride with calcium acetate in the treatment of hyperphosphatemia in hemodialysis patients, Am J Kidney Dis 33:694–701, 1999.

237. Chertow GM, Burke SK, Lazarus JM, et al: Poly[allylamine hydrochloride] (RenaGel): a noncalcemic phosphate binder for the treatment of hyperphosphatemia in chronic renal failure, Am J Kidney Dis 29:66–71, 1997.

238. Chertow GM, Burke SK, Raggi P: Sevelamer attenuates the progression of coronary and aortic calcification in hemodialysis patients, Kidney Int 62:245–252, 2002.

239. Asami T, Kawasaki T, Uchiyama M: Unique form of rickets with low serum 25-hydroxyvitamin D in two normally nourished children, Acta Paediatr Jpn 37:182–188, 1995.

240. Casella SJ, Reiner BJ, Chen TC, et al: A possible genetic defect in 25-hydroxylation as a cause of rickets, J Pediatr 124:929–932, 1994.

241. Nutzenadel W, Mehls O, Klaus G: A new defect in vitamin D metabolism, J Pediatr 126:676–677, 1995.

242. Cheng JB, Levine MA, Bell NH, et al: Genetic evidence that the human CYP2R1 enzyme is a key vitamin D 25-hydroxylase, Proc Natl Acad Sci U S A 101:7711–7715, 2004.

243. Fu G, Lin D, Zang M, et al: Cloning of human 25-hydroxyvitamin D-1-a-hydroxylase and mutations causing vitamin D-dependent rickets type 1, Mol Endocrinol 1961–1970, 1997.

244. Kitnaka S, Takeyama K-I, Muryama A, et al: Inactivating mutations in the 25-hydroxyvitamin D, 1a-hydroxylase gene in patients with pseudovitamin D-deficiency rickets, N Engl J Med 338:653–661, 1998.

245. St-Arnaud R, Messerlian S, Moir J, et al: The 25-hydroxyvitamin D 1-alphahydroxylase gene maps to the pseudovitamin D-deficiency rickets (PDDR) disease locus, J Bone Miner Res 12:1552–1559, 1997.

246. Brooks MH, Bell NH, Love L, et al: Vitamin-D-dependent rickets type II. Resistance of target organs to 1,25-dihydroxyvitamin D, N Engl J Med 298:996–999, 1978.

247. Hughes M, Malloy P, Kieback D, et al: Human vitamin D receptor mutations: identification of molecular defects in hypocalcemic vitamin D resistant rickets, Adv Exp Med Biol 255:491–503, 1989.

248. Balsan S, Garabedian M, Larchet M, et al: Long-term nocturnal calcium infusions can cure rickets and promote normal mineralization in hereditary resistance to 1,25-dihydroxyvitamin D, J Clin Invest 77:1661–1667, 1986.

249. Heaney RP, Dowell MS, Hale CA, et al: Calcium absorption varies within the reference range for serum 25-hydroxyvitamin D, J Am Coll Nutr 22:142–146, 2003.

250. Trivedi DP, Doll R, Khaw KT: Effect of four monthly oral vitamin D₃ (cholecalciferol) supplementation on fractures and mortality in men and women living in the community: randomised double blind controlled trial, BMJ 326:469, 2003.

251. Bischoff-Ferrari HA, Dietrich T, Orav EJ, et al: Positive association between 25-hydroxy vitamin D levels and bone mineral density: a population-based study of younger and older adults, Am J Med 116:634–639, 2004.

252. Heaney RP, Davies KM, Chen TC, et al: Human serum 25-hydroxycholecalciferol response to extended oral dosing with cholecalciferol, Am J Clin Nutr 77:204–210, 2003.

253. Ahonen MH, Tenkanen L, Teppo L, et al: Prostate cancer risk and prediagnostic serum 25-hydroxyvitamin D levels (Finland), Cancer Causes Control 11:847–852, 2000.

254. Grant WB: An ecologic study of dietary and solar ultraviolet-B links to breast carcinoma mortality rates, Cancer 94:272–281, 2002.

255. Mason RS, Lissner D, Posen S, et al: Blood concentrations of dihydroxylated vitamin D metabolites after an oral dose, Br Med J 280:449–450, 1980.

256. Bell NH, Stern PH: Hypercalcemia and increases in serum hormone value during prolonged administration of 1alpha,25-dihydroxyvitamin D, N Engl J Med 298:1241–1243, 1978.

257. Maung HM, Elangovan L, Frazao JM, et al: Efficacy and side effects of intermittent intravenous and oral doxercalciferol (1alpha-hydroxyvitamin D(2)) in dialysis patients with secondary hyperparathyroidism: a sequential comparison, Am J Kidney Dis 37:532–543, 2001.

258. Knutson JC, Hollis BW, LeVan LW, et al: Metabolism of 1 alpha-hydroxyvitamin D₂ to activated dihydroxyvitamin D₂ metabolites decreases endogenous 1 alpha,25-dihydroxyvitamin D₃ in rats and monkeys, Endocrinology 136:4749–4753, 1995.

259. Okonofua F, Gill DS, Alabi ZO, et al: Rickets in Nigerian children: a consequence of calcium malnutrition, Metabolism 40:209–213, 1991.

260. Collins N, Maher J, Cole M, et al: A prospective study to evaluate the dose of vitamin D required to correct low 25-hydroxyvitamin D levels, calcium, and alkaline phosphatase in patients at risk of developing antiepileptic drug-induced osteomalacia, Q J Med 78:113–122, 1991.

261. Hosking DJ, Campbell GA, Kemm JR, et al: Safety of treatment for subclinical osteomalacia in the elderly, Br Med J (Clin Res Ed) 289:785–787, 1984.

262. Paterson CR: Vitamin-D poisoning: survey of causes in 21 patients with hypercalcaemia, Lancet 1:1164–1165, 1980.

263. Rizzoli R, Stoermann C, Ammann P, et al: Hypercalcemia and hyperosteolysis in vitamin D intoxication: effects of clodronate therapy, Bone 15:193–198, 1994.

264. Alon US, Levy-Olomucki R, Moore WV, et al: Calcimimetics as an adjuvant treatment for familial hypophosphatemic rickets, Clin J Am Soc Nephrol 3:658–664, 2008.

265. Geller JL, Khosravi A, Kelly MH, et al: Cinacalcet in the management of tumor-induced osteomalacia, J Bone Miner Res 22:931–937, 2007.

266. Driessen GJ, Gerritsen EJ, Fischer A, et al: Long-term outcome of haematopoietic stem cell transplantation in autosomal recessive osteopetrosis: an EBMT report, Bone Marrow Transplant 32:657–663, 2003.

Chapter 16

PAGET'S DISEASE OF BONE

FREDERICK R. SINGER

Paget's disease of bone (osteitis deformans) is a common disorder of a focal nature that is an example of physiology gone awry. The primary disturbance appears to be an exaggeration of osteoclastic bone resorption that initially produces localized loss of bone. Usually, the disorder is not appreciated until secondary bone formation becomes so pronounced that it results in one or more enlarged and deformed bones. The clinical findings depend on which bones are affected and vary from discovery of an incidental radiologic or biochemical abnormality to devastating muscu-loskeletal disabilities with a variety of neurologic and systemic complications. Great progress has been made in our ability to treat this disorder, and knowledge of its pathogenesis is increasing.

Incidence and Epidemiology

Studies of the incidence of Paget's disease are inherently impre-cise because many affected individuals are asymptomatic and have normal serum total alkaline phosphatase levels.[1] On the basis of autopsy studies[2,3] and review of radiographs, the preva-lence of the disease is believed to be 3% or greater in individuals older than 40 years in countries where the disease is common.[4]

A striking feature of the epidemiology of Paget's disease is the great variability in prevalence estimates in different regions of the world and even within a single country. A survey of hospital radiographs in patients older than 55 years in 31 British towns revealed a prevalence of Paget's disease ranging from 2.3% in Aberdeen, Scotland, to 8.3% in Lancaster, England.[5] A similar survey done throughout Europe found that only in France did the prevalence equal the lowest prevalence rates in Britain.[6] Australia, New Zealand, and the United States[7] have a relatively high prevalence, perhaps because of British migration. The disease appears to be rare in Asia. In Japan, the prevalence has been estimated to be 2.8 per million of the population.[8] In most studies, the prevalence of Paget's disease in men slightly exceeds that in women.[2-7] Several studies suggest that the prevalence rate of Paget's disease is decreasing in Britain,[9] New Zealand,[10] and the United States.[11] Whether a decrease in prevalence has occurred or whether an ascertainment bias has been introduced by the use of automated serum chemistry panels about 30 years ago is unclear.

Much emphasis has been placed on the increase in prevalence of Paget's disease with aging. It has been estimated that the prevalence is nearly 10% by the ninth decade.[2-4] Conversely, the disease has rarely been reported in individuals younger than 20 years. Although Paget's disease is most often recognized after age 50 years, it is probably misleading to conclude that the disease is rare in younger individuals. As is discussed later, the obvious manifestations, such as skeletal deformity, probably evolve over decades. Failure to diagnose the earlier phases of the disease is no doubt due to lack of symptoms and minimal use of the radiologic and biochemical tests that would lead to an early diagnosis in younger individuals.

Since 1883, it has been appreciated that Paget's disease may affect more than one member of a family.[12] In large studies, a family history of the disease has been obtained in 12.3% of 788 cases[13] (United States), 13.8% of 407 cases[14] (Great Britain), and 22.8% of 658 cases[15] (Australia). In the former two studies, a 7- to 10-fold increase in Paget's disease was noted in relatives of patients in comparison with control groups. In a small study in Spain in which relatives of patients were screened with bone scans, 40% of patients had at least one first-degree relative with Paget's disease.[16] Examination of the overall pattern of apparent transmission suggests an autosomal dominant mode of inheritance.[12]

The search for potential environmental factors in the pathogenesis of Paget's disease has led to consideration of whether past ownership of dogs might be a risk factor,[17] but this has not been confirmed by subsequent studies. Occupational exposure to lead has been proposed as a possible factor in Paget's disease.[18] In one study, levels of cortical bone lead were higher than those in control subjects, but trabecular bone lead was lower.[19] The relevance of these findings is unknown.

Pathophysiology

Consideration of the radiologic and pathologic evolution of the lesions of Paget's disease strongly suggests that the primary disturbance is localized acceleration of osteoclastic bone resorption. At the interface of normal bone and an advancing lesion, numerous osteoclasts are found in Howship's lacunae in cortical or trabecular bone.[2] Many of the osteoclasts are larger than normal and may have up to 100 nuclei in cross-section rather than the several found in normal osteoclasts.[20] Examination of the ultrastructure of osteoclasts in specimens of Paget's disease reveals a striking and characteristic feature: the presence of microfilaments in the nucleus and, less frequently, in the cytoplasm.[21,22] These structures have not been observed in osteoclasts from normal subjects or in the bone of patients with primary or secondary hyperparathyroidism, osteoporosis, or osteomalacia. They also have not been observed in osteoblasts, osteocytes, or bone marrow cells in the lesions of Paget's disease. The inclusions have been found in a small percentage of the multinucleated giant cells (osteoclasts) in giant cell tumors of bone and in the osteoclasts of some patients with osteopetrosis and pyknodysostosis.[23] The structure of the microfilaments most closely resembles the nucleocapsids of viruses of the Paramyxoviridae family, a group of RNA viruses known to cause common childhood infections. Evidence of Paramyxoviridae nucleocapsid proteins[24,25] and messenger RNA (mRNA)[26,27] has been found in pagetic lesions. The full-length sequence of the measles virus nucleocapsid gene has been sequenced from a pagetic lesion of one patient.[28] The relevance of these findings to the cause of Paget's disease is discussed later.

As osteoclastic resorption progresses in the cortex, individual osteons widen and become confluent with adjacent osteons. The resorptive area thereby may extend to the endosteal and periosteal surfaces. In trabecular bone of the medullary cavities, the osteolytic process results in a marked reduction in bone volume. Associated with both early cortical and trabecular lesions is a remarkable proliferation of fibrous tissue that replaces normal fatty or hematopoietic bone marrow. The fibrous stroma is highly vascular, and although arteriovenous shunts were previously thought to be present, this feature has not been confirmed with radiolabeled albumin microspheres.[29]

The earliest recognizable radiologic feature of Paget's disease is a focal osteolytic lesion. The skull was first appreciated to be affected by circumscribed osteolytic lesions, and Schuller[30] applied the term **osteoporosis circumscripta** to this finding. One or more osteolytic foci may be present, most often in the frontal and occipital regions, and may be observed to coalesce slowly over a period of years (Fig. 16-1). Pure osteolytic lesions also may be detected in other regions of the skeleton, but less frequently. They are seldom observed in the vertebral column or pelvis. In the long bones, osteolytic lesions usually develop at either end of the bone, less often in the diaphysis.[31] Occasionally, osteolytic foci can be observed simultaneously at both ends of a bone. The junction of normal bone and the osteolytic lesion shows a characteristic appearance that is nearly diagnostic of Paget's disease. The edge of the lesion usually assumes the shape of a flame or an inverted V (Fig. 16-2). Serial radiologic follow-up of untreated lesions has documented an average rate of extension of about 1 cm annually.[31] Bone biopsies taken during this earliest phase of Paget's disease not unexpectedly reveal a marked

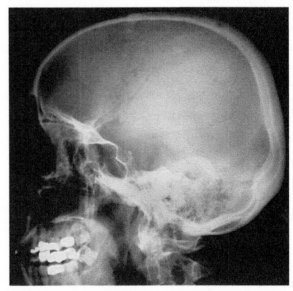

FIGURE 16-1. Radiograph demonstrating osteoporosis circumscripta of the skull affecting the frontal and temporal regions.

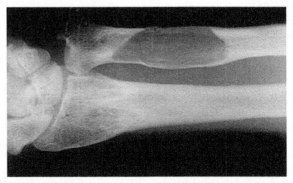

FIGURE 16-2. Radiograph of an osteolytic lesion of Paget's disease that began in the diaphysis of the ulna and exhibits the characteristic flame-shaped or inverted-V extension toward the wrist. Note also the expansile nature of the lesion.

increase in osteoclastic activity and thinning of the trabeculae.[32] Other striking features include a fibrovascular marrow, numerous osteoblasts lining the trabeculae, and prominent woven bone. Thus, a discrepancy is found in the results of radiologic and pathologic examination of an osteolytic lesion. Although focal density is decreased on radiographs, histology demonstrates very active bone formation, but not sufficient to overcome the remarkable degree of osteoclastic bone resorption.

A more commonly observed stage of Paget's disease is the mixed phase, in which osteoblastic (or osteosclerotic) features are intermixed with osteolytic features in an individual bone. This phase is best appreciated in long bones, in which one may observe the advancing osteolytic front adjacent to normal bone and, trailing this front, a heterogeneous region of osteosclerosis superimposed on the region that had previously been dominated by the osteolytic process (Fig. 16-3). Biopsies of the mixed phase reveal a characteristic abnormality of lamellar bone in both cortical and trabecular bone. The matrix is transformed into a bizarre "mosaic" pattern of irregularly juxtaposed pieces of lamellar bone separated by cement lines that have a scalloped outline. The irregularity probably reflects areas of previous osteoclastic resorption. The structure of the involved cortex is so disordered that complete osteons are rare, and the outer and inner circumferential lamellae and the interstitial lamella may be totally disrupted.

The same disordered matrix structure is seen in trabecular bone. Interspersed among the chaotic lamellae are patches of woven bone characterized by a random pattern of deposition of collagen fibers and a larger number of osteocytes per unit area of matrix. It has been suggested that the lacunae surrounding the osteocytes are larger than normal and that this finding represents osteocytic osteolysis.[33] However, it is more likely that the increased size of the periosteocytic lacunae is simply a characteristic of woven bone and not a second type of bone resorption

in Paget's disease. At the surfaces of bone formation, plump osteoblasts are found in great number adjacent to abundant osteoid. This type of bone is seldom found in adults except when associated with rapid remodeling of bone, such as occurs after a fracture or in response to tumor invasion of bone. Studies using quantitative histomorphometry of bone documented the marked degree of cellular activity underlying the dramatic changes in bone structure in Paget's disease.[34] The total amount of osteoid and the percentage of the bone surface covered by osteoid may be increased fourfold to fivefold. The increase in osteoid is not associated with an increase in osteoid seam width because the rate of calcification also is increased, as established by double labeling of bone-forming surfaces with tetracycline. No dynamic means of defining the rate of bone resorption is available, but the extent of the total bone surface exhibiting evidence of bone resorption averages about sixfold that of normal individuals, and the number of osteoclasts may be increased as much as 10-fold. In the medullary cavities, the intense resorptive process may produce hemorrhagic cysts with encircling fibrous marrow containing macrophages filled with hemosiderin. These cysts are believed to result from rupture of multiple dilated vessels and ensuing microinfarctions.[35] In the mixed phase of Paget's disease, not only does patchy sclerosis of bone become apparent on radiography, but a bone also may be enlarged. If the osteolytic process extends to the subperiosteal layer, bone formation may be stimulated to such an extent that the thickness and circumference of the bone are increased as a result of periosteal new bone formation. When the skull is affected, this process can produce as much as a fourfold thickening of the calvarium, as was reported by Paget.[36] A patchy form of sclerosis is often of a "cotton-wool" character (Fig. 16-4). The skull may be so severely affected that platybasia, or basilar impression, may be a complication. Long bones may be shortened, and typically lateral bowing of the femur or anterior bowing of the tibia or both may develop. Later in the course of the disease, the tibia may exhibit severe lateral bowing. The pathogenesis of the slowly progressive deformity is not known but must be related to the state of abnormal remodeling of the bone. Frequently, fissure fractures are associated with the bowing deformity. These fractures are linear transverse radiolucencies that usually are present in the cortex of the convex aspect of the deformed bone. They often are multiple and may remain stable in appearance for years. They can be found in either osteopenic or osteosclerotic cortices and may

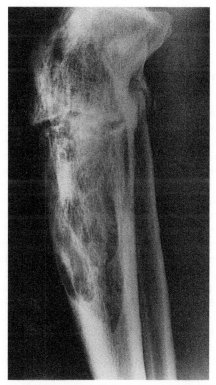

FIGURE 16-3. Radiograph of a tibia exhibiting a distal advancing osteolytic front with proximal sclerotic bone. A partially healed pathologic fracture is present proximally.

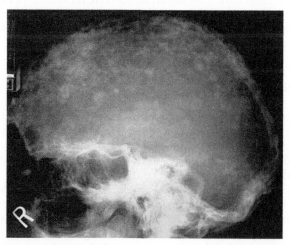

FIGURE 16-4. Radiograph of the sclerotic phase of Paget's disease in the skull exhibiting a "cotton-wool" appearance.

be present even in the absence of deformity. Histologic examination of these lesions suggests that they are incomplete fractures.[2] Only a small percentage of these lesions progress to a complete transverse fracture, which has been seen more often in patients with a sclerotic cortex.

Even after osteosclerotic bone has invaded the previously osteolytic regions of affected bone, evidence of ongoing abnormal bone resorption can be seen in the form of secondary resorption fronts. These secondary fronts are commonly seen as clefts in the cortex of long bones and trail in the path of the primary front.

In the final stage of Paget's disease, termed **osteoblastic** or **sclerotic**, the affected bone remains dense and retains the "mosaic" matrix pattern characteristic of Paget's disease. Tubular bones show a loss of differentiation between cortical and trabecular bone, even with enlargement of the bone as a result of periosteal new bone formation, because the new bone is no longer compact bone. Much less cellular activity is present in sclerotic lesions. Osteoclasts are few or absent, but osteoblasts may still be seen to line bone surfaces. The marrow may remain fibrous, but the numbers of blood vessels are greatly reduced. Scattered chronic inflammatory cells may be present. Occasionally, parts of lesions are totally devoid of bone cells, and for this reason, the concept of "burned-out" Paget's disease has arisen. However, it is very unlikely that extensive lesions of Paget's disease ever achieve an entirely burned-out state. On the contrary, the presence of all stages of the disease in a single bone is much more likely.

The evolution of Paget's disease can also be observed by administration of radioactive tracers and scanning of the entire skeleton or selected regions. Bone scans use technetium-labeled bisphosphonates, which after intravenous injection localize to skeletal sites in proportion to the relative blood flow and the rate of bone formation. The scans usually, but not always, demonstrate high uptake of radioactivity in the areas of the skeleton noted to be radiographically abnormal[37] (Fig. 16-5). In a small proportion of patients, increased uptake may be seen when the radiograph is normal, thus illustrating the great sensitivity of bone scans. On the contrary, a small percentage of sclerotic lesions may not be picked up by a bone scan. These lesions appear to represent areas of inactive disease. Bone scans can be analyzed semiquantitatively or by computer and thus may be used to monitor response to treatment.

Gallium scans, most often used to detect occult infection or tumors, also have been shown to delineate the lesions of Paget's disease.[38] Evidence indicates that tracer gallium is localized to the nuclei of osteoclasts.[39] Therefore, the gallium scan may serve as a direct index of cellular activity in Paget's disease.

Clinical Features

A considerable proportion of individuals with Paget's disease have neither symptoms nor signs of the disease.[1] The disease is accidentally discovered in these cases because of radiologic or biochemical abnormalities uncovered during investigation of another disorder.

The most common clinical problems are pain and deformity. The bone pain of Paget's disease, when present, is seldom severe. Usually it is a dull pain, is located deep below the soft tissues, and often persists during the night. In weight-bearing bone, the pain may be slightly worsened by ambulation, but to a lesser extent than pain originating from the joints or from nerve

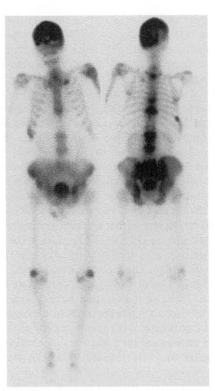

FIGURE 16-5. Anterior and posterior views of a bone scan in a patient with polyostotic Paget's disease. Increased uptake of tracer can be noted in the skull, multiple vertebrae, and the pelvis, areas in which Paget's disease was observed on radiographs. The other abnormal areas probably represent degenerative arthritis and a healed rib fracture.

impingement. Deformity of the skeleton is most often noted in the skull and the lower extremity. Over many years, the hat size of an affected individual may be noted to increase. Bowing and enlargement of the femur and tibia also may evolve over a period of years.

REGIONAL MANIFESTATIONS
The Skull

In the absence of an enlarged cranium, symptoms in the skull are uncommon. Even with an enlarged cranium, symptoms often are absent. Certainly, the most common symptom (30% to 50%) is hearing loss,[40] which is slowly progressive in untreated patients. Vertigo or tinnitus or both are much less common. The main mechanism of hearing loss in Paget's disease has been attributed to a reduction in bone mineral density of the cochlear capsule.[41]

Much more serious complications of Paget's disease may occur in the advanced stage of the disease in a small number of patients. The weight of the skull may be so great that the ability of the patient to keep the head erect is impaired. Muscle spasm may then produce pain in the neck and tension headaches. Neurologic abnormalities may be found in such patients as a consequence of basilar invagination or platybasia. Although they are unusual complications, even in the presence of radiologic evidence of basilar invagination, compression of structures in the posterior fossa or cerebellar tonsillar herniation may produce ataxia, muscle weakness, and impaired respiration. Hydrocephalus also has been noted to be a rare complication and may be manifested by impaired gait, urinary incontinence, and some degree of dementia.

Finally, severe skull disease may be associated with the vague findings of a withdrawn individual who is somnolent and weak. It has been suggested that this manifestation might be a consequence of shunting of blood from the brain vessels to the external carotid artery system, a possible pagetic steal syndrome.[42] These symptoms also could represent a psychological response to disability, inasmuch as nearly 50% of patients in one study have been reported to have depression.[43]

The Jaws

Paget's disease may affect the facial bones and jaws, but such involvement is uncommon. **Leontiasis ossea** is the descriptive term applied to a patient with enlargement of all the facial bones, but such deformity is more likely to be found in fibrous dysplasia.

Involvement of the mandible or maxilla may produce progressive root resorption leading to the loss of teeth.[44] In the more advanced stages of Paget's disease, excessive formation of the cementum is associated with absence of the lamina dura and periodontal membranes. Facial disfigurement may occur from enlargement of the maxilla or mandible or both and is associated with spreading of the teeth and malocclusion. Edentulous patients have difficulty acquiring properly fitting dentures. Oral surgery may be complicated by excessive intraoperative bleeding and postoperative osteomyelitis. Tooth extractions may prove difficult because of ankylosis resulting from hyperplasia of the cementum.

The Spine

Neck pain and back pain are common complaints in an aging population of patients with Paget's disease. Visualization of Paget's disease in one or more vertebrae on radiographic examination often leads clinicians to conclude that they are dealing with bone pain, and treatment is instituted. However, most patients with moderate to severe pain have a complication associated with Paget's disease as the cause of the pain rather than bone pain alone.

Paget's disease affects the lumbar and sacral regions most frequently. One vertebra or many vertebrae may be involved. In the early osteolytic phase, which often is not recognized, the vertebral body appears osteoporotic and, in rare cases, may undergo so much resorption that it takes the shape of a thin transverse rod. Much more often, the vertebral bodies become enlarged overall, with thickened margins and coarse vertical striations centrally. Compression of a sclerotic vertebral body may develop because of the abnormal mechanical properties produced by the chaotic microarchitecture.

Severe pain or impaired neurologic function or both may result from compression of the spinal cord or nerve roots.[45] This complication can arise from enlargement of the vertebral bodies, pedicles, or laminae, as well as from compression fractures. It also has been suggested that shunting of blood may occur from the spinal arteries to the highly vascular bone.[46] Neurologic syndromes are more likely to develop with thoracic involvement. Symptoms include back pain, difficult ambulation, numbness, paresthesias of the feet, and progressive paresis of the legs. Later problems can include impaired bladder and bowel function, as well as spastic paraparesis and loss of sensation. Computed tomography (CT) and magnetic resonance imaging (MRI) are particularly helpful in resolving the anatomic abnormalities producing the disturbed function.

A rare complication in the spine is the development of a discrete paraspinal mass consisting of a central marrow cavity surrounded by pagetic bone that extends from the vertebrae.[47] It may appear that the lesion represents a neoplasm, but careful analysis of prior radiologic studies may reveal the chronic nature of the lesion and may make it unnecessary to perform a biopsy.

The other major causes of back pain in Paget's disease are intervertebral disk disease and degenerative arthritis. No evidence indicates that disk degeneration is more common in patients with Paget's disease, but it has been reported that the pagetic process can invade the disk and produce bony bridging across the disk space.[48] Back pain in the lumbar region is frequently associated with degenerative arthritis,[49] particularly when distortion of the facet joints is associated with Paget's disease. Large osteophytes also may be found in association with enlarged vertebral bodies or where a compression fracture has occurred. A syndrome mimicking ankylosing spondylitis may occur in the presence of extensive osteophyte formation or with ossification of spinal ligaments,[50] but the human leukocyte antigen (HLA)-B27 antigen is absent. However, classic ankylosing spondylitis has been found in association with Paget's disease.[49]

The Pelvis and Extremities

The main symptoms associated with pelvic and lower extremity involvement are pain and impaired ambulation. Pain is seldom a significant symptom in the osteolytic phase of the disease. Hip pain is most common when both the acetabulum and the proximal end of the femur are affected by the sclerotic phase of the disease.[50] Bowing of the femur and protrusio acetabuli are often associated with pain aggravated by weight bearing. Many patients are relatively comfortable when not weight bearing, unlike patients with bone pain, who usually have nocturnal discomfort.

Knee pain and occasionally joint effusions may occur with sclerotic disease affecting the femur or tibia or both. Distortion of the knee joint produced by enlargement of the distal end of the femur or the proximal part of the tibia and severe bowing of either bone can induce mechanical strains on the articular cartilage and thereby accelerate the degenerative process. The pagetic process in subchondral bone also may contribute to joint disease. A similar set of circumstances may account for ankle pain.

Fractures of the lower extremity are more likely to affect the femur than the tibia. In the largest series of reported femoral fractures, the subtrochanteric region was the most common site of fracture (49 of 182), and the rate of nonunion was noted to be 40%, a figure considerably greater than was previously appreciated.[51] Nonunion appears to be less common after tibial fractures.

Involvement of the upper extremity long bones is much less likely to produce symptoms, although deformity may be apparent. At the shoulder, impaired rotator cuff function may be noted when overgrowth of bone leads to anatomic distortion of the glenohumeral joint.

Occasionally, patients who have Paget's disease affecting the foot have pain on weight bearing. Symptoms are seldom encountered in individuals with radiologic evidence of Paget's disease in the hands.

SARCOMA, GIANT CELL TUMORS, AND NONSKELETAL MALIGNANCIES

The most feared complication in Paget's disease is sarcoma. It has been estimated that 10% of patients with extensive disease may experience this problem,[35] but if all affected individuals are considered, the incidence is probably less than 1%.[52] Sarcomas have rarely been reported to develop in multiple members of families with Paget's disease.

Patients in whom sarcomas develop usually have pain and swelling, always in an area previously affected with Paget's disease. Occasionally, fracture at the tumor site may lead to discovery of the neoplasm. Tumors most often arise in the pelvis, femur, humerus, skull, and facial bones.[53] Multifocal sarcomas are found only in patients with advanced and widespread polyostotic disease and are thought to represent tumors of independent origin rather than metastases.[54]

The histology of sarcomas is quite variable. Fibrosarcomas, chondrosarcomas, osteogenic sarcomas, and anaplastic sarcomas may be found.[35] Variable numbers of multinucleated giant cells (probably osteoclasts) may be scattered throughout the tumor stroma and most likely are not neoplastic. The nuclear inclusions typical of Paget's disease have been observed in giant cells but not in the tumor cells.[55] It is not unusual for several histologic patterns to be present in a single tumor, which suggests that a common stem cell may give rise to a variety of better differentiated mesenchymal cells.

Lymphomas and multiple myelomas have been found in association with Paget's disease[52] but probably represent chance occurrence rather than a complication of the pathologic process.

It is difficult to detect early sarcoma formation by radiologic examination because of the underlying distortion of pagetic bone. Because they appear to arise in medullary bone, an early finding may be a subcortical osteolytic lesion. Only when a radiolucent focus with speckled areas of calcification has broken through the confines of the cortex is it apparent that a malignant neoplasm is present. CT or MRI is the best means of determining the extent of the tumor mass.

The rate of change in serum alkaline phosphatase activity has not proved to be a useful marker for the development of sarcomas despite early reports that this might be the case.

The life expectancy for the average patient in whom a sarcoma develops is sadly brief, perhaps because of the difficulty associated with early detection. In one study, only 7.5% of patients survived 5 years, whereas in elderly patients free of underlying Paget's disease, a 37% 5 year survival rate was noted.[56]

Giant cell tumors of bone, which usually follow a benign course and most often are found at the ends of long bones in otherwise normal individuals, may arise in the lesions of Paget's disease.[57] They appear to be much less common than sarcoma in Paget's disease and have frequently been noted to originate in the skull and facial bones. Rarely, these tumors have been reported in multiple family members who have Paget's disease.

These tumors are characterized by spindle-shaped cells with fusiform nuclei and clumped chromatin or nuclei and by scattered multinucleated giant cells. Mitoses are rarely found in either the mononuclear or giant cells. The giant cells contain the nuclear inclusions of Paget's disease, but the stromal cells do not.[57] The opinion has been expressed that many of the reported cases of giant cell tumor in Paget's disease actually represent giant cell reparative granulomas, which are common lesions arising in the jaw.[58]

Surgery and radiation have been used to treat symptomatic giant cell tumors in Paget's disease, and in one patient, high doses of dexamethasone were effective in shrinking an extraskeletal tumor.[59]

Biochemical Features

The intense cellular activity in active lesions of Paget's disease may be reflected in various biochemical markers of bone resorption and bone formation. In most patients who come to clinical attention, biochemical markers do reflect the extent and activity of the disease, although patients with only a small percentage of affected skeleton have no biochemical abnormalities.

INDICES OF BONE RESORPTION

The increased bone resorption typical of active Paget's disease might be expected to produce an increase in serum and urinary calcium levels, but in the absence of fractures or immobilization, hypercalcemia or hypercalciuria is not a prominent feature of Paget's disease.[60] It is generally believed that this finding is explained by a concomitant increase in bone formation that is demonstrable histologically and by kinetic analysis of plasma disappearance rates and skeletal uptake of radiocalcium[60] or other skeletal tracers. A variety of bone collagen matrix breakdown products have been used as indices of bone resorption. These products include urinary hydroxyproline, total and free pyridinoline and deoxypyridinoline, type 1 collagen N-telopeptide, and type 1 collagen C-telopeptide. The telopeptide assays appear to be most specific for bone collagen resorption. Urinary N-telopeptide excretion is sensitive to therapeutic intervention.[61] Measurement of non-isomerized fragments of collagen type 1 C-telopeptide may be the most sensitive means of evaluating bone resorption in patients with Paget's disease.[62]

INDICES OF BONE FORMATION

Since 1929, it has been appreciated that serum total alkaline phosphatase activity may be increased in patients with Paget's disease.[63] The enzyme is localized at the plasma membrane in osteoblasts and may participate in the mineralization of bone matrix. In Paget's disease, enzyme activity in the circulation correlates with the extent of disease on radiographic skeletal surveys,[50] as well as with total urinary hydroxyproline.[50] Effective treatment of Paget's disease reduces total alkaline phosphatase activity by 50% or more.[61]

During long-term follow-up of untreated patients with Paget's disease, alkaline phosphatase activity usually exhibits a gradual increase or no significant change.[64] In some patients, major fluctuations may represent technical errors rather than changes in disease activity. In the presence of liver disease, hepatic alkaline phosphatase activity may interfere with an accurate assessment of Paget's disease activity. In such patients, measurement of bone-specific alkaline phosphatase levels by immunoassay is preferable.[65]

Serum osteocalcin or bone Gla protein is a nearly specific product of osteoblasts that may be elevated in Paget's disease, but not to the same degree as serum alkaline phosphatase activity.[66] Paradoxically, treatment of patients with drugs that reduce turnover may produce a transient increase in osteocalcin levels.[66] A potential explanation for these observations is that osteocalcin gene expression is reduced in active Paget's disease.[67]

Serum levels of procollagen type 1 N-terminal peptide correlate significantly with quantitative bone scintigraphy and decline with treatment of Paget's disease to a greater extent than bone-specific alkaline phosphatase.[61]

Because of the cost-effectiveness of the serum total alkaline phosphatase assay, this remains as a reasonable choice for assessment of the average patient with Paget's disease.

CALCIOTROPIC HORMONES

Calcitonin secretion is normal in patients with Paget's disease.[68] Parathyroid hormone concentrations generally are within the normal range, but in subsets of patients, elevated concentrations have been found.[69,70] This observation could be related to renal failure, vitamin D deficiency, or subtle hypocalcemia related to a higher rate of bone formation than bone resorption.

Patients with adequate vitamin D intake or sufficient ultraviolet light exposure or both have normal 25-hydroxyvitamin D and 1,25-dihydroxyvitamin D levels. In two studies, serum 24,25-dihydroxyvitamin D was reported to be low and to correlate inversely with disease activity.[71,72] The pathogenesis and clinical relevance of this finding are unknown.

Interleukin-6, an important local modulator of osteoclast function, has been reported to be elevated in the bone marrow of patients with Paget's disease[73] and in serum by some[73-75] but not all investigators.[76] Receptor activator of nuclear factor-κ beta ligand (RANK-L) and osteoprotegerin (OPG), a decoy receptor for RANK-L, are key modulators of osteoclast function. Serum measurements in patients with Paget's disease have also been variable, but a recent study indicates that both RANK-L and OPG levels may be highly elevated, and that bisphosphonate therapy can increase OPG and to a lesser extent reduce RANK-L levels, thereby reducing the RANK-L/OPG ratio.[77]

Systemic Complications and Associated Diseases

HYPERCALCIURIA, HYPERCALCEMIA, AND PRIMARY HYPERPARATHYROIDISM

Urinary calcium excretion is usually normal in patients with Paget's disease, and no compelling evidence has been presented that renal stone formation is increased over that in an age- and sex-matched control groups.[60] However, hypercalciuria is readily provoked by immobilization after fracture[78] or neurologic injury. In this setting, bone resorption increases while bone formation decreases.

Hypercalcemia is uncommon in patients with Paget's disease but may occur as a consequence of immobilization,[78] malignancy,[79] or primary hyperparathyroidism.[80] Despite some discussion that an increased incidence of primary hyperparathyroidism may occur in Paget's disease, the presence of both diseases in one individual is very likely coincidental.

HYPERURICEMIA AND GOUT

Serum uric acid concentrations have been reported to be elevated primarily in men with relatively severe Paget's disease.[50] Nearly half of the hyperuricemic men had clinical episodes of gouty arthritis. Paget's disease also was found to be present in 23% of a group of patients with gout.[81] It is possible that a high turnover of nucleic acids in the lesions of Paget's disease could increase the urate pool sufficiently to account for these observations.[82]

CARDIOVASCULAR ABNORMALITIES

Increased cardiac output has been found to be present in patients who have at least 15% of their skeleton affected by Paget's disease.[83] This abnormality is often associated with left ventricular hypertrophy. The excessive vascularity of the soft tissue and adjacent pagetic bone must be factors contributing to these phenomena. In addition, a reduction in peripheral vascular resistance may lead to increased cardiac output.[84] High-output cardiac failure may occur but seems to be unusual.

Calcific aortic stenosis appears to be four to six times more common in patients with Paget's disease than in a control population.[85,86] It is more likely to be found in patients with severe disease, which suggests that increased cardiac output producing turbulence across the valve may induce calcification. Intracardiac calcification also may occur in the interventricular septum and may produce a complete heart block.[86,87]

Drug Treatment

INDICATIONS FOR TREATMENT

Indications for drug treatment of Paget's disease are listed in Table 16-1. Perhaps the most common reason for treatment is bone pain. When Paget's disease occurs adjacent to a joint, it may be difficult to distinguish bone pain from joint pain. In such cases, a therapeutic trial of drug therapy for 1 to 2 months may be particularly useful in clarifying the origin of the pain. Pretreatment of patients who require elective orthopedic surgery may prevent complications such as intraoperative or postoperative hemorrhage and immobilization hypercalcemia. Hypercalciuria and hypercalcemia can be reversed or prevented by drug treatment, but these indications are uncommon.

Some patients with neurologic deficits associated with vertebral disease may experience dramatic remission of their signs and symptoms. Although hearing loss is seldom reversed, preservation of auditory acuity is expected. Reduction of disease activity produces a decrease in cardiac output. It is possible that early treatment could prevent future complications such as skeletal deformity, but no long-term randomized clinical trials have been conducted.

Certainly, many patients do not need to be treated. The decision to treat must take into consideration the present symptoms, the likelihood of future complications, the cost of therapy, and the mode of administration.

PRETREATMENT LABORATORY EVALUATION

Measurement of serum total alkaline phosphatase activity in a reliable laboratory is probably the only biochemical test needed in most patients. Radiographs of known lesions of Paget's disease should be performed to ensure awareness of osteolytic lesions. In patients whose extent of disease is unknown, a bone scan is the best means of defining the regions of the skeleton requiring radiographic evaluation.

CALCITONIN

Salmon calcitonin was introduced into clinical use in the United States in 1975. This peptide hormone binds to calcitonin recep-

Table 16-1. Indications for Drug Treatment in Paget's Disease

Treatment of high-output congestive heart failure
Bone pain
Preparation for orthopedic surgery
Hypercalciuria
Hypercalcemia
Neurologic deficit from vertebral disease
Prevention of hearing loss
Prevention of complications in young patients

tors on osteoclasts and rapidly inhibits bone resorption in vivo and in vitro. Salmon calcitonin, 50 to 100 U subcutaneously, 3 to 7 times per week, relieves bone pain in a high percentage of patients within 2 to 6 weeks, reduces cardiac output and vascularity of affected bones, reverses some neurologic deficits, and stabilizes hearing deficits.[88] Patients treated preoperatively may have less hemorrhage from orthopedic procedures.[89] An immediate decrease in bone resorption parameters is followed by a decrease in alkaline phosphatase activity in 1 month. Both types of parameters decrease by 50% in 3 to 6 months and return toward baseline months after treatment is stopped.

In patients with radiologically defined osteolytic lesions, restoration of a more normal bone structure occurs after long-term treatment.[90] However, treatment must be continued indefinitely, or the osteolytic focus will recur. Bone scans[91] and gallium scans[38] show reduced activity of the pagetic lesions after long-term treatment. Reduced disease activity also is manifested in bone biopsies by a reduction in the number of bone cells, as well as by a decrease in the extent of woven bone and marrow fibrosis.[92]

As many as 26% of patients administered salmon calcitonin exhibit loss of biochemical responsiveness after an initial period of biochemical improvement.[88] Nearly all these patients have high titers of antibodies specific to salmon calcitonin in the circulation. These patients can be treated successfully with any of the bisphosphonates.

Salmon calcitonin may cause a variety of side effects.[88] The most common are nausea and facial flushing (10% to 20%). Less commonly, vomiting, abdominal pain, diarrhea, and polyuria may occur. Tetany and allergic reactions are very rare. Side effects are less common with a nasal spray mode of administration, but efficacy is reduced. Salmon calcitonin is now seldom used because of the availability of potent bisphosphonates.

BISPHOSPHONATES

Bisphosphonates are analogues of inorganic pyrophosphate, a compound thought to participate in the mineralization of bone. By substituting a P-C-P bond for the naturally occurring P-O-P bond, a family of metabolically stable compounds has been produced that bind to hydroxyapatite and inhibit bone resorption and, secondarily, bone formation in experimental animals and humans. The earliest bisphosphonates, such as etidronate, induce osteoclast apoptosis by producing nonhydrolyzable analogues of adenosine triphosphate, whereas the more potent aminobisphosphonates inhibit farnesyl-diphosphate (FPP) synthase in the mevalonate pathway, which produces osteoclast apoptosis by inhibition of protein prenylation.[93]

Four oral bisphosphonates taken daily are etidronate[94] (5 mg/kg body weight for 6 months), alendronate[95] (40 mg for 6 months), tiludronate[96] (400 mg for 3 months), and risedronate[97] (30 mg for 2 months). Pamidronate is available in intravenous form and is commonly infused once over a period of several hours at a dose of 60 mg for patients with less than fivefold elevations of serum total alkaline phosphatase activity[98] and at an intermittent dose of 60 or 90 mg on 2 or more days, depending on the level of alkaline phosphatase and the response to each infusion. Zoledronic acid, the most recently approved agent, is administered as a 5 mg dose intravenously over 15 minutes.[99] Risedronate and the intravenous biphosphonates are probably the most common treatments used in the United States.

The bisphosphonates taken orally must be ingested with water only on an empty stomach because they are poorly absorbed. Generally, side effects are not a major problem and, when present, include abdominal distress, diarrhea, and a temporary increase in bone pain. Patients who receive pamidronate or zoledronic acid intravenously may experience fever and myalgias for about 24 hours. This side effect seldom occurs with subsequent infusions. Allergic reactions are rare and most often are inflammatory eye reactions associated with pamidronate use. Etidronate is the only bisphosphonate reported to produce significant osteomalacia, usually at a dose greater than 5 mg/kg body weight daily. Renal toxicity is not observed with intravenous zoledronic acid if the drug is infused as approved and the creatinine clearance is 35 cc/min or higher.[100] Osteonecrosis of the jaw, an unusual event in cancer patients treated monthly with intravenous bisphosphonates, is extremely uncommon in patients with Paget's disease or osteoporosis.[101]

The potent aminobisphosphonates can induce biochemical remissions in the great majority of patients with mild to moderate disease activity. Only zoledronic acid can consistently normalize biochemical parameters in the most severely affected patients,[99] and the response can persist for at least 2 years.[102] It remains to be seen whether long-term biochemical suppression, an achievable goal in most patients, can reduce the incidence of complications in patients who are most at risk. These individuals include those with skull, vertebral, pelvic, and lower extremity involvement.

Treatment and Posttreatment Laboratory Evaluation

For most patients, measurement of total serum alkaline phosphatase activity is sufficient to determine the success of treatment. In patients with known osteolytic lesions on radiologic examination, an annual evaluation should be adequate.

Surgery

Certainly, the benefits of surgery for the appropriate indications in patients with Paget's disease outweigh the potential complications of excessive hemorrhage and impaired healing. Probably the most common reason for orthopedic surgery is total hip replacement.[103] The rate of success in relieving intractable hip pain and improving mobility is excellent. Heterotopic ossification may be somewhat more common postoperatively but is seldom a major problem. Total knee replacement also is now achieving good clinical results.[104] Tibial and fibular osteotomies to correct varus deformity of the tibia are impressive in relieving knee and ankle pain associated with marked deformity.[89] Because the rate of nonunion is relatively high in femoral fractures, open reduction and fixation of these fractures may prove necessary.

Much less commonly required are suboccipital craniectomy and upper cervical vertebral laminectomy in patients with symptomatic basilar impression. Equally uncommon is the need for ventricular shunting in patients with hydrocephalus. Attempted relief of hearing loss in patients with skull loss by stapes mobilization or stapedectomy has been of questionable benefit. Surgery to correct spinal stenosis or nerve root compression has generally been successful.[4]

Causes

GENETICS

In 2002, a mutation in the sequestosome 1 (SQSTM1) gene on chromosome 5 was reported in 11 of 24 French-Canadian families with Paget's disease and in 18 of 112 patients with apparently sporadic disease (see Chapter 12).[105] This was confirmed in different countries by the finding of at least 14 mutations of this gene.[106] The mutations are mainly clustered around the ubiquitin-binding domain of the SQSTM1 protein. The SQSTM1 protein modulates activity of the nuclear factor kappa B (NF-κB) pathway, an important mediator of osteoclast function. It appears unlikely that mutations of this gene entirely account for a pagetic phenotype, because some of the family members of these pedigrees exhibit no evidence of Paget's disease, yet harbor one of the mutations.[106-108] It is unclear what role SQSTM1 mutations play in patients with sporadic disease, given the uncertainty of defining sporadic cases and the absence of these mutations as recently reported in 23 apparently sporadic cases.[109] Because SQSTM1 mutations are found in only about 20% of Paget's disease pedigrees, other genetic mutations have been sought. Linkage analyses suggest that chromosome 10p13 harbors a major locus in patients of British ancestry.[110]

A rare syndrome of Paget's disease, inclusion body myositis and frontotemporal dementia, also has a genetic association. Mutations in valosine-containing protein are found in this syndrome.[111] This protein also contains a ubiquitin-binding domain. Several rare heritable osteolytic disorders superficially resemble Paget's disease.[112] These are caused by mutations that affect RANK or OPG.

SLOW VIRUS INFECTION

The presence of osteoclast nuclear and cytoplasmic microfilaments essentially identical in structure to nucleocapsids of the Paramyxoviridae virus family initially suggested the possibility that Paget's disease was caused by a slow virus infection.[21,22] Subsequent immunochemical studies[24,25] and sequence analysis of nucleocapsid transcripts[26-28] have added support to the hypothesis, although not all studies have been positive for a viral presence.[113,114]

The most compelling evidence to support a viral role in Paget's disease comes from studies in transgenic mice in which bone histology typical of the disease was induced by inserting the measles virus nucleocapsid gene into precursor cells of the osteoclast lineage.[115] In a separate study of transgenic mice, insertion of a mutated murine SQSTM1 gene into the endogenous mouse SQSTM1 gene increased the osteoclastogenic potential of the bone microenvironment but produced no histologic evidence of Paget's disease.[116]

The findings of clinical studies combined with those of recent studies designed to develop an animal model of Paget's disease continue to support the viral hypothesis of Paget's disease. Integration of genetic and viral interactions may produce a greater understanding of the causes of the disease.

REFERENCES

1. Eekhoff EMW, van der Klift M, Kroon HM, et al: Paget's disease of bone in the Netherlands: a population-based radiological and biochemical survey; the Rotterdam study, J Bone Miner Res 19:566–570, 2004.
2. Schmorl G: Über Osteitis deformans Paget, Virchows Arch 283:694–751, 1932.
3. Collins DH: Paget's disease of bone: incidence and subclinical forms, Lancet 2:51–57, 1956.
4. Pygott F: Paget's disease of bone: The radiological incidence, Lancet 1:1170–1171, 1956.
5. Barker DJP, Chamberlain AT, Guyer PB, et al: Paget's disease of bone: the Lancashire focus, Br Med J 1:1105–1107, 1980.
6. Detheridge FM, Guyer PB, Barker DJP: European distribution of Paget's disease of bone, Br Med J 285:1005–1008, 1982.
7. Altman RD, Bloch DA, Hochberg MC, et al: Prevalence of pelvic Paget's disease of bone in the United States, J Bone Miner Res 15:461–465, 2000.
8. Hashimoto J, Ohno I, Nkatsuka K, et al: Prevalence and clinical features of Paget's disease of bone in Japan, J Bone Miner Metab 24:186–190, 2006.
9. Cooper C, Harvey NC, Dennison E, et al: Update on the epidemiology of Paget's disease of bone, J Bone Miner Res 21(Suppl 2):P3–8, 2006.
10. Cundy T: Is the prevalence of Paget's disease of bone decreasing? J Bone Miner Res 21(Suppl 2):P9–13, 2006.
11. Tiegs RD, Lohse CM, Wollan PC, et al: Long-term trends in the incidence of Paget's disease of bone, Bone 27:423–427, 2000.
12. McKusick VA: Heritable Disorders of Connective Tissue, St. Louis, 1972, Mosby.
13. Siris ES, Ottman R, Flaster E, et al: Familial aggregation of Paget's disease of bone, J Bone Miner Res 6:495–500, 1991.
14. Sofoer JA, Holloway SM, Emery AEH: A family study of Paget's disease of bone, J Epidemiol Community Health 37:226–231, 1983.
15. Posen S: Paget's disease: current concepts, Aust N Z J Surg 62:17–23, 1992.
16. Morales-Piga AA, Rey-Rey JS, Corres-Gonzales J, et al: Frequency and characteristics of familial aggregation of Paget's disease of bone, J Bone Miner Res 10:663–670, 1995.

17. O'Driscoll JB, Anderson DC: Past pets and Paget's disease, Lancet 2:919–921, 1985.
18. Spencer H, O'Sullivan V, Sontag SJ: Does lead play a role in Paget's disease of bone? A hypothesis, J Lab Clin Med 120:798–800, 1992.
19. Adachi JD, Arlen D, Webber CE, et al: Is there any association between the presence of bone disease and cumulative exposure to lead? Calcif Tissue Int 63:429–432, 1998.
20. Rubinstein MA, Smelin A, Freedman AL: Osteoblasts and osteoclasts in bone marrow aspiration, Arch Intern Med 92:684–696, 1953.
21. Rebel A, Malkani K, Basle M: Anomalies nucleaires de la maladie osseuse de Paget, Nouv Presse Med 3:1299–1301, 1974.
22. Mills BG, Singer FR: Nuclear inclusions in Paget's disease of bone, Science 194:201–202, 1976.
23. Singer FR: Paget's disease of bone: possible viral basis, Trends Endocrinol Metab 7:258–261, 1996.
24. Rebel A, Basle M, Pouplard A, et al: Viral antigens in osteoclasts from Paget's disease of bone, Lancet 2:344–346, 1980.
25. Mills BG, Singer FR, Weiner LP, et al: Evidence for both respiratory syncytial virus and measles virus antigens in the osteoclasts of patients with Paget's disease of bone, Clin Orthop 183:303–311, 1984.
26. Basle MF, Fournier JG, Rozenblatt S, et al: Measles virus RNA detected in Paget's disease bone tissue by in situ hybridization, J Gen Virol 67:907–913, 1986.
27. Gordon MT, Sharpe PT, Anderson DC: Canine distemper virus localised in bone cells of patients with Paget's disease, Bone 12:195–201, 1991.
28. Friedrichs WE, Reddy SV, Bruder JM, et al: Sequence analysis of measles virus nucleocapsid transcripts in patients with Paget's disease, J Bone Miner Res 17:145–151, 2002
29. Rhodes BA, Greyson ND, Hamilton CR Jr, et al: Absence of anatomic arteriovenous shunts in Paget's disease of bone, N Engl J Med 287:686–689, 1972.
30. Schuller A: Ueber circumscripte Osteoporose des Schädels, Med Klin 25:631–632, 1929.
31. Maldague B, Malghem J: Dynamic radiologic patterns of Paget's disease of bone, Clin Orthop 217:126–151, 1987.

32. Jacobs P: Osteolytic Paget's disease, Clin Radiol 25:137–144, 1974.
33. Belanger LF, Jarry L, Uhthoff HK: Osteocytic osteolysis in Paget's disease, Rev Can Biol 27:37–44, 1968.
34. Meunier PJ, Coindre JM, Edouard CM, et al: Bone histomorphometry in Paget's disease: quantitative and dynamic analysis of pagetic and non-pagetic bone tissue, Arthritis Rheum 23:1095–1103, 1980.
35. Jaffe HL: Metabolic, Degenerative and Inflammatory Diseases of Bones and Joints, Philadelphia, 1972, Lea & Febiger.
36. Paget J: On a form of chronic inflammation of bones (osteitis deformans), Med Chir Trans 60:37–64, 1877.
37. Vellenga CJLR, Bijuoet OLM, Pauwels EKJ: Bone scintigraphy and radiology in Paget's disease of bone: a review, Am J Physiol 3:154–168, 1988.
38. Waxman AD, McKee D, Siemsen JK, et al: Gallium scanning in Paget's disease of bone: effect of calcitonin, Am J Roentgenol 134:303–306, 1980.
39. Mills BG, Masuoka LS, Graham CC Jr, et al: Gallium-67 citrate localization in osteoclast nuclei of Paget's disease of bone, J Nucl Med 29:1083–1087, 1988.
40. Nager GT: Paget's disease of the temporal bone, Ann Otol Rhinol Laryngol 84(Suppl 22):1–32, 1975.
41. Monsell EM, Cody DD, Bone HG, et al: Hearing loss in Paget's disease of bone: the relationship between pure tone thresholds and mineral density of the cochlear capsule, Hearing Res 83:114–120, 1995.
42. Blotman F, Blard J-M, Labauge R, et al: Exploration ultrasonique de la circulation encephalique chez le Pagetique, Rev Rhum 42:647–651, 1975.
43. Gold DT, Boisture J, Shipp KM, et al: Paget's disease of bone and quality of life, J Bone Miner Res 11:1897–1904, 1996.
44. Smith NHH: Monostotic Paget's disease of the mandible presenting with progressive resorption of the teeth, Oral Surg Oral Med Oral Pathol 46:246–253, 1978.
45. Hadjipavlou A, Lander P: Paget's disease of the spine, J Bone Joint Surg Am 73:1376–1381, 1991.
46. Douglas DL, Duckworth T, Kanis JA, et al: Spinal cord dysfunction in Paget's disease of bone, J Bone Joint Surg Br 63:495–503, 1981.
47. Samuels MA, Schiller AL: Case records of the Massachusetts General Hospital, N Engl J Med 304:1411–1421, 1981.

48. Lander P, Hadjipavlou A: Intradiscal invasion of Paget's disease of the spine, Spine 16:46–51, 1991.

49. Altman RD, Collins B: Musculoskeletal manifestations of Paget's disease of bone, Arthritis Rheum 23:1121–1127, 1980.

50. Franck WA, Bress NM, Singer FR, et al: Rheumatic manifestations of Paget's disease of bone, Am J Med 56:592–603, 1974.

51. Dove J: Complete fractures of the femur in Paget's disease of bone, J Bone Joint Surg Br 62:12–17, 1980.

52. Hadjipavlou A, Lander P, Srolovitz H, et al: Malignant transformation in Paget disease of bone, Cancer 70:2802–2808, 1992.

53. Haibach H, Farrell C, Dittrich BS: Neoplasms arising in Paget's disease of bone: a study of 82 cases, Am J Clin Pathol 83:594–601, 1985.

54. Choquette D, Haraoui B, Altman RD, et al: Simultaneous multifocal sarcomatous degeneration in Paget's disease of bone, Clin Orthop 179:308–311, 1983.

55. Seret P, Basle MF, Rebel A, et al: Sarcomatous degeneration in Paget's bone disease, J Cancer Res Clin Oncol 113:392–399, 1987.

56. Huvos AG: Osteogenic sarcoma of bones and soft tissues in older persons, Cancer 57:1442–1449, 1986.

57. Singer FR, Mills BG: Giant cell tumor in Paget's disease of bone: recurrence after 36 years, Clin Orthop 293:293–301, 1993.

58. Upchurch KS, Simon LS, Schiller AL, et al: Giant cell reparative granuloma of Paget's disease of bone: a unique clinical entity, Ann Intern Med 98:35–40, 1983.

59. Ziambaras K, Totty WA, Teitelbaum SL, et al: Extraskeletal osteoclastomas responsive to dexamethasone treatment in Paget bone disease, J Clin Endocrinol Metab 82:3826–3834, 1997.

60. Nagant de Deuxchaisnes CN, Krane SM: Paget's disease of bone: clinical and metabolic observations, Medicine (Baltimore) 43:233–266, 1964.

61. Alvarez L, Guanabens N, Peris P, et al: Usefulness of biochemical markers of bone turnover in assessing response to the treatment of Paget's disease, Bone 29:447–452, 2001.

62. Alexandersen P, Peris P, Guanabens N, et al: Non-isomerized C-telopeptide fragments are highly sensitive markers for monitoring disease activity and treatment efficacy in Paget's disease of bone, J Bone Miner Res 20:588–595, 2005.

63. Kay HD: Plasma phosphatase in osteitis deformans and in other disease of bone, Br J Exp Pathol 10:253–256, 1929.

64. Woodard HQ: Long term studies of the blood chemistry in Paget's disease of bone, Cancer 12:1226–1237, 1959.

65. Panigrahi K, Delmas PD, Singer F, et al: Characteristics of a two-site immunoradiometric assay for human skeletal alkaline phosphatase in serum, Clin Chem 40:822–828, 1994.

66. Papapoulos SE, Frolich M, Mudde AH, et al: Serum osteocalcin in Paget's disease of bone: basal concentrations and response to bisphosphonate treatment, J Clin Endocrinol Metab 65:189–194, 1987.

67. Naot D, Bava U, Matthews B, et al: Differential gene expression in cultured osteoblasts and bone marrow stromal cells from patients with Paget's disease of bone, J Bone Miner Res 22:298–309, 2007.

68. Kanis JA, Heynen G, Walton RJ: Plasma calcitonin in Paget's disease of bone, Clin Sci 52:329–332, 1977.

69. Chapuy M-C, Zucchelli P, Meunier PJ: Parathyroid function in Paget's disease of bone, Bone Miner Electrolyte Metab 6:112–118, 1981.

70. Siris ES, Clemens TP, McMahon D, et al: Parathyroid function in Paget's disease of bone, J Bone Miner Res 4:75–79, 1989.

71. Guillard-Cumming DF, Beard DJ, Douglas DL, et al: Abnormal vitamin D metabolism in Paget's disease of bone, Clin Endocrinol 22:559–566, 1985.

72. Castro-Errecaborde N, de la Piedra C, Rapado A, et al: Correlation between serum osteocalcin and 24,25-dihydroxyvitamin D levels in Paget's disease of bone, J Clin Endocrinol Metab 72:462–466, 1991.

73. Roodman GD, Kurihara N, Ohsaki Y, et al: Interleukin 6: a potential autocrine/paracrine factor in Paget's disease of bone, J Clin Invest 89:46–52, 1992.

74. Schweitzer DH, Oostendorp-Van de Ruit M, van der Plujim G, et al: Interleukin-6 and the acute phase response during treatment of Paget's disease with the nitrogen-containing bisphosphonate dimethylamino-hydroxypropylidene bisphosphonate, J Bone Miner Res 10:956–962, 1995.

75. Rendina D, Postiglione L, Vuotto P, et al: Clodronate treatment reduces serum levels of interleukin-6 soluble receptor in Paget's disease of bone, Clin Exp Rheumatol 20:359–364, 2002.

76. Neale SD, Schulze E, Smith R, et al: The influence of serum cytokines and growth factors on osteoclast formation in Paget's disease, Q J Med 95:233–240, 2002.

77. Martini G, Gennari, L, Merlotti D, et al: Serum OPG and RANKL levels before and after intravenous bisphosphonate treatment in Paget's disease of bone, Bone 40:457–463, 2007.

78. Reifenstein EC Jr, Albright F: Paget's disease: its pathologic physiology and the importance of this in the complications arising from fracture and immobilization, N Engl J Med 231:343–355, 1944.

79. Rosenkrantz JA, Gluckman EC: Coexistence of Paget's disease of bone and multiple myeloma, Am J Roentgenol 78:30–38, 1957.

80. Gutteridge DH, Gruber HE, Kermode DG, et al: Thirty cases of concurrent Paget's disease and primary hyperparathyroidism: sex distribution, histomorphometry, and prediction of the skeletal response to parathyroidectomy, Calcif Tissue Int 65:427–435, 1999.

81. Lluberas-Acosta G, Hansell JR, Schumacher HR Jr: Paget's disease of bone in patients with gout, Arch Intern Med 146:2389–2392, 1986.

82. Fennelly JJ, Hogan A: Pseudouridine excretion: a reflection of high RNA turnover in Paget's disease, Ir J Med Sci 141:103–107, 1972.

83. Arnalich F, Plaza I, Sobrino JA, et al: Cardiac size and function in Paget's disease of bone, Int J Cardiol 5:491–505, 1984.

84. Morales-Piga AA, Moya JL, Bachiller FJ, et al: Assessment of cardiac function by echocardiography in Paget's disease of bone, Clin Exp Rheumatol 18:31–37, 2000.

85. Strickberger SA, Schulman SP, Hutchins GM: Association of Paget's disease of bone with calcific aortic valve disease, Am J Med 82:953–956, 1987.

86. Hultgren HN: Osteitis deformans (Paget's disease) and calcific disease of the heart valves, Am J Cardiol 81:1461–1464, 1998.

87. Harrison CV, Lennox B: Heart block in osteitis deformans, Br Heart J 10:167–176, 1948.

88. Waxman AD, Ducker S, McKee D, et al: Evaluation of ^{99m}Tc diphosphonate kinetics and bone scans in patients with Paget's disease before and after calcitonin treatment, Radiology 125:761–764, 1977.

89. Meyers M, Singer F: Osteotomy for tibia vara in Paget's disease under cover of calcitonin, J Bone Joint Surg Am 60:810–814, 1978.

90. Nagant de Deuxchaisnes C, Maldague B, Malghem J, et al: The action of the main therapeutic regimes on Paget's disease of bone with a note on the effect of vitamin D deficiency, Arthritis Rheum 23:1215–1234, 1980.

91. Waxman AD, Ducker S, McKee D: Paget's disease of bone. In Avioli LV, Krane SM, editors: Metabolic Bone Disease and Clinically Related Disorders, San Diego, 1998, Academic Press, pp 545–605.

92. Fornasier VL, Stapleton K, Williams CC: Histologic changes in Paget's disease treated with calcitonin, Hum Pathol 9:455–461, 1978.

93. Rogers MJ: New insights into the molecular mechanisms of action of bisphosphonates, Curr Pharm Des 9:2643–2658, 2003.

94. Khairi MRA, Altman RD, DeRosa GP, et al: Sodium etidronate in the treatment of Paget's disease of bone: a study of long-term results, Ann Intern Med 87:656–663, 1977.

95. Siris E, Weinstein RS, Altman R, et al: Comparative study of alendronate versus etidronate for the treatment of Paget's disease of bone, J Clin Endocrinol Metab 81:961–967, 1996.

96. Reginster JY, Calson F, Morlock G, et al: Efficacy and safety of oral tiludronate in Paget's disease of bone: a double-blind, multiple-dosage, placebo-controlled study, Arthritis Rheum 35:967–974, 1992.

97. Siris ES, Chines AA, Altman RD, et al: Risedronate in the treatment of Paget's disease of bone: an open label multicenter study, J Bone Miner Res 13:1032–1038, 1998.

98. Thiebaud D, Jaeger P, Gobelet C, et al: A single infusion of the bisphosphonate AHPrBP (APD) as treatment of Paget's disease of bone, Am J Med 85:207–212, 1988.

99. Reid IR, Miller P, Lyles K, et al: Comparison of a single infusion of zoledronic acid with risedronate for Paget's disease, N Engl J Med 353:898–908, 2005.

100. Boonen S, Sellmayer DE, Lippuner K, et al: Renal safety of annual zoledronic acid infusions in osteoporotic postmenopausal women, Kidney Int 74:641–648, 2008.

101. Rizzoli R, Burlet N, Cahall D, et al: Osteonecrosis of the jaw and bisphophonate treatment for osteoporosis, Bone 42:841–847, 2008.

102. Hosking D, Lyles K, Brown JP, et al: Long-term control of bone turnover in Paget's disease with zoledronic acid and risedronate, J Bone Miner Res 22:142–148, 2007.

103. Sochart DH, Porter ML: Charnley low-friction arthroplasty for Paget's disease of the hip, J Arthroplasty 15:210–219, 2000.

104. Lee GC, Sanchez-Sotelo J, Berry DJ: Total knee arthroplasty in patients with Paget's disease at the knee, J Arthroplasty 20:689–693, 2005.

105. Laurin N, Brown JP, Morissette J, et al: Recurrent mutation of the gene encoding sequestosome 1 (SQSTM1/p62) in Paget's disease of bone, Am J Hum Genet 70:1582–1588, 2002.

106. Morissette J, Laurin N, Brown JP: Sequestosome 1: mutation frequencies, haplotypes, and phenotypes in familial Paget's disease of bone, J Bone Miner Res 21(Suppl 2):P38–44, 2006.

107. Johnson-Pais TL, Wisdom JH, Weldon KS, et al: Three novel mutations in SQSTM1 identified in familial Paget's disease of bone, J Bone Miner Res 18:1748–1753, 2003.

108. Bolland MJ, Tong PC, Naot D, et al: Delayed development of Paget's disease in offspring inheriting SQSTM 1 mutations, J Bone Miner Res 22:411–415, 2007.

109. Matthews BG, Naot D, Bavra U, et al: Absence of somatic SQTM1 mutations in Paget's disease of bone, J Clin Endocrinol Metab 94:691–694, 2009.

110. Lucas GJ, Riches PL, Hocking LJ, et al: Identification of a major locus for Paget's disease on chromosome 10p13 in families of British descent, J Bone Miner Res 23:58–63, 2008.

111. Watts GDJ, Wymer J, Kovach MJ, et al: Inclusion body myositis associated with Paget disease of bone and frontotemporal dementia is caused by a mutant valosin-containing protein, Nat Genet 36:377–381, 2004.

112. Ralston SH: Juvenile Paget's disease, familial expansile osteolysis and other genetic osteolytic disorders, Best Pract Res Clin Rheumatol 22:101–111, 2008.

113. Helfrich MH, Hobson RP, Grabowski PS, et al: A negative search for a paramyxoviral etiology of Paget's disease of bone: molecular, immunological, and ultrastructural studies in UK patients, J Bone Miner Res 15:2315–2329, 2000.

114. Matthews BG, Afzal MA, Minor PD, et al: Failure to detect measles virus ribonucleic acid in bone cells from patients with Paget's disease, J Clin Endocrinol Metab 93:1398–1401, 2008.

115. Kurihara N, Zhou H, Reddy SV, et al: Expression of measles virus nucleocapsid protein in osteoclasts induces Paget's disease–like bone lesions in mice, J Bone Miner Res 21:446–455, 2006.

116. Hiruma Y, Kurihara N, Subler MA, et al: A SQSTM1/p62 mutation linked to Paget's disease increases the osteoclastogenic potential of the bone microenvironment, Hum Mol Genet 17:3708–3719, 2008.

Index

Page numbers followed by 'f' indicate figures and 't' indicate tables

Printed and bound by CPI Group (UK) Ltd, Croydon, CR0 4YY

03/10/2024

01040310-0018